ICD-10-PCS

The complete official code set

Codes valid from October 1, 2018
through September 30, 2019

Power up your coding
optum360coding.com

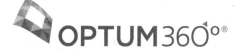

Our Commitment to Accuracy

Optum360 is committed to producing accurate and reliable materials. To report corrections, please visit www.optum360coding.com/accuracy or email accuracy@optum.com. You can also reach customer service by calling 1.800.464.3649, option 1.

Acknowledgments

Marianne Randall, CPC, *Product Manager*

Karen Schmidt, BSN, *Technical Director*

Anita Schmidt, BS, RHIT, AHIMA-approved ICD-10-CM/PCS Trainer, *Clinical Technical Editor*

Peggy Willard, CCS, AHIMA-approved ICD-10-CM/PCS Trainer, *Clinical Technical Editor*

Stacy Perry, *Manager, Desktop Publishing*

Tracy Betzler, *Senior Desktop Publishing Specialist*

Hope M. Dunn, *Senior Desktop Publishing Specialist*

Katie Russell, *Desktop Publishing Specialist*

Kate Holden, *Editor*

Anita Schmidt, BS, RHIT, AHIMA-approved ICD-10-CM/PCS Trainer

Ms. Schmidt has expertise in Level I adult and pediatric trauma hospital coding, specializing in ICD-9-CM, ICD-10-CM/PCS, DRG, and CPT coding. Her experience includes analysis of medical record documentation, assignment of ICD-10-CM and PCS codes, DRG validation, as well as CPT code assignments for same-day surgery cases. She has conducted coding training and auditing, including DRG validation, conducted electronic health record training, and worked with clinical documentation specialists to identify documentation needs and potential areas for physician education. Most recently she has been developing content for resource and educational products related to ICD-10-CM and ICD-10-PCS. Ms. Schmidt is an AHIMA-approved ICD-10-CM/PCS trainer, and is an active member of the American Health Information Management Association (AHIMA) and the Minnesota Health Information Management Association (MHIMA).

Peggy Willard, CCS, AHIMA-approved ICD-10-CM/PCS Trainer

Ms. Willard has 18 years of experience in the healthcare field. Her expertise is in ICD-10-CM and ICD-10-PCS, including in-depth analysis of medical record documentation, ICD-10-CM/PCS code and DRG assignment, as well as clinical documentation improvement (CDI). In recent years Ms. Willard has been responsible for the creation and development of several products for Optum360 Coding Solutions that are designed to assist with appropriate application of the ICD-10-CM and ICD-10-PCS coding systems. She has several years of prior experience in Level I adult and pediatric trauma hospital and inpatient rehabilitation facility (IRF) coding, specializing in ICD-9-CM diagnosis and procedural coding, with emphasis in conducting coding audits, and conducting coding training for coding staff and clinical documentation specialists. Ms. Willard is an AHIMA-approved ICD-10 CM/PCS trainer and is an active member of the American Health Information Management Association (AHIMA) and the Minnesota Health Information Management Association (MHIMA).

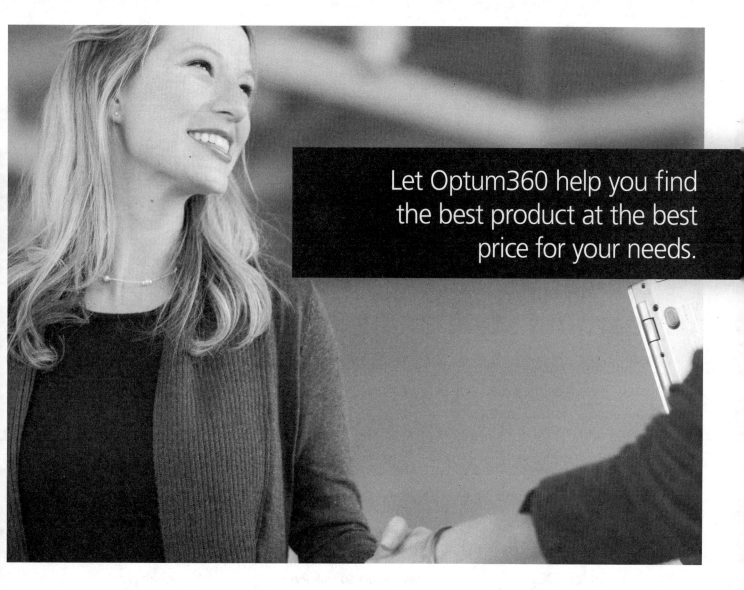

Let Optum360 help you find the best product at the best price for your needs.

Optum360® can help you drive financial results across your organization with industry-leading resources that cut through the complexity of medical coding challenges.

The Price Match Program* is an example of one of the ways in which we can impact your bottom line — to the positive. We're committed to providing you with the best quality product in the market, along with the best price.

Let us help you find the best coding solution, at the best price.

Contact your Medallion representative directly or call Customer Service at 1-800-464-3649, option 1. Or explore online, optum360coding.com/pricematch.

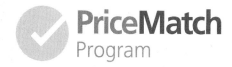

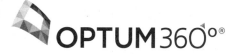

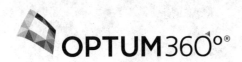

Optum360 Learning

Education suiting your specialty, learning style and schedule

Optum360® Learning is designed to address exactly what you and your learners need. We offer: Several delivery methods developed for various adult learning styles; general public education; and tailor-made programs specific to your organization — all created by our coding and clinical documentation education professionals.

Our strategy is simple — education must be concise, relevant and accurate. Choose the delivery method that works best for you:

eLearning

- **Web-based** courses offered at the most convenient times
- **Interactive**, task-focused and developed around practical scenarios
- **Self-paced** courses include "try-it" functionality, knowledge checks and downloadable resources

Instructor-led training

On-site or remote courses built specifically for your organization and learners
- Providers
- CDI specialists
- Coders

Webinars

Online courses geared toward a broad market of learners and delivered in a live setting

You've worked hard for your credentials, and now you need an easy way to maintain your certification.

WF626270

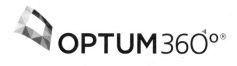
OPTUM360°®

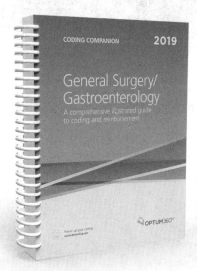
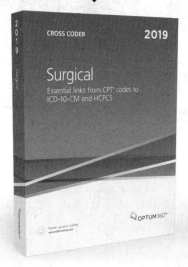
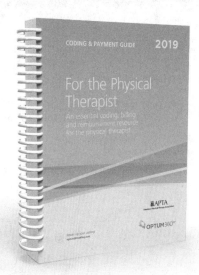
CPT is a registered trademark of the American Medical Association.   © 2018 Optum360, LLC. All rights reserved. WF626533 04/18

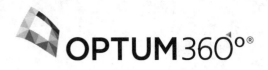

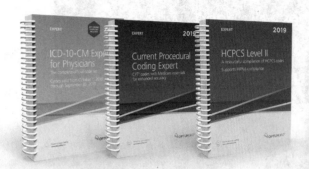

RENEW THIS BOOK
SAVE UP TO 25%
ON 2019 EDITION CODING RESOURCES.*

ITEM #	TITLE INDICATE THE ITEMS YOU WISH TO PURCHASE	QUANTITY	PRICE PER PRODUCT	TOTAL

Subtotal	
(AK, DE, HI, MT, NH & OR are exempt) Sales Tax	
1 item $10.95 • 2–4 items $12.95 • 5+ CALL Shipping & Handling	
TOTAL AMOUNT ENCLOSED	

Save up to 25% when you renew.*

PROMO CODE: **RENEW19B**

 Visit **optum360coding.com** and enter the promo code above at checkout.

 Call **1-800-464-3649, option 1,** and mention the promo code above.

 Fax this order form with purchase order to **1-801-982-4033.** *Optum360 no longer accepts credit cards by fax.*

Mail this order form with payment and/or purchase order to:
Optum360, PO Box 88050, Chicago, IL 60680-9920.
Optum360 no longer accepts credit cards by mail.

Name

Address

Customer Number   Contact Number

○ CHECK ENCLOSED (PAYABLE TO OPTUM360)

○ BILL ME ○ P.O.#

( )
Telephone
( )
Fax
                                    @
Email

Optum360 respects your right to privacy. We will not sell or rent your email address or fax number to anyone outside Optum360 and its business partners. If you would like to remove your name from Optum360 promotions, please call 1-800-464-3649, option 1.

Contents

What's New for 2019

The Centers for Medicare and Medicaid Services is the agency charged with maintaining and updating ICD-10-PCS. CMS released the most current revisions, a summary of which may be found on the CMS website at: https://www.cms.gov/Medicare/Coding/ICD10/2019-ICD-10-PCS-and-GEMs.html

Due to the unique structure of ICD-10-PCS, a change in a character value may affect individual codes and several code tables.

Change Summary Table

2018 Total	New Codes	Revised Titles	Deleted Codes	2019 Total
78,705	392	8	216	78,881

ICD-10-PCS Code FY 2019 Totals, By Section

Medical and Surgical	68,639
Obstetrics	302
Placement	861
Administration	1,445
Measurement and Monitoring	414
Extracorporeal or Systemic Assistance and Performance	45
Extracorporeal or Systemic Therapies	46
Osteopathic	100
Other Procedures	60
Chiropractic	90
Imaging	2,941
Nuclear Medicine	463
Radiation Therapy	1,939
Physical Rehabilitation and Diagnostic Audiology	1,380
Mental Health	30
Substance Abuse Treatment	59
New Technology	67
Total	78,881

ICD-10-PCS Changes Highlights

- In the Medical and Surgical section, body part values revised or streamlined for clarity and usefulness as coded data
- ICD-10-PCS guidelines updated with new and revised guidelines
- Root operation Control was added to the Ear, Nose and Sinus body system for the body part of Nasal Mucosa and Soft Tissue
- Root Operation Extraction was added to the Hepatobiliary System and Pancreas body system
- The No Device value was removed from the Fusion root operation tables
- Unicondylar devices (Medial and Lateral) and Articulating Spacers were added to the Removal table and Replacement table in the Lower Joints body system
- New qualifiers were added to identify:
  - More specificity for Bypass procedures
  - Drug coated balloon use in Dilation procedures
  - Stent Retriever use in Extirpation procedures
  - Use of irreversible electroporation in Destruction procedures

New Definitions Addenda

Section 0 - Medical and Surgical

Body Part Definitions

ICD-10-PCS Value		Definition
Head and Neck Bursa and Ligament	Delete	Interspinous ligament
	Add	Interspinous ligament, cervical
	Add	Intertransverse ligament, cervical
	Add	Ligamentum flavum, cervical
Lower Spine Bursa and Ligament	Delete	Interspinous ligament
	Delete	Intertransverse ligament
	Delete	Ligamentum flavum
	Add	Interspinous ligament, lumbar
	Add	Intertransverse ligament, lumbar
	Add	Ligamentum flavum, lumbar
Add Mediastinum	Add	Mediastinal cavity
	Add	Mediastinal space
Retroperitoneum	Add	Retroperitoneal cavity
Rib(s) Bursa and Ligament	Delete	Costoxiphoid ligament
	Delete	Sternocostal ligament
Sternum Bursa and Ligament	Delete	Costotransverse ligament
Upper Spine Bursa and Ligament	Delete	Interspinous ligament
	Delete	Intertransverse ligament
	Delete	Ligamentum flavum
	Add	Interspinous ligament, thoracic
	Add	Intertransverse ligament, thoracic
	Add	Ligamentum flavum, thoracic

Section 0 - Medical and Surgical

Device Definitions

ICD-10-PCS Value		Definition
Add Articulating Spacer in Lower Joints	Add	Articulating Spacer (Antibiotic)
	Add	Spacer, Articulating (Antibiotic)
Spacer in Lower Joints	Add	Spacer, Static (Antibiotic)
	Add	Static Spacer (Antibiotic)

Section 0 - Medical and Surgical

Device Aggregation Table

Specific Device		for Operation		in Body System		General Device	
Delete	Synthetic Substitute, Unicondylar	Delete	Replacement	Delete	Lower Joints	Delete	J Synthetic Substitute

Section X - New Technology

Root Operation

ICD-10-PCS Value		Definition	
Add	Destruction	Add	Definition: Physical eradication of all or a portion of a body part by the direct use of energy, force, or a destructive agent
		Add	Explanation: None of the body part is physically taken out
		Add	Includes/Examples: Fulguration of rectal polyp, cautery of skin lesion

Section X - New Technology

Approach

ICD-10-PCS Value		Definition	
Add	Via Natural or Artificial Opening Endoscopic	Add	Definition: Entry of instrumentation through a natural or artificial external opening to reach and visualize the site of the procedure

Section X - New Technology

Device / Substance / Technology

ICD-10-PCS Value		Definition	
	Engineered Autologous Chimeric Antigen Receptor T-cell Immunotherapy	Add	KYMRIAH
		Add	Tisagenlecleucel
Add	Synthetic Human Angiotensin II	Add	Angiotensin II
		Add	GIAPREZA™
		Add	Human angiotensin II, synthetic

List of Updated Files

2019 Official ICD-10-PCS Coding Guidelines

- New Guideline B3.17 added in response to public comment.
- Guidelines A10, B3.7, and B6.1a revised in response to public comment and internal review.
- Downloadable PDF, file name pcs_guidelines_2019.pdf

2019 ICD-10-PCS Code Tables and Index (Zip file)

- Code tables for use beginning October 1, 2018
- Downloadable PDF, file name is pcs_2019.pdf
- Downloadable xml files for developers, file names are icd10pcs_tables_2019.xml, icd10pcs_index_2019.xml, icd10pcs_definitions_2019.xml
- Accompanying schema for developers, file names are icd10pcs_tables.xsd, icd10pcs_index.xsd, icd10pcs_definitions.xsd

2019 ICD-10-PCS Codes File (Zip file)

- ICD-10-PCS Codes file is a simple format for non-technical uses, containing the valid FY 2019 ICD-10-PCS codes and their long titles.
- File is in text file format, file name is icd10pcs_codes_2019.txt
- Accompanying documentation for codes file, file name is icd10pcsCodesFile.pdf
- Codes file addenda in text format, file name is codes_addenda_2019.txt

2019 ICD-10-PCS Order File (Long and Abbreviated Titles) (Zip file)

- ICD-10-PCS order file is for developers, provides a unique five-digit "order number" for each ICD-10-PCS table and code, as well as a long and abbreviated code title.
- ICD-10-PCS order file name is icd10pcs_order_2019.txt
- Accompanying documentation for tabular order file, file name is icd10pcsOrderFile.pdf
- Tabular order file addenda in text format, file name is order_addenda_2019.txt

2019 ICD-10-PCS Final Addenda (Zip file)

- Addenda files in downloadable PDF, file names are tables_addenda_2019.pdf, index_addenda_2019.pdf, definitions_addenda_2019.pdf
- Addenda files also in machine readable text format for developers, file names are tables_addenda_2019.txt, index_addenda_2019.txt, definitions_addenda_2019.txt

2019 ICD-10-PCS Conversion Table (Zip file)

- ICD-10-PCS code conversion table is provided to assist users in data retrieval, in downloadable Excel spreadsheet, file name is icd10pcs_conversion_table_2019.xlsx
- Conversion table also in machine readable text format for developers, file name is icd10pcs_conversion_table_2019.txt
- Accompanying documentation for code conversion table, file name is icd10pcsConversionTable.pdf

Introduction

History of ICD-10-PCS

The World Health Organization has maintained the International Classification of Diseases (ICD) for recording cause of death since 1893. It has updated the ICD periodically to reflect new discoveries in epidemiology and changes in medical understanding of disease.

The International Classification of Diseases Tenth Revision (ICD-10), published in 1992, is the latest revision of the ICD. The WHO authorized the National Center for Health Statistics (NCHS) to develop a clinical modification of ICD-10 for use in the United States. This version, called ICD-10-CM, is intended to replace the previous U.S. clinical modification, ICD-9-CM, that has been in use since 1979. ICD-9-CM contains a procedure classification; ICD-10-CM does not.

CMS, the agency responsible for maintaining the inpatient procedure code set in the United States, contracted with 3M Health Information Systems in 1993 to design and then develop a procedure classification system to replace volume 3 of ICD-9-CM.

The result, ICD-10-PCS, was initially completed in 1998. The code set has been updated annually since that time to ensure that ICD-10-PCS includes classifications for new procedures, devices, and technologies.

The development of ICD-10-PCS had as its goal the incorporation of the following major attributes:

- **Completeness:** There should be a unique code for all substantially different procedures.

- **Unique definitions:** Because ICD-10-PCS codes are constructed of individual values rather than lists of fixed codes and text descriptions, the unique, stable definition of a code in the system is retained. New values may be added to the system to represent a specific new approach or device or qualifier, but whole codes by design cannot be given new meanings and reused.

- **Expandability:** As new procedures are developed, the structure of ICD-10-PCS should allow them to be easily incorporated as unique codes.

- **Multi-axial codes:** ICD-10-PCS codes should consist of independent characters, with each individual component retaining its meaning across broad ranges of codes to the extent possible.

- **Standardized terminology:** ICD-10-PCS should include definitions of the terminology used. While the meaning of specific words varies in common usage, ICD-10-PCS should not include multiple meanings for the same term, and each term must be assigned a specific meaning. There are no eponyms or common procedure terms in ICD-10-PCS.

- **Structural integrity:** ICD-10-PCS can be easily expanded without disrupting the structure of the system. ICD-10-PCS allows unique new codes to be added to the system because values for the seven characters that make up a code can be combined as needed. The system can evolve as medical technology and clinical practice evolve, without disrupting the ICD-10-PCS structure.

In the development of ICD-10-PCS, several additional general characteristics were added:

- **Diagnostic information is not included in procedure description:** When procedures are performed for specific diseases or disorders, the disease or disorder is not contained in the procedure code. The diagnosis codes, not the procedure codes, specify the disease or disorder.

- **Explicit not otherwise specified (NOS) options are restricted:** Explicit "not otherwise specified," (NOS) options are restricted in ICD-10-PCS. A minimal level of specificity is required for each component of the procedure.

- **Limited use of not elsewhere classified (NEC) option:** Because all significant components of a procedure are specified in ICD-10-PCS, there is generally no need for a "not elsewhere classified" (NEC) code option. However, limited NEC options are incorporated into ICD-10-PCS where necessary. For example, new devices are frequently developed, and therefore it is necessary to provide an "other device" option for use until the new device can be explicitly added to the coding system.

- **Level of specificity:** All procedures currently performed can be specified in ICD-10-PCS. The frequency with which a procedure is performed was not a consideration in the development of the system. A unique code is available for variations of a procedure that can be performed.

ICD-10-PCS code structure results in qualities that optimize the performance of the system in electronic applications, and maximize the usefulness of the coded healthcare data. These qualities include:

- **Optimal search capability:** ICD-10-PCS is designed for maximum versatility in the ability to aggregate coded data. Values belonging to the same character as defined in a section or sections can be easily compared, since they occupy the same position in a code. This provides a high degree of flexibility and functionality for data mining.

- **Consistent characters and values:** Stability of characters and values across vast ranges of codes provides the maximum degree of functionality and flexibility for the collection and analysis of data. Because the character definition is consistent, and only the individual values assigned to that character differ as needed, meaningful comparisons of data over time can be conducted across a virtually infinite range of procedures.

- **Code readability:** ICD-10-PCS resembles a language in the sense that it is made up of semi-independent values combined by following the rules of the system, much the way a sentence is formed by combining words and following the rules of grammar and syntax. As with words in their context, the meaning of any single value is a combination of its position in the code and any preceding values on which it may be dependent.

ICD-10-PCS Code Structure

ICD-10-PCS has a seven-character alphanumeric code structure. Each character contains up to 34 possible values. Each value represents a specific option for the general character definition. The 10 digits 0–9 and the 24 letters A–H, J–N, and P–Z may be used in each character. The letters O and I are not used so as to avoid confusion with the digits 0 and 1. An ICD-10-PCS code is the result of a process rather than as a single fixed set of digits or alphabetic characters. The process consists of combining semi-independent values from among a selection of values, according to the rules governing the construction of codes.

	Section	Body System	Root Operation	Body Part	Approach	Device	Qualifier
Characters:	1	2	3	4	5	6	7

A code is derived by choosing a specific value for each of the seven characters. Based on details about the procedure performed, values for each character specifying the section, body system, root operation, body part, approach, device, and qualifier are assigned. Because the definition of each character is also a function of its physical position in the code, the same letter or number placed in a different position in the code has a different meaning.

The seven characters that make up a complete code have specific meanings that vary for each of the 17 sections of the manual.

Procedures are then divided into sections that identify the general type of procedure (e.g., Medical and Surgical, Obstetrics, Imaging). The first character of the procedure code always specifies the section. The second through seventh characters have the same meaning within each section, but may mean different things in other sections. In all sections, the third character specifies the general type of procedure performed (e.g., Resection, Transfusion, Fluoroscopy), while the other characters give additional information such as the body part and approach.

In ICD-10-PCS, the term *procedure* refers to the complete specification of the seven characters.

Number of Codes in ICD-10-PCS

The table structure of ICD-10-PCS permits the specification of a large number of codes on a single page. At the time of this publication, there are 78,881 codes in the 2019 ICD-10-PCS.

ICD-10-PCS Manual

Index

Codes may be found in the index based on the general type of procedure (e.g., resection, transfusion, fluoroscopy), or a more commonly used term (e.g., appendectomy). For example, the code for percutaneous intraluminal dilation of the coronary arteries with an intraluminal device can be found in the Index under *Dilation*, or a synonym of *Dilation* (e.g., angioplasty). The Index then specifies the first three or four values of the code or directs the user to see another term.

Example:

> **Dilation**
> Artery
> Coronary
> One Artery 0270

Based on the first three values of the code provided in the Index, the corresponding table can be located. In the example above, the first three values indicate table 027 is to be referenced for code completion.

The tables and characters are arranged first by number and then by letter for each character (tables for 00-, 01-, 02-, etc., are followed by those for 0B-, 0C-, 0D-, etc., followed by 0B1, 0B2, etc., followed by 0BB, 0BC, 0BD, etc.).

Note: The Tables section must be used to construct a complete and valid code by specifying the last three or four values.

Tables

The Tables are composed of rows that specify the valid combinations of code values. In most sections of the system, the upper portion of each table contains a description of the first three characters of the procedure code. In the Medical and Surgical section, for example, the first three characters contain the name of the section, the body system, and the root operation performed.

For instance, the values *027* specify the section *Medical and Surgical* (0), the body system *Heart and Great Vessels* (2) and the root operation *Dilation* (7). As shown in table 027, the root operation (*Dilation*) is accompanied by its definition.

The lower portion of the table specifies all the valid combinations of characters 4 through 7. The four columns in the table specify the last four characters. In the Medical and Surgical section they are labeled body part, approach, device and qualifier, respectively. Each row in the table specifies the valid combination of values for characters 4 through 7.

Table 1: Row from table Ø27

Ø   **Medical and Surgical**
2   **Heart and Great Vessels**
7   **Dilation**   Definition: Expanding an orifice or the lumen of a tubular body part

Explanation: The orifice can be a natural orifice or an artificially created orifice. Accomplished by stretching a tubular body part using intraluminal pressure or by cutting part of the orifice or wall of the tubular body part.

Body Part Character 4	Approach Character 5	Device Character 6	Qualifier Character 7
Ø Coronary Artery, One Artery 1 Coronary Artery, Two Arteries 2 Coronary Artery, Three Arteries 3 Coronary Artery, Four or More Arteries	Ø Open 3 Percutaneous 4 Percutaneous Endoscopic	4 Intraluminal Device, Drug-eluting 5 Intraluminal Device, Drug-eluting, Two 6 Intraluminal Device, Drug-eluting, Three 7 Intraluminal Device, Drug-eluting, Four or More D Intraluminal Device E Intraluminal Device, Two F Intraluminal Device, Three G Intraluminal Device, Four or More T Intraluminal Device, Radioactive Z No Device	6 Bifurcation Z No Qualifier

The rows of this table can be used to construct 240 unique procedure codes. For example, code Ø27Ø3DZ specifies the procedure for dilation of one coronary artery using an intraluminal device via percutaneous approach (i.e., percutaneous transluminal coronary angioplasty with stent).

The valid codes shown in table 2 are constructed using the first body part value in table 1 (i.e., one coronary artery), combined with all the valid approaches and devices listed in the table, and the value "No Qualifier".

Table 2: Code titles for dilation of one coronary artery (Ø27Ø)

Code	Title
Ø27ØØ4Z	Dilation of Coronary Artery, One Artery with Drug-eluting Intraluminal Device, Open Approach
Ø27ØØ5Z	Dilation of Coronary Artery, One Artery with Two Drug-eluting Intraluminal Devices, Open Approach
Ø27ØØ6Z	Dilation of Coronary Artery, One Artery with Three Drug-eluting Intraluminal Devices, Open Approach
Ø27ØØ7Z	Dilation of Coronary Artery, One Artery with Four or More Drug-eluting Intraluminal Devices, Open Approach
Ø27ØØDZ	Dilation of Coronary Artery, One Artery with Intraluminal Device, Open Approach
Ø27ØØEZ	Dilation of Coronary Artery, One Artery with Two Intraluminal Devices, Open Approach
Ø27ØØFZ	Dilation of Coronary Artery, One Artery with Three Intraluminal Devices, Open Approach
Ø27ØØGZ	Dilation of Coronary Artery, One Artery with Four or More Intraluminal Devices, Open Approach
Ø27ØØTZ	Dilation of Coronary Artery, One Artery with Radioactive Intraluminal Device, Open Approach
Ø27ØØZZ	Dilation of Coronary Artery, One Artery, Open Approach
Ø27Ø34Z	Dilation of Coronary Artery, One Artery with Drug-eluting Intraluminal Device, Percutaneous Approach
Ø27Ø35Z	Dilation of Coronary Artery, One Artery with Two Drug-eluting Intraluminal Devices, Percutaneous Approach
Ø27Ø36Z	Dilation of Coronary Artery, One Artery with Three Drug-eluting Intraluminal Devices, Percutaneous Approach
Ø27Ø37Z	Dilation of Coronary Artery, One Artery with Four or More Drug-eluting Intraluminal Devices, Percutaneous Approach
Ø27Ø3DZ	Dilation of Coronary Artery, One Artery with Intraluminal Device, Percutaneous Approach
Ø27Ø3EZ	Dilation of Coronary Artery, One Artery with Two Intraluminal Devices, Percutaneous Approach
Ø27Ø3FZ	Dilation of Coronary Artery, One Artery with Three Intraluminal Devices, Percutaneous Approach
Ø27Ø3GZ	Dilation of Coronary Artery, One Artery with Four or More Intraluminal Devices, Percutaneous Approach
Ø27Ø3TZ	Dilation of Coronary Artery, One Artery with Radioactive Intraluminal Device, Percutaneous Approach
Ø27Ø3ZZ	Dilation of Coronary Artery, One Artery, Percutaneous Approach
Ø27Ø44Z	Dilation of Coronary Artery, One Artery with Drug-eluting Intraluminal Device, Percutaneous Endoscopic Approach
Ø27Ø45Z	Dilation of Coronary Artery, One Artery with Two Drug-eluting Intraluminal Devices, Percutaneous Endoscopic Approach
Ø27Ø46Z	Dilation of Coronary Artery, One Artery with Three Drug-eluting Intraluminal Devices, Percutaneous Endoscopic Approach
Ø27Ø47Z	Dilation of Coronary Artery, One Artery with Four or More Drug-eluting Intraluminal Devices, Percutaneous Endoscopic Approach
Ø27Ø4DZ	Dilation of Coronary Artery, One Artery with Intraluminal Device, Percutaneous Endoscopic Approach
Ø27Ø4EZ	Dilation of Coronary Artery, One Artery with Two Intraluminal Devices, Percutaneous Endoscopic Approach
Ø27Ø4FZ	Dilation of Coronary Artery, One Artery with Three Intraluminal Devices, Percutaneous Endoscopic Approach
Ø27Ø4GZ	Dilation of Coronary Artery, One Artery with Four or More Intraluminal Devices, Percutaneous Endoscopic Approach
Ø27Ø4TZ	Dilation of Coronary Artery, One Artery with Radioactive Intraluminal Device, Percutaneous Endoscopic Approach
Ø27Ø4ZZ	Dilation of Coronary Artery, One Artery, Percutaneous Endoscopic Approach

Table 3: Rows from table 00H

0   Medical and Surgical
0   Central Nervous System and Cranial Nerves
H   Insertion   Definition: Putting in a nonbiological appliance that monitors, assists, performs, or prevents a physiological function but does not physically take the place of a body part

Explanation: None

Body Part Character 4		Approach Character 5	Device Character 6	Qualifier Character 7
0 Brain Cerebrum Corpus callosum Encephalon		**0 Open**	**2 Monitoring Device** **3 Infusion Device** **4 Radioactive Element, Cesium-131 Collagen Implant** **M Neurostimulator Lead** **Y Other Device**	**Z No Qualifier**
0 Brain Cerebrum Corpus callosum Encephalon		**3 Percutaneous** **4 Percutaneous Endoscopic**	**2 Monitoring Device** **3 Infusion Device** **M Neurostimulator Lead** **Y Other Device**	**Z No Qualifier**
6 Cerebral Ventricle Aqueduct of Sylvius Cerebral aqueduct (Sylvius) Choroid plexus Ependyma Foramen of Monro (intraventricular) Fourth ventricle Interventricular foramen (Monro) Left lateral ventricle Right lateral ventricle Third ventricle	**E Cranial Nerve** **U Spinal Canal** Epidural space, spinal Extradural space, spinal Subarachnoid space, spinal Subdural space, spinal Vertebral canal **V Spinal Cord**	**0 Open** **3 Percutaneous** **4 Percutaneous Endoscopic**	**2 Monitoring Device** **3 Infusion Device** **M Neurostimulator Lead** **Y Other Device**	**Z No Qualifier**

Table 3, is split into three rows; values of characters must all be selected from within the same row of the table. Row 1 and 2 indicate that the body part (character 4) value 0 and Qualifier value Z may both be used in combination with device values 2, 3, M or Y. However, the approach (character 5) and device (character 6) values are not exactly the same for both rows. As shown in row 1, Body part value Brain (0) with Device value Radioactive Element, Cesium-131 Collagen Implant (4) can only be used with approach value Open (0). In other words, code 00H034Z would be invalid as the approach value 3 is only applicable to row 2 and the device value 4 is only applicable to row 1. It would be inappropriate to build a code for body part 0 if all of the values are not contained in its own row.

Note: In this manual, there are instances in which some tables due to length must be continued on the next page. Each section must be used separately and value selection must be made within the same row of the table.

Character Meanings

In each section, each character has a specific meaning, and this character meaning remains constant within that section. Character meaning tables have been provided at the beginning of each section or, in the case of the Medical and Surgical section (0), at the beginning of each body system to help the user identify the character members available within that section. These tables have purple headers, unlike the official code tables that have green headers and **SHOULD NOT** be used to build a PCS code. Following is an excerpt of a character meaning table.

Table 4: Rows from Central Nervous System and Cranial Nerves - Character Meanings Table

Operation–Character 3	Body Part–Character 4	Approach–Character 5	Device–Character 6	Qualifier–Character 7
1 Bypass	0 Brain	0 Open	0 Drainage Device	0 Nasopharynx
2 Change	1 Cerebral Meninges	3 Percutaneous	2 Monitoring Device	1 Mastoid Sinus
5 Destruction	2 Dura Mater	4 Percutaneous Endoscopic	3 Infusion Device	2 Atrium
7 Dilation	3 Epidural Space, Intracranial	X External	4 Radioactive Element, Cesium-131 Collagen Implant	3 Blood Vessel
8 Division	4 Subdural Space, Intracranial		7 Autologous Tissue Substitute	4 Pleural Cavity
9 Drainage	5 Subarachnoid Space, Intracranial		J Synthetic Substitute	5 Intestine
B Excision	6 Cerebral Ventricle		K Nonautologous Tissue Substitute	6 Peritoneal Cavity
C Extirpation	7 Cerebral Hemisphere		M Neurostimulator Lead	7 Urinary Tract
D Extraction	8 Basal Ganglia		Y Other Device	8 Bone Marrow
F Fragmentation	9 Thalamus		Z No Device	9 Fallopian Tube
H Insertion	A Hypothalamus			B Cerebral Cisterns
J Inspection	B Pons			F Olfactory Nerve

Sections

Procedures are divided into sections that identify the general type of procedure (e.g., Medical and Surgical, Obstetrics, Imaging). The first character of the procedure code always specifies the section.

The sections are listed below:

Medical and Surgical section
Ø   Medical and Surgical

Medical and Surgical-related sections
1   Obstetrics

2   Placement

3   Administration

4   Measurement and Monitoring

5   Extracorporeal or Systemic Assistance and Performance

6   Extracorporeal or Systemic Therapies

7   Osteopathic

8   Other Procedures

9   Chiropractic

Ancillary Sections
B   Imaging

C   Nuclear Medicine

D   Radiation Therapy

F   Physical Rehabilitation and Diagnostic Audiology

G   Mental Health

H   Substance Abuse Treatment

New Technology Section
X   New Technology

Medical and Surgical Section (Ø)

Character Meaning

The seven characters for Medical and Surgical procedures have the following meaning:

Character	Meaning
1	Section
2	Body System
3	Root Operation
4	Body Part
5	Approach
6	Device
7	Qualifier

The Medical and Surgical section constitutes the vast majority of procedures reported in an inpatient setting. Medical and Surgical procedure codes all have a first character value of Ø. The second character indicates the general body system (e.g., Mouth and Throat, Gastrointestinal). The third character indicates the root operation, or specific objective, of the procedure (e.g., Excision). The fourth character indicates the specific body part on which the procedure was performed (e.g., Tonsils, Duodenum). The fifth character indicates the approach used to reach the procedure site (e.g., Open). The sixth character indicates whether a device was left in place during the procedure (e.g.,

Synthetic Substitute). The seventh character is qualifier, which has a specific meaning for each root operation. For example, the qualifier can be used to identify the destination site of a *Bypass*. The first through fifth characters are always assigned a specific value, but the device (sixth character) and the qualifier (seventh character) are not applicable to all procedures. The value *Z* is used for the sixth and seventh characters to indicate that a specific device or qualifier does not apply to the procedure.

Section (Character 1)

Medical and Surgical procedure codes all have a first character value of Ø.

Body Systems (Character 2)

Body systems for Medical and Surgical section codes are specified in the second character.

Body Systems
Ø   Central Nervous System and Cranial Nerves

1   Peripheral Nervous System

2   Heart and Great Vessels

3   Upper Arteries

4   Lower Arteries

5   Upper Veins

6   Lower Veins

7   Lymphatic and Hemic Systems

8   Eye

9   Ear, Nose, Sinus

B   Respiratory System

C   Mouth and Throat

D   Gastrointestinal System

F   Hepatobiliary System and Pancreas

G   Endocrine System

H   Skin and Breast

J   Subcutaneous Tissue and Fascia

K   Muscles

L   Tendons

M   Bursae and Ligaments

N   Head and Facial Bones

P   Upper Bones

Q   Lower Bones

R   Upper Joints

S   Lower Joints

T   Urinary System

U   Female Reproductive System

V   Male Reproductive System

W   Anatomical Regions, General

X   Anatomical Regions, Upper Extremities

Y   Anatomical Regions, Lower Extremities

Root Operations (Character 3)

The root operation is specified in the third character. In the Medical and Surgical section there are 31 different root operations. The root operation identifies the objective of the procedure. Each root operation has a precise definition.

- *Alteration:* Modifying the natural anatomic structure of a body part without affecting the function of the body part

- *Bypass:* Altering the route of passage of the contents of a tubular body part

- *Change:* Taking out or off a device from a body part and putting back an identical or similar device in or on the same body part without cutting or puncturing the skin or a mucous membrane

- *Control:* Stopping, or attempting to stop, postprocedural or other acute bleeding

- *Creation:* Putting in or on biological or synthetic material to form a new body part that to the extent possible replicates the anatomic structure or function of an absent body part

- *Destruction:* Physical eradication of all or a portion of a body part by the direct use of energy, force, or a destructive agent

- *Detachment:* Cutting off all or a portion of the upper or lower extremities

- *Dilation:* Expanding an orifice or the lumen of a tubular body part

- *Division:* Cutting into a body part without draining fluids and/or gases from the body part in order to separate or transect a body part

- *Drainage:* Taking or letting out fluids and/or gases from a body part

- *Excision:* Cutting out or off, without replacement, a portion of a body part

- *Extirpation:* Taking or cutting out solid matter from a body part

- *Extraction:* Pulling or stripping out or off all or a portion of a body part by the use of force

- *Fragmentation:* Breaking solid matter in a body part into pieces

- *Fusion:* Joining together portions of an articular body part rendering the articular body part immobile

- *Insertion:* Putting in a nonbiological appliance that monitors, assists, performs, or prevents a physiological function but does not physically take the place of a body part

- *Inspection:* Visually and/or manually exploring a body part

- *Map:* Locating the route of passage of electrical impulses and/or locating functional areas in a body part

- *Occlusion:* Completely closing an orifice or lumen of a tubular body part

- *Reattachment:* Putting back in or on all or a portion of a separated body part to its normal location or other suitable location

- *Release:* Freeing a body part from an abnormal physical constraint by cutting or by use of force

- *Removal:* Taking out or off a device from a body part

- *Repair:* Restoring, to the extent possible, a body part to its normal anatomic structure and function

- *Replacement:* Putting in or on biological or synthetic material that physically takes the place and/or function of all or a portion of a body part

- *Reposition:* Moving to its normal location or other suitable location all or a portion of a body part

- *Resection:* Cutting out or off, without replacement, all of a body part

- *Restriction:* Partially closing an orifice or lumen of a tubular body part

- *Revision:* Correcting, to the extent possible, a portion of a malfunctioning device or the position of a displaced device

- *Supplement:* Putting in or on biological or synthetic material that physically reinforces and/or augments the function of a portion of a body part

- *Transfer:* Moving, without taking out, all or a portion of a body part to another location to take over the function of all or a portion of a body part

- *Transplantation:* Putting in or on all or a portion of a living body part taken from another individual or animal to physically take the place and/or function of all or a portion of a similar body part

The above definitions of root operations illustrate the precision of code values defined in the system. There is a clear distinction between each root operation.

A root operation specifies the objective of the procedure. The term *anastomosis* is not a root operation, because it is a means of joining and is always an integral part of another procedure (e.g., Bypass, Resection) with a specific objective. Similarly, *incision* is not a root operation, since it is always part of the objective of another procedure (e.g., Division, Drainage). The root operation *Repair* in the Medical and Surgical section functions as a "not elsewhere classified" option. *Repair* is used when the procedure performed is not one of the other specific root operations.

Appendix B provides additional explanation and representative examples of the Medical and Surgical root operations. Appendix C groups all root operations in the Medical and Surgical section into subcategories and provides an example of each root operation.

Body Part (Character 4)

The body part is specified in the fourth character. The body part indicates the specific anatomical site of the body system on which the procedure was performed (e.g., Duodenum). Tubular body parts are defined in ICD-10-PCS as those hollow body parts that provide a route of passage for solids, liquids, or gases. They include the cardiovascular system and body parts such as those contained in the gastrointestinal tract, genitourinary tract, biliary tract, and respiratory tract.

Approach (Character 5)

The technique used to reach the site of the procedure is specified in the fifth character. There are seven different approaches:

- *Open:* Cutting through the skin or mucous membrane and any other body layers necessary to expose the site of the procedure

- *Percutaneous:* Entry, by puncture or minor incision, of instrumentation through the skin or mucous membrane and any other body layers necessary to reach the site of the procedure

- *Percutaneous Endoscopic:* Entry, by puncture or minor incision, of instrumentation through the skin or mucous membrane and any other body layers necessary to reach and visualize the site of the procedure

- *Via Natural or Artificial Opening:* Entry of instrumentation through a natural or artificial external opening to reach the site of the procedure

- *Via Natural or Artificial Opening Endoscopic:* Entry of instrumentation through a natural or artificial external opening to reach and visualize the site of the procedure

- *Via Natural or Artificial Opening with Percutaneous Endoscopic Assistance:* Entry of instrumentation through a natural or artificial external opening and entry, by puncture or minor incision, of instrumentation through the skin or mucous membrane and any other body layers necessary to aid in the performance of the procedure

- *External*: Procedures performed directly on the skin or mucous membrane and procedures performed indirectly by the application of external force through the skin or mucous membrane

The approach comprises three components: the access location, method, and type of instrumentation.

Access location: For procedures performed on an internal body part, the access location specifies the external site through which the site of the procedure is reached. There are two general types of access locations: skin or mucous membranes, and external orifices. Every approach value except external includes one of these two access locations. The skin or mucous membrane can be cut or punctured to reach the procedure site. All open and percutaneous approach values use this access location. The site of a procedure can also be reached through an external opening. External openings can be natural (e.g., mouth) or artificial (e.g., colostomy stoma).

Method: For procedures performed on an internal body part, the method specifies how the external access location is entered. An open method specifies cutting through the skin or mucous membrane and any other intervening body layers necessary to expose the site of the procedure. An instrumentation method specifies the entry of instrumentation through the access location to the internal procedure site. Instrumentation can be introduced by puncture or minor incision, or through an external opening. The puncture or minor incision does not constitute an open approach because it does not expose the site of the procedure. An approach can define multiple methods. For example, *Via Natural or Artificial Opening with Percutaneous Endoscopic Assistance* includes both the initial entry of instrumentation to reach the site of the procedure, and the placement of additional percutaneous instrumentation into the body part to visualize and assist in the performance of the procedure.

Type of instrumentation: For procedures performed on an internal body part, instrumentation means that specialized equipment is used to perform the procedure. Instrumentation is used in all internal approaches other than the basic open approach. Instrumentation may or may not include the capacity to visualize the procedure site. For example, the instrumentation used to perform a sigmoidoscopy permits the internal site of the procedure to be visualized, while the instrumentation used to perform a needle biopsy of the liver does not. The term "endoscopic" as used in approach values refers to instrumentation that permits a site to be visualized.

Procedures performed directly on the skin or mucous membrane are identified by the external approach (e.g., skin excision). Procedures performed indirectly by the application of external force are also identified by the external approach (e.g., closed reduction of fracture).

Appendix A compares the components (access location, method, and type of instrumentation) of each approach and provides an example and illustration of each approach.

Device (Character 6)
The device is specified in the sixth character and is used only to specify devices that remain after the procedure is completed. There are four general types of devices:

- Biological or synthetic material that takes the place of all or a portion of a body part (e.g, skin graft, joint prosthesis).

- Biological or synthetic material that assists or prevents a physiological function (e.g., IUD).

- Therapeutic material that is not absorbed by, eliminated by, or incorporated into a body part (e.g., radioactive implant).

- Mechanical or electronic appliances used to assist, monitor, take the place of or prevent a physiological function (e.g., cardiac pacemaker, orthopedic pin).

While all devices can be removed, some cannot be removed without putting in another nonbiological appliance or body-part substitute.

When a specific device value is used to identify the device for a root operation, such as *Insertion* and that same device value is not an option for a more broad range root operation such as *Removal*, select the general device value. For example, in the body system Heart and Great Vessels, the specific device character for Cardiac Lead, Pacemaker in root operation *Insertion* is J. For the root operation *Removal*, the general device character M Cardiac Lead would be selected for the pacemaker lead.

ICD-10-PCS contains a PCS Device Aggregation Table (see appendix F) that crosswalks the *specific* device character values that have been created for specific root operations and specific body part character values to the *general* device character value that would be used for root operations that represent a broad range of procedures and general body part character values, such as Removal and Revision.

Instruments used to visualize the procedure site are specified in the approach, not the device, value.

If the objective of the procedure is to put in the device, then the root operation is *Insertion*. If the device is put in to meet an objective other than *Insertion*, then the root operation defining the underlying objective of the procedure is used, with the device specified in the device character. For example, if a procedure to replace the hip joint is performed, the root operation *Replacement* is coded, and the prosthetic device is specified in the device character. Materials that are incidental to a procedure such as clips, ligatures, and sutures are not specified in the device character. Because new devices can be developed, the value *Other Device* is provided as a temporary option for use until a specific device value is added to the system.

Qualifier (Character 7)
The qualifier is specified in the seventh character. The qualifier contains unique values for individual procedures. For example, the qualifier can be used to identify the destination site in a *Bypass*.

Medical and Surgical Section Principles
In developing the Medical and Surgical procedure codes, several specific principles were followed.

Composite Terms Are Not Root Operations
Composite terms such as colonoscopy, sigmoidectomy, or appendectomy do not describe root operations, but they do specify multiple components of a specific root operation. In ICD-10-PCS, the components of a procedure are defined separately by the characters making up the complete code. The only component of a procedure

specified in the root operation is the objective of the procedure. With each complete code the underlying objective of the procedure is specified by the root operation (third character), the precise part is specified by the body part (fourth character), and the method used to reach and visualize the procedure site is specified by the approach (fifth character). While colonoscopy, sigmoidectomy, and appendectomy are included in the Index, they do not constitute root operations in the Tables section. The objective of colonoscopy is the visualization of the colon and the root operation (character 3) is *Inspection*. Character 4 specifies the body part, which in this case is part of the colon. These composite terms, like colonoscopy or appendectomy, are included as cross-reference only. The index provides the correct root operation reference. Examples of other types of composite terms not representative of root operations are *partial* sigmoidectomy, *total* hysterectomy, and *partial* hip replacement. Always refer to the correct root operation in the Index and Tables section.

Root Operation Based on Objective of Procedure

The root operation is based on the objective of the procedure, such as *Resection* of transverse colon or *Dilation* of an artery. The assignment of the root operation is based on the procedure actually performed, which may or may not have been the intended procedure. If the intended procedure is modified or discontinued (e.g., excision instead of resection is performed), the root operation is determined by the procedure actually performed. If the desired result is not attained after completing the procedure (i.e., the artery does not remain expanded after the dilation procedure), the root operation is still determined by the procedure actually performed.

Examples:

* Dilating the urethra is coded as *Dilation* since the objective of the procedure is to dilate the urethra. If dilation of the urethra includes putting in an intraluminal stent, the root operation remains *Dilation* and not *Insertion* of the intraluminal device because the underlying objective of the procedure is dilation of the urethra. The stent is identified by the intraluminal device value in the sixth character of the dilation procedure code.

* If the objective is solely to put a radioactive element in the urethra, then the procedure is coded to the root operation *Insertion*, with the radioactive element identified in the sixth character of the code.

* If the objective of the procedure is to correct a malfunctioning or displaced device, then the procedure is coded to the root operation *Revision*. In the root operation *Revision*, the original device being revised is identified in the device character. *Revision* is typically performed on mechanical appliances (e.g., pacemaker) or materials used in replacement procedures (e.g., synthetic substitute). Typical revision procedures include adjustment of pacemaker position and correction of malfunctioning knee prosthesis.

Combination Procedures Are Coded Separately

If multiple procedures as defined by distinct objectives are performed during an operative episode, then multiple codes are used. For example, obtaining the vein graft used for coronary bypass surgery is coded as a separate procedure from the bypass itself.

Redo of Procedures

The complete or partial redo of the original procedure is coded to the root operation that identifies the procedure performed rather than *Revision*.

Example:

A complete redo of a hip replacement procedure that requires putting in a new prosthesis is coded to the root operation *Replacement* rather than *Revision*.

The correction of complications arising from the original procedure, other than device complications, is coded to the procedure performed. Correction of a malfunctioning or displaced device would be coded to the root operation *Revision*.

Example:

A procedure to control hemorrhage arising from the original procedure is coded to *Control* rather than *Revision*.

Examples of Procedures Coded in the Medical Surgical Section

The following are examples of procedures from the Medical and Surgical section, coded in ICD-10-PCS.

* Suture of skin laceration, left lower arm: ØHQEXZZ

  Medical and Surgical section (Ø), body system *Skin and Breast* (H), root operation *Repair* (Q), body part *Skin, Left Lower Arm* (E), *External* Approach (X) *No device* (Z), and *No qualifier* (Z).

* Laparoscopic appendectomy: ØDTJ4ZZ

  Medical and Surgical section (Ø), body system *Gastrointestinal* (D), root operation *Resection* (T), body part *Appendix* (J), *Percutaneous Endoscopic* approach (4), No Device (Z), and No qualifier (Z).

* Sigmoidoscopy with biopsy: ØDBN8ZX

  Medical and Surgical section (Ø), body system *Gastrointestinal* (D), root operation *Excision* (B), body part *Sigmoid Colon* (N), *Via Natural or Artificial Opening Endoscopic* approach (8), *No Device* (Z), and with qualifier *Diagnostic* (X).

* Tracheostomy with tracheostomy tube: ØB11ØF4

  Medical and Surgical section (Ø), body system *Respiratory* (B), root operation *Bypass* (1), body part *Trachea* (1), *Open* approach (Ø), with *Tracheostomy Device* (F), and qualifier *Cutaneous* (4).

Obstetrics Section (1)

Character Meanings

The seven characters in the Obstetrics section have the same meaning as in the Medical and Surgical section.

Character	Meaning
1	Section
2	Body System
3	Root Operation
4	Body Part
5	Approach
6	Device
7	Qualifier

The Obstetrics section includes procedures performed on the products of conception only. Procedures on the pregnant female are coded in the Medical and Surgical section (e.g., episiotomy). The term "products of conception" refers to all physical components of a pregnancy, including the fetus, amnion, umbilical cord, and placenta. There is no differentiation of the products of conception based on gestational age. Thus, the specification of the products of conception as a zygote, embryo or fetus, or the trimester of the pregnancy is not part of the procedure code but can be found in the diagnosis code.

Section (Character 1)
Obstetrics procedure codes have a first character value of *1*.

Body System (Character 2)
The second character value for body system is *Pregnancy*.

Root Operation (Character 3)
The root operations *Change, Drainage, Extraction, Insertion, Inspection, Removal, Repair, Reposition, Resection,* and *Transplantation* are used in the obstetrics section and have the same meaning as in the Medical and Surgical section.

The Obstetrics section also includes two additional root operations, *Abortion* and *Delivery*, defined below:

- *Abortion*: Artificially terminating a pregnancy

- *Delivery*: Assisting the passage of the products of conception from the genital canal

A cesarean section is not a separate root operation because the underlying objective is *Extraction* (i.e., pulling out all or a portion of a body part).

Body Part (Character 4)
The body part values in the obstetrics section are:

- *Products of conception*

- *Products of conception, retained*

- *Products of conception, ectopic*

Approach (Character 5)
The fifth character specifies approaches and is defined as are those in the Medical and Surgical section. In the case of an abortion procedure that uses a laminaria or an abortifacient, the approach is *Via Natural or Artificial Opening*.

Device (Character 6)
The sixth character is used for devices such as fetal monitoring electrodes.

Qualifier (Character 7)
Qualifier values are specific to the root operation and are used to specify the type of extraction (e.g., low forceps, high forceps, etc.), the type of cesarean section (e.g., classical, low cervical, etc.), or the type of fluid taken out during a drainage procedure (e.g., amniotic fluid, fetal blood, etc.).

Placement Section (2)

Character Meanings
The seven characters in the Placement section have the following meaning:

Character	Meaning
1	Section
2	Body System
3	Root Operation
4	Body Region
5	Approach
6	Device
7	Qualifier

Placement section codes represent procedures for putting a device in or on a body region for the purpose of protection, immobilization, stretching, compression, or packing.

Section (Character 1)
Placement procedure codes have a first character value of *2*.

Body System (Character 2)
The second character contains two values specifying either *Anatomical Regions* or *Anatomical Orifices*.

Root Operation (Character 3)
The root operations in the Placement section include only those procedures that are performed without making an incision or a puncture. The root operations *Change* and *Removal* are in the Placement section and have the same meaning as in the Medical and Surgical section.

The Placement section also includes five additional root operations, defined as follows:

- *Compression*: Putting pressure on a body region

- *Dressing*: Putting material on a body region for protection

- *Immobilization*: Limiting or preventing motion of an external body region

- *Packing*: Putting material in a body region or orifice

- *Traction*: Exerting a pulling force on a body region in a distal direction

Body Region (Character 4)
The fourth character values are either body regions (e.g., *Upper Leg*) or natural orifices (e.g., *Ear*).

Approach (Character 5)
Since all placement procedures are performed directly on the skin or mucous membrane, or performed indirectly by applying external force through the skin or mucous membrane, the approach value is always *External*.

Device (Character 6)
The device character is always specified (except in the case of manual traction) and indicates the device placed during the procedure (e.g., cast, splint, bandage, etc.). Except for casts for fractures and dislocations, devices in the Placement section are off the shelf and do not require any extensive design, fabrication, or fitting. Placement of devices that require extensive design, fabrication, or fitting are coded in the Rehabilitation section.

Qualifier (Character 7)

The qualifier character is not specified in the Placement section; the qualifier value is always *No Qualifier*.

Administration Section (3)

Character Meanings

The seven characters in the Administration section have the following meaning:

Character	Meaning
1	Section
2	Body System
3	Root Operation
4	Body System/Region
5	Approach
6	Substance
7	Qualifier

Administration section codes represent procedures for putting in or on a therapeutic, prophylactic, protective, diagnostic, nutritional, or physiological substance. The section includes transfusions, infusions, and injections, along with other similar services such as irrigation and tattooing.

Section (Character 1)

Administration procedure codes have a first character value of *3*.

Body System (Character 2)

The body system character contains only three values: *Indwelling Device, Physiological Systems and Anatomical Regions,* or *Circulatory System*. The *Circulatory System* is used for transfusion procedures.

Root Operation (Character 3)

There are three root operations in the Administration section.

* *Introduction*: Putting in or on a therapeutic, diagnostic, nutritional, physiological, or prophylactic substance except blood or blood products

* *Irrigation*: Putting in or on a cleansing substance

* *Transfusion*: Putting in blood or blood products

Body/System Region (Character 4)

The fourth character specifies the body system/region. The fourth character identifies the site where the substance is administered, not the site where the substance administered takes effect. Sites include *Skin and Mucous Membranes, Subcutaneous Tissue,* and *Muscle*. These differentiate intradermal, subcutaneous, and intramuscular injections, respectively. Other sites include *Eye, Respiratory Tract, Peritoneal Cavity,* and *Epidural Space*.

The body systems/regions for arteries and veins are *Peripheral Artery, Central Artery, Peripheral Vein,* and *Central Vein*. The *Peripheral Artery or Vein* is typically used when a substance is introduced locally into an artery or vein. For example, chemotherapy is the introduction of an antineoplastic substance into a peripheral artery or vein by a percutaneous approach. In general, the substance introduced into a peripheral artery or vein has a systemic effect.

The *Central Artery* or *Vein* is typically used when the site where the substance is introduced is distant from the point of entry into the artery or vein. For example, the introduction of a substance directly at the site of a clot within an artery or vein using a catheter is coded as an introduction of a thrombolytic substance into a central artery or vein by a percutaneous approach. In general, the substance introduced into a central artery or vein has a local effect.

Approach (Character 5)

The fifth character specifies approaches as defined in the Medical and Surgical section. The approach for intradermal, subcutaneous, and intramuscular introductions (i.e., injections) is *Percutaneous*. If a catheter is placed to introduce a substance into an internal site within the circulatory system, then the approach is also *Percutaneous*. For example, if a catheter is used to introduce contrast directly into the heart for angiography, then the procedure would be coded as a percutaneous introduction of contrast into the heart.

Substance (Character 6)

The sixth character specifies the substance being introduced. Broad categories of substances are defined, such as anesthetic, contrast, dialysate, and blood products such as platelets.

Qualifier (Character 7)

The seventh character is a qualifier and is used to indicate whether the substance is *Autologous* or *Nonautologous*, or to further specify the substance.

Measurement and Monitoring Section (4)

Character Meanings

The seven characters in the Measurement and Monitoring section have the following meaning:

Character	Meaning
1	Section
2	Body System
3	Root Operation
4	Body System
5	Approach
6	Function/Device
7	Qualifier

Measurement and Monitoring section codes represent procedures for determining the level of a physiological or physical function.

Section (Character 1)

Measurement and Monitoring procedure codes have a first character value of *4*.

Body System (Character 2)

The second character values for body system are A, *Physiological Systems* or B, *Physiological Devices*.

Root Operation (Character 3)

There are two root operations in the Measurement and Monitoring section, as defined below:

* *Measurement*: Determining the level of a physiological or physical function at a point in time

- *Monitoring*: Determining the level of a physiological or physical function repetitively over a period of time

Body System (Character 4)

The fourth character specifies the specific body system measured or monitored.

Approach (Character 5)

The fifth character specifies approaches as defined in the Medical and Surgical section.

Function/Device (Character 6)

The sixth character specifies the physiological or physical function being measured or monitored. Examples of physiological or physical functions are *Conductivity, Metabolism, Pulse, Temperature,* and *Volume*. If a device used to perform the measurement or monitoring is inserted and left in, then insertion of the device is coded as a separate Medical and Surgical procedure.

Qualifier (Character 7)

The seventh character qualifier contains specific values as needed to further specify the body part (e.g., central, portal, pulmonary) or a variation of the procedure performed (e.g., ambulatory, stress). Examples of typical procedures coded in this section are EKG, EEG, and cardiac catheterization. An EKG is the measurement of cardiac electrical activity, while an EEG is the measurement of electrical activity of the central nervous system. A cardiac catheterization performed to measure the pressure in the heart is coded as the measurement of cardiac pressure by percutaneous approach.

Extracorporeal or Systemic Assistance and Performance Section (5)

Character Meanings

The seven characters in the Extracorporeal or Systemic Assistance and Performance section have the following meaning:

Character	Meaning
1	Section
2	Body System
3	Root Operation
4	Body System
5	Duration
6	Function
7	Qualifier

In Extracorporeal or Systemic Assistance and Performance procedures, equipment outside the body is used to assist or perform a physiological function. The section includes procedures performed in a critical care setting, such as mechanical ventilation and cardioversion; it also includes other services such as hyperbaric oxygen treatment and hemodialysis.

Section (Character 1)

Extracorporeal or Systemic Assistance and Performance procedure codes have a first character value of *5*.

Body System (Character 2)

The second character value for body system is A, *Physiological Systems*.

Root Operation (Character 3)

There are three root operations in the Extracorporeal or Systemic Assistance and Performance section, as defined below.

- *Assistance*: Taking over a portion of a physiological function by extracorporeal means

- *Performance*: Completely taking over a physiological function by extracorporeal means

- *Restoration*: Returning, or attempting to return, a physiological function to its natural state by extracorporeal means

The root operation *Restoration* contains a single procedure code that identifies extracorporeal cardioversion.

Body System (Character 4)

The fourth character specifies the body system (e.g., cardiac, respiratory) to which extracorporeal or systemic assistance or performance is applied.

Duration (Character 5)

The fifth character specifies the duration of the procedure—*Single, Intermittent,* or *Continuous*. For respiratory ventilation assistance or performance, the duration is specified in hours— *< 24 Consecutive Hours, 24–96 Consecutive Hours,* or *> 96 Consecutive Hours*. For urinary procedures, duration is specified as *Intermittent, Less than 6 Hours Per Day; Prolonged Intermittent, 6-18 hours Per Day;* or *Continuous, Greater than 18 hours Per Day*. Value 6, *Multiple* identifies serial procedure treatment.

Function (Character 6)

The sixth character specifies the physiological function assisted or performed (e.g., oxygenation, ventilation) during the procedure.

Qualifier (Character 7)

The seventh character qualifier specifies the type of equipment used, if any.

Extracorporeal or Systemic Therapies Section (6)

Character Meanings

The seven characters in the Extracorporeal or Systemic Therapies section have the following meaning:

Character	Meaning
1	Section
2	Body System
3	Root Operation
4	Body System
5	Duration
6	Qualifier
7	Qualifier

In extracorporeal or systemic therapy, equipment outside the body is used for a therapeutic purpose that does not involve the assistance or performance of a physiological function.

Section (Character 1)

Extracorporeal or Systemic Therapy procedure codes have a first character value of 6.

Body System (Character 2)

The second character value for body system is *Physiological Systems*.

Root Operation (Character 3)

There are 11 root operations in the Extracorporeal or Systemic Therapy section, as defined below.

- *Atmospheric Control*: Extracorporeal control of atmospheric pressure and composition

- *Decompression*: Extracorporeal elimination of undissolved gas from body fluids

   Coding note: The root operation *Decompression* involves only one type of procedure: treatment for decompression sickness (the bends) in a hyperbaric chamber.

- *Electromagnetic Therapy*: Extracorporeal treatment by electromagnetic rays

- *Hyperthermia*: Extracorporeal raising of body temperature

   Coding note: The term hyperthermia is used to describe both a temperature imbalance treatment and also as an adjunct radiation treatment for cancer. When treating the temperature imbalance, it is coded to this section; for the cancer treatment, it is coded in section *D Radiation Therapy*.

- *Hypothermia*: Extracorporeal lowering of body temperature

- *Perfusion*: Extracorporeal treatment by diffusion of therapeutic fluid

- *Pheresis*: Extracorporeal separation of blood products

   Coding note: Pheresis may be used for two main purposes: to treat diseases when too much of a blood component is produced (e.g., leukemia) and to remove a blood product such as platelets from a donor, for transfusion into another patient.

- *Phototherapy*: Extracorporeal treatment by light rays

   Coding note: Phototherapy involves using a machine that exposes the blood to light rays outside the body, recirculates it, and then returns it to the body.

- *Shock Wave Therapy*: Extracorporeal treatment by shock waves

- *Ultrasound Therapy*: Extracorporeal treatment by ultrasound

- *Ultraviolet Light Therapy*: Extracorporeal treatment by ultraviolet light

Body System (Character 4)

The fourth character specifies the body system on which the extracorporeal or systemic therapy is performed (e.g., skin, circulatory).

Duration (Character 5)

The fifth character specifies the duration of the procedure (e.g., single or intermittent).

Qualifier (Character 6)

The sixth character for Extracorporeal or Systemic Therapies is *No Qualifier*, except for root operation Perfusion which has a sixth character qualifier of *Donor Organ*.

Qualifier (Character 7)

The seventh character qualifier is used in the root operation *Pheresis* to specify the blood component on which pheresis is performed and in the root operation *Ultrasound Therapy* to specify site of treatment.

Osteopathic Section (7)

Character Meanings

The seven characters in the Osteopathic section have the following meaning:

Character	Meaning
1	Section
2	Body System
3	Root Operation
4	Body Region
5	Approach
6	Method
7	Qualifier

Section (Character 1)

Osteopathic procedure codes have a first character value of *7*.

Body System (Character 2)

The body system character contains the value *Anatomical Regions*.

Root Operation (Character 3)

There is only one root operation in the Osteopathic section.

- *Treatment*: Manual treatment to eliminate or alleviate somatic dysfunction and related disorders

Body Region (Character 4)

The fourth character specifies the body region on which the osteopathic treatment is performed.

Approach (Character 5)

The approach for osteopathic treatment is always *External*.

Method (Character 6)

The sixth character specifies the method by which the treatment is accomplished.

Qualifier (Character 7)

The seventh character is not specified in the Osteopathic section and always has the value *None*.

Other Procedures Section (8)

Character Meanings

The seven characters in the Other Procedures section have the following meaning:

Character	Meaning
1	Section
2	Body System
3	Root Operation
4	Body Region
5	Approach
6	Method
7	Qualifier

The Other Procedures section includes acupuncture, suture removal, and in vitro fertilization.

Section (Character 1)

Other Procedure section codes have a first character value of *8*.

Body System (Character 2)

The second character values for body systems are *Physiological Systems and Anatomical Regions* and *Indwelling Device*.

Root Operation (Character 3)

The Other Procedures section has only one root operation, defined as follows:

- *Other Procedures*: Methodologies that attempt to remediate or cure a disorder or disease.

Body Region (Character 4)

The fourth character contains specified body-region values, and also the body-region value *None*.

Approach (Character 5)

The fifth character specifies approaches as defined in the Medical and Surgical section.

Method (Character 6)

The sixth character specifies the method (e.g., *Acupuncture, Therapeutic Massage*).

Qualifier (Character 7)

The seventh character is a qualifier and contains specific values as needed.

Chiropractic Section (9)

Character Meanings

The seven characters in the Chiropractic section have the following meaning:

Character	Meaning
1	Section
2	Body System
3	Root Operation
4	Body Region
5	Approach
6	Method
7	Qualifier

Section (Character 1)

Chiropractic section procedure codes have a first character value of *9*.

Body System (Character 2)

The second character value for body system is *Anatomical Regions*.

Root Operation (Character 3)

There is only one root operation in the *Chiropractic* section.

- *Manipulation:* Manual procedure that involves a directed thrust to move a joint past the physiological range of motion, without exceeding the anatomical limit.

Body Region (Character 4)

The fourth character specifies the body region on which the chiropractic manipulation is performed.

Approach (Character 5)

The approach for chiropractic manipulation is always *External*.

Method (Character 6)

The sixth character is the method by which the manipulation is accomplished.

Qualifier (Character 7)

The seventh character is not specified in the Chiropractic section and always has the value *None*.

Imaging Section (B)

Character Meanings

The seven characters in Imaging procedures have the following meaning:

Character	Meaning
1	Section
2	Body System
3	Type
4	Body Part
5	Contrast
6	Qualifier
7	Qualifier

Imaging procedures include plain radiography, fluoroscopy, CT, MRI, and ultrasound. Nuclear medicine procedures, including PET, uptakes, and scans, are in the nuclear medicine section. Therapeutic radiation procedure codes are in a separate radiation therapy section.

Section (Character 1)
Imaging procedure codes have a first character value of *B*.

Body System (Character 2)
In the Imaging section, the second character defines the body system, such as *Heart* or *Gastrointestinal System*.

Type (Character 3)
The third character defines the type of imaging procedure (e.g., MRI, ultrasound). The following list includes all types in the *Imaging* section with a definition of each type:

- *Computerized Tomography (CT Scan)*: Computer reformatted digital display of multiplanar images developed from the capture of multiple exposures of external ionizing radiation

- *Fluoroscopy*: Single plane or bi-plane real time display of an image developed from the capture of external ionizing radiation on a fluorescent screen. The image may also be stored by either digital or analog means

- *Magnetic Resonance Imaging (MRI)*: Computer reformatted digital display of multiplanar images developed from the capture of radiofrequency signals emitted by nuclei in a body site excited within a magnetic field

- *Plain Radiography*: Planar display of an image developed from the capture of external ionizing radiation on photographic or photoconductive plate

- *Ultrasonography*: Real time display of images of anatomy or flow information developed from the capture of reflected and attenuated high frequency sound waves

Body Part (Character 4)
The fourth character defines the body part with different values for each body system (character 2) value.

Contrast (Character 5)
The fifth character specifies whether the contrast material used in the imaging procedure is *High Osmolar, Low Osmolar*, or *Other Contrast* when applicable.

Qualifier (Character 6)
The sixth character qualifier provides further detail regarding the nature of the substance or technologies used, such as *Unenhanced and Enhanced (contrast), Laser*, or *Intravascular Optical Coherence*.

Qualifier (Character 7)
The seventh character is a qualifier that may be used to specify certain procedural circumstances, the method by which the procedure was performed, or technologies utilized, such as *Intraoperative, Intravascular*, or *Transesophageal*.

Nuclear Medicine Section (C)
Character Meanings
The seven characters in the Nuclear Medicine section have the following meaning:

Character	Meaning
1	Section
2	Body System
3	Type
4	Body Part
5	Radionuclide
6	Qualifier
7	Qualifier

Nuclear Medicine is the introduction of radioactive material into the body to create an image, to diagnose and treat pathologic conditions, or to assess metabolic functions. The Nuclear Medicine section does not include the introduction of encapsulated radioactive material for the treatment of cancer. These procedures are included in the Radiation Therapy section.

Section (Character 1)
Nuclear Medicine procedure codes have a first character value of *C*.

Body System (Character 2)
The second character specifies the body system on which the nuclear medicine procedure is performed.

Type (Character 3)
The third character indicates the type of nuclear medicine procedure (e.g., planar imaging or nonimaging uptake). The following list includes the types of nuclear medicine procedures with a definition of each type.

- *Nonimaging Nuclear Medicine Assay:* Introduction of radioactive materials into the body for the study of body fluids and blood elements, by the detection of radioactive emissions

- *Nonimaging Nuclear Medicine Probe:* Introduction of radioactive materials into the body for the study of distribution and fate of certain substances by the detection of radioactive emissions; or alternatively, measurement of absorption of radioactive emissions from an external source

- *Nonimaging Nuclear Medicine Uptake:* Introduction of radioactive materials into the body for measurements of organ function, from the detection of radioactive emissions

- *Planar Nuclear Medicine Imaging*: Introduction of radioactive materials into the body for single-plane display of images developed from the capture of radioactive emissions

- *Positron Emission Tomography (PET) Imaging:* Introduction of radioactive materials into the body for three dimensional display of images developed from the simultaneous capture, 180 degrees apart, of radioactive emissions

- *Systemic Nuclear Medicine Therapy:* Introduction of unsealed radioactive materials into the body for treatment

- *Tomographic (Tomo) Nuclear Medicine Imaging*: Introduction of radioactive materials into the body for three dimensional display of images developed from the capture of radioactive emissions

Body Part (Character 4)

The fourth character indicates the body part or body region studied; with regional (e.g., *lower extremity veins*) and combination (e.g., *liver and spleen*) body parts commonly used.

Radionuclide (Character 5)

The fifth character specifies the radionuclide, the radiation source. The option *Other Radionuclide* is provided in the nuclear medicine section for newly approved radionuclides until they can be added to the coding system. If more than one radiopharmaceutical is given to perform the procedure, then more than one code is used.

Qualifier (Character 6 and 7)

The sixth and seventh characters are qualifiers but are not specified in the *Nuclear Medicine* section; the value is always *None*.

Radiation Therapy Section (D)

Character Meanings

The seven characters in the Radiation Therapy section have the following meaning:

Character	Meaning
1	Section
2	Body System
3	Modality
4	Treatment Site
5	Modality Qualifier
6	Isotope
7	Qualifier

Section (Character 1)

Radiation therapy procedure codes have a first character value of *D*.

Body System (Character 2)

The second character specifies the body system (e.g., central nervous system, musculoskeletal) irradiated.

Modality (Character 3)

The third character specifies the general modality used (e.g., beam radiation).

Treatment Site (Character 4)

The fourth character specifies the body part that is the focus of the radiation therapy.

Modality Qualifier (Character 5)

The fifth character further specifies the radiation modality used (e.g., photons, electrons).

Isotope (Character 6)

The sixth character specifies the isotopes introduced into the body, if applicable.

Qualifier (Character 7)

The seventh character may specify whether the procedure was performed intraoperatively.

Physical Rehabilitation and Diagnostic Audiology Section (F)

Character Meanings

The seven characters in the Physical Rehabilitation and Diagnostic Audiology section have the following meaning:

Character	Meaning
1	Section
2	Section Qualifier
3	Type
4	Body System/Region
5	Type Qualifier
6	Equipment
7	Qualifier

Physical rehabilitation procedures include physical therapy, occupational therapy, and speech-language pathology. Osteopathic procedures and chiropractic procedures are in separate sections.

Section (Character 1)

Physical Rehabilitation and Diagnostic Audiology procedure codes have a first character value of *F*.

Section Qualifier (Character 2)

The section qualifier *Rehabilitation* or *Diagnostic Audiology* is specified in the second character.

Type (Character 3)

The third character specifies the type. There are 14 different values, which can be classified into four basic types of rehabilitation and diagnostic audiology procedures, defined as follows:

Assessment: Includes a determination of the patient's diagnosis when appropriate, need for treatment, planning for treatment, periodic assessment, and documentation related to these activities

Assessments are further classified into more than 100 different tests or methods. The majority of these focus on the faculties of hearing and speech, but others focus on various aspects of body function, and on the patient's quality of life, such as muscle performance, neuromotor development, and reintegration skills.

- *Speech Assessment*: Measurement of speech and related functions

- *Motor and/or Nerve Function Assessment*: Measurement of motor, nerve, and related functions

- *Activities of Daily Living Assessment*: Measurement of functional level for activities of daily living

- *Hearing Assessment*: Measurement of hearing and related functions

- *Hearing Aid Assessment*: Measurement of the appropriateness and/or effectiveness of a hearing device

- *Vestibular Assessment*: Measurement of the vestibular system and related functions

Caregiver Training: Educating caregiver with the skills and knowledge used to interact with and assist the patient

Caregiver Training is divided into 18 different broad subjects taught to help a caregiver provide proper patient care.

- *Caregiver Training*: Training in activities to support patient's optimal level of function

Fitting(s): Design, fabrication, modification, selection, and/or application of splint, orthosis, prosthesis, hearing aids, and/or other rehabilitation device

The fifth character used in *Device Fitting* procedures describes the device being fitted rather than the method used to fit the device. Definitions of devices, when provided, are located in the definitions portion of the ICD-10-PCS tables and index, under section F, character 5.

- *Device Fitting*: Fitting of a device designed to facilitate or support achievement of a higher level of function

Treatment: Use of specific activities or methods to develop, improve, and/or restore the performance of necessary functions, compensate for dysfunction and/or minimize debilitation

Treatment procedures include swallowing dysfunction exercises, bathing and showering techniques, wound management, gait training, and a host of activities typically associated with rehabilitation.

- *Speech Treatment*: Application of techniques to improve, augment, or compensate for speech and related functional impairment

- *Motor Treatment*: Exercise or activities to increase or facilitate motor function

- *Activities of Daily Living Treatment*: Exercise or activities to facilitate functional competence for activities of daily living

- *Hearing Treatment*: Application of techniques to improve, augment, or compensate for hearing and related functional impairment

- *Cochlear Implant Treatment*: Application of techniques to improve the communication abilities of individuals with cochlear implant

- *Vestibular Treatment*: Application of techniques to improve, augment, or compensate for vestibular and related functional impairment

The type of treatment includes training as well as activities that restore function.

Body System/Region (Character 4)
The fourth character specifies the body region and/or system on which the procedure is performed.

Type Qualifier (Character 5)
The fifth character is a type qualifier that further specifies the procedure performed. Examples include therapy to improve the range of motion and training for bathing techniques. Refer to appendix I for definitions of these types of procedures.

Equipment (Character 6)
The sixth character specifies the equipment used. Specific equipment is not defined in the equipment value. Instead, broad categories of equipment are specified (e.g., aerobic endurance and conditioning, assistive/adaptive/supportive, etc.)

Qualifier (Character 7)
The seventh character is not specified in the Physical Rehabilitation and Diagnostic Audiology section and always has the value *None*.

Mental Health Section (G)
Character Meanings
The seven characters in the Mental Health section have the following meaning:

Character	Meaning
1	Section
2	Body System
3	Type
4	Qualifier
5	Qualifier
6	Qualifier
7	Qualifier

Section (Character 1)
Mental health procedure codes have a first character value of *G*.

Body System (Character 2)
The second character is used to identify the body system elsewhere in ICD-10-PCS. In this section it always has the value *None*.

Type (Character 3)
The third character specifies the procedure type, such as crisis intervention or counseling. There are 12 types of mental health procedures.

- *Psychological Tests:* The administration and interpretation of standardized psychological tests and measurement instruments for the assessment of psychological function

- *Crisis Intervention:* Treatment of a traumatized, acutely disturbed, or distressed individual for the purpose of short-term stabilization

- *Medication Management:* Monitoring and adjusting the use of medications for the treatment of a mental health disorder

- *Individual Psychotherapy:* Treatment of an individual with a mental health disorder by behavioral, cognitive, psychoanalytic, psychodynamic, or psychophysiological means to improve functioning or well-being

- *Counseling:* The application of psychological methods to treat an individual with normal developmental issues and psychological problems in order to increase function, improve well-being, alleviate distress, maladjustment, or resolve crises

- *Family Psychotherapy:* Treatment that includes one or more family members of an individual with a mental health disorder by behavioral, cognitive, psychoanalytic, psychodynamic, or psychophysiological means to improve functioning or well-being

- *Electroconvulsive Therapy:* The application of controlled electrical voltages to treat a mental health disorder

- *Biofeedback:* Provision of information from the monitoring and regulating of physiological processes in conjunction with cognitive-behavioral techniques to improve patient functioning or well-being

- *Hypnosis:* Induction of a state of heightened suggestibility by auditory, visual, and tactile techniques to elicit an emotional or behavioral response

- *Narcosynthesis:* Administration of intravenous barbiturates in order to release suppressed or repressed thoughts

- *Group Psychotherapy:* Treatment of two or more individuals with a mental health disorder by behavioral, cognitive, psychoanalytic, psychodynamic, or psychophysiological means to improve functioning or well-being

- *Light Therapy:* Application of specialized light treatments to improve functioning or well-being

Qualifier (Character 4)
The fourth character is a qualifier to indicate that counseling was educational or vocational or to indicate type of test or method of therapy.

Qualifier (Character 5, 6 and 7)
The fifth, sixth, and seventh characters are not specified and always have the value *None*.

Substance Abuse Treatment Section (H)

Character Meanings
The seven characters in the Substance Abuse Treatment section have the following meaning:

Character	Meaning
1	Section
2	Body System
3	Type
4	Qualifier
5	Qualifier
6	Qualifier
7	Qualifier

Section (Character 1)
Substance Abuse Treatment codes have a first character value of *H*.

Body System (Character 2)
The second character is used to identify the body system elsewhere in ICD-10-PCS. In this section, it always has the value *None*.

Type (Character 3)
The third character specifies the type of procedure. There are seven values classified in this section, as listed below:

- *Detoxification Services:* Detoxification from alcohol and/or drugs

- *Individual Counseling:* The application of psychological methods to treat an individual with addictive behavior

- *Group Counseling:* The application of psychological methods to treat two or more individuals with addictive behavior

- *Individual Psychotherapy:* Treatment of an individual with addictive behavior by behavioral, cognitive, psychoanalytic, psychodynamic, or psychophysiological means

- *Family Counseling:* The application of psychological methods that includes one or more family members to treat an individual with addictive behavior

- *Medication Management:* Monitoring and adjusting the use of replacement medications for the treatment of addiction

- *Pharmacotherapy:* The use of replacement medications for the treatment of addiction

Qualifier (Character 4)
The fourth character further specifies the procedure type. These qualifier values vary dependent upon the Root Type procedure (Character 3). Root type 2, *Detoxification Services* contains only the value Z, *None* and Root type 6, *Family Counseling* contains only the value 3, *Other Family Counseling*, whereas the remainder Root Type procedures include multiple possible values.

Qualifier (Character 5, 6 and 7)
The fifth through seventh characters are designated as qualifiers but are never specified, so they always have the value *None*.

New Technology Section (X)

General Information
Section X New Technology is a section added to ICD-10-PCS beginning October 1, 2015. The new section provides a place for codes that uniquely identify procedures requested via the New Technology Application Process or that capture other new technologies not currently classified in ICD-10-PCS.

Section X does not introduce any new coding concepts or unusual guidelines for correct coding. In fact, Section X codes maintain continuity with the other sections in ICD-10-PCS by using the same root operation and body part values as their closest counterparts in other sections of ICD-10-PCS. For example, the codes for the infusion of ceftazidime-avibactam, use the same root operation (Introduction) and body part values (Central Vein and Peripheral Vein) in section X as the infusion codes in section 3 Administration, which are their closest counterparts in the other sections of ICD-10-PCS.

Character Meanings
The seven characters in the new technology section have the following meaning:

Character	Meaning
1	Section
2	Body System
3	Root Operation
4	Body Part
5	Approach
6	Device/Substance/Technology
7	Qualifier

Section (Character 1)
New technology procedure codes have a first character value of *X*.

Body System (Character 2)
The second character values for body system combine the uses of body system, body region, and physiological system as specified in other sections in ICD-10-PCS.

Root Operation (Character 3)

The third character utilizes the same root operation values as their counterparts in other sections of ICD-10-PCS.

Body Part (Character 4)

The fourth character specifies the same body part values as their closest counterparts in other sections of ICD-10-PCS.

Approach (Character 5)

The fifth character specifies approaches as defined in the Medical and Surgical section.

Device/Substance/Technology (Character 6)

The sixth character specifies the key feature of the new technology procedure. It may be specified as a new device, a new substance, or other new technology. Examples of sixth character values are *blinatumomab antineoplastic immunotherapy, orbital atherectomy technology,* and *intraoperative knee replacement sensor.*

Qualifier (Character 7)

The seventh character qualifier is used exclusively to specify the new technology group, a number or letter that changes each year that new technology codes are added to the system. For example, Section X codes added for the first year have the seventh character value 1, *New Technology Group 1*, and the next year that Section X codes are added have the seventh character value 2, *New Technology Group 2*, and so on. Changing the seventh character value to a unique letter or number every year that there are new codes in the new technology section allows the ICD-10-PCS to "recycle" the values in the third, fourth, and sixth characters as needed.

New Technology Coding Instruction

Section X codes are standalone codes. They are not supplemental codes. Section X codes fully represent the specific procedure described in the code title, and do not require any additional codes from other sections of ICD-10-PCS. When section X contains a code title which describes a specific new technology procedure, only that X code is reported for the procedure. There is no need to report a broader, non-specific code in another section of ICD-10-PCS.

For example, code XW04321 Introduction of Ceftazidime-Avibactam Anti-infective into Central Vein, Percutaneous Approach, New Technology Group 1, would be reported to indicate that Ceftazidime-Avibactam Anti-infective was administered via central vein. A separate code from table 3E0 in the Administration section of ICD-10-PCS would not be reported in addition to this code. The X section code fully identifies the administration of the ceftazidime-avibactam antibiotic, and no additional code is needed.

The New Technology section codes are easily found by looking in the ICD-10-PCS Index or the Tables. In the Index, the name of the new technology device, substance or technology for a section X code is included as a main term. In addition, all codes in section X are listed under the main term New Technology. The new technology code index entry for ceftazidime-avibactam is shown below.

Ceftazidime-Avibactam Anti-infective XW0

New Technology
   Ceftazidime-Avibactam Anti-infective XW0

Appendixes

The resources described below have been included as appendixes for *ICD-10-PCS The Complete Official Code Set*. These resources further instruct the coder on the appropriate application of the ICD-10-PCS code set.

Appendix A: Components of the Medical and Surgical Approach Definitions

This resource further defines the approach characters used in the Medical and Surgical (0) section. Complementing the detailed definition of the approach, additional information includes whether or not instrumentation is a part of the approach, the typical access location, the method used to initiate the approach, related procedural examples, and illustrations all of which will help the user determine the appropriate approach value.

Appendix B: Root Operation Definitions

This resource is a compilation of all root operations found in the Medical and Surgical-related sections (0-9) of this PCS manual. It provides a definition and in some cases a more detailed explanation of the root operation, to better reflect the purpose or objective. Examples of related procedure(s) may also be provided.

Appendix C: Comparison of Medical and Surgical Root Operations

The Medical and Surgical root operations are divided into groups that share similar attributes. These groups, and the root operations in each group, are listed in this resource along with information identifying the target of the root operation, the action used to perform the root operation, any clarification or further explanation on the objective of the root operation, and procedure examples.

Appendix D: Body Part Key

When an anatomical term or description is provided in the documentation but does not have a specific body part character within a table, the user can reference this resource to search for the anatomical description or site noted in the documentation to determine if there is a specific PCS body part character (character 4) to which the anatomical description or site could be coded.

Appendix E: Body Part Definitions

This resource is the reverse look-up of the Body Part Key. Each table in the Medical and Surgical section (0) of the PCS manual contains anatomical terms linked to a body part character or value, for example, in Table 0BB the Body Part (character 4) of 1 is Trachea. The body part Trachea may have anatomical structures or descriptions that may be used in procedure documentation instead of the term trachea. The Body Part Definitions list other anatomical structures or synonyms that are included in specific ICD-10-PCS body part values. According to the body part definitions, in the example above, cricoid cartilage is included in the Trachea (character 1) body part.

Appendix F: Device Key and Aggregation Table

The Device Key relates specific devices used in the medical profession, such as stents or bovine pericardial valves, with the appropriate device character (character 6).

The Aggregation Table crosswalks specific device character value definitions for specific root operations in a specific body system to the more general device character value to be used when the root operation covers a wide range of body parts and the device character represents an entire family of devices.

Appendix G: Device Definitions

This resource is a reverse look-up to the Device Key. The user may reference this resource to see all the specific devices that may be grouped to a particular device character (character 6).

Appendix H: Substance Key/Substance Definitions

The Substance Key lists substances by trade name or synonym and relates them to a PCS character in the Administration (3) or New Technology (X) section in the sixth character Substance or seventh character Qualifier column.

The Substance Definitions table is the reverse look-up of the substance key, relating all substance categories, the sixth- or seventh character values, to all trade name or synonyms that may be classified to that particular character.

Appendix I: Sections B-H Character Definitions

In each ancillary section (B-H) the characters in a particular column may have different meanings depending on which ancillary section the user is working from. This resource provides the values for the characters in that particular ancillary section as well as a definition of the character value.

Appendix J: Hospital Acquired Conditions

This comprehensive table displays codes identifying conditions that are considered reasonably preventable when occurring during the hospital admission and may prevent the case from grouping to a higher-paying MS-DRG. Many of these HACs are conditional and are based on reporting of a specific ICD-10-CM diagnosis code in combination with certain ICD-10-PCS procedure codes, all of which are noted in this table.

Appendix K: Coding Exercises with Answers

This resource provides the coding exercises with answers, and in some cases a brief explanation as to the reason that particular code was used.

Appendix L: Procedure Combination Tables

The procedure combination tables provided in this resource illustrate certain procedure combinations that must occur in order to assign a specific MS-DRG.

Sources

All material contained in this manual is derived from the ICD-10-PCS Coding System files, revised and distributed by the Centers for Medicare and Medicaid Services, FY 2019.

ICD-10-PCS Index and Tabular Format

The *ICD-10-PCS: The Complete Official Code Set* is based on the official version of the International Classification of Diseases, 10th Revision, Procedure Classification System, issued by the U.S. Department of Health and Human Services, Centers for Medicare and Medicaid Services. This book is consistent with the content of the government's version of ICD-10-PCS and follows their official format.

Index

The Alphabetic Index can be used to locate the appropriate table containing all the information necessary to construct a procedure code, however, the PCS tables should always be consulted to find the most appropriate valid code. Users may choose a valid code directly from the tables—he or she need not consult the index before proceeding to the tables to complete the code.

Main Terms

The Alphabetic Index reflects the structure of the tables. Therefore, the index is organized as an alphabetic listing. The index:

- Is based on the value of the third character
- Contains common procedure terms
- Lists anatomic sites
- Uses device terms

The main terms in the Alphabetic Index are root operations, root procedure types, or common procedure names. In addition, anatomic sites from the Body Part Key and device terms from the Device Key have been added for ease of use.

Examples:

Resection (root operation)

Fluoroscopy (root type)

Prostatectomy (common procedure name)

Brachial artery (body part)

Bard® Dulex™ mesh (device)

The index provides at least the first three or four values of the code, and some entries may provide complete valid codes. However, the user should always consult the appropriate table to verify that the most appropriate valid code has been selected.

Root Operation and Procedure Type Main Terms

For the *Medical and Surgical* and related sections, the root operation values are used as main terms in the index. The subterms under the root operation main terms are body parts. For the Ancillary section of the tables, the main terms in the index are the general type of procedure performed.

Examples:

Biofeedback GZC9ZZZ
Destruction
    Acetabulum
        Left 0Q55
        Right 0Q54
    Adenoids 0C5Q
    Ampulla of Vater 0F5C
Planar Nuclear Medicine Imaging
    Abdomen CW10

See Reference

The second type of term in the index uses common procedure names, such as "appendectomy" or "fundoplication." These common terms are listed as main terms with a "see" reference noting the PCS root operations that are possible valid code tables based on the objective of the procedure.

Examples:

Tendonectomy
    see Excision, Tendons 0LB
    see Resection, Tendons 0LT

Use Reference

The index also lists anatomic sites from the Body Part Key and device terms from the Device Key. These terms are listed with a "use" reference. The purpose of these references is to act as an additional reference to the terms located in the Appendix Keys. The term provided is the Body Part value or Device value to be selected when constructing a procedure code using the code tables. This type of index reference is not intended to direct the user to another term in the index, but to provide guidance regarding character value selection. Therefore, "use" references generally do not refer to specific valid code tables.

Examples:

CoAxia NeuroFlo catheter
    use Intraluminal Device
Epitrochlear lymph node
    use Lymphatic, Right Upper Extremity
    use Lymphatic, Left Upper Extremity
SynCardia Total Artificial Heart
    use Synthetic Substitute

Code Tables

ICD-10-PCS contains 17 sections of Code Tables organized by general type of procedure. The first three characters of a procedure code define each table. The tables consist of columns providing the possible last four characters of codes and rows providing valid values for each character. Within a PCS table, valid codes include all combinations of choices in characters 4 through 7 contained in the same row of the table. All seven characters must be specified to form a valid code.

There are three main sections of tables:

- Medical and Surgical section:
  - *Medical and Surgical* (0)
- Medical and Surgical-related sections:
  - *Obstetrics* (1)
  - *Placement* (2)
  - *Administration* (3)
  - *Measurement and Monitoring* (4)
  - *Extracorporeal or Systemic Assistance and Performance* (5)
  - *Extracorporeal or Systemic Therapies* (6)
  - *Osteopathic* (7)
  - *Other Procedures* (8)
  - *Chiropractic* (9)

- Ancillary sections:
  — *Imaging* (B)
  — *Nuclear Medicine* (C)
  — *Radiation Therapy* (D)
  — *Physical Rehabilitation and Diagnostic Audiology* (F)
  — *Mental Health* (G)
  — *Substance Abuse Treatment* (H)
- New Technology section:
  — *New Technology* (X)

The first three character values define each table. The root operation or root type designated for each table is accompanied by its official definition.

Example:

Table 00F provides codes for procedures on the central nervous system that involve breaking up of solid matter into pieces:

Character 1, Section	0: Medical and Surgical
Character 2, Body System	0: Central Nervous System and Cranial Nerves
Character 3, Root Operation	F: Fragmentation: Breaking solid matter in a body part into pieces

Tables are arranged numerically, then alphabetically.

When reviewing tables, the user should keep in mind that:

- Some tables may cover multiple pages in the code book—to ensure maximum clarity about character choices, valid entries do not split rows between pages. For instance, the entire table of valid characters completing a code beginning with 4A1 is split between two pages, but the split is between, not within, rows. This means that all the valid sixth and seventh characters for, say, body system *Arterial* (3) and approach *External* (X) are contained on one page.

- Individual entries may be listed in several horizontal "selection" lines.

- When a table is continued onto another page, a note to this effect has been added in red.

Body Part Definitions:

An exclusive feature in the tables is the incorporation of the body part definitions provided in appendix E into the Medical and Surgical section (0) tables under their appropriate body part characters in the fourth column (character 4). This provides the user a direct reference to all anatomical descriptions, terms, and sites that could be coded to that particular body part value.

Paired body parts typically have values for the right and left side and in some cases a value for bilateral. These paired body parts often have the same list of inclusive body part definitions. When there are paired body parts with the same body part definitions, the first listed body part (usually the right side) contains the list of body part definitions while the second listed body part (usually the left side) contains a **See** instruction. This **See** instruction references the body part value that contains the body part definitions. In the table below, body part value P – Upper Eyelid, Left is followed by a **See** instruction that states **See** N *Upper Eyelid, Right*. All body part descriptions under value N also apply to body part value P.

Example:

0 **Medical and Surgical**
8 **Eye**
M **Reattachment**   Definition: Putting back in or on all or a portion of a separated body part to its normal location or other suitable location
                          Explanation: Vascular circulation and nervous pathways may or may not be reestablished

Body Part Character 4	Approach Character 5	Device Character 6	Qualifier Character 7
N **Upper Eyelid, Right** Lateral canthus Levator palpebrae superioris muscle Orbicularis oculi muscle Superior tarsal plate **P** **Upper Eyelid, Left** *See N Upper Eyelid, Right* **Q** **Lower Eyelid, Right** Inferior tarsal plate Medial canthus **R** **Lower Eyelid, Left** *See Q Lower Eyelid, Right*	**X** External	**Z** No Device	**Z** No Qualifier

ICD-10-PCS Additional Features

Use of Official Sources

The *ICD-10-PCS: The Complete Official Code Set* contains the official U.S. Department of Health and Human Services, Tenth Revision, Procedure Classification System, effective for the current year.

Color-coding, symbol, and other annotations in this manual that identify coding and reimbursement issues are derived from various official federal government sources, including Medicare Code Editor (MCE), version 35, ICD-10 MS-DRG Definitions Manual Files, version 35, and the *Federal Register*, volume 83, number 88, May 7, 2018 ("Hospital Inpatient Prospective Payment Systems for Acute Care Hospitals and the Long Term Care Hospital Prospective Payment System and Proposed Policy Changes and Fiscal Year 2019 Rates; Proposed Rule"). For the most current files related to IPPS, please refer to the following:

https://www.cms.gov/Medicare/Medicare-Fee-for-Service-Payment/AcuteInpatientPPS/IPPS-Regulations-and-Notices.html.

Table Notations

Many tables in ICD-10-PCS contain color or symbol annotations that may aid in code selection, provide clinical or coding information, or alert the coder to reimbursement issues affected by the PCS code assignment. These annotations are most often displayed on or next to a character 4 value. Some character 4 values may have more than one annotation.

Refer to the color/symbol legend at the bottom of each page in the tables section for an abridged description of each color and symbol.

Annotation Box

An annotation box has been appended to all tables that contain color-coding or symbol annotations. The color bar or symbol attached to a character 4 value is provided in the box, as well as a list of the valid PCS code(s) to which that edit applies. The box may also list conditional criteria that must be met to satisfy the edit.

For example, see Table 00F. Four character 4 body part values have a gray color bar. In the annotation box below the table, the gray color bar is defined as "Non-OR," or a nonoperating room procedure edit. Following the Non-OR annotation are the PCS codes that are considered nonoperating room procedures from that row of Table 00F.

Bracketed Code Notation

The use of bracketed codes is an efficient convention to provide all valid character value alternatives for a specific set of circumstances. The character values in the brackets correspond to the valid values for the character in the position the bracket appears.

Examples:

In the annotation box for Table 00F the Noncovered Procedure edit (NC) applies to codes represented in the bracketed code 00F[3,4,5,6]XZZ.

    00F[3,4,5,6]XZZ Fragmentation in (Central Nervous System and Cranial Nerves), External Approach

---

The valid fourth character values (Body Part) that may be selected for this specific circumstance are as follows:

3	Epidural Space, Intracranial
4	Subdural Space, Intracranial
5	Subarachnoid Space, Intracranial
6	Cerebral Ventricle

The fragmentation of matter in the spinal canal, Body Part value U, is not included in the noncovered procedure code edits.

Color-Coding/Symbols

New and Revised Text

To highlight changes to the PCS tables for the current year, the new and revised text is provided in green font.

Medicare Code Edits

Medicare administrative contractors (MACs) and many payers use Medicare code edits to check the coding accuracy on claims. The coding edits in this manual are only those directly related to ICD-10-PCS codes and are used for acute care hospital inpatient admissions.

The PCS related Medicare code edits are listed below:

- Invalid procedure code
- *Sex conflict
- *Noncovered procedure
- *Limited coverage procedure

Starred edits above that are related to PCS issues are identified in this manual by symbols as described below.

Sex Edit Symbols

The sex edit symbols below address MCE and are used to detect inconsistencies between the patient's sex and the procedure. The symbols below most often appear to the right of a character 4 value but may also be found to the right of a character 7 value:

♂   Male procedure only

♀   Female procedure only

NC   **Noncovered Procedure**

Medicare does not cover all procedures. However, some noncovered procedures, due to the presence of certain diagnoses, are reimbursed.

LC   **Limited Coverage**

For certain procedures whose medical complexity and serious nature incur extraordinary associated costs, Medicare limits coverage to a portion of the cost. The limited coverage edit indicates the type of limited coverage.

ICD-10 MS-DRG Definitions Manual Edits

An MS-DRG is assigned based on specific patient attributes, such as principal diagnosis, secondary diagnoses, procedures, and discharge status. The attributes (edits) provided in this manual are only those directly related to ICD-10-PCS codes and are used for acute care hospital inpatient admissions.

Non-Operating Room Procedures Not Affecting MS-DRG Assignment

In the Medical and Surgical section (ØØ1–ØYW) and the Obstetric section (1Ø2–1ØY) tables **only,** ICD-10-PCS procedures codes that DO NOT affect MS-DRG assignment are identified by a **gray color bar** over the character 4 value and are considered non-operating room (non-OR) procedures.

NOTE: The majority of the ICD-10-PCS codes in the Medical and Surgical-Related, Ancillary and New Technology section tables are non-operating room procedures that do not typically affect MS-DRG assignment. Only the Valid Operating Room and DRG Non-Operating Room procedures are highlighted in these sections, *see* Non-Operating Room Procedures Affecting MS-DRG Assignment and Valid OR Procedure description below.

Non-Operating Room Procedures Affecting MS-DRG Assignment

Some ICD-10-PCS procedure codes, although considered non-operating room procedures, may still affect MS-DRG assignment. In all sections of the ICD-10-PCS book, these procedures are identified by a **purple color bar** over the character 4 value.

Valid OR Procedure

In the Medical and Surgical-Related (2WØ–9WB), Ancillary (BØØ–HZ9) and New Technology (X2A–XYØ) section tables **only**, any codes that are considered a valid operating room procedure are identified with a **blue color bar** over the character 4 value and will affect MS-DRG assignment. All codes without a color bar (blue or purple) are considered non-operating room procedures.

Hospital-Acquired Condition Related Procedures

Procedures associated with hospital-acquired conditions (HAC) are identified with the **yellow color bar** over the body part value.

Combination Only

Some ICD-10-PCS procedure codes are considered "noncovered procedures" except when reported in combination with certain other procedure codes. Such codes are designated by a **red color bar** over the character 4 value.

⊞ Combination Member

A combination member is an ICD-10-PCS procedure code that can influence MS-DRG assignment either on its own or in combination with other specific ICD-10-PCS procedure codes. Combination member codes are designated by a plus sign (⊞) to the right of the body part value.

See Appendix L for Procedure Combinations

Under certain circumstances, more than one procedure code is needed in order to group to a specific MS-DRG. When codes within a table have been identified as a Combination Only (**red color bar**) or Combination Member (⊞) code, there is also a footnote instructing the coder to *see Appendix L*. Appendix L contains tables that identify the other procedure codes needed in the combination and the title and number of the MS-DRG to which the combination will group.

Other Table Notations

AHA Coding Clinic:

Official citations from AHA's *Coding Clinic for ICD-10-CM/PCS* have been provided at the beginning of each section, when applicable. Each specific citation is listed below a header identifying the table to which that particular *Coding Clinic* citation applies. The citations appear in purple type with the year, quarter, and page of the reference as well as the title of the question as it appears in that *Coding Clinic's* table of contents. *Coding Clinic* citations included in this edition have been updated through first quarter 2018.

Index Notations

▽ Subterms under main terms may continue to the next column or page. This warning statement is a reminder to always check for additional subterms and information that may continue onto the next page or column before making a final selection.

ICD-10-PCS Official Guidelines for Coding and Reporting 2019

Narrative changes appear in **bold** text.

The Centers for Medicare and Medicaid Services (CMS) and the National Center for Health Statistics (NCHS), two departments within the U.S. Federal Government's Department of Health and Human Services (DHHS) provide the following guidelines for coding and reporting using the International Classification of Diseases, 10th Revision, Procedure Coding System (ICD-10-PCS). These guidelines should be used as a companion document to the official version of the ICD-10-PCS as published on the CMS website. The ICD-10-PCS is a procedure classification published by the United States for classifying procedures performed in hospital inpatient health care settings.

These guidelines have been approved by the four organizations that make up the Cooperating Parties for the ICD-10-PCS: the American Hospital Association (AHA), the American Health Information Management Association (AHIMA), CMS, and NCHS.

These guidelines are a set of rules that have been developed to accompany and complement the official conventions and instructions provided within the ICD-10-PCS itself. The instructions and conventions of the classification take precedence over guidelines. These guidelines are based on the coding and sequencing instructions in the Tables, Index and Definitions of ICD-10-PCS, but provide additional instruction. Adherence to these guidelines when assigning ICD-10-PCS procedure codes is required under the Health Insurance Portability and Accountability Act (HIPAA). The procedure codes have been adopted under HIPAA for hospital inpatient healthcare settings. A joint effort between the healthcare provider and the coder is essential to achieve complete and accurate documentation, code assignment, and reporting of diagnoses and procedures. These guidelines have been developed to assist both the healthcare provider and the coder in identifying those procedures that are to be reported. The importance of consistent, complete documentation in the medical record cannot be overemphasized. Without such documentation accurate coding cannot be achieved.

Conventions

A1. ICD-10-PCS codes are composed of seven characters. Each character is an axis of classification that specifies information about the procedure performed. Within a defined code range, a character specifies the same type of information in that axis of classification.

Example: The fifth axis of classification specifies the approach in sections Ø through 4 and 7 through 9 of the system.

A2. One of 34 possible values can be assigned to each axis of classification in the seven-character code: they are the numbers Ø through 9 and the alphabet (except I and O because they are easily confused with the numbers 1 and Ø). The number of unique values used in an axis of classification differs as needed.

Example: Where the fifth axis of classification specifies the approach, seven different approach values are currently used to specify the approach.

A3. The valid values for an axis of classification can be added to as needed.

Example: If a significantly distinct type of device is used in a new procedure, a new device value can be added to the system.

A4. As with words in their context, the meaning of any single value is a combination of its axis of classification and any preceding values on which it may be dependent.

Example: The meaning of a body part value in the Medical and Surgical section is always dependent on the body system value. The body part value Ø in the Central Nervous body system specifies Brain and the body part value Ø in the Peripheral Nervous body system specifies Cervical Plexus.

A5. As the system is expanded to become increasingly detailed, over time more values will depend on preceding values for their meaning.

Example: In the Lower Joints body system, the device value 3 in the root operation Insertion specifies Infusion Device and the device value 3 in the root operation Replacement specifies Ceramic Synthetic Substitute.

A6. The purpose of the alphabetic index is to locate the appropriate table that contains all information necessary to construct a procedure code. The PCS Tables should always be consulted to find the most appropriate valid code.

A7. It is not required to consult the index first before proceeding to the tables to complete the code. A valid code may be chosen directly from the tables.

A8. All seven characters must be specified to be a valid code. If the documentation is incomplete for coding purposes, the physician should be queried for the necessary information.

A9. Within a PCS table, valid codes include all combinations of choices in characters 4 through 7 contained in the same row of the table. In the example below, ØJHT3VZ is a valid code, and ØJHW3VZ is *not* a valid code.

Section:	Ø	**Medical and Surgical**
Body System:	J	**Subcutaneous Tissue and Fascia**
Operation:	H	**Insertion** Putting in a nonbiological appliance that monitors, assists, performs, or prevents a physiological function but does not physically take the place of a body part

Body Part		Approach		Device		Qualifier	
S Subcutaneous Tissue and Fascia, Head and Neck **V** Subcutaneous Tissue and Fascia, Upper Extremity **W** Subcutaneous Tissue and Fascia, Lower Extremity		**Ø** Open **3** Percutaneous		**1** Radioactive Element **3** Infusion Device		**Z** No Qualifier	
T Subcutaneous Tissue and Fascia, Trunk		**Ø** Open **3** Percutaneous		**1** Radioactive Element **3** Infusion Device **V** Infusion Pump		**Z** No Qualifier	

A10. "And," when used in a code description, means "and/or," **except when used to describe a combination of multiple body parts for which separate values exist for each body part (e.g., Skin and Subcutaneous Tissue used as a qualifier, where there are separate body part values for "Skin" and "Subcutaneous Tissue").**

Example: Lower Arm and Wrist Muscle means lower arm and/or wrist muscle.

A11. Many of the terms used to construct PCS codes are defined within the system. It is the coder's responsibility to determine what the documentation in the medical record equates to in the PCS definitions. The physician is not expected to use the terms used in PCS code descriptions, nor is the coder required to query the physician when the correlation between the documentation and the defined PCS terms is clear.

Example: When the physician documents "partial resection" the coder can independently correlate "partial resection" to the root operation Excision without querying the physician for clarification.

Medical and Surgical Section Guidelines (section 0)

B2. Body System

General guidelines

B2.1a. The procedure codes in the general anatomical regions body systems can be used when the procedure is performed on an anatomical region rather than a specific body part (e.g., root operations Control and Detachment, Drainage of a body cavity) or on the rare occasion when no information is available to support assignment of a code to a specific body part.

Examples: Control of postoperative hemorrhage is coded to the root operation Control found in the general anatomical regions body systems.

Chest tube drainage of the pleural cavity is coded to the root operation Drainage found in the general anatomical regions body systems. Suture repair of the abdominal wall is coded to the root operation Repair in the general anatomical regions body system.

B2.1b. Where the general body part values "upper" and "lower" are provided as an option in the Upper Arteries, Lower Arteries, Upper Veins, Lower Veins, Muscles and Tendons body systems, "upper" or "lower "specifies body parts located above or below the diaphragm respectively.

Example: Vein body parts above the diaphragm are found in the Upper Veins body system; vein body parts below the diaphragm are found in the Lower Veins body system.

B3. Root Operation

General guidelines

B3.1a. In order to determine the appropriate root operation, the full definition of the root operation as contained in the PCS Tables must be applied.

B3.1b. Components of a procedure specified in the root operation definition and explanation are not coded separately. Procedural steps necessary to reach the operative site and close the operative site,

including anastomosis of a tubular body part, are also not coded separately.

Examples: Resection of a joint as part of a joint replacement procedure is included in the root operation definition of Replacement and is not coded separately.

Laparotomy performed to reach the site of an open liver biopsy is not coded separately. In a resection of sigmoid colon with anastomosis of descending colon to rectum, the anastomosis is not coded separately.

Multiple procedures

B3.2. During the same operative episode, multiple procedures are coded if:

    a.   The same root operation is performed on different body parts as defined by distinct values of the body part character.

        Examples: Diagnostic excision of liver and pancreas are coded separately.

        Excision of lesion in the ascending colon and excision of lesion in the transverse colon are coded separately.

    b.   The same root operation is repeated in multiple body parts, and those body parts are separate and distinct body parts classified to a single ICD-10-PCS body part value.

        Examples: Excision of the sartorius muscle and excision of the gracilis muscle are both included in the upper leg muscle body part value, and multiple procedures are coded.

        Extraction of multiple toenails are coded separately.

    c.   Multiple root operations with distinct objectives are performed on the same body part.

        Example: Destruction of sigmoid lesion and bypass of sigmoid colon are coded separately.

    d.   The intended root operation is attempted using one approach, but is converted to a different approach.

        Example: Laparoscopic cholecystectomy converted to an open cholecystectomy is coded as percutaneous endoscopic Inspection and open Resection.

Discontinued or incomplete procedures

B3.3. If the intended procedure is discontinued or otherwise not completed, code the procedure to the root operation performed. If a procedure is discontinued before any other root operation is performed, code the root operation Inspection of the body part or anatomical region inspected.

Example: A planned aortic valve replacement procedure is discontinued after the initial thoracotomy and before any incision is made in the heart muscle, when the patient becomes hemodynamically unstable. This procedure is coded as an open Inspection of the mediastinum.

Biopsy procedures

B3.4a. Biopsy procedures are coded using the root operations Excision, Extraction, or Drainage and the qualifier Diagnostic.

Examples: Fine needle aspiration biopsy of fluid in the lung is coded to the root operation Drainage with the qualifier Diagnostic.

Biopsy of bone marrow is coded to the root operation Extraction with the qualifier Diagnostic.

Lymph node sampling for biopsy is coded to the root operation Excision with the qualifier Diagnostic.

Biopsy followed by more definitive treatment

B3.4b. If a diagnostic Excision, Extraction, or Drainage procedure (biopsy) is followed by a more definitive procedure, such as Destruction, Excision or Resection at the same procedure site, both the biopsy and the more definitive treatment are coded.

Example: Biopsy of breast followed by partial mastectomy at the same procedure site, both the biopsy and the partial mastectomy procedure are coded.

Overlapping body layers

B3.5. If the root operations Excision, Repair or Inspection are performed on overlapping layers of the musculoskeletal system, the body part specifying the deepest layer is coded.

Example: Excisional debridement that includes skin and subcutaneous tissue and muscle is coded to the muscle body part.

Bypass procedures

B3.6a. Bypass procedures are coded by identifying the body part bypassed "from" and the body part bypassed "to." The fourth character body part specifies the body part bypassed from, and the qualifier specifies the body part bypassed to.

Example: Bypass from stomach to jejunum, stomach is the body part and jejunum is the qualifier.

B3.6b. Coronary artery bypass procedures are coded differently than other bypass procedures as described in the previous guideline. Rather than identifying the body part bypassed from, the body part identifies the number of coronary arteries bypassed to, and the qualifier specifies the vessel bypassed from.

Example: Aortocoronary artery bypass of the left anterior descending coronary artery and the obtuse marginal coronary artery is classified in the body part axis of classification as two coronary arteries, and the qualifier specifies the aorta as the body part bypassed from.

B3.6c. If multiple coronary arteries are bypassed, a separate procedure is coded for each coronary artery that uses a different device and/or qualifier.

Example: Aortocoronary artery bypass and internal mammary coronary artery bypass are coded separately.

Control vs. more definitive root operations

B3.7. The root operation Control is defined as, "Stopping, or attempting to stop, postprocedural or other acute bleeding." If an attempt to stop postprocedural or other acute bleeding is **initially** unsuccessful, and to stop the bleeding requires performing a more definitive root operation, such as Bypass, Detachment, Excision, Extraction, Reposition, Replacement, or Resection, then the more definitive root operation is coded instead of Control.

Example: Resection of spleen to stop bleeding is coded to Resection instead of Control.

Excision vs. Resection

B3.8. PCS contains specific body parts for anatomical subdivisions of a body part, such as lobes of the lungs or liver and regions of the intestine. Resection of the specific body part is coded whenever all of the body part is cut out or off, rather than coding Excision of a less specific body part.

Example: Left upper lung lobectomy is coded to Resection of Upper Lung Lobe, Left rather than Excision of Lung, Left.

Excision for graft

B3.9. If an autograft is obtained from a different procedure site in order to complete the objective of the procedure, a separate procedure is coded.

Example: Coronary bypass with excision of saphenous vein graft, excision of saphenous vein is coded separately.

Fusion procedures of the spine

B3.10a. The body part coded for a spinal vertebral joint(s) rendered immobile by a spinal fusion procedure is classified by the level of the spine (e.g. thoracic). There are distinct body part values for a single vertebral joint and for multiple vertebral joints at each spinal level.

Example: Body part values specify Lumbar Vertebral Joint, Lumbar Vertebral Joints, 2 or More and Lumbosacral Vertebral Joint.

B3.10b. If multiple vertebral joints are fused, a separate procedure is coded for each vertebral joint that uses a different device and/or qualifier.

Example: Fusion of lumbar vertebral joint, posterior approach, anterior column and fusion of lumbar vertebral joint, posterior approach, posterior column are coded separately.

B3.10c. Combinations of devices and materials are often used on a vertebral joint to render the joint immobile. When combinations of devices are used on the same vertebral joint, the device value coded for the procedure is as follows:

- If an interbody fusion device is used to render the joint immobile (alone or containing other material like bone graft), the procedure is coded with the device value Interbody Fusion Device

- If bone graft is the *only* device used to render the joint immobile, the procedure is coded with the device value Nonautologous Tissue Substitute or Autologous Tissue Substitute

- If a mixture of autologous and nonautologous bone graft (with or without biological or synthetic extenders or binders) is used to render the joint immobile, code the procedure with the device value Autologous Tissue Substitute

Examples: Fusion of a vertebral joint using a cage style interbody fusion device containing morsellized bone graft is coded to the device Interbody Fusion Device.

Fusion of a vertebral joint using a bone dowel interbody fusion device made of cadaver bone and packed with a mixture of local morsellized bone and demineralized bone matrix is coded to the device Interbody Fusion Device.

Fusion of a vertebral joint using both autologous bone graft and bone bank bone graft is coded to the device Autologous Tissue Substitute.

Inspection procedures

B3.11a. Inspection of a body part(s) performed in order to achieve the objective of a procedure is not coded separately.

Example: Fiberoptic bronchoscopy performed for irrigation of bronchus, only the irrigation procedure is coded.

B3.11b. If multiple tubular body parts are inspected, the most distal body part (the body part furthest from the starting point of the inspection) is coded. If multiple non-tubular body parts in a region are inspected, the body part that specifies the entire area inspected is coded.

Examples: Cystoureteroscopy with inspection of bladder and ureters is coded to the ureter body part value.

Exploratory laparotomy with general inspection of abdominal contents is coded to the peritoneal cavity body part value.

B3.11c. When both an Inspection procedure and another procedure are performed on the same body part during the same episode, if the Inspection procedure is performed using a different approach than the other procedure, the Inspection procedure is coded separately.

Example: Endoscopic Inspection of the duodenum is coded separately when open Excision of the duodenum is performed during the same procedural episode.

Occlusion vs. Restriction for vessel embolization procedures

B3.12. If the objective of an embolization procedure is to completely close a vessel, the root operation Occlusion is coded. If the objective of an embolization procedure is to narrow the lumen of a vessel, the root operation Restriction is coded.

Examples: Tumor embolization is coded to the root operation Occlusion, because the objective of the procedure is to cut off the blood supply to the vessel.

Embolization of a cerebral aneurysm is coded to the root operation Restriction, because the objective of the procedure is not to close off the vessel entirely, but to narrow the lumen of the vessel at the site of the aneurysm where it is abnormally wide.

Release procedures

B3.13. In the root operation Release, the body part value coded is the body part being freed and not the tissue being manipulated or cut to free the body part.

Example: Lysis of intestinal adhesions is coded to the specific intestine body part value.

Release vs. Division

B3.14. If the sole objective of the procedure is freeing a body part without cutting the body part, the root operation is Release. If the sole objective of the procedure is separating or transecting a body part, the root operation is Division.

Examples: Freeing a nerve root from surrounding scar tissue to relieve pain is coded to the root operation Release.

Severing a nerve root to relieve pain is coded to the root operation Division.

Reposition for fracture treatment

B3.15. Reduction of a displaced fracture is coded to the root operation Reposition and the application of a cast or splint in conjunction with the Reposition procedure is not coded separately. Treatment of a nondisplaced fracture is coded to the procedure performed.

Examples: Casting of a nondisplaced fracture is coded to the root operation Immobilization in the Placement section.

Putting a pin in a nondisplaced fracture is coded to the root operation Insertion.

Transplantation vs. Administration

B3.16. Putting in a mature and functioning living body part taken from another individual or animal is coded to the root operation Transplantation. Putting in autologous or nonautologous cells is coded to the Administration section.

Example: Putting in autologous or nonautologous bone marrow, pancreatic islet cells or stem cells is coded to the Administration section.

Transfer procedures using multiple tissue layers

B3.17. The root operation Transfer contains qualifiers that can be used to specify when a transfer flap is composed of more than one tissue layer, such as a musculocutaneous flap. For procedures involving transfer of multiple tissue layers including skin, subcutaneous tissue, fascia or muscle, the procedure is coded to the body part value that describes the deepest tissue layer in the flap, and the qualifier can be used to describe the other tissue layer(s) in the transfer flap.

Example: A **musculocutaneous flap transfer is coded to the appropriate body part value in the body system Muscles, and the qualifier is used to describe the additional tissue layer(s) in the transfer flap.**

B4. Body Part

General guidelines

B4.1a. If a procedure is performed on a portion of a body part that does not have a separate body part value, code the body part value corresponding to the whole body part.

Example: A procedure performed on the alveolar process of the mandible is coded to the mandible body part.

B4.1b. If the prefix "peri" is combined with a body part to identify the site of the procedure, and the site of the procedure is not further specified, then the procedure is coded to the body part named. This guideline applies only when a more specific body part value is not available.

Examples: A procedure site identified as perirenal is coded to the kidney body part when the site of the procedure is not further specified.

A procedure site described in the documentation as peri-urethral, and the documentation also indicates that it is the vulvar tissue and not the urethral tissue that is the site of the procedure, then the procedure is coded to the vulva body part.

B4.1c. If a procedure is performed on a continuous section of a tubular body part, code the body part value corresponding to the furthest anatomical site from the point of entry.

Example: A procedure performed on a continuous section of artery from the femoral artery to the external iliac artery with the point of entry at the femoral artery is coded to the external iliac body part.

Branches of body parts

B4.2. Where a specific branch of a body part does not have its own body part value in PCS, the body part is typically coded to the closest proximal branch that has a specific body part value. In the cardiovascular body systems, if a general body part is available in the correct root operation table, and coding to a proximal branch would require assigning a code in a different body system, the procedure is coded using the general body part value.

Examples: A procedure performed on the mandibular branch of the trigeminal nerve is coded to the trigeminal nerve body part value.

Occlusion of the bronchial artery is coded to the body part value Upper Artery in the body system Upper Arteries, and not to the body part value Thoracic Aorta, Descending in the body system Heart and Great Vessels.

Bilateral body part values

B4.3. Bilateral body part values are available for a limited number of body parts. If the identical procedure is performed on contralateral body parts, and a bilateral body part value exists for that body part, a single procedure is coded using the bilateral body part value. If no bilateral body part value exists, each procedure is coded separately using the appropriate body part value.

Examples: The identical procedure performed on both fallopian tubes is coded once using the body part value Fallopian Tube, Bilateral.

The identical procedure performed on both knee joints is coded twice using the body part values Knee Joint, Right and Knee Joint, Left.

Coronary arteries

B4.4. The coronary arteries are classified as a single body part that is further specified by number of arteries treated. One procedure code specifying multiple arteries is used when the same procedure is performed, including the same device and qualifier values.

Examples: Angioplasty of two distinct coronary arteries with placement of two stents is coded as Dilation of Coronary Artery, Two Arteries with Two Intraluminal Devices.

Angioplasty of two distinct coronary arteries, one with stent placed and one without, is coded separately as Dilation of Coronary Artery, One Artery with Intraluminal Device, and Dilation of Coronary Artery, One Artery with no device.

Tendons, ligaments, bursae and fascia near a joint

B4.5. Procedures performed on tendons, ligaments, bursae and fascia supporting a joint are coded to the body part in the respective body system that is the focus of the procedure. Procedures performed on joint structures themselves are coded to the body part in the joint body systems.

Examples: Repair of the anterior cruciate ligament of the knee is coded to the knee bursa and ligament body part in the bursae and ligaments body system.

Knee arthroscopy with shaving of articular cartilage is coded to the knee joint body part in the Lower Joints body system.

Skin, subcutaneous tissue and fascia overlying a joint

B4.6. If a procedure is performed on the skin, subcutaneous tissue or fascia overlying a joint, the procedure is coded to the following body part:

- Shoulder is coded to Upper Arm
- Elbow is coded to Lower Arm
- Wrist is coded to Lower Arm
- Hip is coded to Upper Leg
- Knee is coded to Lower Leg
- Ankle is coded to Foot

Fingers and toes

B4.7. If a body system does not contain a separate body part value for fingers, procedures performed on the fingers are coded to the body part value for the hand. If a body system does not contain a separate body part value for toes, procedures performed on the toes are coded to the body part value for the foot.

Example: Excision of finger muscle is coded to one of the hand muscle body part values in the Muscles body system.

Upper and lower intestinal tract

B4.8. In the Gastrointestinal body system, the general body part values Upper Intestinal Tract and Lower Intestinal Tract are provided as an option for the root operations Change, Inspection, Removal and Revision. Upper Intestinal Tract includes the portion of the gastrointestinal tract from the esophagus down to and including the duodenum, and Lower Intestinal Tract includes the portion of the gastrointestinal tract from the jejunum down to and including the rectum and anus.

Example: In the root operation Change table, change of a device in the jejunum is coded using the body part Lower Intestinal Tract.

B5. Approach

Open approach with percutaneous endoscopic assistance

B5.2. Procedures performed using the open approach with percutaneous endoscopic assistance are coded to the approach Open.

Example: Laparoscopic-assisted sigmoidectomy is coded to the approach Open.

External approach

B5.3a. Procedures performed within an orifice on structures that are visible without the aid of any instrumentation are coded to the approach External.

Example: Resection of tonsils is coded to the approach External.

B5.3b. Procedures performed indirectly by the application of external force through the intervening body layers are coded to the approach External.

Example: Closed reduction of fracture is coded to the approach External.

Percutaneous procedure via device

B5.4. Procedures performed percutaneously via a device placed for the procedure are coded to the approach Percutaneous.

Example: Fragmentation of kidney stone performed via percutaneous nephrostomy is coded to the approach Percutaneous.

B6. Device

General guidelines

B6.1a. A device is coded only if a device remains after the procedure is completed. If no device remains, the device value No Device is coded. In limited root operations, the classification provides the qualifier values Temporary and Intraoperative, for specific procedures involving clinically significant devices, where the purpose of the device is to be utilized for a brief duration during the procedure or current inpatient stay. **If a device that is intended to remain after the procedure is completed requires removal before the end of the operative episode in which it was inserted (for example, the device size is**

inadequate or a complication occurs), both the insertion and removal of the device should be coded.

B6.1b. Materials such as sutures, ligatures, radiological markers and temporary post-operative wound drains are considered integral to the performance of a procedure and are not coded as devices.

B6.1c. Procedures performed on a device only and not on a body part are specified in the root operations Change, Irrigation, Removal and Revision, and are coded to the procedure performed.

Example: Irrigation of percutaneous nephrostomy tube is coded to the root operation Irrigation of indwelling device in the Administration section.

Drainage device

B6.2. A separate procedure to put in a drainage device is coded to the root operation Drainage with the device value Drainage Device.

Obstetric Section Guidelines (section 1)

C. Obstetrics Section

Products of conception

C1. Procedures performed on the products of conception are coded to the Obstetrics section. Procedures performed on the pregnant female other than the products of conception are coded to the appropriate root operation in the Medical and Surgical section.

Example: Amniocentesis is coded to the products of conception body part in the Obstetrics section. Repair of obstetric urethral laceration is coded to the urethra body part in the Medical and Surgical section.

Procedures following delivery or abortion

C2. Procedures performed following a delivery or abortion for curettage of the endometrium or evacuation of retained products of conception are all coded in the Obstetrics section, to the root operation Extraction and the body part Products of Conception, Retained.

Diagnostic or therapeutic dilation and curettage performed during times other than the postpartum or post-abortion period are all coded in the Medical and Surgical section, to the root operation Extraction and the body part Endometrium.

New Technology Section Guidelines (section X)

D. New Technology Section

General guidelines

D1. Section X codes are standalone codes. They are not supplemental codes. Section X codes fully represent the specific procedure described

in the code title, and do not require any additional codes from other sections of ICD-10-PCS. When section X contains a code title which describes a specific new technology procedure, only that X code is reported for the procedure. There is no need to report a broader, non-specific code in another section of ICD-10-PCS.

Example: XW04321 Introduction of Ceftazidime-Avibactam Anti-infective into Central Vein, Percutaneous Approach, New Technology Group 1, can be coded to indicate that Ceftazidime-Avibactam Anti-infective was administered via a central vein. A separate code from table 3E0 in the Administration section of ICD-10-PCS is not coded in addition to this code.

Selection of Principal Procedure

The following instructions should be applied in the selection of principal procedure and clarification on the importance of the relation to the principal diagnosis when more than one procedure is performed:

1. Procedure performed for definitive treatment of both principal diagnosis and secondary diagnosis

    a. Sequence procedure performed for definitive treatment most related to principal diagnosis as principal procedure.

2. Procedure performed for definitive treatment and diagnostic procedures performed for both principal diagnosis and secondary diagnosis.

    a. Sequence procedure performed for definitive treatment most related to principal diagnosis as principal procedure

3. A diagnostic procedure was performed for the principal diagnosis and a procedure is performed for definitive treatment of a secondary diagnosis.

    a. Sequence diagnostic procedure as principal procedure, since the procedure most related to the principal diagnosis takes precedence.

4. No procedures performed that are related to principal diagnosis; procedures performed for definitive treatment and diagnostic procedures were performed for secondary diagnosis

    a. Sequence procedure performed for definitive treatment of secondary diagnosis as principal procedure, since there are no procedures (definitive or nondefinitive treatment) related to principal diagnosis.

# #

3f (Aortic) Bioprosthesis valve *use* Zooplastic Tissue in Heart and Great Vessels

A

Abdominal aortic plexus *use* Abdominal Sympathetic Nerve
Abdominal esophagus *use* Esophagus, Lower
Abdominohysterectomy *see* Resection, Uterus, ØUT9
Abdominoplasty
  see Alteration, Abdominal Wall, ØWØF
  see Repair, Abdominal Wall, ØWQF
  see Supplement, Abdominal Wall, ØWUF
Abductor hallucis muscle
  use Foot Muscle, Left
  use Foot Muscle, Right
AbioCor® Total Replacement Heart *use* Synthetic Substitute
Ablation *see* Destruction
Abortion
  Abortifacient, 10A07ZX
  Laminaria, 10A07ZW
  Products of Conception, 10A0
  Vacuum, 10A07Z6
Abrasion *see* Extraction
Absolute Pro Vascular (OTW) Self-Expanding Stent System *use* Intraluminal Device
Accessory cephalic vein
  use Cephalic Vein, Left
  use Cephalic Vein, Right
Accessory obturator nerve *use* Lumbar Plexus
Accessory phrenic nerve *use* Phrenic Nerve
Accessory spleen *use* Spleen
Acculink (RX) Carotid Stent System *use* Intraluminal Device
Acellular Hydrated Dermis *use* Nonautologous Tissue Substitute
Acetabular cup *use* Liner in Lower Joints
Acetabulectomy
  see Excision, Lower Bones, ØQB
  see Resection, Lower Bones, ØQT
Acetabulofemoral joint
  use Hip Joint, Left
  use Hip Joint, Right
Acetabuloplasty
  see Repair, Lower Bones, ØQQ
  see Replacement, Lower Bones, ØQR
  see Supplement, Lower Bones, ØQU
Achilles tendon
  use Lower Leg Tendon, Left
  use Lower Leg Tendon, Right
Achillorrhaphy *see* Repair, Tendons, ØLQ
Achillotenotomy, achillotomy
  see Division, Tendons, ØL8
  see Drainage, Tendons, ØL9
Acromioclavicular ligament
  use Shoulder Bursa and Ligament, Left
  use Shoulder Bursa and Ligament, Right
Acromion (process)
  use Scapula, Left
  use Scapula, Right
Acromionectomy
  see Excision, Upper Joints, ØRB
  see Resection, Upper Joints, ØRT
Acromioplasty
  see Repair, Upper Joints, ØRQ
  see Replacement, Upper Joints, ØRR
  see Supplement, Upper Joints, ØRU
Activa PC neurostimulator *use* Stimulator Generator, Multiple Array in, ØJH
Activa RC neurostimulator *use* Stimulator Generator, Multiple Array Rechargeable in, ØJH
Activa SC neurostimulator *use* Stimulator Generator, Single Array in, ØJH
Activities of Daily Living Assessment, F02
Activities of Daily Living Treatment, F08
ACUITY™ Steerable Lead
  use Cardiac Lead, Defibrillator in 02H
  use Cardiac Lead, Pacemaker in 02H
Acupuncture
  Breast
    Anesthesia, 8E0H300
    No Qualifier, 8E0H30Z

Acupuncture — *continued*
  Integumentary System
    Anesthesia, 8E0H300
    No Qualifier, 8E0H30Z
Adductor brevis muscle
  use Upper Leg Muscle, Left
  use Upper Leg Muscle, Right
Adductor hallucis muscle
  use Foot Muscle, Left
  use Foot Muscle, Right
Adductor longus muscle
  use Upper Leg Muscle, Left
  use Upper Leg Muscle, Right
Adductor magnus muscle
  use Upper Leg Muscle, Left
  use Upper Leg Muscle, Right
Adenohypophysis *use* Pituitary Gland
Adenoidectomy
  see Excision, Adenoids, ØCBQ
  see Resection, Adenoids, ØCTQ
Adenoidotomy *see* Drainage, Adenoids, ØC9Q
Adhesiolysis *see* Release
Administration
  Blood products *see* Transfusion
  Other substance *see* Introduction of substance in or on
Adrenalectomy
  see Excision, Endocrine System, ØGB
  see Resection, Endocrine System, ØGT
Adrenalorrhaphy *see* Repair, Endocrine System, ØGQ
Adrenalotomy *see* Drainage, Endocrine System, ØG9
Advancement
  see Reposition
  see Transfer
Advisa (MRI) *use* Pacemaker, Dual Chamber in, ØJH
AFX® Endovascular AAA System *use* Intraluminal Device
AIGISRx Antibacterial Envelope *use* Anti-Infective Envelope
Alar ligament of axis *use* Head and Neck Bursa and Ligament
Alfieri Stitch Valvuloplasty *see* Restriction, Valve, Mitral, 02VG
Alimentation *see* Introduction of substance in or on
Alteration
  Abdominal Wall, ØWØF
  Ankle Region
    Left, ØYØL
    Right, ØYØK
  Arm
    Lower
      Left, ØXØF
      Right, ØXØD
    Upper
      Left, ØXØ9
      Right, ØXØ8
  Axilla
    Left, ØXØ5
    Right, ØXØ4
  Back
    Lower, ØWØL
    Upper, ØWØK
  Breast
    Bilateral, ØHØV
    Left, ØHØU
    Right, ØHØT
  Buttock
    Left, ØYØ1
    Right, ØYØ0
  Chest Wall, ØWØ8
  Ear
    Bilateral, Ø9Ø2
    Left, Ø9Ø1
    Right, Ø9Ø0
  Elbow Region
    Left, ØXØC
    Right, ØXØB
  Extremity
    Lower
      Left, ØYØB
      Right, ØYØ9
    Upper
      Left, ØXØ7
      Right, ØXØ6
  Eyelid
    Lower
      Left, Ø8ØR
      Right, Ø8ØQ

Alteration — *continued*
  Eyelid — *continued*
    Upper
      Left, Ø8ØP
      Right, Ø8ØN
  Face, ØWØ2
  Head, ØWØ0
  Jaw
    Lower, ØWØ5
    Upper, ØWØ4
  Knee Region
    Left, ØYØG
    Right, ØYØF
  Leg
    Lower
      Left, ØYØJ
      Right, ØYØH
    Upper
      Left, ØYØD
      Right, ØYØC
  Lip
    Lower, ØCØ1X
    Upper, ØCØ0X
  Nasal Mucosa and Soft Tissue, Ø90K
  Neck, ØWØ6
  Perineum
    Female, ØWØN
    Male, ØWØM
  Shoulder Region
    Left, ØXØ3
    Right, ØXØ2
  Subcutaneous Tissue and Fascia
    Abdomen, ØJØ8
    Back, ØJØ7
    Buttock, ØJØ9
    Chest, ØJØ6
    Face, ØJØ1
    Lower Arm
      Left, ØJØH
      Right, ØJØG
    Lower Leg
      Left, ØJØP
      Right, ØJØN
    Neck
      Left, ØJØ5
      Right, ØJØ4
    Upper Arm
      Left, ØJØF
      Right, ØJØD
    Upper Leg
      Left, ØJØM
      Right, ØJØL
  Wrist Region
    Left, ØXØH
    Right, ØXØG
Alveolar process of mandible
  use Mandible, Left
  use Mandible, Right
Alveolar process of maxilla *use* Maxilla
Alveolectomy
  see Excision, Head and Facial Bones, ØNB
  see Resection, Head and Facial Bones, ØNT
Alveoloplasty
  see Repair, Head and Facial Bones, ØNQ
  see Replacement, Head and Facial Bones, ØNR
  see Supplement, Head and Facial Bones, ØNU
Alveolotomy
  see Division, Head and Facial Bones, ØN8
  see Drainage, Head and Facial Bones, ØN9
Ambulatory cardiac monitoring, 4A12X45
Amniocentesis *see* Drainage, Products of Conception, 1090
Amnioinfusion *see* Introduction of substance in or on, Products of Conception, 3E0E
Amnioscopy, 10J08ZZ
Amniotomy *see* Drainage, Products of Conception, 1090
AMPLATZER® Muscular VSD Occluder *use* Synthetic Substitute
Amputation *see* Detachment
AMS 800® Urinary Control System *use* Artificial Sphincter in Urinary System
Anal orifice *use* Anus
Analog radiography *see* Plain Radiography
Analog radiology *see* Plain Radiography
Anastomosis *see* Bypass
Anatomical snuffbox
  use Lower Arm and Wrist Muscle, Left
  use Lower Arm and Wrist Muscle, Right

Andexanet Alfa, Factor Xa Inhibitor Reversal Agent
XW0
AneuRx® AAA Advantage® use Intraluminal Device
Angiectomy
see Excision, Heart and Great Vessels, 02B
see Excision, Lower Arteries, 04B
see Excision, Lower Veins, 06B
see Excision, Upper Arteries, 03B
see Excision, Upper Veins, 05B
Angiocardiography
Combined right and left heart see Fluoroscopy, Heart, Right and Left, B216
Left Heart see Fluoroscopy, Heart, Left, B215
Right Heart see Fluoroscopy, Heart, Right, B214
SPY system intravascular fluorescence see Monitoring, Physiological Systems, 4A1
Angiography
see Fluoroscopy, Heart, B21
see Plain Radiography, Heart, B20
Angioplasty
see Dilation, Heart and Great Vessels, 027
see Dilation, Lower Arteries, 047
see Dilation, Upper Arteries, 037
see Repair, Heart and Great Vessels, 02Q
see Repair, Lower Arteries, 04Q
see Repair, Upper Arteries, 03Q
see Replacement, Heart and Great Vessels, 02R
see Replacement, Lower Arteries, 04R
see Replacement, Upper Arteries, 03R
see Supplement, Heart and Great Vessels, 02U
see Supplement, Lower Arteries, 04U
see Supplement, Upper Arteries, 03U
Angiorrhaphy
see Repair, Heart and Great Vessels, 02Q
see Repair, Lower Arteries, 04Q
see Repair, Upper Arteries, 03Q
Angioscopy, 02JY4ZZ, 03JY4ZZ, 04JY4ZZ
Angiotensin II use Synthetic Human Angiotensin II
Angiotripsy
see Occlusion, Lower Arteries, 04L
see Occlusion, Upper Arteries, 03L
Angular artery use Face Artery
Angular vein
use Face Vein, Left
use Face Vein, Right
Annular ligament
use Elbow Bursa and Ligament, Left
use Elbow Bursa and Ligament, Right
Annuloplasty
see Repair, Heart and Great Vessels, 02Q
see Supplement, Heart and Great Vessels, 02U
Annuloplasty ring use Synthetic Substitute
Anoplasty
see Repair, Anus, 0DQQ
see Supplement, Anus, 0DUQ
Anorectal junction use Rectum
Anoscopy, 0DJD8ZZ
Ansa cervicalis use Cervical Plexus
Antabuse therapy, HZ93ZZZ
Antebrachial fascia
use Subcutaneous Tissue and Fascia, Left Lower Arm
use Subcutaneous Tissue and Fascia, Right Lower Arm
Anterior cerebral artery use Intracranial Artery
Anterior cerebral vein use Intracranial Vein
Anterior choroidal artery use Intracranial Artery
Anterior circumflex humeral artery
use Axillary Artery, Left
use Axillary Artery, Right
Anterior communicating artery use Intracranial Artery
Anterior cruciate ligament (ACL)
use Knee Bursa and Ligament, Left
use Knee Bursa and Ligament, Right
Anterior crural nerve use Femoral Nerve
Anterior facial vein
use Face Vein, Left
use Face Vein, Right
Anterior intercostal artery
use Internal Mammary Artery, Left
use Internal Mammary Artery, Right
Anterior interosseous nerve use Median Nerve
Anterior lateral malleolar artery
use Anterior Tibial Artery, Left
use Anterior Tibial Artery, Right
Anterior lingual gland use Minor Salivary Gland
Anterior (pectoral) lymph node
use Lymphatic, Left Axillary

Anterior (pectoral) lymph node — continued
use Lymphatic, Right Axillary
Anterior medial malleolar artery
use Anterior Tibial Artery, Left
use Anterior Tibial Artery, Right
Anterior spinal artery
use Vertebral Artery, Left
use Vertebral Artery, Right
Anterior tibial recurrent artery
use Anterior Tibial Artery, Left
use Anterior Tibial Artery, Right
Anterior ulnar recurrent artery
use Ulnar Artery, Left
use Ulnar Artery, Right
Anterior vagal trunk use Vagus Nerve
Anterior vertebral muscle
use Neck Muscle, Left
use Neck Muscle, Right
Antigen-free air conditioning see Atmospheric Control, Physiological Systems, 6A0
Antihelix
use External Ear, Bilateral
use External Ear, Left
use External Ear, Right
Antimicrobial envelope use Anti-Infective Envelope
Antitragus
use External Ear, Bilateral
use External Ear, Left
use External Ear, Right
Antrostomy see Drainage, Ear, Nose, Sinus, 099
Antrotomy see Drainage, Ear, Nose, Sinus, 099
Antrum of Highmore
use Maxillary Sinus, Left
use Maxillary Sinus, Right
Aortic annulus use Aortic Valve
Aortic arch use Thoracic Aorta, Ascending/Arch
Aortic intercostal artery use Upper Artery
Aortography
see Fluoroscopy, Lower Arteries, B41
see Fluoroscopy, Upper Arteries, B31
see Plain Radiography, Lower Arteries, B40
see Plain Radiography, Upper Arteries, B30
Aortoplasty
see Repair, Aorta, Abdominal, 04Q0
see Repair, Aorta, Thoracic, Ascending/Arch, 02QX
see Repair, Aorta, Thoracic, Descending, 02QW
see Replacement, Aorta, Abdominal, 04R0
see Replacement, Aorta, Thoracic, Ascending/Arch, 02RX
see Replacement, Aorta, Thoracic, Descending, 02RW
see Supplement, Aorta, Abdominal, 04U0
see Supplement, Aorta, Thoracic, Ascending/Arch, 02UX
see Supplement, Aorta, Thoracic, Descending, 02UW
Apical (subclavicular) lymph node
use Lymphatic, Left Axillary
use Lymphatic, Right Axillary
Apneustic center use Pons
Appendectomy
see Excision, Appendix, 0DBJ
see Resection, Appendix, 0DTJ
Appendicolysis see Release, Appendix, 0DNJ
Appendicotomy see Drainage, Appendix, 0D9J
Application see Introduction of substance in or on
Aquablation therapy, prostate, XV508A4
Aquapheresis, 6A550Z3
Aqueduct of Sylvius use Cerebral Ventricle
Aqueous humour
use Anterior Chamber, Left
use Anterior Chamber, Right
Arachnoid mater, intracranial use Cerebral Meninges
Arachnoid mater, spinal use Spinal Meninges
Arcuate artery
use Foot Artery, Left
use Foot Artery, Right
Areola
use Nipple, Left
use Nipple, Right
AROM (artificial rupture of membranes), 10907ZC
Arterial canal (duct) use Pulmonary Artery, Left
Arterial pulse tracing see Measurement, Arterial, 4A03
Arteriectomy
see Excision, Heart and Great Vessels, 02B
see Excision, Lower Arteries, 04B
see Excision, Upper Arteries, 03B

Arteriography
see Fluoroscopy, Heart, B21
see Fluoroscopy, Lower Arteries, B41
see Fluoroscopy, Upper Arteries, B31
see Plain Radiography, Heart, B20
see Plain Radiography, Lower Arteries, B40
see Plain Radiography, Upper Arteries, B30
Arterioplasty
see Repair, Heart and Great Vessels, 02Q
see Repair, Lower Arteries, 04Q
see Repair, Upper Arteries, 03Q
see Replacement, Heart and Great Vessels, 02R
see Replacement, Lower Arteries, 04R
see Replacement, Upper Arteries, 03R
see Supplement, Heart and Great Vessels, 02U
see Supplement, Lower Arteries, 04U
see Supplement, Upper Arteries, 03U
Arteriorrhaphy
see Repair, Heart and Great Vessels, 02Q
see Repair, Lower Arteries, 04Q
see Repair, Upper Arteries, 03Q
Arterioscopy
see Inspection, Artery, Lower, 04JY
see Inspection, Artery, Upper, 03JY
see Inspection, Great Vessel, 02JY
Arthrectomy
see Excision, Lower Joints, 0SB
see Excision, Upper Joints, 0RB
see Resection, Lower Joints, 0ST
see Resection, Upper Joints, 0RT
Arthrocentesis
see Drainage, Lower Joints, 0S9
see Drainage, Upper Joints, 0R9
Arthrodesis
see Fusion, Lower Joints, 0SG
see Fusion, Upper Joints, 0RG
Arthrography
see Plain Radiography, Non-Axial Lower Bones, BQ0
see Plain Radiography, Non-Axial Upper Bones, BP0
see Plain Radiography, Skull and Facial Bones, BN0
Arthrolysis
see Release, Lower Joints, 0SN
see Release, Upper Joints, 0RN
Arthropexy
see Repair, Lower Joints, 0SQ
see Repair, Upper Joints, 0RQ
see Reposition, Lower Joints, 0SS
see Reposition, Upper Joints, 0RS
Arthroplasty
see Repair, Lower Joints, 0SQ
see Repair, Upper Joints, 0RQ
see Replacement, Lower Joints, 0SR
see Replacement, Upper Joints, 0RR
see Supplement, Lower Joints, 0SU
see Supplement, Upper Joints, 0RU
Arthroplasty, radial head
see Replacement, Radius, Left, 0PRJ
see Replacement, Radius, Right, 0PRH
Arthroscopy
see Inspection, Lower Joints, 0SJ
see Inspection, Upper Joints, 0RJ
Arthrotomy
see Drainage, Lower Joints, 0S9
see Drainage, Upper Joints, 0R9
Articulating Spacer (Antibiotic) use Articulating Spacer in Lower Joints
Artificial anal sphincter (AAS) use Artificial Sphincter in Gastrointestinal System
Artificial bowel sphincter (neosphincter) use Artificial Sphincter in Gastrointestinal System
Artificial Sphincter
Insertion of device in
Anus, 0DHQ
Bladder, 0THB
Bladder Neck, 0THC
Urethra, 0THD
Removal of device from
Anus, 0DPQ
Bladder, 0TPB
Urethra, 0TPD
Revision of device in
Anus, 0DWQ
Bladder, 0TWB
Urethra, 0TWD
Artificial urinary sphincter (AUS) use Artificial Sphincter in Urinary System
Aryepiglottic fold use Larynx

Subterms under main terms may continue to next column or page

Arytenoid cartilage *use* Larynx
Arytenoid muscle
  use Neck Muscle, Left
  use Neck Muscle, Right
Arytenoidectomy *see* Excision, Larynx, ØCBS
Arytenoidopexy *see* Repair, Larynx, ØCQS
Ascenda Intrathecal Catheter *use* Infusion Device
Ascending aorta *use* Thoracic Aorta, Ascending/Arch
Ascending palatine artery *use* Face Artery
Ascending pharyngeal artery
  use External Carotid Artery, Left
  use External Carotid Artery, Right
Aspiration, fine needle
  Fluid or gas *see* Drainage
  Tissue biopsy
    see Excision
    see Extraction
Assessment
  Activities of daily living *see* Activities of Daily Living
    Assessment, Rehabilitation, FØ2
  Hearing *see* Hearing Assessment, Diagnostic Audiol-
    ogy, F13
  Hearing aid *see* Hearing Aid Assessment, Diagnostic
    Audiology, F14
  Intravascular perfusion, using indocyanine green (ICG)
    dye *see* Monitoring, Physiological Systems, 4A1
  Motor function *see* Motor Function Assessment, Re-
    habilitation, FØ1
  Nerve function *see* Motor Function Assessment, Re-
    habilitation, FØ1
  Speech *see* Speech Assessment, Rehabilitation, FØØ
  Vestibular *see* Vestibular Assessment, Diagnostic
    Audiology, F15
  Vocational *see* Activities of Daily Living Treatment,
    Rehabilitation, FØ8
Assistance
  Cardiac
    Continuous
      Balloon Pump, 5AØ221Ø
      Impeller Pump, 5AØ221D
      Other Pump, 5AØ2216
      Pulsatile Compression, 5AØ2215
    Intermittent
      Balloon Pump, 5AØ211Ø
      Impeller Pump, 5AØ211D
      Other Pump, 5AØ2116
      Pulsatile Compression, 5AØ2115
  Circulatory
    Continuous
      Hyperbaric, 5AØ5221
      Supersaturated, 5AØ522C
    Intermittent
      Hyperbaric, 5AØ5121
      Supersaturated, 5AØ512C
  Respiratory
    24-96 Consecutive Hours
      Continuous Negative Airway Pressure,
        5AØ9459
      Continuous Positive Airway Pressure,
        5AØ9457
      Intermittent Negative Airway Pressure,
        5AØ945B
      Intermittent Positive Airway Pressure,
        5AØ9458
      No Qualifier, 5AØ945Z
    Continuous, Filtration, 5AØ92ØZ
    Greater than 96 Consecutive Hours
      Continuous Negative Airway Pressure,
        5AØ9559
      Continuous Positive Airway Pressure,
        5AØ9557
      Intermittent Negative Airway Pressure,
        5AØ955B
      Intermittent Positive Airway Pressure,
        5AØ9558
      No Qualifier, 5AØ955Z
    Less than 24 Consecutive Hours
      Continuous Negative Airway Pressure,
        5AØ9359
      Continuous Positive Airway Pressure,
        5AØ9357
      Intermittent Negative Airway Pressure,
        5AØ935B
      Intermittent Positive Airway Pressure,
        5AØ9358
      No Qualifier, 5AØ935Z
Assurant (Cobalt) stent *use* Intraluminal Device

Atherectomy
  see Extirpation, Heart and Great Vessels, Ø2C
  see Extirpation, Lower Arteries, Ø4C
  see Extirpation, Upper Arteries, Ø3C
Atlantoaxial joint *use* Cervical Vertebral Joint
Atmospheric Control, 6AØZ
AtriClip LAA Exclusion System *use* Extraluminal Device
Atrioseptoplasty
  see Repair, Heart and Great Vessels, Ø2Q
  see Replacement, Heart and Great Vessels, Ø2R
  see Supplement, Heart and Great Vessels, Ø2U
Atrioventricular node *use* Conduction Mechanism
Atrium dextrum cordis *use* Atrium, Right
Atrium pulmonale *use* Atrium, Left
Attain Ability® lead, Ø2H
  use Cardiac Lead, Defibrillator in, Ø2H
  use Cardiac Lead, Pacemaker in, Ø2H
Attain Starfix® (OTW) lead
  use Cardiac Lead, Defibrillator in, Ø2H
  use Cardiac Lead, Pacemaker in, Ø2H
Audiology, diagnostic
  see Hearing Aid Assessment, Diagnostic Audiology,
    F14
  see Hearing Assessment, Diagnostic Audiology, F13
  see Vestibular Assessment, Diagnostic Audiology, F15
Audiometry *see* Hearing Assessment, Diagnostic Audiology, F13
Auditory tube
  use Eustachian Tube, Left
  use Eustachian Tube, Right
Auerbach's (myenteric) plexus *use* Abdominal Sympathetic Nerve
Auricle
  use External Ear, Bilateral
  use External Ear, Left
  use External Ear, Right
Auricularis muscle *use* Head Muscle
Autograft *use* Autologous Tissue Substitute
Autologous artery graft
  use Autologous Arterial Tissue in Heart and Great
    Vessels
  use Autologous Arterial Tissue in Lower Arteries
  use Autologous Arterial Tissue in Lower Veins
  use Autologous Arterial Tissue in Upper Arteries
  use Autologous Arterial Tissue in Upper Veins
Autologous vein graft
  use Autologous Venous Tissue in Heart and Great
    Vessels
  use Autologous Venous Tissue in Lower Arteries
  use Autologous Venous Tissue in Lower Veins
  use Autologous Venous Tissue in Upper Arteries
  use Autologous Venous Tissue in Upper Veins
Autotransfusion *see* Transfusion
Autotransplant
  Adrenal tissue *see* Reposition, Endocrine System, ØGS
  Kidney *see* Reposition, Urinary System, ØTS
  Pancreatic tissue *see* Reposition, Pancreas, ØFSG
  Parathyroid tissue *see* Reposition, Endocrine System,
    ØGS
  Thyroid tissue *see* Reposition, Endocrine System, ØGS
  Tooth *see* Reattachment, Mouth and Throat, ØCM
Avulsion *see* Extraction
Axial Lumbar Interbody Fusion System *use* Interbody
  Fusion Device in Lower Joints
AxiaLIF® System *use* Interbody Fusion Device in Lower
  Joints
Axicabtagene Ciloeucel *use* Engineered Autologous
  Chimeric Antigen Receptor T-cell Immunotherapy
Axillary fascia
  use Subcutaneous Tissue and Fascia, Left Upper Arm
  use Subcutaneous Tissue and Fascia, Right Upper Arm
Axillary nerve *use* Brachial Plexus

B

BAK/C® Interbody Cervical Fusion System *use* Inter-
  body Fusion Device in Upper Joints
BAL (bronchial alveolar lavage), diagnostic *see*
  Drainage, Respiratory System, ØB9
Balanoplasty
  see Repair, Penis, ØVQS
  see Supplement, Penis, ØVUS
Balloon atrial septostomy (BAS), Ø2163Z7
Balloon Pump
  Continuous, Output, 5AØ221Ø
  Intermittent, Output, 5AØ211Ø

Bandage, Elastic *see* Compression
Banding
  see Occlusion
  see Restriction
Banding, esophageal varices *see* Occlusion, Vein,
  Esophageal, Ø6L3
Banding, laparoscopic (adjustable) gastric
  Initial procedure, ØDV64CZ
  Surgical correction *see* Revision of device in, Stomach,
    ØDW6
Bard® Composix® Kugel® patch *use* Synthetic Substitute
Bard® Composix® (E/X) (LP) mesh *use* Synthetic Substi-
  tute
Bard® Dulex™ mesh *use* Synthetic Substitute
Bard® Ventralex™ Hernia Patch *use* Synthetic Substitute
Barium swallow *see* Fluoroscopy, Gastrointestinal System,
  BD1
Baroreflex Activation Therapy® (BAT®)
  use Stimulator Generator in Subcutaneous Tissue and
    Fascia
  use Stimulator Lead in Upper Arteries
Bartholin's (greater vestibular) gland *use* Vestibular
  Gland
Basal (internal) cerebral vein *use* Intracranial Vein
Basal metabolic rate (BMR) *see* Measurement, Physio-
  logical Systems, 4AØZ
Basal nuclei *use* Basal Ganglia
Base of Tongue *use* Pharynx
Basilar artery *use* Intracranial Artery
Basis pontis *use* Pons
Beam Radiation
  Abdomen, DWØ3
    Intraoperative, DWØ33ZØ
  Adrenal Gland, DGØ2
    Intraoperative, DGØ23ZØ
  Bile Ducts, DFØ2
    Intraoperative, DFØ23ZØ
  Bladder, DTØ2
    Intraoperative, DTØ23ZØ
  Bone
    Intraoperative, DPØC3ZØ
    Other, DPØC
  Bone Marrow, D7ØØ
    Intraoperative, D7ØØ3ZØ
  Brain, DØØØ
    Intraoperative, DØØØ3ZØ
  Brain Stem, DØØ1
    Intraoperative, DØØ13ZØ
  Breast
    Left, DMØØ
      Intraoperative, DMØØ3ZØ
    Right, DMØ1
      Intraoperative, DMØ13ZØ
  Bronchus, DBØ1
    Intraoperative, DBØ13ZØ
  Cervix, DUØ1
    Intraoperative, DUØ13ZØ
  Chest, DWØ2
    Intraoperative, DWØ23ZØ
  Chest Wall, DBØ7
    Intraoperative, DBØ73ZØ
  Colon, DDØ5
    Intraoperative, DDØ53ZØ
  Diaphragm, DBØ8
    Intraoperative, DBØ83ZØ
  Duodenum, DDØ2
    Intraoperative, DDØ23ZØ
  Ear, D9ØØ
    Intraoperative, D9ØØ3ZØ
  Esophagus, DDØØ
    Intraoperative, DDØØ3ZØ
  Eye, D8ØØ
    Intraoperative, D8ØØ3ZØ
  Femur, DPØ9
    Intraoperative, DPØ93ZØ
  Fibula, DPØB
    Intraoperative, DPØB3ZØ
  Gallbladder, DFØ1
    Intraoperative, DFØ13ZØ
  Gland
    Adrenal, DGØ2
      Intraoperative, DGØ23ZØ
    Parathyroid, DGØ4
      Intraoperative, DGØ43ZØ
    Pituitary, DGØØ
      Intraoperative, DGØØ3ZØ
    Thyroid, DGØ5
      Intraoperative, DGØ53ZØ

Beam Radiation — *continued*
  Glands
    Intraoperative, D9063Z0
    Salivary, D906
  Head and Neck, DW01
    Intraoperative, DW013Z0
  Hemibody, DW04
    Intraoperative, DW043Z0
  Humerus, DP06
    Intraoperative, DP063Z0
  Hypopharynx, D903
    Intraoperative, D9033Z0
  Ileum, DD04
    Intraoperative, DD043Z0
  Jejunum, DD03
    Intraoperative, DD033Z0
  Kidney, DT00
    Intraoperative, DT003Z0
  Larynx, D90B
    Intraoperative, D90B3Z0
  Liver, DF00
    Intraoperative, DF003Z0
  Lung, DB02
    Intraoperative, DB023Z0
  Lymphatics
    Abdomen, D706
      Intraoperative, D7063Z0
    Axillary, D704
      Intraoperative, D7043Z0
    Inguinal, D708
      Intraoperative, D7083Z0
    Neck, D703
      Intraoperative, D7033Z0
    Pelvis, D707
      Intraoperative, D7073Z0
    Thorax, D705
      Intraoperative, D7053Z0
  Mandible, DP03
    Intraoperative, DP033Z0
  Maxilla, DP02
    Intraoperative, DP023Z0
  Mediastinum, DB06
    Intraoperative, DB063Z0
  Mouth, D904
    Intraoperative, D9043Z0
  Nasopharynx, D90D
    Intraoperative, D90D3Z0
  Neck and Head, DW01
    Intraoperative, DW013Z0
  Nerve
    Intraoperative, D0073Z0
    Peripheral, D007
  Nose, D901
    Intraoperative, D9013Z0
  Oropharynx, D90F
    Intraoperative, D90F3Z0
  Ovary, DU00
    Intraoperative, DU003Z0
  Palate
    Hard, D908
      Intraoperative, D9083Z0
    Soft, D909
      Intraoperative, D9093Z0
  Pancreas, DF03
    Intraoperative, DF033Z0
  Parathyroid Gland, DG04
    Intraoperative, DG043Z0
  Pelvic Bones, DP08
    Intraoperative, DP083Z0
  Pelvic Region, DW06
    Intraoperative, DW063Z0
  Pineal Body, DG01
    Intraoperative, DG013Z0
  Pituitary Gland, DG00
    Intraoperative, DG003Z0
  Pleura, DB05
    Intraoperative, DB053Z0
  Prostate, DV00
    Intraoperative, DV003Z0
  Radius, DP07
    Intraoperative, DP073Z0
  Rectum, DD07
    Intraoperative, DD073Z0
  Rib, DP05
    Intraoperative, DP053Z0
  Sinuses, D907
    Intraoperative, D9073Z0
  Skin
    Abdomen, DH08

Beam Radiation — *continued*
  Skin — *continued*
    Abdomen — *continued*
      Intraoperative, DH083Z0
    Arm, DH04
      Intraoperative, DH043Z0
    Back, DH07
      Intraoperative, DH073Z0
    Buttock, DH09
      Intraoperative, DH093Z0
    Chest, DH06
      Intraoperative, DH063Z0
    Face, DH02
      Intraoperative, DH023Z0
    Leg, DH0B
      Intraoperative, DH0B3Z0
    Neck, DH03
      Intraoperative, DH033Z0
  Skull, DP00
    Intraoperative, DP003Z0
  Spinal Cord, D006
    Intraoperative, D0063Z0
  Spleen, D702
    Intraoperative, D7023Z0
  Sternum, DP04
    Intraoperative, DP043Z0
  Stomach, DD01
    Intraoperative, DD013Z0
  Testis, DV01
    Intraoperative, DV013Z0
  Thymus, D701
    Intraoperative, D7013Z0
  Thyroid Gland, DG05
    Intraoperative, DG053Z0
  Tibia, DP0B
    Intraoperative, DP0B3Z0
  Tongue, D905
    Intraoperative, D9053Z0
  Trachea, DB00
    Intraoperative, DB003Z0
  Ulna, DP07
    Intraoperative, DP073Z0
  Ureter, DT01
    Intraoperative, DT013Z0
  Urethra, DT03
    Intraoperative, DT033Z0
  Uterus, DU02
    Intraoperative, DU023Z0
  Whole Body, DW05
    Intraoperative, DW053Z0
Bedside swallow, F00ZJWZ
Berlin Heart Ventricular Assist Device *use* Implantable Heart Assist System in Heart and Great Vessels
Bezlotoxumab Monoclonal Antibody, XW0
Biceps brachii muscle
  use Upper Arm Muscle, Left
  use Upper Arm Muscle, Right
Biceps femoris muscle
  use Upper Leg Muscle, Left
  use Upper Leg Muscle, Right
Bicipital aponeurosis
  use Subcutaneous Tissue and Fascia, Left Lower Arm
  use Subcutaneous Tissue and Fascia, Right Lower Arm
Bicuspid valve *use* Mitral Valve
Bili light therapy *see* Phototherapy, Skin, 6A60
Bioactive embolization coil(s) *use* Intraluminal Device, Bioactive in Upper Arteries
Biofeedback, GZC9ZZZ
Biopsy
  see Drainage with qualifier Diagnostic
  see Excision with qualifier Diagnostic
  see Extraction with qualifier Diagnostic
BiPAP *see* Assistance, Respiratory, 5A09
Bisection *see* Division
Biventricular external heart assist system *use* Short-term External Heart Assist System in Heart and Great Vessels
Blepharectomy
  see Excision, Eye, 08B
  see Resection, Eye, 08T
Blepharoplasty
  see Repair, Eye, 08Q
  see Replacement, Eye, 08R
  see Reposition, Eye, 08S
  see Supplement, Eye, 08U
Blepharorrhaphy *see* Repair, Eye, 08Q
Blepharotomy *see* Drainage, Eye, 089
Blinatumomab Antineoplastic Immunotherapy, XW0

Block, Nerve, anesthetic injection
Blood glucose monitoring system *use* Monitoring Device
Blood pressure *see* Measurement, Arterial, 4A03
BMR (basal metabolic rate) *see* Measurement, Physiological Systems, 4A0Z
Body of femur
  use Femoral Shaft, Left
  use Femoral Shaft, Right
Body of fibula
  use Fibula, Left
  use Fibula, Right
Bone anchored hearing device
  use Hearing Device, Bone Conduction in, 09H
  use Hearing Device in Head and Facial Bones
Bone bank bone graft *use* Nonautologous Tissue Substitute
Bone Growth Stimulator
  Insertion of device in
    Bone
      Facial, 0NHW
      Lower, 0QHY
      Nasal, 0NHB
      Upper, 0PHY
    Skull, 0NH0
  Removal of device from
    Bone
      Facial, 0NPW
      Lower, 0QPY
      Nasal, 0NPB
      Upper, 0PPY
    Skull, 0NP0
  Revision of device in
    Bone
      Facial, 0NWW
      Lower, 0QWY
      Nasal, 0NWB
      Upper, 0PWY
    Skull, 0NW0
Bone marrow transplant *see* Transfusion, Circulatory, 302
Bone morphogenetic protein 2 (BMP 2) *use* Recombinant Bone Morphogenetic Protein
Bone screw (interlocking) (lag) (pedicle) (recessed)
  use Internal Fixation Device in Head and Facial Bones
  use Internal Fixation Device in Lower Bones
  use Internal Fixation Device in Upper Bones
Bony labyrinth
  use Inner Ear, Left
  use Inner Ear, Right
Bony orbit
  use Orbit, Left
  use Orbit, Right
Bony vestibule
  use Inner Ear, Left
  use Inner Ear, Right
Botallo's duct *use* Pulmonary Artery, Left
Bovine pericardial valve *use* Zooplastic Tissue in Heart and Great Vessels
Bovine pericardium graft *use* Zooplastic Tissue in Heart and Great Vessels
BP (blood pressure) *see* Measurement, Arterial, 4A03
Brachial (lateral) lymph node
  use Lymphatic, Left Axillary
  use Lymphatic, Right Axillary
Brachialis muscle
  use Upper Arm Muscle, Left
  use Upper Arm Muscle, Right
Brachiocephalic artery *use* Innominate Artery
Brachiocephalic trunk *use* Innominate Artery
Brachiocephalic vein
  use Innominate Vein, Left
  use Innominate Vein, Right
Brachioradialis muscle
  use Lower Arm and Wrist Muscle, Left
  use Lower Arm and Wrist Muscle, Right
Brachytherapy
  Abdomen, DW13
  Adrenal Gland, DG12
  Bile Ducts, DF12
  Bladder, DT12
  Bone Marrow, D710
  Brain, D010
  Brain Stem, D011
  Breast
    Left, DM10
    Right, DM11

Bypass — *continued*
  Vein — *continued*
    Face — *continued*
      Right, Ø51T
    Femoral
      Left, Ø61N
      Right, Ø61M
    Foot
      Left, Ø61V
      Right, Ø61T
    Gastric, Ø612
    Hand
      Left, Ø51H
      Right, Ø51G
    Hemiazygos, Ø511
    Hepatic, Ø614
    Hypogastric
      Left, Ø61J
      Right, Ø61H
    Inferior Mesenteric, Ø616
    Innominate
      Left, Ø514
      Right, Ø513
    Internal Jugular
      Left, Ø51N
      Right, Ø51M
    Intracranial, Ø51L
    Portal, Ø618
    Renal
      Left, Ø61B
      Right, Ø619
    Saphenous
      Left, Ø61Q
      Right, Ø61P
    Splenic, Ø611
    Subclavian
      Left, Ø516
      Right, Ø515
    Superior Mesenteric, Ø615
    Vertebral
      Left, Ø51S
      Right, Ø51R
    Vena Cava
      Inferior, Ø610
      Superior, Ø21V
    Ventricle
      Left, Ø21L
      Right, Ø21K
Bypass, cardiopulmonary, 5A1221Z

C

Caesarean section *see* Extraction, Products of Conception, 10D0
Calcaneocuboid joint
  use Tarsal Joint, Left
  use Tarsal Joint, Right
Calcaneocuboid ligament
  use Foot Bursa and Ligament, Left
  use Foot Bursa and Ligament, Right
Calcaneofibular ligament
  use Ankle Bursa and Ligament, Left
  use Ankle Bursa and Ligament, Right
Calcaneus
  use Tarsal, Left
  use Tarsal, Right
Cannulation
  see Bypass
  see Dilation
  see Drainage
  see Irrigation
Canthorrhaphy *see* Repair, Eye, Ø8Q
Canthotomy *see* Release, Eye, Ø8N
Capitate bone
  use Carpal, Left
  use Carpal, Right
Capsulectomy, lens *see* Excision, Eye, Ø8B
Capsulorrhaphy, joint
  see Repair, Lower Joints, ØSQ
  see Repair, Upper Joints, ØRQ
Cardia *use* Esophagogastric Junction
Cardiac contractility modulation lead *use* Cardiac Lead in Heart and Great Vessels
Cardiac event recorder *use* Monitoring Device

Cardiac Lead
  Defibrillator
    Atrium
      Left, Ø2H7
      Right, Ø2H6
    Pericardium, Ø2HN
    Vein, Coronary, Ø2H4
    Ventricle
      Left, Ø2HL
      Right, Ø2HK
  Insertion of device in
    Atrium
      Left, Ø2H7
      Right, Ø2H6
    Pericardium, Ø2HN
    Vein, Coronary, Ø2H4
    Ventricle
      Left, Ø2HL
      Right, Ø2HK
  Pacemaker
    Atrium
      Left, Ø2H7
      Right, Ø2H6
    Pericardium, Ø2HN
    Vein, Coronary, Ø2H4
    Ventricle
      Left, Ø2HL
      Right, Ø2HK
  Removal of device from, Heart, Ø2PA
  Revision of device in, Heart, Ø2WA
Cardiac plexus *use* Thoracic Sympathetic Nerve
Cardiac Resynchronization Defibrillator Pulse Generator
  Abdomen, ØJH8
  Chest, ØJH6
Cardiac Resynchronization Pacemaker Pulse Generator
  Abdomen, ØJH8
  Chest, ØJH6
Cardiac resynchronization therapy (CRT) lead
  use Cardiac Lead, Defibrillator in, Ø2H
  use Cardiac Lead, Pacemaker in, Ø2H
Cardiac Rhythm Related Device
  Insertion of device in
    Abdomen, ØJH8
    Chest, ØJH6
  Removal of device from, Subcutaneous Tissue and Fascia, Trunk, ØJPT
  Revision of device in, Subcutaneous Tissue and Fascia, Trunk, ØJWT
Cardiocentesis *see* Drainage, Pericardial Cavity, ØW9D
Cardioesophageal junction *use* Esophagogastric Junction
Cardiolysis *see* Release, Heart and Great Vessels, Ø2N
CardioMEMS® pressure sensor *use* Monitoring Device, Pressure Sensor in, Ø2H
Cardiomyotomy *see* Division, Esophagogastric Junction, ØD84
Cardioplegia *see* Introduction of substance in or on, Heart, 3E08
Cardiorrhaphy *see* Repair, Heart and Great Vessels, Ø2Q
Cardioversion, 5A2204Z
Caregiver Training, FØFZ
Caroticotympanic artery
  use Internal Carotid Artery, Left
  use Internal Carotid Artery, Right
Carotid glomus
  use Carotid Bodies, Bilateral
  use Carotid Body, Left
  use Carotid Body, Right
Carotid sinus
  use Internal Carotid Artery, Left
  use Internal Carotid Artery, Right
Carotid (artery) sinus (baroreceptor) lead *use* Stimulator Lead in Upper Arteries
Carotid sinus nerve *use* Glossopharyngeal Nerve
Carotid WALLSTENT® Monorail® Endoprosthesis *use* Intraluminal Device
Carpectomy
  see Excision, Upper Bones, ØPB
  see Resection, Upper Bones, ØPT
Carpometacarpal ligament
  use Hand Bursa and Ligament, Left
  use Hand Bursa and Ligament, Right
Casting *see* Immobilization
CAT scan *see* Computerized Tomography (CT Scan)

Catheterization
  see Dilation
  see Drainage
  see Insertion of device in
  see Irrigation
  Heart *see* Measurement, Cardiac, 4A02
  Umbilical vein, for infusion, Ø6H033T
Cauda equina *use* Lumbar Spinal Cord
Cauterization
  see Destruction
  see Repair
Cavernous plexus *use* Head and Neck Sympathetic Nerve
CBMA (Concentrated Bone Marrow Aspirate) *use* Concentrated Bone Marrow Aspirate
CBMA (Concentrated Bone Marrow Aspirate) injection, intramuscular, XKØ23Ø3
Cecectomy
  see Excision, Cecum, ØDBH
  see Resection, Cecum, ØDTH
Cecocolostomy
  see Bypass, Gastrointestinal System, ØD1
  see Drainage, Gastrointestinal System, ØD9
Cecopexy
  see Repair, Cecum, ØDQH
  see Reposition, Cecum, ØDSH
Cecoplication *see* Restriction, Cecum, ØDVH
Cecorrhaphy *see* Repair, Cecum, ØDQH
Cecostomy
  see Bypass, Cecum, ØD1H
  see Drainage, Cecum, ØD9H
Cecotomy *see* Drainage, Cecum, ØD9H
Ceftazidime-Avibactam Anti-infective, XWØ
Celiac ganglion *use* Abdominal Sympathetic Nerve
Celiac lymph node *use* Lymphatic, Aortic
Celiac (solar) plexus *use* Abdominal Sympathetic Nerve
Celiac trunk *use* Celiac Artery
Central axillary lymph node
  use Lymphatic, Left Axillary
  use Lymphatic, Right Axillary
Central venous pressure *see* Measurement, Venous, 4A04
Centrimag® Blood Pump *use* Short-term External Heart Assist System in Heart and Great Vessels
Cephalogram, BNØØZZZ
Ceramic on ceramic bearing surface *use* Synthetic Substitute, Ceramic in, ØSR
Cerclage *see* Restriction
Cerebral aqueduct (Sylvius) *use* Cerebral Ventricle
Cerebral Embolic Filtration, Dual Filter, X2A5312
Cerebrum *use* Brain
Cervical esophagus *use* Esophagus, Upper
Cervical facet joint
  use Cervical Vertebral Joint
  use Cervical Vertebral Joint, 2 or more
Cervical ganglion *use* Head and Neck Sympathetic Nerve
Cervical interspinous ligament *use* Head and Neck Bursa and Ligament
Cervical intertransverse ligament *use* Head and Neck Bursa and Ligament
Cervical ligamentum flavum *use* Head and Neck Bursa and Ligament
Cervical lymph node
  use Lymphatic, Left Neck
  use Lymphatic, Right Neck
Cervicectomy
  see Excision, Cervix, ØUBC
  see Resection, Cervix, ØUTC
Cervicothoracic facet joint *use* Cervicothoracic Vertebral Joint
Cesarean section *see* Extraction, Products of Conception, 10D0
Cesium-131 Collagen Implant *use* Radioactive Element, Cesium-131 Collagen Implant in ØØH
Change device in
  Abdominal Wall, ØW2FX
  Back
    Lower, ØW2LX
    Upper, ØW2KX
  Bladder, ØT2BX
  Bone
    Facial, ØN2WX
    Lower, ØQ2YX
    Nasal, ØN2BX
    Upper, ØP2YX
  Bone Marrow, Ø72TX
  Brain, ØØ20X

▽ Subterms under main terms may continue to next column or page

Change device in — *continued*
  Breast
    Left, ØH2UX
    Right, ØH2TX
  Bursa and Ligament
    Lower, ØM2YX
    Upper, ØM2XX
  Cavity, Cranial, ØW21X
  Chest Wall, ØW28X
  Cisterna Chyli, Ø72LX
  Diaphragm, ØB2TX
  Duct
    Hepatobiliary, ØF2BX
    Pancreatic, ØF2DX
  Ear
    Left, Ø92JX
    Right, Ø92HX
  Epididymis and Spermatic Cord, ØV2MX
  Extremity
    Lower
      Left, ØY2BX
      Right, ØY29X
    Upper
      Left, ØX27X
      Right, ØX26X
  Eye
    Left, Ø821X
    Right, Ø820X
  Face, ØW22X
  Fallopian Tube, ØU28X
  Gallbladder, ØF24X
  Gland
    Adrenal, ØG25X
    Endocrine, ØG2SX
    Pituitary, ØG20X
    Salivary, ØC2AX
  Head, ØW20X
  Intestinal Tract
    Lower, ØD2DXUZ
    Upper, ØD20XUZ
  Jaw
    Lower, ØW25X
    Upper, ØW24X
  Joint
    Lower, ØS2YX
    Upper, ØR2YX
  Kidney, ØT25X
  Larynx, ØC2SX
  Liver, ØF20X
  Lung
    Left, ØB2LX
    Right, ØB2KX
  Lymphatic, Ø72NX
    Thoracic Duct, Ø72KX
  Mediastinum, ØW2CX
  Mesentery, ØD2VX
  Mouth and Throat, ØC2YX
  Muscle
    Lower, ØK2YX
    Upper, ØK2XX
  Nasal Mucosa and Soft Tissue, Ø92KX
  Neck, ØW26X
  Nerve
    Cranial, ØØ2EX
    Peripheral, Ø12YX
  Omentum, ØD2UX
  Ovary, ØU23X
  Pancreas, ØF2GX
  Parathyroid Gland, ØG2RX
  Pelvic Cavity, ØW2JX
  Penis, ØV2SX
  Pericardial Cavity, ØW2DX
  Perineum
    Female, ØW2NX
    Male, ØW2MX
  Peritoneal Cavity, ØW2GX
  Peritoneum, ØD2WX
  Pineal Body, ØG21X
  Pleura, ØB2QX
  Pleural Cavity
    Left, ØW2BX
    Right, ØW29X
  Products of Conception, 1Ø207
  Prostate and Seminal Vesicles, ØV24X
  Retroperitoneum, ØW2HX
  Scrotum and Tunica Vaginalis, ØV28X
  Sinus, Ø92YX
  Skin, ØH2PX
  Skull, ØN20X

Change device in — *continued*
  Spinal Canal, ØØ2UX
  Spleen, Ø72PX
  Subcutaneous Tissue and Fascia
    Head and Neck, ØJ2SX
    Lower Extremity, ØJ2WX
    Trunk, ØJ2TX
    Upper Extremity, ØJ2VX
  Tendon
    Lower, ØL2YX
    Upper, ØL2XX
  Testis, ØV2DX
  Thymus, Ø72MX
  Thyroid Gland, ØG2KX
  Trachea, ØB21
  Tracheobronchial Tree, ØB20X
  Ureter, ØT29X
  Urethra, ØT2DX
  Uterus and Cervix, ØU2DXHZ
  Vagina and Cul-de-sac, ØU2HXGZ
  Vas Deferens, ØV2RX
  Vulva, ØU2MX
Change device in or on
  Abdominal Wall, 2WØ3X
  Anorectal, 2YØ3X5Z
  Arm
    Lower
      Left, 2WØDX
      Right, 2WØCX
    Upper
      Left, 2WØBX
      Right, 2WØAX
  Back, 2WØ5X
  Chest Wall, 2WØ4X
  Ear, 2YØ2X5Z
  Extremity
    Lower
      Left, 2WØMX
      Right, 2WØLX
    Upper
      Left, 2WØ9X
      Right, 2WØ8X
  Face, 2WØ1X
  Finger
    Left, 2WØKX
    Right, 2WØJX
  Foot
    Left, 2WØTX
    Right, 2WØSX
  Genital Tract, Female, 2YØ4X5Z
  Hand
    Left, 2WØFX
    Right, 2WØEX
  Head, 2WØØX
  Inguinal Region
    Left, 2WØ7X
    Right, 2WØ6X
  Leg
    Lower
      Left, 2WØRX
      Right, 2WØQX
    Upper
      Left, 2WØPX
      Right, 2WØNX
  Mouth and Pharynx, 2YØØX5Z
  Nasal, 2YØ1X5Z
  Neck, 2WØ2X
  Thumb
    Left, 2WØHX
    Right, 2WØGX
  Toe
    Left, 2WØVX
    Right, 2WØUX
  Urethra, 2YØ5X5Z
Chemoembolization *see* Introduction of substance in or on
Chemosurgery, Skin, 3EØØXTZ
Chemothalamectomy *see* Destruction, Thalamus, ØØ59
Chemotherapy, Infusion for cancer *see* Introduction of substance in or on
Chest x-ray *see* Plain Radiography, Chest, BWØ3
Chiropractic Manipulation
  Abdomen, 9WB9X
  Cervical, 9WB1X
  Extremities
    Lower, 9WB6X
    Upper, 9WB7X
  Head, 9WBØX

Chiropractic Manipulation — *continued*
  Lumbar, 9WB3X
  Pelvis, 9WB5X
  Rib Cage, 9WB8X
  Sacrum, 9WB4X
  Thoracic, 9WB2X
Choana *use* Nasopharynx
Cholangiogram
  see Fluoroscopy, Hepatobiliary System and Pancreas, BF1
  see Plain Radiography, Hepatobiliary System and Pancreas, BFØ
Cholecystectomy
  see Excision, Gallbladder, ØFB4
  see Resection, Gallbladder, ØFT4
Cholecystojejunostomy
  see Bypass, Hepatobiliary System and Pancreas, ØF1
  see Drainage, Hepatobiliary System and Pancreas, ØF9
Cholecystopexy
  see Repair, Gallbladder, ØFQ4
  see Reposition, Gallbladder, ØFS4
Cholecystoscopy, ØFJ44ZZ
Cholecystostomy
  see Bypass, Gallbladder, ØF14
  see Drainage, Gallbladder, ØF94
Cholecystotomy *see* Drainage, Gallbladder, ØF94
Choledochectomy
  see Excision, Hepatobiliary System and Pancreas, ØFB
  see Resection, Hepatobiliary System and Pancreas, ØFT
Choledocholithotomy *see* Extirpation, Duct, Common Bile, ØFC9
Choledochoplasty
  see Repair, Hepatobiliary System and Pancreas, ØFQ
  see Replacement, Hepatobiliary System and Pancreas, ØFR
  see Supplement, Hepatobiliary System and Pancreas, ØFU
Choledochoscopy, ØFJB8ZZ
Choledochotomy *see* Drainage, Hepatobiliary System and Pancreas, ØF9
Cholelithotomy *see* Extirpation, Hepatobiliary System and Pancreas, ØFC
Chondrectomy
  see Excision, Lower Joints, ØSB
  see Excision, Upper Joints, ØRB
  Knee *see* Excision, Lower Joints, ØSB
  Semilunar cartilage *see* Excision, Lower Joints, ØSB
Chondroglossus muscle *use* Tongue, Palate, Pharynx Muscle
Chorda tympani *use* Facial Nerve
Chordotomy *see* Division, Central Nervous System and Cranial Nerves, ØØ8
Choroid plexus *use* Cerebral Ventricle
Choroidectomy
  see Excision, Eye, Ø8B
  see Resection, Eye, Ø8T
Ciliary body
  use Eye, Left
  use Eye, Right
Ciliary ganglion *use* Head and Neck Sympathetic Nerve
Circle of Willis *use* Intracranial Artery
Circumcision, ØVTTXZZ
Circumflex iliac artery
  use Femoral Artery, Left
  use Femoral Artery, Right
Clamp and rod internal fixation system (CRIF)
  use Internal Fixation Device in Lower Bones
  use Internal Fixation Device in Upper Bones
Clamping *see* Occlusion
Claustrum *use* Basal Ganglia
Claviculectomy
  see Excision, Upper Bones, ØPB
  see Resection, Upper Bones, ØPT
Claviculotomy
  see Division, Upper Bones, ØP8
  see Drainage, Upper Bones, ØP9
Clipping, aneurysm
  see Occlusion using Extraluminal Device
  see Restriction using Extraluminal Device
Clitorectomy, clitoridectomy
  see Excision, Clitoris, ØUBJ
  see Resection, Clitoris, ØUTJ
Clolar *use* Clofarabine
Closure
  see Occlusion

Closure — *continued*
  see Repair
Clysis *see* Introduction of substance in or on
Coagulation *see* Destruction
COALESCE® radiolucent interbody fusion device *use*
  Interbody Fusion Device, Radiolucent Porous in New
  Technology
CoAxia NeuroFlo catheter *use* Intraluminal Device
Cobalt/chromium head and polyethylene socket *use*
  Synthetic Substitute, Metal on Polyethylene in, 0SR
Cobalt/chromium head and socket *use* Synthetic Sub-
  stitute, Metal in, 0SR
Coccygeal body *use* Coccygeal Glomus
Coccygeus muscle
  use Trunk Muscle, Left
  use Trunk Muscle, Right
Cochlea
  use Inner Ear, Left
  use Inner Ear, Right
Cochlear implant (CI), multiple channel (electrode)
  use Hearing Device, Multiple Channel Cochlear
  Prosthesis in, 09H
Cochlear implant (CI), single channel (electrode) *use*
  Hearing Device, Single Channel Cochlear Prosthesis
  in, 09H
Cochlear Implant Treatment, F0BZ0
Cochlear nerve *use* Acoustic Nerve
COGNIS® CRT-D *use* Cardiac Resynchronization Defibrilla-
  tor Pulse Generator in, 0JH
COHERE® radiolucent interbody fusion device *use* In-
  terbody Fusion Device, Radiolucent Porous in New
  Technology
Colectomy
  see Excision, Gastrointestinal System, 0DB
  see Resection, Gastrointestinal System, 0DT
Collapse *see* Occlusion
Collection from
  Breast, Breast Milk, 8E0HX62
  Indwelling Device
    Circulatory System
      Blood, 8C02X6K
      Other Fluid, 8C02X6L
    Nervous System
      Cerebrospinal Fluid, 8C01X6J
      Other Fluid, 8C01X6L
  Integumentary System, Breast Milk, 8E0HX62
  Reproductive System, Male, Sperm, 8E0VX63
Colocentesis *see* Drainage, Gastrointestinal System, 0D9
Colofixation
  see Repair, Gastrointestinal System, 0DQ
  see Reposition, Gastrointestinal System, 0DS
Cololysis *see* Release, Gastrointestinal System, 0DN
Colonic Z-Stent® *use* Intraluminal Device
Colonoscopy, 0DJD8ZZ
Colopexy
  see Repair, Gastrointestinal System, 0DQ
  see Reposition, Gastrointestinal System, 0DS
Coloplication *see* Restriction, Gastrointestinal System,
  0DV
Coloproctectomy
  see Excision, Gastrointestinal System, 0DB
  see Resection, Gastrointestinal System, 0DT
Coloproctostomy
  see Bypass, Gastrointestinal System, 0D1
  see Drainage, Gastrointestinal System, 0D9
Colopuncture *see* Drainage, Gastrointestinal System, 0D9
Colorrhaphy *see* Repair, Gastrointestinal System, 0DQ
Colostomy
  see Bypass, Gastrointestinal System, 0D1
  see Drainage, Gastrointestinal System, 0D9
Colpectomy
  see Excision, Vagina, 0UBG
  see Resection, Vagina, 0UTG
Colpocentesis *see* Drainage, Vagina, 0U9G
Colpopexy
  see Repair, Vagina, 0UQG
  see Reposition, Vagina, 0USG
Colpoplasty
  see Repair, Vagina, 0UQG
  see Supplement, Vagina, 0UUG
Colporrhaphy *see* Repair, Vagina, 0UQG
Colposcopy, 0UJH8ZZ
Columella *use* Nasal Mucosa and Soft Tissue
Common digital vein
  use Foot Vein, Left
  use Foot Vein, Right

Common facial vein
  use Face Vein, Left
  use Face Vein, Right
Common fibular nerve *use* Peroneal Nerve
Common hepatic artery *use* Hepatic Artery
Common iliac (subaortic) lymph node *use* Lymphatic,
  Pelvis
Common interosseous artery
  use Ulnar Artery, Left
  use Ulnar Artery, Right
Common peroneal nerve *use* Peroneal Nerve
Complete (SE) stent *use* Intraluminal Device
Compression
  see Restriction
  Abdominal Wall, 2W13X
  Arm
    Lower
      Left, 2W1DX
      Right, 2W1CX
    Upper
      Left, 2W1BX
      Right, 2W1AX
  Back, 2W15X
  Chest Wall, 2W14X
  Extremity
    Lower
      Left, 2W1MX
      Right, 2W1LX
    Upper
      Left, 2W19X
      Right, 2W18X
  Face, 2W11X
  Finger
    Left, 2W1KX
    Right, 2W1JX
  Foot
    Left, 2W1TX
    Right, 2W1SX
  Hand
    Left, 2W1FX
    Right, 2W1EX
  Head, 2W10X
  Inguinal Region
    Left, 2W17X
    Right, 2W16X
  Leg
    Lower
      Left, 2W1RX
      Right, 2W1QX
    Upper
      Left, 2W1PX
      Right, 2W1NX
  Neck, 2W12X
  Thumb
    Left, 2W1HX
    Right, 2W1GX
  Toe
    Left, 2W1VX
    Right, 2W1UX
Computer Assisted Procedure
  Extremity
    Lower
      With Computerized Tomography,
        8E0YXBG
      With Fluoroscopy, 8E0YXBF
      With Magnetic Resonance Imaging,
        8E0YXBH
      No Qualifier, 8E0YXBZ
    Upper
      With Computerized Tomography,
        8E0XXBG
      With Fluoroscopy, 8E0XXBF
      With Magnetic Resonance Imaging,
        8E0XXBH
      No Qualifier, 8E0XXBZ
  Head and Neck Region
    With Computerized Tomography, 8E09XBG
    With Fluoroscopy, 8E09XBF
    With Magnetic Resonance Imaging, 8E09XBH
    No Qualifier, 8E09XBZ
  Trunk Region
    With Computerized Tomography, 8E0WXBG
    With Fluoroscopy, 8E0WXBF
    With Magnetic Resonance Imaging, 8E0WXBH
    No Qualifier, 8E0WXBZ
Computerized Tomography (CT Scan)
  Abdomen, BW20
    Chest and Pelvis, BW25

Computerized Tomography (CT Scan) — *continued*
  Abdomen and Chest, BW24
  Abdomen and Pelvis, BW21
  Airway, Trachea, BB2F
  Ankle
    Left, BQ2H
    Right, BQ2G
  Aorta
    Abdominal, B420
      Intravascular Optical Coherence, B420Z2Z
    Thoracic, B320
      Intravascular Optical Coherence, B320Z2Z
  Arm
    Left, BP2F
    Right, BP2E
  Artery
    Celiac, B421
      Intravascular Optical Coherence, B421Z2Z
    Common Carotid
      Bilateral, B325
      Intravascular Optical Coherence, B325Z2Z
    Coronary
      Bypass Graft
        Intravascular Optical Coherence,
          B223Z2Z
        Multiple, B223
      Multiple, B221
        Intravascular Optical Coherence,
          B221Z2Z
    Internal Carotid
      Bilateral, B328
      Intravascular Optical Coherence, B328Z2Z
    Intracranial, B32R
      Intravascular Optical Coherence, B32RZ2Z
    Lower Extremity
      Bilateral, B42H
        Intravascular Optical Coherence,
          B42HZ2Z
      Left, B42G
        Intravascular Optical Coherence,
          B42GZ2Z
      Right, B42F
        Intravascular Optical Coherence,
          B42FZ2Z
    Pelvic, B42C
      Intravascular Optical Coherence, B42CZ2Z
    Pulmonary
      Left, B32T
        Intravascular Optical Coherence,
          B32TZ2Z
      Right, B32S
        Intravascular Optical Coherence,
          B32SZ2Z
    Renal
      Bilateral, B428
        Intravascular Optical Coherence,
          B428Z2Z
      Transplant, B42M
        Intravascular Optical Coherence,
          B42MZ2Z
    Superior Mesenteric, B424
      Intravascular Optical Coherence, B424Z2Z
    Vertebral
      Bilateral, B32G
      Intravascular Optical Coherence, B32GZ2Z
  Bladder, BT20
  Bone
    Facial, BN25
    Temporal, BN2F
  Brain, B020
  Calcaneus
    Left, BQ2K
    Right, BQ2J
  Cerebral Ventricle, B028
  Chest, Abdomen and Pelvis, BW25
  Chest and Abdomen, BW24
  Cisterna, B027
  Clavicle
    Left, BP25
    Right, BP24
  Coccyx, BR2F
  Colon, BD24
  Ear, B920
  Elbow
    Left, BP2H
    Right, BP2G
  Extremity
    Lower
      Left, BQ2S

Computerized Tomography (CT Scan) — *continued*
  Extremity — *continued*
    Lower — *continued*
      Right, BQ2R
    Upper
      Bilateral, BP2V
      Left, BP2U
      Right, BP2T
  Eye
    Bilateral, B827
    Left, B826
    Right, B825
  Femur
    Left, BQ24
    Right, BQ23
  Fibula
    Left, BQ2C
    Right, BQ2B
  Finger
    Left, BP2S
    Right, BP2R
  Foot
    Left, BQ2M
    Right, BQ2L
  Forearm
    Left, BP2K
    Right, BP2J
  Gland
    Adrenal, Bilateral, BG22
    Parathyroid, BG23
    Parotid, Bilateral, B926
    Salivary, Bilateral, B92D
    Submandibular, Bilateral, B929
    Thyroid, BG24
  Hand
    Left, BP2P
    Right, BP2N
  Hands and Wrists, Bilateral, BP2Q
  Head, BW28
  Head and Neck, BW29
  Heart
    Intravascular Optical Coherence, B226Z2Z
    Right and Left, B226
  Hepatobiliary System, All, BF2C
  Hip
    Left, BQ21
    Right, BQ20
  Humerus
    Left, BP2B
    Right, BP2A
  Intracranial Sinus, B522
    Intravascular Optical Coherence, B522Z2Z
  Joint
    Acromioclavicular, Bilateral, BP23
    Finger
      Left, BP2DZZZ
      Right, BP2CZZZ
    Foot
      Left, BQ2Y
      Right, BQ2X
    Hand
      Left, BP2DZZZ
      Right, BP2CZZZ
    Sacroiliac, BR2D
    Sternoclavicular
      Bilateral, BP22
      Left, BP21
      Right, BP20
    Temporomandibular, Bilateral, BN29
    Toe
      Left, BQ2Y
      Right, BQ2X
  Kidney
    Bilateral, BT23
    Left, BT22
    Right, BT21
    Transplant, BT29
  Knee
    Left, BQ28
    Right, BQ27
  Larynx, B92J
  Leg
    Left, BQ2F
    Right, BQ2D
  Liver, BF25
  Liver and Spleen, BF26
  Lung, Bilateral, BB24
  Mandible, BN26
  Nasopharynx, B92F

Computerized Tomography (CT Scan) — *continued*
  Neck, BW2F
  Neck and Head, BW29
  Orbit, Bilateral, BN23
  Oropharynx, B92F
  Pancreas, BF27
  Patella
    Left, BQ2W
    Right, BQ2V
  Pelvic Region, BW2G
  Pelvis, BR2C
    Chest and Abdomen, BW25
  Pelvis and Abdomen, BW21
  Pituitary Gland, B029
  Prostate, BV23
  Ribs
    Left, BP2Y
    Right, BP2X
  Sacrum, BR2F
  Scapula
    Left, BP27
    Right, BP26
  Sella Turcica, B029
  Shoulder
    Left, BP29
    Right, BP28
  Sinus
    Intracranial, B522
      Intravascular Optical Coherence, B522Z2Z
    Paranasal, B922
  Skull, BN20
  Spinal Cord, B02B
  Spine
    Cervical, BR20
    Lumbar, BR29
    Thoracic, BR27
  Spleen and Liver, BF26
  Thorax, BP2W
  Tibia
    Left, BQ2C
    Right, BQ2B
  Toe
    Left, BQ2Q
    Right, BQ2P
  Trachea, BB2F
  Tracheobronchial Tree
    Bilateral, BB29
    Left, BB28
    Right, BB27
  Vein
    Pelvic (Iliac)
      Left, B52G
        Intravascular Optical Coherence,
          B52GZ2Z
      Right, B52F
        Intravascular Optical Coherence,
          B52FZ2Z
    Pelvic (Iliac) Bilateral, B52H
      Intravascular Optical Coherence, B52HZ2Z
    Portal, B52T
      Intravascular Optical Coherence, B52TZ2Z
    Pulmonary
      Bilateral, B52S
        Intravascular Optical Coherence,
          B52SZ2Z
      Left, B52R
        Intravascular Optical Coherence,
          B52RZ2Z
      Right, B52Q
        Intravascular Optical Coherence,
          B52QZ2Z
    Renal
      Bilateral, B52L
        Intravascular Optical Coherence,
          B52LZ2Z
      Left, B52K
        Intravascular Optical Coherence,
          B52KZ2Z
      Right, B52J
        Intravascular Optical Coherence,
          B52JZ2Z
    Spanchnic, B52T
      Intravascular Optical Coherence, B52TZ2Z
  Vena Cava
    Inferior, B529
      Intravascular Optical Coherence, B529Z2Z
    Superior, B528
      Intravascular Optical Coherence, B528Z2Z
  Ventricle, Cerebral, B028

Computerized Tomography (CT Scan) — *continued*
  Wrist
    Left, BP2M
    Right, BP2L
Concentrated Bone Marrow Aspirate (CBMA) injection, intramuscular, XK02303
Concerto II CRT-D *use* Cardiac Resynchronization Defibrillator Pulse Generator in, 0JH
Condylectomy
  see Excision, Head and Facial Bones, 0NB
  see Excision, Lower Bones, 0QB
  see Excision, Upper Bones, 0PB
Condyloid process
  use Mandible, Left
  use Mandible, Right
Condylotomy
  see Division, Head and Facial Bones, 0N8
  see Division, Lower Bones, 0Q8
  see Division, Upper Bones, 0P8
  see Drainage, Head and Facial Bones, 0N9
  see Drainage, Lower Bones, 0Q9
  see Drainage, Upper Bones, 0P9
Condylysis
  see Release, Head and Facial Bones, 0NN
  see Release, Lower Bones, 0QN
  see Release, Upper Bones, 0PN
Conization, cervix *see* Excision, Cervix, 0UBC
Conjunctivoplasty
  see Repair, Eye, 08Q
  see Replacement, Eye, 08R
CONSERVE® PLUS Total Resurfacing Hip System *use* Resurfacing Device in Lower Joints
Construction
  Auricle, ear *see* Replacement, Ear, Nose, Sinus, 09R
  Ileal conduit *see* Bypass, Urinary System, 0T1
Consulta CRT-D *use* Cardiac Resynchronization Defibrillator Pulse Generator in, 0JH
Consulta CRT-P *use* Cardiac Resynchronization Pacemaker Pulse Generator in, 0JH
Contact Radiation
  Abdomen, DWY37ZZ
  Adrenal Gland, DGY27ZZ
  Bile Ducts, DFY27ZZ
  Bladder, DTY27ZZ
  Bone, Other, DPYC7ZZ
  Brain, D0Y07ZZ
  Brain Stem, D0Y17ZZ
  Breast
    Left, DMY07ZZ
    Right, DMY17ZZ
  Bronchus, DBY17ZZ
  Cervix, DUY17ZZ
  Chest, DWY27ZZ
  Chest Wall, DBY77ZZ
  Colon, DDY57ZZ
  Diaphragm, DBY87ZZ
  Duodenum, DDY27ZZ
  Ear, D9Y07ZZ
  Esophagus, DDY07ZZ
  Eye, D8Y07ZZ
  Femur, DPY97ZZ
  Fibula, DPYB7ZZ
  Gallbladder, DFY17ZZ
  Gland
    Adrenal, DGY27ZZ
    Parathyroid, DGY47ZZ
    Pituitary, DGY07ZZ
    Thyroid, DGY57ZZ
  Glands, Salivary, D9Y67ZZ
  Head and Neck, DWY17ZZ
  Hemibody, DWY47ZZ
  Humerus, DPY67ZZ
  Hypopharynx, D9Y37ZZ
  Ileum, DDY47ZZ
  Jejunum, DDY37ZZ
  Kidney, DTY07ZZ
  Larynx, D9YB7ZZ
  Liver, DFY07ZZ
  Lung, DBY27ZZ
  Mandible, DPY37ZZ
  Maxilla, DPY27ZZ
  Mediastinum, DBY67ZZ
  Mouth, D9Y47ZZ
  Nasopharynx, D9YD7ZZ
  Neck and Head, DWY17ZZ
  Nerve, Peripheral, D0Y77ZZ
  Nose, D9Y17ZZ
  Oropharynx, D9YF7ZZ

Contact Radiation — *continued*
- Ovary, DUYØ7ZZ
- Palate
  - Hard, D9Y87ZZ
  - Soft, D9Y97ZZ
- Pancreas, DFY37ZZ
- Parathyroid Gland, DGY47ZZ
- Pelvic Bones, DPY87ZZ
- Pelvic Region, DWY67ZZ
- Pineal Body, DGY17ZZ
- Pituitary Gland, DGYØ7ZZ
- Pleura, DBY57ZZ
- Prostate, DVYØ7ZZ
- Radius, DPY77ZZ
- Rectum, DDY77ZZ
- Rib, DPY57ZZ
- Sinuses, D9Y77ZZ
- Skin
  - Abdomen, DHY87ZZ
  - Arm, DHY47ZZ
  - Back, DHY77ZZ
  - Buttock, DHY97ZZ
  - Chest, DHY67ZZ
  - Face, DHY27ZZ
  - Leg, DHYB7ZZ
  - Neck, DHY37ZZ
- Skull, DPYØ7ZZ
- Spinal Cord, DØY67ZZ
- Sternum, DPY47ZZ
- Stomach, DDY17ZZ
- Testis, DVY17ZZ
- Thyroid Gland, DGY57ZZ
- Tibia, DPYB7ZZ
- Tongue, D9Y57ZZ
- Trachea, DBYØ7ZZ
- Ulna, DPY77ZZ
- Ureter, DTY17ZZ
- Urethra, DTY37ZZ
- Uterus, DUY27ZZ
- Whole Body, DWY57ZZ

CONTAK RENEWAL® 3 RF (HE) CRT-D *use* Cardiac Resynchronization Defibrillator Pulse Generator in, ØJH

Contegra Pulmonary Valved Conduit *use* Zooplastic Tissue in Heart and Great Vessels

Continuous Glucose Monitoring (CGM) device *use* Monitoring Device

Continuous Negative Airway Pressure
- 24-96 Consecutive Hours, Ventilation, 5AØ9459
- Greater than 96 Consecutive Hours, Ventilation, 5AØ9559
- Less than 24 Consecutive Hours, Ventilation, 5AØ9359

Continuous Positive Airway Pressure
- 24-96 Consecutive Hours, Ventilation, 5AØ9457
- Greater than 96 Consecutive Hours, Ventilation, 5AØ9557
- Less than 24 Consecutive Hours, Ventilation, 5AØ9357

Continuous renal replacement therapy (CRRT), 5A1D9ØZ

Contraceptive Device
- Change device in, Uterus and Cervix, ØU2DXHZ
- Insertion of device in
  - Cervix, ØUHC
  - Subcutaneous Tissue and Fascia
    - Abdomen, ØJH8
    - Chest, ØJH6
    - Lower Arm
      - Left, ØJHH
      - Right, ØJHG
    - Lower Leg
      - Left, ØJHP
      - Right, ØJHN
    - Upper Arm
      - Left, ØJHF
      - Right, ØJHD
    - Upper Leg
      - Left, ØJHM
      - Right, ØJHL
  - Uterus, ØUH9
- Removal of device from
  - Subcutaneous Tissue and Fascia
    - Lower Extremity, ØJPW
    - Trunk, ØJPT
    - Upper Extremity, ØJPV
  - Uterus and Cervix, ØUPD
- Revision of device in
  - Subcutaneous Tissue and Fascia
    - Lower Extremity, ØJWW

Contraceptive Device — *continued*
- Revision of device in — *continued*
  - Subcutaneous Tissue and Fascia — *continued*
    - Trunk, ØJWT
    - Upper Extremity, ØJWV
  - Uterus and Cervix, ØUWD

Contractility Modulation Device
- Abdomen, ØJH8
- Chest, ØJH6

Control bleeding in
- Abdominal Wall, ØW3F
- Ankle Region
  - Left, ØY3L
  - Right, ØY3K
- Arm
  - Lower
    - Left, ØX3F
    - Right, ØX3D
  - Upper
    - Left, ØX39
    - Right, ØX38
- Axilla
  - Left, ØX35
  - Right, ØX34
- Back
  - Lower, ØW3L
  - Upper, ØW3K
- Buttock
  - Left, ØY31
  - Right, ØY3Ø
- Cavity, Cranial, ØW31
- Chest Wall, ØW38
- Elbow Region
  - Left, ØX3C
  - Right, ØX3B
- Extremity
  - Lower
    - Left, ØY3B
    - Right, ØY39
  - Upper
    - Left, ØX37
    - Right, ØX36
- Face, ØW32
- Femoral Region
  - Left, ØY38
  - Right, ØY37
- Foot
  - Left, ØY3N
  - Right, ØY3M
- Gastrointestinal Tract, ØW3P
- Genitourinary Tract, ØW3R
- Hand
  - Left, ØX3K
  - Right, ØX3J
- Head, ØW3Ø
- Inguinal Region
  - Left, ØY36
  - Right, ØY35
- Jaw
  - Lower, ØW35
  - Upper, ØW34
- Knee Region
  - Left, ØY3G
  - Right, ØY3F
- Leg
  - Lower
    - Left, ØY3J
    - Right, ØY3H
  - Upper
    - Left, ØY3D
    - Right, ØY3C
- Mediastinum, ØW3C
- Nasal Mucosa and Soft Tissue, Ø93K
- Neck, ØW36
- Oral Cavity and Throat, ØW33
- Pelvic Cavity, ØW3J
- Pericardial Cavity, ØW3D
- Perineum
  - Female, ØW3N
  - Male, ØW3M
- Peritoneal Cavity, ØW3G
- Pleural Cavity
  - Left, ØW3B
  - Right, ØW39
- Respiratory Tract, ØW3Q
- Retroperitoneum, ØW3H
- Shoulder Region
  - Left, ØX33
  - Right, ØX32

Control bleeding in — *continued*
- Wrist Region
  - Left, ØX3H
  - Right, ØX3G

Control, Epistaxis *see* Control bleeding in, Nasal Mucosa and Soft Tissue, Ø93K

Conus arteriosus *use* Ventricle, Right

Conus medullaris *use* Lumbar Spinal Cord

Conversion
- Cardiac rhythm, 5A22Ø4Z
- Gastrostomy to jejunostomy feeding device *see* Insertion of device in, Jejunum, ØDHA

Cook Biodesign® Fistula Plug(s) *use* Nonautologous Tissue Substitute

Cook Biodesign® Hernia Graft(s) *use* Nonautologous Tissue Substitute

Cook Biodesign® Layered Graft(s) *use* Nonautologous Tissue Substitute

Cook Zenaprom™ Layered Graft(s) *use* Nonautologous Tissue Substitute

Cook Zenith AAA Endovascular Graft
- *use* Intraluminal Device
- *use* Intraluminal Device, Branched or Fenestrated, One or Two Arteries in, Ø4V
- *use* Intraluminal Device, Branched or Fenestrated, Three or More Arteries in, Ø4V

Coracoacromial ligament
- *use* Shoulder Bursa and Ligament, Left
- *use* Shoulder Bursa and Ligament, Right

Coracobrachialis muscle
- *use* Upper Arm Muscle, Left
- *use* Upper Arm Muscle, Right

Coracoclavicular ligament
- *use* Shoulder Bursa and Ligament, Left
- *use* Shoulder Bursa and Ligament, Right

Coracohumeral ligament
- *use* Shoulder Bursa and Ligament, Left
- *use* Shoulder Bursa and Ligament, Right

Coracoid process
- *use* Scapula, Left
- *use* Scapula, Right

Cordotomy *see* Division, Central Nervous System and Cranial Nerves, ØØ8

Core needle biopsy *see* Excision with qualifier Diagnostic

CoreValve transcatheter aortic valve *use* Zooplastic Tissue in Heart and Great Vessels

Cormet Hip Resurfacing System *use* Resurfacing Device in Lower Joints

Corniculate cartilage *use* Larynx

CoRoent® XL *use* Interbody Fusion Device in Lower Joints

Coronary arteriography
- *see* Fluoroscopy, Heart, B21
- *see* Plain Radiography, Heart, B2Ø

Corox (OTW) Bipolar Lead
- *use* Cardiac Lead, Defibrillator in, Ø2H
- *use* Cardiac Lead, Pacemaker in, Ø2H

Corpus callosum *use* Brain

Corpus cavernosum *use* Penis

Corpus spongiosum *use* Penis

Corpus striatum *use* Basal Ganglia

Corrugator supercilii muscle *use* Facial Muscle

Cortical strip neurostimulator lead *use* Neurostimulator Lead in Central Nervous System and Cranial Nerves

Costatectomy
- *see* Excision, Upper Bones, ØPB
- *see* Resection, Upper Bones, ØPT

Costectomy
- *see* Excision, Upper Bones, ØPB
- *see* Resection, Upper Bones, ØPT

Costocervical trunk
- *use* Subclavian Artery, Left
- *use* Subclavian Artery, Right

Costochondrectomy
- *see* Excision, Upper Bones, ØPB
- *see* Resection, Upper Bones, ØPT

Costoclavicular ligament
- *use* Shoulder Bursa and Ligament, Left
- *use* Shoulder Bursa and Ligament, Right

Costosternoplasty
- *see* Repair, Upper Bones, ØPQ
- *see* Replacement, Upper Bones, ØPR
- *see* Supplement, Upper Bones, ØPU

Costotomy
- *see* Division, Upper Bones, ØP8
- *see* Drainage, Upper Bones, ØP9

Costotransverse joint *use* Thoracic Vertebral Joint

Costotransverse ligament *use* Rib(s) Bursa and Ligament

Costovertebral joint *use* Thoracic Vertebral Joint
Costoxiphoid ligament *use* Sternum Bursa and Ligament
Counseling
   Family, for substance abuse, Other Family Counseling,
      HZ63ZZZ
   Group
      12-Step, HZ43ZZZ
      Behavioral, HZ41ZZZ
      Cognitive, HZ40ZZZ
      Cognitive-Behavioral, HZ42ZZZ
      Confrontational, HZ48ZZZ
      Continuing Care, HZ49ZZZ
      Infectious Disease
         Post-Test, HZ4CZZZ
         Pre-Test, HZ4CZZZ
      Interpersonal, HZ44ZZZ
      Motivational Enhancement, HZ47ZZZ
      Psychoeducation, HZ46ZZZ
      Spiritual, HZ4BZZZ
      Vocational, HZ45ZZZ
   Individual
      12-Step, HZ33ZZZ
      Behavioral, HZ31ZZZ
      Cognitive, HZ30ZZZ
      Cognitive-Behavioral, HZ32ZZZ
      Confrontational, HZ38ZZZ
      Continuing Care, HZ39ZZZ
      Infectious Disease
         Post-Test, HZ3CZZZ
         Pre-Test, HZ3CZZZ
      Interpersonal, HZ34ZZZ
      Motivational Enhancement, HZ37ZZZ
      Psychoeducation, HZ36ZZZ
      Spiritual, HZ3BZZZ
      Vocational, HZ35ZZZ
   Mental Health Services
      Educational, GZ60ZZZ
      Other Counseling, GZ63ZZZ
      Vocational, GZ61ZZZ
Countershock, cardiac, 5A2204Z
Cowper's (bulbourethral) gland *use* Urethra
CPAP (continuous positive airway pressure) *see* Assistance, Respiratory, 5A09
Craniectomy
   see Excision, Head and Facial Bones, ØNB
   see Resection, Head and Facial Bones, ØNT
Cranioplasty
   see Repair, Head and Facial Bones, ØNQ
   see Replacement, Head and Facial Bones, ØNR
   see Supplement, Head and Facial Bones, ØNU
Craniotomy
   see Division, Head and Facial Bones, ØN8
   see Drainage, Central Nervous System and Cranial
      Nerves, ØØ9
   see Drainage, Head and Facial Bones, ØN9
Creation
   Perineum
      Female, ØW4NØ
      Male, ØW4MØ
   Valve
      Aortic, Ø24FØ
      Mitral, Ø24GØ
      Tricuspid, Ø24JØ
Cremaster muscle *use* Perineum Muscle
Cribriform plate
   use Ethmoid Bone, Left
   use Ethmoid Bone, Right
Cricoid cartilage *use* Trachea
Cricoidectomy *see* Excision, Larynx, ØCBS
Cricothyroid artery
   use Thyroid Artery, Left
   use Thyroid Artery, Right
Cricothyroid muscle
   use Neck Muscle, Left
   use Neck Muscle, Right
Crisis Intervention, GZ2ZZZZ
CRRT (Continuous renal replacement therapy),
   5A1D90Z
Crural fascia
   use Subcutaneous Tissue and Fascia, Left Upper Leg
   use Subcutaneous Tissue and Fascia, Right Upper Leg
Crushing, nerve
   Cranial *see* Destruction, Central Nervous System and
      Cranial Nerves, ØØ5
   Peripheral *see* Destruction, Peripheral Nervous System, Ø15
Cryoablation *see* Destruction

Cryotherapy *see* Destruction
Cryptorchidectomy
   see Excision, Male Reproductive System, ØVB
   see Resection, Male Reproductive System, ØVT
Cryptorchiectomy
   see Excision, Male Reproductive System, ØVB
   see Resection, Male Reproductive System, ØVT
Cryptotomy
   see Division, Gastrointestinal System, ØD8
   see Drainage, Gastrointestinal System, ØD9
CT scan *see* Computerized Tomography (CT Scan)
CT sialogram *see* Computerized Tomography (CT Scan),
   Ear, Nose, Mouth and Throat, B92
Cubital lymph node
   use Lymphatic, Left Upper Extremity
   use Lymphatic, Right Upper Extremity
Cubital nerve *use* Ulnar Nerve
Cuboid bone
   use Tarsal, Left
   use Tarsal, Right
Cuboideonavicular joint
   use Tarsal Joint, Left
   use Tarsal Joint, Right
Culdocentesis *see* Drainage, Cul-de-sac, ØU9F
Culdoplasty
   see Repair, Cul-de-sac, ØUQF
   see Supplement, Cul-de-sac, ØUUF
Culdoscopy, ØUJH8ZZ
Culdotomy *see* Drainage, Cul-de-sac, ØU9F
Culmen *use* Cerebellum
Cultured epidermal cell autograft *use* Autologous Tissue Substitute
Cuneiform cartilage *use* Larynx
Cuneonavicular joint
   use Joint, Tarsal, Left
   use Joint, Tarsal, Right
Cuneonavicular ligament
   use Foot Bursa and Ligament, Left
   use Foot Bursa and Ligament, Right
Curettage
   see Excision
   see Extraction
Cutaneous (transverse) cervical nerve *use* Cervical
   Plexus
CVP (central venous pressure) *see* Measurement, Venous, 4A04
Cyclodiathermy *see* Destruction, Eye, Ø85
Cyclophotocoagulation *see* Destruction, Eye, Ø85
CYPHER® Stent *use* Intraluminal Device, Drug-eluting in
   Heart and Great Vessels
Cystectomy
   see Excision, Bladder, ØTBB
   see Resection, Bladder, ØTTB
Cystocele repair *see* Repair, Subcutaneous Tissue and
   Fascia, Pelvic Region, ØJQC
Cystography
   see Fluoroscopy, Urinary System, BT1
   see Plain Radiography, Urinary System, BTØ
Cystolithotomy *see* Extirpation, Bladder, ØTCB
Cystopexy
   see Repair, Bladder, ØTQB
   see Reposition, Bladder, ØTSB
Cystoplasty
   see Repair, Bladder, ØTQB
   see Replacement, Bladder, ØTRB
   see Supplement, Bladder, ØTUB
Cystorrhaphy *see* Repair, Bladder, ØTQB
Cystoscopy, ØTJB8ZZ
Cystostomy *see* Bypass, Bladder, ØT1B
Cystostomy tube *use* Drainage Device
Cystotomy *see* Drainage, Bladder, ØT9B
Cystourethrography
   see Fluoroscopy, Urinary System, BT1
   see Plain Radiography, Urinary System, BTØ
Cystourethroplasty
   see Repair, Urinary System, ØTQ
   see Replacement, Urinary System, ØTR
   see Supplement, Urinary System, ØTU
Cytarabine and Daunorubicin Liposome Antineoplastic, XWØ

D

DBS lead *use* Neurostimulator Lead in Central Nervous
   System and Cranial Nerves

DeBakey Left Ventricular Assist Device *use* Implantable
   Heart Assist System in Heart and Great Vessels
Debridement
   Excisional *see* Excision
   Non-excisional *see* Extraction
Decompression, Circulatory, 6A15
Decortication, lung
   see Extirpation, Respiratory System, ØBC
   see Release, Respiratory System, ØBN
Deep brain neurostimulator lead *use* Neurostimulator
   Lead in Central Nervous System and Cranial Nerves
Deep cervical fascia
   use Subcutaneous Tissue and Fascia, Left Neck
   use Subcutaneous Tissue and Fascia, Right Neck
Deep cervical vein
   use Vertebral Vein, Left
   use Vertebral Vein, Right
Deep circumflex iliac artery
   use External Iliac Artery, Left
   use External Iliac Artery, Right
Deep facial vein
   use Face Vein, Left
   use Face Vein, Right
Deep femoral artery
   use Femoral Artery, Left
   use Femoral Artery, Right
Deep femoral (profunda femoris) vein
   use Femoral Vein, Left
   use Femoral Vein, Right
Deep Inferior Epigastric Artery Perforator Flap
   Replacement
      Bilateral, ØHRVØ77
      Left, ØHRUØ77
      Right, ØHRTØ77
   Transfer
      Left, ØKXG
      Right, ØKXF
Deep palmar arch
   use Hand Artery, Left
   use Hand Artery, Right
Deep transverse perineal muscle *use* Perineum Muscle
Deferential artery
   use Internal Iliac Artery, Left
   use Internal Iliac Artery, Right
Defibrillator Generator
   Abdomen, ØJH8
   Chest, ØJH6
Defibrotide Sodium Anticoagulant, XWØ
Defitelio *use* Defibrotide Sodium Anticoagulant
Delivery
   Cesarean *see* Extraction, Products of Conception,
      10DØ
   Forceps *see* Extraction, Products of Conception, 10DØ
   Manually assisted, 10E0XZZ
   Products of Conception, 10E0XZZ
   Vacuum assisted *see* Extraction, Products of Conception, 10DØ
Delta frame external fixator
   use External Fixation Device, Hybrid in, ØPH
   use External Fixation Device, Hybrid in, ØPS
   use External Fixation Device, Hybrid in, ØQH
   use External Fixation Device, Hybrid in, ØQS
Delta III Reverse shoulder prosthesis *use* Synthetic
   Substitute, Reverse Ball and Socket in, ØRR
Deltoid fascia
   use Subcutaneous Tissue and Fascia, Left Upper Arm
   use Subcutaneous Tissue and Fascia, Right Upper Arm
Deltoid ligament
   use Ankle Bursa and Ligament, Left
   use Ankle Bursa and Ligament, Right
Deltoid muscle
   use Shoulder Muscle, Left
   use Shoulder Muscle, Right
Deltopectoral (infraclavicular) lymph node
   use Lymphatic, Left Upper Extremity
   use Lymphatic, Right Upper Extremity
Denervation
   Cranial nerve *see* Destruction, Central Nervous System
      and Cranial Nerves, ØØ5
   Peripheral nerve *see* Destruction, Peripheral Nervous
      System, Ø15
Dens *use* Cervical Vertebra
Densitometry
   Plain Radiography
      Femur
         Left, BQ04ZZ1
         Right, BQ03ZZ1

 Subterms under main terms may continue to next column or page

Index

Densitometry — Destruction

Densitometry — *continued*
  Plain Radiography — *continued*
    Hip
      Left, BQ01ZZ1
      Right, BQ00ZZ1
    Spine
      Cervical, BR00ZZ1
      Lumbar, BR09ZZ1
      Thoracic, BR07ZZ1
      Whole, BR0GZZ1
  Ultrasonography
    Elbow
      Left, BP4HZZ1
      Right, BP4GZZ1
    Hand
      Left, BP4PZZ1
      Right, BP4NZZ1
    Shoulder
      Left, BP49ZZ1
      Right, BP48ZZ1
    Wrist
      Left, BP4MZZ1
      Right, BP4LZZ1
Denticulate (dentate) ligament *use* Spinal Meninges
Depressor anguli oris muscle *use* Facial Muscle
Depressor labii inferioris muscle *use* Facial Muscle
Depressor septi nasi muscle *use* Facial Muscle
Depressor supercilii muscle *use* Facial Muscle
Dermabrasion *see* Extraction, Skin and Breast, 0HD
Dermis *use* Skin
Descending genicular artery
    use Femoral Artery, Left
    use Femoral Artery, Right
Destruction
  Acetabulum
    Left, 0Q55
    Right, 0Q54
  Adenoids, 0C5Q
  Ampulla of Vater, 0F5C
  Anal Sphincter, 0D5R
  Anterior Chamber
    Left, 08533ZZ
    Right, 08523ZZ
  Anus, 0D5Q
  Aorta
    Abdominal
    Thoracic
      Ascending/Arch, 025X
      Descending, 025W
  Aortic Body, 0G5D
  Appendix, 0D5J
  Artery
    Anterior Tibial
      Left, 045Q
      Right, 045P
    Axillary
      Left, 0356
      Right, 0355
    Brachial
      Left, 0358
      Right, 0357
    Celiac, 0451
    Colic
      Left, 0457
      Middle, 0458
      Right, 0456
    Common Carotid
      Left, 035J
      Right, 035H
    Common Iliac
      Left, 045D
      Right, 045C
    External Carotid
      Left, 035N
      Right, 035M
    External Iliac
      Left, 045J
      Right, 045H
    Face, 035R
    Femoral
      Left, 045L
      Right, 045K
    Foot
      Left, 045W
      Right, 045V
    Gastric, 0452
    Hand
      Left, 035F

Destruction — *continued*
  Artery — *continued*
    Hand — *continued*
      Right, 035D
    Hepatic, 0453
    Inferior Mesenteric, 045B
    Innominate, 0352
    Internal Carotid
      Left, 035L
      Right, 035K
    Internal Iliac
      Left, 045F
      Right, 045E
    Internal Mammary
      Left, 0351
      Right, 0350
    Intracranial, 035G
    Lower, 045Y
    Peroneal
      Left, 045U
      Right, 045T
    Popliteal
      Left, 045N
      Right, 045M
    Posterior Tibial
      Left, 045S
      Right, 045R
    Pulmonary
      Left, 025R
      Right, 025Q
    Pulmonary Trunk, 025P
    Radial
      Left, 035C
      Right, 035B
    Renal
      Left, 045A
      Right, 0459
    Splenic, 0454
    Subclavian
      Left, 0354
      Right, 0353
    Superior Mesenteric, 0455
    Temporal
      Left, 035T
      Right, 035S
    Thyroid
      Left, 035V
      Right, 035U
    Ulnar
      Left, 035A
      Right, 0359
    Upper, 035Y
    Vertebral
      Left, 035Q
      Right, 035P
  Atrium
    Left, 0257
    Right, 0256
  Auditory Ossicle
    Left, 095A
    Right, 0959
  Basal Ganglia, 0058
  Bladder, 0T5B
  Bladder Neck, 0T5C
  Bone
    Ethmoid
      Left, 0N5G
      Right, 0N5F
    Frontal, 0N51
    Hyoid, 0N5X
    Lacrimal
      Left, 0N5J
      Right, 0N5H
    Nasal, 0N5B
    Occipital, 0N57
    Palatine
      Left, 0N5L
      Right, 0N5K
    Parietal
      Left, 0N54
      Right, 0N53
    Pelvic
      Left, 0Q53
      Right, 0Q52
    Sphenoid, 0N5C
    Temporal
      Left, 0N56
      Right, 0N55

Destruction — *continued*
  Bone — *continued*
    Zygomatic
      Left, 0N5N
      Right, 0N5M
  Brain, 0050
  Breast
    Bilateral, 0H5V
    Left, 0H5U
    Right, 0H5T
  Bronchus
    Lingula, 0B59
    Lower Lobe
      Left, 0B5B
      Right, 0B56
    Main
      Left, 0B57
      Right, 0B53
    Middle Lobe, Right, 0B55
    Upper Lobe
      Left, 0B58
      Right, 0B54
  Buccal Mucosa, 0C54
  Bursa and Ligament
    Abdomen
      Left, 0M5J
      Right, 0M5H
    Ankle
      Left, 0M5R
      Right, 0M5Q
    Elbow
      Left, 0M54
      Right, 0M53
    Foot
      Left, 0M5T
      Right, 0M5S
    Hand
      Left, 0M58
      Right, 0M57
    Head and Neck, 0M50
    Hip
      Left, 0M5M
      Right, 0M5L
    Knee
      Left, 0M5P
      Right, 0M5N
    Lower Extremity
      Left, 0M5W
      Right, 0M5V
    Perineum, 0M5K
    Rib(s), 0M5G
    Shoulder
      Left, 0M52
      Right, 0M51
    Spine
      Lower, 0M5D
      Upper, 0M5C
    Sternum, 0M5F
    Upper Extremity
      Left, 0M5B
      Right, 0M59
    Wrist
      Left, 0M56
      Right, 0M55
  Carina, 0B52
  Carotid Bodies, Bilateral, 0G58
  Carotid Body
    Left, 0G56
    Right, 0G57
  Carpal
    Left, 0P5N
    Right, 0P5M
  Cecum, 0D5H
  Cerebellum, 005C
  Cerebral Hemisphere, 0057
  Cerebral Meninges, 0051
  Cerebral Ventricle, 0056
  Cervix, 0U5C
  Chordae Tendineae, 0259
  Choroid
    Left, 085B
    Right, 085A
  Cisterna Chyli, 075L
  Clavicle
    Left, 0P5B
    Right, 0P59
  Clitoris, 0U5J
  Coccygeal Glomus, 0G5B
  Coccyx, 0Q5S

Destruction — *continued*
- Colon
  - Ascending, ØD5K
  - Descending, ØD5M
  - Sigmoid, ØD5N
  - Transverse, ØD5L
- Conduction Mechanism, Ø258
- Conjunctiva
  - Left, Ø85TXZZ
  - Right, Ø85SXZZ
- Cord
  - Bilateral, ØV5H
  - Left, ØV5G
  - Right, ØV5F
- Cornea
  - Left, Ø859XZZ
  - Right, Ø858XZZ
- Cul-de-sac, ØU5F
- Diaphragm, ØB5T
- Disc
  - Cervical Vertebral, ØR53
  - Cervicothoracic Vertebral, ØR55
  - Lumbar Vertebral, ØS52
  - Lumbosacral, ØS54
  - Thoracic Vertebral, ØR59
  - Thoracolumbar Vertebral, ØR5B
- Duct
  - Common Bile, ØF59
  - Cystic, ØF58
  - Hepatic
    - Common, ØF57
    - Left, ØF56
    - Right, ØF55
  - Lacrimal
    - Left, Ø85Y
    - Right, Ø85X
  - Pancreatic, ØF5D
    - Accessory, ØF5F
  - Parotid
    - Left, ØC5C
    - Right, ØC5B
- Duodenum, ØD59
- Dura Mater, ØØ52
- Ear
  - External
    - Left, Ø951
    - Right, Ø950
  - External Auditory Canal
    - Left, Ø954
    - Right, Ø953
  - Inner
    - Left, Ø95E
    - Right, Ø95D
  - Middle
    - Left, Ø956
    - Right, Ø955
- Endometrium, ØU5B
- Epididymis
  - Bilateral, ØV5L
  - Left, ØV5K
  - Right, ØV5J
- Epiglottis, ØC5R
- Esophagogastric Junction, ØD54
- Esophagus, ØD55
  - Lower, ØD53
  - Middle, ØD52
  - Upper, ØD51
- Eustachian Tube
  - Left, Ø95G
  - Right, Ø95F
- Eye
  - Left, Ø851XZZ
  - Right, Ø850XZZ
- Eyelid
  - Lower
    - Left, Ø85R
    - Right, Ø85Q
  - Upper
    - Left, Ø85P
    - Right, Ø85N
- Fallopian Tube
  - Left, ØU56
  - Right, ØU55
- Fallopian Tubes, Bilateral, ØU57
- Femoral Shaft
  - Left, ØQ59
  - Right, ØQ58

Destruction — *continued*
- Femur
  - Lower
    - Left, ØQ5C
    - Right, ØQ5B
  - Upper
    - Left, ØQ57
    - Right, ØQ56
- Fibula
  - Left, ØQ5K
  - Right, ØQ5J
- Finger Nail, ØH5QXZZ
- Gallbladder, ØF54
- Gingiva
  - Lower, ØC56
  - Upper, ØC55
- Gland
  - Adrenal
    - Bilateral, ØG54
    - Left, ØG52
    - Right, ØG53
  - Lacrimal
    - Left, Ø85W
    - Right, Ø85V
  - Minor Salivary, ØC5J
  - Parotid
    - Left, ØC59
    - Right, ØC58
  - Pituitary, ØG50
  - Sublingual
    - Left, ØC5F
    - Right, ØC5D
  - Submaxillary
    - Left, ØC5H
    - Right, ØC5G
  - Vestibular, ØU5L
- Glenoid Cavity
  - Left, ØP58
  - Right, ØP57
- Glomus Jugulare, ØG5C
- Humeral Head
  - Left, ØP5D
  - Right, ØP5C
- Humeral Shaft
  - Left, ØP5G
  - Right, ØP5F
- Hymen, ØU5K
- Hypothalamus, ØØ5A
- Ileocecal Valve, ØD5C
- Ileum, ØD5B
- Intestine
  - Large, ØD5E
    - Left, ØD5G
    - Right, ØD5F
  - Small, ØD58
- Iris
  - Left, Ø85D3ZZ
  - Right, Ø85C3ZZ
- Jejunum, ØD5A
- Joint
  - Acromioclavicular
    - Left, ØR5H
    - Right, ØR5G
  - Ankle
    - Left, ØS5G
    - Right, ØS5F
  - Carpal
    - Left, ØR5R
    - Right, ØR5Q
  - Carpometacarpal
    - Left, ØR5T
    - Right, ØR5S
  - Cervical Vertebral, ØR51
  - Cervicothoracic Vertebral, ØR54
  - Coccygeal, ØS56
  - Elbow
    - Left, ØR5M
    - Right, ØR5L
  - Finger Phalangeal
    - Left, ØR5X
    - Right, ØR5W
  - Hip
    - Left, ØS5B
    - Right, ØS59
  - Knee
    - Left, ØS5D
    - Right, ØS5C
  - Lumbar Vertebral, ØS50
  - Lumbosacral, ØS53

Destruction — *continued*
- Joint — *continued*
  - Metacarpophalangeal
    - Left, ØR5V
    - Right, ØR5U
  - Metatarsal-Phalangeal
    - Left, ØS5N
    - Right, ØS5M
  - Occipital-cervical, ØR50
  - Sacrococcygeal, ØS55
  - Sacroiliac
    - Left, ØS58
    - Right, ØS57
  - Shoulder
    - Left, ØR5K
    - Right, ØR5J
  - Sternoclavicular
    - Left, ØR5F
    - Right, ØR5E
  - Tarsal
    - Left, ØS5J
    - Right, ØS5H
  - Tarsometatarsal
    - Left, ØS5L
    - Right, ØS5K
  - Temporomandibular
    - Left, ØR5D
    - Right, ØR5C
  - Thoracic Vertebral, ØR56
  - Thoracolumbar Vertebral, ØR5A
  - Toe Phalangeal
    - Left, ØS5Q
    - Right, ØS5P
  - Wrist
    - Left, ØR5P
    - Right, ØR5N
- Kidney
  - Left, ØT51
  - Right, ØT50
- Kidney Pelvis
  - Left, ØT54
  - Right, ØT53
- Larynx, ØC5S
- Lens
  - Left, Ø85K3ZZ
  - Right, Ø85J3ZZ
- Lip
  - Lower, ØC51
  - Upper, ØC50
- Liver, ØF50
  - Left Lobe, ØF52
  - Right Lobe, ØF51
- Lung
  - Bilateral, ØB5M
  - Left, ØB5L
  - Lower Lobe
    - Left, ØB5J
    - Right, ØB5F
  - Middle Lobe, Right, ØB5D
  - Right, ØB5K
  - Upper Lobe
    - Left, ØB5G
    - Right, ØB5C
- Lung Lingula, ØB5H
- Lymphatic
  - Aortic, Ø75D
  - Axillary
    - Left, Ø756
    - Right, Ø755
  - Head, Ø750
  - Inguinal
    - Left, Ø75J
    - Right, Ø75H
  - Internal Mammary
    - Left, Ø759
    - Right, Ø758
  - Lower Extremity
    - Left, Ø75G
    - Right, Ø75F
  - Mesenteric, Ø75B
  - Neck
    - Left, Ø752
    - Right, Ø751
  - Pelvis, Ø75C
  - Thoracic Duct, Ø75K
  - Thorax, Ø757
  - Upper Extremity
    - Left, Ø754
    - Right, Ø753

Destruction — *continued*
  Mandible
    Left, ØN5V
    Right, ØN5T
  Maxilla, ØN5R
  Medulla Oblongata, ØØ5D
  Mesentery, ØD5V
  Metacarpal
    Left, ØP5Q
    Right, ØP5P
  Metatarsal
    Left, ØQ5P
    Right, ØQ5N
  Muscle
    Abdomen
      Left, ØK5L
      Right, ØK5K
    Extraocular
      Left, Ø85M
      Right, Ø85L
    Facial, ØK51
    Foot
      Left, ØK5W
      Right, ØK5V
    Hand
      Left, ØK5D
      Right, ØK5C
    Head, ØK5Ø
    Hip
      Left, ØK5P
      Right, ØK5N
    Lower Arm and Wrist
      Left, ØK5B
      Right, ØK59
    Lower Leg
      Left, ØK5T
      Right, ØK5S
    Neck
      Left, ØK53
      Right, ØK52
    Papillary, Ø25D
    Perineum, ØK5M
    Shoulder
      Left, ØK56
      Right, ØK55
    Thorax
      Left, ØK5J
      Right, ØK5H
    Tongue, Palate, Pharynx, ØK54
    Trunk
      Left, ØK5G
      Right, ØK5F
    Upper Arm
      Left, ØK58
      Right, ØK57
    Upper Leg
      Left, ØK5R
      Right, ØK5Q
  Nasal Mucosa and Soft Tissue, Ø95K
  Nasopharynx, Ø95N
  Nerve
    Abdominal Sympathetic, Ø15M
    Abducens, ØØ5L
    Accessory, ØØ5R
    Acoustic, ØØ5N
    Brachial Plexus, Ø153
    Cervical, Ø151
    Cervical Plexus, Ø15Ø
    Facial, ØØ5M
    Femoral, Ø15D
    Glossopharyngeal, ØØ5P
    Head and Neck Sympathetic, Ø15K
    Hypoglossal, ØØ5S
    Lumbar, Ø15B
    Lumbar Plexus, Ø159
    Lumbar Sympathetic, Ø15N
    Lumbosacral Plexus, Ø15A
    Median, Ø155
    Oculomotor, ØØ5H
    Olfactory, ØØ5F
    Optic, ØØ5G
    Peroneal, Ø15H
    Phrenic, Ø152
    Pudendal, Ø15C
    Radial, Ø156
    Sacral, Ø15R
    Sacral Plexus, Ø15Q
    Sacral Sympathetic, Ø15P
    Sciatic, Ø15F

Destruction — *continued*
  Nerve — *continued*
    Thoracic, Ø158
    Thoracic Sympathetic, Ø15L
    Tibial, Ø15G
    Trigeminal, ØØ5K
    Trochlear, ØØ5J
    Ulnar, Ø154
    Vagus, ØØ5Q
  Nipple
    Left, ØH5X
    Right, ØH5W
  Omentum, ØD5U
  Orbit
    Left, ØN5Q
    Right, ØN5P
  Ovary
    Bilateral, ØU52
    Left, ØU51
    Right, ØU5Ø
  Palate
    Hard, ØC52
    Soft, ØC53
  Pancreas, ØF5G
  Para-aortic Body, ØG59
  Paraganglion Extremity, ØG5F
  Parathyroid Gland, ØG5R
    Inferior
      Left, ØG5P
      Right, ØG5N
    Multiple, ØG5Q
    Superior
      Left, ØG5M
      Right, ØG5L
  Patella
    Left, ØQ5F
    Right, ØQ5D
  Penis, ØV5S
  Pericardium, Ø25N
  Peritoneum, ØD5W
  Phalanx
    Finger
      Left, ØP5V
      Right, ØP5T
    Thumb
      Left, ØP5S
      Right, ØP5R
    Toe
      Left, ØQ5R
      Right, ØQ5Q
  Pharynx, ØC5M
  Pineal Body, ØG51
  Pleura
    Left, ØB5P
    Right, ØB5N
  Pons, ØØ5B
  Prepuce, ØV5T
  Prostate, ØV5Ø
    Robotic Waterjet Ablation, XV5Ø8A4
  Radius
    Left, ØP5J
    Right, ØP5H
  Rectum, ØD5P
  Retina
    Left, Ø85F3ZZ
    Right, Ø85E3ZZ
  Retinal Vessel
    Left, Ø85H3ZZ
    Right, Ø85G3ZZ
  Ribs
    1 to 2, ØP51
    3 or More, ØP52
  Sacrum, ØQ51
  Scapula
    Left, ØP56
    Right, ØP55
  Sclera
    Left, Ø857XZZ
    Right, Ø856XZZ
  Scrotum, ØV55
  Septum
    Atrial, Ø255
    Nasal, Ø95M
    Ventricular, Ø25M
  Sinus
    Accessory, Ø95P
    Ethmoid
      Left, Ø95V
      Right, Ø95U

Destruction — *continued*
  Sinus — *continued*
    Frontal
      Left, Ø95T
      Right, Ø95S
    Mastoid
      Left, Ø95C
      Right, Ø95B
    Maxillary
      Left, Ø95R
      Right, Ø95Q
    Sphenoid
      Left, Ø95X
      Right, Ø95W
  Skin
    Abdomen, ØH57XZ
    Back, ØH56XZ
    Buttock, ØH58XZ
    Chest, ØH55XZ
    Ear
      Left, ØH53XZ
      Right, ØH52XZ
    Face, ØH51XZ
    Foot
      Left, ØH5NXZ
      Right, ØH5MXZ
    Hand
      Left, ØH5GXZ
      Right, ØH5FXZ
    Inguinal, ØH5AXZ
    Lower Arm
      Left, ØH5EXZ
      Right, ØH5DXZ
    Lower Leg
      Left, ØH5LXZ
      Right, ØH5KXZ
    Neck, ØH54XZ
    Perineum, ØH59XZ
    Scalp, ØH5ØXZ
    Upper Arm
      Left, ØH5CXZ
      Right, ØH5BXZ
    Upper Leg
      Left, ØH5JXZ
      Right, ØH5HXZ
  Skull, ØN5Ø
  Spinal Cord
    Cervical, ØØ5W
    Lumbar, ØØ5Y
    Thoracic, ØØ5X
  Spinal Meninges, ØØ5T
  Spleen, Ø75P
  Sternum, ØP5Ø
  Stomach, ØD56
    Pylorus, ØD57
  Subcutaneous Tissue and Fascia
    Abdomen, ØJ58
    Back, ØJ57
    Buttock, ØJ59
    Chest, ØJ56
    Face, ØJ51
    Foot
      Left, ØJ5R
      Right, ØJ5Q
    Hand
      Left, ØJ5K
      Right, ØJ5J
    Lower Arm
      Left, ØJ5H
      Right, ØJ5G
    Lower Leg
      Left, ØJ5P
      Right, ØJ5N
    Neck
      Left, ØJ55
      Right, ØJ54
    Pelvic Region, ØJ5C
    Perineum, ØJ5B
    Scalp, ØJ5Ø
    Upper Arm
      Left, ØJ5F
      Right, ØJ5D
    Upper Leg
      Left, ØJ5M
      Right, ØJ5L
  Tarsal
    Left, ØQ5M
    Right, ØQ5L

▽ **Subterms under main terms may continue to next column or page**

Destruction — *continued*
  Tendon
    Abdomen
      Left, ØL5G
      Right, ØI 5F
    Ankle
      Left, ØL5T
      Right, ØL5S
    Foot
      Left, ØL5W
      Right, ØL5V
    Hand
      Left, ØL58
      Right, ØL57
    Head and Neck, ØL50
    Hip
      Left, ØL5K
      Right, ØL5J
    Knee
      Left, ØL5R
      Right, ØL5Q
    Lower Arm and Wrist
      Left, ØL56
      Right, ØL55
    Lower Leg
      Left, ØL5P
      Right, ØL5N
    Perineum, ØL5H
    Shoulder
      Left, ØL52
      Right, ØL51
    Thorax
      Left, ØL5D
      Right, ØL5C
    Trunk
      Left, ØL5B
      Right, ØL59
    Upper Arm
      Left, ØL54
      Right, ØL53
    Upper Leg
      Left, ØL5M
      Right, ØL5L
  Testis
    Bilateral, ØV5C
    Left, ØV5B
    Right, ØV59
  Thalamus, ØØ59
  Thymus, Ø75M
  Thyroid Gland, ØG5K
    Left Lobe, ØG5G
    Right Lobe, ØG5H
  Tibia
    Left, ØQ5H
    Right, ØQ5G
  Toe Nail, ØH5RXZZ
  Tongue, ØC57
  Tonsils, ØC5P
  Tooth
    Lower, ØC5X
    Upper, ØC5W
  Trachea, ØB51
  Tunica Vaginalis
    Left, ØV57
    Right, ØV56
  Turbinate, Nasal, Ø95L
  Tympanic Membrane
    Left, Ø958
    Right, Ø957
  Ulna
    Left, ØP5L
    Right, ØP5K
  Ureter
    Left, ØT57
    Right, ØT56
  Urethra, ØT5D
  Uterine Supporting Structure, ØU54
  Uterus, ØU59
  Uvula, ØC5N
  Vagina, ØU5G
  Valve
    Aortic, Ø25F
    Mitral, Ø25G
    Pulmonary, Ø25H
    Tricuspid, Ø25J
  Vas Deferens
    Bilateral, ØV5Q
    Left, ØV5P
    Right, ØV5N

Destruction — *continued*
  Vein
    Axillary
      Left, Ø558
      Right, Ø557
    Azygos, Ø55Ø
    Basilic
      Left, Ø55C
      Right, Ø55B
    Brachial
      Left, Ø55A
      Right, Ø559
    Cephalic
      Left, Ø55F
      Right, Ø55D
    Colic, Ø657
    Common Iliac
      Left, Ø65D
      Right, Ø65C
    Coronary, Ø254
    Esophageal, Ø653
    External Iliac
      Left, Ø65G
      Right, Ø65F
    External Jugular
      Left, Ø55Q
      Right, Ø55P
    Face
      Left, Ø55V
      Right, Ø55T
    Femoral
      Left, Ø65N
      Right, Ø65M
    Foot
      Left, Ø65V
      Right, Ø65T
    Gastric, Ø652
    Hand
      Left, Ø55H
      Right, Ø55G
    Hemiazygos, Ø551
    Hepatic, Ø654
    Hypogastric
      Left, Ø65J
      Right, Ø65H
    Inferior Mesenteric, Ø656
    Innominate
      Left, Ø554
      Right, Ø553
    Internal Jugular
      Left, Ø55N
      Right, Ø55M
    Intracranial, Ø55L
    Lower, Ø65Y
    Portal, Ø658
    Pulmonary
      Left, Ø25T
      Right, Ø25S
    Renal
      Left, Ø65B
      Right, Ø659
    Saphenous
      Left, Ø65Q
      Right, Ø65P
    Splenic, Ø651
    Subclavian
      Left, Ø556
      Right, Ø555
    Superior Mesenteric, Ø655
    Upper, Ø55Y
    Vertebral
      Left, Ø55S
      Right, Ø55R
  Vena Cava
    Inferior, Ø65Ø
    Superior, Ø25V
  Ventricle
    Left, Ø25L
    Right, Ø25K
  Vertebra
    Cervical, ØP53
    Lumbar, ØQ53
    Thoracic, ØP54
  Vesicle
    Bilateral, ØV53
    Left, ØV52
    Right, ØV51
  Vitreous
    Left, Ø8553ZZ

Destruction — *continued*
  Vitreous — *continued*
    Right, Ø8543ZZ
  Vocal Cord
    Left, ØC5V
    Right, ØC5T
  Vulva, ØU5M
Detachment
  Arm
    Lower
      Left, ØX6FØZ
      Right, ØX6DØZ
    Upper
      Left, ØX69ØZ
      Right, ØX68ØZ
  Elbow Region
    Left, ØX6CØZZ
    Right, ØX6BØZZ
  Femoral Region
    Left, ØY68ØZZ
    Right, ØY67ØZZ
  Finger
    Index
      Left, ØX6PØZ
      Right, ØX6NØZ
    Little
      Left, ØX6WØZ
      Right, ØX6VØZ
    Middle
      Left, ØX6RØZ
      Right, ØX6QØZ
    Ring
      Left, ØX6TØZ
      Right, ØX6SØZ
  Foot
    Left, ØY6NØZ
    Right, ØY6MØZ
  Forequarter
    Left, ØX61ØZZ
    Right, ØX60ØZZ
  Hand
    Left, ØX6KØZ
    Right, ØX6JØZ
  Hindquarter
    Bilateral, ØY64ØZZ
    Left, ØY63ØZZ
    Right, ØY62ØZZ
  Knee Region
    Left, ØY6GØZZ
    Right, ØY6FØZZ
  Leg
    Lower
      Left, ØY6JØZ
      Right, ØY6HØZ
    Upper
      Left, ØY6DØZ
      Right, ØY6CØZ
  Shoulder Region
    Left, ØX63ØZZ
    Right, ØX62ØZZ
  Thumb
    Left, ØX6MØZ
    Right, ØX6LØZ
  Toe
    1st
      Left, ØY6QØZ
      Right, ØY6PØZ
    2nd
      Left, ØY6SØZ
      Right, ØY6RØZ
    3rd
      Left, ØY6UØZ
      Right, ØY6TØZ
    4th
      Left, ØY6WØZ
      Right, ØY6VØZ
    5th
      Left, ØY6YØZ
      Right, ØY6XØZ
Determination, Mental status, GZ14ZZZ
Detorsion
  see Release
  see Reposition
Detoxification Services, for substance abuse, HZ2ZZZZ
Device Fitting, FØDZ
Diagnostic Audiology *see* Audiology, Diagnostic
Diagnostic imaging *see* Imaging, Diagnostic
Diagnostic radiology *see* Imaging, Diagnostic

Dialysis
Hemodialysis *see* Performance, Urinary, 5A1D
Peritoneal, 3E1M39Z
Diaphragma sellae *use* Dura Mater
Diaphragmatic pacemaker generator *use* Stimulator
Generator in Subcutaneous Tissue and Fascia
Diaphragmatic Pacemaker Lead
Insertion of device in, Diaphragm, ØBHT
Removal of device from, Diaphragm, ØBPT
Revision of device in, Diaphragm, ØBWT
Digital radiography, plain *see* Plain Radiography
Dilation
Ampulla of Vater, ØF7C
Anus, ØD7Q
Aorta
Abdominal
Thoracic
Ascending/Arch, Ø27X
Descending, Ø27W
Artery
Anterior Tibial
Left, Ø47Q
Right, Ø47P
Axillary
Left, Ø376
Right, Ø375
Brachial
Left, Ø378
Right, Ø377
Celiac, Ø471
Colic
Left, Ø477
Middle, Ø478
Right, Ø476
Common Carotid
Left, Ø37J
Right, Ø37H
Common Iliac
Left, Ø47D
Right, Ø47C
Coronary
Four or More Arteries, Ø273
One Artery, Ø270
Three Arteries, Ø272
Two Arteries, Ø271
External Carotid
Left, Ø37N
Right, Ø37M
External Iliac
Left, Ø47J
Right, Ø47H
Face, Ø37R
Femoral
Left, Ø47L
Right, Ø47K
Foot
Left, Ø47W
Right, Ø47V
Gastric, Ø472
Hand
Left, Ø37F
Right, Ø37D
Hepatic, Ø473
Inferior Mesenteric, Ø47B
Innominate, Ø372
Internal Carotid
Left, Ø37L
Right, Ø37K
Internal Iliac
Left, Ø47F
Right, Ø47E
Internal Mammary
Left, Ø371
Right, Ø370
Intracranial, Ø37G
Lower, Ø47Y
Peroneal
Left, Ø47U
Right, Ø47T
Popliteal
Left, Ø47N
Right, Ø47M
Posterior Tibial
Left, Ø47S
Right, Ø47R
Pulmonary
Left, Ø27R
Right, Ø27Q
Pulmonary Trunk, Ø27P

Dilation — *continued*
Artery — *continued*
Radial
Left, Ø37C
Right, Ø37B
Renal
Left, Ø47A
Right, Ø479
Splenic, Ø474
Subclavian
Left, Ø374
Right, Ø373
Superior Mesenteric, Ø475
Temporal
Left, Ø37T
Right, Ø37S
Thyroid
Left, Ø37V
Right, Ø37U
Ulnar
Left, Ø37A
Right, Ø379
Upper, Ø37Y
Vertebral
Left, Ø37Q
Right, Ø37P
Bladder, ØT7B
Bladder Neck, ØT7C
Bronchus
Lingula, ØB79
Lower Lobe
Left, ØB7B
Right, ØB76
Main
Left, ØB77
Right, ØB73
Middle Lobe, Right, ØB75
Upper Lobe
Left, ØB78
Right, ØB74
Carina, ØB72
Cecum, ØD7H
Cerebral Ventricle, ØØ76
Cervix, ØU7C
Colon
Ascending, ØD7K
Descending, ØD7M
Sigmoid, ØD7N
Transverse, ØD7L
Duct
Common Bile, ØF79
Cystic, ØF78
Hepatic
Common, ØF77
Left, ØF76
Right, ØF75
Lacrimal
Left, Ø87Y
Right, Ø87X
Pancreatic, ØF7D
Accessory, ØF7F
Parotid
Left, ØC7C
Right, ØC7B
Duodenum, ØD79
Esophagogastric Junction, ØD74
Esophagus, ØD75
Lower, ØD73
Middle, ØD72
Upper, ØD71
Eustachian Tube
Left, Ø97G
Right, Ø97F
Fallopian Tube
Left, ØU76
Right, ØU75
Fallopian Tubes, Bilateral, ØU77
Hymen, ØU7K
Ileocecal Valve, ØD7C
Ileum, ØD7B
Intestine
Large, ØD7E
Left, ØD7G
Right, ØD7F
Small, ØD78
Jejunum, ØD7A
Kidney Pelvis
Left, ØT74
Right, ØT73

Dilation — *continued*
Larynx, ØC7S
Pharynx, ØC7M
Rectum, ØD7P
Stomach, ØD76
Pylorus, ØD77
Trachea, ØB71
Ureter
Left, ØT77
Right, ØT76
Ureters, Bilateral, ØT78
Urethra, ØT7D
Uterus, ØU79
Vagina, ØU7G
Valve
Aortic, Ø27F
Mitral, Ø27G
Pulmonary, Ø27H
Tricuspid, Ø27J
Vas Deferens
Bilateral, ØV7Q
Left, ØV7P
Right, ØV7N
Vein
Axillary
Left, Ø578
Right, Ø577
Azygos, Ø570
Basilic
Left, Ø57C
Right, Ø57B
Brachial
Left, Ø57A
Right, Ø579
Cephalic
Left, Ø57F
Right, Ø57D
Colic, Ø677
Common Iliac
Left, Ø67D
Right, Ø67C
Esophageal, Ø673
External Iliac
Left, Ø67G
Right, Ø67F
External Jugular
Left, Ø57Q
Right, Ø57P
Face
Left, Ø57V
Right, Ø57T
Femoral
Left, Ø67N
Right, Ø67M
Foot
Left, Ø67V
Right, Ø67T
Gastric, Ø672
Hand
Left, Ø57H
Right, Ø57G
Hemiazygos, Ø571
Hepatic, Ø674
Hypogastric
Left, Ø67J
Right, Ø67H
Inferior Mesenteric, Ø676
Innominate
Left, Ø574
Right, Ø573
Internal Jugular
Left, Ø57N
Right, Ø57M
Intracranial, Ø57L
Lower, Ø67Y
Portal, Ø678
Pulmonary
Left, Ø27T
Right, Ø27S
Renal
Left, Ø67B
Right, Ø679
Saphenous
Left, Ø67Q
Right, Ø67P
Splenic, Ø671
Subclavian
Left, Ø576
Right, Ø575

Dilation — *continued*
  Vein — *continued*
    Superior Mesenteric, Ø675
    Upper, Ø57Y
    Vertebral
      Left, Ø57S
      Right, Ø57R
  Vena Cava
    Inferior, Ø67Ø
    Superior, Ø27V
  Ventricle
    Left, Ø27L
    Right, Ø27K

Direct Lateral Interbody Fusion (DLIF) device *use* Interbody Fusion Device in Lower Joints

Disarticulation *see* Detachment

Discectomy, diskectomy
  see Excision, Lower Joints, ØSB
  see Excision, Upper Joints, ØRB
  see Resection, Lower Joints, ØST
  see Resection, Upper Joints, ØRT

Discography
  see Fluoroscopy, Axial Skeleton, Except Skull and Facial Bones, BR1
  see Plain Radiography, Axial Skeleton, Except Skull and Facial Bones, BRØ

Distal humerus
  use Humeral Shaft, Left
  use Humeral Shaft, Right

Distal humerus, involving joint
  use Elbow Joint, Left
  use Elbow Joint, Right

Distal radioulnar joint
  use Wrist Joint, Left
  use Wrist Joint, Right

Diversion *see* Bypass

Diverticulectomy *see* Excision, Gastrointestinal System, ØDB

Division
  Acetabulum
    Left, ØQ85
    Right, ØQ84
  Anal Sphincter, ØD8R
  Basal Ganglia, ØØ88
  Bladder Neck, ØT8C
  Bone
    Ethmoid
      Left, ØN8G
      Right, ØN8F
    Frontal, ØN81
    Hyoid, ØN8X
    Lacrimal
      Left, ØN8J
      Right, ØN8H
    Nasal, ØN8B
    Occipital, ØN87
    Palatine
      Left, ØN8L
      Right, ØN8K
    Parietal
      Left, ØN84
      Right, ØN83
    Pelvic
      Left, ØQ83
      Right, ØQ82
    Sphenoid, ØN8C
    Temporal
      Left, ØN86
      Right, ØN85
    Zygomatic
      Left, ØN8N
      Right, ØN8M
  Brain, ØØ8Ø
  Bursa and Ligament
    Abdomen
      Left, ØM8J
      Right, ØM8H
    Ankle
      Left, ØM8R
      Right, ØM8Q
    Elbow
      Left, ØM84
      Right, ØM83
    Foot
      Left, ØM8T
      Right, ØM8S
    Hand
      Left, ØM88

Division — *continued*
  Bursa and Ligament — *continued*
    Hand — *continued*
      Right, ØM87
    Head and Neck, ØM8Ø
    Hip
      Left, ØM8M
      Right, ØM8L
    Knee
      Left, ØM8P
      Right, ØM8N
    Lower Extremity
      Left, ØM8W
      Right, ØM8V
    Perineum, ØM8K
    Rib(s), ØM8G
    Shoulder
      Left, ØM82
      Right, ØM81
    Spine
      Lower, ØM8D
      Upper, ØM8C
    Sternum, ØM8F
    Upper Extremity
      Left, ØM8B
      Right, ØM89
    Wrist
      Left, ØM86
      Right, ØM85
  Carpal
    Left, ØP8N
    Right, ØP8M
  Cerebral Hemisphere, ØØ87
  Chordae Tendineae, Ø289
  Clavicle
    Left, ØP8B
    Right, ØP89
  Coccyx, ØQ8S
  Conduction Mechanism, Ø288
  Esophagogastric Junction, ØD84
  Femoral Shaft
    Left, ØQ89
    Right, ØQ88
  Femur
    Lower
      Left, ØQ8C
      Right, ØQ8B
    Upper
      Left, ØQ87
      Right, ØQ86
  Fibula
    Left, ØQ8K
    Right, ØQ8J
  Gland, Pituitary, ØG8Ø
  Glenoid Cavity
    Left, ØP88
    Right, ØP87
  Humeral Head
    Left, ØP8D
    Right, ØP8C
  Humeral Shaft
    Left, ØP8G
    Right, ØP8F
  Hymen, ØU8K
  Kidneys, Bilateral, ØT82
  Mandible
    Left, ØN8V
    Right, ØN8T
  Maxilla, ØN8R
  Metacarpal
    Left, ØP8Q
    Right, ØP8P
  Metatarsal
    Left, ØQ8P
    Right, ØQ8N
  Muscle
    Abdomen
      Left, ØK8L
      Right, ØK8K
    Facial, ØK81
    Foot
      Left, ØK8W
      Right, ØK8V
    Hand
      Left, ØK8D
      Right, ØK8C
    Head, ØK8Ø
    Hip
      Left, ØK8P

Division — *continued*
  Muscle — *continued*
    Hip — *continued*
      Right, ØK8N
    Lower Arm and Wrist
      Left, ØK8B
      Right, ØK89
    Lower Leg
      Left, ØK8T
      Right, ØK8S
    Neck
      Left, ØK83
      Right, ØK82
    Papillary, Ø28D
    Perineum, ØK8M
    Shoulder
      Left, ØK86
      Right, ØK85
    Thorax
      Left, ØK8J
      Right, ØK8H
    Tongue, Palate, Pharynx, ØK84
    Trunk
      Left, ØK8G
      Right, ØK8F
    Upper Arm
      Left, ØK88
      Right, ØK87
    Upper Leg
      Left, ØK8R
      Right, ØK8Q
  Nerve
    Abdominal Sympathetic, Ø18M
    Abducens, ØØ8L
    Accessory, ØØ8R
    Acoustic, ØØ8N
    Brachial Plexus, Ø183
    Cervical, Ø181
    Cervical Plexus, Ø18Ø
    Facial, ØØ8M
    Femoral, Ø18D
    Glossopharyngeal, ØØ8P
    Head and Neck Sympathetic, Ø18K
    Hypoglossal, ØØ8S
    Lumbar, Ø18B
    Lumbar Plexus, Ø189
    Lumbar Sympathetic, Ø18N
    Lumbosacral Plexus, Ø18A
    Median, Ø185
    Oculomotor, ØØ8H
    Olfactory, ØØ8F
    Optic, ØØ8G
    Peroneal, Ø18H
    Phrenic, Ø182
    Pudendal, Ø18C
    Radial, Ø186
    Sacral, Ø18R
    Sacral Plexus, Ø18Q
    Sacral Sympathetic, Ø18P
    Sciatic, Ø18F
    Thoracic, Ø188
    Thoracic Sympathetic, Ø18L
    Tibial, Ø18G
    Trigeminal, ØØ8K
    Trochlear, ØØ8J
    Ulnar, Ø184
    Vagus, ØØ8Q
  Orbit
    Left, ØN8Q
    Right, ØN8P
  Ovary
    Bilateral, ØU82
    Left, ØU81
    Right, ØU8Ø
  Pancreas, ØF8G
  Patella
    Left, ØQ8F
    Right, ØQ8D
  Perineum, Female, ØW8NXZZ
  Phalanx
    Finger
      Left, ØP8V
      Right, ØP8T
    Thumb
      Left, ØP8S
      Right, ØP8R
    Toe
      Left, ØQ8R
      Right, ØQ8Q

Division — continued
Radius
  Left, ØP8J
  Right, ØP8H
Ribs
  1 to 2, ØP81
  3 or More, ØP82
Sacrum, ØQ81
Scapula
  Left, ØP86
  Right, ØP85
Skin
  Abdomen, ØH87XZZ
  Back, ØH86XZZ
  Buttock, ØH88XZZ
  Chest, ØH85XZZ
  Ear
    Left, ØH83XZZ
    Right, ØH82XZZ
  Face, ØH81XZZ
  Foot
    Left, ØH8NXZZ
    Right, ØH8MXZZ
  Hand
    Left, ØH8GXZZ
    Right, ØH8FXZZ
  Inguinal, ØH8AXZZ
  Lower Arm
    Left, ØH8EXZZ
    Right, ØH8DXZZ
  Lower Leg
    Left, ØH8LXZZ
    Right, ØH8KXZZ
  Neck, ØH84XZZ
  Perineum, ØH89XZZ
  Scalp, ØH80XZZ
  Upper Arm
    Left, ØH8CXZZ
    Right, ØH8BXZZ
  Upper Leg
    Left, ØH8JXZZ
    Right, ØH8HXZZ
Skull, ØN80
Spinal Cord
  Cervical, 008W
  Lumbar, 008Y
  Thoracic, 008X
Sternum, ØP80
Stomach, Pylorus, ØD87
Subcutaneous Tissue and Fascia
  Abdomen, ØJ88
  Back, ØJ87
  Buttock, ØJ89
  Chest, ØJ86
  Face, ØJ81
  Foot
    Left, ØJ8R
    Right, ØJ8Q
  Hand
    Left, ØJ8K
    Right, ØJ8J
  Head and Neck, ØJ8S
  Lower Arm
    Left, ØJ8H
    Right, ØJ8G
  Lower Extremity, ØJ8W
  Lower Leg
    Left, ØJ8P
    Right, ØJ8N
  Neck
    Left, ØJ85
    Right, ØJ84
  Pelvic Region, ØJ8C
  Perineum, ØJ8B
  Scalp, ØJ80
  Trunk, ØJ8T
  Upper Arm
    Left, ØJ8F
    Right, ØJ8D
  Upper Extremity, ØJ8V
  Upper Leg
    Left, ØJ8M
    Right, ØJ8L
Tarsal
  Left, ØQ8M
  Right, ØQ8L
Tendon
  Abdomen
    Left, ØL8G

Division — continued
Tendon — continued
  Abdomen — continued
    Right, ØL8F
  Ankle
    Left, ØL8T
    Right, ØL8S
  Foot
    Left, ØL8W
    Right, ØL8V
  Hand
    Left, ØL88
    Right, ØL87
  Head and Neck, ØL80
  Hip
    Left, ØL8K
    Right, ØL8J
  Knee
    Left, ØL8R
    Right, ØL8Q
  Lower Arm and Wrist
    Left, ØL86
    Right, ØL85
  Lower Leg
    Left, ØL8P
    Right, ØL8N
  Perineum, ØL8H
  Shoulder
    Left, ØL82
    Right, ØL81
  Thorax
    Left, ØL8D
    Right, ØL8C
  Trunk
    Left, ØL8B
    Right, ØL89
  Upper Arm
    Left, ØL84
    Right, ØL83
  Upper Leg
    Left, ØL8M
    Right, ØL8L
Thyroid Gland Isthmus, ØG8J
Tibia
  Left, ØQ8H
  Right, ØQ8G
Turbinate, Nasal, Ø98L
Ulna
  Left, ØP8L
  Right, ØP8K
Uterine Supporting Structure, ØU84
Vertebra
  Cervical, ØP83
  Lumbar, ØQ80
  Thoracic, ØP84
Doppler study see Ultrasonography
Dorsal digital nerve use Radial Nerve
Dorsal metacarpal vein
  use Hand Vein, Left
  use Hand Vein, Right
Dorsal metatarsal artery
  use Foot Artery, Left
  use Foot Artery, Right
Dorsal metatarsal vein
  use Foot Vein, Left
  use Foot Vein, Right
Dorsal scapular artery
  use Subclavian Artery, Left
  use Subclavian Artery, Right
Dorsal scapular nerve use Brachial Plexus
Dorsal venous arch
  use Foot Vein, Left
  use Foot Vein, Right
Dorsalis pedis artery
  use Anterior Tibial Artery, Left
  use Anterior Tibial Artery, Right
DownStream® System, 5A0512C, 5A0522C
Drainage
  Abdominal Wall, ØW9F
  Acetabulum
    Left, ØQ95
    Right, ØQ94
  Adenoids, ØC9Q
  Ampulla of Vater, ØF9C
  Anal Sphincter, ØD9R
  Ankle Region
    Left, ØY9L
    Right, ØY9K

Drainage — continued
Anterior Chamber
  Left, Ø893
  Right, Ø892
Anus, ØD9Q
Aorta, Abdominal, Ø490
Aortic Body, ØG9D
Appendix, ØD9J
Arm
  Lower
    Left, ØX9F
    Right, ØX9D
  Upper
    Left, ØX99
    Right, ØX98
Artery
  Anterior Tibial
    Left, Ø49Q
    Right, Ø49P
  Axillary
    Left, Ø396
    Right, Ø395
  Brachial
    Left, Ø398
    Right, Ø397
  Celiac, Ø491
  Colic
    Left, Ø497
    Middle, Ø498
    Right, Ø496
  Common Carotid
    Left, Ø39J
    Right, Ø39H
  Common Iliac
    Left, Ø49D
    Right, Ø49C
  External Carotid
    Left, Ø39N
    Right, Ø39M
  External Iliac
    Left, Ø49J
    Right, Ø49H
  Face, Ø39R
  Femoral
    Left, Ø49L
    Right, Ø49K
  Foot
    Left, Ø49W
    Right, Ø49V
  Gastric, Ø492
  Hand
    Left, Ø39F
    Right, Ø39D
  Hepatic, Ø493
  Inferior Mesenteric, Ø49B
  Innominate, Ø392
  Internal Carotid
    Left, Ø39L
    Right, Ø39K
  Internal Iliac
    Left, Ø49F
    Right, Ø49E
  Internal Mammary
    Left, Ø391
    Right, Ø390
  Intracranial, Ø39G
  Lower, Ø49Y
  Peroneal
    Left, Ø49U
    Right, Ø49T
  Popliteal
    Left, Ø49N
    Right, Ø49M
  Posterior Tibial
    Left, Ø49S
    Right, Ø49R
  Radial
    Left, Ø39C
    Right, Ø39B
  Renal
    Left, Ø49A
    Right, Ø499
  Splenic, Ø494
  Subclavian
    Left, Ø394
    Right, Ø393
  Superior Mesenteric, Ø495
  Temporal
    Left, Ø39T

Subterms under main terms may continue to next column or page

Drainage — *continued*
  Artery — *continued*
    Temporal — *continued*
      Right, Ø39S
    Thyroid
      Left, Ø39V
      Right, Ø39U
    Ulnar
      Left, Ø39A
      Right, Ø399
    Upper, Ø39Y
    Vertebral
      Left, Ø39Q
      Right, Ø39P
  Auditory Ossicle
    Left, Ø99A
    Right, Ø999
  Axilla
    Left, ØX95
    Right, ØX94
  Back
    Lower, ØW9L
    Upper, ØW9K
  Basal Ganglia, ØØ98
  Bladder, ØT9B
  Bladder Neck, ØT9C
  Bone
    Ethmoid
      Left, ØN9G
      Right, ØN9F
    Frontal, ØN91
    Hyoid, ØN9X
    Lacrimal
      Left, ØN9J
      Right, ØN9H
    Nasal, ØN9B
    Occipital, ØN97
    Palatine
      Left, ØN9L
      Right, ØN9K
    Parietal
      Left, ØN94
      Right, ØN93
    Pelvic
      Left, ØQ93
      Right, ØQ92
    Sphenoid, ØN9C
    Temporal
      Left, ØN96
      Right, ØN95
    Zygomatic
      Left, ØN9N
      Right, ØN9M
  Bone Marrow, Ø79T
  Brain, ØØ9Ø
  Breast
    Bilateral, ØH9V
    Left, ØH9U
    Right, ØH9T
  Bronchus
    Lingula, ØB99
    Lower Lobe
      Left, ØB9B
      Right, ØB96
    Main
      Left, ØB97
      Right, ØB93
    Middle Lobe, Right, ØB95
    Upper Lobe
      Left, ØB98
      Right, ØB94
  Buccal Mucosa, ØC94
  Bursa and Ligament
    Abdomen
      Left, ØM9J
      Right, ØM9H
    Ankle
      Left, ØM9R
      Right, ØM9Q
    Elbow
      Left, ØM94
      Right, ØM93
    Foot
      Left, ØM9T
      Right, ØM9S
    Hand
      Left, ØM98
      Right, ØM97
    Head and Neck, ØM9Ø

Drainage — *continued*
  Bursa and Ligament — *continued*
    Hip
      Left, ØM9M
      Right, ØM9L
    Knee
      Left, ØM9P
      Right, ØM9N
    Lower Extremity
      Left, ØM9W
      Right, ØM9V
    Perineum, ØM9K
    Rib(s), ØM9G
    Shoulder
      Left, ØM92
      Right, ØM91
    Spine
      Lower, ØM9D
      Upper, ØM9C
    Sternum, ØM9F
    Upper Extremity
      Left, ØM9B
      Right, ØM99
    Wrist
      Left, ØM96
      Right, ØM95
  Buttock
    Left, ØY91
    Right, ØY9Ø
  Carina, ØB92
  Carotid Bodies, Bilateral, ØG98
  Carotid Body
    Left, ØG96
    Right, ØG97
  Carpal
    Left, ØP9N
    Right, ØP9M
  Cavity, Cranial, ØW91
  Cecum, ØD9H
  Cerebellum, ØØ9C
  Cerebral Hemisphere, ØØ97
  Cerebral Meninges, ØØ91
  Cerebral Ventricle, ØØ96
  Cervix, ØU9C
  Chest Wall, ØW98
  Choroid
    Left, Ø89B
    Right, Ø89A
  Cisterna Chyli, Ø79L
  Clavicle
    Left, ØP9B
    Right, ØP99
  Clitoris, ØU9J
  Coccygeal Glomus, ØG9B
  Coccyx, ØQ9S
  Colon
    Ascending, ØD9K
    Descending, ØD9M
    Sigmoid, ØD9N
    Transverse, ØD9L
  Conjunctiva
    Left, Ø89T
    Right, Ø89S
  Cord
    Bilateral, ØV9H
    Left, ØV9G
    Right, ØV9F
  Cornea
    Left, Ø899
    Right, Ø898
  Cul-de-sac, ØU9F
  Diaphragm, ØB9T
  Disc
    Cervical Vertebral, ØR93
    Cervicothoracic Vertebral, ØR95
    Lumbar Vertebral, ØS92
    Lumbosacral, ØS94
    Thoracic Vertebral, ØR99
    Thoracolumbar Vertebral, ØR9B
  Duct
    Common Bile, ØF99
    Cystic, ØF98
    Hepatic
      Common, ØF97
      Left, ØF96
      Right, ØF95
    Lacrimal
      Left, Ø89Y
      Right, Ø89X

Drainage — *continued*
  Duct — *continued*
    Pancreatic, ØF9D
      Accessory, ØF9F
    Parotid
      Left, ØC9C
      Right, ØC9B
  Duodenum, ØD99
  Dura Mater, ØØ92
  Ear
    External
      Left, Ø991
      Right, Ø990
    External Auditory Canal
      Left, Ø994
      Right, Ø993
    Inner
      Left, Ø99E
      Right, Ø99D
    Middle
      Left, Ø996
      Right, Ø995
  Elbow Region
    Left, ØX9C
    Right, ØX9B
  Epididymis
    Bilateral, ØV9L
    Left, ØV9K
    Right, ØV9J
  Epidural Space, Intracranial, ØØ93
  Epiglottis, ØC9R
  Esophagogastric Junction, ØD94
  Esophagus, ØD95
    Lower, ØD93
    Middle, ØD92
    Upper, ØD91
  Eustachian Tube
    Left, Ø99G
    Right, Ø99F
  Extremity
    Lower
      Left, ØY9B
      Right, ØY99
    Upper
      Left, ØX97
      Right, ØX96
  Eye
    Left, Ø891
    Right, Ø890
  Eyelid
    Lower
      Left, Ø89R
      Right, Ø89Q
    Upper
      Left, Ø89P
      Right, Ø89N
  Face, ØW92
  Fallopian Tube
    Left, ØU96
    Right, ØU95
  Fallopian Tubes, Bilateral, ØU97
  Femoral Region
    Left, ØY98
    Right, ØY97
  Femoral Shaft
    Left, ØQ99
    Right, ØQ98
  Femur
    Lower
      Left, ØQ9C
      Right, ØQ9B
    Upper
      Left, ØQ97
      Right, ØQ96
  Fibula
    Left, ØQ9K
    Right, ØQ9J
  Finger Nail, ØH9Q
  Foot
    Left, ØY9N
    Right, ØY9M
  Gallbladder, ØF94
  Gingiva
    Lower, ØC96
    Upper, ØC95
  Gland
    Adrenal
      Bilateral, ØG94
      Left, ØG92

Drainage — *continued*
  Gland — *continued*
    Adrenal — *continued*
      Right, ØG93
    Lacrimal
      Left, Ø89W
      Right, Ø89V
    Minor Salivary, ØC9J
    Parotid
      Left, ØC99
      Right, ØC98
    Pituitary, ØG90
    Sublingual
      Left, ØC9F
      Right, ØC9D
    Submaxillary
      Left, ØC9H
      Right, ØC9G
    Vestibular, ØU9L
  Glenoid Cavity
    Left, ØP98
    Right, ØP97
  Glomus Jugulare, ØG9C
  Hand
    Left, ØX9K
    Right, ØX9J
  Head, ØW90
  Humeral Head
    Left, ØP9D
    Right, ØP9C
  Humeral Shaft
    Left, ØP9G
    Right, ØP9F
  Hymen, ØU9K
  Hypothalamus, ØØ9A
  Ileocecal Valve, ØD9C
  Ileum, ØD9B
  Inguinal Region
    Left, ØY96
    Right, ØY95
  Intestine
    Large, ØD9E
      Left, ØD9G
      Right, ØD9F
    Small, ØD98
  Iris
    Left, Ø89D
    Right, Ø89C
  Jaw
    Lower, ØW95
    Upper, ØW94
  Jejunum, ØD9A
  Joint
    Acromioclavicular
      Left, ØR9H
      Right, ØR9G
    Ankle
      Left, ØS9G
      Right, ØS9F
    Carpal
      Left, ØR9R
      Right, ØR9Q
    Carpometacarpal
      Left, ØR9T
      Right, ØR9S
    Cervical Vertebral, ØR91
    Cervicothoracic Vertebral, ØR94
    Coccygeal, ØS96
    Elbow
      Left, ØR9M
      Right, ØR9L
    Finger Phalangeal
      Left, ØR9X
      Right, ØR9W
    Hip
      Left, ØS9B
      Right, ØS99
    Knee
      Left, ØS9D
      Right, ØS9C
    Lumbar Vertebral, ØS90
    Lumbosacral, ØS93
    Metacarpophalangeal
      Left, ØR9V
      Right, ØR9U
    Metatarsal-Phalangeal
      Left, ØS9N
      Right, ØS9M
    Occipital-cervical, ØR90

Drainage — *continued*
  Joint — *continued*
    Sacrococcygeal, ØS95
    Sacroiliac
      Left, ØS98
      Right, ØS97
    Shoulder
      Left, ØR9K
      Right, ØR9J
    Sternoclavicular
      Left, ØR9F
      Right, ØR9E
    Tarsal
      Left, ØS9J
      Right, ØS9H
    Tarsometatarsal
      Left, ØS9L
      Right, ØS9K
    Temporomandibular
      Left, ØR9D
      Right, ØR9C
    Thoracic Vertebral, ØR96
    Thoracolumbar Vertebral, ØR9A
    Toe Phalangeal
      Left, ØS9Q
      Right, ØS9P
    Wrist
      Left, ØR9P
      Right, ØR9N
  Kidney
    Left, ØT91
    Right, ØT90
  Kidney Pelvis
    Left, ØT94
    Right, ØT93
  Knee Region
    Left, ØY9G
    Right, ØY9F
  Larynx, ØC9S
  Leg
    Lower
      Left, ØY9J
      Right, ØY9H
    Upper
      Left, ØY9D
      Right, ØY9C
  Lens
    Left, Ø89K
    Right, Ø89J
  Lip
    Lower, ØC91
    Upper, ØC90
  Liver, ØF90
    Left Lobe, ØF92
    Right Lobe, ØF91
  Lung
    Bilateral, ØB9M
    Left, ØB9L
    Lower Lobe
      Left, ØB9J
      Right, ØB9F
    Middle Lobe, Right, ØB9D
    Right, ØB9K
    Upper Lobe
      Left, ØB9G
      Right, ØB9C
  Lung Lingula, ØB9H
  Lymphatic
    Aortic, Ø79D
    Axillary
      Left, Ø796
      Right, Ø795
    Head, Ø790
    Inguinal
      Left, Ø79J
      Right, Ø79H
    Internal Mammary
      Left, Ø799
      Right, Ø798
    Lower Extremity
      Left, Ø79G
      Right, Ø79F
    Mesenteric, Ø79B
    Neck
      Left, Ø792
      Right, Ø791
    Pelvis, Ø79C
    Thoracic Duct, Ø79K
    Thorax, Ø797

Drainage — *continued*
  Lymphatic — *continued*
    Upper Extremity
      Left, Ø794
      Right, Ø793
  Mandible
    Left, ØN9V
    Right, ØN9T
  Maxilla, ØN9R
  Mediastinum, ØW9C
  Medulla Oblongata, ØØ9D
  Mesentery, ØD9V
  Metacarpal
    Left, ØP9Q
    Right, ØP9P
  Metatarsal
    Left, ØQ9P
    Right, ØQ9N
  Muscle
    Abdomen
      Left, ØK9L
      Right, ØK9K
    Extraocular
      Left, Ø89M
      Right, Ø89L
    Facial, ØK91
    Foot
      Left, ØK9W
      Right, ØK9V
    Hand
      Left, ØK9D
      Right, ØK9C
    Head, ØK90
    Hip
      Left, ØK9P
      Right, ØK9N
    Lower Arm and Wrist
      Left, ØK9B
      Right, ØK99
    Lower Leg
      Left, ØK9T
      Right, ØK9S
    Neck
      Left, ØK93
      Right, ØK92
    Perineum, ØK9M
    Shoulder
      Left, ØK96
      Right, ØK95
    Thorax
      Left, ØK9J
      Right, ØK9H
    Tongue, Palate, Pharynx, ØK94
    Trunk
      Left, ØK9G
      Right, ØK9F
    Upper Arm
      Left, ØK98
      Right, ØK97
    Upper Leg
      Left, ØK9R
      Right, ØK9Q
  Nasal Mucosa and Soft Tissue, Ø99K
  Nasopharynx, Ø99N
  Neck, ØW96
  Nerve
    Abdominal Sympathetic, Ø19M
    Abducens, ØØ9L
    Accessory, ØØ9R
    Acoustic, ØØ9N
    Brachial Plexus, Ø193
    Cervical, Ø191
    Cervical Plexus, Ø190
    Facial, ØØ9M
    Femoral, Ø19D
    Glossopharyngeal, ØØ9P
    Head and Neck Sympathetic, Ø19K
    Hypoglossal, ØØ9S
    Lumbar, Ø19B
    Lumbar Plexus, Ø199
    Lumbar Sympathetic, Ø19N
    Lumbosacral Plexus, Ø19A
    Median, Ø195
    Oculomotor, ØØ9H
    Olfactory, ØØ9F
    Optic, ØØ9G
    Peroneal, Ø19H
    Phrenic, Ø192
    Pudendal, Ø19C

Drainage — *continued*
  Nerve — *continued*
    Radial, 0196
    Sacral, 019R
    Sacral Plexus, 019Q
    Sacral Sympathetic, 019P
    Sciatic, 019F
    Thoracic, 0198
    Thoracic Sympathetic, 019L
    Tibial, 019G
    Trigeminal, 009K
    Trochlear, 009J
    Ulnar, 0194
    Vagus, 009Q
  Nipple
    Left, 0H9X
    Right, 0H9W
  Omentum, 0D9U
  Oral Cavity and Throat, 0W93
  Orbit
    Left, 0N9Q
    Right, 0N9P
  Ovary
    Bilateral, 0U92
    Left, 0U91
    Right, 0U90
  Palate
    Hard, 0C92
    Soft, 0C93
  Pancreas, 0F9G
  Para-aortic Body, 0G99
  Paraganglion Extremity, 0G9F
  Parathyroid Gland, 0G9R
    Inferior
      Left, 0G9P
      Right, 0G9N
    Multiple, 0G9Q
    Superior
      Left, 0G9M
      Right, 0G9L
  Patella
    Left, 0Q9F
    Right, 0Q9D
  Pelvic Cavity, 0W9J
  Penis, 0V9S
  Pericardial Cavity, 0W9D
  Perineum
    Female, 0W9N
    Male, 0W9M
  Peritoneal Cavity, 0W9G
  Peritoneum, 0D9W
  Phalanx
    Finger
      Left, 0P9V
      Right, 0P9T
    Thumb
      Left, 0P9S
      Right, 0P9R
    Toe
      Left, 0Q9R
      Right, 0Q9Q
  Pharynx, 0C9M
  Pineal Body, 0G91
  Pleura
    Left, 0B9P
    Right, 0B9N
  Pleural Cavity
    Left, 0W9B
    Right, 0W99
  Pons, 009B
  Prepuce, 0V9T
  Products of Conception
    Amniotic Fluid
      Diagnostic, 1090
      Therapeutic, 1090
    Fetal Blood, 1090
    Fetal Cerebrospinal Fluid, 1090
    Fetal Fluid, Other, 1090
    Fluid, Other, 1090
  Prostate, 0V90
  Radius
    Left, 0P9J
    Right, 0P9H
  Rectum, 0D9P
  Retina
    Left, 089F
    Right, 089E
  Retinal Vessel
    Left, 089H

Drainage — *continued*
  Retinal Vessel — *continued*
    Right, 089G
  Retroperitoneum, 0W9H
  Ribs
    1 to 2, 0P91
    3 or More, 0P92
  Sacrum, 0Q91
  Scapula
    Left, 0P96
    Right, 0P95
  Sclera
    Left, 0897
    Right, 0896
  Scrotum, 0V95
  Septum, Nasal, 099M
  Shoulder Region
    Left, 0X93
    Right, 0X92
  Sinus
    Accessory, 099P
    Ethmoid
      Left, 099V
      Right, 099U
    Frontal
      Left, 099T
      Right, 099S
    Mastoid
      Left, 099C
      Right, 099B
    Maxillary
      Left, 099R
      Right, 099Q
    Sphenoid
      Left, 099X
      Right, 099W
  Skin
    Abdomen, 0H97
    Back, 0H96
    Buttock, 0H98
    Chest, 0H95
    Ear
      Left, 0H93
      Right, 0H92
    Face, 0H91
    Foot
      Left, 0H9N
      Right, 0H9M
    Hand
      Left, 0H9G
      Right, 0H9F
    Inguinal, 0H9A
    Lower Arm
      Left, 0H9E
      Right, 0H9D
    Lower Leg
      Left, 0H9L
      Right, 0H9K
    Neck, 0H94
    Perineum, 0H99
    Scalp, 0H90
    Upper Arm
      Left, 0H9C
      Right, 0H9B
    Upper Leg
      Left, 0H9J
      Right, 0H9H
  Skull, 0N90
  Spinal Canal, 009U
  Spinal Cord
    Cervical, 009W
    Lumbar, 009Y
    Thoracic, 009X
  Spinal Meninges, 009T
  Spleen, 079P
  Sternum, 0P90
  Stomach, 0D96
    Pylorus, 0D97
  Subarachnoid Space, Intracranial, 0095
  Subcutaneous Tissue and Fascia
    Abdomen, 0J98
    Back, 0J97
    Buttock, 0J99
    Chest, 0J96
    Face, 0J91
    Foot
      Left, 0J9R
      Right, 0J9Q

Drainage — *continued*
  Subcutaneous Tissue and Fascia — *continued*
    Hand
      Left, 0J9K
      Right, 0J9J
    Lower Arm
      Left, 0J9H
      Right, 0J9G
    Lower Leg
      Left, 0J9P
      Right, 0J9N
    Neck
      Left, 0J95
      Right, 0J94
    Pelvic Region, 0J9C
    Perineum, 0J9B
    Scalp, 0J90
    Upper Arm
      Left, 0J9F
      Right, 0J9D
    Upper Leg
      Left, 0J9M
      Right, 0J9L
  Subdural Space, Intracranial, 0094
  Tarsal
    Left, 0Q9M
    Right, 0Q9L
  Tendon
    Abdomen
      Left, 0L9G
      Right, 0L9F
    Ankle
      Left, 0L9T
      Right, 0L9S
    Foot
      Left, 0L9W
      Right, 0L9V
    Hand
      Left, 0L98
      Right, 0L97
    Head and Neck, 0L90
    Hip
      Left, 0L9K
      Right, 0L9J
    Knee
      Left, 0L9R
      Right, 0L9Q
    Lower Arm and Wrist
      Left, 0L96
      Right, 0L95
    Lower Leg
      Left, 0L9P
      Right, 0L9N
    Perineum, 0L9H
    Shoulder
      Left, 0L92
      Right, 0L91
    Thorax
      Left, 0L9D
      Right, 0L9C
    Trunk
      Left, 0L9B
      Right, 0L99
    Upper Arm
      Left, 0L94
      Right, 0L93
    Upper Leg
      Left, 0L9M
      Right, 0L9L
  Testis
    Bilateral, 0V9C
    Left, 0V9B
    Right, 0V99
  Thalamus, 0099
  Thymus, 079M
  Thyroid Gland, 0G9K
    Left Lobe, 0G9G
    Right Lobe, 0G9H
  Tibia
    Left, 0Q9H
    Right, 0Q9G
  Toe Nail, 0H9R
  Tongue, 0C97
  Tonsils, 0C9P
  Tooth
    Lower, 0C9X
    Upper, 0C9W
  Trachea, 0B91

Drainage — *continued*
  Tunica Vaginalis
    Left, ØV97
    Right, ØV96
  Turbinate, Nasal, Ø99L
  Tympanic Membrane
    Left, Ø998
    Right, Ø997
  Ulna
    Left, ØP9L
    Right, ØP9K
  Ureter
    Left, ØT97
    Right, ØT96
  Ureters, Bilateral, ØT98
  Urethra, ØT9D
  Uterine Supporting Structure, ØU94
  Uterus, ØU99
  Uvula, ØC9N
  Vagina, ØU9G
  Vas Deferens
    Bilateral, ØV9Q
    Left, ØV9P
    Right, ØV9N
  Vein
    Axillary
      Left, Ø598
      Right, Ø597
    Azygos, Ø59Ø
    Basilic
      Left, Ø59C
      Right, Ø59B
    Brachial
      Left, Ø59A
      Right, Ø599
    Cephalic
      Left, Ø59F
      Right, Ø59D
    Colic, Ø697
    Common Iliac
      Left, Ø69D
      Right, Ø69C
    Esophageal, Ø693
    External Iliac
      Left, Ø69G
      Right, Ø69F
    External Jugular
      Left, Ø59Q
      Right, Ø59P
    Face
      Left, Ø59V
      Right, Ø59T
    Femoral
      Left, Ø69N
      Right, Ø69M
    Foot
      Left, Ø69V
      Right, Ø69T
    Gastric, Ø692
    Hand
      Left, Ø59H
      Right, Ø59G
    Hemiazygos, Ø591
    Hepatic, Ø694
    Hypogastric
      Left, Ø69J
      Right, Ø69H
    Inferior Mesenteric, Ø696
    Innominate
      Left, Ø594
      Right, Ø593
    Internal Jugular
      Left, Ø59N
      Right, Ø59M
    Intracranial, Ø59L
    Lower, Ø69Y
    Portal, Ø698
    Renal
      Left, Ø69B
      Right, Ø699
    Saphenous
      Left, Ø69Q
      Right, Ø69P
    Splenic, Ø691
    Subclavian
      Left, Ø596
      Right, Ø595
    Superior Mesenteric, Ø695
    Upper, Ø59Y

Drainage — *continued*
  Vein — *continued*
    Vertebral
      Left, Ø59S
      Right, Ø59R
    Vena Cava, Inferior, Ø69Ø
    Vertebra
      Cervical, ØP93
      Lumbar, ØQ9Ø
      Thoracic, ØP94
    Vesicle
      Bilateral, ØV93
      Left, ØV92
      Right, ØV91
    Vitreous
      Left, Ø895
      Right, Ø894
    Vocal Cord
      Left, ØC9V
      Right, ØC9T
    Vulva, ØU9M
    Wrist Region
      Left, ØX9H
      Right, ØX9G
Dressing
  Abdominal Wall, 2W23X4Z
  Arm
    Lower
      Left, 2W2DX4Z
      Right, 2W2CX4Z
    Upper
      Left, 2W2BX4Z
      Right, 2W2AX4Z
  Back, 2W25X4Z
  Chest Wall, 2W24X4Z
  Extremity
    Lower
      Left, 2W2MX4Z
      Right, 2W2LX4Z
    Upper
      Left, 2W29X4Z
      Right, 2W28X4Z
  Face, 2W21X4Z
  Finger
    Left, 2W2KX4Z
    Right, 2W2JX4Z
  Foot
    Left, 2W2TX4Z
    Right, 2W2SX4Z
  Hand
    Left, 2W2FX4Z
    Right, 2W2EX4Z
  Head, 2W20X4Z
  Inguinal Region
    Left, 2W27X4Z
    Right, 2W26X4Z
  Leg
    Lower
      Left, 2W2RX4Z
      Right, 2W2QX4Z
    Upper
      Left, 2W2PX4Z
      Right, 2W2NX4Z
  Neck, 2W22X4Z
  Thumb
    Left, 2W2HX4Z
    Right, 2W2GX4Z
  Toe
    Left, 2W2VX4Z
    Right, 2W2UX4Z
Driver stent (RX) (OTW) *use* Intraluminal Device
Drotrecogin alfa, infusion *see* Introduction of Recombinant Human-activated Protein C
Duct of Santorini *use* Pancreatic Duct, Accessory
Duct of Wirsung *use* Pancreatic Duct
Ductogram, mammary *see* Plain Radiography, Skin, Subcutaneous Tissue and Breast, BHØ
Ductography, mammary *see* Plain Radiography, Skin, Subcutaneous Tissue and Breast, BHØ
Ductus deferens
  use Vas Deferens
  use Vas Deferens, Bilateral
  use Vas Deferens, Left
  use Vas Deferens, Right
Duodenal ampulla *use* Ampulla of Vater
Duodenectomy
  see Excision, Duodenum, ØDB9
  see Resection, Duodenum, ØDT9

Duodenocholedochotomy *see* Drainage, Gallbladder, ØF94
Duodenocystostomy
  see Bypass, Gallbladder, ØF14
  see Drainage, Gallbladder, ØF94
Duodenoenterostomy
  see Bypass, Gastrointestinal System, ØD1
  see Drainage, Gastrointestinal System, ØD9
Duodenojejunal flexure *use* Jejunum
Duodenolysis *see* Release, Duodenum, ØDN9
Duodenorrhaphy *see* Repair, Duodenum, ØDQ9
Duodenostomy
  see Bypass, Duodenum, ØD19
  see Drainage, Duodenum, ØD99
Duodenotomy *see* Drainage, Duodenum, ØD99
Dura mater, intracranial *use* Dura Mater
Dura mater, spinal *use* Spinal Meninges
DuraGraft® Endothelial Damage Inhibitor *use* Endothelial Damage Inhibitor
DuraHeart Left Ventricular Assist System *use* Implantable Heart Assist System in Heart and Great Vessels
Dural venous sinus *use* Intracranial Vein
Durata® Defibrillation Lead *use* Cardiac Lead, Defibrillator in, Ø2H
Dynesys® Dynamic Stabilization System
  use Spinal Stabilization Device, Pedicle-Based in, ØRH
  use Spinal Stabilization Device, Pedicle-Based in, ØSH

E

Earlobe
  use Ear, External, Bilateral
  use Ear, External, Left
  use Ear, External, Right
ECCO2R (Extracorporeal Carbon Dioxide Removal), 5A0920Z
Echocardiogram *see* Ultrasonography, Heart, B24
Echography *see* Ultrasonography
ECMO *see* Performance, Circulatory, 5A15
EDWARDS INTUITY Elite valve system *use* Zooplastic Tissue, Rapid Deployment Technique in New Technology
EEG (electroencephalogram) *see* Measurement, Central Nervous, 4A00
EGD (esophagogastroduodenoscopy), ØDJ08ZZ
Eighth cranial nerve *use* Acoustic Nerve
Ejaculatory duct
  use Vas Deferens
  use Vas Deferens, Bilateral
  use Vas Deferens, Left
  use Vas Deferens, Right
EKG (electrocardiogram) *see* Measurement, Cardiac, 4A02
Electrical bone growth stimulator (EBGS)
  use Bone Growth Stimulator in Head and Facial Bones
  use Bone Growth Stimulator in Lower Bones
  use Bone Growth Stimulator in Upper Bones
Electrical muscle stimulation (EMS) lead *use* Stimulator Lead in Muscles
Electrocautery
  Destruction *see* Destruction
  Repair *see* Repair
Electroconvulsive Therapy
  Bilateral-Multiple Seizure, GZB3ZZZ
  Bilateral-Single Seizure, GZB2ZZZ
  Electroconvulsive Therapy, Other, GZB4ZZZ
  Unilateral-Multiple Seizure, GZB1ZZZ
  Unilateral-Single Seizure, GZB0ZZZ
Electroencephalogram (EEG) *see* Measurement, Central Nervous, 4A00
Electromagnetic Therapy
  Central Nervous, 6A22
  Urinary, 6A21
Electronic muscle stimulator lead *use* Stimulator Lead in Muscles
Electrophysiologic stimulation (EPS) *see* Measurement, Cardiac, 4A02
Electroshock therapy *see* Electroconvulsive Therapy
Elevation, bone fragments, skull *see* Reposition, Head and Facial Bones, ØNS
Eleventh cranial nerve *use* Accessory Nerve
E-Luminexx™ (Biliary) (Vascular) Stent *use* Intraluminal Device
Embolectomy *see* Extirpation

Embolization
   see Occlusion
   see Restriction
Embolization coil(s) *use* Intraluminal Device
EMG (electromyogram) *see* Measurement, Musculoskele-
   tal, 4A0F
Encephalon *use* Brain
Endarterectomy
   see Extirpation, Lower Arteries, 04C
   see Extirpation, Upper Arteries, 03C
Endeavor® (III) (IV) (Sprint) Zotarolimus-eluting
   Coronary Stent System *use* Intraluminal Device,
   Drug-eluting in Heart and Great Vessels
Endologix® AFX Endovascular AAA System *use* Intralu-
   minal Device
EndoSure® sensor *use* Monitoring Device, Pressure Sensor
   in, 02H
ENDOTAK RELIANCE® (G) Defibrillation Lead *use* Car-
   diac Lead, Defibrillator in, 02H
Endothelial damage inhibitor, applied to vein graft,
   XY0VX83
Endotracheal tube (cuffed) (double-lumen) *use* Intra-
   luminal Device, Endotracheal Airway in Respiratory
   System
Endurant® Endovascular Stent Graft *use* Intraluminal
   Device
Endurant® II AAA stent graft system *use* Intraluminal
   Device
Engineered Autologous Chimeric Antigen Receptor
   T-cell Immunotherapy, XW0
Enlargement
   see Dilation
   see Repair
EnRhythm *use* Pacemaker, Dual Chamber in, 0JH
Enterorrhaphy *see* Repair, Gastrointestinal System, 0DQ
Enterra gastric neurostimulator *use* Stimulator Gener-
   ator, Multiple Array in, 0JH
Enucleation
   Eyeball *see* Resection, Eye, 08T
   Eyeball with prosthetic implant *see* Replacement,
     Eye, 08R
Ependyma *use* Cerebral Ventricle
Epicel® cultured epidermal autograft *use* Autologous
   Tissue Substitute
Epic™ Stented Tissue Valve (aortic) *use* Zooplastic Tis-
   sue in Heart and Great Vessels
Epidermis *use* Skin
Epididymectomy
   see Excision, Male Reproductive System, 0VB
   see Resection, Male Reproductive System, 0VT
Epididymoplasty
   see Repair, Male Reproductive System, 0VQ
   see Supplement, Male Reproductive System, 0VU
Epididymorrhaphy *see* Repair, Male Reproductive System,
   0VQ
Epididymotomy *see* Drainage, Male Reproductive System,
   0V9
Epidural space, spinal *use* Spinal Canal
Epiphysiodesis
   see Insertion of device in, Lower Bones, 0QH
   see Insertion of device in, Upper Bones, 0PH
   see Repair, Lower Bones, 0QQ
   see Repair, Upper Bones, 0PQ
Epiploic foramen *use* Peritoneum
Epiretinal Visual Prosthesis
   Left, 08H105Z
   Right, 08H005Z
Episiorrhaphy *see* Repair, Perineum, Female, 0WQN
Episiotomy *see* Division, Perineum, Female, 0W8N
Epithalamus *use* Thalamus
Epitrochlear lymph node
   use Lymphatic, Left Upper Extremity
   use Lymphatic, Right Upper Extremity
EPS (electrophysiologic stimulation) *see* Measurement,
   Cardiac, 4A02
Eptifibatide, infusion *see* Introduction of Platelet In-
   hibitor
ERCP (endoscopic retrograde cholangiopancreatog-
   raphy) *see* Fluoroscopy, Hepatobiliary System and
   Pancreas, BF1
Erector spinae muscle
   use Trunk Muscle, Left
   use Trunk Muscle, Right
Esophageal artery *use* Upper Artery
Esophageal obturator airway (EOA) *use* Intraluminal
   Device, Airway in Gastrointestinal System
Esophageal plexus *use* Thoracic Sympathetic Nerve

Esophagectomy
   see Excision, Gastrointestinal System, 0DB
   see Resection, Gastrointestinal System, 0DT
Esophagocoloplasty
   see Repair, Gastrointestinal System, 0DQ
   see Supplement, Gastrointestinal System, 0DU
Esophagoenterostomy
   see Bypass, Gastrointestinal System, 0D1
   see Drainage, Gastrointestinal System, 0D9
Esophagoesophagostomy
   see Bypass, Gastrointestinal System, 0D1
   see Drainage, Gastrointestinal System, 0D9
Esophagogastrectomy
   see Excision, Gastrointestinal System, 0DB
   see Resection, Gastrointestinal System, 0DT
Esophagogastroduodenoscopy (EGD), 0DJ08ZZ
Esophagogastroplasty
   see Repair, Gastrointestinal System, 0DQ
   see Supplement, Gastrointestinal System, 0DU
Esophagogastroscopy, 0DJ68ZZ
Esophagogastrostomy
   see Bypass, Gastrointestinal System, 0D1
   see Drainage, Gastrointestinal System, 0D9
Esophagojejunoplasty *see* Supplement, Gastrointestinal
   System, 0DU
Esophagojejunostomy
   see Bypass, Gastrointestinal System, 0D1
   see Drainage, Gastrointestinal System, 0D9
Esophagomyotomy *see* Division, Esophagogastric Junction, 0D84
Esophagoplasty
   see Repair, Gastrointestinal System, 0DQ
   see Replacement, Esophagus, 0DR5
   see Supplement, Gastrointestinal System, 0DU
Esophagoplication *see* Restriction, Gastrointestinal System, 0DV
Esophagorrhaphy *see* Repair, Gastrointestinal System,
   0DQ
Esophagoscopy, 0DJ08ZZ
Esophagotomy *see* Drainage, Gastrointestinal System,
   0D9
Esteem® implantable hearing system *use* Hearing Device in Ear, Nose, Sinus
ESWL (extracorporeal shock wave lithotripsy) *see*
   Fragmentation
Ethmoidal air cell
   use Ethmoid Sinus, Left
   use Ethmoid Sinus, Right
Ethmoidectomy
   see Excision, Ear, Nose, Sinus, 09B
   see Excision, Head and Facial Bones, 0NB
   see Resection, Ear, Nose, Sinus, 09T
   see Resection, Head and Facial Bones, 0NT
Ethmoidotomy *see* Drainage, Ear, Nose, Sinus, 099
Evacuation
   Hematoma *see* Extirpation
   Other Fluid *see* Drainage
Evera (XT) (S) (DR/VR) *use* Defibrillator Generator in, 0JH
Everolimus-eluting coronary stent *use* Intraluminal
   Device, Drug-eluting in Heart and Great Vessels
Evisceration
   Eyeball *see* Resection, Eye, 08T
   Eyeball with prosthetic implant *see* Replacement,
     Eye, 08R
Examination *see* Inspection
Exchange *see* Change device in
Excision
   Abdominal Wall, 0WBF
   Acetabulum
     Left, 0QB5
     Right, 0QB4
   Adenoids, 0CBQ
   Ampulla of Vater, 0FBC
   Anal Sphincter, 0DBR
   Ankle Region
     Left, 0YBL
     Right, 0YBK
   Anus, 0DBQ
   Aorta
     Abdominal
     Thoracic
       Ascending/Arch, 02BX
       Descending, 02BW
   Aortic Body, 0GBD
   Appendix, 0DBJ

Excision — *continued*
   Arm
     Lower
       Left, 0XBF
       Right, 0XBD
     Upper
       Left, 0XB9
       Right, 0XB8
   Artery
     Anterior Tibial
       Left, 04BQ
       Right, 04BP
     Axillary
       Left, 03B6
       Right, 03B5
     Brachial
       Left, 03B8
       Right, 03B7
     Celiac, 04B1
     Colic
       Left, 04B7
       Middle, 04B8
       Right, 04B6
     Common Carotid
       Left, 03BJ
       Right, 03BH
     Common Iliac
       Left, 04BD
       Right, 04BC
     External Carotid
       Left, 03BN
       Right, 03BM
     External Iliac
       Left, 04BJ
       Right, 04BH
     Face, 03BR
     Femoral
       Left, 04BL
       Right, 04BK
     Foot
       Left, 04BW
       Right, 04BV
     Gastric, 04B2
     Hand
       Left, 03BF
       Right, 03BD
     Hepatic, 04B3
     Inferior Mesenteric, 04BB
     Innominate, 03B2
     Internal Carotid
       Left, 03BL
       Right, 03BK
     Internal Iliac
       Left, 04BF
       Right, 04BE
     Internal Mammary
       Left, 03B1
       Right, 03B0
     Intracranial, 03BG
     Lower, 04BY
     Peroneal
       Left, 04BU
       Right, 04BT
     Popliteal
       Left, 04BN
       Right, 04BM
     Posterior Tibial
       Left, 04BS
       Right, 04BR
     Pulmonary
       Left, 02BR
       Right, 02BQ
     Pulmonary Trunk, 02BP
     Radial
       Left, 03BC
       Right, 03BB
     Renal
       Left, 04BA
       Right, 04B9
     Splenic, 04B4
     Subclavian
       Left, 03B4
       Right, 03B3
     Superior Mesenteric, 04B5
     Temporal
       Left, 03BT
       Right, 03BS
     Thyroid
       Left, 03BV

▽ **Subterms under main terms may continue to next column or page**

Excision — continued
Gland
Adrenal
Bilateral, 0GB4
Left, 0GB2
Right, 0GB3
Lacrimal
Left, 08BW
Right, 08BV
Minor Salivary, 0CBJ
Parotid
Left, 0CB9
Right, 0CB8
Pituitary, 0GB0
Sublingual
Left, 0CBF
Right, 0CBD
Submaxillary
Left, 0CBH
Right, 0CBG
Vestibular, 0UBL
Glenoid Cavity
Left, 0PB8
Right, 0PB7
Glomus Jugulare, 0GBC
Hand
Left, 0XBK
Right, 0XBJ
Head, 0WB0
Humeral Head
Left, 0PBD
Right, 0PBC
Humeral Shaft
Left, 0PBG
Right, 0PBF
Hymen, 0UBK
Hypothalamus, 00BA
Ileocecal Valve, 0DBC
Ileum, 0DBB
Inguinal Region
Left, 0YB6
Right, 0YB5
Intestine
Large, 0DBE
Left, 0DBG
Right, 0DBF
Small, 0DB8
Iris
Left, 08BD3Z
Right, 08BC3Z
Jaw
Lower, 0WB5
Upper, 0WB4
Jejunum, 0DBA
Joint
Acromioclavicular
Left, 0RBH
Right, 0RBG
Ankle
Left, 0SBG
Right, 0SBF
Carpal
Left, 0RBR
Right, 0RBQ
Carpometacarpal
Left, 0RBT
Right, 0RBS
Cervical Vertebral, 0RB1
Cervicothoracic Vertebral, 0RB4
Coccygeal, 0SB6
Elbow
Left, 0RBM
Right, 0RBL
Finger Phalangeal
Left, 0RBX
Right, 0RBW
Hip
Left, 0SBB
Right, 0SB9
Knee
Left, 0SBD
Right, 0SBC
Lumbar Vertebral, 0SB0
Lumbosacral, 0SB3
Metacarpophalangeal
Left, 0RBV
Right, 0RBU
Metatarsal-Phalangeal
Left, 0SBN

Excision — continued
Joint — continued
Metatarsal-Phalangeal — continued
Right, 0SBM
Occipital-cervical, 0RB0
Sacrococcygeal, 0SB5
Sacroiliac
Left, 0SB8
Right, 0SB7
Shoulder
Left, 0RBK
Right, 0RBJ
Sternoclavicular
Left, 0RBF
Right, 0RBE
Tarsal
Left, 0SBJ
Right, 0SBH
Tarsometatarsal
Left, 0SBL
Right, 0SBK
Temporomandibular
Left, 0RBD
Right, 0RBC
Thoracic Vertebral, 0RB6
Thoracolumbar Vertebral, 0RBA
Toe Phalangeal
Left, 0SBQ
Right, 0SBP
Wrist
Left, 0RBP
Right, 0RBN
Kidney
Left, 0TB1
Right, 0TB0
Kidney Pelvis
Left, 0TB4
Right, 0TB3
Knee Region
Left, 0YBG
Right, 0YBF
Larynx, 0CBS
Leg
Lower
Left, 0YBJ
Right, 0YBH
Upper
Left, 0YBD
Right, 0YBC
Lens
Left, 08BK3Z
Right, 08BJ3Z
Lip
Lower, 0CB1
Upper, 0CB0
Liver, 0FB0
Left Lobe, 0FB2
Right Lobe, 0FB1
Lung
Bilateral, 0BBM
Left, 0BBL
Lower Lobe
Left, 0BBJ
Right, 0BBF
Middle Lobe, Right, 0BBD
Right, 0BBK
Upper Lobe
Left, 0BBG
Right, 0BBC
Lung Lingula, 0BBH
Lymphatic
Aortic, 07BD
Axillary
Left, 07B6
Right, 07B5
Head, 07B0
Inguinal
Left, 07BJ
Right, 07BH
Internal Mammary
Left, 07B9
Right, 07B8
Lower Extremity
Left, 07BG
Right, 07BF
Mesenteric, 07BB
Neck
Left, 07B2
Right, 07B1

Excision — continued
Lymphatic — continued
Pelvis, 07BC
Thoracic Duct, 07BK
Thorax, 07B7
Upper Extremity
Left, 07B4
Right, 07B3
Mandible
Left, 0NBV
Right, 0NBT
Maxilla, 0NBR
Mediastinum, 0WBC
Medulla Oblongata, 00BD
Mesentery, 0DBV
Metacarpal
Left, 0PBQ
Right, 0PBP
Metatarsal
Left, 0QBP
Right, 0QBN
Muscle
Abdomen
Left, 0KBL
Right, 0KBK
Extraocular
Left, 08BM
Right, 08BL
Facial, 0KB1
Foot
Left, 0KBW
Right, 0KBV
Hand
Left, 0KBD
Right, 0KBC
Head, 0KB0
Hip
Left, 0KBP
Right, 0KBN
Lower Arm and Wrist
Left, 0KBB
Right, 0KB9
Lower Leg
Left, 0KBT
Right, 0KBS
Neck
Left, 0KB3
Right, 0KB2
Papillary, 02BD
Perineum, 0KBM
Shoulder
Left, 0KB6
Right, 0KB5
Thorax
Left, 0KBJ
Right, 0KBH
Tongue, Palate, Pharynx, 0KB4
Trunk
Left, 0KBG
Right, 0KBF
Upper Arm
Left, 0KB8
Right, 0KB7
Upper Leg
Left, 0KBR
Right, 0KBQ
Nasal Mucosa and Soft Tissue, 09BK
Nasopharynx, 09BN
Neck, 0WB6
Nerve
Abdominal Sympathetic, 01BM
Abducens, 00BL
Accessory, 00BR
Acoustic, 00BN
Brachial Plexus, 01B3
Cervical, 01B1
Cervical Plexus, 01B0
Facial, 00BM
Femoral, 01BD
Glossopharyngeal, 00BP
Head and Neck Sympathetic, 01BK
Hypoglossal, 00BS
Lumbar, 01BB
Lumbar Plexus, 01B9
Lumbar Sympathetic, 01BN
Lumbosacral Plexus, 01BA
Median, 01B5
Oculomotor, 00BH
Olfactory, 00BF

▽ Subterms under main terms may continue to next column or page

▽ **Subterms under main terms may continue to next column or page**

Excision — *continued*

Uterine Supporting Structure, ØUB4
Uterus, ØUB9
Uvula, ØCBN
Vagina, ØUBG
Valve
  Aortic, Ø2BF
  Mitral, Ø2BG
  Pulmonary, Ø2BH
  Tricuspid, Ø2BJ
Vas Deferens
  Bilateral, ØVBQ
  Left, ØVBP
  Right, ØVBN
Vein
  Axillary
    Left, Ø5B8
    Right, Ø5B7
  Azygos, Ø5BØ
  Basilic
    Left, Ø5BC
    Right, Ø5BB
  Brachial
    Left, Ø5BA
    Right, Ø5B9
  Cephalic
    Left, Ø5BF
    Right, Ø5BD
  Colic, Ø6B7
  Common Iliac
    Left, Ø6BD
    Right, Ø6BC
  Coronary, Ø2B4
  Esophageal, Ø6B3
  External Iliac
    Left, Ø6BG
    Right, Ø6BF
  External Jugular
    Left, Ø5BQ
    Right, Ø5BP
  Face
    Left, Ø5BV
    Right, Ø5BT
  Femoral
    Left, Ø6BN
    Right, Ø6BM
  Foot
    Left, Ø6BV
    Right, Ø6BT
  Gastric, Ø6B2
  Hand
    Left, Ø5BH
    Right, Ø5BG
  Hemiazygos, Ø5B1
  Hepatic, Ø6B4
  Hypogastric
    Left, Ø6BJ
    Right, Ø6BH
  Inferior Mesenteric, Ø6B6
  Innominate
    Left, Ø5B4
    Right, Ø5B3
  Internal Jugular
    Left, Ø5BN
    Right, Ø5BM
  Intracranial, Ø5BL
  Lower, Ø6BY
  Portal, Ø6B8
  Pulmonary
    Left, Ø2BT
    Right, Ø2BS
  Renal
    Left, Ø6BB
    Right, Ø6B9
  Saphenous
    Left, Ø6BQ
    Right, Ø6BP
  Splenic, Ø6B1
  Subclavian
    Left, Ø5B6
    Right, Ø5B5
  Superior Mesenteric, Ø6B5
  Upper, Ø5BY
  Vertebral
    Left, Ø5BS
    Right, Ø5BR
Vena Cava
  Inferior, Ø6BØ
  Superior, Ø2BV

Excision — *continued*

Ventricle
  Left, Ø2BL
  Right, Ø2BK
Vertebra
  Cervical, ØPB3
  Lumbar, ØQBØ
  Thoracic, ØPB4
Vesicle
  Bilateral, ØVB3
  Left, ØVB2
  Right, ØVB1
Vitreous
  Left, Ø8B53Z
  Right, Ø8B43Z
Vocal Cord
  Left, ØCBV
  Right, ØCBT
Vulva, ØUBM
Wrist Region
  Left, ØXBH
  Right, ØXBG
EXCLUDER® AAA Endoprosthesis
  use Intraluminal Device
  use Intraluminal Device, Branched or Fenestrated, One or Two Arteries in, Ø4V
  use Intraluminal Device, Branched or Fenestrated, Three or More Arteries in, Ø4V
EXCLUDER® IBE Endoprosthesis *use* Intraluminal Device, Branched or Fenestrated, One or Two Arteries in, Ø4V
Exclusion, Left atrial appendage (LAA) *see* Occlusion, Atrium, Left, Ø2L7
Exercise, rehabilitation *see* Motor Treatment, Rehabilitation, FØ7
Exploration *see* Inspection
Express® Biliary SD Monorail® Premounted Stent System *use* Intraluminal Device
Express® (LD) Premounted Stent System *use* Intraluminal Device
Express® SD Renal Monorail® Premounted Stent System *use* Intraluminal Device
Ex-PRESS™ mini glaucoma shunt *use* Synthetic Substitute
Extensor carpi radialis muscle
  use Lower Arm and Wrist Muscle, Left
  use Lower Arm and Wrist Muscle, Right
Extensor carpi ulnaris muscle
  use Lower Arm and Wrist Muscle, Left
  use Lower Arm and Wrist Muscle, Right
Extensor digitorum brevis muscle
  use Foot Muscle, Left
  use Foot Muscle, Right
Extensor digitorum longus muscle
  use Lower Leg Muscle, Left
  use Lower Leg Muscle, Right
Extensor hallucis brevis muscle
  use Foot Muscle, Left
  use Foot Muscle, Right
Extensor hallucis longus muscle
  use Lower Leg Muscle, Left
  use Lower Leg Muscle, Right
External anal sphincter *use* Anal Sphincter
External auditory meatus
  use External Auditory Canal, Left
  use External Auditory Canal, Right
External fixator
  use External Fixation Device in Head and Facial Bones
  use External Fixation Device in Lower Bones
  use External Fixation Device in Lower Joints
  use External Fixation Device in Upper Bones
  use External Fixation Device in Upper Joints
External maxillary artery *use* Face Artery
External naris *use* Nasal Mucosa and Soft Tissue
External oblique aponeurosis *use* Subcutaneous Tissue and Fascia, Trunk
External oblique muscle
  use Abdomen Muscle, Left
  use Abdomen Muscle, Right
External popliteal nerve *use* Peroneal Nerve
External pudendal artery
  use Femoral Artery, Left
  use Femoral Artery, Right
External pudendal vein
  use Saphenous Vein, Left
  use Saphenous Vein, Right
External urethral sphincter *use* Urethra

Extirpation

Acetabulum
  Left, ØQC5
  Right, ØQC4
Adenoids, ØCCQ
Ampulla of Vater, ØFCC
Anal Sphincter, ØDCR
Anterior Chamber
  Left, Ø8C3
  Right, Ø8C2
Anus, ØDCQ
Aorta
  Abdominal, Ø4CØ
  Thoracic
    Ascending/Arch, Ø2CX
    Descending, Ø2CW
Aortic Body, ØGCD
Appendix, ØDCJ
Artery
  Anterior Tibial
    Left, Ø4CQ
    Right, Ø4CP
  Axillary
    Left, Ø3C6
    Right, Ø3C5
  Brachial
    Left, Ø3C8
    Right, Ø3C7
  Celiac, Ø4C1
  Colic
    Left, Ø4C7
    Middle, Ø4C8
    Right, Ø4C6
  Common Carotid
    Left, Ø3CJ
    Right, Ø3CH
  Common Iliac
    Left, Ø4CD
    Right, Ø4CC
  Coronary
    Four or More Arteries, Ø2C3
    One Artery, Ø2CØ
    Three Arteries, Ø2C2
    Two Arteries, Ø2C1
  External Carotid
    Left, Ø3CN
    Right, Ø3CM
  External Iliac
    Left, Ø4CJ
    Right, Ø4CH
  Face, Ø3CR
  Femoral
    Left, Ø4CL
    Right, Ø4CK
  Foot
    Left, Ø4CW
    Right, Ø4CV
  Gastric, Ø4C2
  Hand
    Left, Ø3CF
    Right, Ø3CD
  Hepatic, Ø4C3
  Inferior Mesenteric, Ø4CB
  Innominate, Ø3C2
  Internal Carotid
    Left, Ø3CL
    Right, Ø3CK
  Internal Iliac
    Left, Ø4CF
    Right, Ø4CE
  Internal Mammary
    Left, Ø3C1
    Right, Ø3CØ
  Intracranial, Ø3CG
  Lower, Ø4CY
  Peroneal
    Left, Ø4CU
    Right, Ø4CT
  Popliteal
    Left, Ø4CN
    Right, Ø4CM
  Posterior Tibial
    Left, Ø4CS
    Right, Ø4CR
  Pulmonary
    Left, Ø2CR
    Right, Ø2CQ
  Pulmonary Trunk, Ø2CP

Extirpation — *continued*
    Artery — *continued*
        Radial
            Left, Ø3CC
            Right, Ø3CB
        Renal
            Left, Ø4CA
            Right, Ø4C9
        Splenic, Ø4C4
        Subclavian
            Left, Ø3C4
            Right, Ø3C3
        Superior Mesenteric, Ø4C5
        Temporal
            Left, Ø3CT
            Right, Ø3CS
        Thyroid
            Left, Ø3CV
            Right, Ø3CU
        Ulnar
            Left, Ø3CA
            Right, Ø3C9
        Upper, Ø3CY
        Vertebral
            Left, Ø3CQ
            Right, Ø3CP
    Atrium
        Left, Ø2C7
        Right, Ø2C6
    Auditory Ossicle
        Left, Ø9CA
        Right, Ø9C9
    Basal Ganglia, ØØC8
    Bladder, ØTCB
    Bladder Neck, ØTCC
    Bone
        Ethmoid
            Left, ØNCG
            Right, ØNCF
        Frontal, ØNC1
        Hyoid, ØNCX
        Lacrimal
            Left, ØNCJ
            Right, ØNCH
        Nasal, ØNCB
        Occipital, ØNC7
        Palatine
            Left, ØNCL
            Right, ØNCK
        Parietal
            Left, ØNC4
            Right, ØNC3
        Pelvic
            Left, ØQC3
            Right, ØQC2
        Sphenoid, ØNCC
        Temporal
            Left, ØNC6
            Right, ØNC5
        Zygomatic
            Left, ØNCN
            Right, ØNCM
    Brain, ØØCØ
    Breast
        Bilateral, ØHCV
        Left, ØHCU
        Right, ØHCT
    Bronchus
        Lingula, ØBC9
        Lower Lobe
            Left, ØBCB
            Right, ØBC6
        Main
            Left, ØBC7
            Right, ØBC3
        Middle Lobe, Right, ØBC5
        Upper Lobe
            Left, ØBC8
            Right, ØBC4
    Buccal Mucosa, ØCC4
    Bursa and Ligament
        Abdomen
            Left, ØMCJ
            Right, ØMCH
        Ankle
            Left, ØMCR
            Right, ØMCQ
        Elbow
            Left, ØMC4

Extirpation — *continued*
    Bursa and Ligament — *continued*
        Elbow — *continued*
            Right, ØMC3
        Foot
            Left, ØMCT
            Right, ØMCS
        Hand
            Left, ØMC8
            Right, ØMC7
        Head and Neck, ØMCØ
        Hip
            Left, ØMCM
            Right, ØMCL
        Knee
            Left, ØMCP
            Right, ØMCN
        Lower Extremity
            Left, ØMCW
            Right, ØMCV
        Perineum, ØMCK
        Rib(s), ØMCG
        Shoulder
            Left, ØMC2
            Right, ØMC1
        Spine
            Lower, ØMCD
            Upper, ØMCC
        Sternum, ØMCF
        Upper Extremity
            Left, ØMCB
            Right, ØMC9
        Wrist
            Left, ØMC6
            Right, ØMC5
    Carina, ØBC2
    Carotid Bodies, Bilateral, ØGC8
    Carotid Body
        Left, ØGC6
        Right, ØGC7
    Carpal
        Left, ØPCN
        Right, ØPCM
    Cavity, Cranial, ØWC1
    Cecum, ØDCH
    Cerebellum, ØØCC
    Cerebral Hemisphere, ØØC7
    Cerebral Meninges, ØØC1
    Cerebral Ventricle, ØØC6
    Cervix, ØUCC
    Chordae Tendineae, Ø2C9
    Choroid
        Left, Ø8CB
        Right, Ø8CA
    Cisterna Chyli, Ø7CL
    Clavicle
        Left, ØPCB
        Right, ØPC9
    Clitoris, ØUCJ
    Coccygeal Glomus, ØGCB
    Coccyx, ØQCS
    Colon
        Ascending, ØDCK
        Descending, ØDCM
        Sigmoid, ØDCN
        Transverse, ØDCL
    Conduction Mechanism, Ø2C8
    Conjunctiva
        Left, Ø8CTXZZ
        Right, Ø8CSXZZ
    Cord
        Bilateral, ØVCH
        Left, ØVCG
        Right, ØVCF
    Cornea
        Left, Ø8C9XZZ
        Right, Ø8C8XZZ
    Cul-de-sac, ØUCF
    Diaphragm, ØBCT
    Disc
        Cervical Vertebral, ØRC3
        Cervicothoracic Vertebral, ØRC5
        Lumbar Vertebral, ØSC2
        Lumbosacral, ØSC4
        Thoracic Vertebral, ØRC9
        Thoracolumbar Vertebral, ØRCB
    Duct
        Common Bile, ØFC9
        Cystic, ØFC8

Extirpation — *continued*
    Duct — *continued*
        Hepatic
            Common, ØFC7
            Left, ØFC6
            Right, ØFC5
        Lacrimal
            Left, Ø8CY
            Right, Ø8CX
        Pancreatic, ØFCD
            Accessory, ØFCF
        Parotid
            Left, ØCCC
            Right, ØCCB
    Duodenum, ØDC9
    Dura Mater, ØØC2
    Ear
        External
            Left, Ø9C1
            Right, Ø9CØ
        External Auditory Canal
            Left, Ø9C4
            Right, Ø9C3
        Inner
            Left, Ø9CE
            Right, Ø9CD
        Middle
            Left, Ø9C6
            Right, Ø9C5
    Endometrium, ØUCB
    Epididymis
        Bilateral, ØVCL
        Left, ØVCK
        Right, ØVCJ
    Epidural Space, Intracranial, ØØC3
    Epiglottis, ØCCR
    Esophagogastric Junction, ØDC4
    Esophagus, ØDC5
        Lower, ØDC3
        Middle, ØDC2
        Upper, ØDC1
    Eustachian Tube
        Left, Ø9CG
        Right, Ø9CF
    Eye
        Left, Ø8C1XZZ
        Right, Ø8CØXZZ
    Eyelid
        Lower
            Left, Ø8CR
            Right, Ø8CQ
        Upper
            Left, Ø8CP
            Right, Ø8CN
    Fallopian Tube
        Left, ØUC6
        Right, ØUC5
    Fallopian Tubes, Bilateral, ØUC7
    Femoral Shaft
        Left, ØQC9
        Right, ØQC8
    Femur
        Lower
            Left, ØQCC
            Right, ØQCB
        Upper
            Left, ØQC7
            Right, ØQC6
    Fibula
        Left, ØQCK
        Right, ØQCJ
    Finger Nail, ØHCQXZZ
    Gallbladder, ØFC4
    Gastrointestinal Tract, ØWCP
    Genitourinary Tract, ØWCR
    Gingiva
        Lower, ØCC6
        Upper, ØCC5
    Gland
        Adrenal
            Bilateral, ØGC4
            Left, ØGC2
            Right, ØGC3
        Lacrimal
            Left, Ø8CW
            Right, Ø8CV
        Minor Salivary, ØCCJ
        Parotid
            Left, ØCC9

▼ **Subterms under main terms may continue to next column or page**

Extirpation — *continued*
  Gland — *continued*
    Parotid — *continued*
      Right, ØCC8
    Pituitary, ØGCØ
    Sublingual
      Left, ØCCF
      Right, ØCCD
    Submaxillary
      Left, ØCCH
      Right, ØCCG
    Vestibular, ØUCL
  Glenoid Cavity
    Left, ØPC8
    Right, ØPC7
  Glomus Jugulare, ØGCC
  Humeral Head
    Left, ØPCD
    Right, ØPCC
  Humeral Shaft
    Left, ØPCG
    Right, ØPCF
  Hymen, ØUCK
  Hypothalamus, ØØCA
  Ileocecal Valve, ØDCC
  Ileum, ØDCB
  Intestine
    Large, ØDCE
      Left, ØDCG
      Right, ØDCF
    Small, ØDC8
  Iris
    Left, Ø8CD
    Right, Ø8CC
  Jejunum, ØDCA
  Joint
    Acromioclavicular
      Left, ØRCH
      Right, ØRCG
    Ankle
      Left, ØSCG
      Right, ØSCF
    Carpal
      Left, ØRCR
      Right, ØRCQ
    Carpometacarpal
      Left, ØRCT
      Right, ØRCS
    Cervical Vertebral, ØRC1
    Cervicothoracic Vertebral, ØRC4
    Coccygeal, ØSC6
    Elbow
      Left, ØRCM
      Right, ØRCL
    Finger Phalangeal
      Left, ØRCX
      Right, ØRCW
    Hip
      Left, ØSCB
      Right, ØSC9
    Knee
      Left, ØSCD
      Right, ØSCC
    Lumbar Vertebral, ØSCØ
    Lumbosacral, ØSC3
    Metacarpophalangeal
      Left, ØRCV
      Right, ØRCU
    Metatarsal-Phalangeal
      Left, ØSCN
      Right, ØSCM
    Occipital-cervical, ØRCØ
    Sacrococcygeal, ØSC5
    Sacroiliac
      Left, ØSC8
      Right, ØSC7
    Shoulder
      Left, ØRCK
      Right, ØRCJ
    Sternoclavicular
      Left, ØRCF
      Right, ØRCE
    Tarsal
      Left, ØSCJ
      Right, ØSCH
    Tarsometatarsal
      Left, ØSCL
      Right, ØSCK

Extirpation — *continued*
  Joint — *continued*
    Temporomandibular
      Left, ØRCD
      Right, ØRCC
    Thoracic Vertebral, ØRC6
    Thoracolumbar Vertebral, ØRCA
    Toe Phalangeal
      Left, ØSCQ
      Right, ØSCP
    Wrist
      Left, ØRCP
      Right, ØRCN
  Kidney
    Left, ØTC1
    Right, ØTCØ
  Kidney Pelvis
    Left, ØTC4
    Right, ØTC3
  Larynx, ØCCS
  Lens
    Left, Ø8CK
    Right, Ø8CJ
  Lip
    Lower, ØCC1
    Upper, ØCCØ
  Liver, ØFCØ
    Left Lobe, ØFC2
    Right Lobe, ØFC1
  Lung
    Bilateral, ØBCM
    Left, ØBCL
    Lower Lobe
      Left, ØBCJ
      Right, ØBCF
    Middle Lobe, Right, ØBCD
    Right, ØBCK
    Upper Lobe
      Left, ØBCG
      Right, ØBCC
  Lung Lingula, ØBCH
  Lymphatic
    Aortic, Ø7CD
    Axillary
      Left, Ø7C6
      Right, Ø7C5
    Head, Ø7CØ
    Inguinal
      Left, Ø7CJ
      Right, Ø7CH
    Internal Mammary
      Left, Ø7C9
      Right, Ø7C8
    Lower Extremity
      Left, Ø7CG
      Right, Ø7CF
    Mesenteric, Ø7CB
    Neck
      Left, Ø7C2
      Right, Ø7C1
    Pelvis, Ø7CC
    Thoracic Duct, Ø7CK
    Thorax, Ø7C7
    Upper Extremity
      Left, Ø7C4
      Right, Ø7C3
  Mandible
    Left, ØNCV
    Right, ØNCT
  Maxilla, ØNCR
  Mediastinum, ØWCC
  Medulla Oblongata, ØØCD
  Mesentery, ØDCV
  Metacarpal
    Left, ØPCQ
    Right, ØPCP
  Metatarsal
    Left, ØQCP
    Right, ØQCN
  Muscle
    Abdomen
      Left, ØKCL
      Right, ØKCK
    Extraocular
      Left, Ø8CM
      Right, Ø8CL
    Facial, ØKC1
    Foot
      Left, ØKCW

Extirpation — *continued*
  Muscle — *continued*
    Foot — *continued*
      Right, ØKCV
    Hand
      Left, ØKCD
      Right, ØKCC
    Head, ØKCØ
    Hip
      Left, ØKCP
      Right, ØKCN
    Lower Arm and Wrist
      Left, ØKCB
      Right, ØKC9
    Lower Leg
      Left, ØKCT
      Right, ØKCS
    Neck
      Left, ØKC3
      Right, ØKC2
    Papillary, Ø2CD
    Perineum, ØKCM
    Shoulder
      Left, ØKC6
      Right, ØKC5
    Thorax
      Left, ØKCJ
      Right, ØKCH
    Tongue, Palate, Pharynx, ØKC4
    Trunk
      Left, ØKCG
      Right, ØKCF
    Upper Arm
      Left, ØKC8
      Right, ØKC7
    Upper Leg
      Left, ØKCR
      Right, ØKCQ
  Nasal Mucosa and Soft Tissue, Ø9CK
  Nasopharynx, Ø9CN
  Nerve
    Abdominal Sympathetic, Ø1CM
    Abducens, ØØCL
    Accessory, ØØCR
    Acoustic, ØØCN
    Brachial Plexus, Ø1C3
    Cervical, Ø1C1
    Cervical Plexus, Ø1CØ
    Facial, ØØCM
    Femoral, Ø1CD
    Glossopharyngeal, ØØCP
    Head and Neck Sympathetic, Ø1CK
    Hypoglossal, ØØCS
    Lumbar, Ø1CB
    Lumbar Plexus, Ø1C9
    Lumbar Sympathetic, Ø1CN
    Lumbosacral Plexus, Ø1CA
    Median, Ø1C5
    Oculomotor, ØØCH
    Olfactory, ØØCF
    Optic, ØØCG
    Peroneal, Ø1CH
    Phrenic, Ø1C2
    Pudendal, Ø1CC
    Radial, Ø1C6
    Sacral, Ø1CR
    Sacral Plexus, Ø1CQ
    Sacral Sympathetic, Ø1CP
    Sciatic, Ø1CF
    Thoracic, Ø1C8
    Thoracic Sympathetic, Ø1CL
    Tibial, Ø1CG
    Trigeminal, ØØCK
    Trochlear, ØØCJ
    Ulnar, Ø1C4
    Vagus, ØØCQ
  Nipple
    Left, ØHCX
    Right, ØHCW
  Omentum, ØDCU
  Oral Cavity and Throat, ØWC3
  Orbit
    Left, ØNCQ
    Right, ØNCP
  Orbital Atherectomy Technology, X2C
  Ovary
    Bilateral, ØUC2
    Left, ØUC1
    Right, ØUCØ

Extirpation

⬙ **Subterms under main terms may continue to next column or page**

Extirpation — continued
  Vein — continued
    Brachial — continued
      Right, 05C9
    Cephalic
      Left, 05CF
      Right, 05CD
    Colic, 06C7
    Common Iliac
      Left, 06CD
      Right, 06CC
    Coronary, 02C4
    Esophageal, 06C3
    External Iliac
      Left, 06CG
      Right, 06CF
    External Jugular
      Left, 05CQ
      Right, 05CP
    Face
      Left, 05CV
      Right, 05CT
    Femoral
      Left, 06CN
      Right, 06CM
    Foot
      Left, 06CV
      Right, 06CT
    Gastric, 06C2
    Hand
      Left, 05CH
      Right, 05CG
    Hemiazygos, 05C1
    Hepatic, 06C4
    Hypogastric
      Left, 06CJ
      Right, 06CH
    Inferior Mesenteric, 06C6
    Innominate
      Left, 05C4
      Right, 05C3
    Internal Jugular
      Left, 05CN
      Right, 05CM
    Intracranial, 05CL
    Lower, 06CY
    Portal, 06C8
    Pulmonary
      Left, 02CT
      Right, 02CS
    Renal
      Left, 06CB
      Right, 06C9
    Saphenous
      Left, 06CQ
      Right, 06CP
    Splenic, 06C1
    Subclavian
      Left, 05C6
      Right, 05C5
    Superior Mesenteric, 06C5
    Upper, 05CY
    Vertebral
      Left, 05CS
      Right, 05CR
  Vena Cava
    Inferior, 06C0
    Superior, 02CV
  Ventricle
    Left, 02CL
    Right, 02CK
  Vertebra
    Cervical, 0PC3
    Lumbar, 0QC0
    Thoracic, 0PC4
  Vesicle
    Bilateral, 0VC3
    Left, 0VC2
    Right, 0VC1
  Vitreous
    Left, 08C5
    Right, 08C4
  Vocal Cord
    Left, 0CCV
    Right, 0CCT
  Vulva, 0UCM

Extracorporeal Carbon Dioxide Removal (ECCO2R),
  5A0920Z

Extracorporeal shock wave lithotripsy see Fragmentation

Extracranial-intracranial bypass (EC-IC) see Bypass,
  Upper Arteries, 031

Extraction
  Acetabulum
    Left, 0QD50ZZ
    Right, 0QD40ZZ
  Ampulla of Vater, 0FDC
  Anus, 0DDQ
  Appendix, 0DDJ
  Auditory Ossicle
    Left, 09DA0ZZ
    Right, 09D90ZZ
  Bone
    Ethmoid
      Left, 0NDG0ZZ
      Right, 0NDF0ZZ
    Frontal, 0ND10ZZ
    Hyoid, 0NDX0ZZ
    Lacrimal
      Left, 0NDJ0ZZ
      Right, 0NDH0ZZ
    Nasal, 0NDB0ZZ
    Occipital, 0ND70ZZ
    Palatine
      Left, 0NDL0ZZ
      Right, 0NDK0ZZ
    Parietal
      Left, 0ND40ZZ
      Right, 0ND30ZZ
    Pelvic
      Left, 0QD30ZZ
      Right, 0QD20ZZ
    Sphenoid, 0NDC0ZZ
    Temporal
      Left, 0ND60ZZ
      Right, 0ND50ZZ
    Zygomatic
      Left, 0NDN0ZZ
      Right, 0NDM0ZZ
  Bone Marrow
    Iliac, 07DR
    Sternum, 07DQ
    Vertebral, 07DS
  Bronchus
    Lingula, 0BD9
    Lower Lobe
      Left, 0BDB
      Right, 0BD6
    Main
      Left, 0BD7
      Right, 0BD3
    Middle Lobe, Right, 0BD5
    Upper Lobe
      Left, 0BD8
      Right, 0BD4
  Bursa and Ligament
    Abdomen
      Left, 0MDJ
      Right, 0MDH
    Ankle
      Left, 0MDR
      Right, 0MDQ
    Elbow
      Left, 0MD4
      Right, 0MD3
    Foot
      Left, 0MDT
      Right, 0MDS
    Hand
      Left, 0MD8
      Right, 0MD7
    Head and Neck, 0MD0
    Hip
      Left, 0MDM
      Right, 0MDL
    Knee
      Left, 0MDP
      Right, 0MDN
    Lower Extremity
      Left, 0MDW
      Right, 0MDV
    Perineum, 0MDK
    Rib(s), 0MDG
    Shoulder
      Left, 0MD2
      Right, 0MD1

Extraction — continued
  Bursa and Ligament — continued
    Spine
      Lower, 0MDD
      Upper, 0MDC
    Sternum, 0MDF
    Upper Extremity
      Left, 0MDB
      Right, 0MD9
    Wrist
      Left, 0MD6
      Right, 0MD5
  Carina, 0BD2
  Carpal
    Left, 0PDN0ZZ
    Right, 0PDM0ZZ
  Cecum, 0DDH
  Cerebral Meninges, 00D1
  Cisterna Chyli, 07DL
  Clavicle
    Left, 0PDB0ZZ
    Right, 0PD90ZZ
  Coccyx, 0QDS0ZZ
  Colon
    Ascending, 0DDK
    Descending, 0DDM
    Sigmoid, 0DDN
    Transverse, 0DDL
  Cornea
    Left, 08D9XZ
    Right, 08D8XZ
  Duct
    Common Bile, 0FD9
    Cystic, 0FD8
    Hepatic
      Common, 0FD7
      Left, 0FD6
      Right, 0FD5
    Pancreatic, 0FDD
      Accessory, 0FDF
  Duodenum, 0DD9
  Dura Mater, 00D2
  Endometrium, 0UDB
  Esophagogastric Junction, 0DD4
  Esophagus, 0DD5
    Lower, 0DD3
    Middle, 0DD2
    Upper, 0DD1
  Femoral Shaft
    Left, 0QD90ZZ
    Right, 0QD80ZZ
  Femur
    Lower
      Left, 0QDC0ZZ
      Right, 0QDB0ZZ
    Upper
      Left, 0QD70ZZ
      Right, 0QD60ZZ
  Fibula
    Left, 0QDK0ZZ
    Right, 0QDJ0ZZ
  Finger Nail, 0HDQXZZ
  Gallbladder, 0FD4
  Glenoid Cavity
    Left, 0PD80ZZ
    Right, 0PD70ZZ
  Hair, 0HDSXZZ
  Humeral Head
    Left, 0PDD0ZZ
    Right, 0PDC0ZZ
  Humeral Shaft
    Left, 0PDG0ZZ
    Right, 0PDF0ZZ
  Ileocecal Valve, 0DDC
  Ileum, 0DDB
  Intestine
    Large, 0DDE
      Left, 0DDG
      Right, 0DDF
    Small, 0DD8
  Jejunum, 0DDA
  Kidney
    Left, 0TD1
    Right, 0TD0
  Lens
    Left, 08DK3ZZ
    Right, 08DJ3ZZ
  Liver, 0FD0
    Left Lobe, 0FD2

Extraction — *continued*
  Liver — *continued*
    Right Lobe, ØFD1
  Lung
    Bilateral, ØBDM
    Left, ØBDL
    Lower Lobe
      Left, ØBDJ
      Right, ØBDF
    Middle Lobe, Right, ØBDD
    Right, ØBDK
    Upper Lobe
      Left, ØBDG
      Right, ØBDC
  Lung Lingula, ØBDH
  Lymphatic
    Aortic, Ø7DD
    Axillary
      Left, Ø7D6
      Right, Ø7D5
    Head, Ø7DØ
    Inguinal
      Left, Ø7DJ
      Right, Ø7DH
    Internal Mammary
      Left, Ø7D9
      Right, Ø7D8
    Lower Extremity
      Left, Ø7DG
      Right, Ø7DF
    Mesenteric, Ø7DB
    Neck
      Left, Ø7D2
      Right, Ø7D1
    Pelvis, Ø7DC
    Thoracic Duct, Ø7DK
    Thorax, Ø7D7
    Upper Extremity
      Left, Ø7D4
      Right, Ø7D3
  Mandible
    Left, ØNDVØZZ
    Right, ØNDTØZZ
  Maxilla, ØNDRØZZ
  Metacarpal
    Left, ØPDQØZZ
    Right, ØPDPØZZ
  Metatarsal
    Left, ØQDPØZZ
    Right, ØQDNØZZ
  Muscle
    Abdomen
      Left, ØKDLØZZ
      Right, ØKDKØZZ
    Facial, ØKD1ØZZ
    Foot
      Left, ØKDWØZZ
      Right, ØKDVØZZ
    Hand
      Left, ØKDDØZZ
      Right, ØKDCØZZ
    Head, ØKDØØZZ
    Hip
      Left, ØKDPØZZ
      Right, ØKDNØZZ
    Lower Arm and Wrist
      Left, ØKDBØZZ
      Right, ØKD9ØZZ
    Lower Leg
      Left, ØKDTØZZ
      Right, ØKDSØZZ
    Neck
      Left, ØKD3ØZZ
      Right, ØKD2ØZZ
    Perineum, ØKDMØZZ
    Shoulder
      Left, ØKD6ØZZ
      Right, ØKD5ØZZ
    Thorax
      Left, ØKDJØZZ
      Right, ØKDHØZZ
    Tongue, Palate, Pharynx, ØKD4ØZZ
    Trunk
      Left, ØKDGØZZ
      Right, ØKDFØZZ
    Upper Arm
      Left, ØKD8ØZZ
      Right, ØKD7ØZZ

Extraction — *continued*
  Muscle — *continued*
    Upper Leg
      Left, ØKDRØZZ
      Right, ØKDQØZZ
  Nerve
    Abdominal Sympathetic, Ø1DM
    Abducens, ØØDL
    Accessory, ØØDR
    Acoustic, ØØDN
    Brachial Plexus, Ø1D3
    Cervical, Ø1D1
    Cervical Plexus, Ø1DØ
    Facial, ØØDM
    Femoral, Ø1DD
    Glossopharyngeal, ØØDP
    Head and Neck Sympathetic, Ø1DK
    Hypoglossal, ØØDS
    Lumbar, Ø1DB
    Lumbar Plexus, Ø1D9
    Lumbar Sympathetic, Ø1DN
    Lumbosacral Plexus, Ø1DA
    Median, Ø1D5
    Oculomotor, ØØDH
    Olfactory, ØØDF
    Optic, ØØDG
    Peroneal, Ø1DH
    Phrenic, Ø1D2
    Pudendal, Ø1DC
    Radial, Ø1D6
    Sacral, Ø1DR
    Sacral Plexus, Ø1DQ
    Sacral Sympathetic, Ø1DP
    Sciatic, Ø1DF
    Thoracic, Ø1D8
    Thoracic Sympathetic, Ø1DL
    Tibial, Ø1DG
    Trigeminal, ØØDK
    Trochlear, ØØDJ
    Ulnar, Ø1D4
    Vagus, ØØDQ
  Orbit
    Left, ØNDQØZZ
    Right, ØNDPØZZ
  Ova, ØUDN
  Pancreas, ØFDG
  Patella
    Left, ØQDFØZZ
    Right, ØQDDØZZ
  Phalanx
    Finger
      Left, ØPDVØZZ
      Right, ØPDTØZZ
    Thumb
      Left, ØPDSØZZ
      Right, ØPDRØZZ
    Toe
      Left, ØQDRØZZ
      Right, ØQDQØZZ
  Pleura
    Left, ØBDP
    Right, ØBDN
  Products of Conception
    Ectopic, 1ØD2
    Extraperitoneal, 1ØDØØZ2
    High, 1ØDØØZØ
    High Forceps, 1ØDØ7Z5
    Internal Version, 1ØDØ7Z7
    Low, 1ØDØØZ1
    Low Forceps, 1ØDØ7Z3
    Mid Forceps, 1ØDØ7Z4
    Other, 1ØDØ7Z8
    Retained, 1ØD1
    Vacuum, 1ØDØ7Z6
  Radius
    Left, ØPDJØZZ
    Right, ØPDHØZZ
  Rectum, ØDDP
  Ribs
    1 to 2, ØPD1ØZZ
    3 or More, ØPD2ØZZ
  Sacrum, ØQD1ØZZ
  Scapula
    Left, ØPD6ØZZ
    Right, ØPD5ØZZ
  Septum, Nasal, Ø9DM
  Sinus
    Accessory, Ø9DP

Extraction — *continued*
  Sinus — *continued*
    Ethmoid
      Left, Ø9DV
      Right, Ø9DU
    Frontal
      Left, Ø9DT
      Right, Ø9DS
    Mastoid
      Left, Ø9DC
      Right, Ø9DB
    Maxillary
      Left, Ø9DR
      Right, Ø9DQ
    Sphenoid
      Left, Ø9DX
      Right, Ø9DW
  Skin
    Abdomen, ØHD7XZZ
    Back, ØHD6XZZ
    Buttock, ØHD8XZZ
    Chest, ØHD5XZZ
    Ear
      Left, ØHD3XZZ
      Right, ØHD2XZZ
    Face, ØHD1XZZ
    Foot
      Left, ØHDNXZZ
      Right, ØHDMXZZ
    Hand
      Left, ØHDGXZZ
      Right, ØHDFXZZ
    Inguinal, ØHDAXZZ
    Lower Arm
      Left, ØHDEXZZ
      Right, ØHDDXZZ
    Lower Leg
      Left, ØHDLXZZ
      Right, ØHDKXZZ
    Neck, ØHD4XZZ
    Perineum, ØHD9XZZ
    Scalp, ØHDØXZZ
    Upper Arm
      Left, ØHDCXZZ
      Right, ØHDBXZZ
    Upper Leg
      Left, ØHDJXZZ
      Right, ØHDHXZZ
  Skull, ØNDØØZZ
  Spinal Meninges, ØØDT
  Spleen, Ø7DP
  Sternum, ØPDØØZZ
  Stomach, ØDD6
    Pylorus, ØDD7
  Subcutaneous Tissue and Fascia
    Abdomen, ØJD8
    Back, ØJD7
    Buttock, ØJD9
    Chest, ØJD6
    Face, ØJD1
    Foot
      Left, ØJDR
      Right, ØJDQ
    Hand
      Left, ØJDK
      Right, ØJDJ
    Lower Arm
      Left, ØJDH
      Right, ØJDG
    Lower Leg
      Left, ØJDP
      Right, ØJDN
    Neck
      Left, ØJD5
      Right, ØJD4
    Pelvic Region, ØJDC
    Perineum, ØJDB
    Scalp, ØJDØ
    Upper Arm
      Left, ØJDF
      Right, ØJDD
    Upper Leg
      Left, ØJDM
      Right, ØJDL
  Tarsal
    Left, ØQDMØZZ
    Right, ØQDLØZZ

Subterms under main terms may continue to next column or page

Extraction — *continued*
  Tendon
    Abdomen
      Left, ØLDGØZZ
      Right, ØLDFØZZ
    Ankle
      Left, ØLDTØZZ
      Right, ØLDSØZZ
    Foot
      Left, ØLDWØZZ
      Right, ØLDVØZZ
    Hand
      Left, ØLD8ØZZ
      Right, ØLD7ØZZ
    Head and Neck, ØLD00ZZ
    Hip
      Left, ØLDKØZZ
      Right, ØLDJØZZ
    Knee
      Left, ØLDRØZZ
      Right, ØLDQØZZ
    Lower Arm and Wrist
      Left, ØLD6ØZZ
      Right, ØLD5ØZZ
    Lower Leg
      Left, ØLDPØZZ
      Right, ØLDNØZZ
    Perineum, ØLDHØZZ
    Shoulder
      Left, ØLD2ØZZ
      Right, ØLD1ØZZ
    Thorax
      Left, ØLDDØZZ
      Right, ØLDCØZZ
    Trunk
      Left, ØLDBØZZ
      Right, ØLD9ØZZ
    Upper Arm
      Left, ØLD4ØZZ
      Right, ØLD3ØZZ
    Upper Leg
      Left, ØLDMØZZ
      Right, ØDLLØZZ
  Thymus, Ø7DM
  Tibia
    Left, ØQDHØZZ
    Right, ØQDGØZZ
  Toe Nail, ØHDRXZZ
  Tooth
    Lower, ØCDXXZ
    Upper, ØCDWXZ
  Trachea, ØBD1
  Turbinate, Nasal, Ø9DL
  Tympanic Membrane
    Left, Ø9D8
    Right, Ø9D7
  Ulna
    Left, ØPDLØZZ
    Right, ØPDKØZZ
  Vein
    Basilic
      Left, Ø5DC
      Right, Ø5DB
    Brachial
      Left, Ø5DA
      Right, Ø5D9
    Cephalic
      Left, Ø5DF
      Right, Ø5DD
    Femoral
      Left, Ø6DN
      Right, Ø6DM
    Foot
      Left, Ø6DV
      Right, Ø6DT
    Hand
      Left, Ø5DH
      Right, Ø5DG
    Lower, Ø6DY
    Saphenous
      Left, Ø6DQ
      Right, Ø6DP
    Upper, Ø5DY
  Vertebra
    Cervical, ØPD3ØZZ
    Lumbar, ØQD00ZZ
    Thoracic, ØPD4ØZZ
  Vocal Cord
    Left, ØCDV

Extraction — *continued*
  Vocal Cord — *continued*
    Right, ØCDT
Extradural space, intracranial *use* Epidural Space, Intracranial
Extradural space, spinal *use* Spinal Canal
EXtreme Lateral Interbody Fusion (XLIF) device *use*
  Interbody Fusion Device in Lower Joints

F

Face lift *see* Alteration, Face, ØW02
Facet replacement spinal stabilization device
  use Spinal Stabilization Device, Facet Replacement
    in, ØRH
  use Spinal Stabilization Device, Facet Replacement
    in, ØSH
Facial artery *use* Face Artery
Factor Xa Inhibitor Reversal Agent, Andexanet Alfa
  use Andexanet Alfa, Factor Xa Inhibitor Reversal
    Agent
False vocal cord *use* Larynx
Falx cerebri *use* Dura Mater
Fascia lata
  use Subcutaneous Tissue and Fascia, Left Upper Leg
  use Subcutaneous Tissue and Fascia, Right Upper Leg
Fasciaplasty, fascioplasty
  see Repair, Subcutaneous Tissue and Fascia, ØJQ
  see Replacement, Subcutaneous Tissue and Fascia,
    ØJR
Fasciectomy *see* Excision, Subcutaneous Tissue and Fascia,
  ØJB
Fasciorrhaphy *see* Repair, Subcutaneous Tissue and Fascia, ØJQ
Fasciotomy
  see Division, Subcutaneous Tissue and Fascia, ØJ8
  see Drainage, Subcutaneous Tissue and Fascia, ØJ9
  see Release
Feeding Device
  Change device in
    Lower, ØD2DXUZ
    Upper, ØD20XUZ
  Insertion of device in
    Duodenum, ØDH9
    Esophagus, ØDH5
    Ileum, ØDHB
    Intestine, Small, ØDH8
    Jejunum, ØDHA
    Stomach, ØDH6
  Removal of device from
    Esophagus, ØDP5
    Intestinal Tract
      Lower, ØDPD
      Upper, ØDPØ
    Stomach, ØDP6
  Revision of device in
    Intestinal Tract
      Lower, ØDWD
      Upper, ØDWØ
    Stomach, ØDW6
Femoral head
  use Upper Femur, Left
  use Upper Femur, Right
Femoral lymph node
  use Lymphatic, Left Lower Extremity
  use Lymphatic, Right Lower Extremity
Femoropatellar joint
  use Knee Joint, Left
  use Knee Joint, Left, Tibial Surface
  use Knee Joint, Right
  use Knee Joint, Right, Femoral Surface
Femorotibial joint
  use Knee Joint, Left
  use Knee Joint, Left, Tibial Surface
  use Knee Joint, Right
  use KneeJoint, Right, Tibial Surface
Fibular artery
  use Peroneal Artery, Left
  use Peroneal Artery, Right
Fibularis brevis muscle
  use Lower Leg Muscle, Left
  use Lower Leg Muscle, Right
Fibularis longus muscle
  use Lower Leg Muscle, Left
  use Lower Leg Muscle, Right
Fifth cranial nerve *use* Trigeminal Nerve

Filum terminale *use* Spinal Meninges
Fimbriectomy
  see Excision, Female Reproductive System, ØUB
  see Resection, Female Reproductive System, ØUT
Fine needle aspiration
  Fluid or gas *see* Drainage
  Tissue biopsy
    see Excision
    see Extraction
First cranial nerve *use* Olfactory Nerve
First intercostal nerve *use* Brachial Plexus
Fistulization
  see Bypass
  see Drainage
  see Repair
Fitting
  Arch bars, for fracture reduction *see* Reposition,
    Mouth and Throat, ØCS
  Arch bars, for immobilization *see* Immobilization,
    Face, 2W31
  Artificial limb *see* Device Fitting, Rehabilitation, FØD
  Hearing aid *see* Device Fitting, Rehabilitation, FØD
  Ocular prosthesis, FØDZ8UZ
  Prosthesis, limb *see* Device Fitting, Rehabilitation,
    FØD
  Prosthesis, ocular, FØDZ8UZ
Fixation, bone
  External, with fracture reduction *see* Reposition
  External, without fracture reduction *see* Insertion
  Internal, with fracture reduction *see* Reposition
  Internal, without fracture reduction *see* Insertion
FLAIR® Endovascular Stent Graft *use* Intraluminal Device
Flexible Composite Mesh *use* Synthetic Substitute
Flexor carpi radialis muscle
  use Lower Arm and Wrist Muscle, Left
  use Lower Arm and Wrist Muscle, Right
Flexor carpi ulnaris muscle
  use Lower Arm and Wrist Muscle, Left
  use Lower Arm and Wrist Muscle, Right
Flexor digitorum brevis muscle
  use Foot Muscle, Left
  use Foot Muscle, Right
Flexor digitorum longus muscle
  use Lower Leg Muscle, Left
  use Lower Leg Muscle, Right
Flexor hallucis brevis muscle
  use Foot Muscle, Left
  use Foot Muscle, Right
Flexor hallucis longus muscle
  use Lower Leg Muscle, Left
  use Lower Leg Muscle, Right
Flexor pollicis longus muscle
  use Lower Arm and Wrist Muscle, Left
  use Lower Arm and Wrist Muscle, Right
Fluoroscopy
  Abdomen and Pelvis, BW11
  Airway, Upper, BB1DZZZ
  Ankle
    Left, BQ1H
    Right, BQ1G
  Aorta
    Abdominal, B41Ø
      Laser, Intraoperative, B41Ø
    Thoracic, B31Ø
      Laser, Intraoperative, B31Ø
    Thoraco-Abdominal, B31P
      Laser, Intraoperative, B31P
  Aorta and Bilateral Lower Extremity Arteries, B41D
    Laser, Intraoperative, B41D
  Arm
    Left, BP1FZZZ
    Right, BP1EZZZ
  Artery
    Brachiocephalic-Subclavian
      Laser, Intraoperative, B311
      Right, B311
    Bronchial, B31L
      Laser, Intraoperative, B31L
    Bypass Graft, Other, B21F
    Cervico-Cerebral Arch, B31Q
      Laser, Intraoperative, B31Q
    Common Carotid
      Bilateral, B315
        Laser, Intraoperative, B315
      Left, B314
        Laser, Intraoperative, B314
      Right, B313

Fluoroscopy — *continued*
  Artery — *continued*
    Common Carotid — *continued*
      Right — *continued*
        Laser, Intraoperative, B313
    Coronary
      Bypass Graft
        Multiple, B213
          Laser, Intraoperative, B213
        Single, B212
          Laser, Intraoperative, B212
      Multiple, B211
        Laser, Intraoperative, B211
      Single, B210
        Laser, Intraoperative, B210
    External Carotid
      Bilateral, B31C
        Laser, Intraoperative, B31C
      Left, B31B
        Laser, Intraoperative, B31B
      Right, B319
        Laser, Intraoperative, B319
    Hepatic, B412
      Laser, Intraoperative, B412
    Inferior Mesenteric, B415
      Laser, Intraoperative, B415
    Intercostal, B31L
      Laser, Intraoperative, B31L
    Internal Carotid
      Bilateral, B318
        Laser, Intraoperative, B318
      Left, B317
        Laser, Intraoperative, B317
      Right, B316
        Laser, Intraoperative, B316
    Internal Mammary Bypass Graft
      Left, B218
      Right, B217
    Intra-Abdominal
      Laser, Intraoperative, B41B
      Other, B41B
    Intracranial, B31R
      Laser, Intraoperative, B31R
    Lower
      Laser, Intraoperative, B41J
      Other, B41J
    Lower Extremity
      Bilateral and Aorta, B41D
        Laser, Intraoperative, B41D
      Left, B41G
        Laser, Intraoperative, B41G
      Right, B41F
        Laser, Intraoperative, B41F
    Lumbar, B419
      Laser, Intraoperative, B419
    Pelvic, B41C
      Laser, Intraoperative, B41C
    Pulmonary
      Left, B31T
        Laser, Intraoperative, B31T
      Right, B31S
        Laser, Intraoperative, B31S
    Pulmonary Trunk, B31U
      Laser, Intraoperative, B31U
    Renal
      Bilateral, B418
        Laser, Intraoperative, B418
      Left, B417
        Laser, Intraoperative, B417
      Right, B416
        Laser, Intraoperative, B416
    Spinal, B31M
      Laser, Intraoperative, B31M
    Splenic, B413
      Laser, Intraoperative, B413
    Subclavian
      Laser, Intraoperative, B312
      Left, B312
    Superior Mesenteric, B414
      Laser, Intraoperative, B414
    Upper
      Laser, Intraoperative, B31N
      Other, B31N
    Upper Extremity
      Bilateral, B31K
        Laser, Intraoperative, B31K
      Left, B31J
        Laser, Intraoperative, B31J
      Right, B31H

Fluoroscopy — *continued*
  Artery — *continued*
    Upper Extremity — *continued*
      Right — *continued*
        Laser, Intraoperative, B31H
    Vertebral
      Bilateral, B31G
        Laser, Intraoperative, B31G
      Left, B31F
        Laser, Intraoperative, B31F
      Right, B31D
        Laser, Intraoperative, B31D
  Bile Duct, BF10
    Pancreatic Duct and Gallbladder, BF14
  Bile Duct and Gallbladder, BF13
  Biliary Duct, BF11
  Bladder, BT10
    Kidney and Ureter, BT14
      Left, BT1F
      Right, BT1D
  Bladder and Urethra, BT1B
  Bowel, Small, BD1
  Calcaneus
    Left, BQ1KZZZ
    Right, BQ1JZZZ
  Clavicle
    Left, BP15ZZZ
    Right, BP14ZZZ
  Coccyx, BR1F
  Colon, BD14
  Corpora Cavernosa, BV10
  Dialysis Fistula, B51W
  Dialysis Shunt, B51W
  Diaphragm, BB16ZZZ
  Disc
    Cervical, BR11
    Lumbar, BR13
    Thoracic, BR12
  Duodenum, BD19
  Elbow
    Left, BP1H
    Right, BP1G
  Epiglottis, B91G
  Esophagus, BD11
  Extremity
    Lower, BW1C
    Upper, BW1J
  Facet Joint
    Cervical, BR14
    Lumbar, BR16
    Thoracic, BR15
  Fallopian Tube
    Bilateral, BU12
    Left, BU11
    Right, BU10
  Fallopian Tube and Uterus, BU18
  Femur
    Left, BQ14ZZZ
    Right, BQ13ZZZ
  Finger
    Left, BP1SZZZ
    Right, BP1RZZZ
  Foot
    Left, BQ1MZZZ
    Right, BQ1LZZZ
  Forearm
    Left, BP1KZZZ
    Right, BP1JZZZ
  Gallbladder, BF12
    Bile Duct and Pancreatic Duct, BF14
  Gallbladder and Bile Duct, BF13
  Gastrointestinal, Upper, BD1
  Hand
    Left, BP1PZZZ
    Right, BP1NZZZ
  Head and Neck, BW19
  Heart
    Left, B215
    Right, B214
    Right and Left, B216
  Hip
    Left, BQ11
    Right, BQ10
  Humerus
    Left, BP1BZZZ
    Right, BP1AZZZ
  Ileal Diversion Loop, BT1C
  Ileal Loop, Ureters and Kidney, BT1G
  Intracranial Sinus, B512

Fluoroscopy — *continued*
  Joint
    Acromioclavicular, Bilateral, BP13ZZZ
    Finger
      Left, BP1D
      Right, BP1C
    Foot
      Left, BQ1Y
      Right, BQ1X
    Hand
      Left, BP1D
      Right, BP1C
    Lumbosacral, BR1B
    Sacroiliac, BR1D
    Sternoclavicular
      Bilateral, BP12ZZZ
      Left, BP11ZZZ
      Right, BP10ZZZ
    Temporomandibular
      Bilateral, BN19
      Left, BN18
      Right, BN17
    Thoracolumbar, BR18
    Toe
      Left, BQ1Y
      Right, BQ1X
  Kidney
    Bilateral, BT13
    Ileal Loop and Ureter, BT1G
    Left, BT12
    Right, BT11
    Ureter and Bladder, BT14
      Left, BT1F
      Right, BT1D
  Knee
    Left, BQ18
    Right, BQ17
  Larynx, B91J
  Leg
    Left, BQ1FZZZ
    Right, BQ1DZZZ
  Lung
    Bilateral, BB14ZZZ
    Left, BB13ZZZ
    Right, BB12ZZZ
  Mediastinum, BB1CZZZ
  Mouth, BD1B
  Neck and Head, BW19
  Oropharynx, BD1B
  Pancreatic Duct, BF1
    Gallbladder and Bile Buct, BF14
  Patella
    Left, BQ1WZZZ
    Right, BQ1VZZZ
  Pelvis, BR1C
  Pelvis and Abdomen, BW11
  Pharynix, B91G
  Ribs
    Left, BP1YZZZ
    Right, BP1XZZZ
  Sacrum, BR1F
  Scapula
    Left, BP17ZZZ
    Right, BP16ZZZ
  Shoulder
    Left, BP19
    Right, BP18
  Sinus, Intracranial, B512
  Spinal Cord, B01B
  Spine
    Cervical, BR10
    Lumbar, BR19
    Thoracic, BR17
    Whole, BR1G
  Sternum, BR1H
  Stomach, BD12
  Toe
    Left, BQ1QZZZ
    Right, BQ1PZZZ
  Tracheobronchial Tree
    Bilateral, BB19YZZ
    Left, BB18YZZ
    Right, BB17YZZ
  Ureter
    Ileal Loop and Kidney, BT1G
    Kidney and Bladder, BT14
      Left, BT1F
      Right, BT1D
    Left, BT17

▼ **Subterms under main terms may continue to next column or page**

Fluoroscopy — *continued*
  Ureter — *continued*
    Right, BT16
  Urethra, BT15
  Urethra and Bladder, BT1B
  Uterus, BU16
  Uterus and Fallopian Tube, BU18
  Vagina, BU19
  Vasa Vasorum, BV18
  Vein
    Cerebellar, B511
    Cerebral, B511
    Epidural, B510
    Jugular
      Bilateral, B515
      Left, B514
      Right, B513
    Lower Extremity
      Bilateral, B51D
      Left, B51C
      Right, B51B
    Other, B51V
    Pelvic (Iliac)
      Left, B51G
      Right, B51F
    Pelvic (Iliac) Bilateral, B51H
    Portal, B51T
    Pulmonary
      Bilateral, B51S
      Left, B51R
      Right, B51Q
    Renal
      Bilateral, B51L
      Left, B51K
      Right, B51J
    Spanchnic, B51T
    Subclavian
      Left, B517
      Right, B516
    Upper Extremity
      Bilateral, B51P
      Left, B51N
      Right, B51M
  Vena Cava
    Inferior, B519
    Superior, B518
  Wrist
    Left, BP1M
    Right, BP1L
Fluoroscopy, laser intraoperative
  see Fluoroscopy, Heart, B21
  see Fluoroscopy, Lower Arteries, B41
  see Fluoroscopy, Upper Arteries, B31
Flushing *see* Irrigation
Foley catheter *use* Drainage Device
Fontan completion procedure Stage II *see* Bypass, Vena Cava, Inferior, 0610
Foramen magnum *use* Occipital Bone
Foramen of Monro (intraventricular) *use* Cerebral Ventricle
Foreskin *use* Prepuce
Formula™ Balloon-Expandable Renal Stent System *use* Intraluminal Device
Fossa of Rosenmuller *use* Nasopharynx
Fourth cranial nerve *use* Trochlear Nerve
Fourth ventricle *use* Cerebral Ventricle
Fovea
  use Retina, Left
  use Retina, Right
Fragmentation
  Ampulla of Vater, 0FFC
  Anus, 0DFQ
  Appendix, 0DFJ
  Bladder, 0TFB
  Bladder Neck, 0TFC
  Bronchus
    Lingula, 0BF9
    Lower Lobe
      Left, 0BFB
      Right, 0BF6
    Main
      Left, 0BF7
      Right, 0BF3
    Middle Lobe, Right, 0BF5
    Upper Lobe
      Left, 0BF8
      Right, 0BF4
  Carina, 0BF2

Fragmentation — *continued*
  Cavity, Cranial, 0WF1
  Cecum, 0DFH
  Cerebral Ventricle, 00F6
  Colon
    Ascending, 0DFK
    Descending, 0DFM
    Sigmoid, 0DFN
    Transverse, 0DFL
  Duct
    Common Bile, 0FF9
    Cystic, 0FF8
    Hepatic
      Common, 0FF7
      Left, 0FF6
      Right, 0FF5
    Pancreatic, 0FFD
      Accessory, 0FFF
    Parotid
      Left, 0CFC
      Right, 0CFB
  Duodenum, 0DF9
  Epidural Space, Intracranial, 00F3
  Esophagus, 0DF5
  Fallopian Tube
    Left, 0UF6
    Right, 0UF5
  Fallopian Tubes, Bilateral, 0UF7
  Gallbladder, 0FF4
  Gastrointestinal Tract, 0WFP
  Genitourinary Tract, 0WFR
  Ileum, 0DFB
  Intestine
    Large, 0DFE
      Left, 0DFG
      Right, 0DFF
    Small, 0DF8
  Jejunum, 0DFA
  Kidney Pelvis
    Left, 0TF4
    Right, 0TF3
  Mediastinum, 0WFC
  Oral Cavity and Throat, 0WF3
  Pelvic Cavity, 0WFJ
  Pericardial Cavity, 0WFD
  Pericardium, 02FN
  Peritoneal Cavity, 0WFG
  Pleural Cavity
    Left, 0WFB
    Right, 0WF9
  Rectum, 0DFP
  Respiratory Tract, 0WFQ
  Spinal Canal, 00FU
  Stomach, 0DF6
  Subarachnoid Space, Intracranial, 00F5
  Subdural Space, Intracranial, 00F4
  Trachea, 0BF1
  Ureter
    Left, 0TF7
    Right, 0TF6
  Urethra, 0TFD
  Uterus, 0UF9
  Vitreous
    Left, 08F5
    Right, 08F4
Freestyle (Stentless) Aortic Root Bioprosthesis *use* Zooplastic Tissue in Heart and Great Vessels
Frenectomy
  see Excision, Mouth and Throat, 0CB
  see Resection, Mouth and Throat, 0CT
Frenoplasty, frenuloplasty
  see Repair, Mouth and Throat, 0CQ
  see Replacement, Mouth and Throat, 0CR
  see Supplement, Mouth and Throat, 0CU
Frenotomy
  see Drainage, Mouth and Throat, 0C9
  see Release, Mouth and Throat, 0CN
Frenulotomy
  see Drainage, Mouth and Throat, 0C9
  see Release, Mouth and Throat, 0CN
Frenulum labii inferioris *use* Lower Lip
Frenulum labii superioris *use* Upper Lip
Frenulum linguae *use* Tongue
Frenulumectomy
  see Excision, Mouth and Throat, 0CB
  see Resection, Mouth and Throat, 0CT
Frontal lobe *use* Cerebral Hemisphere

Frontal vein
  use Face Vein, Left
  use Face Vein, Right
Fulguration *see* Destruction
Fundoplication, gastroesophageal *see* Restriction, Esophagogastric Junction, 0DV4
Fundus uteri *use* Uterus
Fusion
  Acromioclavicular
    Left, 0RGH
    Right, 0RGG
  Ankle
    Left, 0SGG
    Right, 0SGF
  Carpal
    Left, 0RGR
    Right, 0RGQ
  Carpometacarpal
    Left, 0RGT
    Right, 0RGS
  Cervical Vertebral, 0RG1
    2 or more, 0RG2
      Interbody Fusion Device
        Nanotextured Surface, XRG2092
        Radiolucent Porous, XRG20F3
      Interbody Fusion Device
        Nanotextured Surface, XRG1092
        Radiolucent Porous, XRG10F3
  Cervicothoracic Vertebral, 0RG4
    Interbody Fusion Device
      Nanotextured Surface, XRG4092
      Radiolucent Porous, XRG40F3
  Coccygeal, 0SG6
  Elbow
    Left, 0RGM
    Right, 0RGL
  Finger Phalangeal
    Left, 0RGX
    Right, 0RGW
  Hip
    Left, 0SGB
    Right, 0SG9
  Knee
    Left, 0SGD
    Right, 0SGC
  Lumbar Vertebral, 0SG0
    2 or more, 0SG1
      Interbody Fusion Device
        Nanotextured Surface, XRGC092
        Radiolucent Porous, XRGC0F3
      Interbody Fusion Device
        Nanotextured Surface, XRGB092
        Radiolucent Porous, XRGB0F3
  Lumbosacral, 0SG3
    Interbody Fusion Device
      Nanotextured Surface, XRGD092
      Radiolucent Porous, XRGD0F3
  Metacarpophalangeal
    Left, 0RGV
    Right, 0RGU
  Metatarsal-Phalangeal
    Left, 0SGN
    Right, 0SGM
  Occipital-cervical, 0RG0
    Interbody Fusion Device
      Nanotextured Surface, XRG0092
      Radiolucent Porous, XRG00F3
  Sacrococcygeal, 0SG5
  Sacroiliac
    Left, 0SG8
    Right, 0SG7
  Shoulder
    Left, 0RGK
    Right, 0RGJ
  Sternoclavicular
    Left, 0RGF
    Right, 0RGE
  Tarsal
    Left, 0SGJ
    Right, 0SGH
  Tarsometatarsal
    Left, 0SGL
    Right, 0SGK
  Temporomandibular
    Left, 0RGD
    Right, 0RGC
  Thoracic Vertebral, 0RG6
    2 to 7, 0RG7

Fusion

Fusion — *continued*
Thoracic Vertebral — *continued*
2 to 7 — *continued*
Interbody Fusion Device
Nanotextured Surface, XRG7Ø92
Radiolucent Porous, XRG7ØF3
8 or more, ØRG8
Interbody Fusion Device
Nanotextured Surface, XRG8Ø92
Radiolucent Porous, XRG8ØF3
Interbody Fusion Device
Nanotextured Surface, XRG6Ø92
Radiolucent Porous, XRG6ØF3
Thoracolumbar Vertebral, ØRGA
Interbody Fusion Device
Nanotextured Surface, XRGAØ92
Radiolucent Porous, XRGAØF3
Toe Phalangeal
Left, ØSGQ
Right, ØSGP
Wrist
Left, ØRGP
Right, ØRGN
Fusion screw (compression) (lag) (locking)
use Internal Fixation Device in Lower Joints
use Internal Fixation Device in Upper Joints

G

Gait training *see* Motor Treatment, Rehabilitation, FØ7
Galea aponeurotica *use* Subcutaneous Tissue and Fascia, Scalp
GammaTile™ *use* Radioactive Element, Cesium-131 Collagen Implant in ØØH
Ganglion impar (ganglion of Walther) *use* Sacral Sympathetic Nerve
Ganglionectomy
Destruction of lesion *see* Destruction
Excision of lesion *see* Excision
Gasserian ganglion *use* Trigeminal Nerve
Gastrectomy
Partial *see* Excision, Stomach, ØDB6
Total *see* Resection, Stomach, ØDT6
Vertical (sleeve) *see* Excision, Stomach, ØDB6
Gastric electrical stimulation (GES) lead *use* Stimulator Lead in Gastrointestinal System
Gastric lymph node *use* Lymphatic, Aortic
Gastric pacemaker lead *use* Stimulator Lead in Gastrointestinal System
Gastric plexus *use* Abdominal Sympathetic Nerve
Gastrocnemius muscle
use Lower Leg Muscle, Left
use Lower Leg Muscle, Right
Gastrocolic ligament *use* Omentum
Gastrocolic omentum *use* Omentum
Gastrocolostomy
see Bypass, Gastrointestinal System, ØD1
see Drainage, Gastrointestinal System, ØD9
Gastroduodenal artery *use* Hepatic Artery
Gastroduodenectomy
see Excision, Gastrointestinal System, ØDB
see Resection, Gastrointestinal System, ØDT
Gastroduodenoscopy, ØDJØ8ZZ
Gastroenteroplasty
see Repair, Gastrointestinal System, ØDQ
see Supplement, Gastrointestinal System, ØDU
Gastroenterostomy
see Bypass, Gastrointestinal System, ØD1
see Drainage, Gastrointestinal System, ØD9
Gastroesophageal (GE) junction *use* Esophagogastric Junction
Gastrogastrostomy
see Bypass, Stomach, ØD16
see Drainage, Stomach, ØD96
Gastrohepatic omentum *use* Omentum
Gastrojejunostomy
see Bypass, Stomach, ØD16
see Drainage, Stomach, ØD96
Gastrolysis *see* Release, Stomach, ØDN6
Gastropexy
see Repair, Stomach, ØDQ6
see Reposition, Stomach, ØDS6
Gastrophrenic ligament *use* Omentum
Gastroplasty
see Repair, Stomach, ØDQ6
see Supplement, Stomach, ØDU6

Gastroplication *see* Restriction, Stomach, ØDV6
Gastropylorectomy *see* Excision, Gastrointestinal System, ØDB
Gastrorrhaphy *see* Repair, Stomach, ØDQ6
Gastroscopy, ØDJ68ZZ
Gastrosplenic ligament *use* Omentum
Gastrostomy
see Bypass, Stomach, ØD16
see Drainage, Stomach, ØD96
Gastrotomy *see* Drainage, Stomach, ØD96
Gemellus muscle
use Hip Muscle, Left
use Hip Muscle, Right
Geniculate ganglion *use* Facial Nerve
Geniculate nucleus *use* Thalamus
Genioglossus muscle *use* Tongue, Palate, Pharynx Muscle
Genioplasty *see* Alteration, Jaw, Lower, ØWØ5
Genitofemoral nerve *use* Lumbar Plexus
GIAPREZA™ *use* Synthetic Human Angiotensin II
Gingivectomy *see* Excision, Mouth and Throat, ØCB
Gingivoplasty
see Repair, Mouth and Throat, ØCQ
see Replacement, Mouth and Throat, ØCR
see Supplement, Mouth and Throat, ØCU
Glans penis *use* Prepuce
Glenohumeral joint
use Shoulder Joint, Left
use Shoulder Joint, Right
Glenohumeral ligament
use Shoulder Bursa and Ligament, Left
use Shoulder Bursa and Ligament, Right
Glenoid fossa (of scapula)
use Glenoid Cavity, Left
use Glenoid Cavity, Right
Glenoid ligament (labrum)
use Shoulder Joint, Left
use Shoulder Joint, Right
Globus pallidus *use* Basal Ganglia
Glomectomy
see Excision, Endocrine System, ØGB
see Resection, Endocrine System, ØGT
Glossectomy
see Excision, Tongue, ØCB7
see Resection, Tongue, ØCT7
Glossoepiglottic fold *use* Epiglottis
Glossopexy
see Repair, Tongue, ØCQ7
see Reposition, Tongue, ØCS7
Glossoplasty
see Repair, Tongue, ØCQ7
see Replacement, Tongue, ØCR7
see Supplement, Tongue, ØCU7
Glossorrhaphy *see* Repair, Tongue, ØCQ7
Glossotomy *see* Drainage, Tongue, ØC97
Glottis *use* Larynx
Gluteal Artery Perforator Flap
Replacement
Bilateral, ØHRVØ79
Left, ØHRUØ79
Right, ØHRTØ79
Transfer
Left, ØKXG
Right, ØKXF
Gluteal lymph node *use* Lymphatic, Pelvis
Gluteal vein
use Hypogastric Vein, Left
use Hypogastric Vein, Right
Gluteus maximus muscle
use Hip Muscle, Left
use Hip Muscle, Right
Gluteus medius muscle
use Hip Muscle, Left
use Hip Muscle, Right
Gluteus minimus muscle
use Hip Muscle, Left
use Hip Muscle, Right
GORE EXCLUDER® AAA Endoprosthesis
use Intraluminal Device
use Intraluminal Device, Branched or Fenestrated, One or Two Arteries in, Ø4V
use Intraluminal Device, Branched or Fenestrated, Three or More Arteries in, Ø4V
GORE EXCLUDER® IBE Endoprosthesis *use* Intraluminal Device, Branched or Fenestrated, One or Two Arteries in, Ø4V

GORE TAG® Thoracic Endoprosthesis *use* Intraluminal Device
GORE® DUALMESH® *use* Synthetic Substitute
Gracilis muscle
use Upper Leg Muscle, Left
use Upper Leg Muscle, Right
Graft
see Replacement
see Supplement
Great auricular nerve *use* Cervical Plexus
Great cerebral vein *use* Intracranial Vein
Great(er) saphenous vein
use Saphenous Vein, Left
use Saphenous Vein, Right
Greater alar cartilage *use* Nasal Mucosa and Soft Tissue
Greater occipital nerve *use* Cervical Nerve
Greater Omentum *use* Omentum
Greater splanchnic nerve *use* Thoracic Sympathetic Nerve
Greater superficial petrosal nerve *use* Facial Nerve
Greater trochanter
use Upper Femur, Left
use Upper Femur, Right
Greater tuberosity
use Humeral Head, Left
use Humeral Head, Right
Greater vestibular (Bartholin's) gland *use* Vestibular Gland
Greater wing *use* Sphenoid Bone
Guedel airway *use* Intraluminal Device, Airway in Mouth and Throat
Guidance, catheter placement
EKG *see* Measurement, Physiological Systems, 4AØ
Fluoroscopy *see* Fluoroscopy, Veins, B51
Ultrasound *see* Ultrasonography, Veins, B54

H

Hallux
use 1st Toe, Left
use 1st Toe, Right
Hamate bone
use Carpal, Left
use Carpal, Right
Hancock Bioprosthesis (aortic) (mitral) valve *use* Zooplastic Tissue in Heart and Great Vessels
Hancock Bioprosthetic Valved Conduit *use* Zooplastic Tissue in Heart and Great Vessels
Harvesting, stem cells *see* Pheresis, Circulatory, 6A55
Head of fibula
use Fibula, Left
use Fibula, Right
Hearing Aid Assessment, F14Z
Hearing Assessment, F13Z
Hearing Device
Bone Conduction
Left, Ø9HE
Right, Ø9HD
Insertion of device in
Left, ØNH6
Right, ØNH5
Multiple Channel Cochlear Prosthesis
Left, Ø9HE
Right, Ø9HD
Removal of device from, Skull, ØNPØ
Revision of device in, Skull, ØNWØ
Single Channel Cochlear Prosthesis
Left, Ø9HE
Right, Ø9HD
Hearing Treatment, FØ9Z
Heart Assist System
Implantable
Insertion of device in, Heart, Ø2HA
Removal of device from, Heart, Ø2PA
Revision of device in, Heart, Ø2WA
Short-term External
Insertion of device in, Heart, Ø2HA
Removal of device from, Heart, Ø2PA
Revision of device in, Heart, Ø2WA
HeartMate 3™ LVAS *use* Implantable Heart Assist System in Heart and Great Vessels
HeartMate II® Left Ventricular Assist Device (LVAD)
use Implantable Heart Assist System in Heart and Great Vessels

  Subterms under main terms may continue to next column or page

HeartMate XVE® Left Ventricular Assist Device (LVAD) *use* Implantable Heart Assist System in Heart and Great Vessels

HeartMate® implantable heart assist system *see* Insertion of device in, Heart, 02HA

Helix
use Ear, External, Bilateral
use Ear, External, Left
use Ear, External, Right

Hematopoietic cell transplant (HCT) *see* Transfusion, Circulatory, 302

Hemicolectomy *see* Resection, Gastrointestinal System, 0DT

Hemicystectomy *see* Excision, Urinary System, 0TB

Hemigastrectomy *see* Excision, Gastrointestinal System, 0DB

Hemiglossectomy *see* Excision, Mouth and Throat, 0CB

Hemilaminectomy
see Excision, Lower Bones, 0QB
see Excision, Upper Bones, 0PB

Hemilaminotomy
see Drainage, Lower Bones, 0Q9
see Drainage, Upper Bones, 0P9
see Excision, Lower Bones, 0QB
see Excision, Upper Bones, 0PB
see Release, Central Nervous System and Cranial Nerves, 00N
see Release, Lower Bones, 0QN
see Release, Peripheral Nervous System, 01N
see Release, Upper Bones, 0PN

Hemilaryngectomy *see* Excision, Larynx, 0CBS

Hemimandibulectomy *see* Excision, Head and Facial Bones, 0NB

Hemimaxillectomy *see* Excision, Head and Facial Bones, 0NB

Hemipylorectomy *see* Excision, Gastrointestinal System, 0DB

Hemispherectomy
see Excision, Central Nervous System and Cranial Nerves, 00B
see Resection, Central Nervous System and Cranial Nerves, 00T

Hemithyroidectomy
see Excision, Endocrine System, 0GB
see Resection, Endocrine System, 0GT

Hemodialysis *see* Performance, Urinary, 5A1D

Hemolung® Respiratory Assist System (RAS), 5A0920Z

Hepatectomy
see Excision, Hepatobiliary System and Pancreas, 0FB
see Resection, Hepatobiliary System and Pancreas, 0FT

Hepatic artery proper *use* Hepatic Artery

Hepatic flexure *use* Transverse Colon

Hepatic lymph node *use* Lymphatic, Aortic

Hepatic plexus *use* Abdominal Sympathetic Nerve

Hepatic portal vein *use* Portal Vein

Hepaticoduodenostomy
see Bypass, Hepatobiliary System and Pancreas, 0F1
see Drainage, Hepatobiliary System and Pancreas, 0F9

Hepaticotomy *see* Drainage, Hepatobiliary System and Pancreas, 0F9

Hepatocholedochostomy *see* Drainage, Duct, Common Bile, 0F99

Hepatogastric ligament *use* Omentum

Hepatopancreatic ampulla *use* Ampulla of Vater

Hepatopexy
see Repair, Hepatobiliary System and Pancreas, 0FQ
see Reposition, Hepatobiliary System and Pancreas, 0FS

Hepatorrhaphy *see* Repair, Hepatobiliary System and Pancreas, 0FQ

Hepatotomy *see* Drainage, Hepatobiliary System and Pancreas, 0F9

Herculink (RX) Elite Renal Stent System *use* Intraluminal Device

Herniorrhaphy
With synthetic substitute
see Supplement, Anatomical Regions, General, 0WU
see Supplement, Anatomical Regions, Lower Extremities, 0YU
see Repair, Anatomical Regions, General, 0WQ
see Repair, Anatomical Regions, Lower Extremities, 0YQ

Hip (joint) liner *use* Liner in Lower Joints

Holter monitoring, 4A12X45

Holter valve ventricular shunt *use* Synthetic Substitute

Human angiotensin II, synthetic *use* Synthetic Human Angiotensin II

Humeroradial joint
use Elbow Joint, Left
use Elbow Joint, Right

Humeroulnar joint
use Elbow Joint, Left
use Elbow Joint, Right

Humerus, distal
use Humeral Shaft, Left
use Humeral Shaft, Right

Hydrocelectomy *see* Excision, Male Reproductive System, 0VB

Hydrotherapy
Assisted exercise in pool *see* Motor Treatment, Rehabilitation, F07
Whirlpool *see* Activities of Daily Living Treatment, Rehabilitation, F08

Hymenectomy
see Excision, Hymen, 0UBK
see Resection, Hymen, 0UTK

Hymenoplasty
see Repair, Hymen, 0UQK
see Supplement, Hymen, 0UUK

Hymenorrhaphy *see* Repair, Hymen, 0UQK

Hymenotomy
see Division, Hymen, 0U8K
see Drainage, Hymen, 0U9K

Hyoglossus muscle *use* Tongue, Palate, Pharynx Muscle

Hyoid artery
use Thyroid Artery, Left
use Thyroid Artery, Right

Hyperalimentation *see* Introduction of substance in or on

Hyperbaric oxygenation
Decompression sickness treatment *see* Decompression, Circulatory, 6A15
Wound treatment *see* Assistance, Circulatory, 5A05

Hyperthermia
Radiation Therapy
Abdomen, DWY38ZZ
Adrenal Gland, DGY28ZZ
Bile Ducts, DFY28ZZ
Bladder, DTY28ZZ
Bone Marrow, D7Y08ZZ
Bone, Other, DPYC8ZZ
Brain, D0Y08ZZ
Brain Stem, D0Y18ZZ
Breast
Left, DMY08ZZ
Right, DMY18ZZ
Bronchus, DBY18ZZ
Cervix, DUY18ZZ
Chest, DWY28ZZ
Chest Wall, DBY78ZZ
Colon, DDY58ZZ
Diaphragm, DBY88ZZ
Duodenum, DDY28ZZ
Ear, D9Y08ZZ
Esophagus, DDY08ZZ
Eye, D8Y08ZZ
Femur, DPY98ZZ
Fibula, DPYB8ZZ
Gallbladder, DFY18ZZ
Gland
Adrenal, DGY28ZZ
Parathyroid, DGY48ZZ
Pituitary, DGY08ZZ
Thyroid, DGY58ZZ
Glands, Salivary, D9Y68ZZ
Head and Neck, DWY18ZZ
Hemibody, DWY48ZZ
Humerus, DPY68ZZ
Hypopharynx, D9Y38ZZ
Ileum, DDY48ZZ
Jejunum, DDY38ZZ
Kidney, DTY08ZZ
Larynx, D9YB8ZZ
Liver, DFY08ZZ
Lung, DBY28ZZ
Lymphatics
Abdomen, D7Y68ZZ
Axillary, D7Y48ZZ
Inguinal, D7Y78ZZ
Neck, D7Y38ZZ
Pelvis, D7Y78ZZ
Thorax, D7Y58ZZ

Hyperthermia — *continued*
Radiation Therapy — *continued*
Mandible, DPY38ZZ
Maxilla, DPY28ZZ
Mediastinum, DBY68ZZ
Mouth, D9Y48ZZ
Nasopharynx, D9YD8ZZ
Neck and Head, DWY18ZZ
Nerve, Peripheral, D0Y78ZZ
Nose, D9Y18ZZ
Oropharynx, D9YF8ZZ
Ovary, DUY08ZZ
Palate
Hard, D9Y88ZZ
Soft, D9Y98ZZ
Pancreas, DFY38ZZ
Parathyroid Gland, DGY48ZZ
Pelvic Bones, DPY88ZZ
Pelvic Region, DWY68ZZ
Pineal Body, DGY18ZZ
Pituitary Gland, DGY08ZZ
Pleura, DBY58ZZ
Prostate, DVY08ZZ
Radius, DPY78ZZ
Rectum, DDY78ZZ
Rib, DPY58ZZ
Sinuses, D9Y78ZZ
Skin
Abdomen, DHY88ZZ
Arm, DHY48ZZ
Back, DHY78ZZ
Buttock, DHY98ZZ
Chest, DHY68ZZ
Face, DHY28ZZ
Leg, DHYB8ZZ
Neck, DHY38ZZ
Skull, DPY08ZZ
Spinal Cord, D0Y68ZZ
Spleen, D7Y28ZZ
Sternum, DPY48ZZ
Stomach, DDY18ZZ
Testis, DVY18ZZ
Thymus, D7Y18ZZ
Thyroid Gland, DGY58ZZ
Tibia, DPYB8ZZ
Tongue, D9Y58ZZ
Trachea, DBY08ZZ
Ulna, DPY78ZZ
Ureter, DTY18ZZ
Urethra, DTY38ZZ
Uterus, DUY28ZZ
Whole Body, DWY58ZZ
Whole Body, 6A3Z

Hypnosis, GZFZZZZ

Hypogastric artery
use Internal Iliac Artery, Left
use Internal Iliac Artery, Right

Hypopharynx *use* Pharynx

Hypophysectomy
see Excision, Gland, Pituitary, 0GB0
see Resection, Gland, Pituitary, 0GT0

Hypophysis *use* Pituitary Gland

Hypothalamotomy *see* Destruction, Thalamus, 0059

Hypothenar muscle
use Hand Muscle, Left
use Hand Muscle, Right

Hypothermia, Whole Body, 6A4Z

Hysterectomy
Supracervical *see* Resection, Uterus, 0UT9
Total *see* Resection, Uterus, 0UT9

Hysterolysis *see* Release, Uterus, 0UN9

Hysteropexy
see Repair, Uterus, 0UQ9
see Reposition, Uterus, 0US9

Hysteroplasty *see* Repair, Uterus, 0UQ9

Hysterorrhaphy *see* Repair, Uterus, 0UQ9

Hysteroscopy, 0UJD8ZZ

Hysterotomy *see* Drainage, Uterus, 0U99

Hysterotrachelectomy
see Resection, Cervix, 0UTC
see Resection, Uterus, 0UT9

Hysterotracheloplasty *see* Repair, Uterus, 0UQ9

Hysterotrachelorrhaphy *see* Repair, Uterus, 0UQ9

I

IABP (Intra-aortic balloon pump) *see* Assistance, Cardiac, 5A02
IAEMT (Intraoperative anesthetic effect monitoring and titration) *see* Monitoring, Central Nervous, 4A10
Idarucizumab, Dabigatran Reversal Agent, XW0
IHD (Intermittent hemodialysis), 5A1D70Z
Ileal artery *use* Superior Mesenteric Artery
Ileectomy
  see Excision, Ileum, 0DBB
  see Resection, Ileum, 0DTB
Ileocolic artery *use* Superior Mesenteric Artery
Ileocolic vein *use* Colic Vein
Ileopexy
  see Repair, Ileum, 0DQB
  see Reposition, Ileum, 0DSB
Ileorrhaphy *see* Repair, Ileum, 0DQB
Ileoscopy, 0DJD8ZZ
Ileostomy
  see Bypass, Ileum, 0D1B
  see Drainage, Ileum, 0D9B
Ileotomy *see* Drainage, Ileum, 0D9B
Ileoureterostomy *see* Bypass, Urinary System, 0T1
Iliac crest
  use Pelvic Bone, Left
  use Pelvic Bone, Right
Iliac fascia
  use Subcutaneous Tissue and Fascia, Left Upper Leg
  use Subcutaneous Tissue and Fascia, Right Upper Leg
Iliac lymph node *use* Lymphatic, Pelvis
Iliacus muscle
  use Hip Muscle, Left
  use Hip Muscle, Right
Iliofemoral ligament
  use Hip Bursa and Ligament, Left
  use Hip Bursa and Ligament, Right
Iliohypogastric nerve *use* Lumbar Plexus
Ilioinguinal nerve *use* Lumbar Plexus
Iliolumbar artery
  use Internal Iliac Artery, Left
  use Internal Iliac Artery, Right
Iliolumbar ligament *use* Lower Spine Bursa and Ligament
Iliotibial tract (band)
  use Subcutaneous Tissue and Fascia, Left Upper Leg
  use Subcutaneous Tissue and Fascia, Right Upper Leg
Ilium
  use Pelvic Bone, Left
  use Pelvic Bone, Right
Ilizarov external fixator
  use External Fixation Device, Ring in, 0PH
  use External Fixation Device, Ring in, 0PS
  use External Fixation Device, Ring in, 0QH
  use External Fixation Device, Ring in, 0QS
Ilizarov-Vecklich device
  use External Fixation Device, Limb Lengthening in, 0PH
  use External Fixation Device, Limb Lengthening in, 0QH
Imaging, diagnostic
  see Computerized Tomography (CT Scan)
  see Fluoroscopy
  see Magnetic Resonance Imaging (MRI)
  see Plain Radiography
  see Ultrasonography
Immobilization
  Abdominal Wall, 2W33X
  Arm
    Lower
      Left, 2W3DX
      Right, 2W3CX
    Upper
      Left, 2W3BX
      Right, 2W3AX
  Back, 2W35X
  Chest Wall, 2W34X
  Extremity
    Lower
      Left, 2W3MX
      Right, 2W3LX
    Upper
      Left, 2W39X
      Right, 2W38X
  Face, 2W31X

Immobilization — *continued*
  Finger
    Left, 2W3KX
    Right, 2W3JX
  Foot
    Left, 2W3TX
    Right, 2W3SX
  Hand
    Left, 2W3FX
    Right, 2W3EX
  Head, 2W30X
  Inguinal Region
    Left, 2W37X
    Right, 2W36X
  Leg
    Lower
      Left, 2W3RX
      Right, 2W3QX
    Upper
      Left, 2W3PX
      Right, 2W3NX
  Neck, 2W32X
  Thumb
    Left, 2W3HX
    Right, 2W3GX
  Toe
    Left, 2W3VX
    Right, 2W3UX
Immunization *see* Introduction of Serum, Toxoid, and Vaccine
Immunotherapy *see* Introduction of Immunotherapeutic Substance
Immunotherapy, antineoplastic
  Interferon *see* Introduction of Low-dose Interleukin-2
  Interleukin-2, high-dose *see* Introduction of High-dose Interleukin-2
  Interleukin-2, low-dose *see* Introduction of Low-dose Interleukin-2
  Monoclonal antibody *see* Introduction of Monoclonal Antibody
  Proleukin, high-dose *see* Introduction of High-dose Interleukin-2
  Proleukin, low-dose *see* Introduction of Low-dose Interleukin-2
Impella® heart pump *use* Short-term External Heart Assist System in Heart and Great Vessels
Impeller Pump
  Continuous, Output, 5A0221D
  Intermittent, Output, 5A0211D
Implantable cardioverter-defibrillator (ICD) *use* Defibrillator Generator in, 0JH
Implantable drug infusion pump (anti-spasmodic) (chemotherapy) (pain) *use* Infusion Device, Pump in Subcutaneous Tissue and Fascia
Implantable glucose monitoring device *use* Monitoring Device
Implantable hemodynamic monitor (IHM) *use* Monitoring Device, Hemodynamic in, 0JH
Implantable hemodynamic monitoring system (IHMS) *use* Monitoring Device, Hemodynamic in, 0JH
Implantable Miniature Telescope™ (IMT) *use* Synthetic Substitute, Intraocular Telescope in, 08R
Implantation
  see Insertion
  see Replacement
Implanted (venous)(access) port *use* Vascular Access Device, Totally Implantable in Subcutaneous Tissue and Fascia
IMV (intermittent mandatory ventilation) *see* Assistance, Respiratory, 5A09
In Vitro Fertilization, 8E0ZXY1
Incision, abscess *see* Drainage
Incudectomy
  see Excision, Ear, Nose, Sinus, 09B
  see Resection, Ear, Nose, Sinus, 09T
Incudopexy
  see Repair, Ear, Nose, Sinus, 09Q
  see Reposition, Ear, Nose, Sinus, 09S
Incus
  use Auditory Ossicle, Left
  use Auditory Ossicle, Right
Induction of labor
  Artificial rupture of membranes *see* Drainage, Pregnancy, 109
  Oxytocin *see* Introduction of Hormone

InDura, intrathecal catheter (1P) (spinal) *use* Infusion Device
Inferior cardiac nerve *use* Thoracic Sympathetic Nerve
Inferior cerebellar vein *use* Intracranial Vein
Inferior cerebral vein *use* Intracranial Vein
Inferior epigastric artery
  use External Iliac Artery, Left
  use External Iliac Artery, Right
Inferior epigastric lymph node *use* Lymphatic, Pelvis
Inferior genicular artery
  use Popliteal Artery, Left
  use Popliteal Artery, Right
Inferior gluteal artery
  use Internal Iliac Artery, Left
  use Internal Iliac Artery, Right
Inferior gluteal nerve *use* Sacral Plexus
Inferior hypogastric plexus *use* Abdominal Sympathetic Nerve
Inferior labial artery *use* Face Artery
Inferior longitudinal muscle *use* Tongue, Palate, Pharynx Muscle
Inferior mesenteric ganglion *use* Abdominal Sympathetic Nerve
Inferior mesenteric lymph node *use* Lymphatic, Mesenteric
Inferior mesenteric plexus *use* Abdominal Sympathetic Nerve
Inferior oblique muscle
  use Extraocular Muscle, Left
  use Extraocular Muscle, Right
Inferior pancreaticoduodenal artery *use* Superior Mesenteric Artery
Inferior phrenic artery *use* Abdominal Aorta
Inferior rectus muscle
  use Extraocular Muscle, Left
  use Extraocular Muscle, Right
Inferior suprarenal artery
  use Renal Artery, Left
  use Renal Artery, Right
Inferior tarsal plate
  use Lower Eyelid, Left
  use Lower Eyelid, Right
Inferior thyroid vein
  use Innominate Vein, Left
  use Innominate Vein, Right
Inferior tibiofibular joint
  use Ankle Joint, Left
  use Ankle Joint, Right
Inferior turbinate *use* Nasal Turbinate
Inferior ulnar collateral artery
  use Brachial Artery, Left
  use Brachial Artery, Right
Inferior vesical artery
  use Internal Iliac Artery, Left
  use Internal Iliac Artery, Right
Infraauricular lymph node *use* Lymphatic, Head
Infraclavicular (deltopectoral) lymph node
  use Lymphatic, Left Upper Extremity
  use Lymphatic, Right Upper Extremity
Infrahyoid muscle
  use Neck Muscle, Left
  use Neck Muscle, Right
Infraparotid lymph node *use* Lymphatic, Head
Infraspinatus fascia
  use Subcutaneous Tissue and Fascia, Left Upper Arm
  use Subcutaneous Tissue and Fascia, Right Upper Arm
Infraspinatus muscle
  use Shoulder Muscle, Left
  use Shoulder Muscle, Right
Infundibulopelvic ligament *use* Uterine Supporting Structure
Infusion *see* Introduction of substance in or on
Infusion Device, Pump
  Insertion of device in
    Abdomen, 0JH8
    Back, 0JH7
    Chest, 0JH6
    Lower Arm
      Left, 0JHH
      Right, 0JHG
    Lower Leg
      Left, 0JHP
      Right, 0JHN
    Trunk, 0JHT
    Upper Arm
      Left, 0JHF
      Right, 0JHD

Subterms under main terms may continue to next column or page

Infusion Device, Pump — continued
  Insertion of device in — continued
    Upper Leg
      Left, ØJHM
      Right, ØJHL
  Removal of device from
    Lower Extremity, ØJPW
    Trunk, ØJPT
    Upper Extremity, ØJPV
  Revision of device in
    Lower Extremity, ØJWW
    Trunk, ØJWT
    Upper Extremity, ØJWV
Infusion, glucarpidase
  Central Vein, 3E043GQ
  Peripheral Vein, 3E033GQ
Inguinal canal
  use Inguinal Region, Bilateral
  use Inguinal Region, Left
  use Inguinal Region, Right
Inguinal triangle
  use Inguinal Region, Bilateral
  use Inguinal Region, Left
  use Inguinal Region, Right
Injection *see* Introduction of substance in or on
Injection, Concentrated Bone Marrow Aspirate (CB-MA), intramuscular, XK02303
Injection reservoir, port *use* Vascular Access Device, Totally Implantable in Subcutaneous Tissue and Fascia
Injection reservoir, pump *use* Infusion Device, Pump in Subcutaneous Tissue and Fascia
Insemination, artificial, 3E0P7LZ
Insertion
  Antimicrobial envelope *see* Introduction of Anti-infective
  Aqueous drainage shunt
    see Bypass, Eye, Ø81
    see Drainage, Eye, Ø89
  Products of Conception, 10H0
  Spinal Stabilization Device
    see Insertion of device in, Lower Joints, ØSH
    see Insertion of device in, Upper Joints, ØRH
Insertion of device in
  Abdominal Wall, ØWHF
  Acetabulum
    Left, ØQH5
    Right, ØQH4
  Anal Sphincter, ØDHR
  Ankle Region
    Left, ØYHL
    Right, ØYHK
  Anus, ØDHQ
  Aorta
    Abdominal, 04H0
    Thoracic
      Ascending/Arch, 02HX
      Descending, 02HW
  Arm
    Lower
      Left, ØXHF
      Right, ØXHD
    Upper
      Left, ØXH9
      Right, ØXH8
  Artery
    Anterior Tibial
      Left, 04HQ
      Right, 04HP
    Axillary
      Left, 03H6
      Right, 03H5
    Brachial
      Left, 03H8
      Right, 03H7
    Celiac, 04H1
    Colic
      Left, 04H7
      Middle, 04H8
      Right, 04H6
    Common Carotid
      Left, 03HJ
      Right, 03HH
    Common Iliac
      Left, 04HD
      Right, 04HC
    External Carotid
      Left, 03HN

Insertion of device in — continued
  Artery — continued
    External Carotid — continued
      Right, 03HM
    External Iliac
      Left, 04HJ
      Right, 04HH
    Face, 03HR
    Femoral
      Left, 04HL
      Right, 04HK
    Foot
      Left, 04HW
      Right, 04HV
    Gastric, 04H2
    Hand
      Left, 03HF
      Right, 03HD
    Hepatic, 04H3
    Inferior Mesenteric, 04HB
    Innominate, 03H2
    Internal Carotid
      Left, 03HL
      Right, 03HK
    Internal Iliac
      Left, 04HF
      Right, 04HE
    Internal Mammary
      Left, 03H1
      Right, 03H0
    Intracranial, 03HG
    Lower, 04HY
    Peroneal
      Left, 04HU
      Right, 04HT
    Popliteal
      Left, 04HN
      Right, 04HM
    Posterior Tibial
      Left, 04HS
      Right, 04HR
    Pulmonary
      Left, 02HR
      Right, 02HQ
    Pulmonary Trunk, 02HP
    Radial
      Left, 03HC
      Right, 03HB
    Renal
      Left, 04HA
      Right, 04H9
    Splenic, 04H4
    Subclavian
      Left, 03H4
      Right, 03H3
    Superior Mesenteric, 04H5
    Temporal
      Left, 03HT
      Right, 03HS
    Thyroid
      Left, 03HV
      Right, 03HU
    Ulnar
      Left, 03HA
      Right, 03H9
    Upper, 03HY
    Vertebral
      Left, 03HQ
      Right, 03HP
  Atrium
    Left, 02H7
    Right, 02H6
  Axilla
    Left, ØXH5
    Right, ØXH4
  Back
    Lower, ØWHL
    Upper, ØWHK
  Bladder, ØTHB
  Bladder Neck, ØTHC
  Bone
    Ethmoid
      Left, ØNHG
      Right, ØNHF
    Facial, ØNHW
    Frontal, ØNH1
    Hyoid, ØNHX
    Lacrimal
      Left, ØNHJ

Insertion of device in — continued
  Bone — continued
    Lacrimal — continued
      Right, ØNHH
    Lower, ØQHY
    Nasal, ØNHB
    Occipital, ØNH7
    Palatine
      Left, ØNHL
      Right, ØNHK
    Parietal
      Left, ØNH4
      Right, ØNH3
    Pelvic
      Left, ØQH3
      Right, ØQH2
    Sphenoid, ØNHC
    Temporal
      Left, ØNH6
      Right, ØNH5
    Upper, ØPHY
    Zygomatic
      Left, ØNHN
      Right, ØNHM
  Brain, 00H0
  Breast
    Bilateral, ØHHV
    Left, ØHHU
    Right, ØHHT
  Bronchus
    Lingula, ØBH9
    Lower Lobe
      Left, ØBHB
      Right, ØBH6
    Main
      Left, ØBH7
      Right, ØBH3
    Middle Lobe, Right, ØBH5
    Upper Lobe
      Left, ØBH8
      Right, ØBH4
  Bursa and Ligament
    Lower, ØMHY
    Upper, ØMHX
  Buttock
    Left, ØYH1
    Right, ØYH0
  Carpal
    Left, ØPHN
    Right, ØPHM
  Cavity, Cranial, ØWH1
  Cerebral Ventricle, 00H6
  Cervix, ØUHC
  Chest Wall, ØWH8
  Cisterna Chyli, 07HL
  Clavicle
    Left, ØPHB
    Right, ØPH9
  Coccyx, ØQHS
  Cul-de-sac, ØUHF
  Diaphragm, ØBHT
  Disc
    Cervical Vertebral, ØRH3
    Cervicothoracic Vertebral, ØRH5
    Lumbar Vertebral, ØSH2
    Lumbosacral, ØSH4
    Thoracic Vertebral, ØRH9
    Thoracolumbar Vertebral, ØRHB
  Duct
    Hepatobiliary, ØFHB
    Pancreatic, ØFHD
  Duodenum, ØDH9
  Ear
    Inner
      Left, 09HE
      Right, 09HD
    Left, 09HJ
    Right, 09HH
  Elbow Region
    Left, ØXHC
    Right, ØXHB
  Epididymis and Spermatic Cord, ØVHM
  Esophagus, ØDH5
  Extremity
    Lower
      Left, ØYHB
      Right, ØYH9
    Upper
      Left, ØXH7

Insertion of device in

Insertion of device in — *continued*

Extremity — *continued*
  Upper — *continued*
    Right, ØXH6

Eye
  Left, 08H1
  Right, 08H0
Face, ØWH2
Fallopian Tube, ØUH8
Femoral Region
  Left, ØYH8
  Right, ØYH7
Femoral Shaft
  Left, ØQH9
  Right, ØQH8
Femur
  Lower
    Left, ØQHC
    Right, ØQHB
  Upper
    Left, ØQH7
    Right, ØQH6
Fibula
  Left, ØQHK
  Right, ØQHJ
Foot
  Left, ØYHN
  Right, ØYHM
Gallbladder, ØFH4
Gastrointestinal Tract, ØWHP
Genitourinary Tract, ØWHR
Gland
  Endocrine, ØGHS
  Salivary, ØCHA
Glenoid Cavity
  Left, ØPH8
  Right, ØPH7
Hand
  Left, ØXHK
  Right, ØXHJ
Head, ØWH0
Heart, Ø2HA
Humeral Head
  Left, ØPHD
  Right, ØPHC
Humeral Shaft
  Left, ØPHG
  Right, ØPHF
Ileum, ØDHB
Inguinal Region
  Left, ØYH6
  Right, ØYH5
Intestinal Tract
  Lower, ØDHD
  Upper, ØDH0
Intestine
  Large, ØDHE
  Small, ØDH8
Jaw
  Lower, ØWH5
  Upper, ØWH4
Jejunum, ØDHA
Joint
  Acromioclavicular
    Left, ØRHH
    Right, ØRHG
  Ankle
    Left, ØSHG
    Right, ØSHF
  Carpal
    Left, ØRHR
    Right, ØRHQ
  Carpometacarpal
    Left, ØRHT
    Right, ØRHS
  Cervical Vertebral, ØRH1
  Cervicothoracic Vertebral, ØRH4
  Coccygeal, ØSH6
  Elbow
    Left, ØRHM
    Right, ØRHL
  Finger Phalangeal
    Left, ØRHX
    Right, ØRHW
  Hip
    Left, ØSHB
    Right, ØSH9
  Knee
    Left, ØSHD

Insertion of device in — *continued*

Joint — *continued*
  Knee — *continued*
    Right, ØSHC
  Lumbar Vertebral, ØSH0
  Lumbosacral, ØSH3
  Metacarpophalangeal
    Left, ØRHV
    Right, ØRHU
  Metatarsal-Phalangeal
    Left, ØSHN
    Right, ØSHM
  Occipital-cervical, ØRH0
  Sacrococcygeal, ØSH5
  Sacroiliac
    Left, ØSH8
    Right, ØSH7
  Shoulder
    Left, ØRHK
    Right, ØRHJ
  Sternoclavicular
    Left, ØRHF
    Right, ØRHE
  Tarsal
    Left, ØSHJ
    Right, ØSHH
  Tarsometatarsal
    Left, ØSHL
    Right, ØSHK
  Temporomandibular
    Left, ØRHD
    Right, ØRHC
  Thoracic Vertebral, ØRH6
  Thoracolumbar Vertebral, ØRHA
  Toe Phalangeal
    Left, ØSHQ
    Right, ØSHP
  Wrist
    Left, ØRHP
    Right, ØRHN
Kidney, ØTH5
Knee Region
  Left, ØYHG
  Right, ØYHF
Larynx, ØCHS
Leg
  Lower
    Left, ØYHJ
    Right, ØYHH
  Upper
    Left, ØYHD
    Right, ØYHC
Liver, ØFH0
  Left Lobe, ØFH2
  Right Lobe, ØFH1
Lung
  Left, ØBHL
  Right, ØBHK
Lymphatic, Ø7HN
  Thoracic Duct, Ø7HK
Mandible
  Left, ØNHV
  Right, ØNHT
Maxilla, ØNHR
Mediastinum, ØWHC
Metacarpal
  Left, ØPHQ
  Right, ØPHP
Metatarsal
  Left, ØQHP
  Right, ØQHN
Mouth and Throat, ØCHY
Muscle
  Lower, ØKHY
  Upper, ØKHX
Nasal Mucosa and Soft Tissue, Ø9HK
Nasopharynx, Ø9HN
Neck, ØWH6
Nerve
  Cranial, ØØHE
  Peripheral, Ø1HY
Nipple
  Left, ØHHX
  Right, ØHHW
Oral Cavity and Throat, ØWH3
Orbit
  Left, ØNHQ
  Right, ØNHP
Ovary, ØUH3

Insertion of device in — *continued*

Pancreas, ØFHG
Patella
  Left, ØQHF
  Right, ØQHD
Pelvic Cavity, ØWHJ
Penis, ØVHS
Pericardial Cavity, ØWHD
Pericardium, Ø2HN
Perineum
  Female, ØWHN
  Male, ØWHM
Peritoneal Cavity, ØWHG
Phalanx
  Finger
    Left, ØPHV
    Right, ØPHT
  Thumb
    Left, ØPHS
    Right, ØPHR
  Toe
    Left, ØQHR
    Right, ØQHQ
Pleura, ØBHQ
Pleural Cavity
  Left, ØWHB
  Right, ØWH9
Prostate, ØVH0
Prostate and Seminal Vesicles, ØVH4
Radius
  Left, ØPHJ
  Right, ØPHH
Rectum, ØDHP
Respiratory Tract, ØWHQ
Retroperitoneum, ØWHH
Ribs
  1 to 2, ØPH1
  3 or More, ØPH2
Sacrum, ØQH1
Scapula
  Left, ØPH6
  Right, ØPH5
Scrotum and Tunica Vaginalis, ØVH8
Shoulder Region
  Left, ØXH3
  Right, ØXH2
Sinus, Ø9HY
Skin, ØHHPXYZ
Skull, ØNH0
Spinal Canal, ØØHU
Spinal Cord, ØØHV
Spleen, Ø7HP
Sternum, ØPH0
Stomach, ØDH6
Subcutaneous Tissue and Fascia
  Abdomen, ØJH8
  Back, ØJH7
  Buttock, ØJH9
  Chest, ØJH6
  Face, ØJH1
  Foot
    Left, ØJHR
    Right, ØJHQ
  Hand
    Left, ØJHK
    Right, ØJHJ
  Head and Neck, ØJHS
  Lower Arm
    Left, ØJHH
    Right, ØJHG
  Lower Extremity, ØJHW
  Lower Leg
    Left, ØJHP
    Right, ØJHN
  Neck
    Left, ØJH5
    Right, ØJH4
  Pelvic Region, ØJHC
  Perineum, ØJHB
  Scalp, ØJH0
  Trunk, ØJHT
  Upper Arm
    Left, ØJHF
    Right, ØJHD
  Upper Extremity, ØJHV
  Upper Leg
    Left, ØJHM
    Right, ØJHL

▽ **Subterms under main terms may continue to next column or page**

Insertion of device in — *continued*

Tarsal
  Left, ØQHM
  Right, ØQHL
Tendon
  Lower, ØLHY
  Upper, ØLHX
Testis, ØVHD
Thymus, Ø7HM
Tibia
  Left, ØQHH
  Right, ØQHG
Tongue, ØCH7
Trachea, ØBH1
Tracheobronchial Tree, ØBHØ
Ulna
  Left, ØPHL
  Right, ØPHK
Ureter, ØTH9
Urethra, ØTHD
Uterus, ØUH9
Uterus and Cervix, ØUHD
Vagina, ØUHG
Vagina and Cul-de-sac, ØUHH
Vas Deferens, ØVHR
Vein
  Axillary
    Left, Ø5H8
    Right, Ø5H7
  Azygos, Ø5HØ
  Basilic
    Left, Ø5HC
    Right, Ø5HB
  Brachial
    Left, Ø5HA
    Right, Ø5H9
  Cephalic
    Left, Ø5HF
    Right, Ø5HD
  Colic, Ø6H7
  Common Iliac
    Left, Ø6HD
    Right, Ø6HC
  Coronary, Ø2H4
  Esophageal, Ø6H3
  External Iliac
    Left, Ø6HG
    Right, Ø6HF
  External Jugular
    Left, Ø5HQ
    Right, Ø5HP
  Face
    Left, Ø5HV
    Right, Ø5HT
  Femoral
    Left, Ø6HN
    Right, Ø6HM
  Foot
    Left, Ø6HV
    Right, Ø6HT
  Gastric, Ø6H2
  Hand
    Left, Ø5HH
    Right, Ø5HG
  Hemiazygos, Ø5H1
  Hepatic, Ø6H4
  Hypogastric
    Left, Ø6HJ
    Right, Ø6HH
  Inferior Mesenteric, Ø6H6
  Innominate
    Left, Ø5H4
    Right, Ø5H3
  Internal Jugular
    Left, Ø5HN
    Right, Ø5HM
  Intracranial, Ø5HL
  Lower, Ø6HY
  Portal, Ø6H8
  Pulmonary
    Left, Ø2HT
    Right, Ø2HS
  Renal
    Left, Ø6HB
    Right, Ø6H9
  Saphenous
    Left, Ø6HQ
    Right, Ø6HP
  Splenic, Ø6H1

Insertion of device in — *continued*

Vein — *continued*
  Subclavian
    Left, Ø5H6
    Right, Ø5H5
  Superior Mesenteric, Ø6H5
  Upper, Ø5HY
  Vertebral
    Left, Ø5HS
    Right, Ø5HR
Vena Cava
  Inferior, Ø6HØ
  Superior, Ø2HV
Ventricle
  Left, Ø2HL
  Right, Ø2HK
Vertebra
  Cervical, ØPH3
  Lumbar, ØQHØ
  Thoracic, ØPH4
Wrist Region
  Left, ØXHH
  Right, ØXHG

Inspection

Abdominal Wall, ØWJF
Ankle Region
  Left, ØYJL
  Right, ØYJK
Arm
  Lower
    Left, ØXJF
    Right, ØXJD
  Upper
    Left, ØXJ9
    Right, ØXJ8
Artery
  Lower, Ø4JY
  Upper, Ø3JY
Axilla
  Left, ØXJ5
  Right, ØXJ4
Back
  Lower, ØWJL
  Upper, ØWJK
Bladder, ØTJB
Bone
  Facial, ØNJW
  Lower, ØQJY
  Nasal, ØNJB
  Upper, ØPJY
Bone Marrow, Ø7JT
Brain, ØØJØ
Breast
  Left, ØHJU
  Right, ØHJT
Bursa and Ligament
  Lower, ØMJY
  Upper, ØMJX
Buttock
  Left, ØYJ1
  Right, ØYJØ
Cavity, Cranial, ØWJ1
Chest Wall, ØWJ8
Cisterna Chyli, Ø7JL
Diaphragm, ØBJT
Disc
  Cervical Vertebral, ØRJ3
  Cervicothoracic Vertebral, ØRJ5
  Lumbar Vertebral, ØSJ2
  Lumbosacral, ØSJ4
  Thoracic Vertebral, ØRJ9
  Thoracolumbar Vertebral, ØRJB
Duct
  Hepatobiliary, ØFJB
  Pancreatic, ØFJD
Ear
  Inner
    Left, Ø9JE
    Right, Ø9JD
  Left, Ø9JJ
  Right, Ø9JH
Elbow Region
  Left, ØXJC
  Right, ØXJB
Epididymis and Spermatic Cord, ØVJM
Extremity
  Lower
    Left, ØYJB
    Right, ØYJ9

Inspection — *continued*

Extremity — *continued*
  Upper
    Left, ØXJ7
    Right, ØXJ6
Eye
  Left, Ø8J1XZZ
  Right, Ø8JØXZZ
Face, ØWJ2
Fallopian Tube, ØUJ8
Femoral Region
  Bilateral, ØYJE
  Left, ØYJ8
  Right, ØYJ7
Finger Nail, ØHJQXZZ
Foot
  Left, ØYJN
  Right, ØYJM
Gallbladder, ØFJ4
Gastrointestinal Tract, ØWJP
Genitourinary Tract, ØWJR
Gland
  Adrenal, ØGJ5
  Endocrine, ØGJS
  Pituitary, ØGJØ
  Salivary, ØCJA
Great Vessel, Ø2JY
Hand
  Left, ØXJK
  Right, ØXJJ
Head, ØWJØ
Heart, Ø2JA
Inguinal Region
  Bilateral, ØYJA
  Left, ØYJ6
  Right, ØYJ5
Intestinal Tract
  Lower, ØDJD
  Upper, ØDJØ
Jaw
  Lower, ØWJ5
  Upper, ØWJ4
Joint
  Acromioclavicular
    Left, ØRJH
    Right, ØRJG
  Ankle
    Left, ØSJG
    Right, ØSJF
  Carpal
    Left, ØRJR
    Right, ØRJQ
  Carpometacarpal
    Left, ØRJT
    Right, ØRJS
  Cervical Vertebral, ØRJ1
  Cervicothoracic Vertebral, ØRJ4
  Coccygeal, ØSJ6
  Elbow
    Left, ØRJM
    Right, ØRJL
  Finger Phalangeal
    Left, ØRJX
    Right, ØRJW
  Hip
    Left, ØSJB
    Right, ØSJ9
  Knee
    Left, ØSJD
    Right, ØSJC
  Lumbar Vertebral, ØSJØ
  Lumbosacral, ØSJ3
  Metacarpophalangeal
    Left, ØRJV
    Right, ØRJU
  Metatarsal-Phalangeal
    Left, ØSJN
    Right, ØSJM
  Occipital-cervical, ØRJØ
  Sacrococcygeal, ØSJ5
  Sacroiliac
    Left, ØSJ8
    Right, ØSJ7
  Shoulder
    Left, ØRJK
    Right, ØRJJ
  Sternoclavicular
    Left, ØRJF
    Right, ØRJE

▽ **Subterms under main terms may continue to next column or page**

Inspection — continued

Joint — continued
Tarsal
Left, 0SJJ
Right, 0SJH
Tarsometatarsal
Left, 0SJL
Right, 0SJK
Temporomandibular
Left, 0RJD
Right, 0RJC
Thoracic Vertebral, 0RJ6
Thoracolumbar Vertebral, 0RJA
Toe Phalangeal
Left, 0SJQ
Right, 0SJP
Wrist
Left, 0RJP
Right, 0RJN
Kidney, 0TJ5
Knee Region
Left, 0YJG
Right, 0YJF
Larynx, 0CJS
Leg
Lower
Left, 0YJJ
Right, 0YJH
Upper
Left, 0YJD
Right, 0YJC
Lens
Left, 08JKXZZ
Right, 08JJXZZ
Liver, 0FJ0
Lung
Left, 0BJL
Right, 0BJK
Lymphatic, 07JN
Thoracic Duct, 07JK
Mediastinum, 0WJC
Mesentery, 0DJV
Mouth and Throat, 0CJY
Muscle
Extraocular
Left, 08JM
Right, 08JL
Lower, 0KJY
Upper, 0KJX
Nasal Mucosa and Soft Tissue, 09JK
Neck, 0WJ6
Nerve
Cranial, 00JE
Peripheral, 01JY
Omentum, 0DJU
Oral Cavity and Throat, 0WJ3
Ovary, 0UJ3
Pancreas, 0FJG
Parathyroid Gland, 0GJR
Pelvic Cavity, 0WJJ
Penis, 0VJS
Pericardial Cavity, 0WJD
Perineum
Female, 0WJN
Male, 0WJM
Peritoneal Cavity, 0WJG
Peritoneum, 0DJW
Pineal Body, 0GJ1
Pleura, 0BJQ
Pleural Cavity
Left, 0WJB
Right, 0WJ9
Products of Conception, 10J0
Ectopic, 10J2
Retained, 10J1
Prostate and Seminal Vesicles, 0VJ4
Respiratory Tract, 0WJQ
Retroperitoneum, 0WJH
Scrotum and Tunica Vaginalis, 0VJ8
Shoulder Region
Left, 0XJ3
Right, 0XJ2
Sinus, 09JY
Skin, 0HJPXZZ
Skull, 0NJ0
Spinal Canal, 00JU
Spinal Cord, 00JV
Spleen, 07JP
Stomach, 0DJ6

Inspection — continued

Subcutaneous Tissue and Fascia
Head and Neck, 0JJS
Lower Extremity, 0JJW
Trunk, 0JJT
Upper Extremity, 0JJV
Tendon
Lower, 0LJY
Upper, 0LJX
Testis, 0VJD
Thymus, 07JM
Thyroid Gland, 0GJK
Toe Nail, 0HJRXZZ
Trachea, 0BJ1
Tracheobronchial Tree, 0BJ0
Tympanic Membrane
Left, 09J8
Right, 09J7
Ureter, 0TJ9
Urethra, 0TJD
Uterus and Cervix, 0UJD
Vagina and Cul-de-sac, 0UJH
Vas Deferens, 0VJR
Vein
Lower, 06JY
Upper, 05JY
Vulva, 0UJM
Wrist Region
Left, 0XJH
Right, 0XJG
Installation see Introduction of substance in or on
Insufflation see Introduction of substance in or on
Interatrial septum use Atrial Septum
Interbody fusion (spine) cage
use Interbody Fusion Device in Lower Joints
use Interbody Fusion Device in Upper Joints
Interbody Fusion Device
Nanotextured Surface
Cervical Vertebral, XRG1092
2 or more, XRG2092
Cervicothoracic Vertebral, XRG4092
Lumbar Vertebral, XRGB092
2 or more, XRGC092
Lumbosacral, XRGD092
Occipital-cervical, XRG0092
Thoracic Vertebral, XRG6092
2 to 7, XRG7092
8 or more, XRG8092
Thoracolumbar Vertebral, XRGA092
Radiolucent Porous
Cervical Vertebral, XRG10F3
2 or more, XRG20F3
Cervicothoracic Vertebral, XRG40F3
Lumbar Vertebral, XRGB0F3
2 or more, XRGC0F3
Lumbosacral, XRGD0F3
Occipital-cervical, XRG00F3
Thoracic Vertebral, XRG60F3
2 to 7, XRG70F3
8 or more, XRG80F3
Thoracolumbar Vertebral, XRGA0F3
Intercarpal joint
use Carpal Joint, Left
use Carpal Joint, Right
Intercarpal ligament
use Hand Bursa and Ligament, Left
use Hand Bursa and Ligament, Right
Interclavicular ligament
use Shoulder Bursa and Ligament, Left
use Shoulder Bursa and Ligament, Right
Intercostal lymph node use Lymphatic, Thorax
Intercostal muscle
use Thorax Muscle, Left
use Thorax Muscle, Right
Intercostal nerve use Thoracic Nerve
Intercostobrachial nerve use Thoracic Nerve
Intercuneiform joint
use Tarsal Joint, Left
use Tarsal Joint, Right
Intercuneiform ligament
use Foot Bursa and Ligament, Left
use Foot Bursa and Ligament, Right
Intermediate bronchus use Main Bronchus, Right
Intermediate cuneiform bone
use Tarsal, Left
use Tarsal, Right
Intermittent hemodialysis (IHD), 5A1D70Z

Intermittent mandatory ventilation see Assistance, Respiratory, 5A09
Intermittent Negative Airway Pressure
24-96 Consecutive Hours, Ventilation, 5A0945B
Greater than 96 Consecutive Hours, Ventilation, 5A0955B
Less than 24 Consecutive Hours, Ventilation, 5A0935B
Intermittent Positive Airway Pressure
24-96 Consecutive Hours, Ventilation, 5A09458
Greater than 96 Consecutive Hours, Ventilation, 5A09558
Less than 24 Consecutive Hours, Ventilation, 5A09358
Intermittent positive pressure breathing see Assistance, Respiratory, 5A09
Internal anal sphincter use Anal Sphincter
Internal carotid artery, intracranial portion use Intracranial Artery
Internal carotid plexus use Head and Neck Sympathetic Nerve
Internal (basal) cerebral vein use Intracranial Vein
Internal iliac vein
use Hypogastric Vein, Left
use Hypogastric Vein, Right
Internal maxillary artery
use External Carotid Artery, Left
use External Carotid Artery, Right
Internal naris use Nasal Mucosa and Soft Tissue
Internal oblique muscle
use Abdomen Muscle, Left
use Abdomen Muscle, Right
Internal pudendal artery
use Internal Iliac Artery, Left
use Internal Iliac Artery, Right
Internal pudendal vein
use Hypogastric Vein, Left
use Hypogastric Vein, Right
Internal thoracic artery
use Internal Mammary Artery, Left
use Internal Mammary Artery, Right
use Subclavian Artery, Left
use Subclavian Artery, Right
Internal urethral sphincter use Urethra
Interphalangeal (IP) joint
use Finger Phalangeal Joint, Left
use Finger Phalangeal Joint, Right
use Toe Phalangeal Joint, Left
use Toe Phalangeal Joint, Right
Interphalangeal ligament
use Foot Bursa and Ligament, Left
use Foot Bursa and Ligament, Right
use Hand Bursa and Ligament, Left
use Hand Bursa and Ligament, Right
Interrogation, cardiac rhythm related device
With cardiac function testing see Measurement, Cardiac, 4A02
Interrogation only see Measurement, Cardiac, 4B02
Interruption see Occlusion
Interspinalis muscle
use Trunk Muscle, Left
use Trunk Muscle, Right
Interspinous ligament, cervical use Head and Neck Bursa and Ligament
Interspinous ligament, lumbar use Lower Spine Bursa and Ligament
Interspinous ligament, thoracic use Upper Spine Bursa and Ligament
Interspinous process spinal stabilization device
use Spinal Stabilization Device, Interspinous Process in, 0RH
use Spinal Stabilization Device, Interspinous Process in, 0SH
InterStim® Therapy lead use Neurostimulator Lead in Peripheral Nervous System
InterStim® Therapy neurostimulator use Stimulator Generator, Single Array in, 0JH
Intertransversarius muscle
use Trunk Muscle, Left
use Trunk Muscle, Right
Intertransverse ligament, cervical use Head and Neck Bursa and Ligament
Intertransverse ligament, lumbar use Lower Spine Bursa and Ligament
Intertransverse ligament, thoracic use Upper Spine Bursa and Ligament
Interventricular foramen (Monro) use Cerebral Ventricle
Interventricular septum use Ventricular Septum
Intestinal lymphatic trunk use Cisterna Chyli

▽ **Subterms under main terms may continue to next column or page**

Intraluminal Device

Airway
  Esophagus, ØDH5
  Mouth and Throat, ØCHY
  Nasopharynx, Ø9HN
Bioactive
  Occlusion
    Common Carotid
      Left, Ø3LJ
      Right, Ø3LH
    External Carotid
      Left, Ø3LN
      Right, Ø3LM
    Internal Carotid
      Left, Ø3LL
      Right, Ø3LK
    Intracranial, Ø3LG
    Vertebral
      Left, Ø3LQ
      Right, Ø3LP
  Restriction
    Common Carotid
      Left, Ø3VJ
      Right, Ø3VH
    External Carotid
      Left, Ø3VN
      Right, Ø3VM
    Internal Carotid
      Left, Ø3VL
      Right, Ø3VK
    Intracranial, Ø3VG
    Vertebral
      Left, Ø3VQ
      Right, Ø3VP
Endobronchial Valve
  Lingula, ØBH9
  Lower Lobe
    Left, ØBHB
    Right, ØBH6
  Main
    Left, ØBH7
    Right, ØBH3
  Middle Lobe, Right, ØBH5
  Upper Lobe
    Left, ØBH8
    Right, ØBH4
Endotracheal Airway
  Change device in, Trachea, ØB21XEZ
  Insertion of device in, Trachea, ØBH1
Pessary
  Change device in, Vagina and Cul-de-sac, ØU2HXGZ
  Insertion of device in
    Cul-de-sac, ØUHF
    Vagina, ØUHG

Intramedullary (IM) rod (nail)
  use Internal Fixation Device, Intramedullary in Lower Bones
  use Internal Fixation Device, Intramedullary in Upper Bones

Intramedullary skeletal kinetic distractor (ISKD)
  use Internal Fixation Device, Intramedullary in Lower Bones
  use Internal Fixation Device, Intramedullary in Upper Bones

Intraocular Telescope
  Left, Ø8RK3ØZ
  Right, Ø8RJ3ØZ

Intraoperative Knee Replacement Sensor, XR2

Intraoperative Radiation Therapy (IORT)
  Anus, DDY8CZZ
  Bile Ducts, DFY2CZZ
  Bladder, DTY2CZZ
  Cervix, DUY1CZZ
  Colon, DDY5CZZ
  Duodenum, DDY2CZZ
  Gallbladder, DFY1CZZ
  Ileum, DDY4CZZ
  Jejunum, DDY3CZZ
  Kidney, DTYØCZZ
  Larynx, D9YBCZZ
  Liver, DFYØCZZ
  Mouth, D9Y4CZZ
  Nasopharynx, D9YDCZZ
  Ovary, DUYØCZZ
  Pancreas, DFY3CZZ
  Pharynx, D9YCCZZ
  Prostate, DVYØCZZ

Intraoperative Radiation Therapy — *continued*
  Rectum, DDY7CZZ
  Stomach, DDY1CZZ
  Ureter, DTY1CZZ
  Urethra, DTY3CZZ
  Uterus, DUY2CZZ

Intrauterine Device (IUD) *use* Contraceptive Device in Female Reproductive System

Intravascular fluorescence angiography (IFA) *see*
  Monitoring, Physiological Systems, 4A1

Introduction of substance in or on
Artery
  Central, 3EØ6
    Analgesics, 3EØ6
    Anesthetic, Intracirculatory, 3EØ6
    Antiarrhythmic, 3EØ6
    Anti-infective, 3EØ6
    Anti-inflammatory, 3EØ6
    Antineoplastic, 3EØ6
    Destructive Agent, 3EØ6
    Diagnostic Substance, Other, 3EØ6
    Electrolytic Substance, 3EØ6
    Hormone, 3EØ6
    Hypnotics, 3EØ6
    Immunotherapeutic, 3EØ6
    Nutritional Substance, 3EØ6
    Platelet Inhibitor, 3EØ6
    Radioactive Substance, 3EØ6
    Sedatives, 3EØ6
    Serum, 3EØ6
    Thrombolytic, 3EØ6
    Toxoid, 3EØ6
    Vaccine, 3EØ6
    Vasopressor, 3EØ6
    Water Balance Substance, 3EØ6
  Coronary, 3EØ7
    Diagnostic Substance, Other, 3EØ7
    Platelet Inhibitor, 3EØ7
    Thrombolytic, 3EØ7
  Peripheral, 3EØ5
    Analgesics, 3EØ5
    Anesthetic, Intracirculatory, 3EØ5
    Antiarrhythmic, 3EØ5
    Anti-infective, 3EØ5
    Anti-inflammatory, 3EØ5
    Antineoplastic, 3EØ5
    Destructive Agent, 3EØ5
    Diagnostic Substance, Other, 3EØ5
    Electrolytic Substance, 3EØ5
    Hormone, 3EØ5
    Hypnotics, 3EØ5
    Immunotherapeutic, 3EØ5
    Nutritional Substance, 3EØ5
    Platelet Inhibitor, 3EØ5
    Radioactive Substance, 3EØ5
    Sedatives, 3EØ5
    Serum, 3EØ5
    Thrombolytic, 3EØ5
    Toxoid, 3EØ5
    Vaccine, 3EØ5
    Vasopressor, 3EØ5
    Water Balance Substance, 3EØ5
Biliary Tract, 3EØJ
  Analgesics, 3EØJ
  Anesthetic Agent, 3EØJ
  Anti-infective, 3EØJ
  Anti-inflammatory, 3EØJ
  Antineoplastic, 3EØJ
  Destructive Agent, 3EØJ
  Diagnostic Substance, Other, 3EØJ
  Electrolytic Substance, 3EØJ
  Gas, 3EØJ
  Hypnotics, 3EØJ
  Islet Cells, Pancreatic, 3EØJ
  Nutritional Substance, 3EØJ
  Radioactive Substance, 3EØJ
  Sedatives, 3EØJ
  Water Balance Substance, 3EØJ
Bone, 3EØV
  Analgesics, 3EØV3NZ
  Anesthetic Agent, 3EØV3BZ
  Anti-infective, 3EØV32
  Anti-inflammatory, 3EØV33Z
  Antineoplastic, 3EØV3Ø
  Destructive Agent, 3EØV3TZ
  Diagnostic Substance, Other, 3EØV3KZ
  Electrolytic Substance, 3EØV37Z
  Hypnotics, 3EØV3NZ
  Nutritional Substance, 3EØV36Z

Introduction of substance in or on — *continued*
Bone — *continued*
  Radioactive Substance, 3EØV3HZ
  Sedatives, 3EØV3NZ
  Water Balance Substance, 3EØV37Z
Bone Marrow, 3EØA3GC
  Antineoplastic, 3EØA3Ø
Brain, 3EØQ
  Analgesics, 3EØQ
  Anesthetic Agent, 3EØQ
  Anti-infective, 3EØQ
  Anti-inflammatory, 3EØQ
  Antineoplastic, 3EØQ
  Destructive Agent, 3EØQ
  Diagnostic Substance, Other, 3EØQ
  Electrolytic Substance, 3EØQ
  Gas, 3EØQ
  Hypnotics, 3EØQ
  Nutritional Substance, 3EØQ
  Radioactive Substance, 3EØQ
  Sedatives, 3EØQ
  Stem Cells
    Embryonic, 3EØQ
    Somatic, 3EØQ
  Water Balance Substance, 3EØQ
Cranial Cavity, 3EØQ
  Analgesics, 3EØQ
  Anesthetic Agent, 3EØQ
  Anti-infective, 3EØQ
  Anti-inflammatory, 3EØQ
  Antineoplastic, 3EØQ
  Destructive Agent, 3EØQ
  Diagnostic Substance, Other, 3EØQ
  Electrolytic Substance, 3EØQ
  Gas, 3EØQ
  Hypnotics, 3EØQ
  Nutritional Substance, 3EØQ
  Radioactive Substance, 3EØQ
  Sedatives, 3EØQ
  Stem Cells
    Embryonic, 3EØQ
    Somatic, 3EØQ
  Water Balance Substance, 3EØQ
Ear, 3EØB
  Analgesics, 3EØB
  Anesthetic Agent, 3EØB
  Anti-infective, 3EØB
  Anti-inflammatory, 3EØB
  Antineoplastic, 3EØB
  Destructive Agent, 3EØB
  Diagnostic Substance, Other, 3EØB
  Hypnotics, 3EØB
  Radioactive Substance, 3EØB
  Sedatives, 3EØB
Epidural Space, 3EØS3GC
  Analgesics, 3EØS3NZ
  Anesthetic Agent, 3EØS3BZ
  Anti-infective, 3EØS32
  Anti-inflammatory, 3EØS33Z
  Antineoplastic, 3EØS3Ø
  Destructive Agent, 3EØS3TZ
  Diagnostic Substance, Other, 3EØS3KZ
  Electrolytic Substance, 3EØS37Z
  Gas, 3EØS
  Hypnotics, 3EØS3NZ
  Nutritional Substance, 3EØS36Z
  Radioactive Substance, 3EØS3HZ
  Sedatives, 3EØS3NZ
  Water Balance Substance, 3EØS37Z
Eye, 3EØC
  Analgesics, 3EØC
  Anesthetic Agent, 3EØC
  Anti-infective, 3EØC
  Anti-inflammatory, 3EØC
  Antineoplastic, 3EØC
  Destructive Agent, 3EØC
  Diagnostic Substance, Other, 3EØC
  Gas, 3EØC
  Hypnotics, 3EØC
  Pigment, 3EØC
  Radioactive Substance, 3EØC
  Sedatives, 3EØC
Gastrointestinal Tract
  Lower, 3EØH
    Analgesics, 3EØH
    Anesthetic Agent, 3EØH
    Anti-infective, 3EØH
    Anti-inflammatory, 3EØH
    Antineoplastic, 3EØH

Introduction of substance in or on

Introduction of substance in or on — *continued*
  Gastrointestinal Tract — *continued*
    Lower — *continued*
      Destructive Agent, 3E0H
      Diagnostic Substance, Other, 3E0H
      Electrolytic Substance, 3E0H
      Gas, 3E0H
      Hypnotics, 3E0H
      Nutritional Substance, 3E0H
      Radioactive Substance, 3E0H
      Sedatives, 3E0H
      Water Balance Substance, 3E0H
    Upper, 3E0G
      Analgesics, 3E0G
      Anesthetic Agent, 3E0G
      Anti-infective, 3E0G
      Anti-inflammatory, 3E0G
      Antineoplastic, 3E0G
      Destructive Agent, 3E0G
      Diagnostic Substance, Other, 3E0G
      Electrolytic Substance, 3E0G
      Gas, 3E0G
      Hypnotics, 3E0G
      Nutritional Substance, 3E0G
      Radioactive Substance, 3E0G
      Sedatives, 3E0G
      Water Balance Substance, 3E0G
  Genitourinary Tract, 3E0K
    Analgesics, 3E0K
    Anesthetic Agent, 3E0K
    Anti-infective, 3E0K
    Anti-inflammatory, 3E0K
    Antineoplastic, 3E0K
    Destructive Agent, 3E0K
    Diagnostic Substance, Other, 3E0K
    Electrolytic Substance, 3E0K
    Gas, 3E0K
    Hypnotics, 3E0K
    Nutritional Substance, 3E0K
    Radioactive Substance, 3E0K
    Sedatives, 3E0K
    Water Balance Substance, 3E0K
  Heart, 3E08
    Diagnostic Substance, Other, 3E08
    Platelet Inhibitor, 3E08
    Thrombolytic, 3E08
  Joint, 3E0U
    Analgesics, 3E0U3NZ
    Anesthetic Agent, 3E0U3BZ
    Anti-infective, 3E0U
    Anti-inflammatory, 3E0U33Z
    Antineoplastic, 3E0U30
    Destructive Agent, 3E0U3TZ
    Diagnostic Substance, Other, 3E0U3KZ
    Electrolytic Substance, 3E0U37Z
    Gas, 3E0U3SF
    Hypnotics, 3E0U3NZ
    Nutritional Substance, 3E0U36Z
    Radioactive Substance, 3E0U3HZ
    Sedatives, 3E0U3NZ
    Water Balance Substance, 3E0U37Z
  Lymphatic, 3E0W3GC
    Analgesics, 3E0W3NZ
    Anesthetic Agent, 3E0W3BZ
    Anti-infective, 3E0W32
    Anti-inflammatory, 3E0W33Z
    Antineoplastic, 3E0W30
    Destructive Agent, 3E0W3TZ
    Diagnostic Substance, Other, 3E0W3KZ
    Electrolytic Substance, 3E0W37Z
    Hypnotics, 3E0W3NZ
    Nutritional Substance, 3E0W36Z
    Radioactive Substance, 3E0W3HZ
    Sedatives, 3E0W3NZ
    Water Balance Substance, 3E0W37Z
  Mouth, 3E0D
    Analgesics, 3E0D
    Anesthetic Agent, 3E0D
    Antiarrhythmic, 3E0D
    Anti-infective, 3E0D
    Anti-inflammatory, 3E0D
    Antineoplastic, 3E0D
    Destructive Agent, 3E0D
    Diagnostic Substance, Other, 3E0D
    Electrolytic Substance, 3E0D
    Hypnotics, 3E0D
    Nutritional Substance, 3E0D
    Radioactive Substance, 3E0D
    Sedatives, 3E0D

Introduction of substance in or on — *continued*
  Mouth — *continued*
    Serum, 3E0D
    Toxoid, 3E0D
    Vaccine, 3E0D
    Water Balance Substance, 3E0D
  Mucous Membrane, 3E00XGC
    Analgesics, 3E00XNZ
    Anesthetic Agent, 3E00XBZ
    Anti-infective, 3E00X2
    Anti-inflammatory, 3E00X3Z
    Antineoplastic, 3E00X0
    Destructive Agent, 3E00XTZ
    Diagnostic Substance, Other, 3E00XKZ
    Hypnotics, 3E00XNZ
    Pigment, 3E00XMZ
    Sedatives, 3E00XNZ
    Serum, 3E00X4Z
    Toxoid, 3E00X4Z
    Vaccine, 3E00X4Z
  Muscle, 3E023GC
    Analgesics, 3E023NZ
    Anesthetic Agent, 3E023BZ
    Anti-infective, 3E0232
    Anti-inflammatory, 3E0233Z
    Antineoplastic, 3E0230
    Destructive Agent, 3E023TZ
    Diagnostic Substance, Other, 3E023KZ
    Electrolytic Substance, 3E0237Z
    Hypnotics, 3E023NZ
    Nutritional Substance, 3E0236Z
    Radioactive Substance, 3E023HZ
    Sedatives, 3E023NZ
    Serum, 3E0234Z
    Toxoid, 3E0234Z
    Vaccine, 3E0234Z
    Water Balance Substance, 3E0237Z
  Nerve
    Cranial, 3E0X3GC
      Anesthetic Agent, 3E0X3BZ
      Anti-inflammatory, 3E0X33Z
      Destructive Agent, 3E0X3TZ
    Peripheral, 3E0T3GC
      Anesthetic Agent, 3E0T3BZ
      Anti-inflammatory, 3E0T33Z
      Destructive Agent, 3E0T3TZ
    Plexus, 3E0T3GC
      Anesthetic Agent, 3E0T3BZ
      Anti-inflammatory, 3E0T33Z
      Destructive Agent, 3E0T3TZ
  Nose, 3E09
    Analgesics, 3E09
    Anesthetic Agent, 3E09
    Anti-infective, 3E09
    Anti-inflammatory, 3E09
    Antineoplastic, 3E09
    Destructive Agent, 3E09
    Diagnostic Substance, Other, 3E09
    Hypnotics, 3E09
    Radioactive Substance, 3E09
    Sedatives, 3E09
    Serum, 3E09
    Toxoid, 3E09
    Vaccine, 3E09
  Pancreatic Tract, 3E0J
    Analgesics, 3E0J
    Anesthetic Agent, 3E0J
    Anti-infective, 3E0J
    Anti-inflammatory, 3E0J
    Antineoplastic, 3E0J
    Destructive Agent, 3E0J
    Diagnostic Substance, Other, 3E0J
    Electrolytic Substance, 3E0J
    Gas, 3E0J
    Hypnotics, 3E0J
    Islet Cells, Pancreatic, 3E0J
    Nutritional Substance, 3E0J
    Radioactive Substance, 3E0J
    Sedatives, 3E0J
    Water Balance Substance, 3E0J
  Pericardial Cavity, 3E0Y
    Analgesics, 3E0Y3NZ
    Anesthetic Agent, 3E0Y3BZ
    Anti-infective, 3E0Y32
    Anti-inflammatory, 3E0Y33Z
    Antineoplastic, 3E0Y
    Destructive Agent, 3E0Y3TZ
    Diagnostic Substance, Other, 3E0Y3KZ
    Electrolytic Substance, 3E0Y37Z

Introduction of substance in or on — *continued*
  Pericardial Cavity — *continued*
    Gas, 3E0Y
    Hypnotics, 3E0Y3NZ
    Nutritional Substance, 3E0Y36Z
    Radioactive Substance, 3E0Y3HZ
    Sedatives, 3E0Y3NZ
    Water Balance Substance, 3E0Y37Z
  Peritoneal Cavity, 3E0M
    Adhesion Barrier, 3E0M
    Analgesics, 3E0M3NZ
    Anesthetic Agent, 3E0M3BZ
    Anti-infective, 3E0M32
    Anti-inflammatory, 3E0M33Z
    Antineoplastic, 3E0M
    Destructive Agent, 3E0M3TZ
    Diagnostic Substance, Other, 3E0M3KZ
    Electrolytic Substance, 3E0M37Z
    Gas, 3E0M
    Hypnotics, 3E0M3NZ
    Nutritional Substance, 3E0M36Z
    Radioactive Substance, 3E0M3HZ
    Sedatives, 3E0M3NZ
    Water Balance Substance, 3E0M37Z
  Pharynx, 3E0D
    Analgesics, 3E0D
    Anesthetic Agent, 3E0D
    Antiarrhythmic, 3E0D
    Anti-infective, 3E0D
    Anti-inflammatory, 3E0D
    Antineoplastic, 3E0D
    Destructive Agent, 3E0D
    Diagnostic Substance, Other, 3E0D
    Electrolytic Substance, 3E0D
    Hypnotics, 3E0D
    Nutritional Substance, 3E0D
    Radioactive Substance, 3E0D
    Sedatives, 3E0D
    Serum, 3E0D
    Toxoid, 3E0D
    Vaccine, 3E0D
    Water Balance Substance, 3E0D
  Pleural Cavity, 3E0L
    Adhesion Barrier, 3E0L
    Analgesics, 3E0L3NZ
    Anesthetic Agent, 3E0L3BZ
    Anti-infective, 3E0L32
    Anti-inflammatory, 3E0L33Z
    Antineoplastic, 3E0L
    Destructive Agent, 3E0L3TZ
    Diagnostic Substance, Other, 3E0L3KZ
    Electrolytic Substance, 3E0L37Z
    Gas, 3E0L
    Hypnotics, 3E0L3NZ
    Nutritional Substance, 3E0L36Z
    Radioactive Substance, 3E0L3HZ
    Sedatives, 3E0L3NZ
    Water Balance Substance, 3E0L37Z
  Products of Conception, 3E0E
    Analgesics, 3E0E
    Anesthetic Agent, 3E0E
    Anti-infective, 3E0E
    Anti-inflammatory, 3E0E
    Antineoplastic, 3E0E
    Destructive Agent, 3E0E
    Diagnostic Substance, Other, 3E0E
    Electrolytic Substance, 3E0E
    Gas, 3E0E
    Hypnotics, 3E0E
    Nutritional Substance, 3E0E
    Radioactive Substance, 3E0E
    Sedatives, 3E0E
    Water Balance Substance, 3E0E
  Reproductive
    Female, 3E0P
      Adhesion Barrier, 3E0P
      Analgesics, 3E0P
      Anesthetic Agent, 3E0P
      Anti-infective, 3E0P
      Anti-inflammatory, 3E0P
      Antineoplastic, 3E0P
      Destructive Agent, 3E0P
      Diagnostic Substance, Other, 3E0P
      Electrolytic Substance, 3E0P
      Gas, 3E0P
      Hormone, 3E0P
      Hypnotics, 3E0P
      Nutritional Substance, 3E0P
      Ovum, Fertilized, 3E0P

Introduction of substance in or on — *continued*
  Reproductive — *continued*
    Female — *continued*
      Radioactive Substance, 3E0P
      Sedatives, 3E0P
      Sperm, 3E0P
      Water Balance Substance, 3E0P
    Male, 3E0N
      Analgesics, 3E0N
      Anesthetic Agent, 3E0N
      Anti-infective, 3E0N
      Anti-inflammatory, 3E0N
      Antineoplastic, 3E0N
      Destructive Agent, 3E0N
      Diagnostic Substance, Other, 3E0N
      Electrolytic Substance, 3E0N
      Gas, 3E0N
      Hypnotics, 3E0N
      Nutritional Substance, 3E0N
      Radioactive Substance, 3E0N
      Sedatives, 3E0N
      Water Balance Substance, 3E0N
  Respiratory Tract, 3E0F
    Analgesics, 3E0F
    Anesthetic Agent, 3E0F
    Anti-infective, 3E0F
    Anti-inflammatory, 3E0F
    Antineoplastic, 3E0F
    Destructive Agent, 3E0F
    Diagnostic Substance, Other, 3E0F
    Electrolytic Substance, 3E0F
    Gas, 3E0F
    Hypnotics, 3E0F
    Nutritional Substance, 3E0F
    Radioactive Substance, 3E0F
    Sedatives, 3E0F
    Water Balance Substance, 3E0F
  Skin, 3E00XGC
    Analgesics, 3E00XNZ
    Anesthetic Agent, 3E00XBZ
    Anti-infective, 3E00X2
    Anti-inflammatory, 3E00X3Z
    Antineoplastic, 3E00X0
    Destructive Agent, 3E00XTZ
    Diagnostic Substance, Other, 3E00XKZ
    Hypnotics, 3E00XNZ
    Pigment, 3E00XMZ
    Sedatives, 3E00XNZ
    Serum, 3E00X4Z
    Toxoid, 3E00X4Z
    Vaccine, 3E00X4Z
  Spinal Canal, 3E0R3GC
    Analgesics, 3E0R3NZ
    Anesthetic Agent, 3E0R3BZ
    Anti-infective, 3E0R32
    Anti-inflammatory, 3E0R33Z
    Antineoplastic, 3E0R30
    Destructive Agent, 3E0R3TZ
    Diagnostic Substance, Other, 3E0R3KZ
    Electrolytic Substance, 3E0R37Z
    Gas, 3E0R
    Hypnotics, 3E0R3NZ
    Nutritional Substance, 3E0R36Z
    Radioactive Substance, 3E0R3HZ
    Sedatives, 3E0R3NZ
    Stem Cells
      Embryonic, 3E0R
      Somatic, 3E0R
    Water Balance Substance, 3E0R37Z
  Subcutaneous Tissue, 3E013GC
    Analgesics, 3E013NZ
    Anesthetic Agent, 3E013BZ
    Anti-infective, 3E01
    Anti-inflammatory, 3E0133Z
    Antineoplastic, 3E0130
    Destructive Agent, 3E013TZ
    Diagnostic Substance, Other, 3E013KZ
    Electrolytic Substance, 3E0137Z
    Hormone, 3E013V
    Hypnotics, 3E013NZ
    Nutritional Substance, 3E0136Z
    Radioactive Substance, 3E013HZ
    Sedatives, 3E013NZ
    Serum, 3E0134Z
    Toxoid, 3E0134Z
    Vaccine, 3E0134Z
    Water Balance Substance, 3E0137Z
  Vein
    Central, 3E04

Introduction of substance in or on — *continued*
  Vein — *continued*
    Central — *continued*
      Analgesics, 3E04
      Anesthetic, Intracirculatory, 3E04
      Antiarrhythmic, 3E04
      Anti-infective, 3E04
      Anti-inflammatory, 3E04
      Antineoplastic, 3E04
      Destructive Agent, 3E04
      Diagnostic Substance, Other, 3E04
      Electrolytic Substance, 3E04
      Hormone, 3E04
      Hypnotics, 3E04
      Immunotherapeutic, 3E04
      Nutritional Substance, 3E04
      Platelet Inhibitor, 3E04
      Radioactive Substance, 3E04
      Sedatives, 3E04
      Serum, 3E04
      Thrombolytic, 3E04
      Toxoid, 3E04
      Vaccine, 3E04
      Vasopressor, 3E04
      Water Balance Substance, 3E04
    Peripheral, 3E03
      Analgesics, 3E03
      Anesthetic, Intracirculatory, 3E03
      Antiarrhythmic, 3E03
      Anti-infective, 3E03
      Anti-inflammatory, 3E03
      Antineoplastic, 3E03
      Destructive Agent, 3E03
      Diagnostic Substance, Other, 3E03
      Electrolytic Substance, 3E03
      Hormone, 3E03
      Hypnotics, 3E03
      Immunotherapeutic, 3E03
      Islet Cells, Pancreatic, 3E03
      Nutritional Substance, 3E03
      Platelet Inhibitor, 3E03
      Radioactive Substance, 3E03
      Sedatives, 3E03
      Serum, 3E03
      Thrombolytic, 3E03
      Toxoid, 3E03
      Vaccine, 3E03
      Vasopressor, 3E03
      Water Balance Substance, 3E03
Intubation
  Airway
    see Insertion of device in, Esophagus, 0DH5
    see Insertion of device in, Mouth and Throat, 0CHY
    see Insertion of device in, Trachea, 0BH1
  Drainage device *see* Drainage
  Feeding Device *see* Insertion of device in, Gastrointestinal System, 0DH
INTUITY Elite valve system, EDWARDS *use* Zooplastic Tissue, Rapid Deployment Technique in New Technology
IPPB (intermittent positive pressure breathing) *see* Assistance, Respiratory, 5A09
IRE (Irreversible Electroporation) *see* Destruction, Hepatobiliary System and Pancreas, 0F5
Iridectomy
  see Excision, Eye, 08B
  see Resection, Eye, 08T
Iridoplasty
  see Repair, Eye, 08Q
  see Replacement, Eye, 08R
  see Supplement, Eye, 08U
Iridotomy *see* Drainage, Eye, 089
Irreversible Electroporation (IRE) *see* Destruction, Hepatobiliary System and Pancreas, 0F5
Irrigation
  Biliary Tract, Irrigating Substance, 3E1J
  Brain, Irrigating Substance, 3E1Q38Z
  Cranial Cavity, Irrigating Substance, 3E1Q38Z
  Ear, Irrigating Substance, 3E1B
  Epidural Space, Irrigating Substance, 3E1S38Z
  Eye, Irrigating Substance, 3E1C
  Gastrointestinal Tract
    Lower, Irrigating Substance, 3E1H
    Upper, Irrigating Substance, 3E1G
  Genitourinary Tract, Irrigating Substance, 3E1K
  Irrigating Substance, 3C1ZX8Z
  Joint, Irrigating Substance, 3E1U38Z

Irrigation — *continued*
  Mucous Membrane, Irrigating Substance, 3E10
  Nose, Irrigating Substance, 3E19
  Pancreatic Tract, Irrigating Substance, 3E1J
  Pericardial Cavity, Irrigating Substance, 3E1Y38Z
  Peritoneal Cavity
    Dialysate, 3E1M39Z
    Irrigating Substance, 3E1M38Z
  Pleural Cavity, Irrigating Substance, 3E1L38Z
  Reproductive
    Female, Irrigating Substance, 3E1P
    Male, Irrigating Substance, 3E1N
  Respiratory Tract, Irrigating Substance, 3E1F
  Skin, Irrigating Substance, 3E10
  Spinal Canal, Irrigating Substance, 3E1R38Z
Isavuconazole Anti-infective, XW0
Ischiatic nerve *use* Sciatic Nerve
Ischiocavernosus muscle *use* Perineum Muscle
Ischiofemoral ligament
  use Hiip Bursa and Ligament, Left
  use Hip Bursa and Ligament, Right
Ischium
  use Pelvic Bone, Left
  use Pelvic Bone, Right
Isolation, 8E0ZXY6
Isotope Administration, Whole Body, DWY5G
Itrel (3) (4) neurostimulator *use* Stimulator Generator, Single Array in, 0JH

J

Jejunal artery *use* Superior Mesenteric Artery
Jejunectomy
  see Excision, Jejunum, 0DBA
  see Resection, Jejunum, 0DTA
Jejunocolostomy
  see Bypass, Gastrointestinal System, 0D1
  see Drainage, Gastrointestinal System, 0D9
Jejunopexy
  see Repair, Jejunum, 0DQA
  see Reposition, Jejunum, 0DSA
Jejunostomy
  see Bypass, Jejunum, 0D1A
  see Drainage, Jejunum, 0D9A
Jejunotomy *see* Drainage, Jejunum, 0D9A
Joint fixation plate
  use Internal Fixation Device in Lower Joints
  use Internal Fixation Device in Upper Joints
Joint liner (insert) *use* Liner in Lower Joints
Joint spacer (antibiotic)
  use Spacer in Lower Joints
  use Spacer in Upper Joints
Jugular body *use* Glomus Jugulare
Jugular lymph node
  use Lymphatic, Left Neck
  use Lymphatic, Right Neck

K

Kappa *use* Pacemaker, Dual Chamber in, 0JH
Kcentra *use* 4-Factor Prothrombin Complex Concentrate
Keratectomy, kerectomy
  see Excision, Eye, 08B
  see Resection, Eye, 08T
Keratocentesis *see* Drainage, Eye, 089
Keratoplasty
  see Repair, Eye, 08Q
  see Replacement, Eye, 08R
  see Supplement, Eye, 08U
Keratotomy
  see Drainage, Eye, 089
  see Repair, Eye, 08Q
Kirschner wire (K-wire)
  use Internal Fixation Device in Head and Facial Bones
  use Internal Fixation Device in Lower Bones
  use Internal Fixation Device in Lower Joints
  use Internal Fixation Device in Upper Bones
  use Internal Fixation Device in Upper Joints
Knee (implant) insert *use* Liner in Lower Joints
KUB x-ray *see* Plain Radiography, Kidney, Ureter and Bladder, BT04
Kuntscher nail
  use Internal Fixation Device, Intramedullary in Lower Bones

L

Kuntscher nail — *continued*
  use Internal Fixation Device, Intramedullary in Upper Bones
KYMRIAH *use* Engineered Autologous Chimeric Antigen Receptor T-cell Immunotherapy

Labia majora *use* Vulva
Labia minora *use* Vulva
Labial gland
  use Lower Lip
  use Upper Lip
Labiectomy
  see Excision, Female Reproductive System, ØUB
  see Resection, Female Reproductive System, ØUT
Lacrimal canaliculus
  use Lacrimal Duct, Left
  use Lacrimal Duct, Right
Lacrimal punctum
  use Lacrimal Duct, Left
  use Lacrimal Duct, Right
Lacrimal sac
  use Lacrimal Duct, Left
  use Lacrimal Duct, Right
LAGB (laparoscopic adjustable gastric banding)
  Initial procedure, ØDV64CZ
  Surgical correction *see* Revision of device in, Stomach, ØDW6
Laminectomy
  see Excision, Lower Bones, ØQB
  see Excision, Upper Bones, ØPB
  see Release, Central Nervous System and Cranial Nerves, ØØN
  see Release, Peripheral Nervous System, Ø1N
Laminotomy
  see Drainage, Lower Bones, ØQ9
  see Drainage, Upper Bones, ØP9
  see Excision, Lower Bones, ØQB
  see Excision, Upper Bones, ØPB
  see Release, Central Nervous System and Cranial Nerves, ØØN
  see Release, Lower Bones, ØQN
  see Release, Peripheral Nervous System, Ø1N
  see Release, Upper Bones, ØPN
Laparoscopic-assisted transanal pull-through
  see Excision, Gastrointestinal System, ØDB
  see Resection, Gastrointestinal System, ØDT
Laparoscopy *see* Inspection
Laparotomy
  Drainage *see* Drainage, Peritoneal Cavity, ØW9G
  Exploratory *see* Inspection, Peritoneal Cavity, ØWJG
LAP-BAND® Adjustable Gastric Banding System *use* Extraluminal Device
Laryngectomy
  see Excision, Larynx, ØCBS
  see Resection, Larynx, ØCTS
Laryngocentesis *see* Drainage, Larynx, ØC9S
Laryngogram *see* Fluoroscopy, Larynx, B91J
Laryngopexy *see* Repair, Larynx, ØCQS
Laryngopharynx *use* Pharynx
Laryngoplasty
  see Repair, Larynx, ØCQS
  see Replacement, Larynx, ØCRS
  see Supplement, Larynx, ØCUS
Laryngorrhaphy *see* Repair, Larynx, ØCQS
Laryngoscopy, ØCJS8ZZ
Laryngotomy *see* Drainage, Larynx, ØC9S
Laser Interstitial Thermal Therapy
  Adrenal Gland, DGY2KZZ
  Anus, DDY8KZZ
  Bile Ducts, DFY2KZZ
  Brain, DØYØKZZ
  Brain Stem, DØY1KZZ
  Breast
    Left, DMYØKZZ
    Right, DMY1KZZ
  Bronchus, DBY1KZZ
  Chest Wall, DBY7KZZ
  Colon, DDY5KZZ
  Diaphragm, DBY8KZZ
  Duodenum, DDY2KZZ
  Esophagus, DDYØKZZ
  Gallbladder, DFY1KZZ
  Gland
    Adrenal, DGY2KZZ

Laser Interstitial Thermal Therapy — *continued*
  Gland — *continued*
    Parathyroid, DGY4KZZ
    Pituitary, DGYØKZZ
    Thyroid, DGY5KZZ
  Ileum, DDY4KZZ
  Jejunum, DDY3KZZ
  Liver, DFYØKZZ
  Lung, DBY2KZZ
  Mediastinum, DBY6KZZ
  Nerve, Peripheral, DØY7KZZ
  Pancreas, DFY3KZZ
  Parathyroid Gland, DGY4KZZ
  Pineal Body, DGY1KZZ
  Pituitary Gland, DGYØKZZ
  Pleura, DBY5KZZ
  Prostate, DVYØKZZ
  Rectum, DDY7KZZ
  Spinal Cord, DØY6KZZ
  Stomach, DDY1KZZ
  Thyroid Gland, DGY5KZZ
  Trachea, DBYØKZZ
Lateral canthus
  use Upper Eyelid, Left
  use Upper Eyelid, Right
Lateral collateral ligament (LCL)
  use Knee Bursa and Ligament, Left
  use Knee Bursa and Ligament, Right
Lateral condyle of femur
  use Lower Femur, Left
  use Lower Femur, Right
Lateral condyle of tibia
  use Tibia, Left
  use Tibia, Right
Lateral cuneiform bone
  use Tarsal, Left
  use Tarsal, Right
Lateral epicondyle of femur
  use Lower Femur, Left
  use Lower Femur, Right
Lateral epicondyle of humerus
  use Humeral Shaft, Left
  use Humeral Shaft, Right
Lateral femoral cutaneous nerve *use* Lumbar Plexus
Lateral (brachial) lymph node
  use Lymphatic, Left Axillary
  use Lymphatic, Right Axillary
Lateral malleolus
  use Fibula, Left
  use Fibula, Right
Lateral meniscus
  use Knee Joint, Left
  use Knee Joint, Right
Lateral nasal cartilage *use* Nasal Mucosa and Soft Tissue
Lateral plantar artery
  use Foot Artery, Left
  use Foot Artery, Right
Lateral plantar nerve *use* Tibial Nerve
Lateral rectus muscle
  use Extraocular Muscle, Left
  use Extraocular Muscle, Right
Lateral sacral artery
  use Internal Iliac Artery, Left
  use Internal Iliac Artery, Right
Lateral sacral vein
  use Hypogastric Vein, Left
  use Hypogastric Vein, Right
Lateral sural cutaneous nerve *use* Peroneal Nerve
Lateral tarsal artery
  use Foot Artery, Left
  use Foot Artery, Right
Lateral temporomandibular ligament *use* Head and Neck Bursa and Ligament
Lateral thoracic artery
  use Axillary Artery, Left
  use Axillary Artery, Right
Latissimus dorsi muscle
  use Trunk Muscle, Left
  use Trunk Muscle, Right
Latissimus Dorsi Myocutaneous Flap
  Replacement
    Bilateral, ØHRVØ75
    Left, ØHRUØ75
    Right, ØHRTØ75
  Transfer
    Left, ØKXG
    Right, ØKXF

Lavage
  see Irrigation
  Bronchial alveolar, diagnostic *see* Drainage, Respiratory System, ØB9
Least splanchnic nerve *use* Thoracic Sympathetic Nerve
Left ascending lumbar vein *use* Hemiazygos Vein
Left atrioventricular valve *use* Mitral Valve
Left auricular appendix *use* Atrium, Left
Left colic vein *use* Colic Vein
Left coronary sulcus *use* Heart, Left
Left gastric artery *use* Gastric Artery
Left gastroepiploic artery *use* Splenic Artery
Left gastroepiploic vein *use* Splenic Vein
Left inferior phrenic vein *use* Renal Vein, Left
Left inferior pulmonary vein *use* Pulmonary Vein, Left
Left jugular trunk *use* Thoracic Duct
Left lateral ventricle *use* Cerebral Ventricle
Left ovarian vein *use* Renal Vein, Left
Left second lumbar vein *use* Renal Vein, Left
Left subclavian trunk *use* Thoracic Duct
Left subcostal vein *use* Hemiazygos Vein
Left superior pulmonary vein *use* Pulmonary Vein, Left
Left suprarenal vein *use* Renal Vein, Left
Left testicular vein *use* Renal Vein, Left
Lengthening
  Bone, with device *see* Insertion of Limb Lengthening Device
  Muscle, by incision *see* Division, Muscles, ØK8
  Tendon, by incision *see* Division, Tendons, ØL8
Leptomeninges, intracranial *use* Cerebral Meninges
Leptomeninges, spinal *use* Spinal Meninges
Lesser alar cartilage *use* Nasal Mucosa and Soft Tissue
Lesser occipital nerve *use* Cervical Plexus
Lesser Omentum *use* Omentum
Lesser saphenous vein
  use Saphenous Vein, Left
  use Saphenous Vein, Right
Lesser splanchnic nerve *use* Thoracic Sympathetic Nerve
Lesser trochanter
  use Upper Femur, Left
  use Upper Femur, Right
Lesser tuberosity
  use Humeral Head, Left
  use Humeral Head, Right
Lesser wing *use* Sphenoid Bone
Leukopheresis, therapeutic *see* Pheresis, Circulatory, 6A55
Levator anguli oris muscle *use* Facial Muscle
Levator ani muscle *use* Perineum Muscle
Levator labii superioris alaeque nasi muscle *use* Facial Muscle
Levator labii superioris muscle *use* Facial Muscle
Levator palpebrae superioris muscle
  use Upper Eyelid, Left
  use Upper Eyelid, Right
Levator scapulae muscle
  use Neck Muscle, Left
  use Neck Muscle, Right
Levator veli palatini muscle *use* Tongue, Palate, Pharynx Muscle
Levatores costarum muscle
  use Thorax Muscle, Left
  use Thorax Muscle, Right
LifeStent® (Flexstar) (XL) Vascular Stent System *use* Intraluminal Device
Ligament of head of fibula
  use Knee Bursa and Ligament, Left
  use Knee Bursa and Ligament, Right
Ligament of the lateral malleolus
  use Ankle Bursa and Ligament, Left
  use Ankle Bursa and Ligament, Right
Ligamentum flavum, cervical *use* Head and Neck Bursa and Ligament
Ligamentum flavum, lumbar *use* Lower Spine Bursa and Ligament
Ligamentum flavum, thoracic *use* Upper Spine Bursa and Ligament
Ligation *see* Occlusion
Ligation, hemorrhoid *see* Occlusion, Lower Veins, Hemorrhoidal Plexus
Light Therapy, GZJZZZZ
Liner
  Removal of device from
    Hip
      Left, ØSPB09Z
      Right, ØSP909Z

▼ Subterms under main terms may continue to next column or page

Liner — *continued*
Removal of device from — *continued*
Knee
Left, ØSPDØ9Z
Right, ØSPCØ9Z
Revision of device in
Hip
Left, ØSWBØ9Z
Right, ØSW9Ø9Z
Knee
Left, ØSWDØ9Z
Right, ØSWCØ9Z
Supplement
Hip
Left, ØSUBØ9Z
Acetabular Surface, ØSUEØ9Z
Femoral Surface, ØSUSØ9Z
Right, ØSU9Ø9Z
Acetabular Surface, ØSUAØ9Z
Femoral Surface, ØSURØ9Z
Knee
Left, ØSUDØ9
Femoral Surface, ØSUUØ9Z
Tibial Surface, ØSUWØ9Z
Right, ØSUCØ9
Femoral Surface, ØSUTØ9Z
Tibial Surface, ØSUVØ9Z
Lingual artery
use External Carotid Artery, Left
use External Carotid Artery, Right
Lingual tonsil *use* Pharynx
Lingulectomy, lung
see Excision, Lung Lingula, ØBBH
see Resection, Lung Lingula, ØBTH
Lithotripsy
With removal of fragments *see* Extirpation
see Fragmentation
LITT (laser interstitial thermal therapy) *see* Laser Interstitial Thermal Therapy
LIVIAN™ CRT-D *use* Cardiac Resynchronization Defibrillator Pulse Generator in, ØJH
Lobectomy
see Excision, Central Nervous System and Cranial Nerves, ØØB
see Excision, Endocrine System, ØGB
see Excision, Hepatobiliary System and Pancreas, ØFB
see Excision, Respiratory System, ØBB
see Resection, Endocrine System, ØGT
see Resection, Hepatobiliary System and Pancreas, ØFT
see Resection, Respiratory System, ØBT
Lobotomy *see* Division, Brain, ØØ8Ø
Localization
see Imaging
see Map
Locus ceruleus *use* Pons
Long thoracic nerve *use* Brachial Plexus
Loop ileostomy *see* Bypass, Ileum, ØD1B
Loop recorder, implantable *use* Monitoring Device
Lower GI series *see* Fluoroscopy, Colon, BD14
Lumbar artery *use* Abdominal Aorta
Lumbar facet joint *use* Lumbar Vertebral Joint
Lumbar ganglion *use* Lumbar Sympathetic Nerve
Lumbar lymph node *use* Lymphatic, Aortic
Lumbar lymphatic trunk *use* Cisterna Chyli
Lumbar splanchnic nerve *use* Lumbar Sympathetic Nerve
Lumbosacral facet joint *use* Lumbosacral Joint
Lumbosacral trunk *use* Lumbar Nerve
Lumpectomy *see* Excision
Lunate bone
use Carpal, Left
use Carpal, Right
Lunotriquetral ligament
use Hand Bursa and Ligament, Left
use Hand Bursa and Ligament, Right
Lymphadenectomy
see Excision, Lymphatic and Hemic Systems, Ø7B
see Resection, Lymphatic and Hemic Systems, Ø7T
Lymphadenotomy *see* Drainage, Lymphatic and Hemic Systems, Ø79
Lymphangiectomy
see Excision, Lymphatic and Hemic Systems, Ø7B
see Resection, Lymphatic and Hemic Systems, Ø7T
Lymphangiogram *see* Plain Radiography, Lymphatic System, B7Ø
Lymphangioplasty
see Repair, Lymphatic and Hemic Systems, Ø7Q

Lymphangioplasty — *continued*
see Supplement, Lymphatic and Hemic Systems, Ø7U
Lymphangiorrhaphy *see* Repair, Lymphatic and Hemic Systems, Ø7Q
Lymphangiotomy *see* Drainage, Lymphatic and Hemic Systems, Ø79
Lysis *see* Release

M

Macula
use Retina, Left
use Retina, Right
MAGEC® Spinal Bracing and Distraction System *use* Magnetically Controlled Growth Rod(s) in New Technology
Magnet extraction, ocular foreign body *see* Extirpation, Eye, Ø8C
Magnetic Resonance Imaging (MRI)
Abdomen, BW3Ø
Ankle
Left, BQ3H
Right, BQ3G
Aorta
Abdominal, B43Ø
Thoracic, B33Ø
Arm
Left, BP3F
Right, BP3E
Artery
Celiac, B431
Cervico-Cerebral Arch, B33Q
Common Carotid, Bilateral, B335
Coronary
Bypass Graft, Multiple, B233
Multiple, B231
Internal Carotid, Bilateral, B338
Intracranial, B33R
Lower Extremity
Bilateral, B43H
Left, B43G
Right, B43F
Pelvic, B43C
Renal, Bilateral, B438
Spinal, B33M
Superior Mesenteric, B434
Upper Extremity
Bilateral, B33K
Left, B33J
Right, B33H
Vertebral, Bilateral, B33G
Bladder, BT3Ø
Brachial Plexus, BW3P
Brain, BØ3Ø
Breast
Bilateral, BH32
Left, BH31
Right, BH3Ø
Calcaneus
Left, BQ3K
Right, BQ3J
Chest, BW33Y
Coccyx, BR3F
Connective Tissue
Lower Extremity, BL31
Upper Extremity, BL3Ø
Corpora Cavernosa, BV3Ø
Disc
Cervical, BR31
Lumbar, BR33
Thoracic, BR32
Ear, B93Ø
Elbow
Left, BP3H
Right, BP3G
Eye
Bilateral, B837
Left, B836
Right, B835
Femur
Left, BQ34
Right, BQ33
Fetal Abdomen, BY33
Fetal Extremity, BY35
Fetal Head, BY3Ø
Fetal Heart, BY31
Fetal Spine, BY34
Fetal Thorax, BY32

Magnetic Resonance Imaging (MRI) — *continued*
Fetus, Whole, BY36
Foot
Left, BQ3M
Right, BQ3L
Forearm
Left, BP3K
Right, BP3J
Gland
Adrenal, Bilateral, BG32
Parathyroid, BG33
Parotid, Bilateral, B936
Salivary, Bilateral, B93D
Submandibular, Bilateral, B939
Thyroid, BG34
Head, BW38
Heart, Right and Left, B236
Hip
Left, BQ31
Right, BQ3Ø
Intracranial Sinus, B532
Joint
Finger
Left, BP3D
Right, BP3C
Hand
Left, BP3D
Right, BP3C
Temporomandibular, Bilateral, BN39
Kidney
Bilateral, BT33
Left, BT32
Right, BT31
Transplant, BT39
Knee
Left, BQ38
Right, BQ37
Larynx, B93J
Leg
Left, BQ3F
Right, BQ3D
Liver, BF35
Liver and Spleen, BF36
Lung Apices, BB3G
Nasopharynx, B93F
Neck, BW3F
Nerve
Acoustic, BØ3C
Brachial Plexus, BW3P
Oropharynx, B93F
Ovary
Bilateral, BU35
Left, BU34
Right, BU33
Ovary and Uterus, BU3C
Pancreas, BF37
Patella
Left, BQ3W
Right, BQ3V
Pelvic Region, BW3G
Pelvis, BR3C
Pituitary Gland, BØ39
Plexus, Brachial, BW3P
Prostate, BV33
Retroperitoneum, BW3H
Sacrum, BR3F
Scrotum, BV34
Sella Turcica, BØ39
Shoulder
Left, BP39
Right, BP38
Sinus
Intracranial, B532
Paranasal, B932
Spinal Cord, BØ3B
Spine
Cervical, BR3Ø
Lumbar, BR39
Thoracic, BR37
Spleen and Liver, BF36
Subcutaneous Tissue
Abdomen, BH3H
Extremity
Lower, BH3J
Upper, BH3F
Head, BH3D
Neck, BH3D
Pelvis, BH3H
Thorax, BH3G

Magnetic Resonance Imaging (MRI)

Magnetic Resonance Imaging (MRI) — continued

Tendon
- Lower Extremity, BL33
- Upper Extremity, BL32

Testicle
- Bilateral, BV37
- Left, BV36
- Right, BV35

Toe
- Left, BQ3Q
- Right, BQ3P

Uterus, BU36
- Pregnant, BU3B

Uterus and Ovary, BU3C

Vagina, BU39

Vein
- Cerebellar, B531
- Cerebral, B531
- Jugular, Bilateral, B535
- Lower Extremity
  - Bilateral, B53D
  - Left, B53C
  - Right, B53B
- Other, B53V
- Pelvic (Iliac) Bilateral, B53H
- Portal, B53T
- Pulmonary, Bilateral, B53S
- Renal, Bilateral, B53L
- Spanchnic, B53T
- Upper Extremity
  - Bilateral, B53P
  - Left, B53N
  - Right, B53M
- Vena Cava
  - Inferior, B539
  - Superior, B538
- Wrist
  - Left, BP3M
  - Right, BP3L

Magnetically Controlled Growth Rod(s)
- Cervical, XNS3
- Lumbar, XNS0
- Thoracic, XNS4

Malleotomy see Drainage, Ear, Nose, Sinus, 099

Malleus
- use Auditory Ossicle, Left
- use Auditory Ossicle, Right

Mammaplasty, mammoplasty
- see Alteration, Skin and Breast, 0H0
- see Repair, Skin and Breast, 0HQ
- see Replacement, Skin and Breast, 0HR
- see Supplement, Skin and Breast, 0HU

Mammary duct
- use Breast, Bilateral
- use Breast, Left
- use Breast, Right

Mammary gland
- use Breast, Bilateral
- use Breast, Left
- use Breast, Right

Mammectomy
- see Excision, Skin and Breast, 0HB
- see Resection, Skin and Breast, 0HT

Mammillary body use Hypothalamus

Mammography see Plain Radiography, Skin, Subcutaneous Tissue and Breast, BH0

Mammotomy see Drainage, Skin and Breast, 0H9

Mandibular nerve use Trigeminal Nerve

Mandibular notch
- use Mandible, Left
- use Mandible, Right

Mandibulectomy
- see Excision, Head and Facial Bones, 0NB
- see Resection, Head and Facial Bones, 0NT

Manipulation
- Adhesions see Release
- Chiropractic see Chiropractic Manipulation

Manual removal, retained placenta see Extraction, Products of Conception, Retained, 10D1

Manubrium use Sternum

Map
- Basal Ganglia, 00K8
- Brain, 00K0
- Cerebellum, 00KC
- Cerebral Hemisphere, 00K7
- Conduction Mechanism, 02K8
- Hypothalamus, 00KA
- Medulla Oblongata, 00KD

Map — continued
- Pons, 00KB
- Thalamus, 00K9

Mapping
- Doppler ultrasound see Ultrasonography
- Electrocardiogram only see Measurement, Cardiac, 4A02

Mark IV Breathing Pacemaker System use Stimulator Generator in Subcutaneous Tissue and Fascia

Marsupialization
- see Drainage
- see Excision

Massage, cardiac
- External, 5A12012
- Open, 02QA0ZZ

Masseter muscle use Head Muscle

Masseteric fascia use Subcutaneous Tissue and Fascia, Face

Mastectomy
- see Excision, Skin and Breast, 0HB
- see Resection, Skin and Breast, 0HT

Mastoid air cells
- use Mastoid Sinus, Left
- use Mastoid Sinus, Right

Mastoid (postauricular) lymph node
- use Lymphatic, Left Neck
- use Lymphatic, Right Neck

Mastoid process
- use Temporal Bone, Left
- use Temporal Bone, Right

Mastoidectomy
- see Excision, Ear, Nose, Sinus, 09B
- see Resection, Ear, Nose, Sinus, 09T

Mastoidotomy see Drainage, Ear, Nose, Sinus, 099

Mastopexy
- see Repair, Skin and Breast, 0HQ
- see Reposition, Skin and Breast, 0HS

Mastorrhaphy see Repair, Skin and Breast, 0HQ

Mastotomy see Drainage, Skin and Breast, 0H9

Maxillary artery
- use External Carotid Artery, Left
- use External Carotid Artery, Right

Maxillary nerve use Trigeminal Nerve

Maximo II DR (VR) use Defibrillator Generator in, 0JH

Maximo II DR CRT-D use Cardiac Resynchronization Defibrillator Pulse Generator in, 0JH

Measurement
- Arterial
  - Flow
    - Coronary, 4A03
    - Peripheral, 4A03
    - Pulmonary, 4A03
  - Pressure
    - Coronary, 4A03
    - Peripheral, 4A03
    - Pulmonary, 4A03
    - Thoracic, Other, 4A03
  - Pulse
    - Coronary, 4A03
    - Peripheral, 4A03
    - Pulmonary, 4A03
  - Saturation, Peripheral, 4A03
  - Sound, Peripheral, 4A03
- Biliary
  - Flow, 4A0C
  - Pressure, 4A0C
- Cardiac
  - Action Currents, 4A02
  - Defibrillator, 4B02XTZ
  - Electrical Activity, 4A02
    - Guidance, 4A02X4A
    - No Qualifier, 4A02X4Z
  - Output, 4A02
  - Pacemaker, 4B02XSZ
  - Rate, 4A02
  - Rhythm, 4A02
  - Sampling and Pressure
    - Bilateral, 4A02
    - Left Heart, 4A02
    - Right Heart, 4A02
  - Sound, 4A02
  - Total Activity, Stress, 4A02XM4
- Central Nervous
  - Conductivity, 4A00
  - Electrical Activity, 4A00
  - Pressure, 4A000BZ
    - Intracranial, 4A00
  - Saturation, Intracranial, 4A00

Measurement — continued
- Central Nervous — continued
  - Stimulator, 4B00XVZ
  - Temperature, Intracranial, 4A00
- Circulatory, Volume, 4A05XLZ
- Gastrointestinal
  - Motility, 4A0B
  - Pressure, 4A0B
  - Secretion, 4A0B
- Lymphatic
  - Flow, 4A06
  - Pressure, 4A06
- Metabolism, 4A0Z
- Musculoskeletal
  - Contractility, 4A0F
  - Stimulator, 4B0FXVZ
- Olfactory, Acuity, 4A08X0Z
- Peripheral Nervous
  - Conductivity
    - Motor, 4A01
    - Sensory, 4A01
  - Electrical Activity, 4A01
  - Stimulator, 4B01XVZ
- Products of Conception
  - Cardiac
    - Electrical Activity, 4A0H
    - Rate, 4A0H
    - Rhythm, 4A0H
    - Sound, 4A0H
  - Nervous
    - Conductivity, 4A0J
    - Electrical Activity, 4A0J
    - Pressure, 4A0J
- Respiratory
  - Capacity, 4A09
  - Flow, 4A09
  - Pacemaker, 4B09XSZ
  - Rate, 4A09
  - Resistance, 4A09
  - Total Activity, 4A09
  - Volume, 4A09
- Sleep, 4A0ZXQZ
- Temperature, 4A0Z
- Urinary
  - Contractility, 4A0D
  - Flow, 4A0D
  - Pressure, 4A0D
  - Resistance, 4A0D
  - Volume, 4A0D
- Venous
  - Flow
    - Central, 4A04
    - Peripheral, 4A04
    - Portal, 4A04
    - Pulmonary, 4A04
  - Pressure
    - Central, 4A04
    - Peripheral, 4A04
    - Portal, 4A04
    - Pulmonary, 4A04
  - Pulse
    - Central, 4A04
    - Peripheral, 4A04
    - Portal, 4A04
    - Pulmonary, 4A04
  - Saturation, Peripheral, 4A04
- Visual
  - Acuity, 4A07X0Z
  - Mobility, 4A07X7Z
  - Pressure, 4A07XBZ

Meatoplasty, urethra see Repair, Urethra, 0TQD

Meatotomy see Drainage, Urinary System, 0T9

Mechanical ventilation see Performance, Respiratory, 5A19

Medial canthus
- use Lower Eyelid, Left
- use Lower Eyelid, Right

Medial collateral ligament (MCL)
- use Knee Bursa and Ligament, Left
- use Knee Bursa and Ligament, Right

Medial condyle of femur
- use Lower Femur, Left
- use Lower Femur, Right

Medial condyle of tibia
- use Tibia, Left
- use Tibia, Right

Medial cuneiform bone
- use Tarsal, Left

Medial cuneiform bone — *continued*
  use Tarsal, Right
Medial epicondyle of femur
  use Lower Femur, Left
  use Lower Femur, Right
Medial epicondyle of humerus
  use Humeral Shaft, Left
  use Humeral Shaft, Right
Medial malleolus
  use Tibia, Left
  use Tibia, Right
Medial meniscus
  use Knee Joint, Left
  use Knee Joint, Right
Medial plantar artery
  use Foot Artery, Left
  use Foot Artery, Right
Medial plantar nerve *use* Tibial Nerve
Medial popliteal nerve *use* Tibial Nerve
Medial rectus muscle
  use Extraocular Muscle, Left
  use Extraocular Muscle, Right
Medial sural cutaneous nerve *use* Tibial Nerve
Median antebrachial vein
  use Basilic Vein, Left
  use Basilic Vein, Right
Median cubital vein
  use Basilic Vein, Left
  use Basilic Vein, Right
Median sacral artery *use* Abdominal Aorta
Mediastinal cavity *use* Mediastinum
Mediastinal lymph node *use* Lymphatic, Thorax
Mediastinal space *use* Mediastinum
Mediastinoscopy, 0WJC4ZZ
Medication Management, GZ3ZZZZ
  for substance abuse
    Antabuse, HZ83ZZZ
    Bupropion, HZ87ZZZ
    Clonidine, HZ86ZZZ
    Levo-alpha-acetyl-methadol (LAAM), HZ82ZZZ
    Methadone Maintenance, HZ81ZZZ
    Naloxone, HZ85ZZZ
    Naltrexone, HZ84ZZZ
    Nicotine Replacement, HZ80ZZZ
    Other Replacement Medication, HZ89ZZZ
    Psychiatric Medication, HZ88ZZZ
Meditation, 8E0ZXY5
Medtronic Endurant® II AAA stent graft system *use* Intraluminal Device
Meissner's (submucous) plexus *use* Abdominal Sympathetic Nerve
Melody® transcatheter pulmonary valve *use* Zooplastic Tissue in Heart and Great Vessels
Membranous urethra *use* Urethra
Meningeorrhaphy
  see Repair, Cerebral Meninges, 00Q1
  see Repair, Spinal Meninges, 00QT
Meniscectomy, knee
  see Excision, Joint, Knee, Left, 0SBD
  see Excision, Joint, Knee, Right, 0SBC
Mental foramen
  use Mandible, Left
  use Mandible, Right
Mentalis muscle *use* Facial Muscle
Mentoplasty *see* Alteration, Jaw, Lower, 0W05
Mesenterectomy *see* Excision, Mesentery, 0DBV
Mesenteriorrhaphy, mesenterorrhaphy *see* Repair, Mesentery, 0DQV
Mesenteriplication *see* Repair, Mesentery, 0DQV
Mesoappendix *use* Mesentery
Mesocolon *use* Mesentery
Metacarpal ligament
  use Hand Bursa and Ligament, Left
  use Hand Bursa and Ligament, Right
Metacarpophalangeal ligament
  use Hand Bursa and Ligament, Left
  use Hand Bursa and Ligament, Right
Metal on metal bearing surface *use* Synthetic Substitute, Metal in, 0SR
Metatarsal ligament
  use Foot Bursa and Ligament, Left
  use Foot Bursa and Ligament, Right
Metatarsectomy
  see Excision, Lower Bones, 0QB
  see Resection, Lower Bones, 0QT
Metatarsophalangeal (MTP) joint
  use Metatarsal-Phalangeal Joint, Left

Metatarsophalangeal (MTP) joint — *continued*
  use Metatarsal-Phalangeal Joint, Right
Metatarsophalangeal ligament
  use Foot Bursa and Ligament, Left
  use Foot Bursa and Ligament, Right
Metathalamus *use* Thalamus
Micro-Driver stent (RX) (OTW) *use* Intraluminal Device
MicroMed HeartAssist *use* Implantable Heart Assist System in Heart and Great Vessels
Micrus CERECYTE Microcoil *use* Intraluminal Device, Bioactive in Upper Arteries
Midcarpal joint
  use Carpal Joint, Left
  use Carpal Joint, Right
Middle cardiac nerve *use* Thoracic Sympathetic Nerve
Middle cerebral artery *use* Intracranial Artery
Middle cerebral vein *use* Intracranial Vein
Middle colic vein *use* Colic Vein
Middle genicular artery
  use Popliteal Artery, Left
  use Popliteal Artery, Right
Middle hemorrhoidal vein
  use Hypogastric Vein, Left
  use Hypogastric Vein, Right
Middle rectal artery
  use Internal Iliac Artery, Left
  use Internal Iliac Artery, Right
Middle suprarenal artery *use* Abdominal Aorta
Middle temporal artery
  use Temporal Artery, Left
  use Temporal Artery, Right
Middle turbinate *use* Nasal Turbinate
MIRODERM™ Biologic Wound Matrix *use* Skin Substitute, Porcine Liver Derived in New Technology
MitraClip valve repair system *use* Synthetic Substitute
Mitral annulus *use* Mitral Valve
Mitroflow® Aortic Pericardial Heart Valve *use* Zooplastic Tissue in Heart and Great Vessels
Mobilization, adhesions *see* Release
Molar gland *use* Buccal Mucosa
Monitoring
  Arterial
    Flow
      Coronary, 4A13
      Peripheral, 4A13
      Pulmonary, 4A13
    Pressure
      Coronary, 4A13
      Peripheral, 4A13
      Pulmonary, 4A13
    Pulse
      Coronary, 4A13
      Peripheral, 4A13
      Pulmonary, 4A13
    Saturation, Peripheral, 4A13
    Sound, Peripheral, 4A13
  Cardiac
    Electrical Activity, 4A12
      Ambulatory, 4A12X45
      No Qualifier, 4A12X4Z
    Output, 4A12
    Rate, 4A12
    Rhythm, 4A12
    Sound, 4A12
    Total Activity, Stress, 4A12XM4
    Vascular Perfusion, Indocyanine Green Dye, 4A12XSH
  Central Nervous
    Conductivity, 4A10
    Electrical Activity
      Intraoperative, 4A10
      No Qualifier, 4A10
    Pressure, 4A100BZ
      Intracranial, 4A10
    Saturation, Intracranial, 4A10
    Temperature, Intracranial, 4A10
  Gastrointestinal
    Motility, 4A1B
    Pressure, 4A1B
    Secretion, 4A1B
    Vascular Perfusion, Indocyanine Green Dye, 4A1BXSH
  Intraoperative Knee Replacement Sensor, XR2
  Lymphatic
    Flow, 4A16
    Pressure, 4A16

Monitoring — *continued*
  Peripheral Nervous
    Conductivity
      Motor, 4A11
      Sensory, 4A11
    Electrical Activity
      Intraoperative, 4A11
      No Qualifier, 4A11
  Products of Conception
    Cardiac
      Electrical Activity, 4A1H
      Rate, 4A1H
      Rhythm, 4A1H
      Sound, 4A1H
    Nervous
      Conductivity, 4A1J
      Electrical Activity, 4A1J
      Pressure, 4A1J
  Respiratory
    Capacity, 4A19
    Flow, 4A19
    Rate, 4A19
    Resistance, 4A19
    Volume, 4A19
  Skin and Breast, Vascular Perfusion, Indocyanine Green Dye, 4A1GXSH
  Sleep, 4A1ZXQZ
  Temperature, 4A1Z
  Urinary
    Contractility, 4A1D
    Flow, 4A1D
    Pressure, 4A1D
    Resistance, 4A1D
    Volume, 4A1D
  Venous
    Flow
      Central, 4A14
      Peripheral, 4A14
      Portal, 4A14
      Pulmonary, 4A14
    Pressure
      Central, 4A14
      Peripheral, 4A14
      Portal, 4A14
      Pulmonary, 4A14
    Pulse
      Central, 4A14
      Peripheral, 4A14
      Portal, 4A14
      Pulmonary, 4A14
    Saturation
      Central, 4A14
      Portal, 4A14
      Pulmonary, 4A14
Monitoring Device, Hemodynamic
  Abdomen, 0JH8
  Chest, 0JH6
Mosaic Bioprosthesis (aortic) (mitral) valve *use* Zooplastic Tissue in Heart and Great Vessels
Motor Function Assessment, F01
Motor Treatment, F07
MR Angiography
  see Magnetic Resonance Imaging (MRI), Heart, B23
  see Magnetic Resonance Imaging (MRI), Lower Arteries, B43
  see Magnetic Resonance Imaging (MRI), Upper Arteries, B33
MULTI-LINK (VISION) (MINI-VISION) (ULTRA) Coronary Stent System *use* Intraluminal Device
Multiple sleep latency test, 4A0ZXQZ
Musculocutaneous nerve *use* Brachial Plexus
Musculopexy
  see Repair, Muscles, 0KQ
  see Reposition, Muscles, 0KS
Musculophrenic artery
  use Internal Mammary Artery, Left
  use Internal Mammary Artery, Right
Musculoplasty
  see Repair, Muscles, 0KQ
  see Supplement, Muscles, 0KU
Musculorrhaphy *see* Repair, Muscles, 0KQ
Musculospiral nerve *use* Radial Nerve
Myectomy
  see Excision, Muscles, 0KB
  see Resection, Muscles, 0KT
Myelencephalon *use* Medulla Oblongata

Myelogram
  CT *see* Computerized Tomography (CT Scan), Central Nervous System, B02
  MRI *see* Magnetic Resonance Imaging (MRI), Central Nervous System, B03
Myenteric (Auerbach's) plexus *use* Abdominal Sympathetic Nerve
Myocardial Bridge Release *see* Release, Artery, Coronary
Myomectomy *see* Excision, Female Reproductive System, 0UB
Myometrium *use* Uterus
Myopexy
  see Repair, Muscles, 0KQ
  see Reposition, Muscles, 0KS
Myoplasty
  see Repair, Muscles, 0KQ
  see Supplement, Muscles, 0KU
Myorrhaphy *see* Repair, Muscles, 0KQ
Myoscopy *see* Inspection, Muscles, 0KJ
Myotomy
  see Division, Muscles, 0K8
  see Drainage, Muscles, 0K9
Myringectomy
  see Excision, Ear, Nose, Sinus, 09B
  see Resection, Ear, Nose, Sinus, 09T
Myringoplasty
  see Repair, Ear, Nose, Sinus, 09Q
  see Replacement, Ear, Nose, Sinus, 09R
  see Supplement, Ear, Nose, Sinus, 09U
Myringostomy *see* Drainage, Ear, Nose, Sinus, 099
Myringotomy *see* Drainage, Ear, Nose, Sinus, 099

N

Nail bed
  use Finger Nail
  use Toe Nail
Nail plate
  use Finger Nail
  use Toe Nail
nanoLOCK™ interbody fusion device *use* Interbody Fusion Device, Nanotextured Surface in New Technology
Narcosynthesis, GZGZZZZ
Nasal cavity *use* Nasal Mucosa and Soft Tissue
Nasal concha *use* Nasal Turbinate
Nasalis muscle *use* Facial Muscle
Nasolacrimal duct
  use Lacrimal Duct, Left
  use Lacrimal Duct, Right
Nasopharyngeal airway (NPA) *use* Intraluminal Device, Airway in Ear, Nose, Sinus
Navicular bone
  use Tarsal, Left
  use Tarsal, Right
Near Infrared Spectroscopy, Circulatory System, 8E023DZ
Neck of femur
  use Upper Femur, Left
  use Upper Femur, Right
Neck of humerus (anatomical) (surgical)
  use Humeral Head, Left
  use Humeral Head, Right
Nephrectomy
  see Excision, Urinary System, 0TB
  see Resection, Urinary System, 0TT
Nephrolithotomy *see* Extirpation, Urinary System, 0TC
Nephrolysis *see* Release, Urinary System, 0TN
Nephropexy
  see Repair, Urinary System, 0TQ
  see Reposition, Urinary System, 0TS
Nephroplasty
  see Repair, Urinary System, 0TQ
  see Supplement, Urinary System, 0TU
Nephropyeloureterostomy
  see Bypass, Urinary System, 0T1
  see Drainage, Urinary System, 0T9
Nephrorrhaphy *see* Repair, Urinary System, 0TQ
Nephroscopy, transurethral, 0TJ58ZZ
Nephrostomy
  see Bypass, Urinary System, 0T1
  see Drainage, Urinary System, 0T9
Nephrotomography
  see Fluoroscopy, Urinary System, BT1
  see Plain Radiography, Urinary System, BT0

Nephrotomy
  see Division, Urinary System, 0T8
  see Drainage, Urinary System, 0T9
Nerve conduction study
  see Measurement, Central Nervous, 4A00
  see Measurement, Peripheral Nervous, 4A01
Nerve Function Assessment, F01
Nerve to the stapedius *use* Facial Nerve
Nesiritide *use* Human B-Type Natriuretic Peptide
Neurectomy
  see Excision, Central Nervous System and Cranial Nerves, 00B
  see Excision, Peripheral Nervous System, 01B
Neurexeresis
  see Extraction, Central Nervous System and Cranial Nerves, 00D
  see Extraction, Peripheral Nervous System, 01D
Neurohypophysis *use* Pituitary Gland
Neurolysis
  see Release, Central Nervous System and Cranial Nerves, 00N
  see Release, Peripheral Nervous System, 01N
Neuromuscular electrical stimulation (NEMS) lead
  use Stimulator Lead in Muscles
Neurophysiologic monitoring *see* Monitoring, Central Nervous, 4A10
Neuroplasty
  see Repair, Central Nervous System and Cranial Nerves, 00Q
  see Repair, Peripheral Nervous System, 01Q
  see Supplement, Central Nervous System and Cranial Nerves, 00U
  see Supplement, Peripheral Nervous System, 01U
Neurorrhaphy
  see Repair, Central Nervous System and Cranial Nerves, 00Q
  see Repair, Peripheral Nervous System, 01Q
Neurostimulator Generator
  Insertion of device in, Skull, 0NH00NZ
  Removal of device from, Skull, 0NP00NZ
  Revision of device in, Skull, 0NW00NZ
Neurostimulator generator, multiple channel *use* Stimulator Generator, Multiple Array in, 0JH
Neurostimulator generator, multiple channel rechargeable *use* Stimulator Generator, Multiple Array Rechargeable in, 0JH
Neurostimulator generator, single channel *use* Stimulator Generator, Single Array in, 0JH
Neurostimulator generator, single channel rechargeable *use* Stimulator Generator, Single Array Rechargeable in, 0JH
Neurostimulator Lead
  Insertion of device in
    Brain, 00H0
    Cerebral Ventricle, 00H6
    Nerve
      Cranial, 00HE
      Peripheral, 01HY
    Spinal Canal, 00HU
    Spinal Cord, 00HV
    Vein
      Azygos, 05H0
      Innominate
        Left, 05H4
        Right, 05H3
  Removal of device from
    Brain, 00P0
    Cerebral Ventricle, 00P6
    Nerve
      Cranial, 00PE
      Peripheral, 01PY
    Spinal Canal, 00PU
    Spinal Cord, 00PV
    Vein
      Azygos, 05P0
      Innominate
        Left, 05P4
        Right, 05P3
  Revision of device in
    Brain, 00W0
    Cerebral Ventricle, 00W6
    Nerve
      Cranial, 00WE
      Peripheral, 01WY
    Spinal Canal, 00WU
    Spinal Cord, 00WV
    Vein
      Azygos, 05W0

Neurostimulator Lead — *continued*
  Revision of device in — *continued*
    Vein — *continued*
      Innominate
        Left, 05W4
        Right, 05W3
Neurotomy
  see Division, Central Nervous System and Cranial Nerves, 008
  see Division, Peripheral Nervous System, 018
Neurotripsy
  see Destruction, Central Nervous System and Cranial Nerves, 005
  see Destruction, Peripheral Nervous System, 015
Neutralization plate
  use Internal Fixation Device in Head and Facial Bones
  use Internal Fixation Device in Lower Bones
  use Internal Fixation Device in Upper Bones
New Technology
  Andexanet Alfa, Factor Xa Inhibitor Reversal Agent, XW0
  Bezlotoxumab Monoclonal Antibody, XW0
  Blinatumomab Antineoplastic Immunotherapy, XW0
  Ceftazidime-Avibactam Anti-infective, XW0
  Cerebral Embolic Filtration, Dual Filter, X2A5312
  Concentrated Bone Marrow Aspirate, XK02303
  Cytarabine and Daunorubicin Liposome Antineoplastic, XW0
  Defibrotide Sodium Anticoagulant, XW0
  Destruction, Prostate, Robotic Waterjet Ablation, XV508A4
  Endothelial Damage Inhibitor, XY0VX83
  Engineered Autologous Chimeric Antigen Receptor T-cell Immunotherapy, XW0
  Fusion
    Cervical Vertebral
      2 or more
        Nanotextured Surface, XRG2092
        Radiolucent Porous, XRG20F3
      Interbody Fusion Device
        Nanotextured Surface, XRG1092
        Radiolucent Porous, XRG10F3
    Cervicothoracic Vertebral
      Nanotextured Surface, XRG4092
      Radiolucent Porous, XRG40F3
    Lumbar Vertebral
      2 or more
        Nanotextured Surface, XRGC092
        Radiolucent Porous, XRGC0F3
      Interbody Fusion Device
        Nanotextured Surface, XRGB092
        Radiolucent Porous, XRGB0F3
    Lumbosacral
      Nanotextured Surface, XRGD092
      Radiolucent Porous, XRGD0F3
    Occipital-cervical
      Nanotextured Surface, XRG0092
      Radiolucent Porous, XRG00F3
    Thoracic Vertebral
      2 to 7
        Nanotextured Surface, XRG7092
        Radiolucent Porous, XRG70F3
      8 or more
        Nanotextured Surface, XRG8092
        Radiolucent Porous, XRG80F3
      Interbody Fusion Device
        Nanotextured Surface, XRG6092
        Radiolucent Porous, XRG60F3
    Thoracolumbar Vertebral
      Nanotextured Surface, XRGA092
      Radiolucent Porous, XRGA0F3
  Idarucizumab, Dabigatran Reversal Agent, XW0
  Intraoperative Knee Replacement Sensor, XR2
  Isavuconazole Anti-infective, XW0
  Orbital Atherectomy Technology, X2C
  Other New Technology Therapeutic Substance, XW0
  Plazomicin Anti-infective, XW0
  Replacement
    Skin Substitute, Porcine Liver Derived, XHRPXL2
    Zooplastic Tissue, Rapid Deployment Technique, X2RF
  Reposition
    Cervical, Magnetically Controlled Growth Rod(s), XNS3
    Lumbar, Magnetically Controlled Growth Rod(s), XNS0
    Thoracic, Magnetically Controlled Growth Rod(s), XNS4

New Technology — *continued*
  Synthetic Human Angiotensin II, XWØ
  Uridine Triacetate, XWØDX82
Ninth cranial nerve *use* Glossopharyngeal Nerve
Nitinol framed polymer mesh *use* Synthetic Substitute
Nonimaging Nuclear Medicine Assay
  Bladder, Kidneys and Ureters, CT63
  Blood, C763
  Kidneys, Ureters and Bladder, CT63
  Lymphatics and Hematologic System, C76YYZZ
  Ureters, Kidneys and Bladder, CT63
  Urinary System, CT6YYZZ
Nonimaging Nuclear Medicine Probe
  Abdomen, CW5Ø
  Abdomen and Chest, CW54
  Abdomen and Pelvis, CW51
  Brain, CØ5Ø
  Central Nervous System, CØ5YYZZ
  Chest, CW53
  Chest and Abdomen, CW54
  Chest and Neck, CW56
  Extremity
    Lower, CP5PZZZ
    Upper, CP5NZZZ
  Head and Neck, CW5B
  Heart, C25YYZZ
    Right and Left, C256
  Lymphatics
    Head, C75J
    Head and Neck, C755
    Lower Extremity, C75P
    Neck, C75K
    Pelvic, C75D
    Trunk, C75M
    Upper Chest, C75L
    Upper Extremity, C75N
  Lymphatics and Hematologic System, C75YYZZ
  Musculoskeletal System, Other, CP5YYZZ
  Neck and Chest, CW56
  Neck and Head, CW5B
  Pelvic Region, CW5J
  Pelvis and Abdomen, CW51
  Spine, CP55ZZZ
Nonimaging Nuclear Medicine Uptake
  Endocrine System, CG4YYZZ
  Gland, Thyroid, CG42
Non-tunneled central venous catheter *use* Infusion
  Device
Nostril *use* Nasal Mucosa and Soft Tissue
Novacor Left Ventricular Assist Device *use* Implantable
  Heart Assist System in Heart and Great Vessels
Novation® Ceramic AHS® (Articulation Hip System)
  use Synthetic Substitute, Ceramic in, ØSR
Nuclear medicine
  see Nonimaging Nuclear Medicine Assay
  see Nonimaging Nuclear Medicine Probe
  see Nonimaging Nuclear Medicine Uptake
  see Planar Nuclear Medicine Imaging
  see Positron Emission Tomographic (PET) Imaging
  see Systemic Nuclear Medicine Therapy
  see Tomographic (Tomo) Nuclear Medicine Imaging
Nuclear scintigraphy *see* Nuclear Medicine
Nutrition, concentrated substances
  Enteral infusion, 3E0G36Z
  Parenteral (peripheral) infusion *see* Introduction of
    Nutritional Substance

O

Obliteration *see* Destruction
Obturator artery
  use Internal Iliac Artery, Left
  use Internal Iliac Artery, Right
Obturator lymph node *use* Lymphatic, Pelvis
Obturator muscle
  use Hip Muscle, Left
  use Hip Muscle, Right
Obturator nerve *use* Lumbar Plexus
Obturator vein
  use Hypogastric Vein, Left
  use Hypogastric Vein, Right
Obtuse margin *use* Heart, Left
Occipital artery
  use External Carotid Artery, Left
  use External Carotid Artery, Right
Occipital lobe *use* Cerebral Hemisphere

Occipital lymph node
  use Lymphatic, Left Neck
  use Lymphatic, Right Neck
Occipitofrontalis muscle *use* Facial Muscle
Occlusion
  Ampulla of Vater, ØFLC
  Anus, ØDLQ
  Aorta
    Abdominal, 04L0
    Thoracic, Descending, 02LW3DJ
  Artery
    Anterior Tibial
      Left, 04LQ
      Right, 04LP
    Axillary
      Left, 03L6
      Right, 03L5
    Brachial
      Left, 03L8
      Right, 03L7
    Celiac, 04L1
    Colic
      Left, 04L7
      Middle, 04L8
      Right, 04L6
    Common Carotid
      Left, 03LJ
      Right, 03LH
    Common Iliac
      Left, 04LD
      Right, 04LC
    External Carotid
      Left, 03LN
      Right, 03LM
    External Iliac
      Left, 04LJ
      Right, 04LH
    Face, 03LR
    Femoral
      Left, 04LL
      Right, 04LK
    Foot
      Left, 04LW
      Right, 04LV
    Gastric, 04L2
    Hand
      Left, 03LF
      Right, 03LD
    Hepatic, 04L3
    Inferior Mesenteric, 04LB
    Innominate, 03L2
    Internal Carotid
      Left, 03LL
      Right, 03LK
    Internal Iliac
      Left, 04LF
      Right, 04LE
    Internal Mammary
      Left, 03L1
      Right, 03L0
    Intracranial, 03LG
    Lower, 04LY
    Peroneal
      Left, 04LU
      Right, 04LT
    Popliteal
      Left, 04LN
      Right, 04LM
    Posterior Tibial
      Left, 04LS
      Right, 04LR
    Pulmonary
      Left, 02LR
      Right, 02LQ
    Pulmonary Trunk, 02LP
    Radial
      Left, 03LC
      Right, 03LB
    Renal
      Left, 04LA
      Right, 04L9
    Splenic, 04L4
    Subclavian
      Left, 03L4
      Right, 03L3
    Superior Mesenteric, 04L5
    Temporal
      Left, 03LT
      Right, 03LS

Occlusion — *continued*
  Artery — *continued*
    Thyroid
      Left, 03LV
      Right, 03LU
    Ulnar
      Left, 03LA
      Right, 03L9
    Upper, 03LY
    Vertebral
      Left, 03LQ
      Right, 03LP
  Atrium, Left, 02L7
  Bladder, ØTLB
  Bladder Neck, ØTLC
  Bronchus
    Lingula, ØBL9
    Lower Lobe
      Left, ØBLB
      Right, ØBL6
    Main
      Left, ØBL7
      Right, ØBL3
    Middle Lobe, Right, ØBL5
    Upper Lobe
      Left, ØBL8
      Right, ØBL4
  Carina, ØBL2
  Cecum, ØDLH
  Cisterna Chyli, 07LL
  Colon
    Ascending, ØDLK
    Descending, ØDLM
    Sigmoid, ØDLN
    Transverse, ØDLL
  Cord
    Bilateral, ØVLH
    Left, ØVLG
    Right, ØVLF
  Cul-de-sac, ØULF
  Duct
    Common Bile, ØFL9
    Cystic, ØFL8
    Hepatic
      Common, ØFL7
      Left, ØFL6
      Right, ØFL5
    Lacrimal
      Left, 08LY
      Right, 08LX
    Pancreatic, ØFLD
      Accessory, ØFLF
    Parotid
      Left, ØCLC
      Right, ØCLB
  Duodenum, ØDL9
  Esophagogastric Junction, ØDL4
  Esophagus, ØDL5
    Lower, ØDL3
    Middle, ØDL2
    Upper, ØDL1
  Fallopian Tube
    Left, ØUL6
    Right, ØUL5
  Fallopian Tubes, Bilateral, ØUL7
  Ileocecal Valve, ØDLC
  Ileum, ØDLB
  Intestine
    Large, ØDLE
      Left, ØDLG
      Right, ØDLF
    Small, ØDL8
  Jejunum, ØDLA
  Kidney Pelvis
    Left, ØTL4
    Right, ØTL3
  Left atrial appendage (LAA) *see* Occlusion, Atrium,
    Left, 02L7
  Lymphatic
    Aortic, 07LD
    Axillary
      Left, 07L6
      Right, 07L5
    Head, 07L0
    Inguinal
      Left, 07LJ
      Right, 07LH
    Internal Mammary
      Left, 07L9

▽ Subterms under main terms may continue to next column or page

Osteoplasty
see Repair, Head and Facial Bones, ØNQ
see Repair, Lower Bones, ØQQ
see Repair, Upper Bones, ØPQ
see Replacement, Head and Facial Bones, ØNR
see Replacement, Lower Bones, ØQR
see Replacement, Upper Bones, ØPR
see Supplement, Head and Facial Bones, ØNU
see Supplement, Lower Bones, ØQU
see Supplement, Upper Bones, ØPU

Osteorrhaphy
see Repair, Head and Facial Bones, ØNQ
see Repair, Lower Bones, ØQQ
see Repair, Upper Bones, ØPQ

Osteotomy, ostotomy
see Division, Head and Facial Bones, ØN8
see Division, Lower Bones, ØQ8
see Division, Upper Bones, ØP8
see Drainage, Head and Facial Bones, ØN9
see Drainage, Lower Bones, ØQ9
see Drainage, Upper Bones, ØP9

Otic ganglion use Head and Neck Sympathetic Nerve

Otoplasty
see Repair, Ear, Nose, Sinus, Ø9Q
see Replacement, Ear, Nose, Sinus, Ø9R
see Supplement, Ear, Nose, Sinus, Ø9U

Otoscopy see Inspection, Ear, Nose, Sinus, Ø9J

Oval window
use Middle Ear, Left
use Middle Ear, Right

Ovarian artery use Abdominal Aorta
Ovarian ligament use Uterine Supporting Structure

Ovariectomy
see Excision, Female Reproductive System, ØUB
see Resection, Female Reproductive System, ØUT

Ovariocentesis see Drainage, Female Reproductive System, ØU9

Ovariopexy
see Repair, Female Reproductive System, ØUQ
see Reposition, Female Reproductive System, ØUS

Ovariotomy
see Division, Female Reproductive System, ØU8
see Drainage, Female Reproductive System, ØU9

Ovatio™ CRT-D use Cardiac Resynchronization Defibrillator Pulse Generator in, ØJH

Oversewing
Gastrointestinal ulcer see Repair, Gastrointestinal System, ØDQ
Pleural bleb see Repair, Respiratory System, ØBQ

Oviduct
use Fallopian Tube, Left
use Fallopian Tube, Right

Oximetry, Fetal pulse, 1ØHØ73Z
OXINIUM use Synthetic Substitute, Oxidized Zirconium on Polyethylene in, ØSR

Oxygenation
Extracorporeal membrane (ECMO) see Performance, Circulatory, 5A15
Hyperbaric see Assistance, Circulatory, 5AØ5
Supersaturated see Assistance, Circulatory, 5AØ5

P

Pacemaker
Dual Chamber
  Abdomen, ØJH8
  Chest, ØJH6
Intracardiac
  Insertion of device in
    Atrium
      Left, Ø2H7
      Right, Ø2H6
    Vein, Coronary, Ø2H4
    Ventricle
      Left, Ø2HL
      Right, Ø2HK
  Removal of device from, Heart, Ø2PA
  Revision of device in, Heart, Ø2WA
Single Chamber
  Abdomen, ØJH8
  Chest, ØJH6
Single Chamber Rate Responsive
  Abdomen, ØJH8
  Chest, ØJH6

Packing
Abdominal Wall, 2W43X5Z

Packing — continued
Anorectal, 2Y43X5Z
Arm
  Lower
    Left, 2W4DX5Z
    Right, 2W4CX5Z
  Upper
    Left, 2W4BX5Z
    Right, 2W4AX5Z
Back, 2W45X5Z
Chest Wall, 2W44X5Z
Ear, 2Y42X5Z
Extremity
  Lower
    Left, 2W4MX5Z
    Right, 2W4LX5Z
  Upper
    Left, 2W49X5Z
    Right, 2W48X5Z
Face, 2W41X5Z
Finger
  Left, 2W4KX5Z
  Right, 2W4JX5Z
Foot
  Left, 2W4TX5Z
  Right, 2W4SX5Z
Genital Tract, Female, 2Y44X5Z
Hand
  Left, 2W4FX5Z
  Right, 2W4EX5Z
Head, 2W40X5Z
Inguinal Region
  Left, 2W47X5Z
  Right, 2W46X5Z
Leg
  Lower
    Left, 2W4RX5Z
    Right, 2W4QX5Z
  Upper
    Left, 2W4PX5Z
    Right, 2W4NX5Z
Mouth and Pharynx, 2Y40X5Z
Nasal, 2Y41X5Z
Neck, 2W42X5Z
Thumb
  Left, 2W4HX5Z
  Right, 2W4GX5Z
Toe
  Left, 2W4VX5Z
  Right, 2W4UX5Z
Urethra, 2Y45X5Z

Paclitaxel-eluting coronary stent use Intraluminal Device, Drug-eluting in Heart and Great Vessels

Paclitaxel-eluting peripheral stent
use Intraluminal Device, Drug-eluting in Lower Arteries
use Intraluminal Device, Drug-eluting in Upper Arteries

Palatine gland use Buccal Mucosa
Palatine tonsil use Tonsils
Palatine uvula use Uvula
Palatoglossal muscle use Tongue, Palate, Pharynx Muscle
Palatopharyngeal muscle use Tongue, Palate, Pharynx Muscle

Palatoplasty
see Repair, Mouth and Throat, ØCQ
see Replacement, Mouth and Throat, ØCR
see Supplement, Mouth and Throat, ØCU

Palatorrhaphy see Repair, Mouth and Throat, ØCQ

Palmar cutaneous nerve
use Median Nerve
use Radial Nerve

Palmar (volar) digital vein
use Hand Vein, Left
use Hand Vein, Right

Palmar fascia (aponeurosis)
use Subcutaneous Tissue and Fascia, Left Hand
use Subcutaneous Tissue and Fascia, Right Hand

Palmar interosseous muscle
use Hand Muscle, Left
use Hand Muscle, Right

Palmar (volar) metacarpal vein
use Hand Vein, Left
use Hand Vein, Right

Palmar ulnocarpal ligament
use Wrist Bursa and Ligament, Left
use Wrist Bursa and Ligament, Right

Palmaris longus muscle
use Lower Arm and Wrist Muscle, Left
use Lower Arm and Wrist Muscle, Right

Pancreatectomy
see Excision, Pancreas, ØFBG
see Resection, Pancreas, ØFTG

Pancreatic artery use Splenic Artery
Pancreatic plexus use Abdominal Sympathetic Nerve
Pancreatic vein use Splenic Vein
Pancreaticoduodenostomy see Bypass, Hepatobiliary System and Pancreas, ØF1
Pancreaticosplenic lymph node use Lymphatic, Aortic
Pancreatogram, endoscopic retrograde see Fluoroscopy, Pancreatic Duct, BF18
Pancreatolithotomy see Extirpation, Pancreas, ØFCG

Pancreatotomy
see Division, Pancreas, ØF8G
see Drainage, Pancreas, ØF9G

Panniculectomy
see Excision, Abdominal Wall, ØWBF
see Excision, Skin, Abdomen, ØHB7

Paraaortic lymph node use Lymphatic, Aortic

Paracentesis
Eye see Drainage, Eye, Ø89
Peritoneal Cavity see Drainage, Peritoneal Cavity, ØW9G
Tympanum see Drainage, Ear, Nose, Sinus, Ø99

Pararectal lymph node use Lymphatic, Mesenteric
Parasternal lymph node use Lymphatic, Thorax

Parathyroidectomy
see Excision, Endocrine System, ØGB
see Resection, Endocrine System, ØGT

Paratracheal lymph node use Lymphatic, Thorax
Paraurethral (Skene's) gland use Vestibular Gland
Parenteral nutrition, total see Introduction of Nutritional Substance
Parietal lobe use Cerebral Hemisphere
Parotid lymph node use Lymphatic, Head
Parotid plexus use Facial Nerve

Parotidectomy
see Excision, Mouth and Throat, ØCB
see Resection, Mouth and Throat, ØCT

Pars flaccida
use Tympanic Membrane, Left
use Tympanic Membrane, Right

Partial joint replacement
Hip see Replacement, Lower Joints, ØSR
Knee see Replacement, Lower Joints, ØSR
Shoulder see Replacement, Upper Joints, ØRR

Partially absorbable mesh use Synthetic Substitute
Patch, blood, spinal, 3EØR3GC

Patellapexy
see Repair, Lower Bones, ØQQ
see Reposition, Lower Bones, ØQS

Patellaplasty
see Repair, Lower Bones, ØQQ
see Replacement, Lower Bones, ØQR
see Supplement, Lower Bones, ØQU

Patellar ligament
use Knee Bursa and Ligament, Left
use Knee Bursa and Ligament, Right

Patellar tendon
use Knee Tendon, Left
use Knee Tendon, Right

Patellectomy
see Excision, Lower Bones, ØQB
see Resection, Lower Bones, ØQT

Patellofemoral joint
use Knee Joint, Left
use Knee Joint, Left, Femoral Surface
use Knee Joint, Right
use Knee Joint, Right, Femoral Surface

Pectineus muscle
use Upper Leg Muscle, Left
use Upper Leg Muscle, Right

Pectoral fascia use Subcutaneous Tissue and Fascia, Chest

Pectoral (anterior) lymph node
use Lymphatic Left, Axillary
use Lymphatic Right, Axillary

Pectoralis major muscle
use Thorax Muscle, Left
use Thorax Muscle, Right

Pectoralis minor muscle
use Thorax Muscle, Left
use Thorax Muscle, Right

Pedicle-based dynamic stabilization device
use Spinal Stabilization Device, Pedicle-Based in, ØSH
use Spinal Stabilization Device, Pedicle-Based in, ØRH
PEEP (positive end expiratory pressure) *see* Assistance, Respiratory, 5AØ9
PEG (percutaneous endoscopic gastrostomy), ØDH63UZ
PEJ (percutaneous endoscopic jejunostomy), ØDHA3UZ
Pelvic splanchnic nerve
use Abdominal Sympathetic Nerve
use Sacral Sympathetic Nerve
Penectomy
see Excision, Male Reproductive System, ØVB
see Resection, Male Reproductive System, ØVT
Penile urethra *use* Urethra
Perceval sutureless valve *use* Zooplastic Tissue, Rapid Deployment Technique in New Technology
Percutaneous endoscopic gastrojejunostomy (PEG/J) tube *use* Feeding Device in Gastrointestinal System
Percutaneous endoscopic gastrostomy (PEG) tube
use Feeding Device in Gastrointestinal System
Percutaneous nephrostomy catheter *use* Drainage Device
Percutaneous transluminal coronary angioplasty (PTCA) *see* Dilation, Heart and Great Vessels, Ø27
Performance
Biliary
Multiple, Filtration, 5A1C6ØZ
Single, Filtration, 5A1CØØZ
Cardiac
Continuous
Output, 5A1221Z
Pacing, 5A1223Z
Intermittent, Pacing, 5A1213Z
Single, Output, Manual, 5A12Ø12
Circulatory
Central Membrane, 5A1522F
Peripheral Veno-arterial Membrane, 5A1522G
Peripheral Veno-venous Membrane, 5A1522H
Respiratory
24-96 Consecutive Hours, Ventilation, 5A1945Z
Greater than 96 Consecutive Hours, Ventilation, 5A1955Z
Less than 24 Consecutive Hours, Ventilation, 5A1935Z
Single, Ventilation, Nonmechanical, 5A19Ø54
Urinary
Continuous, Greater than 18 hours per day, Filtration, 5A1D9ØZ
Intermittent, Less than 6 Hours Per Day, Filtration, 5A1D7ØZ
Prolonged Intermittent, 6-18 hours per day, Filtration, 5A1D8ØZ
Perfusion *see* Introduction of substance in or on
Perfusion, donor organ
Heart, 6AB5ØBZ
Kidney(s), 6ABTØBZ
Liver, 6ABFØBZ
Lung(s), 6ABBØBZ
Pericardiectomy
see Excision, Pericardium, Ø2BN
see Resection, Pericardium, Ø2TN
Pericardiocentesis *see* Drainage, Pericardial Cavity, ØW9D
Pericardiolysis *see* Release, Pericardium, Ø2NN
Pericardiophrenic artery
use Internal Mammary Artery, Left
use Internal Mammary Artery, Right
Pericardioplasty
see Repair, Pericardium, Ø2QN
see Replacement, Pericardium, Ø2RN
see Supplement, Pericardium, Ø2UN
Pericardiorrhaphy *see* Repair, Pericardium, Ø2QN
Pericardiostomy *see* Drainage, Pericardial Cavity, ØW9D
Pericardiotomy *see* Drainage, Pericardial Cavity, ØW9D
Perimetrium *use* Uterus
Peripheral parenteral nutrition *see* Introduction of Nutritional Substance
Peripherally inserted central catheter (PICC) *use* Infusion Device
Peritoneal dialysis, 3E1M39Z
Peritoneocentesis
see Drainage, Peritoneal Cavity, ØW9G
see Drainage, Peritoneum, ØD9W
Peritoneoplasty
see Repair, Peritoneum, ØDQW
see Replacement, Peritoneum, ØDRW

Peritoneoplasty — *continued*
see Supplement, Peritoneum, ØDUW
Peritoneoscopy, ØDJW4ZZ
Peritoneotomy *see* Drainage, Peritoneum, ØD9W
Peritoneumectomy *see* Excision, Peritoneum, ØDBW
Peroneus brevis muscle
use Lower Leg Muscle, Left
use Lower Leg Muscle, Right
Peroneus longus muscle
use Lower Leg Muscle, Left
use Lower Leg Muscle, Right
Pessary ring *use* Intraluminal Device, Pessary in Female Reproductive System
PET scan *see* Positron Emission Tomographic (PET) Imaging
Petrous part of temporal bone
use Temporal Bone, Left
use Temporal Bone, Right
Phacoemulsification, lens
With IOL implant *see* Replacement, Eye, Ø8R
Without IOL implant *see* Extraction, Eye, Ø8D
Phalangectomy
see Excision, Lower Bones, ØQB
see Excision, Upper Bones, ØPB
see Resection, Lower Bones, ØQT
see Resection, Upper Bones, ØPT
Phallectomy
see Excision, Penis, ØVBS
see Resection, Penis, ØVTS
Phalloplasty
see Repair, Penis, ØVQS
see Supplement, Penis, ØVUS
Phallotomy *see* Drainage, Penis, ØV9S
Pharmacotherapy, for substance abuse
Antabuse, HZ93ZZZ
Bupropion, HZ97ZZZ
Clonidine, HZ96ZZZ
Levo-alpha-acetyl-methadol (LAAM), HZ92ZZZ
Methadone Maintenance, HZ91ZZZ
Naloxone, HZ95ZZZ
Naltrexone, HZ94ZZZ
Nicotine Replacement, HZ9ØZZZ
Psychiatric Medication, HZ98ZZZ
Replacement Medication, Other, HZ99ZZZ
Pharyngeal constrictor muscle *use* Tongue, Palate, Pharynx Muscle
Pharyngeal plexus *use* Vagus Nerve
Pharyngeal recess *use* Nasopharynx
Pharyngeal tonsil *use* Adenoids
Pharyngogram *see* Fluoroscopy, Pharynix, B91G
Pharyngoplasty
see Repair, Mouth and Throat, ØCQ
see Replacement, Mouth and Throat, ØCR
see Supplement, Mouth and Throat, ØCU
Pharyngorrhaphy *see* Repair, Mouth and Throat, ØCQ
Pharyngotomy *see* Drainage, Mouth and Throat, ØC9
Pharyngotympanic tube
use Eustachian Tube, Left
use Eustachian Tube, Right
Pheresis
Erythrocytes, 6A55
Leukocytes, 6A55
Plasma, 6A55
Platelets, 6A55
Stem Cells
Cord Blood, 6A55
Hematopoietic, 6A55
Phlebectomy
see Excision, Lower Veins, Ø6B
see Excision, Upper Veins, Ø5B
see Extraction, Lower Veins, Ø6D
see Extraction, Upper Veins, Ø5D
Phlebography
see Plain Radiography, Veins, B5Ø
Impedance, 4AØ4X51
Phleborrhaphy
see Repair, Lower Veins, Ø6Q
see Repair, Upper Veins, Ø5Q
Phlebotomy
see Drainage, Lower Veins, Ø69
see Drainage, Upper Veins, Ø59
Photocoagulation
For Destruction *see* Destruction
For Repair *see* Repair
Photopheresis, therapeutic *see* Phototherapy, Circulatory, 6A65

Phototherapy
Circulatory, 6A65
Skin, 6A6Ø
Ultraviolet light *see* Ultraviolet Light Therapy, Physiological Systems, 6A8
Phrenectomy, phrenoneurectomy *see* Excision, Nerve, Phrenic, Ø1B2
Phrenemphraxis *see* Destruction, Nerve, Phrenic, Ø152
Phrenic nerve stimulator generator *use* Stimulator Generator in Subcutaneous Tissue and Fascia
Phrenic nerve stimulator lead *use* Diaphragmatic Pacemaker Lead in Respiratory System
Phreniclasis *see* Destruction, Nerve, Phrenic, Ø152
Phrenicoexeresis *see* Extraction, Nerve, Phrenic, Ø1D2
Phrenicotomy *see* Division, Nerve, Phrenic, Ø182
Phrenicotripsy *see* Destruction, Nerve, Phrenic, Ø152
Phrenoplasty
see Repair, Respiratory System, ØBQ
see Supplement, Respiratory System, ØBU
Phrenotomy *see* Drainage, Respiratory System, ØB9
Physiatry *see* Motor Treatment, Rehabilitation, FØ7
Physical medicine *see* Motor Treatment, Rehabilitation, FØ7
Physical therapy *see* Motor Treatment, Rehabilitation, FØ7
PHYSIOMESH™ Flexible Composite Mesh *use* Synthetic Substitute
Pia mater, intracranial *use* Cerebral Meninges
Pia mater, spinal *use* Spinal Meninges
Pinealectomy
see Excision, Pineal Body, ØGB1
see Resection, Pineal Body, ØGT1
Pinealoscopy, ØGJ14ZZ
Pinealotomy *see* Drainage, Pineal Body, ØG91
Pinna
use External Ear, Bilateral
use External Ear, Left
use External Ear, Right
Pipeline™ Embolization device (PED) *use* Intraluminal Device
Piriform recess (sinus) *use* Pharynx
Piriformis muscle
use Hip Muscle, Left
use Hip Muscle, Right
PIRRT (Prolonged intermittent renal replacement therapy), 5A1D8ØZ
Pisiform bone
use Carpal, Left
use Carpal, Right
Pisohamate ligament
use Hand Bursa and Ligament, Left
use Hand Bursa and Ligament, Right
Pisometacarpal ligament
use Hand Bursa and Ligament, Left
use Hand Bursa and Ligament, Right
Pituitectomy
see Excision, Gland, Pituitary, ØGBØ
see Resection, Gland, Pituitary, ØGTØ
Plain film radiology *see* Plain Radiography
Plain Radiography
Abdomen, BWØØZZZ
Abdomen and Pelvis, BWØ1ZZZ
Abdominal Lymphatic
Bilateral, B7Ø1
Unilateral, B7ØØ
Airway, Upper, BBØDZZZ
Ankle
Left, BQØH
Right, BQØG
Aorta
Abdominal, B4ØØ
Thoracic, B3ØØ
Thoraco-Abdominal, B3ØP
Aorta and Bilateral Lower Extremity Arteries, B4ØD
Arch
Bilateral, BNØDZZZ
Left, BNØCZZZ
Right, BNØBZZZ
Arm
Left, BPØFZZZ
Right, BPØEZZZ
Artery
Brachiocephalic-Subclavian, Right, B3Ø1
Bronchial, B3ØL
Bypass Graft, Other, B2ØF
Cervico-Cerebral Arch, B3ØQ

Plain Radiography — continued

Tracheobronchial Tree
Bilateral, BB09YZZ
Left, BB08YZZ
Right, BB07YZZ
Ureter
Bilateral, BT08
Kidney and Bladder, BT04
Left, BT07
Right, BT06
Urethra, BT05
Urethra and Bladder, BT0B
Uterus, BU06
Uterus and Fallopian Tube, BU08
Vagina, BU09
Vasa Vasorum, BV08
Vein
Cerebellar, B501
Cerebral, B501
Epidural, B500
Jugular
Bilateral, B505
Left, B504
Right, B503
Lower Extremity
Bilateral, B50D
Left, B50C
Right, B50B
Other, B50V
Pelvic (Iliac)
Left, B50G
Right, B50F
Pelvic (Iliac) Bilateral, B50H
Portal, B50T
Pulmonary
Bilateral, B50S
Left, B50R
Right, B50Q
Renal
Bilateral, B50L
Left, B50K
Right, B50J
Spanchnic, B50T
Subclavian
Left, B507
Right, B506
Upper Extremity
Bilateral, B50P
Left, B50N
Right, B50M
Vena Cava
Inferior, B509
Superior, B508
Whole Body, BW0KZZZ
Infant, BW0MZZZ
Whole Skeleton, BW0LZZZ
Wrist
Left, BP0M
Right, BP0L

Planar Nuclear Medicine Imaging

Abdomen, CW10
Abdomen and Chest, CW14
Abdomen and Pelvis, CW11
Anatomical Region, Other, CW1ZZZZ
Anatomical Regions, Multiple, CW1YYZZ
Bladder and Ureters, CT1H
Bladder, Kidneys and Ureters, CT13
Blood, C713
Bone Marrow, C710
Brain, C010
Breast, CH1YYZZ
Bilateral, CH12
Left, CH11
Right, CH10
Bronchi and Lungs, CB12
Central Nervous System, C01YYZZ
Cerebrospinal Fluid, C015
Chest, CW13
Chest and Abdomen, CW14
Chest and Neck, CW16
Digestive System, CD1YYZZ
Ducts, Lacrimal, Bilateral, C819
Ear, Nose, Mouth and Throat, C91YYZZ
Endocrine System, CG1YYZZ
Extremity
Lower, CW1D
Bilateral, CP1F
Left, CP1D
Right, CP1C

Planar Nuclear Medicine Imaging — continued

Extremity — continued
Upper, CW1M
Bilateral, CP1B
Left, CP19
Right, CP18
Eye, C81YYZZ
Gallbladder, CF14
Gastrointestinal Tract, CD17
Upper, CD15
Gland
Adrenal, Bilateral, CG14
Parathyroid, CG11
Thyroid, CG12
Glands, Salivary, Bilateral, C91B
Head and Neck, CW1B
Heart, C21YYZZ
Right and Left, C216
Hepatobiliary System, All, CF1C
Hepatobiliary System and Pancreas, CF1YYZZ
Kidneys, Ureters and Bladder, CT13
Liver, CF15
Liver and Spleen, CF16
Lungs and Bronchi, CB12
Lymphatics
Head, C71J
Head and Neck, C715
Lower Extremity, C71P
Neck, C71K
Pelvic, C71D
Trunk, C71M
Upper Chest, C71L
Upper Extremity, C71N
Lymphatics and Hematologic System, C71YYZZ
Musculoskeletal System
All, CP1Z
Other, CP1YYZZ
Myocardium, C21G
Neck and Chest, CW16
Neck and Head, CW1B
Pancreas and Hepatobiliary System, CF1YYZZ
Pelvic Region, CW1J
Pelvis, CP16
Pelvis and Abdomen, CW11
Pelvis and Spine, CP17
Reproductive System, Male, CV1YYZZ
Respiratory System, CB1YYZZ
Skin, CH1YYZZ
Skull, CP11
Spine, CP15
Spine and Pelvis, CP17
Spleen, C712
Spleen and Liver, CF16
Subcutaneous Tissue, CH1YYZZ
Testicles, Bilateral, CV19
Thorax, CP14
Ureters and Bladder, CT1H
Ureters, Kidneys and Bladder, CT13
Urinary System, CT1YYZZ
Veins, C51YYZZ
Central, C51R
Lower Extremity
Bilateral, C51D
Left, C51C
Right, C51B
Upper Extremity
Bilateral, C51Q
Left, C51P
Right, C51N
Whole Body, CW1N

Plantar digital vein
use Foot Vein, Left
use Foot Vein, Right

Plantar fascia (aponeurosis)
use Subcutaneous Tissue and Fascia, Left Foot
use Subcutaneous Tissue and Fascia, Right Foot

Plantar metatarsal vein
use Foot Vein, Left
use Foot Vein, Right

Plantar venous arch
use Foot Vein, Left
use Foot Vein, Right

Plaque Radiation

Abdomen, DWY3FZZ
Adrenal Gland, DGY2FZZ
Anus, DDY8FZZ
Bile Ducts, DFY2FZZ
Bladder, DTY2FZZ

Plaque Radiation — continued

Bone Marrow, D7Y0FZZ
Bone, Other, DPYCFZZ
Brain, D0Y0FZZ
Brain Stem, D0Y1FZZ
Breast
Left, DMY0FZZ
Right, DMY1FZZ
Bronchus, DBY1FZZ
Cervix, DUY1FZZ
Chest, DWY2FZZ
Chest Wall, DBY7FZZ
Colon, DDY5FZZ
Diaphragm, DBY8FZZ
Duodenum, DDY2FZZ
Ear, D9Y0FZZ
Esophagus, DDY0FZZ
Eye, D8Y0FZZ
Femur, DPY9FZZ
Fibula, DPYBFZZ
Gallbladder, DFY1FZZ
Gland
Adrenal, DGY2FZZ
Parathyroid, DGY4FZZ
Pituitary, DGY0FZZ
Thyroid, DGY5FZZ
Glands, Salivary, D9Y6FZZ
Head and Neck, DWY1FZZ
Hemibody, DWY4FZZ
Humerus, DPY6FZZ
Ileum, DDY4FZZ
Jejunum, DDY3FZZ
Kidney, DTY0FZZ
Larynx, D9YBFZZ
Liver, DFY0FZZ
Lung, DBY2FZZ
Lymphatics
Abdomen, D7Y6FZZ
Axillary, D7Y4FZZ
Inguinal, D7Y8FZZ
Neck, D7Y3FZZ
Pelvis, D7Y7FZZ
Thorax, D7Y5FZZ
Mandible, DPY3FZZ
Maxilla, DPY2FZZ
Mediastinum, DBY6FZZ
Mouth, D9Y4FZZ
Nasopharynx, D9YDFZZ
Neck and Head, DWY1FZZ
Nerve, Peripheral, D0Y7FZZ
Nose, D9Y1FZZ
Ovary, DUY0FZZ
Palate
Hard, D9Y8FZZ
Soft, D9Y9FZZ
Pancreas, DFY3FZZ
Parathyroid Gland, DGY4FZZ
Pelvic Bones, DPY8FZZ
Pelvic Region, DWY6FZZ
Pharynx, D9YCFZZ
Pineal Body, DGY1FZZ
Pituitary Gland, DGY0FZZ
Pleura, DBY5FZZ
Prostate, DVY0FZZ
Radius, DPY7FZZ
Rectum, DDY7FZZ
Rib, DPY5FZZ
Sinuses, D9Y7FZZ
Skin
Abdomen, DHY8FZZ
Arm, DHY4FZZ
Back, DHY7FZZ
Buttock, DHY9FZZ
Chest, DHY6FZZ
Face, DHY2FZZ
Foot, DHYCFZZ
Hand, DHY5FZZ
Leg, DHYBFZZ
Neck, DHY3FZZ
Skull, DPY0FZZ
Spinal Cord, D0Y6FZZ
Spleen, D7Y2FZZ
Sternum, DPY4FZZ
Stomach, DDY1FZZ
Testis, DVY1FZZ
Thymus, D7Y1FZZ
Thyroid Gland, DGY5FZZ
Tibia, DPYBFZZ
Tongue, D9Y5FZZ

Plaque Radiation — *continued*
- Trachea, DBY0FZZ
- Ulna, DPY7FZZ
- Ureter, DTY1FZZ
- Urethra, DTY3FZZ
- Uterus, DUY2FZZ
- Whole Body, DWY5FZZ

Plasmapheresis, therapeutic *see* Pheresis, Physiological Systems, 6A5

Plateletpheresis, therapeutic *see* Pheresis, Physiological Systems, 6A5

Platysma muscle
- *use* Neck Muscle, Left
- *use* Neck Muscle, Right

Plazomicin Anti-infective, XW0

Pleurectomy
- *see* Excision, Respiratory System, 0BB
- *see* Resection, Respiratory System, 0BT

Pleurocentesis *see* Drainage, Anatomical Regions, General, 0W9

Pleurodesis, pleurosclerosis
- Chemical injection *see* Introduction of Substance in or on, Pleural Cavity, 3E0L
- Surgical *see* Destruction, Respiratory System, 0B5

Pleurolysis *see* Release, Respiratory System, 0BN

Pleuroscopy, 0BJQ4ZZ

Pleurotomy *see* Drainage, Respiratory System, 0B9

Plica semilunaris
- *use* Conjunctiva, Left
- *use* Conjunctiva, Right

Plication *see* Restriction

Pneumectomy
- *see* Excision, Respiratory System, 0BB
- *see* Resection, Respiratory System, 0BT

Pneumocentesis *see* Drainage, Respiratory System, 0B9

Pneumogastric nerve *use* Vagus Nerve

Pneumolysis *see* Release, Respiratory System, 0BN

Pneumonectomy *see* Resection, Respiratory System, 0BT

Pneumonolysis *see* Release, Respiratory System, 0BN

Pneumonopexy
- *see* Repair, Respiratory System, 0BQ
- *see* Reposition, Respiratory System, 0BS

Pneumonorrhaphy *see* Repair, Respiratory System, 0BQ

Pneumonotomy *see* Drainage, Respiratory System, 0B9

Pneumotaxic center *use* Pons

Pneumotomy *see* Drainage, Respiratory System, 0B9

Pollicization *see* Transfer, Anatomical Regions, Upper Extremities, 0XX

Polyethylene socket *use* Synthetic Substitute, Polyethylene in, 0SR

Polymethylmethacrylate (PMMA) *use* Synthetic Substitute

Polypectomy, gastrointestinal *see* Excision, Gastrointestinal System, 0DB

Polypropylene mesh *use* Synthetic Substitute

Polysomnogram, 4A1ZXQZ

Pontine tegmentum *use* Pons

Popliteal ligament
- *use* Knee Bursa and Ligament, Left
- *use* Knee Bursa and Ligament, Right

Popliteal lymph node
- *use* Lymphatic, Left Lower Extremity
- *use* Lymphatic, Right Lower Extremity

Popliteal vein
- *use* Femoral Vein, Left
- *use* Femoral Vein, Right

Popliteus muscle
- *use* Lower Leg Muscle, Left
- *use* Lower Leg Muscle, Right

Porcine (bioprosthetic) valve *use* Zooplastic Tissue in Heart and Great Vessels

Positive end expiratory pressure *see* Performance, Respiratory, 5A19

Positron Emission Tomographic (PET) Imaging
- Brain, C030
- Bronchi and Lungs, CB32
- Central Nervous System, C03YYZZ
- Heart, C23YYZZ
- Lungs and Bronchi, CB32
- Myocardium, C23G
- Respiratory System, CB3YYZZ
- Whole Body, CW3NYZZ

Positron emission tomography *see* Positron Emission Tomographic (PET) Imaging

Postauricular (mastoid) lymph node
- *use* Lymphatic, Left Neck
- *use* Lymphatic, Right Neck

Postcava *use* Inferior Vena Cava

Posterior auricular artery
- *use* External Carotid Artery, Left
- *use* External Carotid Artery, Right

Posterior auricular nerve *use* Facial Nerve

Posterior auricular vein
- *use* External Jugular Vein, Left
- *use* External Jugular Vein, Right

Posterior cerebral artery *use* Intracranial Artery

Posterior chamber
- *use* Eye, Left
- *use* Eye, Right

Posterior circumflex humeral artery
- *use* Axillary Artery, Left
- *use* Axillary Artery, Right

Posterior communicating artery *use* Intracranial Artery

Posterior cruciate ligament (PCL)
- *use* Knee Bursa and Ligament, Left
- *use* Knee Bursa and Ligament, Right

Posterior facial (retromandibular) vein
- *use* Face Vein, Left
- *use* Face Vein, Right

Posterior femoral cutaneous nerve *use* Sacral Plexus

Posterior inferior cerebellar artery (PICA) *use* Intracranial Artery

Posterior interosseous nerve *use* Radial Nerve

Posterior labial nerve *use* Pudendal Nerve

Posterior (subscapular) lymph node
- *use* Lymphatic, Left Axillary
- *use* Lymphatic, Right Axillary

Posterior scrotal nerve *use* Pudendal Nerve

Posterior spinal artery
- *use* Vertebral Artery, Left
- *use* Vertebral Artery, Right

Posterior tibial recurrent artery
- *use* Anterior Tibial Artery, Left
- *use* Anterior Tibial Artery, Right

Posterior ulnar recurrent artery
- *use* Ulnar Artery, Left
- *use* Ulnar Artery, Right

Posterior vagal trunk *use* Vagus Nerve

PPN (peripheral parenteral nutrition) *see* Introduction of Nutritional Substance

Preauricular lymph node *use* Lymphatic, Head

Precava *use* Superior Vena Cava

Prepatellar bursa
- *use* Knee Bursa and Ligament, Left
- *use* Knee Bursa and Ligament, Right

Preputiotomy *see* Drainage, Male Reproductive System, 0V9

Pressure support ventilation *see* Performance, Respiratory, 5A19

PRESTIGE® Cervical Disc *use* Synthetic Substitute

Pretracheal fascia
- *use* Subcutaneous Tissue and Fascia, Left Neck
- *use* Subcutaneous Tissue and Fascia, Right Neck

Prevertebral fascia
- *use* Subcutaneous Tissue and Fascia, Left Neck
- *use* Subcutaneous Tissue and Fascia, Right Neck

PrimeAdvanced neurostimulator (SureScan) (MRI Safe) *use* Stimulator Generator, Multiple Array in, 0JH

Princeps pollicis artery
- *use* Hand Artery, Left
- *use* Hand Artery, Right

Probing, duct
- Diagnostic *see* Inspection
- Dilation *see* Dilation

PROCEED™ Ventral Patch *use* Synthetic Substitute

Procerus muscle *use* Facial Muscle

Proctectomy
- *see* Excision, Rectum, 0DBP
- *see* Resection, Rectum, 0DTP

Proctoclysis *see* Introduction of substance in or on, Gastrointestinal Tract, Lower, 3E0H

Proctocolectomy
- *see* Excision, Gastrointestinal System, 0DB
- *see* Resection, Gastrointestinal System, 0DT

Proctocolpoplasty
- *see* Repair, Gastrointestinal System, 0DQ
- *see* Supplement, Gastrointestinal System, 0DU

Proctoperineoplasty
- *see* Repair, Gastrointestinal System, 0DQ
- *see* Supplement, Gastrointestinal System, 0DU

Proctoperineorrhaphy *see* Repair, Gastrointestinal System, 0DQ

Proctopexy
- *see* Repair, Rectum, 0DQP
- *see* Reposition, Rectum, 0DSP

Proctoplasty
- *see* Repair, Rectum, 0DQP
- *see* Supplement, Rectum, 0DUP

Proctorrhaphy *see* Repair, Rectum, 0DQP

Proctoscopy, 0DJD8ZZ

Proctosigmoidectomy
- *see* Excision, Gastrointestinal System, 0DB
- *see* Resection, Gastrointestinal System, 0DT

Proctosigmoidoscopy, 0DJD8ZZ

Proctostomy *see* Drainage, Rectum, 0D9P

Proctotomy *see* Drainage, Rectum, 0D9P

Prodisc-C *use* Synthetic Substitute

Prodisc-L *use* Synthetic Substitute

Production, atrial septal defect *see* Excision, Septum, Atrial, 02B5

Profunda brachii
- *use* Brachial Artery, Left
- *use* Brachial Artery, Right

Profunda femoris (deep femoral) vein
- *use* Femoral Vein, Left
- *use* Femoral Vein, Right

PROLENE Polypropylene Hernia System (PHS) *use* Synthetic Substitute

Prolonged intermittent renal replacement therapy (PIRRT), 5A1D80Z

Pronator quadratus muscle
- *use* Lower Arm and Wrist Muscle, Left
- *use* Lower Arm and Wrist Muscle, Right

Pronator teres muscle
- *use* Lower Arm and Wrist Muscle, Left
- *use* Lower Arm and Wrist Muscle, Right

Prostatectomy
- *see* Excision, Prostate, 0VB0
- *see* Resection, Prostate, 0VT0

Prostatic urethra *use* Urethra

Prostatomy, prostatotomy *see* Drainage, Prostate, 0V90

Protecta XT CRT-D *use* Cardiac Resynchronization Defibrillator Pulse Generator in, 0JH

Protecta XT DR (XT VR) *use* Defibrillator Generator in, 0JH

Protégé® RX Carotid Stent System *use* Intraluminal Device

Proximal radioulnar joint
- *use* Elbow Joint, Left
- *use* Elbow Joint, Right

Psoas muscle
- *use* Hip Muscle, Left
- *use* Hip Muscle, Right

PSV (pressure support ventilation) *see* Performance, Respiratory, 5A19

Psychoanalysis, GZ54ZZZ

Psychological Tests
- Cognitive Status, GZ14ZZZ
- Developmental, GZ10ZZZ
- Intellectual and Psychoeducational, GZ12ZZZ
- Neurobehavioral Status, GZ14ZZZ
- Neuropsychological, GZ13ZZZ
- Personality and Behavioral, GZ11ZZZ

Psychotherapy
- Family, Mental Health Services, GZ72ZZZ
- Group, GZHZZZZ
  - Mental Health Services, GZHZZZZ
- Individual
  - *see* Psychotherapy, Individual, Mental Health Services
  - for substance abuse
    - 12-Step, HZ53ZZZ
    - Behavioral, HZ51ZZZ
    - Cognitive, HZ50ZZZ
    - Cognitive-Behavioral, HZ52ZZZ
    - Confrontational, HZ58ZZZ
    - Interactive, HZ55ZZZ
    - Interpersonal, HZ54ZZZ
    - Motivational Enhancement, HZ57ZZZ
    - Psychoanalysis, HZ5BZZZ
    - Psychodynamic, HZ5CZZZ
    - Psychoeducation, HZ56ZZZ
    - Psychophysiological, HZ5DZZZ
    - Supportive, HZ59ZZZ
- Mental Health Services
  - Behavioral, GZ51ZZZ
  - Cognitive, GZ52ZZZ
  - Cognitive-Behavioral, GZ58ZZZ
  - Interactive, GZ50ZZZ

Psychotherapy — *continued*
  Individual — *continued*
    Mental Health Services — *continued*
      Interpersonal, GZ53ZZZ
      Psychoanalysis, GZ54ZZZ
      Psychodynamic, GZ55ZZZ
      Psychophysiological, GZ59ZZZ
      Supportive, GZ56ZZZ
PTCA (percutaneous transluminal coronary angioplasty) *see* Dilation, Heart and Great Vessels, Ø27
Pterygoid muscle *use* Head Muscle
Pterygoid process *use* Sphenoid Bone
Pterygopalatine (sphenopalatine) ganglion *use* Head and Neck Sympathetic Nerve
Pubis
  use Pelvic Bone, Left
  use Pelvic Bone, Right
Pubofemoral ligament
  use Hip Bursa and Ligament, Left
  use Hip Bursa and Ligament, Right
Pudendal nerve *use* Sacral Plexus
Pull-through, laparoscopic-assisted transanal
  see Excision, Gastrointestinal System, ØDB
  see Resection, Gastrointestinal System, ØDT
Pull-through, rectal *see* Resection, Rectum, ØDTP
Pulmoaortic canal *use* Pulmonary Artery, Left
Pulmonary annulus *use* Pulmonary Valve
Pulmonary artery wedge monitoring *see* Monitoring, Arterial, 4A13
Pulmonary plexus
  use Thoracic Sympathetic Nerve
  use Vagus Nerve
Pulmonic valve *use* Pulmonary Valve
Pulpectomy *see* Excision, Mouth and Throat, ØCB
Pulverization *see* Fragmentation
Pulvinar *use* Thalamus
Pump reservoir *use* Infusion Device, Pump in Subcutaneous Tissue and Fascia
Punch biopsy *see* Excision with qualifier Diagnostic
Puncture *see* Drainage
Puncture, lumbar *see* Drainage, Spinal Canal, ØØ9U
Pyelography
  see Fluoroscopy, Urinary System, BT1
  see Plain Radiography, Urinary System, BTØ
Pyeloileostomy, urinary diversion *see* Bypass, Urinary System, ØT1
Pyeloplasty
  see Repair, Urinary System, ØTQ
  see Replacement, Urinary System, ØTR
  see Supplement, Urinary System, ØTU
Pyelorrhaphy *see* Repair, Urinary System, ØTQ
Pyeloscopy, ØTJ58ZZ
Pyelostomy
  see Bypass, Urinary System, ØT1
  see Drainage, Urinary System, ØT9
Pyelotomy *see* Drainage, Urinary System, ØT9
Pylorectomy
  see Excision, Stomach, Pylorus, ØDB7
  see Resection, Stomach, Pylorus, ØDT7
Pyloric antrum *use* Stomach, Pylorus
Pyloric canal *use* Stomach, Pylorus
Pyloric sphincter *use* Stomach, Pylorus
Pylorodiosis *see* Dilation, Stomach, Pylorus, ØD77
Pylorogastrectomy
  see Excision, Gastrointestinal System, ØDB
  see Resection, Gastrointestinal System, ØDT
Pyloroplasty
  see Repair, Stomach, Pylorus, ØDQ7
  see Supplement, Stomach, Pylorus, ØDU7
Pyloroscopy, ØDJ68ZZ
Pylorotomy *see* Drainage, Stomach, Pylorus, ØD97
Pyramidalis muscle
  use Abdomen Muscle, Left
  use Abdomen Muscle, Right

Q

Quadrangular cartilage *use* Nasal Septum
Quadrant resection of breast *see* Excision, Skin and Breast, ØHB
Quadrate lobe *use* Liver
Quadratus femoris muscle
  use Hip Muscle, Left
  use Hip Muscle, Right
Quadratus lumborum muscle
  use Trunk Muscle, Left

Quadratus lumborum muscle — *continued*
  use Trunk Muscle, Right
Quadratus plantae muscle
  use Foot Muscle, Left
  use Foot Muscle, Right
Quadriceps (femoris)
  use Upper Leg Muscle, Left
  use Upper Leg Muscle, Right
Quarantine, 8EØZXY6

R

Radial collateral carpal ligament
  use Wrist Bursa and Ligament, Left
  use Wrist Bursa and Ligament, Right
Radial collateral ligament
  use Elbow Bursa and Ligament, Left
  use Elbow Bursa and Ligament, Right
Radial notch
  use Ulna, Left
  use Ulna, Right
Radial recurrent artery
  use Radial Artery, Left
  use Radial Artery, Right
Radial vein
  use Brachial Vein, Left
  use Brachial Vein, Right
Radialis indicis
  use Hand Artery, Left
  use Hand Artery, Right
Radiation Therapy
  see Beam Radiation
  see Brachytherapy
  see Stereotactic Radiosurgery
Radiation treatment *see* Radiation Therapy
Radiocarpal joint
  use Wrist Joint, Left
  use Wrist Joint, Right
Radiocarpal ligament
  use Wrist Bursa and Ligament, Left
  use Wrist Bursa and Ligament, Right
Radiography *see* Plain Radiography
Radiology, analog *see* Plain Radiography
Radiology, diagnostic *see* Imaging, Diagnostic
Radioulnar ligament
  use Wrist Bursa and Ligament, Left
  use Wrist Bursa and Ligament, Right
Range of motion testing *see* Motor Function Assessment, Rehabilitation, FØ1
REALIZE® Adjustable Gastric Band *use* Extraluminal Device
Reattachment
  Abdominal Wall, ØWMFØZZ
  Ampulla of Vater, ØFMC
  Ankle Region
    Left, ØYMLØZZ
    Right, ØYMKØZZ
  Arm
    Lower
      Left, ØXMFØZZ
      Right, ØXMDØZZ
    Upper
      Left, ØXM9ØZZ
      Right, ØXM8ØZZ
  Axilla
    Left, ØXM5ØZZ
    Right, ØXM4ØZZ
  Back
    Lower, ØWMLØZZ
    Upper, ØWMKØZZ
  Bladder, ØTMB
  Bladder Neck, ØTMC
  Breast
    Bilateral, ØHMVXZZ
    Left, ØHMUXZZ
    Right, ØHMTXZZ
  Bronchus
    Lingula, ØBM9ØZZ
    Lower Lobe
      Left, ØBMBØZZ
      Right, ØBM6ØZZ
    Main
      Left, ØBM7ØZZ
      Right, ØBM3ØZZ
    Middle Lobe, Right, ØBM5ØZZ

Reattachment — *continued*
  Bronchus — *continued*
    Upper Lobe
      Left, ØBM8ØZZ
      Right, ØBM4ØZZ
  Bursa and Ligament
    Abdomen
      Left, ØMMJ
      Right, ØMMH
    Ankle
      Left, ØMMR
      Right, ØMMQ
    Elbow
      Left, ØMM4
      Right, ØMM3
    Foot
      Left, ØMMT
      Right, ØMMS
    Hand
      Left, ØMM8
      Right, ØMM7
    Head and Neck, ØMMØ
    Hip
      Left, ØMMM
      Right, ØMML
    Knee
      Left, ØMMP
      Right, ØMMN
    Lower Extremity
      Left, ØMMW
      Right, ØMMV
    Perineum, ØMMK
    Rib(s), ØMMG
    Shoulder
      Left, ØMM2
      Right, ØMM1
    Spine
      Lower, ØMMD
      Upper, ØMMC
    Sternum, ØMMF
    Upper Extremity
      Left, ØMMB
      Right, ØMM9
    Wrist
      Left, ØMM6
      Right, ØMM5
  Buttock
    Left, ØYM1ØZZ
    Right, ØYMØØZZ
  Carina, ØBM2ØZZ
  Cecum, ØDMH
  Cervix, ØUMC
  Chest Wall, ØWM8ØZZ
  Clitoris, ØUMJXZZ
  Colon
    Ascending, ØDMK
    Descending, ØDMM
    Sigmoid, ØDMN
    Transverse, ØDML
  Cord
    Bilateral, ØVMH
    Left, ØVMG
    Right, ØVMF
  Cul-de-sac, ØUMF
  Diaphragm, ØBMTØZZ
  Duct
    Common Bile, ØFM9
    Cystic, ØFM8
    Hepatic
      Common, ØFM7
      Left, ØFM6
      Right, ØFM5
    Pancreatic, ØFMD
      Accessory, ØFMF
  Duodenum, ØDM9
  Ear
    Left, Ø9M1XZZ
    Right, Ø9MØXZZ
  Elbow Region
    Left, ØXMCØZZ
    Right, ØXMBØZZ
  Esophagus, ØDM5
  Extremity
    Lower
      Left, ØYMBØZZ
      Right, ØYM9ØZZ
    Upper
      Left, ØXM7ØZZ
      Right, ØXM6ØZZ

▼ **Subterms under main terms may continue to next column or page**

Reattachment — *continued*
- Eyelid
  - Lower
    - Left, 08MRXZZ
    - Right, 08MQXZZ
  - Upper
    - Left, 08MPXZZ
    - Right, 08MNXZZ
- Face, 0WM20ZZ
- Fallopian Tube
  - Left, 0UM6
  - Right, 0UM5
- Fallopian Tubes, Bilateral, 0UM7
- Femoral Region
  - Left, 0YM80ZZ
  - Right, 0YM70ZZ
- Finger
  - Index
    - Left, 0XMP0ZZ
    - Right, 0XMN0ZZ
  - Little
    - Left, 0XMW0ZZ
    - Right, 0XMV0ZZ
  - Middle
    - Left, 0XMR0ZZ
    - Right, 0XMQ0ZZ
  - Ring
    - Left, 0XMT0ZZ
    - Right, 0XMS0ZZ
- Foot
  - Left, 0YMN0ZZ
  - Right, 0YMM0ZZ
- Forequarter
  - Left, 0XM10ZZ
  - Right, 0XM00ZZ
- Gallbladder, 0FM4
- Gland
  - Left, 0GM2
  - Right, 0GM3
- Hand
  - Left, 0XMK0ZZ
  - Right, 0XMJ0ZZ
- Hindquarter
  - Bilateral, 0YM40ZZ
  - Left, 0YM30ZZ
  - Right, 0YM20ZZ
- Hymen, 0UMK
- Ileum, 0DMB
- Inguinal Region
  - Left, 0YM60ZZ
  - Right, 0YM50ZZ
- Intestine
  - Large, 0DME
    - Left, 0DMG
    - Right, 0DMF
  - Small, 0DM8
- Jaw
  - Lower, 0WM50ZZ
  - Upper, 0WM40ZZ
- Jejunum, 0DMA
- Kidney
  - Left, 0TM1
  - Right, 0TM0
- Kidney Pelvis
  - Left, 0TM4
  - Right, 0TM3
- Kidneys, Bilateral, 0TM2
- Knee Region
  - Left, 0YMG0ZZ
  - Right, 0YMF0ZZ
- Leg
  - Lower
    - Left, 0YMJ0ZZ
    - Right, 0YMH0ZZ
  - Upper
    - Left, 0YMD0ZZ
    - Right, 0YMC0ZZ
- Lip
  - Lower, 0CM10ZZ
  - Upper, 0CM00ZZ
- Liver, 0FM0
  - Left Lobe, 0FM2
  - Right Lobe, 0FM1
- Lung
  - Left, 0BML0ZZ
  - Lower Lobe
    - Left, 0BMJ0ZZ
    - Right, 0BMF0ZZ
  - Middle Lobe, Right, 0BMD0ZZ

Reattachment — *continued*
- Lung — *continued*
  - Right, 0BMK0ZZ
  - Upper Lobe
    - Left, 0BMG0ZZ
    - Right, 0BMC0ZZ
- Lung Lingula, 0BMH0ZZ
- Muscle
  - Abdomen
    - Left, 0KML
    - Right, 0KMK
  - Facial, 0KM1
  - Foot
    - Left, 0KMW
    - Right, 0KMV
  - Hand
    - Left, 0KMD
    - Right, 0KMC
  - Head, 0KM0
  - Hip
    - Left, 0KMP
    - Right, 0KMN
  - Lower Arm and Wrist
    - Left, 0KMB
    - Right, 0KM9
  - Lower Leg
    - Left, 0KMT
    - Right, 0KMS
  - Neck
    - Left, 0KM3
    - Right, 0KM2
  - Perineum, 0KMM
  - Shoulder
    - Left, 0KM6
    - Right, 0KM5
  - Thorax
    - Left, 0KMJ
    - Right, 0KMH
  - Tongue, Palate, Pharynx, 0KM4
  - Trunk
    - Left, 0KMG
    - Right, 0KMF
  - Upper Arm
    - Left, 0KM8
    - Right, 0KM7
  - Upper Leg
    - Left, 0KMR
    - Right, 0KMQ
- Nasal Mucosa and Soft Tissue, 09MKXZZ
- Neck, 0WM60ZZ
- Nipple
  - Left, 0HMXXZZ
  - Right, 0HMWXZZ
- Ovary
  - Bilateral, 0UM2
  - Left, 0UM1
  - Right, 0UM0
- Palate, Soft, 0CM30ZZ
- Pancreas, 0FMG
- Parathyroid Gland, 0GMR
  - Inferior
    - Left, 0GMP
    - Right, 0GMN
  - Multiple, 0GMQ
  - Superior
    - Left, 0GMM
    - Right, 0GML
- Penis, 0VMSXZZ
- Perineum
  - Female, 0WMN0ZZ
  - Male, 0WMM0ZZ
- Rectum, 0DMP
- Scrotum, 0VM5XZZ
- Shoulder Region
  - Left, 0XM30ZZ
  - Right, 0XM20ZZ
- Skin
  - Abdomen, 0HM7XZZ
  - Back, 0HM6XZZ
  - Buttock, 0HM8XZZ
  - Chest, 0HM5XZZ
  - Ear
    - Left, 0HM3XZZ
    - Right, 0HM2XZZ
  - Face, 0HM1XZZ
  - Foot
    - Left, 0HMNXZZ
    - Right, 0HMMXZZ

Reattachment — *continued*
- Skin — *continued*
  - Hand
    - Left, 0HMGXZZ
    - Right, 0HMFXZZ
  - Inguinal, 0HMAXZZ
  - Lower Arm
    - Left, 0HMEXZZ
    - Right, 0HMDXZZ
  - Lower Leg
    - Left, 0HMLXZZ
    - Right, 0HMKXZZ
  - Neck, 0HM4XZZ
  - Perineum, 0HM9XZZ
  - Scalp, 0HM0XZZ
  - Upper Arm
    - Left, 0HMCXZZ
    - Right, 0HMBXZZ
  - Upper Leg
    - Left, 0HMJXZZ
    - Right, 0HMHXZZ
- Stomach, 0DM6
- Tendon
  - Abdomen
    - Left, 0LMG
    - Right, 0LMF
  - Ankle
    - Left, 0LMT
    - Right, 0LMS
  - Foot
    - Left, 0LMW
    - Right, 0LMV
  - Hand
    - Left, 0LM8
    - Right, 0LM7
  - Head and Neck, 0LM0
  - Hip
    - Left, 0LMK
    - Right, 0LMJ
  - Knee
    - Left, 0LMR
    - Right, 0LMQ
  - Lower Arm and Wrist
    - Left, 0LM6
    - Right, 0LM5
  - Lower Leg
    - Left, 0LMP
    - Right, 0LMN
  - Perineum, 0LMH
  - Shoulder
    - Left, 0LM2
    - Right, 0LM1
  - Thorax
    - Left, 0LMD
    - Right, 0LMC
  - Trunk
    - Left, 0LMB
    - Right, 0LM9
  - Upper Arm
    - Left, 0LM4
    - Right, 0LM3
  - Upper Leg
    - Left, 0LMM
    - Right, 0LML
- Testis
  - Bilateral, 0VMC
  - Left, 0VMB
  - Right, 0VM9
- Thumb
  - Left, 0XMM0ZZ
  - Right, 0XML0ZZ
- Thyroid Gland
  - Left Lobe, 0GMG
  - Right Lobe, 0GMH
- Toe
  - 1st
    - Left, 0YMQ0ZZ
    - Right, 0YMP0ZZ
  - 2nd
    - Left, 0YMS0ZZ
    - Right, 0YMR0ZZ
  - 3rd
    - Left, 0YMU0ZZ
    - Right, 0YMT0ZZ
  - 4th
    - Left, 0YMW0ZZ
    - Right, 0YMV0ZZ
  - 5th
    - Left, 0YMY0ZZ

Reattachment — *continued*
Toe — *continued*
5th — *continued*
Right, ØYMXØZZ
Tongue, ØCM7ØZZ
Tooth
Lower, ØCMX
Upper, ØCMW
Trachea, ØBM1ØZZ
Tunica Vaginalis
Left, ØVM7
Right, ØVM6
Ureter
Left, ØTM7
Right, ØTM6
Ureters, Bilateral, ØTM8
Urethra, ØTMD
Uterine Supporting Structure, ØUM4
Uterus, ØUM9
Uvula, ØCMNØZZ
Vagina, ØUMG
Vulva, ØUMMXZZ
Wrist Region
Left, ØXMHØZZ
Right, ØXMGØZZ
REBOA (resuscitative endovascular balloon occlusion of the aorta)
Ø2LW3DJ
Ø4LØ3DJ
Rebound HRD® (Hernia Repair Device) *use* Synthetic Substitute
Recession
see Repair
see Reposition
Reclosure, disrupted abdominal wall, ØWQFXZZ
Reconstruction
see Repair
see Replacement
see Supplement
Rectectomy
see Excision, Rectum, ØDBP
see Resection, Rectum, ØDTP
Rectocele repair *see* Repair, Subcutaneous Tissue and Fascia, Pelvic Region, ØJQC
Rectopexy
see Repair, Gastrointestinal System, ØDQ
see Reposition, Gastrointestinal System, ØDS
Rectoplasty
see Repair, Gastrointestinal System, ØDQ
see Supplement, Gastrointestinal System, ØDU
Rectorrhaphy *see* Repair, Gastrointestinal System, ØDQ
Rectoscopy, ØDJD8ZZ
Rectosigmoid junction *use* Sigmoid Colon
Rectosigmoidectomy
see Excision, Gastrointestinal System, ØDB
see Resection, Gastrointestinal System, ØDT
Rectostomy *see* Drainage, Rectum, ØD9P
Rectotomy *see* Drainage, Rectum, ØD9P
Rectus abdominis muscle
use Abdomen Muscle, Left
use Abdomen Muscle, Right
Rectus femoris muscle
use Upper Leg Muscle, Left
use Upper Leg Muscle, Right
Recurrent laryngeal nerve *use* Vagus Nerve
Reduction
Dislocation *see* Reposition
Fracture *see* Reposition
Intussusception, intestinal *see* Reposition, Gastrointestinal System, ØDS
Mammoplasty *see* Excision, Skin and Breast, ØHB
Prolapse *see* Reposition
Torsion *see* Reposition
Volvulus, gastrointestinal *see* Reposition, Gastrointestinal System, ØDS
Refusion *see* Fusion
Rehabilitation
see Activities of Daily Living Assessment, Rehabilitation, FØ2
see Activities of Daily Living Treatment, Rehabilitation, FØ8
see Caregiver Training, Rehabilitation, FØF
see Cochlear Implant Treatment, Rehabilitation, FØB
see Device Fitting, Rehabilitation, FØD
see Hearing Treatment, Rehabilitation, FØ9
see Motor Function Assessment, Rehabilitation, FØ1
see Motor Treatment, Rehabilitation, FØ7

Rehabilitation — *continued*
see Speech Assessment, Rehabilitation, FØØ
see Speech Treatment, Rehabilitation, FØ6
see Vestibular Treatment, Rehabilitation, FØC
Reimplantation
see Reattachment
see Reposition
see Transfer
Reinforcement
see Repair
see Supplement
Relaxation, scar tissue *see* Release
Release
Acetabulum
Left, ØQN5
Right, ØQN4
Adenoids, ØCNQ
Ampulla of Vater, ØFNC
Anal Sphincter, ØDNR
Anterior Chamber
Left, Ø8N33ZZ
Right, Ø8N23ZZ
Anus, ØDNQ
Aorta
Abdominal, Ø4NØ
Thoracic
Ascending/Arch, Ø2NX
Descending, Ø2NW
Aortic Body, ØGND
Appendix, ØDNJ
Artery
Anterior Tibial
Left, Ø4NQ
Right, Ø4NP
Axillary
Left, Ø3N6
Right, Ø3N5
Brachial
Left, Ø3N8
Right, Ø3N7
Celiac, Ø4N1
Colic
Left, Ø4N7
Middle, Ø4N8
Right, Ø4N6
Common Carotid
Left, Ø3NJ
Right, Ø3NH
Common Iliac
Left, Ø4ND
Right, Ø4NC
Coronary
Four or More Arteries, Ø2N3
One Artery, Ø2NØ
Three Arteries, Ø2N2
Two Arteries, Ø2N1
External Carotid
Left, Ø3NN
Right, Ø3NM
External Iliac
Left, Ø4NJ
Right, Ø4NH
Face, Ø3NR
Femoral
Left, Ø4NL
Right, Ø4NK
Foot
Left, Ø4NW
Right, Ø4NV
Gastric, Ø4N2
Hand
Left, Ø3NF
Right, Ø3ND
Hepatic, Ø4N3
Inferior Mesenteric, Ø4NB
Innominate, Ø3N2
Internal Carotid
Left, Ø3NL
Right, Ø3NK
Internal Iliac
Left, Ø4NF
Right, Ø4NE
Internal Mammary
Left, Ø3N1
Right, Ø3NØ
Intracranial, Ø3NG
Lower, Ø4NY

Release — *continued*
Artery — *continued*
Peroneal
Left, Ø4NU
Right, Ø4NT
Popliteal
Left, Ø4NN
Right, Ø4NM
Posterior Tibial
Left, Ø4NS
Right, Ø4NR
Pulmonary
Left, Ø2NR
Right, Ø2NQ
Pulmonary Trunk, Ø2NP
Radial
Left, Ø3NC
Right, Ø3NB
Renal
Left, Ø4NA
Right, Ø4N9
Splenic, Ø4N4
Subclavian
Left, Ø3N4
Right, Ø3N3
Superior Mesenteric, Ø4N5
Temporal
Left, Ø3NT
Right, Ø3NS
Thyroid
Left, Ø3NV
Right, Ø3NU
Ulnar
Left, Ø3NA
Right, Ø3N9
Upper, Ø3NY
Vertebral
Left, Ø3NQ
Right, Ø3NP
Atrium
Left, Ø2N7
Right, Ø2N6
Auditory Ossicle
Left, Ø9NA
Right, Ø9N9
Basal Ganglia, ØØN8
Bladder, ØTNB
Bladder Neck, ØTNC
Bone
Ethmoid
Left, ØNNG
Right, ØNNF
Frontal, ØNN1
Hyoid, ØNNX
Lacrimal
Left, ØNNJ
Right, ØNNH
Nasal, ØNNB
Occipital, ØNN7
Palatine
Left, ØNNL
Right, ØNNK
Parietal
Left, ØNN4
Right, ØNN3
Pelvic
Left, ØQN3
Right, ØQN2
Sphenoid, ØNNC
Temporal
Left, ØNN6
Right, ØNN5
Zygomatic
Left, ØNNN
Right, ØNNM
Brain, ØØNØ
Breast
Bilateral, ØHNV
Left, ØHNU
Right, ØHNT
Bronchus
Lingula, ØBN9
Lower Lobe
Left, ØBNB
Right, ØBN6
Main
Left, ØBN7
Right, ØBN3
Middle Lobe, Right, ØBN5

Release — *continued*
  Bronchus — *continued*
    Upper Lobe
      Left, 0BN8
      Right, 0BN4
  Buccal Mucosa, 0CN4
  Bursa and Ligament
    Abdomen
      Left, 0MNJ
      Right, 0MNH
    Ankle
      Left, 0MNR
      Right, 0MNQ
    Elbow
      Left, 0MN4
      Right, 0MN3
    Foot
      Left, 0MNT
      Right, 0MNS
    Hand
      Left, 0MN8
      Right, 0MN7
    Head and Neck, 0MN0
    Hip
      Left, 0MNM
      Right, 0MNL
    Knee
      Left, 0MNP
      Right, 0MNN
    Lower Extremity
      Left, 0MNW
      Right, 0MNV
    Perineum, 0MNK
    Rib(s), 0MNG
    Shoulder
      Left, 0MN2
      Right, 0MN1
    Spine
      Lower, 0MND
      Upper, 0MNC
    Sternum, 0MNF
    Upper Extremity
      Left, 0MNB
      Right, 0MN9
    Wrist
      Left, 0MN6
      Right, 0MN5
  Carina, 0BN2
  Carotid Bodies, Bilateral, 0GN8
  Carotid Body
    Left, 0GN6
    Right, 0GN7
  Carpal
    Left, 0PNN
    Right, 0PNM
  Cecum, 0DNH
  Cerebellum, 00NC
  Cerebral Hemisphere, 00N7
  Cerebral Meninges, 00N1
  Cerebral Ventricle, 00N6
  Cervix, 0UNC
  Chordae Tendineae, 02N9
  Choroid
    Left, 08NB
    Right, 08NA
  Cisterna Chyli, 07NL
  Clavicle
    Left, 0PNB
    Right, 0PN9
  Clitoris, 0UNJ
  Coccygeal Glomus, 0GNB
  Coccyx, 0QNS
  Colon
    Ascending, 0DNK
    Descending, 0DNM
    Sigmoid, 0DNN
    Transverse, 0DNL
  Conduction Mechanism, 02N8
  Conjunctiva
    Left, 08NTXZZ
    Right, 08NSXZZ
  Cord
    Bilateral, 0VNH
    Left, 0VNG
    Right, 0VNF
  Cornea
    Left, 08N9XZZ
    Right, 08N8XZZ
  Cul-de-sac, 0UNF

Release — *continued*
  Diaphragm, 0BNT
  Disc
    Cervical Vertebral, 0RN3
    Cervicothoracic Vertebral, 0RN5
    Lumbar Vertebral, 0SN2
    Lumbosacral, 0SN4
    Thoracic Vertebral, 0RN9
    Thoracolumbar Vertebral, 0RNB
  Duct
    Common Bile, 0FN9
    Cystic, 0FN8
    Hepatic
      Common, 0FN7
      Left, 0FN6
      Right, 0FN5
    Lacrimal
      Left, 08NY
      Right, 08NX
    Pancreatic, 0FND
      Accessory, 0FNF
    Parotid
      Left, 0CNC
      Right, 0CNB
  Duodenum, 0DN9
  Dura Mater, 00N2
  Ear
    External
      Left, 09N1
      Right, 09N0
    External Auditory Canal
      Left, 09N4
      Right, 09N3
    Inner
      Left, 09NE
      Right, 09ND
    Middle
      Left, 09N6
      Right, 09N5
  Epididymis
    Bilateral, 0VNL
    Left, 0VNK
    Right, 0VNJ
  Epiglottis, 0CNR
  Esophagogastric Junction, 0DN4
  Esophagus, 0DN5
    Lower, 0DN3
    Middle, 0DN2
    Upper, 0DN1
  Eustachian Tube
    Left, 09NG
    Right, 09NF
  Eye
    Left, 08N1XZZ
    Right, 08N0XZZ
  Eyelid
    Lower
      Left, 08NR
      Right, 08NQ
    Upper
      Left, 08NP
      Right, 08NN
  Fallopian Tube
    Left, 0UN6
    Right, 0UN5
  Fallopian Tubes, Bilateral, 0UN7
  Femoral Shaft
    Left, 0QN9
    Right, 0QN8
  Femur
    Lower
      Left, 0QNC
      Right, 0QNB
    Upper
      Left, 0QN7
      Right, 0QN6
  Fibula
    Left, 0QNK
    Right, 0QNJ
  Finger Nail, 0HNQXZZ
  Gallbladder, 0FN4
  Gingiva
    Lower, 0CN6
    Upper, 0CN5
  Gland
    Adrenal
      Bilateral, 0GN4
      Left, 0GN2
      Right, 0GN3

Release — *continued*
  Gland — *continued*
    Lacrimal
      Left, 08NW
      Right, 08NV
    Minor Salivary, 0CNJ
    Parotid
      Left, 0CN9
      Right, 0CN8
    Pituitary, 0GN0
    Sublingual
      Left, 0CNF
      Right, 0CND
    Submaxillary
      Left, 0CNH
      Right, 0CNG
    Vestibular, 0UNL
  Glenoid Cavity
    Left, 0PN8
    Right, 0PN7
  Glomus Jugulare, 0GNC
  Humeral Head
    Left, 0PND
    Right, 0PNC
  Humeral Shaft
    Left, 0PNG
    Right, 0PNF
  Hymen, 0UNK
  Hypothalamus, 00NA
  Ileocecal Valve, 0DNC
  Ileum, 0DNB
  Intestine
    Large, 0DNE
      Left, 0DNG
      Right, 0DNF
    Small, 0DN8
  Iris
    Left, 08ND3ZZ
    Right, 08NC3ZZ
  Jejunum, 0DNA
  Joint
    Acromioclavicular
      Left, 0RNH
      Right, 0RNG
    Ankle
      Left, 0SNG
      Right, 0SNF
    Carpal
      Left, 0RNR
      Right, 0RNQ
    Carpometacarpal
      Left, 0RNT
      Right, 0RNS
    Cervical Vertebral, 0RN1
    Cervicothoracic Vertebral, 0RN4
    Coccygeal, 0SN6
    Elbow
      Left, 0RNM
      Right, 0RNL
    Finger Phalangeal
      Left, 0RNX
      Right, 0RNW
    Hip
      Left, 0SNB
      Right, 0SN9
    Knee
      Left, 0SND
      Right, 0SNC
    Lumbar Vertebral, 0SN0
    Lumbosacral, 0SN3
    Metacarpophalangeal
      Left, 0RNV
      Right, 0RNU
    Metatarsal-Phalangeal
      Left, 0SNN
      Right, 0SNM
    Occipital-cervical, 0RN0
    Sacrococcygeal, 0SN5
    Sacroiliac
      Left, 0SN8
      Right, 0SN7
    Shoulder
      Left, 0RNK
      Right, 0RNJ
    Sternoclavicular
      Left, 0RNF
      Right, 0RNE
    Tarsal
      Left, 0SNJ

▽ **Subterms under main terms may continue to next column or page**

Release — continued
Joint — continued
Tarsal — continued
Right, ØSNH
Tarsometatarsal
Left, ØSNL
Right, ØSNK
Temporomandibular
Left, ØRND
Right, ØRNC
Thoracic Vertebral, ØRN6
Thoracolumbar Vertebral, ØRNA
Toe Phalangeal
Left, ØSNQ
Right, ØSNP
Wrist
Left, ØRNP
Right, ØRNN
Kidney
Left, ØTN1
Right, ØTNØ
Kidney Pelvis
Left, ØTN4
Right, ØTN3
Larynx, ØCNS
Lens
Left, Ø8NK3ZZ
Right, Ø8NJ3ZZ
Lip
Lower, ØCN1
Upper, ØCNØ
Liver, ØFNØ
Left Lobe, ØFN2
Right Lobe, ØFN1
Lung
Bilateral, ØBNM
Left, ØBNL
Lower Lobe
Left, ØBNJ
Right, ØBNF
Middle Lobe, Right, ØBND
Right, ØBNK
Upper Lobe
Left, ØBNG
Right, ØBNC
Lung Lingula, ØBNH
Lymphatic
Aortic, Ø7ND
Axillary
Left, Ø7N6
Right, Ø7N5
Head, Ø7NØ
Inguinal
Left, Ø7NJ
Right, Ø7NH
Internal Mammary
Left, Ø7N9
Right, Ø7N8
Lower Extremity
Left, Ø7NG
Right, Ø7NF
Mesenteric, Ø7NB
Neck
Left, Ø7N2
Right, Ø7N1
Pelvis, Ø7NC
Thoracic Duct, Ø7NK
Thorax, Ø7N7
Upper Extremity
Left, Ø7N4
Right, Ø7N3
Mandible
Left, ØNNV
Right, ØNNT
Maxilla, ØNNR
Medulla Oblongata, ØØND
Mesentery, ØDNV
Metacarpal
Left, ØPNQ
Right, ØPNP
Metatarsal
Left, ØQNP
Right, ØQNN
Muscle
Abdomen
Left, ØKNL
Right, ØKNK
Extraocular
Left, Ø8NM

Release — continued
Muscle — continued
Extraocular — continued
Right, Ø8NL
Facial, ØKN1
Foot
Left, ØKNW
Right, ØKNV
Hand
Left, ØKND
Right, ØKNC
Head, ØKNØ
Hip
Left, ØKNP
Right, ØKNN
Lower Arm and Wrist
Left, ØKNB
Right, ØKN9
Lower Leg
Left, ØKNT
Right, ØKNS
Neck
Left, ØKN3
Right, ØKN2
Papillary, Ø2ND
Perineum, ØKNM
Shoulder
Left, ØKN6
Right, ØKN5
Thorax
Left, ØKNJ
Right, ØKNH
Tongue, Palate, Pharynx, ØKN4
Trunk
Left, ØKNG
Right, ØKNF
Upper Arm
Left, ØKN8
Right, ØKN7
Upper Leg
Left, ØKNR
Right, ØKNQ
Myocardial Bridge see Release, Artery, Coronary
Nasal Mucosa and Soft Tissue, Ø9NK
Nasopharynx, Ø9NN
Nerve
Abdominal Sympathetic, Ø1NM
Abducens, ØØNL
Accessory, ØØNR
Acoustic, ØØNN
Brachial Plexus, Ø1N3
Cervical, Ø1N1
Cervical Plexus, Ø1NØ
Facial, ØØNM
Femoral, Ø1ND
Glossopharyngeal, ØØNP
Head and Neck Sympathetic, Ø1NK
Hypoglossal, ØØNS
Lumbar, Ø1NB
Lumbar Plexus, Ø1N9
Lumbar Sympathetic, Ø1NN
Lumbosacral Plexus, Ø1NA
Median, Ø1N5
Oculomotor, ØØNH
Olfactory, ØØNF
Optic, ØØNG
Peroneal, Ø1NH
Phrenic, Ø1N2
Pudendal, Ø1NC
Radial, Ø1N6
Sacral, Ø1NR
Sacral Plexus, Ø1NQ
Sacral Sympathetic, Ø1NP
Sciatic, Ø1NF
Thoracic, Ø1N8
Thoracic Sympathetic, Ø1NL
Tibial, Ø1NG
Trigeminal, ØØNK
Trochlear, ØØNJ
Ulnar, Ø1N4
Vagus, ØØNQ
Nipple
Left, ØHNX
Right, ØHNW
Omentum, ØDNU
Orbit
Left, ØNNQ
Right, ØNNP

Release — continued
Ovary
Bilateral, ØUN2
Left, ØUN1
Right, ØUNØ
Palate
Hard, ØCN2
Soft, ØCN3
Pancreas, ØFNG
Para-aortic Body, ØGN9
Paraganglion Extremity, ØGNF
Parathyroid Gland, ØGNR
Inferior
Left, ØGNP
Right, ØGNN
Multiple, ØGNQ
Superior
Left, ØGNM
Right, ØGNL
Patella
Left, ØQNF
Right, ØQND
Penis, ØVNS
Pericardium, Ø2NN
Peritoneum, ØDNW
Phalanx
Finger
Left, ØPNV
Right, ØPNT
Thumb
Left, ØPNS
Right, ØPNR
Toe
Left, ØQNR
Right, ØQNQ
Pharynx, ØCNM
Pineal Body, ØGN1
Pleura
Left, ØBNP
Right, ØBNN
Pons, ØØNB
Prepuce, ØVNT
Prostate, ØVNØ
Radius
Left, ØPNJ
Right, ØPNH
Rectum, ØDNP
Retina
Left, Ø8NF3ZZ
Right, Ø8NE3ZZ
Retinal Vessel
Left, Ø8NH3ZZ
Right, Ø8NG3ZZ
Ribs
1 to 2, ØPN1
3 or More, ØPN2
Sacrum, ØQN1
Scapula
Left, ØPN6
Right, ØPN5
Sclera
Left, Ø8N7XZZ
Right, Ø8N6XZZ
Scrotum, ØVN5
Septum
Atrial, Ø2N5
Nasal, Ø9NM
Ventricular, Ø2NM
Sinus
Accessory, Ø9NP
Ethmoid
Left, Ø9NV
Right, Ø9NU
Frontal
Left, Ø9NT
Right, Ø9NS
Mastoid
Left, Ø9NC
Right, Ø9NB
Maxillary
Left, Ø9NR
Right, Ø9NQ
Sphenoid
Left, Ø9NX
Right, Ø9NW
Skin
Abdomen, ØHN7XZZ
Back, ØHN6XZZ
Buttock, ØHN8XZZ

▽ **Subterms under main terms may continue to next column or page**

Release — continued
  Skin — continued
    Chest, ØHN5XZZ
    Ear
      Left, ØHN3XZZ
      Right, ØHN2XZZ
    Face, ØHN1XZZ
    Foot
      Left, ØHNNXZZ
      Right, ØHNMXZZ
    Hand
      Left, ØHNGXZZ
      Right, ØHNFXZZ
    Inguinal, ØHNAXZZ
    Lower Arm
      Left, ØHNEXZZ
      Right, ØHNDXZZ
    Lower Leg
      Left, ØHNLXZZ
      Right, ØHNKXZZ
    Neck, ØHN4XZZ
    Perineum, ØHN9XZZ
    Scalp, ØHN0XZZ
    Upper Arm
      Left, ØHNCXZZ
      Right, ØHNBXZZ
    Upper Leg
      Left, ØHNJXZZ
      Right, ØHNHXZZ
  Spinal Cord
    Cervical, ØØNW
    Lumbar, ØØNY
    Thoracic, ØØNX
  Spinal Meninges, ØØNT
  Spleen, Ø7NP
  Sternum, ØPNØ
  Stomach, ØDN6
    Pylorus, ØDN7
  Subcutaneous Tissue and Fascia
    Abdomen, ØJN8
    Back, ØJN7
    Buttock, ØJN9
    Chest, ØJN6
    Face, ØJN1
    Foot
      Left, ØJNR
      Right, ØJNQ
    Hand
      Left, ØJNK
      Right, ØJNJ
    Lower Arm
      Left, ØJNH
      Right, ØJNG
    Lower Leg
      Left, ØJNP
      Right, ØJNN
    Neck
      Left, ØJN5
      Right, ØJN4
    Pelvic Region, ØJNC
    Perineum, ØJNB
    Scalp, ØJNØ
    Upper Arm
      Left, ØJNF
      Right, ØJND
    Upper Leg
      Left, ØJNM
      Right, ØJNL
  Tarsal
    Left, ØQNM
    Right, ØQNL
  Tendon
    Abdomen
      Left, ØLNG
      Right, ØLNF
    Ankle
      Left, ØLNT
      Right, ØLNS
    Foot
      Left, ØLNW
      Right, ØLNV
    Hand
      Left, ØLN8
      Right, ØLN7
    Head and Neck, ØLNØ
    Hip
      Left, ØLNK
      Right, ØLNJ

Release — continued
  Tendon — continued
    Knee
      Left, ØLNR
      Right, ØLNQ
    Lower Arm and Wrist
      Left, ØLN6
      Right, ØLN5
    Lower Leg
      Left, ØLNP
      Right, ØLNN
    Perineum, ØLNH
    Shoulder
      Left, ØLN2
      Right, ØLN1
    Thorax
      Left, ØLND
      Right, ØLNC
    Trunk
      Left, ØLNB
      Right, ØLN9
    Upper Arm
      Left, ØLN4
      Right, ØLN3
    Upper Leg
      Left, ØLNM
      Right, ØLNL
  Testis
    Bilateral, ØVNC
    Left, ØVNB
    Right, ØVN9
  Thalamus, ØØN9
  Thymus, Ø7NM
  Thyroid Gland, ØGNK
    Left Lobe, ØGNG
    Right Lobe, ØGNH
  Tibia
    Left, ØQNH
    Right, ØQNG
  Toe Nail, ØHNRXZZ
  Tongue, ØCN7
  Tonsils, ØCNP
  Tooth
    Lower, ØCNX
    Upper, ØCNW
  Trachea, ØBN1
  Tunica Vaginalis
    Left, ØVN7
    Right, ØVN6
  Turbinate, Nasal, Ø9NL
  Tympanic Membrane
    Left, Ø9N8
    Right, Ø9N7
  Ulna
    Left, ØPNL
    Right, ØPNK
  Ureter
    Left, ØTN7
    Right, ØTN6
  Urethra, ØTND
  Uterine Supporting Structure, ØUN4
  Uterus, ØUN9
  Uvula, ØCNN
  Vagina, ØUNG
  Valve
    Aortic, Ø2NF
    Mitral, Ø2NG
    Pulmonary, Ø2NH
    Tricuspid, Ø2NJ
  Vas Deferens
    Bilateral, ØVNQ
    Left, ØVNP
    Right, ØVNN
  Vein
    Axillary
      Left, Ø5N8
      Right, Ø5N7
    Azygos, Ø5NØ
    Basilic
      Left, Ø5NC
      Right, Ø5NB
    Brachial
      Left, Ø5NA
      Right, Ø5N9
    Cephalic
      Left, Ø5NF
      Right, Ø5ND
    Colic, Ø6N7

Release — continued
  Vein — continued
    Common Iliac
      Left, Ø6ND
      Right, Ø6NC
    Coronary, Ø2N4
    Esophageal, Ø6N3
    External Iliac
      Left, Ø6NG
      Right, Ø6NF
    External Jugular
      Left, Ø5NQ
      Right, Ø5NP
    Face
      Left, Ø5NV
      Right, Ø5NT
    Femoral
      Left, Ø6NN
      Right, Ø6NM
    Foot
      Left, Ø6NV
      Right, Ø6NT
    Gastric, Ø6N2
    Hand
      Left, Ø5NH
      Right, Ø5NG
    Hemiazygos, Ø5N1
    Hepatic, Ø6N4
    Hypogastric
      Left, Ø6NJ
      Right, Ø6NH
    Inferior Mesenteric, Ø6N6
    Innominate
      Left, Ø5N4
      Right, Ø5N3
    Internal Jugular
      Left, Ø5NN
      Right, Ø5NM
    Intracranial, Ø5NL
    Lower, Ø6NY
    Portal, Ø6N8
    Pulmonary
      Left, Ø2NT
      Right, Ø2NS
    Renal
      Left, Ø6NB
      Right, Ø6N9
    Saphenous
      Left, Ø6NQ
      Right, Ø6NP
    Splenic, Ø6N1
    Subclavian
      Left, Ø5N6
      Right, Ø5N5
    Superior Mesenteric, Ø6N5
    Upper, Ø5NY
    Vertebral
      Left, Ø5NS
      Right, Ø5NR
  Vena Cava
    Inferior, Ø6NØ
    Superior, Ø2NV
  Ventricle
    Left, Ø2NL
    Right, Ø2NK
  Vertebra
    Cervical, ØPN3
    Lumbar, ØQNØ
    Thoracic, ØPN4
  Vesicle
    Bilateral, ØVN3
    Left, ØVN2
    Right, ØVN1
  Vitreous
    Left, Ø8N53ZZ
    Right, Ø8N43ZZ
  Vocal Cord
    Left, ØCNV
    Right, ØCNT
  Vulva, ØUNM
Relocation see Reposition
Removal
  Abdominal Wall, 2W53X
  Anorectal, 2Y53X5Z
  Arm
    Lower
      Left, 2W5DX
      Right, 2W5CX

Removal — *continued*
  Arm — *continued*
    Upper
      Left, 2W5BX
      Right, 2W5AX
  Back, 2W55X
  Chest Wall, 2W54X
  Ear, 2Y52X5Z
  Extremity
    Lower
      Left, 2W5MX
      Right, 2W5LX
    Upper
      Left, 2W59X
      Right, 2W58X
  Face, 2W51X
  Finger
    Left, 2W5KX
    Right, 2W5JX
  Foot
    Left, 2W5TX
    Right, 2W5SX
  Genital Tract, Female, 2Y54X5Z
  Hand
    Left, 2W5FX
    Right, 2W5EX
  Head, 2W50X
  Inguinal Region
    Left, 2W57X
    Right, 2W56X
  Leg
    Lower
      Left, 2W5RX
      Right, 2W5QX
    Upper
      Left, 2W5PX
      Right, 2W5NX
  Mouth and Pharynx, 2Y50X5Z
  Nasal, 2Y51X5Z
  Neck, 2W52X
  Thumb
    Left, 2W5HX
    Right, 2W5GX
  Toe
    Left, 2W5VX
    Right, 2W5UX
  Urethra, 2Y55X5Z
Removal of device from
  Abdominal Wall, 0WPF
  Acetabulum
    Left, 0QP5
    Right, 0QP4
  Anal Sphincter, 0DPR
  Anus, 0DPQ
  Artery
    Lower, 04PY
    Upper, 03PY
  Back
    Lower, 0WPL
    Upper, 0WPK
  Bladder, 0TPB
  Bone
    Facial, 0NPW
    Lower, 0QPY
    Nasal, 0NPB
    Pelvic
      Left, 0QP3
      Right, 0QP2
    Upper, 0PPY
  Bone Marrow, 07PT
  Brain, 00P0
  Breast
    Left, 0HPU
    Right, 0HPT
  Bursa and Ligament
    Lower, 0MPY
    Upper, 0MPX
  Carpal
    Left, 0PPN
    Right, 0PPM
  Cavity, Cranial, 0WP1
  Cerebral Ventricle, 00P6
  Chest Wall, 0WP8
  Cisterna Chyli, 07PL
  Clavicle
    Left, 0PPB
    Right, 0PP9
  Coccyx, 0QPS
  Diaphragm, 0BPT

Removal of device from — *continued*
  Disc
    Cervical Vertebral, 0RP3
    Cervicothoracic Vertebral, 0RP5
    Lumbar Vertebral, 0SP2
    Lumbosacral, 0SP4
    Thoracic Vertebral, 0RP9
    Thoracolumbar Vertebral, 0RPB
  Duct
    Hepatobiliary, 0FPB
    Pancreatic, 0FPD
  Ear
    Inner
      Left, 09PJ
      Right, 09PD
    Left, 09PJ
    Right, 09PH
  Epididymis and Spermatic Cord, 0VPM
  Esophagus, 0DP5
  Extremity
    Lower
      Left, 0YPB
      Right, 0YP9
    Upper
      Left, 0XP7
      Right, 0XP6
  Eye
    Left, 08P1
    Right, 08P0
  Face, 0WP2
  Fallopian Tube, 0UP8
  Femoral Shaft
    Left, 0QP9
    Right, 0QP8
  Femur
    Lower
      Left, 0QPC
      Right, 0QPB
    Upper
      Left, 0QP7
      Right, 0QP6
  Fibula
    Left, 0QPK
    Right, 0QPJ
  Finger Nail, 0HPQX
  Gallbladder, 0FP4
  Gastrointestinal Tract, 0WPP
  Genitourinary Tract, 0WPR
  Gland
    Adrenal, 0GP5
    Endocrine, 0GPS
    Pituitary, 0GP0
    Salivary, 0CPA
  Glenoid Cavity
    Left, 0PP8
    Right, 0PP7
  Great Vessel, 02PY
  Hair, 0HPSX
  Head, 0WP0
  Heart, 02PA
  Humeral Head
    Left, 0PPD
    Right, 0PPC
  Humeral Shaft
    Left, 0PPG
    Right, 0PPF
  Intestinal Tract
    Lower, 0DPD
    Upper, 0DP0
  Jaw
    Lower, 0WP5
    Upper, 0WP4
  Joint
    Acromioclavicular
      Left, 0RPH
      Right, 0RPG
    Ankle
      Left, 0SPG
      Right, 0SPF
    Carpal
      Left, 0RPR
      Right, 0RPQ
    Carpometacarpal
      Left, 0RPT
      Right, 0RPS
    Cervical Vertebral, 0RP1
    Cervicothoracic Vertebral, 0RP4
    Coccygeal, 0SP6

Removal of device from — *continued*
  Joint — *continued*
    Elbow
      Left, 0RPM
      Right, 0RPL
    Finger Phalangeal
      Left, 0RPX
      Right, 0RPW
    Hip
      Left, 0SPB
        Acetabular Surface, 0SPE
        Femoral Surface, 0SPS
      Right, 0SP9
        Acetabular Surface, 0SPA
        Femoral Surface, 0SPR
    Knee
      Left, 0SPD
        Femoral Surface, 0SPU
        Tibial Surface, 0SPW
      Right, 0SPC
        Femoral Surface, 0SPT
        Tibial Surface, 0SPV
    Lumbar Vertebral, 0SP0
    Lumbosacral, 0SP3
    Metacarpophalangeal
      Left, 0RPV
      Right, 0RPU
    Metatarsal-Phalangeal
      Left, 0SPN
      Right, 0SPM
    Occipital-cervical, 0RP0
    Sacrococcygeal, 0SP5
    Sacroiliac
      Left, 0SP8
      Right, 0SP7
    Shoulder
      Left, 0RPK
      Right, 0RPJ
    Sternoclavicular
      Left, 0RPF
      Right, 0RPE
    Tarsal
      Left, 0SPJ
      Right, 0SPH
    Tarsometatarsal
      Left, 0SPL
      Right, 0SPK
    Temporomandibular
      Left, 0RPD
      Right, 0RPC
    Thoracic Vertebral, 0RP6
    Thoracolumbar Vertebral, 0RPA
    Toe Phalangeal
      Left, 0SPQ
      Right, 0SPP
    Wrist
      Left, 0RPP
      Right, 0RPN
  Kidney, 0TP5
  Larynx, 0CPS
  Lens
    Left, 08PK3
    Right, 08PJ3
  Liver, 0FP0
  Lung
    Left, 0BPL
    Right, 0BPK
  Lymphatic, 07PN
    Thoracic Duct, 07PK
  Mediastinum, 0WPC
  Mesentery, 0DPV
  Metacarpal
    Left, 0PPQ
    Right, 0PPP
  Metatarsal
    Left, 0QPP
    Right, 0QPN
  Mouth and Throat, 0CPY
  Muscle
    Extraocular
      Left, 08PM
      Right, 08PL
    Lower, 0KPY
    Upper, 0KPX
  Nasal Mucosa and Soft Tissue, 09PK
  Neck, 0WP6
  Nerve
    Cranial, 00PE
    Peripheral, 01PY

▼ **Subterms under main terms may continue to next column or page**

Removal of device from — continued
Omentum, ØDPU
Ovary, ØUP3
Pancreas, ØFPG
Parathyroid Gland, ØGPR
Patella
Left, ØQPF
Right, ØQPD
Pelvic Cavity, ØWPJ
Penis, ØVPS
Pericardial Cavity, ØWPD
Perineum
Female, ØWPN
Male, ØWPM
Peritoneal Cavity, ØWPG
Peritoneum, ØDPW
Phalanx
Finger
Left, ØPPV
Right, ØPPT
Thumb
Left, ØPPS
Right, ØPPR
Toe
Left, ØQPR
Right, ØQPQ
Pineal Body, ØGP1
Pleura, ØBPQ
Pleural Cavity
Left, ØWPB
Right, ØWP9
Products of Conception, 10P0
Prostate and Seminal Vesicles, ØVP4
Radius
Left, ØPPJ
Right, ØPPH
Rectum, ØDPP
Respiratory Tract, ØWPQ
Retroperitoneum, ØWPH
Ribs
1 to 2, ØPP1
3 or More, ØPP2
Sacrum, ØQP1
Scapula
Left, ØPP6
Right, ØPP5
Scrotum and Tunica Vaginalis, ØVP8
Sinus, Ø9PY
Skin, ØHPPX
Skull, ØNPØ
Spinal Canal, ØØPU
Spinal Cord, ØØPV
Spleen, Ø7PP
Sternum, ØPPØ
Stomach, ØDP6
Subcutaneous Tissue and Fascia
Head and Neck, ØJPS
Lower Extremity, ØJPW
Trunk, ØJPT
Upper Extremity, ØJPV
Tarsal
Left, ØQPM
Right, ØQPL
Tendon
Lower, ØLPY
Upper, ØLPX
Testis, ØVPD
Thymus, Ø7PM
Thyroid Gland, ØGPK
Tibia
Left, ØQPH
Right, ØQPG
Toe Nail, ØHPRX
Trachea, ØBP1
Tracheobronchial Tree, ØBPØ
Tympanic Membrane
Left, Ø9P8
Right, Ø9P7
Ulna
Left, ØPPL
Right, ØPPK
Ureter, ØTP9
Urethra, ØTPD
Uterus and Cervix, ØUPD
Vagina and Cul-de-sac, ØUPH
Vas Deferens, ØVPR
Vein
Azygos, Ø5PØ

Removal of device from — continued
Vein — continued
Innominate
Left, Ø5P4
Right, Ø5P3
Lower, Ø6PY
Upper, Ø5PY
Vertebra
Cervical, ØPP3
Lumbar, ØQPØ
Thoracic, ØPP4
Vulva, ØUPM
Renal calyx
use Kidney
use Kidney, Left
use Kidney, Right
use Kidneys, Bilateral
Renal capsule
use Kidney
use Kidney, Left
use Kidney, Right
use Kidneys, Bilateral
Renal cortex
use Kidney
use Kidney, Left
use Kidney, Right
use Kidneys, Bilateral
Renal dialysis *see* Performance, Urinary, 5A1D
Renal plexus *use* Abdominal Sympathetic Nerve
Renal segment
use Kidney
use Kidney, Left
use Kidney, Right
use Kidneys, Bilateral
Renal segmental artery
use Renal Artery, Left
use Renal Artery, Right
Reopening, operative site
Control of bleeding *see* Control bleeding in
Inspection only *see* Inspection
Repair
Abdominal Wall, ØWQF
Acetabulum
Left, ØQQ5
Right, ØQQ4
Adenoids, ØCQQ
Ampulla of Vater, ØFQC
Anal Sphincter, ØDQR
Ankle Region
Left, ØYQL
Right, ØYQK
Anterior Chamber
Left, Ø8Q33ZZ
Right, Ø8Q23ZZ
Anus, ØDQQ
Aorta
Abdominal, Ø4QØ
Thoracic
Ascending/Arch, Ø2QX
Descending, Ø2QW
Aortic Body, ØGQD
Appendix, ØDQJ
Arm
Lower
Left, ØXQF
Right, ØXQD
Upper
Left, ØXQ9
Right, ØXQ8
Artery
Anterior Tibial
Left, Ø4QQ
Right, Ø4QP
Axillary
Left, Ø3Q6
Right, Ø3Q5
Brachial
Left, Ø3Q8
Right, Ø3Q7
Celiac, Ø4Q1
Colic
Left, Ø4Q7
Middle, Ø4Q8
Right, Ø4Q6
Common Carotid
Left, Ø3QJ
Right, Ø3QH

Repair — continued
Artery — continued
Common Iliac
Left, Ø4QD
Right, Ø4QC
Coronary
Four or More Arteries, Ø2Q3
One Artery, Ø2QØ
Three Arteries, Ø2Q2
Two Arteries, Ø2Q1
External Carotid
Left, Ø3QN
Right, Ø3QM
External Iliac
Left, Ø4QJ
Right, Ø4QH
Face, Ø3QR
Femoral
Left, Ø4QL
Right, Ø4QK
Foot
Left, Ø4QW
Right, Ø4QV
Gastric, Ø4Q2
Hand
Left, Ø3QF
Right, Ø3QD
Hepatic, Ø4Q3
Inferior Mesenteric, Ø4QB
Innominate, Ø3Q2
Internal Carotid
Left, Ø3QL
Right, Ø3QK
Internal Iliac
Left, Ø4QF
Right, Ø4QE
Internal Mammary
Left, Ø3Q1
Right, Ø3QØ
Intracranial, Ø3QG
Lower, Ø4QY
Peroneal
Left, Ø4QU
Right, Ø4QT
Popliteal
Left, Ø4QN
Right, Ø4QM
Posterior Tibial
Left, Ø4QS
Right, Ø4QR
Pulmonary
Left, Ø2QR
Right, Ø2QQ
Pulmonary Trunk, Ø2QP
Radial
Left, Ø3QC
Right, Ø3QB
Renal
Left, Ø4QA
Right, Ø4Q9
Splenic, Ø4Q4
Subclavian
Left, Ø3Q4
Right, Ø3Q3
Superior Mesenteric, Ø4Q5
Temporal
Left, Ø3QT
Right, Ø3QS
Thyroid
Left, Ø3QV
Right, Ø3QU
Ulnar
Left, Ø3QA
Right, Ø3Q9
Upper, Ø3QY
Vertebral
Left, Ø3QQ
Right, Ø3QP
Atrium
Left, Ø2Q7
Right, Ø2Q6
Auditory Ossicle
Left, Ø9QA
Right, Ø9Q9
Axilla
Left, ØXQ5
Right, ØXQ4
Back
Lower, ØWQL

Repair — *continued*
Back — *continued*
Upper, ØWQK
Basal Ganglia, ØØQ8
Bladder, ØTQB
Bladder Neck, ØTQC
Bone
Ethmoid
Left, ØNQG
Right, ØNQF
Frontal, ØNQ1
Hyoid, ØNQX
Lacrimal
Left, ØNQJ
Right, ØNQH
Nasal, ØNQB
Occipital, ØNQ7
Palatine
Left, ØNQL
Right, ØNQK
Parietal
Left, ØNQ4
Right, ØNQ3
Pelvic
Left, ØQQ3
Right, ØQQ2
Sphenoid, ØNQC
Temporal
Left, ØNQ6
Right, ØNQ5
Zygomatic
Left, ØNQN
Right, ØNQM
Brain, ØØQ0
Breast
Bilateral, ØHQV
Left, ØHQU
Right, ØHQT
Supernumerary, ØHQY
Bronchus
Lingula, ØBQ9
Lower Lobe
Left, ØBQB
Right, ØBQ6
Main
Left, ØBQ7
Right, ØBQ3
Middle Lobe, Right, ØBQ5
Upper Lobe
Left, ØBQ8
Right, ØBQ4
Buccal Mucosa, ØCQ4
Bursa and Ligament
Abdomen
Left, ØMQJ
Right, ØMQH
Ankle
Left, ØMQR
Right, ØMQQ
Elbow
Left, ØMQ4
Right, ØMQ3
Foot
Left, ØMQT
Right, ØMQS
Hand
Left, ØMQ8
Right, ØMQ7
Head and Neck, ØMQ0
Hip
Left, ØMQM
Right, ØMQL
Knee
Left, ØMQP
Right, ØMQN
Lower Extremity
Left, ØMQW
Right, ØMQV
Perineum, ØMQK
Rib(s), ØMQG
Shoulder
Left, ØMQ2
Right, ØMQ1
Spine
Lower, ØMQD
Upper, ØMQC
Sternum, ØMQF
Upper Extremity
Left, ØMQB

Repair — *continued*
Bursa and Ligament — *continued*
Upper Extremity — *continued*
Right, ØMQ9
Wrist
Left, ØMQ6
Right, ØMQ5
Buttock
Left, ØYQ1
Right, ØYQ0
Carina, ØBQ2
Carotid Bodies, Bilateral, ØGQ8
Carotid Body
Left, ØGQ6
Right, ØGQ7
Carpal
Left, ØPQN
Right, ØPQM
Cecum, ØDQH
Cerebellum, ØØQC
Cerebral Hemisphere, ØØQ7
Cerebral Meninges, ØØQ1
Cerebral Ventricle, ØØQ6
Cervix, ØUQC
Chest Wall, ØWQ8
Chordae Tendineae, Ø2Q9
Choroid
Left, Ø8QB
Right, Ø8QA
Cisterna Chyli, Ø7QL
Clavicle
Left, ØPQB
Right, ØPQ9
Clitoris, ØUQJ
Coccygeal Glomus, ØGQB
Coccyx, ØQQS
Colon
Ascending, ØDQK
Descending, ØDQM
Sigmoid, ØDQN
Transverse, ØDQL
Conduction Mechanism, Ø2Q8
Conjunctiva
Left, Ø8QTXZZ
Right, Ø8QSXZZ
Cord
Bilateral, ØVQH
Left, ØVQG
Right, ØVQF
Cornea
Left, Ø8Q9XZZ
Right, Ø8Q8XZZ
Cul-de-sac, ØUQF
Diaphragm, ØBQT
Disc
Cervical Vertebral, ØRQ3
Cervicothoracic Vertebral, ØRQ5
Lumbar Vertebral, ØSQ2
Lumbosacral, ØSQ4
Thoracic Vertebral, ØRQ9
Thoracolumbar Vertebral, ØRQB
Duct
Common Bile, ØFQ9
Cystic, ØFQ8
Hepatic
Common, ØFQ7
Left, ØFQ6
Right, ØFQ5
Lacrimal
Left, Ø8QY
Right, Ø8QX
Pancreatic, ØFQD
Accessory, ØFQF
Parotid
Left, ØCQC
Right, ØCQB
Duodenum, ØDQ9
Dura Mater, ØØQ2
Ear
External
Bilateral, Ø9Q2
Left, Ø9Q1
Right, Ø9Q0
External Auditory Canal
Left, Ø9Q4
Right, Ø9Q3
Inner
Left, Ø9QE
Right, Ø9QD

Repair — *continued*
Ear — *continued*
Middle
Left, Ø9Q6
Right, Ø9Q5
Elbow Region
Left, ØXQC
Right, ØXQB
Epididymis
Bilateral, ØVQL
Left, ØVQK
Right, ØVQJ
Epiglottis, ØCQR
Esophagogastric Junction, ØDQ4
Esophagus, ØDQ5
Lower, ØDQ3
Middle, ØDQ2
Upper, ØDQ1
Eustachian Tube
Left, Ø9QG
Right, Ø9QF
Extremity
Lower
Left, ØYQB
Right, ØYQ9
Upper
Left, ØXQ7
Right, ØXQ6
Eye
Left, Ø8Q1XZZ
Right, Ø8Q0XZZ
Eyelid
Lower
Left, Ø8QR
Right, Ø8QQ
Upper
Left, Ø8QP
Right, Ø8QN
Face, ØWQ2
Fallopian Tube
Left, ØUQ6
Right, ØUQ5
Fallopian Tubes, Bilateral, ØUQ7
Femoral Region
Bilateral, ØYQE
Left, ØYQ8
Right, ØYQ7
Femoral Shaft
Left, ØQQ9
Right, ØQQ8
Femur
Lower
Left, ØQQC
Right, ØQQB
Upper
Left, ØQQ7
Right, ØQQ6
Fibula
Left, ØQQK
Right, ØQQJ
Finger
Index
Left, ØXQP
Right, ØXQN
Little
Left, ØXQW
Right, ØXQV
Middle
Left, ØXQR
Right, ØXQQ
Ring
Left, ØXQT
Right, ØXQS
Finger Nail, ØHQQXZZ
Floor of mouth *see* Repair, Oral Cavity and Throat, ØWQ3
Foot
Left, ØYQN
Right, ØYQM
Gallbladder, ØFQ4
Gingiva
Lower, ØCQ6
Upper, ØCQ5
Gland
Adrenal
Bilateral, ØGQ4
Left, ØGQ2
Right, ØGQ3

Subterms under main terms may continue to next column or page

Repair — *continued*
  Gland — *continued*
    Lacrimal
      Left, 08QW
      Right, 08QV
    Minor Salivary, 0CQJ
    Parotid
      Left, 0CQ9
      Right, 0CQ8
    Pituitary, 0GQ0
    Sublingual
      Left, 0CQF
      Right, 0CQD
    Submaxillary
      Left, 0CQH
      Right, 0CQG
    Vestibular, 0UQL
  Glenoid Cavity
    Left, 0PQ8
    Right, 0PQ7
  Glomus Jugulare, 0GQC
  Hand
    Left, 0XQK
    Right, 0XQJ
  Head, 0WQ0
  Heart, 02QA
    Left, 02QC
    Right, 02QB
  Humeral Head
    Left, 0PQD
    Right, 0PQC
  Humeral Shaft
    Left, 0PQG
    Right, 0PQF
  Hymen, 0UQK
  Hypothalamus, 00QA
  Ileocecal Valve, 0DQC
  Ileum, 0DQB
  Inguinal Region
    Bilateral, 0YQA
    Left, 0YQ6
    Right, 0YQ5
  Intestine
    Large, 0DQE
      Left, 0DQG
      Right, 0DQF
    Small, 0DQ8
  Iris
    Left, 08QD3ZZ
    Right, 08QC3ZZ
  Jaw
    Lower, 0WQ5
    Upper, 0WQ4
  Jejunum, 0DQA
  Joint
    Acromioclavicular
      Left, 0RQH
      Right, 0RQG
    Ankle
      Left, 0SQG
      Right, 0SQF
    Carpal
      Left, 0RQR
      Right, 0RQQ
    Carpometacarpal
      Left, 0RQT
      Right, 0RQS
    Cervical Vertebral, 0RQ1
    Cervicothoracic Vertebral, 0RQ4
    Coccygeal, 0SQ6
    Elbow
      Left, 0RQM
      Right, 0RQL
    Finger Phalangeal
      Left, 0RQX
      Right, 0RQW
    Hip
      Left, 0SQB
      Right, 0SQ9
    Knee
      Left, 0SQD
      Right, 0SQC
    Lumbar Vertebral, 0SQ0
    Lumbosacral, 0SQ3
    Metacarpophalangeal
      Left, 0RQV
      Right, 0RQU
    Metatarsal-Phalangeal
      Left, 0SQN

Repair — *continued*
  Joint — *continued*
    Metatarsal-Phalangeal — *continued*
      Right, 0SQM
    Occipital-cervical, 0RQ0
    Sacrococcygeal, 0SQ5
    Sacroiliac
      Left, 0SQ8
      Right, 0SQ7
    Shoulder
      Left, 0RQK
      Right, 0RQJ
    Sternoclavicular
      Left, 0RQF
      Right, 0RQE
    Tarsal
      Left, 0SQJ
      Right, 0SQH
    Tarsometatarsal
      Left, 0SQL
      Right, 0SQK
    Temporomandibular
      Left, 0RQD
      Right, 0RQC
    Thoracic Vertebral, 0RQ6
    Thoracolumbar Vertebral, 0RQA
    Toe Phalangeal
      Left, 0SQQ
      Right, 0SQP
    Wrist
      Left, 0RQP
      Right, 0RQN
  Kidney
    Left, 0TQ1
    Right, 0TQ0
  Kidney Pelvis
    Left, 0TQ4
    Right, 0TQ3
  Knee Region
    Left, 0YQG
    Right, 0YQF
  Larynx, 0CQS
  Leg
    Lower
      Left, 0YQJ
      Right, 0YQH
    Upper
      Left, 0YQD
      Right, 0YQC
  Lens
    Left, 08QK3ZZ
    Right, 08QJ3ZZ
  Lip
    Lower, 0CQ1
    Upper, 0CQ0
  Liver, 0FQ0
    Left Lobe, 0FQ2
    Right Lobe, 0FQ1
  Lung
    Bilateral, 0BQM
    Left, 0BQL
    Lower Lobe
      Left, 0BQJ
      Right, 0BQF
    Middle Lobe, Right, 0BQD
    Right, 0BQK
    Upper Lobe
      Left, 0BQG
      Right, 0BQC
  Lung Lingula, 0BQH
  Lymphatic
    Aortic, 07QD
    Axillary
      Left, 07Q6
      Right, 07Q5
    Head, 07Q0
    Inguinal
      Left, 07QJ
      Right, 07QH
    Internal Mammary
      Left, 07Q9
      Right, 07Q8
    Lower Extremity
      Left, 07QG
      Right, 07QF
    Mesenteric, 07QB
    Neck
      Left, 07Q2
      Right, 07Q1

Repair — *continued*
  Lymphatic — *continued*
    Pelvis, 07QC
    Thoracic Duct, 07QK
    Thorax, 07Q7
    Upper Extremity
      Left, 07Q4
      Right, 07Q3
  Mandible
    Left, 0NQV
    Right, 0NQT
  Maxilla, 0NQR
  Mediastinum, 0WQC
  Medulla Oblongata, 00QD
  Mesentery, 0DQV
  Metacarpal
    Left, 0PQQ
    Right, 0PQP
  Metatarsal
    Left, 0QQP
    Right, 0QQN
  Muscle
    Abdomen
      Left, 0KQL
      Right, 0KQK
    Extraocular
      Left, 08QM
      Right, 08QL
    Facial, 0KQ1
    Foot
      Left, 0KQW
      Right, 0KQV
    Hand
      Left, 0KQD
      Right, 0KQC
    Head, 0KQ0
    Hip
      Left, 0KQP
      Right, 0KQN
    Lower Arm and Wrist
      Left, 0KQB
      Right, 0KQ9
    Lower Leg
      Left, 0KQT
      Right, 0KQS
    Neck
      Left, 0KQ3
      Right, 0KQ2
    Papillary, 02QD
    Perineum, 0KQM
    Shoulder
      Left, 0KQ6
      Right, 0KQ5
    Thorax
      Left, 0KQJ
      Right, 0KQH
    Tongue, Palate, Pharynx, 0KQ4
    Trunk
      Left, 0KQG
      Right, 0KQF
    Upper Arm
      Left, 0KQ8
      Right, 0KQ7
    Upper Leg
      Left, 0KQR
      Right, 0KQQ
  Nasal Mucosa and Soft Tissue, 09QK
  Nasopharynx, 09QN
  Neck, 0WQ6
  Nerve
    Abdominal Sympathetic, 01QM
    Abducens, 00QL
    Accessory, 00QR
    Acoustic, 00QN
    Brachial Plexus, 01Q3
    Cervical, 01Q1
    Cervical Plexus, 01Q0
    Facial, 00QM
    Femoral, 01QD
    Glossopharyngeal, 00QP
    Head and Neck Sympathetic, 01QK
    Hypoglossal, 00QS
    Lumbar, 01QB
    Lumbar Plexus, 01Q9
    Lumbar Sympathetic, 01QN
    Lumbosacral Plexus, 01QA
    Median, 01Q5
    Oculomotor, 00QH
    Olfactory, 00QF

Repair — continued
Nerve — continued
Optic, 00QG
Peroneal, 01QH
Phrenic, 01Q2
Pudendal, 01QC
Radial, 01Q6
Sacral, 01QR
Sacral Plexus, 01QQ
Sacral Sympathetic, 01QP
Sciatic, 01QF
Thoracic, 01Q8
Thoracic Sympathetic, 01QL
Tibial, 01QG
Trigeminal, 00QK
Trochlear, 00QJ
Ulnar, 01Q4
Vagus, 00QQ
Nipple
Left, 0HQX
Right, 0HQW
Omentum, 0DQU
Oral Cavity and Throat, 0WQ3
Orbit
Left, 0NQQ
Right, 0NQP
Ovary
Bilateral, 0UQ2
Left, 0UQ1
Right, 0UQ0
Palate
Hard, 0CQ2
Soft, 0CQ3
Pancreas, 0FQG
Para-aortic Body, 0GQ9
Paraganglion Extremity, 0GQF
Parathyroid Gland, 0GQR
Inferior
Left, 0GQP
Right, 0GQN
Multiple, 0GQQ
Superior
Left, 0GQM
Right, 0GQL
Patella
Left, 0QQF
Right, 0QQD
Penis, 0VQS
Pericardium, 02QN
Perineum
Female, 0WQN
Male, 0WQM
Peritoneum, 0DQW
Phalanx
Finger
Left, 0PQV
Right, 0PQT
Thumb
Left, 0PQS
Right, 0PQR
Toe
Left, 0QQR
Right, 0QQQ
Pharynx, 0CQM
Pineal Body, 0GQ1
Pleura
Left, 0BQP
Right, 0BQN
Pons, 00QB
Prepuce, 0VQT
Products of Conception, 10Q0
Prostate, 0VQ0
Radius
Left, 0PQJ
Right, 0PQH
Rectum, 0DQP
Retina
Left, 08QF3ZZ
Right, 08QE3ZZ
Retinal Vessel
Left, 08QH3ZZ
Right, 08QG3ZZ
Ribs
1 to 2, 0PQ1
3 or More, 0PQ2
Sacrum, 0QQ1
Scapula
Left, 0PQ6
Right, 0PQ5

Repair — continued
Sclera
Left, 08Q7XZZ
Right, 08Q6XZZ
Scrotum, 0VQ5
Septum
Atrial, 02Q5
Nasal, 09QM
Ventricular, 02QM
Shoulder Region
Left, 0XQ3
Right, 0XQ2
Sinus
Accessory, 09QP
Ethmoid
Left, 09QV
Right, 09QU
Frontal
Left, 09QT
Right, 09QS
Mastoid
Left, 09QC
Right, 09QB
Maxillary
Left, 09QR
Right, 09QQ
Sphenoid
Left, 09QX
Right, 09QW
Skin
Abdomen, 0HQ7XZZ
Back, 0HQ6XZZ
Buttock, 0HQ8XZZ
Chest, 0HQ5XZZ
Ear
Left, 0HQ3XZZ
Right, 0HQ2XZZ
Face, 0HQ1XZZ
Foot
Left, 0HQNXZZ
Right, 0HQMXZZ
Hand
Left, 0HQGXZZ
Right, 0HQFXZZ
Inguinal, 0HQAXZZ
Lower Arm
Left, 0HQEXZZ
Right, 0HQDXZZ
Lower Leg
Left, 0HQLXZZ
Right, 0HQKXZZ
Neck, 0HQ4XZZ
Perineum, 0HQ9XZZ
Scalp, 0HQ0XZZ
Upper Arm
Left, 0HQCXZZ
Right, 0HQBXZZ
Upper Leg
Left, 0HQJXZZ
Right, 0HQHXZZ
Skull, 0NQ0
Spinal Cord
Cervical, 00QW
Lumbar, 00QY
Thoracic, 00QX
Spinal Meninges, 00QT
Spleen, 07QP
Sternum, 0PQ0
Stomach, 0DQ6
Pylorus, 0DQ7
Subcutaneous Tissue and Fascia
Abdomen, 0JQ8
Back, 0JQ7
Buttock, 0JQ9
Chest, 0JQ6
Face, 0JQ1
Foot
Left, 0JQR
Right, 0JQQ
Hand
Left, 0JQK
Right, 0JQJ
Lower Arm
Left, 0JQH
Right, 0JQG
Lower Leg
Left, 0JQP
Right, 0JQN

Repair — continued
Subcutaneous Tissue and Fascia — continued
Neck
Left, 0JQ5
Right, 0JQ4
Pelvic Region, 0JQC
Perineum, 0JQB
Scalp, 0JQ0
Upper Arm
Left, 0JQF
Right, 0JQD
Upper Leg
Left, 0JQM
Right, 0JQL
Tarsal
Left, 0QQM
Right, 0QQL
Tendon
Abdomen
Left, 0LQG
Right, 0LQF
Ankle
Left, 0LQT
Right, 0LQS
Foot
Left, 0LQW
Right, 0LQV
Hand
Left, 0LQ8
Right, 0LQ7
Head and Neck, 0LQ0
Hip
Left, 0LQK
Right, 0LQJ
Knee
Left, 0LQR
Right, 0LQQ
Lower Arm and Wrist
Left, 0LQ6
Right, 0LQ5
Lower Leg
Left, 0LQP
Right, 0LQN
Perineum, 0LQH
Shoulder
Left, 0LQ2
Right, 0LQ1
Thorax
Left, 0LQD
Right, 0LQC
Trunk
Left, 0LQB
Right, 0LQ9
Upper Arm
Left, 0LQ4
Right, 0LQ3
Upper Leg
Left, 0LQM
Right, 0LQL
Testis
Bilateral, 0VQC
Left, 0VQB
Right, 0VQ9
Thalamus, 00Q9
Thumb
Left, 0XQM
Right, 0XQL
Thymus, 07QM
Thyroid Gland, 0GQK
Left Lobe, 0GQG
Right Lobe, 0GQH
Thyroid Gland Isthmus, 0GQJ
Tibia
Left, 0QQH
Right, 0QQG
Toe
1st
Left, 0YQQ
Right, 0YQP
2nd
Left, 0YQS
Right, 0YQR
3rd
Left, 0YQU
Right, 0YQT
4th
Left, 0YQW
Right, 0YQV

Index

Repair — Replacement

Repair — *continued*
  Toe — *continued*
    5th
      Left, ØYQY
      Right, ØYQX
  Toe Nail, ØHQRXZZ
  Tongue, ØCQ7
  Tonsils, ØCQP
  Tooth
    Lower, ØCQX
    Upper, ØCQW
  Trachea, ØBQ1
  Tunica Vaginalis
    Left, ØVQ7
    Right, ØVQ6
  Turbinate, Nasal, Ø9QL
  Tympanic Membrane
    Left, Ø9Q8
    Right, Ø9Q7
  Ulna
    Left, ØPQL
    Right, ØPQK
  Ureter
    Left, ØTQ7
    Right, ØTQ6
  Urethra, ØTQD
  Uterine Supporting Structure, ØUQ4
  Uterus, ØUQ9
  Uvula, ØCQN
  Vagina, ØUQG
  Valve
    Aortic, Ø2QF
    Mitral, Ø2QG
    Pulmonary, Ø2QH
    Tricuspid, Ø2QJ
  Vas Deferens
    Bilateral, ØVQQ
    Left, ØVQP
    Right, ØVQN
  Vein
    Axillary
      Left, Ø5Q8
      Right, Ø5Q7
    Azygos, Ø5Q0
    Basilic
      Left, Ø5QC
      Right, Ø5QB
    Brachial
      Left, Ø5QA
      Right, Ø5Q9
    Cephalic
      Left, Ø5QF
      Right, Ø5QD
    Colic, Ø6Q7
    Common Iliac
      Left, Ø6QD
      Right, Ø6QC
    Coronary, Ø2Q4
    Esophageal, Ø6Q3
    External Iliac
      Left, Ø6QG
      Right, Ø6QF
    External Jugular
      Left, Ø5QQ
      Right, Ø5QP
    Face
      Left, Ø5QV
      Right, Ø5QT
    Femoral
      Left, Ø6QN
      Right, Ø6QM
    Foot
      Left, Ø6QV
      Right, Ø6QT
    Gastric, Ø6Q2
    Hand
      Left, Ø5QH
      Right, Ø5QG
    Hemiazygos, Ø5Q1
    Hepatic, Ø6Q4
    Hypogastric
      Left, Ø6QJ
      Right, Ø6QH
    Inferior Mesenteric, Ø6Q6
    Innominate
      Left, Ø5Q4
      Right, Ø5Q3
    Internal Jugular
      Left, Ø5QN

Repair — *continued*
  Vein — *continued*
    Internal Jugular — *continued*
      Right, Ø5QM
    Intracranial, Ø5QL
    Lower, Ø6QY
    Portal, Ø6Q8
    Pulmonary
      Left, Ø2QT
      Right, Ø2QS
    Renal
      Left, Ø6QB
      Right, Ø6Q9
    Saphenous
      Left, Ø6QQ
      Right, Ø6QP
    Splenic, Ø6Q1
    Subclavian
      Left, Ø5Q6
      Right, Ø5Q5
    Superior Mesenteric, Ø6Q5
    Upper, Ø5QY
    Vertebral
      Left, Ø5QS
      Right, Ø5QR
  Vena Cava
    Inferior, Ø6Q0
    Superior, Ø2QV
  Ventricle
    Left, Ø2QL
    Right, Ø2QK
  Vertebra
    Cervical, ØPQ3
    Lumbar, ØQQ0
    Thoracic, ØPQ4
  Vesicle
    Bilateral, ØVQ3
    Left, ØVQ2
    Right, ØVQ1
  Vitreous
    Left, Ø8Q53ZZ
    Right, Ø8Q43ZZ
  Vocal Cord
    Left, ØCQV
    Right, ØCQT
  Vulva, ØUQM
  Wrist Region
    Left, ØXQH
    Right, ØXQG
Repair, obstetric laceration, periurethral, ØUQMXZZ
Replacement
  Acetabulum
    Left, ØQR5
    Right, ØQR4
  Ampulla of Vater, ØFRC
  Anal Sphincter, ØDRR
  Aorta
    Abdominal, Ø4R0
    Thoracic
      Ascending/Arch, Ø2RX
      Descending, Ø2RW
  Artery
    Anterior Tibial
      Left, Ø4RQ
      Right, Ø4RP
    Axillary
      Left, Ø3R6
      Right, Ø3R5
    Brachial
      Left, Ø3R8
      Right, Ø3R7
    Celiac, Ø4R1
    Colic
      Left, Ø4R7
      Middle, Ø4R8
      Right, Ø4R6
    Common Carotid
      Left, Ø3RJ
      Right, Ø3RH
    Common Iliac
      Left, Ø4RD
      Right, Ø4RC
    External Carotid
      Left, Ø3RN
      Right, Ø3RM
    External Iliac
      Left, Ø4RJ
      Right, Ø4RH
    Face, Ø3RR

Replacement — *continued*
  Artery — *continued*
    Femoral
      Left, Ø4RL
      Right, Ø4RK
    Foot
      Left, Ø4RW
      Right, Ø4RV
    Gastric, Ø4R2
    Hand
      Left, Ø3RF
      Right, Ø3RD
    Hepatic, Ø4R3
    Inferior Mesenteric, Ø4RB
    Innominate, Ø3R2
    Internal Carotid
      Left, Ø3RL
      Right, Ø3RK
    Internal Iliac
      Left, Ø4RF
      Right, Ø4RE
    Internal Mammary
      Left, Ø3R1
      Right, Ø3R0
    Intracranial, Ø3RG
    Lower, Ø4RY
    Peroneal
      Left, Ø4RU
      Right, Ø4RT
    Popliteal
      Left, Ø4RN
      Right, Ø4RM
    Posterior Tibial
      Left, Ø4RS
      Right, Ø4RR
    Pulmonary
      Left, Ø2RR
      Right, Ø2RQ
    Pulmonary Trunk, Ø2RP
    Radial
      Left, Ø3RC
      Right, Ø3RB
    Renal
      Left, Ø4RA
      Right, Ø4R9
    Splenic, Ø4R4
    Subclavian
      Left, Ø3R4
      Right, Ø3R3
    Superior Mesenteric, Ø4R5
    Temporal
      Left, Ø3RT
      Right, Ø3RS
    Thyroid
      Left, Ø3RV
      Right, Ø3RU
    Ulnar
      Left, Ø3RA
      Right, Ø3R9
    Upper, Ø3RY
    Vertebral
      Left, Ø3RQ
      Right, Ø3RP
  Atrium
    Left, Ø2R7
    Right, Ø2R6
  Auditory Ossicle
    Left, Ø9RA0
    Right, Ø9R90
  Bladder, ØTRB
  Bladder Neck, ØTRC
  Bone
    Ethmoid
      Left, ØNRG
      Right, ØNRF
    Frontal, ØNR1
    Hyoid, ØNRX
    Lacrimal
      Left, ØNRJ
      Right, ØNRH
    Nasal, ØNRB
    Occipital, ØNR7
    Palatine
      Left, ØNRL
      Right, ØNRK
    Parietal
      Left, ØNR4
      Right, ØNR3

Replacement — *continued*
  Bone — *continued*
    Pelvic
      Left, 0QR3
      Right, 0QR2
    Sphenoid, 0NRC
    Temporal
      Left, 0NR6
      Right, 0NR5
    Zygomatic
      Left, 0NRN
      Right, 0NRM
  Breast
    Bilateral, 0HRV
    Left, 0HRU
    Right, 0HRT
  Bronchus
    Lingula, 0BR9
    Lower Lobe
      Left, 0BRB
      Right, 0BR6
    Main
      Left, 0BR7
      Right, 0BR3
    Middle Lobe, Right, 0BR5
    Upper Lobe
      Left, 0BR8
      Right, 0BR4
  Buccal Mucosa, 0CR4
  Bursa and Ligament
    Abdomen
      Left, 0MRJ
      Right, 0MRH
    Ankle
      Left, 0MRR
      Right, 0MRQ
    Elbow
      Left, 0MR4
      Right, 0MR3
    Foot
      Left, 0MRT
      Right, 0MRS
    Hand
      Left, 0MR8
      Right, 0MR7
    Head and Neck, 0MR0
    Hip
      Left, 0MRM
      Right, 0MRL
    Knee
      Left, 0MRP
      Right, 0MRN
    Lower Extremity
      Left, 0MRW
      Right, 0MRV
    Perineum, 0MRK
    Rib(s), 0MRG
    Shoulder
      Left, 0MR2
      Right, 0MR1
    Spine
      Lower, 0MRD
      Upper, 0MRC
    Sternum, 0MRF
    Upper Extremity
      Left, 0MRB
      Right, 0MR9
    Wrist
      Left, 0MR6
      Right, 0MR5
  Carina, 0BR2
  Carpal
    Left, 0PRN
    Right, 0PRM
  Cerebral Meninges, 00R1
  Cerebral Ventricle, 00R6
  Chordae Tendineae, 02R9
  Choroid
    Left, 08RB
    Right, 08RA
  Clavicle
    Left, 0PRB
    Right, 0PR9
  Coccyx, 0QRS
  Conjunctiva
    Left, 08RTX
    Right, 08RSX
  Cornea
    Left, 08R9

Replacement — *continued*
  Cornea — *continued*
    Right, 08R8
  Diaphragm, 0BRT
  Disc
    Cervical Vertebral, 0RR30
    Cervicothoracic Vertebral, 0RR50
    Lumbar Vertebral, 0SR20
    Lumbosacral, 0SR40
    Thoracic Vertebral, 0RR90
    Thoracolumbar Vertebral, 0RRB0
  Duct
    Common Bile, 0FR9
    Cystic, 0FR8
    Hepatic
      Common, 0FR7
      Left, 0FR6
      Right, 0FR5
    Lacrimal
      Left, 08RY
      Right, 08RX
    Pancreatic, 0FRD
      Accessory, 0FRF
    Parotid
      Left, 0CRC
      Right, 0CRB
  Dura Mater, 00R2
  Ear
    External
      Bilateral, 09R2
      Left, 09R1
      Right, 09R0
    Inner
      Left, 09RE0
      Right, 09RD0
    Middle
      Left, 09R60
      Right, 09R50
  Epiglottis, 0CRR
  Esophagus, 0DR5
  Eye
    Left, 08R1
    Right, 08R0
  Eyelid
    Lower
      Left, 08RR
      Right, 08RQ
    Upper
      Left, 08RP
      Right, 08RN
  Femoral Shaft
    Left, 0QR9
    Right, 0QR8
  Femur
    Lower
      Left, 0QRC
      Right, 0QRB
    Upper
      Left, 0QR7
      Right, 0QR6
  Fibula
    Left, 0QRK
    Right, 0QRJ
  Finger Nail, 0HRQX
  Gingiva
    Lower, 0CR6
    Upper, 0CR5
  Glenoid Cavity
    Left, 0PR8
    Right, 0PR7
  Hair, 0HRSX
  Humeral Head
    Left, 0PRD
    Right, 0PRC
  Humeral Shaft
    Left, 0PRG
    Right, 0PRF
  Iris
    Left, 08RD3
    Right, 08RC3
  Joint
    Acromioclavicular
      Left, 0RRH0
      Right, 0RRG0
    Ankle
      Left, 0SRG
      Right, 0SRF
    Carpal
      Left, 0RRR0

Replacement — *continued*
  Joint — *continued*
    Carpal — *continued*
      Right, 0RRQ0
    Carpometacarpal
      Left, 0RRT0
      Right, 0RRS0
    Cervical Vertebral, 0RR10
    Cervicothoracic Vertebral, 0RR40
    Coccygeal, 0SR60
    Elbow
      Left, 0RRM0
      Right, 0RRL0
    Finger Phalangeal
      Left, 0RRX0
      Right, 0RRW0
    Hip
      Left, 0SRB
        Acetabular Surface, 0SRE
        Femoral Surface, 0SRS
      Right, 0SR9
        Acetabular Surface, 0SRA
        Femoral Surface, 0SRR
    Knee
      Left, 0SRD
        Femoral Surface, 0SRU
        Tibial Surface, 0SRW
      Right, 0SRC
        Femoral Surface, 0SRT
        Tibial Surface, 0SRV
    Lumbar Vertebral, 0SR00
    Lumbosacral, 0SR30
    Metacarpophalangeal
      Left, 0RRV0
      Right, 0RRU0
    Metatarsal-Phalangeal
      Left, 0SRN0
      Right, 0SRM0
    Occipital-cervical, 0RR00
    Sacrococcygeal, 0SR50
    Sacroiliac
      Left, 0SR80
      Right, 0SR70
    Shoulder
      Left, 0RRK
      Right, 0RRJ
    Sternoclavicular
      Left, 0RRF0
      Right, 0RRE0
    Tarsal
      Left, 0SRJ0
      Right, 0SRH0
    Tarsometatarsal
      Left, 0SRL0
      Right, 0SRK0
    Temporomandibular
      Left, 0RRD0
      Right, 0RRC0
    Thoracic Vertebral, 0RR60
    Thoracolumbar Vertebral, 0RRA0
    Toe Phalangeal
      Left, 0SRQ0
      Right, 0SRP0
    Wrist
      Left, 0RRP0
      Right, 0RRN0
  Kidney Pelvis
    Left, 0TR4
    Right, 0TR3
  Larynx, 0CRS
  Lens
    Left, 08RK30Z
    Right, 08RJ30Z
  Lip
    Lower, 0CR1
    Upper, 0CR0
  Mandible
    Left, 0NRV
    Right, 0NRT
  Maxilla, 0NRR
  Mesentery, 0DRV
  Metacarpal
    Left, 0PRQ
    Right, 0PRP
  Metatarsal
    Left, 0QRP
    Right, 0QRN

▽ **Subterms under main terms may continue to next column or page**

Replacement — *continued*
- Muscle
  - Abdomen
    - Left, ØKRL
    - Right, ØKRK
  - Facial, ØKR1
  - Foot
    - Left, ØKRW
    - Right, ØKRV
  - Hand
    - Left, ØKRD
    - Right, ØKRC
  - Head, ØKRØ
  - Hip
    - Left, ØKRP
    - Right, ØKRN
  - Lower Arm and Wrist
    - Left, ØKRB
    - Right, ØKR9
  - Lower Leg
    - Left, ØKRT
    - Right, ØKRS
  - Neck
    - Left, ØKR3
    - Right, ØKR2
  - Papillary, Ø2RD
  - Perineum, ØKRM
  - Shoulder
    - Left, ØKR6
    - Right, ØKR5
  - Thorax
    - Left, ØKRJ
    - Right, ØKRH
  - Tongue, Palate, Pharynx, ØKR4
  - Trunk
    - Left, ØKRG
    - Right, ØKRF
  - Upper Arm
    - Left, ØKR8
    - Right, ØKR7
  - Upper Leg
    - Left, ØKRR
    - Right, ØKRQ
- Nasal Mucosa and Soft Tissue, Ø9RK
- Nasopharynx, Ø9RN
- Nerve
  - Abducens, ØØRL
  - Accessory, ØØRR
  - Acoustic, ØØRN
  - Cervical, Ø1R1
  - Facial, ØØRM
  - Femoral, Ø1RD
  - Glossopharyngeal, ØØRP
  - Hypoglossal, ØØRS
  - Lumbar, Ø1RB
  - Median, Ø1R5
  - Oculomotor, ØØRH
  - Olfactory, ØØRF
  - Optic, ØØRG
  - Peroneal, Ø1RH
  - Phrenic, Ø1R2
  - Pudendal, Ø1RC
  - Radial, Ø1R6
  - Sacral, Ø1RR
  - Sciatic, Ø1RF
  - Thoracic, Ø1R8
  - Tibial, Ø1RG
  - Trigeminal, ØØRK
  - Trochlear, ØØRJ
  - Ulnar, Ø1R4
  - Vagus, ØØRQ
- Nipple
  - Left, ØHRX
  - Right, ØHRW
- Omentum, ØDRU
- Orbit
  - Left, ØNRQ
  - Right, ØNRP
- Palate
  - Hard, ØCR2
  - Soft, ØCR3
- Patella
  - Left, ØQRF
  - Right, ØQRD
- Pericardium, Ø2RN
- Peritoneum, ØDRW
- Phalanx
  - Finger
    - Left, ØPRV

Replacement — *continued*
- Phalanx — *continued*
  - Finger — *continued*
    - Right, ØPRT
  - Thumb
    - Left, ØPRS
    - Right, ØPRR
  - Toe
    - Left, ØQRR
    - Right, ØQRQ
- Pharynx, ØCRM
- Radius
  - Left, ØPRJ
  - Right, ØPRH
- Retinal Vessel
  - Left, Ø8RH3
  - Right, Ø8RG3
- Ribs
  - 1 to 2, ØPR1
  - 3 or More, ØPR2
- Sacrum, ØQR1
- Scapula
  - Left, ØPR6
  - Right, ØPR5
- Sclera
  - Left, Ø8R7X
  - Right, Ø8R6X
- Septum
  - Atrial, Ø2R5
  - Nasal, Ø9RM
  - Ventricular, Ø2RM
- Skin
  - Abdomen, ØHR7
  - Back, ØHR6
  - Buttock, ØHR8
  - Chest, ØHR5
  - Ear
    - Left, ØHR3
    - Right, ØHR2
  - Face, ØHR1
  - Foot
    - Left, ØHRN
    - Right, ØHRM
  - Hand
    - Left, ØHRG
    - Right, ØHRF
  - Inguinal, ØHRA
  - Lower Arm
    - Left, ØHRE
    - Right, ØHRD
  - Lower Leg
    - Left, ØHRL
    - Right, ØHRK
  - Neck, ØHR4
  - Perineum, ØHR9
  - Scalp, ØHRØ
  - Upper Arm
    - Left, ØHRC
    - Right, ØHRB
  - Upper Leg
    - Left, ØHRJ
    - Right, ØHRH
- Skin Substitute, Porcine Liver Derived, XHRPXL2
- Skull, ØNRØ
- Spinal Meninges, ØØRT
- Sternum, ØPRØ
- Subcutaneous Tissue and Fascia
  - Abdomen, ØJR8
  - Back, ØJR7
  - Buttock, ØJR9
  - Chest, ØJR6
  - Face, ØJR1
  - Foot
    - Left, ØJRR
    - Right, ØJRQ
  - Hand
    - Left, ØJRK
    - Right, ØJRJ
  - Lower Arm
    - Left, ØJRH
    - Right, ØJRG
  - Lower Leg
    - Left, ØJRP
    - Right, ØJRN
  - Neck
    - Left, ØJR5
    - Right, ØJR4
  - Pelvic Region, ØJRC
  - Perineum, ØJRB

Replacement — *continued*
- Subcutaneous Tissue and Fascia — *continued*
  - Scalp, ØJRØ
  - Upper Arm
    - Left, ØJRF
    - Right, ØJRD
  - Upper Leg
    - Left, ØJRM
    - Right, ØJRL
- Tarsal
  - Left, ØQRM
  - Right, ØQRL
- Tendon
  - Abdomen
    - Left, ØLRG
    - Right, ØLRF
  - Ankle
    - Left, ØLRT
    - Right, ØLRS
  - Foot
    - Left, ØLRW
    - Right, ØLRV
  - Hand
    - Left, ØLR8
    - Right, ØLR7
  - Head and Neck, ØLRØ
  - Hip
    - Left, ØLRK
    - Right, ØLRJ
  - Knee
    - Left, ØLRR
    - Right, ØLRQ
  - Lower Arm and Wrist
    - Left, ØLR6
    - Right, ØLR5
  - Lower Leg
    - Left, ØLRP
    - Right, ØLRN
  - Perineum, ØLRH
  - Shoulder
    - Left, ØLR2
    - Right, ØLR1
  - Thorax
    - Left, ØLRD
    - Right, ØLRC
  - Trunk
    - Left, ØLRB
    - Right, ØLR9
  - Upper Arm
    - Left, ØLR4
    - Right, ØLR3
  - Upper Leg
    - Left, ØLRM
    - Right, ØLRL
- Testis
  - Bilateral, ØVRCØJZ
  - Left, ØVRBØJZ
  - Right, ØVR9ØJZ
- Thumb
  - Left, ØXRM
  - Right, ØXRL
- Tibia
  - Left, ØQRH
  - Right, ØQRG
- Toe Nail, ØHRRX
- Tongue, ØCR7
- Tooth
  - Lower, ØCRX
  - Upper, ØCRW
- Trachea, ØBR1
- Turbinate, Nasal, Ø9RL
- Tympanic Membrane
  - Left, Ø9R8
  - Right, Ø9R7
- Ulna
  - Left, ØPRL
  - Right, ØPRK
- Ureter
  - Left, ØTR7
  - Right, ØTR6
- Urethra, ØTRD
- Uvula, ØCRN
- Valve
  - Aortic, Ø2RF
  - Mitral, Ø2RG
  - Pulmonary, Ø2RH
  - Tricuspid, Ø2RJ

Replacement — continued

Vein
- Axillary
  - Left, Ø5R8
  - Right, Ø5R7
- Azygos, Ø5RØ
- Basilic
  - Left, Ø5RC
  - Right, Ø5RB
- Brachial
  - Left, Ø5RA
  - Right, Ø5R9
- Cephalic
  - Left, Ø5RF
  - Right, Ø5RD
- Colic, Ø6R7
- Common Iliac
  - Left, Ø6RD
  - Right, Ø6RC
- Esophageal, Ø6R3
- External Iliac
  - Left, Ø6RG
  - Right, Ø6RF
- External Jugular
  - Left, Ø5RQ
  - Right, Ø5RP
- Face
  - Left, Ø5RV
  - Right, Ø5RT
- Femoral
  - Left, Ø6RN
  - Right, Ø6RM
- Foot
  - Left, Ø6RV
  - Right, Ø6RT
- Gastric, Ø6R2
- Hand
  - Left, Ø5RH
  - Right, Ø5RG
- Hemiazygos, Ø5R1
- Hepatic, Ø6R4
- Hypogastric
  - Left, Ø6RJ
  - Right, Ø6RH
- Inferior Mesenteric, Ø6R6
- Innominate
  - Left, Ø5R4
  - Right, Ø5R3
- Internal Jugular
  - Left, Ø5RN
  - Right, Ø5RM
- Intracranial, Ø5RL
- Lower, Ø6RY
- Portal, Ø6R8
- Pulmonary
  - Left, Ø2RT
  - Right, Ø2RS
- Renal
  - Left, Ø6RB
  - Right, Ø6R9
- Saphenous
  - Left, Ø6RQ
  - Right, Ø6RP
- Splenic, Ø6R1
- Subclavian
  - Left, Ø5R6
  - Right, Ø5R5
- Superior Mesenteric, Ø6R5
- Upper, Ø5RY
- Vertebral
  - Left, Ø5RS
  - Right, Ø5RR

Vena Cava
- Inferior, Ø6RØ
- Superior, Ø2RV

Ventricle
- Left, Ø2RL
- Right, Ø2RK

Vertebra
- Cervical, ØPR3
- Lumbar, ØQRØ
- Thoracic, ØPR4

Vitreous
- Left, Ø8R53
- Right, Ø8R43

Vocal Cord
- Left, ØCRV
- Right, ØCRT

Zooplastic Tissue, Rapid Deployment Technique, X2RF

Replacement, hip
Partial or total *see* Replacement, Lower Joints, ØSR
Resurfacing only *see* Supplement, Lower Joints, ØSU

Replantation *see* Reposition
Replantation, scalp *see* Reattachment, Skin, Scalp, ØHMØ

Reposition
- Acetabulum
  - Left, ØQS5
  - Right, ØQS4
- Ampulla of Vater, ØFSC
- Anus, ØDSQ
- Aorta
  - Abdominal, Ø4SØ
  - Thoracic
    - Ascending/Arch, Ø2SXØZZ
    - Descending, Ø2SWØZZ
- Artery
  - Anterior Tibial
    - Left, Ø4SQ
    - Right, Ø4SP
  - Axillary
    - Left, Ø3S6
    - Right, Ø3S5
  - Brachial
    - Left, Ø3S8
    - Right, Ø3S7
  - Celiac, Ø4S1
  - Colic
    - Left, Ø4S7
    - Middle, Ø4S8
    - Right, Ø4S6
  - Common Carotid
    - Left, Ø3SJ
    - Right, Ø3SH
  - Common Iliac
    - Left, Ø4SD
    - Right, Ø4SC
  - Coronary
    - One Artery, Ø2SØØZZ
    - Two Arteries, Ø2S1ØZZ
  - External Carotid
    - Left, Ø3SN
    - Right, Ø3SM
  - External Iliac
    - Left, Ø4SJ
    - Right, Ø4SH
  - Face, Ø3SR
  - Femoral
    - Left, Ø4SL
    - Right, Ø4SK
  - Foot
    - Left, Ø4SW
    - Right, Ø4SV
  - Gastric, Ø4S2
  - Hand
    - Left, Ø3SF
    - Right, Ø3SD
  - Hepatic, Ø4S3
  - Inferior Mesenteric, Ø4SB
  - Innominate, Ø3S2
  - Internal Carotid
    - Left, Ø3SL
    - Right, Ø3SK
  - Internal Iliac
    - Left, Ø4SF
    - Right, Ø4SE
  - Internal Mammary
    - Left, Ø3S1
    - Right, Ø3SØ
  - Intracranial, Ø3SG
  - Lower, Ø4SY
  - Peroneal
    - Left, Ø4SU
    - Right, Ø4ST
  - Popliteal
    - Left, Ø4SN
    - Right, Ø4SM
  - Posterior Tibial
    - Left, Ø4SS
    - Right, Ø4SR
  - Pulmonary
    - Left, Ø2SRØZZ
    - Right, Ø2SQØZZ
  - Pulmonary Trunk, Ø2SPØZZ
  - Radial
    - Left, Ø3SC
    - Right, Ø3SB
  - Renal
    - Left, Ø4SA

Reposition — continued
- Artery — continued
  - Renal — continued
    - Right, Ø4S9
  - Splenic, Ø4S4
  - Subclavian
    - Left, Ø3S4
    - Right, Ø3S3
  - Superior Mesenteric, Ø4S5
  - Temporal
    - Left, Ø3ST
    - Right, Ø3SS
  - Thyroid
    - Left, Ø3SV
    - Right, Ø3SU
  - Ulnar
    - Left, Ø3SA
    - Right, Ø3S9
  - Upper, Ø3SY
  - Vertebral
    - Left, Ø3SQ
    - Right, Ø3SP
- Auditory Ossicle
  - Left, Ø9SA
  - Right, Ø9S9
- Bladder, ØTSB
- Bladder Neck, ØTSC
- Bone
  - Ethmoid
    - Left, ØNSG
    - Right, ØNSF
  - Frontal, ØNS1
  - Hyoid, ØNSX
  - Lacrimal
    - Left, ØNSJ
    - Right, ØNSH
  - Nasal, ØNSB
  - Occipital, ØNS7
  - Palatine
    - Left, ØNSL
    - Right, ØNSK
  - Parietal
    - Left, ØNS4
    - Right, ØNS3
  - Pelvic
    - Left, ØQS3
    - Right, ØQS2
  - Sphenoid, ØNSC
  - Temporal
    - Left, ØNS6
    - Right, ØNS5
  - Zygomatic
    - Left, ØNSN
    - Right, ØNSM
- Breast
  - Bilateral, ØHSVØZZ
  - Left, ØHSUØZZ
  - Right, ØHSTØZZ
- Bronchus
  - Lingula, ØBS9ØZZ
  - Lower Lobe
    - Left, ØBSBØZZ
    - Right, ØBS6ØZZ
  - Main
    - Left, ØBS7ØZZ
    - Right, ØBS3ØZZ
  - Middle Lobe, Right, ØBS5ØZZ
  - Upper Lobe
    - Left, ØBS8ØZZ
    - Right, ØBS4ØZZ
- Bursa and Ligament
  - Abdomen
    - Left, ØMSJ
    - Right, ØMSH
  - Ankle
    - Left, ØMSR
    - Right, ØMSQ
  - Elbow
    - Left, ØMS4
    - Right, ØMS3
  - Foot
    - Left, ØMST
    - Right, ØMSS
  - Hand
    - Left, ØMS8
    - Right, ØMS7
  - Head and Neck, ØMSØ
  - Hip
    - Left, ØMSM

Reposition — *continued*
  Bursa and Ligament — *continued*
    Hip — *continued*
      Right, ØMSL
    Knee
      Left, ØMSP
      Right, ØMSN
    Lower Extremity
      Left, ØMSW
      Right, ØMSV
    Perineum, ØMSK
    Rib(s), ØMSG
    Shoulder
      Left, ØMS2
      Right, ØMS1
    Spine
      Lower, ØMSD
      Upper, ØMSC
    Sternum, ØMSF
    Upper Extremity
      Left, ØMSB
      Right, ØMS9
    Wrist
      Left, ØMS6
      Right, ØMS5
  Carina, ØBS2ØZZ
  Carpal
    Left, ØPSN
    Right, ØPSM
  Cecum, ØDSH
  Cervix, ØUSC
  Clavicle
    Left, ØPSB
    Right, ØPS9
  Coccyx, ØQSS
  Colon
    Ascending, ØDSK
    Descending, ØDSM
    Sigmoid, ØDSN
    Transverse, ØDSL
  Cord
    Bilateral, ØVSH
    Left, ØVSG
    Right, ØVSF
  Cul-de-sac, ØUSF
  Diaphragm, ØBSTØZZ
  Duct
    Common Bile, ØFS9
    Cystic, ØFS8
    Hepatic
      Common, ØFS7
      Left, ØFS6
      Right, ØFS5
    Lacrimal
      Left, Ø8SY
      Right, Ø8SX
    Pancreatic, ØFSD
      Accessory, ØFSF
    Parotid
      Left, ØCSC
      Right, ØCSB
  Duodenum, ØDS9
  Ear
    Bilateral, Ø9S2
    Left, Ø9S1
    Right, Ø9SØ
  Epiglottis, ØCSR
  Esophagus, ØDS5
  Eustachian Tube
    Left, Ø9SG
    Right, Ø9SF
  Eyelid
    Lower
      Left, Ø8SR
      Right, Ø8SQ
    Upper
      Left, Ø8SP
      Right, Ø8SN
  Fallopian Tube
    Left, ØUS6
    Right, ØUS5
  Fallopian Tubes, Bilateral, ØUS7
  Femoral Shaft
    Left, ØQS9
    Right, ØQS8
  Femur
    Lower
      Left, ØQSC
      Right, ØQSB

Reposition — *continued*
  Femur — *continued*
    Upper
      Left, ØQS7
      Right, ØQS6
  Fibula
    Left, ØQSK
    Right, ØQSJ
  Gallbladder, ØFS4
  Gland
    Adrenal
      Left, ØGS2
      Right, ØGS3
    Lacrimal
      Left, Ø8SW
      Right, Ø8SV
  Glenoid Cavity
    Left, ØPS8
    Right, ØPS7
  Hair, ØHSSXZZ
  Humeral Head
    Left, ØPSD
    Right, ØPSC
  Humeral Shaft
    Left, ØPSG
    Right, ØPSF
  Ileum, ØDSB
  Intestine
    Large, ØDSE
    Small, ØDS8
  Iris
    Left, Ø8SD3ZZ
    Right, Ø8SC3ZZ
  Jejunum, ØDSA
  Joint
    Acromioclavicular
      Left, ØRSH
      Right, ØRSG
    Ankle
      Left, ØSSG
      Right, ØSSF
    Carpal
      Left, ØRSR
      Right, ØRSQ
    Carpometacarpal
      Left, ØRST
      Right, ØRSS
    Cervical Vertebral, ØRS1
    Cervicothoracic Vertebral, ØRS4
    Coccygeal, ØSS6
    Elbow
      Left, ØRSM
      Right, ØRSL
    Finger Phalangeal
      Left, ØRSX
      Right, ØRSW
    Hip
      Left, ØSSB
      Right, ØSS9
    Knee
      Left, ØSSD
      Right, ØSSC
    Lumbar Vertebral, ØSSØ
    Lumbosacral, ØSS3
    Metacarpophalangeal
      Left, ØRSV
      Right, ØRSU
    Metatarsal-Phalangeal
      Left, ØSSN
      Right, ØSSM
    Occipital-cervical, ØRSØ
    Sacrococcygeal, ØSS5
    Sacroiliac
      Left, ØSS8
      Right, ØSS7
    Shoulder
      Left, ØRSK
      Right, ØRSJ
    Sternoclavicular
      Left, ØRSF
      Right, ØRSE
    Tarsal
      Left, ØSSJ
      Right, ØSSH
    Tarsometatarsal
      Left, ØSSL
      Right, ØSSK
    Temporomandibular
      Left, ØRSD

Reposition — *continued*
  Joint — *continued*
    Temporomandibular — *continued*
      Right, ØRSC
    Thoracic Vertebral, ØRS6
    Thoracolumbar Vertebral, ØRSA
    Toe Phalangeal
      Left, ØSSQ
      Right, ØSSP
    Wrist
      Left, ØRSP
      Right, ØRSN
  Kidney
    Left, ØTS1
    Right, ØTSØ
  Kidney Pelvis
    Left, ØTS4
    Right, ØTS3
  Kidneys, Bilateral, ØTS2
  Lens
    Left, Ø8SK3ZZ
    Right, Ø8SJ3ZZ
  Lip
    Lower, ØCS1
    Upper, ØCSØ
  Liver, ØFSØ
  Lung
    Left, ØBSLØZZ
    Lower Lobe
      Left, ØBSJØZZ
      Right, ØBSFØZZ
    Middle Lobe, Right, ØBSDØZZ
    Right, ØBSKØZZ
    Upper Lobe
      Left, ØBSGØZZ
      Right, ØBSCØZZ
  Lung Lingula, ØBSHØZZ
  Mandible
    Left, ØNSV
    Right, ØNST
  Maxilla, ØNSR
  Metacarpal
    Left, ØPSQ
    Right, ØPSP
  Metatarsal
    Left, ØQSP
    Right, ØQSN
  Muscle
    Abdomen
      Left, ØKSL
      Right, ØKSK
    Extraocular
      Left, Ø8SM
      Right, Ø8SL
    Facial, ØKS1
    Foot
      Left, ØKSW
      Right, ØKSV
    Hand
      Left, ØKSD
      Right, ØKSC
    Head, ØKSØ
    Hip
      Left, ØKSP
      Right, ØKSN
    Lower Arm and Wrist
      Left, ØKSB
      Right, ØKS9
    Lower Leg
      Left, ØKST
      Right, ØKSS
    Neck
      Left, ØKS3
      Right, ØKS2
    Perineum, ØKSM
    Shoulder
      Left, ØKS6
      Right, ØKS5
    Thorax
      Left, ØKSJ
      Right, ØKSH
    Tongue, Palate, Pharynx, ØKS4
    Trunk
      Left, ØKSG
      Right, ØKSF
    Upper Arm
      Left, ØKS8
      Right, ØKS7

Reposition

Reposition — *continued*
- Muscle — *continued*
  - Upper Leg
    - Left, ØKSR
    - Right, ØKSQ
- Nasal Mucosa and Soft Tissue, Ø9SK
- Nerve
  - Abducens, ØØSL
  - Accessory, ØØSR
  - Acoustic, ØØSN
  - Brachial Plexus, Ø1S3
  - Cervical, Ø1S1
  - Cervical Plexus, Ø1SØ
  - Facial, ØØSM
  - Femoral, Ø1SD
  - Glossopharyngeal, ØØSP
  - Hypoglossal, ØØSS
  - Lumbar, Ø1SB
  - Lumbar Plexus, Ø1S9
  - Lumbosacral Plexus, Ø1SA
  - Median, Ø1S5
  - Oculomotor, ØØSH
  - Olfactory, ØØSF
  - Optic, ØØSG
  - Peroneal, Ø1SH
  - Phrenic, Ø1S2
  - Pudendal, Ø1SC
  - Radial, Ø1S6
  - Sacral, Ø1SR
  - Sacral Plexus, Ø1SQ
  - Sciatic, Ø1SF
  - Thoracic, Ø1S8
  - Tibial, Ø1SG
  - Trigeminal, ØØSK
  - Trochlear, ØØSJ
  - Ulnar, Ø1S4
  - Vagus, ØØSQ
- Nipple
  - Left, ØHSXXZZ
  - Right, ØHSWXZZ
- Orbit
  - Left, ØNSQ
  - Right, ØNSP
- Ovary
  - Bilateral, ØUS2
  - Left, ØUS1
  - Right, ØUSØ
- Palate
  - Hard, ØCS2
  - Soft, ØCS3
- Pancreas, ØFSG
- Parathyroid Gland, ØGSR
  - Inferior
    - Left, ØGSP
    - Right, ØGSN
  - Multiple, ØGSQ
  - Superior
    - Left, ØGSM
    - Right, ØGSL
- Patella
  - Left, ØQSF
  - Right, ØQSD
- Phalanx
  - Finger
    - Left, ØPSV
    - Right, ØPST
  - Thumb
    - Left, ØPSS
    - Right, ØPSR
  - Toe
    - Left, ØQSR
    - Right, ØQSQ
- Products of Conception, 1ØSØ
  - Ectopic, 1ØS2
- Radius
  - Left, ØPSJ
  - Right, ØPSH
- Rectum, ØDSP
- Retinal Vessel
  - Left, Ø8SH3ZZ
  - Right, Ø8SG3ZZ
- Ribs
  - 1 to 2, ØPS1
  - 3 or More, ØPS2
- Sacrum, ØQS1
- Scapula
  - Left, ØPS6
  - Right, ØPS5
- Septum, Nasal, Ø9SM

Reposition — *continued*
- Sesamoid Bone(s) 1st Toe
  - *see* Reposition, Metatarsal, Left, ØQSP
  - *see* Reposition, Metatarsal, Right, ØQSN
- Skull, ØNSØ
- Spinal Cord
  - Cervical, ØØSW
  - Lumbar, ØØSY
  - Thoracic, ØØSX
- Spleen, Ø7SPØZZ
- Sternum, ØPSØ
- Stomach, ØDS6
- Tarsal
  - Left, ØQSM
  - Right, ØQSL
- Tendon
  - Abdomen
    - Left, ØLSG
    - Right, ØLSF
  - Ankle
    - Left, ØLST
    - Right, ØLSS
  - Foot
    - Left, ØLSW
    - Right, ØLSV
  - Hand
    - Left, ØLS8
    - Right, ØLS7
  - Head and Neck, ØLSØ
  - Hip
    - Left, ØLSK
    - Right, ØLSJ
  - Knee
    - Left, ØLSR
    - Right, ØLSQ
  - Lower Arm and Wrist
    - Left, ØLS6
    - Right, ØLS5
  - Lower Leg
    - Left, ØLSP
    - Right, ØLSN
  - Perineum, ØLSH
  - Shoulder
    - Left, ØLS2
    - Right, ØLS1
  - Thorax
    - Left, ØLSD
    - Right, ØLSC
  - Trunk
    - Left, ØLSB
    - Right, ØLS9
  - Upper Arm
    - Left, ØLS4
    - Right, ØLS3
  - Upper Leg
    - Left, ØLSM
    - Right, ØLSL
- Testis
  - Bilateral, ØVSC
  - Left, ØVSB
  - Right, ØVS9
- Thymus, Ø7SMØZZ
- Thyroid Gland
  - Left Lobe, ØGSG
  - Right Lobe, ØGSH
- Tibia
  - Left, ØQSH
  - Right, ØQSG
- Tongue, ØCS7
- Tooth
  - Lower, ØCSX
  - Upper, ØCSW
- Trachea, ØBS1ØZZ
- Turbinate, Nasal, Ø9SL
- Tympanic Membrane
  - Left, Ø9S8
  - Right, Ø9S7
- Ulna
  - Left, ØPSL
  - Right, ØPSK
- Ureter
  - Left, ØTS7
  - Right, ØTS6
- Ureters, Bilateral, ØTS8
- Urethra, ØTSD
- Uterine Supporting Structure, ØUS4
- Uterus, ØUS9
- Uvula, ØCSN
- Vagina, ØUSG

Reposition — *continued*
- Vein
  - Axillary
    - Left, Ø5S8
    - Right, Ø5S7
  - Azygos, Ø5SØ
  - Basilic
    - Left, Ø5SC
    - Right, Ø5SB
  - Brachial
    - Left, Ø5SA
    - Right, Ø5S9
  - Cephalic
    - Left, Ø5SF
    - Right, Ø5SD
  - Colic, Ø6S7
  - Common Iliac
    - Left, Ø6SD
    - Right, Ø6SC
  - Esophageal, Ø6S3
  - External Iliac
    - Left, Ø6SG
    - Right, Ø6SF
  - External Jugular
    - Left, Ø5SQ
    - Right, Ø5SP
  - Face
    - Left, Ø5SV
    - Right, Ø5ST
  - Femoral
    - Left, Ø6SN
    - Right, Ø6SM
  - Foot
    - Left, Ø6SV
    - Right, Ø6ST
  - Gastric, Ø6S2
  - Hand
    - Left, Ø5SH
    - Right, Ø5SG
  - Hemiazygos, Ø5S1
  - Hepatic, Ø6S4
  - Hypogastric
    - Left, Ø6SJ
    - Right, Ø6SH
  - Inferior Mesenteric, Ø6S6
  - Innominate
    - Left, Ø5S4
    - Right, Ø5S3
  - Internal Jugular
    - Left, Ø5SN
    - Right, Ø5SM
  - Intracranial, Ø5SL
  - Lower, Ø6SY
  - Portal, Ø6S8
  - Pulmonary
    - Left, Ø2STØZZ
    - Right, Ø2SSØZZ
  - Renal
    - Left, Ø6SB
    - Right, Ø6S9
  - Saphenous
    - Left, Ø6SQ
    - Right, Ø6SP
  - Splenic, Ø6S1
  - Subclavian
    - Left, Ø5S6
    - Right, Ø5S5
  - Superior Mesenteric, Ø6S5
  - Upper, Ø5SY
  - Vertebral
    - Left, Ø5SS
    - Right, Ø5SR
- Vena Cava
  - Inferior, Ø6SØ
  - Superior, Ø2SVØZZ
- Vertebra
  - Cervical, ØPS3
    - Magnetically Controlled Growth Rod(s), XNS3
  - Lumbar, ØQSØ
    - Magnetically Controlled Growth Rod(s), XNSØ
  - Thoracic, ØPS4
    - Magnetically Controlled Growth Rod(s), XNS4
- Vocal Cord
  - Left, ØCSV
  - Right, ØCST

▼ **Subterms under main terms may continue to next column or page**

Resection

Acetabulum
  Left, ØQT5ØZZ
  Right, ØQT4ØZZ
Adenoids, ØCTQ
Ampulla of Vater, ØFTC
Anal Sphincter, ØDTR
Anus, ØDTQ
Aortic Body, ØGTD
Appendix, ØDTJ
Auditory Ossicle
  Left, Ø9TA
  Right, Ø9T9
Bladder, ØTTB
Bladder Neck, ØTTC
Bone
  Ethmoid
    Left, ØNTGØZZ
    Right, ØNTFØZZ
  Frontal, ØNT1ØZZ
  Hyoid, ØNTXØZZ
  Lacrimal
    Left, ØNTJØZZ
    Right, ØNTHØZZ
  Nasal, ØNTBØZZ
  Occipital, ØNT7ØZZ
  Palatine
    Left, ØNTLØZZ
    Right, ØNTKØZZ
  Parietal
    Left, ØNT4ØZZ
    Right, ØNT3ØZZ
  Pelvic
    Left, ØQT3ØZZ
    Right, ØQT2ØZZ
  Sphenoid, ØNTCØZZ
  Temporal
    Left, ØNT6ØZZ
    Right, ØNT5ØZZ
  Zygomatic
    Left, ØNTNØZZ
    Right, ØNTMØZZ
Breast
  Bilateral, ØHTVØZZ
  Left, ØHTUØZZ
  Right, ØHTTØZZ
  Supernumerary, ØHTYØZZ
Bronchus
  Lingula, ØBT9
  Lower Lobe
    Left, ØBTB
    Right, ØBT6
  Main
    Left, ØBT7
    Right, ØBT3
  Middle Lobe, Right, ØBT5
  Upper Lobe
    Left, ØBT8
    Right, ØBT4
Bursa and Ligament
  Abdomen
    Left, ØMTJ
    Right, ØMTH
  Ankle
    Left, ØMTR
    Right, ØMTQ
  Elbow
    Left, ØMT4
    Right, ØMT3
  Foot
    Left, ØMTT
    Right, ØMTS
  Hand
    Left, ØMT8
    Right, ØMT7
  Head and Neck, ØMTØ
  Hip
    Left, ØMTM
    Right, ØMTL
  Knee
    Left, ØMTP
    Right, ØMTN
  Lower Extremity
    Left, ØMTW
    Right, ØMTV
  Perineum, ØMTK
  Rib(s), ØMTG
  Shoulder
    Left, ØMT2

Resection — continued
Bursa and Ligament — continued
  Shoulder — continued
    Right, ØMT1
  Spine
    Lower, ØMTD
    Upper, ØMTC
  Sternum, ØMTF
  Upper Extremity
    Left, ØMTB
    Right, ØMT9
  Wrist
    Left, ØMT6
    Right, ØMT5
Carina, ØBT2
Carotid Bodies, Bilateral, ØGT8
Carotid Body
  Left, ØGT6
  Right, ØGT7
Carpal
  Left, ØPTNØZZ
  Right, ØPTMØZZ
Cecum, ØDTH
Cerebral Hemisphere, ØØT7
Cervix, ØUTC
Chordae Tendineae, Ø2T9
Cisterna Chyli, Ø7TL
Clavicle
  Left, ØPTBØZZ
  Right, ØPT9ØZZ
Clitoris, ØUTJ
Coccygeal Glomus, ØGTB
Coccyx, ØQTSØZZ
Colon
  Ascending, ØDTK
  Descending, ØDTM
  Sigmoid, ØDTN
  Transverse, ØDTL
Conduction Mechanism, Ø2T8
Cord
  Bilateral, ØVTH
  Left, ØVTG
  Right, ØVTF
Cornea
  Left, Ø8T9XZZ
  Right, Ø8T8XZZ
Cul-de-sac, ØUTF
Diaphragm, ØBTT
Disc
  Cervical Vertebral, ØRT3ØZZ
  Cervicothoracic Vertebral, ØRT5ØZZ
  Lumbar Vertebral, ØST2ØZZ
  Lumbosacral, ØST4ØZZ
  Thoracic Vertebral, ØRT9ØZZ
  Thoracolumbar Vertebral, ØRTBØZZ
Duct
  Common Bile, ØFT9
  Cystic, ØFT8
  Hepatic
    Common, ØFT7
    Left, ØFT6
    Right, ØFT5
  Lacrimal
    Left, Ø8TY
    Right, Ø8TX
  Pancreatic, ØFTD
    Accessory, ØFTF
  Parotid
    Left, ØCTCØZZ
    Right, ØCTBØZZ
Duodenum, ØDT9
Ear
  External
    Left, Ø9T1
    Right, Ø9TØ
  Inner
    Left, Ø9TE
    Right, Ø9TD
  Middle
    Left, Ø9T6
    Right, Ø9T5
Epididymis
  Bilateral, ØVTL
  Left, ØVTK
  Right, ØVTJ
Epiglottis, ØCTR
Esophagogastric Junction, ØDT4
Esophagus, ØDT5
  Lower, ØDT3

Resection — continued
Esophagus — continued
  Middle, ØDT2
  Upper, ØDT1
Eustachian Tube
  Left, Ø9TG
  Right, Ø9TF
Eye
  Left, Ø8T1XZZ
  Right, Ø8TØXZZ
Eyelid
  Lower
    Left, Ø8TR
    Right, Ø8TQ
  Upper
    Left, Ø8TP
    Right, Ø8TN
Fallopian Tube
  Left, ØUT6
  Right, ØUT5
Fallopian Tubes, Bilateral, ØUT7
Femoral Shaft
  Left, ØQT9ØZZ
  Right, ØQT8ØZZ
Femur
  Lower
    Left, ØQTCØZZ
    Right, ØQTBØZZ
  Upper
    Left, ØQT7ØZZ
    Right, ØQT6ØZZ
Fibula
  Left, ØQTKØZZ
  Right, ØQTJØZZ
Finger Nail, ØHTQXZZ
Gallbladder, ØFT4
Gland
  Adrenal
    Bilateral, ØGT4
    Left, ØGT2
    Right, ØGT3
  Lacrimal
    Left, Ø8TW
    Right, Ø8TV
  Minor Salivary, ØCTJØZZ
  Parotid
    Left, ØCT9ØZZ
    Right, ØCT8ØZZ
  Pituitary, ØGTØ
  Sublingual
    Left, ØCTFØZZ
    Right, ØCTDØZZ
  Submaxillary
    Left, ØCTHØZZ
    Right, ØCTGØZZ
  Vestibular, ØUTL
Glenoid Cavity
  Left, ØPT8ØZZ
  Right, ØPT7ØZZ
Glomus Jugulare, ØGTC
Humeral Head
  Left, ØPTDØZZ
  Right, ØPTCØZZ
Humeral Shaft
  Left, ØPTGØZZ
  Right, ØPTFØZZ
Hymen, ØUTK
Ileocecal Valve, ØDTC
Ileum, ØDTB
Intestine
  Large, ØDTE
    Left, ØDTG
    Right, ØDTF
  Small, ØDT8
Iris
  Left, Ø8TD3ZZ
  Right, Ø8TC3ZZ
Jejunum, ØDTA
Joint
  Acromioclavicular
    Left, ØRTHØZZ
    Right, ØRTGØZZ
  Ankle
    Left, ØSTGØZZ
    Right, ØSTFØZZ
  Carpal
    Left, ØRTRØZZ
    Right, ØRTQØZZ

Resection — *continued*
Joint — *continued*
Carpometacarpal
  Left, ØRTTØZZ
  Right, ØRTSØZZ
Cervicothoracic Vertebral, ØRT4ØZZ
Coccygeal, ØST6ØZZ
Elbow
  Left, ØRTMØZZ
  Right, ØRTLØZZ
Finger Phalangeal
  Left, ØRTXØZZ
  Right, ØRTWØZZ
Hip
  Left, ØSTBØZZ
  Right, ØST9ØZZ
Knee
  Left, ØSTDØZZ
  Right, ØSTCØZZ
Metacarpophalangeal
  Left, ØRTVØZZ
  Right, ØRTUØZZ
Metatarsal-Phalangeal
  Left, ØSTNØZZ
  Right, ØSTMØZZ
Sacrococcygeal, ØST5ØZZ
Sacroiliac
  Left, ØST8ØZZ
  Right, ØST7ØZZ
Shoulder
  Left, ØRTKØZZ
  Right, ØRTJØZZ
Sternoclavicular
  Left, ØRTFØZZ
  Right, ØRTEØZZ
Tarsal
  Left, ØSTJØZZ
  Right, ØSTHØZZ
Tarsometatarsal
  Left, ØSTLØZZ
  Right, ØSTKØZZ
Temporomandibular
  Left, ØRTDØZZ
  Right, ØRTCØZZ
Toe Phalangeal
  Left, ØSTQØZZ
  Right, ØSTPØZZ
Wrist
  Left, ØRTPØZZ
  Right, ØRTNØZZ
Kidney
  Left, ØTT1
  Right, ØTTØ
Kidney Pelvis
  Left, ØTT4
  Right, ØTT3
Kidneys, Bilateral, ØTT2
Larynx, ØCTS
Lens
  Left, Ø8TK3ZZ
  Right, Ø8TJ3ZZ
Lip
  Lower, ØCT1
  Upper, ØCTØ
Liver, ØFTØ
  Left Lobe, ØFT2
  Right Lobe, ØFT1
Lung
  Bilateral, ØBTM
  Left, ØBTL
  Lower Lobe
    Left, ØBTJ
    Right, ØBTF
  Middle Lobe, Right, ØBTD
  Right, ØBTK
  Upper Lobe
    Left, ØBTG
    Right, ØBTC
Lung Lingula, ØBTH
Lymphatic
  Aortic, Ø7TD
  Axillary
    Left, Ø7T6
    Right, Ø7T5
  Head, Ø7TØ
  Inguinal
    Left, Ø7TJ
    Right, Ø7TH

Lymphatic — *continued*
  Internal Mammary
    Left, Ø7T9
    Right, Ø7T8
  Lower Extremity
    Left, Ø7TG
    Right, Ø7TF
  Mesenteric, Ø7TB
  Neck
    Left, Ø7T2
    Right, Ø7T1
  Pelvis, Ø7TC
  Thoracic Duct, Ø7TK
  Thorax, Ø7T7
  Upper Extremity
    Left, Ø7T4
    Right, Ø7T3
Mandible
  Left, ØNTVØZZ
  Right, ØNTTØZZ
Maxilla, ØNTRØZZ
Metacarpal
  Left, ØPTQØZZ
  Right, ØPTPØZZ
Metatarsal
  Left, ØQTPØZZ
  Right, ØQTNØZZ
Muscle
  Abdomen
    Left, ØKTL
    Right, ØKTK
  Extraocular
    Left, Ø8TM
    Right, Ø8TL
  Facial, ØKT1
  Foot
    Left, ØKTW
    Right, ØKTV
  Hand
    Left, ØKTD
    Right, ØKTC
  Head, ØKTØ
  Hip
    Left, ØKTP
    Right, ØKTN
  Lower Arm and Wrist
    Left, ØKTB
    Right, ØKT9
  Lower Leg
    Left, ØKTT
    Right, ØKTS
  Neck
    Left, ØKT3
    Right, ØKT2
  Papillary, Ø2TD
  Perineum, ØKTM
  Shoulder
    Left, ØKT6
    Right, ØKT5
  Thorax
    Left, ØKTJ
    Right, ØKTH
  Tongue, Palate, Pharynx, ØKT4
  Trunk
    Left, ØKTG
    Right, ØKTF
  Upper Arm
    Left, ØKT8
    Right, ØKT7
  Upper Leg
    Left, ØKTR
    Right, ØKTQ
Nasal Mucosa and Soft Tissue, Ø9TK
Nasopharynx, Ø9TN
Nipple
  Left, ØHTXXZZ
  Right, ØHTWXZZ
Omentum, ØDTU
Orbit
  Left, ØNTQØZZ
  Right, ØNTPØZZ
Ovary
  Bilateral, ØUT2
  Left, ØUT1
  Right, ØUTØ
Palate
  Hard, ØCT2
  Soft, ØCT3

Resection — *continued*
Pancreas, ØFTG
Para-aortic Body, ØGT9
Paraganglion Extremity, ØGTF
Parathyroid Gland, ØGTR
  Inferior
    Left, ØGTP
    Right, ØGTN
  Multiple, ØGTQ
  Superior
    Left, ØGTM
    Right, ØGTL
Patella
  Left, ØQTFØZZ
  Right, ØQTDØZZ
Penis, ØVTS
Pericardium, Ø2TN
Phalanx
  Finger
    Left, ØPTVØZZ
    Right, ØPTTØZZ
  Thumb
    Left, ØPTSØZZ
    Right, ØPTRØZZ
  Toe
    Left, ØQTRØZZ
    Right, ØQTQØZZ
Pharynx, ØCTM
Pineal Body, ØGT1
Prepuce, ØVTT
Products of Conception, Ectopic, 1ØT2
Prostate, ØVTØ
Radius
  Left, ØPTJØZZ
  Right, ØPTHØZZ
Rectum, ØDTP
Ribs
  1 to 2, ØPT1ØZZ
  3 or More, ØPT2ØZZ
Scapula
  Left, ØPT6ØZZ
  Right, ØPT5ØZZ
Scrotum, ØVT5
Septum
  Atrial, Ø2T5
  Nasal, Ø9TM
  Ventricular, Ø2TM
Sinus
  Accessory, Ø9TP
  Ethmoid
    Left, Ø9TV
    Right, Ø9TU
  Frontal
    Left, Ø9TT
    Right, Ø9TS
  Mastoid
    Left, Ø9TC
    Right, Ø9TB
  Maxillary
    Left, Ø9TR
    Right, Ø9TQ
  Sphenoid
    Left, Ø9TX
    Right, Ø9TW
Spleen, Ø7TP
Sternum, ØPTØØZZ
Stomach, ØDT6
  Pylorus, ØDT7
Tarsal
  Left, ØQTMØZZ
  Right, ØQTLØZZ
Tendon
  Abdomen
    Left, ØLTG
    Right, ØLTF
  Ankle
    Left, ØLTT
    Right, ØLTS
  Foot
    Left, ØLTW
    Right, ØLTV
  Hand
    Left, ØLT8
    Right, ØLT7
  Head and Neck, ØLTØ
  Hip
    Left, ØLTK
    Right, ØLTJ

Resection — *continued*
Tendon — *continued*
Knee
Left, ØLTR
Right, ØLTQ
Lower Arm and Wrist
Left, ØLT6
Right, ØLT5
Lower Leg
Left, ØLTP
Right, ØLTN
Perineum, ØLTH
Shoulder
Left, ØLT2
Right, ØLT1
Thorax
Left, ØLTD
Right, ØLTC
Trunk
Left, ØLTB
Right, ØLT9
Upper Arm
Left, ØLT4
Right, ØLT3
Upper Leg
Left, ØLTM
Right, ØLTL
Testis
Bilateral, ØVTC
Left, ØVTB
Right, ØVT9
Thymus, Ø7TM
Thyroid Gland, ØGTK
Left Lobe, ØGTG
Right Lobe, ØGTH
Thyroid Gland Isthmus, ØGTJ
Tibia
Left, ØQTHØZZ
Right, ØQTGØZZ
Toe Nail, ØHTRXZZ
Tongue, ØCT7
Tonsils, ØCTP
Tooth
Lower, ØCTXØZ
Upper, ØCTWØZ
Trachea, ØBT1
Tunica Vaginalis
Left, ØVT7
Right, ØVT6
Turbinate, Nasal, Ø9TL
Tympanic Membrane
Left, Ø9T8
Right, Ø9T7
Ulna
Left, ØPTLØZZ
Right, ØPTKØZZ
Ureter
Left, ØTT7
Right, ØTT6
Urethra, ØTTD
Uterine Supporting Structure, ØUT4
Uterus, ØUT9
Uvula, ØCTN
Vagina, ØUTG
Valve, Pulmonary, Ø2TH
Vas Deferens
Bilateral, ØVTQ
Left, ØVTP
Right, ØVTN
Vesicle
Bilateral, ØVT3
Left, ØVT2
Right, ØVT1
Vitreous
Left, Ø8T53ZZ
Right, Ø8T43ZZ
Vocal Cord
Left, ØCTV
Right, ØCTT
Vulva, ØUTM

Resection, Left ventricular outflow tract obstruction (LVOT) *see* Dilation, Ventricle, Left, Ø27L

Resection, Subaortic membrane (Left ventricular outflow tract obstruction) *see* Dilation, Ventricle, Left, Ø27L

Restoration, Cardiac, Single, Rhythm, 5A22Ø4Z

RestoreAdvanced neurostimulator (SureScan) (MRI Safe) *use* Stimulator Generator, Multiple Array Rechargeable in, ØJH

RestoreSensor neurostimulator (SureScan) (MRI Safe) *use* Stimulator Generator, Multiple Array Rechargeable in, ØJH

RestoreUltra neurostimulator (SureScan) (MRI Safe) *use* Simulator Generator, Multiple Array Rechargeable in, ØJH

Restriction
Ampulla of Vater, ØFVC
Anus, ØDVQ
Aorta
Abdominal, Ø4VØ
Intraluminal Device, Branched or Fenestrated, Ø4VØ
Thoracic
Ascending/Arch, Intraluminal Device, Branched or Fenestrated, Ø2VX
Descending, Intraluminal Device, Branched or Fenestrated, Ø2VW
Artery
Anterior Tibial
Left, Ø4VQ
Right, Ø4VP
Axillary
Left, Ø3V6
Right, Ø3V5
Brachial
Left, Ø3V8
Right, Ø3V7
Celiac, Ø4V1
Colic
Left, Ø4V7
Middle, Ø4V8
Right, Ø4V6
Common Carotid
Left, Ø3VJ
Right, Ø3VH
Common Iliac
Left, Ø4VD
Right, Ø4VC
External Carotid
Left, Ø3VN
Right, Ø3VM
External Iliac
Left, Ø4VJ
Right, Ø4VH
Face, Ø3VR
Femoral
Left, Ø4VL
Right, Ø4VK
Foot
Left, Ø4VW
Right, Ø4VV
Gastric, Ø4V2
Hand
Left, Ø3VF
Right, Ø3VD
Hepatic, Ø4V3
Inferior Mesenteric, Ø4VB
Innominate, Ø3V2
Internal Carotid
Left, Ø3VL
Right, Ø3VK
Internal Iliac
Left, Ø4VF
Right, Ø4VE
Internal Mammary
Left, Ø3V1
Right, Ø3VØ
Intracranial, Ø3VG
Lower, Ø4VY
Peroneal
Left, Ø4VU
Right, Ø4VT
Popliteal
Left, Ø4VN
Right, Ø4VM
Posterior Tibial
Left, Ø4VS
Right, Ø4VR
Pulmonary
Left, Ø2VR
Right, Ø2VQ
Pulmonary Trunk, Ø2VP
Radial
Left, Ø3VC
Right, Ø3VB

Restriction — *continued*
Artery — *continued*
Renal
Left, Ø4VA
Right, Ø4V9
Splenic, Ø4V4
Subclavian
Left, Ø3V4
Right, Ø3V3
Superior Mesenteric, Ø4V5
Temporal
Left, Ø3VT
Right, Ø3VS
Thyroid
Left, Ø3VV
Right, Ø3VU
Ulnar
Left, Ø3VA
Right, Ø3V9
Upper, Ø3VY
Vertebral
Left, Ø3VQ
Right, Ø3VP
Bladder, ØTVB
Bladder Neck, ØTVC
Bronchus
Lingula, ØBV9
Lower Lobe
Left, ØBVB
Right, ØBV6
Main
Left, ØBV7
Right, ØBV3
Middle Lobe, Right, ØBV5
Upper Lobe
Left, ØBV8
Right, ØBV4
Carina, ØBV2
Cecum, ØDVH
Cervix, ØUVC
Cisterna Chyli, Ø7VL
Colon
Ascending, ØDVK
Descending, ØDVM
Sigmoid, ØDVN
Transverse, ØDVL
Duct
Common Bile, ØFV9
Cystic, ØFV8
Hepatic
Common, ØFV7
Left, ØFV6
Right, ØFV5
Lacrimal
Left, Ø8VY
Right, Ø8VX
Pancreatic, ØFVD
Accessory, ØFVF
Parotid
Left, ØCVC
Right, ØCVB
Duodenum, ØDV9
Esophagogastric Junction, ØDV4
Esophagus, ØDV5
Lower, ØDV3
Middle, ØDV2
Upper, ØDV1
Heart, Ø2VA
Ileocecal Valve, ØDVC
Ileum, ØDVB
Intestine
Large, ØDVE
Left, ØDVG
Right, ØDVF
Small, ØDV8
Jejunum, ØDVA
Kidney Pelvis
Left, ØTV4
Right, ØTV3
Lymphatic
Aortic, Ø7VD
Axillary
Left, Ø7V6
Right, Ø7V5
Head, Ø7VØ
Inguinal
Left, Ø7VJ
Right, Ø7VH

Restriction — *continued*
  Lymphatic — *continued*
    Internal Mammary
      Left, 07V9
      Right, 07V8
    Lower Extremity
      Left, 07VG
      Right, 07VF
    Mesenteric, 07VB
    Neck
      Left, 07V2
      Right, 07V1
    Pelvis, 07VC
    Thoracic Duct, 07VK
    Thorax, 07V7
    Upper Extremity
      Left, 07V4
      Right, 07V3
  Rectum, 0DVP
  Stomach, 0DV6
    Pylorus, 0DV7
  Trachea, 0BV1
  Ureter
    Left, 0TV7
    Right, 0TV6
  Urethra, 0TVD
  Valve, Mitral, 02VG
  Vein
    Axillary
      Left, 05V8
      Right, 05V7
    Azygos, 05V0
    Basilic
      Left, 05VC
      Right, 05VB
    Brachial
      Left, 05VA
      Right, 05V9
    Cephalic
      Left, 05VF
      Right, 05VD
    Colic, 06V7
    Common Iliac
      Left, 06VD
      Right, 06VC
    Esophageal, 06V3
    External Iliac
      Left, 06VG
      Right, 06VF
    External Jugular
      Left, 05VQ
      Right, 05VP
    Face
      Left, 05VV
      Right, 05VT
    Femoral
      Left, 06VN
      Right, 06VM
    Foot
      Left, 06VV
      Right, 06VT
    Gastric, 06V2
    Hand
      Left, 05VH
      Right, 05VG
    Hemiazygos, 05V1
    Hepatic, 06V4
    Hypogastric
      Left, 06VJ
      Right, 06VH
    Inferior Mesenteric, 06V6
    Innominate
      Left, 05V4
      Right, 05V3
    Internal Jugular
      Left, 05VN
      Right, 05VM
    Intracranial, 05VL
    Lower, 06VY
    Portal, 06V8
    Pulmonary
      Left, 02VT
      Right, 02VS
    Renal
      Left, 06VB
      Right, 06V9
    Saphenous
      Left, 06VQ
      Right, 06VP

Restriction — *continued*
  Vein — *continued*
    Splenic, 06V1
    Subclavian
      Left, 05V6
      Right, 05V5
    Superior Mesenteric, 06V5
    Upper, 05VY
    Vertebral
      Left, 05VS
      Right, 05VR
  Vena Cava
    Inferior, 06V0
    Superior, 02VV
Resurfacing Device
  Removal of device from
    Left, 0SPB0BZ
    Right, 0SP90BZ
  Revision of device in
    Left, 0SWB0BZ
    Right, 0SW90BZ
  Supplement
    Left, 0SUB0BZ
      Acetabular Surface, 0SUE0BZ
      Femoral Surface, 0SUS0BZ
    Right, 0SU90BZ
      Acetabular Surface, 0SUA0BZ
      Femoral Surface, 0SUR0BZ
Resuscitation
  Cardiopulmonary *see* Assistance, Cardiac, 5A02
  Cardioversion, 5A2204Z
  Defibrillation, 5A2204Z
  Endotracheal intubation *see* Insertion of device in, Trachea, 0BH1
  External chest compression, 5A12012
  Pulmonary, 5A19054
Resuscitative endovascular balloon occlusion of the aorta (REBOA)
  02LW3DJ
  04L03DJ
Resuture, Heart valve prosthesis *see* Revision of device in, Heart and Great Vessels, 02W
Retained placenta, manual removal *see* Extraction, Products of Conception, Retained, 10D1
Retraining
  Cardiac *see* Motor Treatment, Rehabilitation, F07
  Vocational *see* Activities of Daily Living Treatment, Rehabilitation, F08
Retrogasserian rhizotomy *see* Division, Nerve, Trigeminal, 008K
Retroperitoneal cavity *use* Retroperitoneum
Retroperitoneal lymph node *use* Lymphatic, Aortic
Retroperitoneal space *use* Retroperitoneum
Retropharyngeal lymph node
  use Lymphatic, Left Neck
  use Lymphatic, Right Neck
Retropubic space *use* Pelvic Cavity
Reveal (DX) (XT) *use* Monitoring Device
Reverse total shoulder replacement *see* Replacement, Upper Joints, 0RR
Reverse® Shoulder Prosthesis *use* Synthetic Substitute, Reverse Ball and Socket in, 0RR
Revision
  Correcting a portion of existing device *see* Revision of device in
  Removal of device without replacement *see* Removal of device from
  Replacement of existing device
    see Removal of device from
    see Root operation to place new device, e.g., Insertion, Replacement, Supplement
Revision of device in
  Abdominal Wall, 0WWF
  Acetabulum
    Left, 0QW5
    Right, 0QW4
  Anal Sphincter, 0DWR
  Anus, 0DWQ
  Artery
    Lower, 04WY
    Upper, 03WY
  Auditory Ossicle
    Left, 09WA
    Right, 09W9
  Back
    Lower, 0WWL
    Upper, 0WWK
  Bladder, 0TWB

Revision of device in — *continued*
  Bone
    Facial, 0NWW
    Lower, 0QWY
    Nasal, 0NWB
    Pelvic
      Left, 0QW3
      Right, 0QW2
    Upper, 0PWY
  Bone Marrow, 07WT
  Brain, 00W0
  Breast
    Left, 0HWU
    Right, 0HWT
  Bursa and Ligament
    Lower, 0MWY
    Upper, 0MWX
  Carpal
    Left, 0PWN
    Right, 0PWM
  Cavity, Cranial, 0WW1
  Cerebral Ventricle, 00W6
  Chest Wall, 0WW8
  Cisterna Chyli, 07WL
  Clavicle
    Left, 0PWB
    Right, 0PW9
  Coccyx, 0QWS
  Diaphragm, 0BWT
  Disc
    Cervical Vertebral, 0RW3
    Cervicothoracic Vertebral, 0RW5
    Lumbar Vertebral, 0SW2
    Lumbosacral, 0SW4
    Thoracic Vertebral, 0RW9
    Thoracolumbar Vertebral, 0RWB
  Duct
    Hepatobiliary, 0FWB
    Pancreatic, 0FWD
  Ear
    Inner
      Left, 09WE
      Right, 09WD
    Left, 09WJ
    Right, 09WH
  Epididymis and Spermatic Cord, 0VWM
  Esophagus, 0DW5
  Extremity
    Lower
      Left, 0YWB
      Right, 0YW9
    Upper
      Left, 0XW7
      Right, 0XW6
  Eye
    Left, 08W1
    Right, 08W0
  Face, 0WW2
  Fallopian Tube, 0UW8
  Femoral Shaft
    Left, 0QW9
    Right, 0QW8
  Femur
    Lower
      Left, 0QWC
      Right, 0QWB
    Upper
      Left, 0QW7
      Right, 0QW6
  Fibula
    Left, 0QWK
    Right, 0QWJ
  Finger Nail, 0HWQX
  Gallbladder, 0FW4
  Gastrointestinal Tract, 0WWP
  Genitourinary Tract, 0WWR
  Gland
    Adrenal, 0GW5
    Endocrine, 0GWS
    Pituitary, 0GW0
    Salivary, 0CWA
  Glenoid Cavity
    Left, 0PW8
    Right, 0PW7
  Great Vessel, 02WY
  Hair, 0HWSX
  Head, 0WW0
  Heart, 02WA

Revision of device in — continued

Humeral Head
  Left, 0PWD
  Right, 0PWC
Humeral Shaft
  Left, 0PWG
  Right, 0PWF
Intestinal Tract
  Lower, 0DWD
  Upper, 0DW0
Intestine
  Large, 0DWE
  Small, 0DW8
Jaw
  Lower, 0WW5
  Upper, 0WW4
Joint
  Acromioclavicular
    Left, 0RWH
    Right, 0RWG
  Ankle
    Left, 0SWG
    Right, 0SWF
  Carpal
    Left, 0RWR
    Right, 0RWQ
  Carpometacarpal
    Left, 0RWT
    Right, 0RWS
  Cervical Vertebral, 0RW1
  Cervicothoracic Vertebral, 0RW4
  Coccygeal, 0SW6
  Elbow
    Left, 0RWM
    Right, 0RWL
  Finger Phalangeal
    Left, 0RWX
    Right, 0RWW
  Hip
    Left, 0SWB
      Acetabular Surface, 0SWE
      Femoral Surface, 0SWS
    Right, 0SW9
      Acetabular Surface, 0SWA
      Femoral Surface, 0SWR
  Knee
    Left, 0SWD
      Femoral Surface, 0SWU
      Tibial Surface, 0SWW
    Right, 0SWC
      Femoral Surface, 0SWT
      Tibial Surface, 0SWV
  Lumbar Vertebral, 0SW0
  Lumbosacral, 0SW3
  Metacarpophalangeal
    Left, 0RWV
    Right, 0RWU
  Metatarsal-Phalangeal
    Left, 0SWN
    Right, 0SWM
  Occipital-cervical, 0RW0
  Sacrococcygeal, 0SW5
  Sacroiliac
    Left, 0SW8
    Right, 0SW7
  Shoulder
    Left, 0RWK
    Right, 0RWJ
  Sternoclavicular
    Left, 0RWF
    Right, 0RWE
  Tarsal
    Left, 0SWJ
    Right, 0SWH
  Tarsometatarsal
    Left, 0SWL
    Right, 0SWK
  Temporomandibular
    Left, 0RWD
    Right, 0RWC
  Thoracic Vertebral, 0RW6
  Thoracolumbar Vertebral, 0RWA
  Toe Phalangeal
    Left, 0SWQ
    Right, 0SWP
  Wrist
    Left, 0RWP
    Right, 0RWN
Kidney, 0TW5

Revision of device in — continued

Larynx, 0CWS
Lens
  Left, 08WK
  Right, 08WJ
Liver, 0FW0
Lung
  Left, 0BWL
  Right, 0BWN
Lymphatic, 07WN
  Thoracic Duct, 07WK
Mediastinum, 0WWC
Mesentery, 0DWV
Metacarpal
  Left, 0PWQ
  Right, 0PWP
Metatarsal
  Left, 0QWP
  Right, 0QWN
Mouth and Throat, 0CWY
Muscle
  Extraocular
    Left, 08WM
    Right, 08WL
  Lower, 0KWY
  Upper, 0KWX
Nasal Mucosa and Soft Tissue, 09WK
Neck, 0WW6
Nerve
  Cranial, 00WE
  Peripheral, 01WY
Omentum, 0DWU
Ovary, 0UW3
Pancreas, 0FWG
Parathyroid Gland, 0GWR
Patella
  Left, 0QWF
  Right, 0QWD
Pelvic Cavity, 0WWJ
Penis, 0VWS
Pericardial Cavity, 0WWD
Perineum
  Female, 0WWN
  Male, 0WWM
Peritoneal Cavity, 0WWG
Peritoneum, 0DWW
Phalanx
  Finger
    Left, 0PWV
    Right, 0PWT
  Thumb
    Left, 0PWS
    Right, 0PWR
  Toe
    Left, 0QWR
    Right, 0QWQ
Pineal Body, 0GW1
Pleura, 0BWQ
Pleural Cavity
  Left, 0WWB
  Right, 0WW9
Prostate and Seminal Vesicles, 0VW4
Radius
  Left, 0PWJ
  Right, 0PWH
Respiratory Tract, 0WWQ
Retroperitoneum, 0WWH
Ribs
  1 to 2, 0PW1
  3 or More, 0PW2
Sacrum, 0QW1
Scapula
  Left, 0PW6
  Right, 0PW5
Scrotum and Tunica Vaginalis, 0VW8
Septum
  Atrial, 02W5
  Ventricular, 02WM
Sinus, 09WY
Skin, 0HWPX
Skull, 0NW0
Spinal Canal, 00WU
Spinal Cord, 00WV
Spleen, 07WP
Sternum, 0PW0
Stomach, 0DW6
Subcutaneous Tissue and Fascia
  Head and Neck, 0JWS
  Lower Extremity, 0JWW

Revision of device in — continued

Subcutaneous Tissue and Fascia — continued
  Trunk, 0JWT
  Upper Extremity, 0JWV
Tarsal
  Left, 0QWM
  Right, 0QWL
Tendon
  Lower, 0LWY
  Upper, 0LWX
Testis, 0VWD
Thymus, 07WM
Thyroid Gland, 0GWK
Tibia
  Left, 0QWH
  Right, 0QWG
Toe Nail, 0HWRX
Trachea, 0BW1
Tracheobronchial Tree, 0BW0
Tympanic Membrane
  Left, 09W8
  Right, 09W7
Ulna
  Left, 0PWL
  Right, 0PWK
Ureter, 0TW9
Urethra, 0TWD
Uterus and Cervix, 0UWD
Vagina and Cul-de-sac, 0UWH
Valve
  Aortic, 02WF
  Mitral, 02WG
  Pulmonary, 02WH
  Tricuspid, 02WJ
Vas Deferens, 0VWR
Vein
  Azygos, 05W0
  Innominate
    Left, 05W4
    Right, 05W3
  Lower, 06WY
  Upper, 05WY
Vertebra
  Cervical, 0PW3
  Lumbar, 0QW0
  Thoracic, 0PW4
Vulva, 0UWM

Revo MRI™ SureScan® pacemaker use Pacemaker, Dual Chamber in, 0JH

rhBMP-2 use Recombinant Bone Morphogenetic Protein

Rheos® System device use Stimulator Generator in Subcutaneous Tissue and Fascia

Rheos® System lead use Stimulator Lead in Upper Arteries

Rhinopharynx use Nasopharynx

Rhinoplasty
  see Alteration, Nasal Mucosa and Soft Tissue, 090K
  see Repair, Nasal Mucosa and Soft Tissue, 090K
  see Replacement, Nasal Mucosa and Soft Tissue, 09RK
  see Supplement, Nasal Mucosa and Soft Tissue, 09UK

Rhinorrhaphy see Repair, Nasal Mucosa and Soft Tissue, 090K

Rhinoscopy, 09JKXZZ

Rhizotomy
  see Division, Central Nervous System and Cranial Nerves, 008
  see Division, Peripheral Nervous System, 018

Rhomboid major muscle
  use Trunk Muscle, Left
  use Trunk Muscle, Right

Rhomboid minor muscle
  use Trunk Muscle, Left
  use Trunk Muscle, Right

Rhythm electrocardiogram see Measurement, Cardiac, 4A02

Rhytidectomy see Alteration, Face, 0W02

Right ascending lumbar vein use Azygos Vein

Right atrioventricular valve use Tricuspid Valve

Right auricular appendix use Atrium, Right

Right colic vein use Colic Vein

Right coronary sulcus use Heart, Right

Right gastric artery use Gastric Artery

Right gastroepiploic vein use Superior Mesenteric Vein

Right inferior phrenic vein use Inferior Vena Cava

Right inferior pulmonary vein use Pulmonary Vein, Right

Right jugular trunk use Lymphatic, Right Neck

Right lateral ventricle use Cerebral Ventricle

Right lymphatic duct use Lymphatic, Right Neck

Right ovarian vein *use* Inferior Vena Cava
Right second lumbar vein *use* Inferior Vena Cava
Right subclavian trunk *use* Lymphatic, Right Neck
Right subcostal vein *use* Azygos Vein
Right superior pulmonary vein *use* Pulmonary Vein, Right
Right suprarenal vein *use* Inferior Vena Cava
Right testicular vein *use* Inferior Vena Cava
Rima glottidis *use* Larynx
Risorius muscle *use* Facial Muscle
RNS System lead *use* Neurostimulator Lead in Central Nervous System and Cranial Nerves
RNS system neurostimulator generator *use* Neurostimulator Generator in Head and Facial Bones
Robotic Assisted Procedure
    Extremity
        Lower, 8E0Y
        Upper, 8E0X
    Head and Neck Region, 8E09
    Trunk Region, 8E0W
Robotic Waterjet Ablation, Destruction, Prostate, XV508A4
Rotation of fetal head
    Forceps, 10S07ZZ
    Manual, 10S0XZZ
Round ligament of uterus *use* Uterine Supporting Structure
Round window
    use Inner Ear, Left
    use Inner Ear, Right
Roux-en-Y operation
    see Bypass, Gastrointestinal System, 0D1
    see Bypass, Hepatobiliary System and Pancreas, 0F1
Rupture
    Adhesions *see* Release
    Fluid collection *see* Drainage

S

Sacral ganglion *use* Sacral Sympathetic Nerve
Sacral lymph node *use* Lymphatic, Pelvis
Sacral nerve modulation (SNM) lead *use* Stimulator Lead in Urinary System
Sacral neuromodulation lead *use* Stimulator Lead in Urinary System
Sacral splanchnic nerve *use* Sacral Sympathetic Nerve
Sacrectomy *see* Excision, Lower Bones, 0QB
Sacrococcygeal ligament *use* Lower Spine Bursa and Ligament
Sacrococcygeal symphysis *use* Sacrococcygeal Joint
Sacroiliac ligament *use* Lower Spine Bursa and Ligament
Sacrospinous ligament *use* Lower Spine Bursa and Ligament
Sacrotuberous ligament *use* Lower Spine Bursa and Ligament
Salpingectomy
    see Excision, Female Reproductive System, 0UB
    see Resection, Female Reproductive System, 0UT
Salpingolysis *see* Release, Female Reproductive System, 0UN
Salpingopexy
    see Repair, Female Reproductive System, 0UQ
    see Reposition, Female Reproductive System, 0US
Salpingopharyngeus muscle *use* Tongue, Palate, Pharynx Muscle
Salpingoplasty
    see Repair, Female Reproductive System, 0UQ
    see Supplement, Female Reproductive System, 0UU
Salpingorrhaphy *see* Repair, Female Reproductive System, 0UQ
Salpingoscopy, 0UJ88ZZ
Salpingostomy *see* Drainage, Female Reproductive System, 0U9
Salpingotomy *see* Drainage, Female Reproductive System, 0U9
Salpinx
    use Fallopian Tube, Left
    use Fallopian Tube, Right
Saphenous nerve *use* Femoral Nerve
SAPIEN transcatheter aortic valve *use* Zooplastic Tissue in Heart and Great Vessels
Sartorius muscle
    use Upper Leg Muscle, Left
    use Upper Leg Muscle, Right
Scalene muscle
    use Neck Muscle, Left

Scalene muscle — *continued*
    use Neck Muscle, Right
Scan
    Computerized Tomography (CT) *see* Computerized Tomography (CT Scan)
    Radioisotope *see* Planar Nuclear Medicine Imaging
Scaphoid bone
    use Carpal, Left
    use Carpal, Right
Scapholunate ligament
    use Hand Bursa and Ligament, Left
    use Hand Bursa and Ligament, Right
Scaphotrapezium ligament
    use Hand Bursa and Ligament, Left
    use Hand Bursa and Ligament, Right
Scapulectomy
    see Excision, Upper Bones, 0PB
    see Resection, Upper Bones, 0PT
Scapulopexy
    see Repair, Upper Bones, 0PQ
    see Reposition, Upper Bones, 0PS
Scarpa's (vestibular) ganglion *use* Acoustic Nerve
Sclerectomy *see* Excision, Eye, 08B
Sclerotherapy, mechanical *see* Destruction
Sclerotherapy, via injection of sclerosing agent *see* Introduction, Destructive Agent
Sclerotomy *see* Drainage, Eye, 089
Scrotectomy
    see Excision, Male Reproductive System, 0VB
    see Resection, Male Reproductive System, 0VT
Scrotoplasty
    see Repair, Male Reproductive System, 0VQ
    see Supplement, Male Reproductive System, 0VU
Scrotorrhaphy *see* Repair, Male Reproductive System, 0VQ
Scrototomy *see* Drainage, Male Reproductive System, 0V9
Sebaceous gland *use* Skin
Second cranial nerve *use* Optic Nerve
Section, cesarean *see* Extraction, Pregnancy, 10D
Secura (DR) (VR) *use* Defibrillator Generator in, 0JH
Sella turcica *use* Sphenoid Bone
Semicircular canal
    use Inner Ear, Left
    use Inner Ear, Right
Semimembranosus muscle
    use Upper Leg Muscle, Left
    use Upper Leg Muscle, Right
Semitendinosus muscle
    use Upper Leg Muscle, Left
    use Upper Leg Muscle, Right
Seprafilm *use* Adhesion Barrier
Septal cartilage *use* Nasal Septum
Septectomy
    see Excision, Ear, Nose, Sinus, 09B
    see Excision, Heart and Great Vessels, 02B
    see Resection, Ear, Nose, Sinus, 09T
    see Resection, Heart and Great Vessels, 02T
Septoplasty
    see Repair, Ear, Nose, Sinus, 09Q
    see Repair, Heart and Great Vessels, 02Q
    see Replacement, Ear, Nose, Sinus, 09R
    see Replacement, Heart and Great Vessels, 02R
    see Reposition, Ear, Nose, Sinus, 09S
    see Supplement, Ear, Nose, Sinus, 09U
    see Supplement, Heart and Great Vessels, 02U
Septostomy, balloon atrial, 02163Z7
Septotomy *see* Drainage, Ear, Nose, Sinus, 099
Sequestrectomy, bone *see* Extirpation
Serratus anterior muscle
    use Thorax Muscle, Left
    use Thorax Muscle, Right
Serratus posterior muscle
    use Trunk Muscle, Left
    use Trunk Muscle, Right
Seventh cranial nerve *use* Facial Nerve
Sheffield hybrid external fixator
    use External Fixation Device, Hybrid in, 0PH
    use External Fixation Device, Hybrid in, 0PS
    use External Fixation Device, Hybrid in, 0QH
    use External Fixation Device, Hybrid in, 0QS
Sheffield ring external fixator
    use External Fixation Device, Ring in, 0PH
    use External Fixation Device, Ring in, 0PS
    use External Fixation Device, Ring in, 0QH
    use External Fixation Device, Ring in, 0QS
Shirodkar cervical cerclage, 0UVC7ZZ

Shock Wave Therapy, Musculoskeletal, 6A93
Short gastric artery *use* Splenic Artery
Shortening
    see Excision
    see Repair
    see Reposition
Shunt creation *see* Bypass
Sialoadenectomy
    Complete *see* Resection, Mouth and Throat, 0CT
    Partial *see* Excision, Mouth and Throat, 0CB
Sialodochoplasty
    see Repair, Mouth and Throat, 0CQ
    see Replacement, Mouth and Throat, 0CR
    see Supplement, Mouth and Throat, 0CU
Sialoectomy
    see Excision, Mouth and Throat, 0CB
    see Resection, Mouth and Throat, 0CT
Sialography *see* Plain Radiography, Ear, Nose, Mouth and Throat, B90
Sialolithotomy *see* Extirpation, Mouth and Throat, 0CC
Sigmoid artery *use* Inferior Mesenteric Artery
Sigmoid flexure *use* Sigmoid Colon
Sigmoid vein *use* Inferior Mesenteric Vein
Sigmoidectomy
    see Excision, Gastrointestinal System, 0DB
    see Resection, Gastrointestinal System, 0DT
Sigmoidorrhaphy *see* Repair, Gastrointestinal System, 0DQ
Sigmoidoscopy, 0DJD8ZZ
Sigmoidotomy *see* Drainage, Gastrointestinal System, 0D9
Single lead pacemaker (atrium) (ventricle) *use* Pacemaker, Single Chamber in, 0JH
Single lead rate responsive pacemaker (atrium) (ventricle) *use* Pacemaker, Single Chamber Rate Responsive in, 0JH
Sinoatrial node *use* Conduction Mechanism
Sinogram
    Abdominal Wall *see* Fluoroscopy, Abdomen and Pelvis, BW11
    Chest Wall *see* Plain Radiography, Chest, BW03
    Retroperitoneum *see* Fluoroscopy, Abdomen and Pelvis, BW11
Sinus venosus *use* Atrium, Right
Sinusectomy
    see Excision, Ear, Nose, Sinus, 09B
    see Resection, Ear, Nose, Sinus, 09T
Sinusoscopy, 09JY4ZZ
Sinusotomy *see* Drainage, Ear, Nose, Sinus, 099
Sirolimus-eluting coronary stent *use* Intraluminal Device, Drug-eluting in Heart and Great Vessels
Sixth cranial nerve *use* Abducens Nerve
Size reduction, breast *see* Excision, Skin and Breast, 0HB
SJM Biocor® Stented Valve System *use* Zooplastic Tissue in Heart and Great Vessels
Skene's (paraurethral) gland *use* Vestibular Gland
Skin Substitute, Porcine Liver Derived, Replacement, XHRPXL2
Sling
    Fascial, orbicularis muscle (mouth) *see* Supplement, Muscle, Facial, 0KU1
    Levator muscle, for urethral suspension *see* Reposition, Bladder Neck, 0TSC
    Pubococcygeal, for urethral suspension *see* Reposition, Bladder Neck, 0TSC
    Rectum *see* Reposition, Rectum, 0DSP
Small bowel series *see* Fluoroscopy, Bowel, Small, BD13
Small saphenous vein
    use Saphenous Vein, Left
    use Saphenous Vein, Right
Snaring, polyp, colon *see* Excision, Gastrointestinal System, 0DB
Solar (celiac) plexus *use* Abdominal Sympathetic Nerve
Soleus muscle
    use Lower Leg Muscle, Left
    use Lower Leg Muscle, Right
Spacer
    Insertion of device in
        Disc
            Lumbar Vertebral, 0SH2
            Lumbosacral, 0SH4
        Joint
            Acromioclavicular
                Left, 0RHH
                Right, 0RHG
            Ankle
                Left, 0SHG

Subterms under main terms may continue to next column or page

Spacer — *continued*
Insertion of device in — *continued*
  Joint — *continued*
    Ankle — *continued*
      Right, ØSHF
    Carpal
      Left, ØRHR
      Right, ØRHQ
    Carpometacarpal
      Left, ØRHT
      Right, ØRHS
    Cervical Vertebral, ØRH1
    Cervicothoracic Vertebral, ØRH4
    Coccygeal, ØSH6
    Elbow
      Left, ØRHM
      Right, ØRHL
    Finger Phalangeal
      Left, ØRHX
      Right, ØRHW
    Hip
      Left, ØSHB
      Right, ØSH9
    Knee
      Left, ØSHD
      Right, ØSHC
    Lumbar Vertebral, ØSHØ
    Lumbosacral, ØSH3
    Metacarpophalangeal
      Left, ØRHV
      Right, ØRHU
    Metatarsal-Phalangeal
      Left, ØSHN
      Right, ØSHM
    Occipital-cervical, ØRHØ
    Sacrococcygeal, ØSH5
    Sacroiliac
      Left, ØSH8
      Right, ØSH7
    Shoulder
      Left, ØRHK
      Right, ØRHJ
    Sternoclavicular
      Left, ØRHF
      Right, ØRHE
    Tarsal
      Left, ØSHJ
      Right, ØSHH
    Tarsometatarsal
      Left, ØSHL
      Right, ØSHK
    Temporomandibular
      Left, ØRHD
      Right, ØRHC
    Thoracic Vertebral, ØRH6
    Thoracolumbar Vertebral, ØRHA
    Toe Phalangeal
      Left, ØSHQ
      Right, ØSHP
    Wrist
      Left, ØRHP
      Right, ØRHN
Removal of device from
  Acromioclavicular
    Left, ØRPH
    Right, ØRPG
  Ankle
    Left, ØSPG
    Right, ØSPF
  Carpal
    Left, ØRPR
    Right, ØRPQ
  Carpometacarpal
    Left, ØRPT
    Right, ØRPS
  Cervical Vertebral, ØRP1
  Cervicothoracic Vertebral, ØRP4
  Coccygeal, ØSP6
  Elbow
    Left, ØRPM
    Right, ØRPL
  Finger Phalangeal
    Left, ØRPX
    Right, ØRPW
  Hip
    Left, ØSPB
    Right, ØSP9
  Knee
    Left, ØSPD

Spacer — *continued*
Removal of device from — *continued*
  Knee — *continued*
    Right, ØSPC
  Lumbar Vertebral, ØSPØ
  Lumbosacral, ØSP3
  Metacarpophalangeal
    Left, ØRPV
    Right, ØRPU
  Metatarsal-Phalangeal
    Left, ØSPN
    Right, ØSPM
  Occipital-cervical, ØRPØ
  Sacrococcygeal, ØSP5
  Sacroiliac
    Left, ØSP8
    Right, ØSP7
  Shoulder
    Left, ØRPK
    Right, ØRPJ
  Sternoclavicular
    Left, ØRPF
    Right, ØRPE
  Tarsal
    Left, ØSPJ
    Right, ØSPH
  Tarsometatarsal
    Left, ØSPL
    Right, ØSPK
  Temporomandibular
    Left, ØRPD
    Right, ØRPC
  Thoracic Vertebral, ØRP6
  Thoracolumbar Vertebral, ØRPA
  Toe Phalangeal
    Left, ØSPQ
    Right, ØSPP
  Wrist
    Left, ØRPP
    Right, ØRPN
Revision of device in
  Acromioclavicular
    Left, ØRWH
    Right, ØRWG
  Ankle
    Left, ØSWG
    Right, ØSWF
  Carpal
    Left, ØRWR
    Right, ØRWQ
  Carpometacarpal
    Left, ØRWT
    Right, ØRWS
  Cervical Vertebral, ØRW1
  Cervicothoracic Vertebral, ØRW4
  Coccygeal, ØSW6
  Elbow
    Left, ØRWM
    Right, ØRWL
  Finger Phalangeal
    Left, ØRWX
    Right, ØRWW
  Hip
    Left, ØSWB
    Right, ØSW9
  Knee
    Left, ØSWD
    Right, ØSWC
  Lumbar Vertebral, ØSWØ
  Lumbosacral, ØSW3
  Metacarpophalangeal
    Left, ØRWV
    Right, ØRWU
  Metatarsal-Phalangeal
    Left, ØSWN
    Right, ØSWM
  Occipital-cervical, ØRWØ
  Sacrococcygeal, ØSW5
  Sacroiliac
    Left, ØSW8
    Right, ØSW7
  Shoulder
    Left, ØRWK
    Right, ØRWJ
  Sternoclavicular
    Left, ØRWF
    Right, ØRWE
  Tarsal
    Left, ØSWJ

Spacer — *continued*
Revision of device in — *continued*
  Tarsal — *continued*
    Right, ØSWH
  Tarsometatarsal
    Left, ØSWL
    Right, ØSWK
  Temporomandibular
    Left, ØRWD
    Right, ØRWC
  Thoracic Vertebral, ØRW6
  Thoracolumbar Vertebral, ØRWA
  Toe Phalangeal
    Left, ØSWQ
    Right, ØSWP
  Wrist
    Left, ØRWP
    Right, ØRWN
Spacer, Articulating (Antibiotic) *use* Articulating Spacer in Lower Joints
Spacer, Static (Antibiotic) *use* Spacer in Lower Joints
Spectroscopy
  Intravascular, 8E023DZ
  Near infrared, 8E023DZ
Speech Assessment, FØØ
Speech therapy *see* Speech Treatment, Rehabilitation, FØ6
Speech Treatment, FØ6
Sphenoidectomy
  see Excision, Ear, Nose, Sinus, Ø9B
  see Excision, Head and Facial Bones, ØNB
  see Resection, Ear, Nose, Sinus, Ø9T
  see Resection, Head and Facial Bones, ØNT
Sphenoidotomy *see* Drainage, Ear, Nose, Sinus, Ø99
Sphenomandibular ligament *use* Head and Neck Bursa and Ligament
Sphenopalatine (pterygopalatine) ganglion *use* Head and Neck Sympathetic Nerve
Sphincterorrhaphy, anal *see* Repair, Anal Sphincter, ØDQR
Sphincterotomy, anal
  see Division, Anal Sphincter, ØD8R
  see Drainage, Anal Sphincter, ØD9R
Spinal cord neurostimulator lead *use* Neurostimulator Lead in Central Nervous System and Cranial Nerves
Spinal growth rods, magnetically controlled *use* Magnetically Controlled Growth Rod(s) in New Technology
Spinal nerve, cervical *use* Cervical Nerve
Spinal nerve, lumbar *use* Lumbar Nerve
Spinal nerve, sacral *use* Sacral Nerve
Spinal nerve, thoracic *use* Thoracic Nerve
Spinal Stabilization Device
  Facet Replacement
    Cervical Vertebral, ØRH1
    Cervicothoracic Vertebral, ØRH4
    Lumbar Vertebral, ØSHØ
    Lumbosacral, ØSH3
    Occipital-cervical, ØRHØ
    Thoracic Vertebral, ØRH6
    Thoracolumbar Vertebral, ØRHA
  Interspinous Process
    Cervical Vertebral, ØRH1
    Cervicothoracic Vertebral, ØRH4
    Lumbar Vertebral, ØSHØ
    Lumbosacral, ØSH3
    Occipital-cervical, ØRHØ
    Thoracic Vertebral, ØRH6
    Thoracolumbar Vertebral, ØRHA
  Pedicle-Based
    Cervical Vertebral, ØRH1
    Cervicothoracic Vertebral, ØRH4
    Lumbar Vertebral, ØSHØ
    Lumbosacral, ØSH3
    Occipital-cervical, ØRHØ
    Thoracic Vertebral, ØRH6
    Thoracolumbar Vertebral, ØRHA
Spinous process
  use Cervical Vertebra
  use Lumbar Vertebra
  use Thoracic Vertebra
Spiral ganglion *use* Acoustic Nerve
Spiration IBV™ Valve System *use* Intraluminal Device, Endobronchial Valve in Respiratory System
Splenectomy
  see Excision, Lymphatic and Hemic Systems, Ø7B
  see Resection, Lymphatic and Hemic Systems, Ø7T
Splenic flexure *use* Transverse Colon

Splenic plexus *use* Abdominal Sympathetic Nerve
Splenius capitis muscle *use* Head Muscle
Splenius cervicis muscle
   use Neck Muscle, Left
   use Neck Muscle, Right
Splenolysis *see* Release, Lymphatic and Hemic Systems, Ø7N
Splenopexy
   see Repair, Lymphatic and Hemic Systems, Ø7Q
   see Reposition, Lymphatic and Hemic Systems, Ø7S
Splenoplasty *see* Repair, Lymphatic and Hemic Systems, Ø7Q
Splenorrhaphy *see* Repair, Lymphatic and Hemic Systems, Ø7Q
Splenotomy *see* Drainage, Lymphatic and Hemic Systems, Ø79
Splinting, musculoskeletal *see* Immobilization, Anatomical Regions, 2W3
SPY system intravascular fluorescence angiography *see* Monitoring, Physiological Systems, 4A1
Stapedectomy
   see Excision, Ear, Nose, Sinus, Ø9B
   see Resection, Ear, Nose, Sinus, Ø9T
Stapediolysis *see* Release, Ear, Nose, Sinus, Ø9N
Stapedioplasty
   see Repair, Ear, Nose, Sinus, Ø9Q
   see Replacement, Ear, Nose, Sinus, Ø9R
   see Supplement, Ear, Nose, Sinus, Ø9U
Stapedotomy *see* Drainage, Ear, Nose, Sinus, Ø99
Stapes
   use Auditory Ossicle, Left
   use Auditory Ossicle, Right
Static Spacer (Antibiotic) *use* Spacer in Lower Joints
STELARA® *use* Other New Technology Therapeutic Substance
Stellate ganglion *use* Head and Neck Sympathetic Nerve
Stem cell transplant *see* Transfusion, Circulatory, 3Ø2
Stensen's duct
   use Parotid Duct, Left
   use Parotid Duct, Right
Stent, intraluminal (cardiovascular) (gastrointestinal) (hepatobiliary) (urinary) *use* Intraluminal Device
Stent retriever thrombectomy *see* Extirpation, Upper Arteries, Ø3C
Stented tissue valve *use* Zooplastic Tissue in Heart and Great Vessels
Stereotactic Radiosurgery
   Abdomen, DW23
   Adrenal Gland, DG22
   Bile Ducts, DF22
   Bladder, DT22
   Bone Marrow, D72Ø
   Brain, DØ2Ø
   Brain Stem, DØ21
   Breast
      Left, DM2Ø
      Right, DM21
   Bronchus, DB21
   Cervix, DU21
   Chest, DW22
   Chest Wall, DB27
   Colon, DD25
   Diaphragm, DB28
   Duodenum, DD22
   Ear, D92Ø
   Esophagus, DD2Ø
   Eye, D82Ø
   Gallbladder, DF21
   Gamma Beam
      Abdomen, DW23JZZ
      Adrenal Gland, DG22JZZ
      Bile Ducts, DF22JZZ
      Bladder, DT22JZZ
      Bone Marrow, D72ØJZZ
      Brain, DØ2ØJZZ
      Brain Stem, DØ21JZZ
      Breast
         Left, DM2ØJZZ
         Right, DM21JZZ
      Bronchus, DB21JZZ
      Cervix, DU21JZZ
      Chest, DW22JZZ
      Chest Wall, DB27JZZ
      Colon, DD25JZZ
      Diaphragm, DB28JZZ
      Duodenum, DD22JZZ
      Ear, D92ØJZZ
      Esophagus, DD2ØJZZ

Stereotactic Radiosurgery — *continued*
   Gamma Beam — *continued*
      Eye, D82ØJZZ
      Gallbladder, DF21JZZ
      Gland
         Adrenal, DG22JZZ
         Parathyroid, DG24JZZ
         Pituitary, DG2ØJZZ
         Thyroid, DG25JZZ
      Glands, Salivary, D926JZZ
      Head and Neck, DW21JZZ
      Ileum, DD24JZZ
      Jejunum, DD23JZZ
      Kidney, DT2ØJZZ
      Larynx, D92BJZZ
      Liver, DF2ØJZZ
      Lung, DB22JZZ
      Lymphatics
         Abdomen, D726JZZ
         Axillary, D724JZZ
         Inguinal, D728JZZ
         Neck, D723JZZ
         Pelvis, D727JZZ
         Thorax, D725JZZ
      Mediastinum, DB26JZZ
      Mouth, D924JZZ
      Nasopharynx, D92DJZZ
      Neck and Head, DW21JZZ
      Nerve, Peripheral, DØ27JZZ
      Nose, D921JZZ
      Ovary, DU2ØJZZ
      Palate
         Hard, D928JZZ
         Soft, D929JZZ
      Pancreas, DF23JZZ
      Parathyroid Gland, DG24JZZ
      Pelvic Region, DW26JZZ
      Pharynx, D92CJZZ
      Pineal Body, DG21JZZ
      Pituitary Gland, DG2ØJZZ
      Pleura, DB25JZZ
      Prostate, DV2ØJZZ
      Rectum, DD27JZZ
      Sinuses, D927JZZ
      Spinal Cord, DØ26JZZ
      Spleen, D722JZZ
      Stomach, DD21JZZ
      Testis, DV21JZZ
      Thymus, D721JZZ
      Thyroid Gland, DG25JZZ
      Tongue, D925JZZ
      Trachea, DB2ØJZZ
      Ureter, DT21JZZ
      Urethra, DT23JZZ
      Uterus, DU22JZZ
   Gland
      Adrenal, DG22
      Parathyroid, DG24
      Pituitary, DG2Ø
      Thyroid, DG25
   Glands, Salivary, D926
   Head and Neck, DW21
   Ileum, DD24
   Jejunum, DD23
   Kidney, DT2Ø
   Larynx, D92B
   Liver, DF2Ø
   Lung, DB22
   Lymphatics
      Abdomen, D726
      Axillary, D724
      Inguinal, D728
      Neck, D723
      Pelvis, D727
      Thorax, D725
   Mediastinum, DB26
   Mouth, D924
   Nasopharynx, D92D
   Neck and Head, DW21
   Nerve, Peripheral, DØ27
   Nose, D921
   Other Photon
      Abdomen, DW23DZZ
      Adrenal Gland, DG22DZZ
      Bile Ducts, DF22DZZ
      Bladder, DT22DZZ
      Bone Marrow, D72ØDZZ
      Brain, DØ2ØDZZ
      Brain Stem, DØ21DZZ

Stereotactic Radiosurgery — *continued*
   Other Photon — *continued*
      Breast
         Left, DM2ØDZZ
         Right, DM21DZZ
      Bronchus, DB21DZZ
      Cervix, DU21DZZ
      Chest, DW22DZZ
      Chest Wall, DB27DZZ
      Colon, DD25DZZ
      Diaphragm, DB28DZZ
      Duodenum, DD22DZZ
      Ear, D92ØDZZ
      Esophagus, DD2ØDZZ
      Eye, D82ØDZZ
      Gallbladder, DF21DZZ
      Gland
         Adrenal, DG22DZZ
         Parathyroid, DG24DZZ
         Pituitary, DG2ØDZZ
         Thyroid, DG25DZZ
      Glands, Salivary, D926DZZ
      Head and Neck, DW21DZZ
      Ileum, DD24DZZ
      Jejunum, DD23DZZ
      Kidney, DT2ØDZZ
      Larynx, D92BDZZ
      Liver, DF2ØDZZ
      Lung, DB22DZZ
      Lymphatics
         Abdomen, D726DZZ
         Axillary, D724DZZ
         Inguinal, D728DZZ
         Neck, D723DZZ
         Pelvis, D727DZZ
         Thorax, D725DZZ
      Mediastinum, DB26DZZ
      Mouth, D924DZZ
      Nasopharynx, D92DDZZ
      Neck and Head, DW21DZZ
      Nerve, Peripheral, DØ27DZZ
      Nose, D921DZZ
      Ovary, DU2ØDZZ
      Palate
         Hard, D928DZZ
         Soft, D929DZZ
      Pancreas, DF23DZZ
      Parathyroid Gland, DG24DZZ
      Pelvic Region, DW26DZZ
      Pharynx, D92CDZZ
      Pineal Body, DG21DZZ
      Pituitary Gland, DG2ØDZZ
      Pleura, DB25DZZ
      Prostate, DV2ØDZZ
      Rectum, DD27DZZ
      Sinuses, D927DZZ
      Spinal Cord, DØ26DZZ
      Spleen, D722DZZ
      Stomach, DD21DZZ
      Testis, DV21DZZ
      Thymus, D721DZZ
      Thyroid Gland, DG25DZZ
      Tongue, D925DZZ
      Trachea, DB2ØDZZ
      Ureter, DT21DZZ
      Urethra, DT23DZZ
      Uterus, DU22DZZ
   Ovary, DU2Ø
   Palate
      Hard, D928
      Soft, D929
   Pancreas, DF23
   Parathyroid Gland, DG24
   Particulate
      Abdomen, DW23HZZ
      Adrenal Gland, DG22HZZ
      Bile Ducts, DF22HZZ
      Bladder, DT22HZZ
      Bone Marrow, D72ØHZZ
      Brain, DØ2ØHZZ
      Brain Stem, DØ21HZZ
      Breast
         Left, DM2ØHZZ
         Right, DM21HZZ
      Bronchus, DB21HZZ
      Cervix, DU21HZZ
      Chest, DW22HZZ
      Chest Wall, DB27HZZ
      Colon, DD25HZZ

△ Subterms under main terms may continue to next column or page

Substance Abuse Treatment — *continued*
  Counseling — *continued*
    Individual — *continued*
      Infectious Disease — *continued*
        Pre-Test, HZ3CZZZ
      Interpersonal, HZ34ZZZ
      Motivational Enhancement, HZ37ZZZ
      Psychoeducation, HZ36ZZZ
      Spiritual, HZ3BZZZ
      Vocational, HZ35ZZZ
  Detoxification Services, for substance abuse, HZ2ZZZZ
  Medication Management
    Antabuse, HZ83ZZZ
    Bupropion, HZ87ZZZ
    Clonidine, HZ86ZZZ
    Levo-alpha-acetyl-methadol (LAAM), HZ82ZZZ
    Methadone Maintenance, HZ81ZZZ
    Naloxone, HZ85ZZZ
    Naltrexone, HZ84ZZZ
    Nicotine Replacement, HZ80ZZZ
    Other Replacement Medication, HZ89ZZZ
    Psychiatric Medication, HZ88ZZZ
  Pharmacotherapy
    Antabuse, HZ93ZZZ
    Bupropion, HZ97ZZZ
    Clonidine, HZ96ZZZ
    Levo-alpha-acetyl-methadol (LAAM), HZ92ZZZ
    Methadone Maintenance, HZ91ZZZ
    Naloxone, HZ95ZZZ
    Naltrexone, HZ94ZZZ
    Nicotine Replacement, HZ90ZZZ
    Psychiatric Medication, HZ98ZZZ
    Replacement Medication, Other, HZ99ZZZ
  Psychotherapy
    12-Step, HZ53ZZZ
    Behavioral, HZ51ZZZ
    Cognitive, HZ50ZZZ
    Cognitive-Behavioral, HZ52ZZZ
    Confrontational, HZ58ZZZ
    Interactive, HZ55ZZZ
    Interpersonal, HZ54ZZZ
    Motivational Enhancement, HZ57ZZZ
    Psychoanalysis, HZ5BZZZ
    Psychodynamic, HZ5CZZZ
    Psychoeducation, HZ56ZZZ
    Psychophysiological, HZ5DZZZ
    Supportive, HZ59ZZZ
Substantia nigra *use* Basal Ganglia
Subtalar (talocalcaneal) joint
  use Tarsal Joint, Left
  use Tarsal Joint, Right
Subtalar ligament
  use Foot Bursa and Ligament, Left
  use Foot Bursa and Ligament, Right
Subthalamic nucleus *use* Basal Ganglia
Suction curettage (D&C), nonobstetric *see* Extraction, Endometrium, ØUDB
Suction curettage, obstetric post-delivery *see* Extraction, Products of Conception, Retained, 1ØD1
Superficial circumflex iliac vein
  use Saphenous Vein, Left
  use Saphenous Vein, Right
Superficial epigastric artery
  use Femoral Artery, Left
  use Femoral Artery, Right
Superficial epigastric vein
  use Saphenous Vein, Left
  use Saphenous Vein, Right
Superficial Inferior Epigastric Artery Flap
  Replacement
    Bilateral, ØHRVØ78
    Left, ØHRUØ78
    Right, ØHRTØ78
  Transfer
    Left, ØKXG
    Right, ØKXF
Superficial palmar arch
  use Hand Artery, Left
  use Hand Artery, Right
Superficial palmar venous arch
  use Hand Vein, Left
  use Hand Vein, Right
Superficial temporal artery
  use Temporal Artery, Left
  use Temporal Artery, Right
Superficial transverse perineal muscle *use* Perineum Muscle
Superior cardiac nerve *use* Thoracic Sympathetic Nerve

Superior cerebellar vein *use* Intracranial Vein
Superior cerebral vein *use* Intracranial Vein
Superior clunic (cluneal) nerve *use* Lumbar Nerve
Superior epigastric artery
  use Internal Mammary Artery, Left
  use Internal Mammary Artery, Right
Superior genicular artery
  use Popliteal Artery, Left
  use Popliteal Artery, Right
Superior gluteal artery
  use Internal Iliac Artery, Left
  use Internal Iliac Artery, Right
Superior gluteal nerve *use* Lumbar Plexus
Superior hypogastric plexus *use* Abdominal Sympathetic Nerve
Superior labial artery *use* Face Artery
Superior laryngeal artery
  use Thyroid Artery, Left
  use Thyroid Artery, Right
Superior laryngeal nerve *use* Vagus Nerve
Superior longitudinal muscle *use* Tongue, Palate, Pharynx Muscle
Superior mesenteric ganglion *use* Abdominal Sympathetic Nerve
Superior mesenteric lymph node *use* Lymphatic, Mesenteric
Superior mesenteric plexus *use* Abdominal Sympathetic Nerve
Superior oblique muscle
  use Extraocular Muscle, Left
  use Extraocular Muscle, Right
Superior olivary nucleus *use* Pons
Superior rectal artery *use* Inferior Mesenteric Artery
Superior rectal vein *use* Inferior Mesenteric Vein
Superior rectus muscle
  use Extraocular Muscle, Left
  use Extraocular Muscle, Right
Superior tarsal plate
  use Upper Eyelid, Left
  use Upper Eyelid, Right
Superior thoracic artery
  use Axillary Artery, Left
  use Axillary Artery, Right
Superior thyroid artery
  use External Carotid Artery, Left
  use External Carotid Artery, Right
  use Thyroid Artery, Left
  use Thyroid Artery, Right
Superior turbinate *use* Nasal Turbinate
Superior ulnar collateral artery
  use Brachial Artery, Left
  use Brachial Artery, Right
Supersaturated Oxygen therapy, 5AØ512C, 5AØ522C
Supplement
  Abdominal Wall, ØWUF
  Acetabulum
    Left, ØQU5
    Right, ØQU4
  Ampulla of Vater, ØFUC
  Anal Sphincter, ØDUR
  Ankle Region
    Left, ØYUL
    Right, ØYUK
  Anus, ØDUQ
  Aorta
    Abdominal, Ø4UØ
    Thoracic
      Ascending/Arch, Ø2UX
      Descending, Ø2UW
  Arm
    Lower
      Left, ØXUF
      Right, ØXUD
    Upper
      Left, ØXU9
      Right, ØXU8
  Artery
    Anterior Tibial
      Left, Ø4UQ
      Right, Ø4UP
    Axillary
      Left, Ø3U6
      Right, Ø3U5
    Brachial
      Left, Ø3U8
      Right, Ø3U7
    Celiac, Ø4U1

Supplement — *continued*
  Artery — *continued*
    Colic
      Left, Ø4U7
      Middle, Ø4U8
      Right, Ø4U6
    Common Carotid
      Left, Ø3UJ
      Right, Ø3UH
    Common Iliac
      Left, Ø4UD
      Right, Ø4UC
    External Carotid
      Left, Ø3UN
      Right, Ø3UM
    External Iliac
      Left, Ø4UJ
      Right, Ø4UH
    Face, Ø3UR
    Femoral
      Left, Ø4UL
      Right, Ø4UK
    Foot
      Left, Ø4UW
      Right, Ø4UV
    Gastric, Ø4U2
    Hand
      Left, Ø3UF
      Right, Ø3UD
    Hepatic, Ø4U3
    Inferior Mesenteric, Ø4UB
    Innominate, Ø3U2
    Internal Carotid
      Left, Ø3UL
      Right, Ø3UK
    Internal Iliac
      Left, Ø4UF
      Right, Ø4UE
    Internal Mammary
      Left, Ø3U1
      Right, Ø3UØ
    Intracranial, Ø3UG
    Lower, Ø4UY
    Peroneal
      Left, Ø4UU
      Right, Ø4UT
    Popliteal
      Left, Ø4UN
      Right, Ø4UM
    Posterior Tibial
      Left, Ø4US
      Right, Ø4UR
    Pulmonary
      Left, Ø2UR
      Right, Ø2UQ
    Pulmonary Trunk, Ø2UP
    Radial
      Left, Ø3UC
      Right, Ø3UB
    Renal
      Left, Ø4UA
      Right, Ø4U9
    Splenic, Ø4U4
    Subclavian
      Left, Ø3U4
      Right, Ø3U3
    Superior Mesenteric, Ø4U5
    Temporal
      Left, Ø3UT
      Right, Ø3US
    Thyroid
      Left, Ø3UV
      Right, Ø3UU
    Ulnar
      Left, Ø3UA
      Right, Ø3U9
    Upper, Ø3UY
    Vertebral
      Left, Ø3UQ
      Right, Ø3UP
  Atrium
    Left, Ø2U7
    Right, Ø2U6
  Auditory Ossicle
    Left, Ø9UA
    Right, Ø9U9
  Axilla
    Left, ØXU5
    Right, ØXU4

Supplement

▼ **Subterms under main terms may continue to next column or page**

Supplement — *continued*
  Subcutaneous Tissue and Fascia — *continued*
    Chest, ØJU6
    Face, ØJU1
    Foot
      Left, ØJUR
      Right, ØJUQ
    Hand
      Left, ØJUK
      Right, ØJUJ
    Lower Arm
      Left, ØJUH
      Right, ØJUG
    Lower Leg
      Left, ØJUP
      Right, ØJUN
    Neck
      Left, ØJU5
      Right, ØJU4
    Pelvic Region, ØJUC
    Perineum, ØJUB
    Scalp, ØJUØ
    Upper Arm
      Left, ØJUF
      Right, ØJUD
    Upper Leg
      Left, ØJUM
      Right, ØJUL
  Tarsal
    Left, ØQUM
    Right, ØQUL
  Tendon
    Abdomen
      Left, ØLUG
      Right, ØLUF
    Ankle
      Left, ØLUT
      Right, ØLUS
    Foot
      Left, ØLUW
      Right, ØLUV
    Hand
      Left, ØLU8
      Right, ØLU7
    Head and Neck, ØLUØ
    Hip
      Left, ØLUK
      Right, ØLUJ
    Knee
      Left, ØLUR
      Right, ØLUQ
    Lower Arm and Wrist
      Left, ØLU6
      Right, ØLU5
    Lower Leg
      Left, ØLUP
      Right, ØLUN
    Perineum, ØLUH
    Shoulder
      Left, ØLU2
      Right, ØLU1
    Thorax
      Left, ØLUD
      Right, ØLUC
    Trunk
      Left, ØLUB
      Right, ØLU9
    Upper Arm
      Left, ØLU4
      Right, ØLU3
    Upper Leg
      Left, ØLUM
      Right, ØLUL
  Testis
    Bilateral, ØVUCØ
    Left, ØVUBØ
    Right, ØVU9Ø
  Thumb
    Left, ØXUM
    Right, ØXUL
  Tibia
    Left, ØQUH
    Right, ØQUG
  Toe
    1st
      Left, ØYUQ
      Right, ØYUP
    2nd
      Left, ØYUS

Supplement — *continued*
  Toe — *continued*
    2nd — *continued*
      Right, ØYUR
    3rd
      Left, ØYUU
      Right, ØYUT
    4th
      Left, ØYUW
      Right, ØYUV
    5th
      Left, ØYUY
      Right, ØYUX
  Tongue, ØCU7
  Trachea, ØBU1
  Tunica Vaginalis
    Left, ØVU7
    Right, ØVU6
  Turbinate, Nasal, Ø9UL
  Tympanic Membrane
    Left, Ø9U8
    Right, Ø9U7
  Ulna
    Left, ØPUL
    Right, ØPUK
  Ureter
    Left, ØTU7
    Right, ØTU6
  Urethra, ØTUD
  Uterine Supporting Structure, ØUU4
  Uvula, ØCUN
  Vagina, ØUUG
  Valve
    Aortic, Ø2UF
    Mitral, Ø2UG
    Pulmonary, Ø2UH
    Tricuspid, Ø2UJ
  Vas Deferens
    Bilateral, ØVUQ
    Left, ØVUP
    Right, ØVUN
  Vein
    Axillary
      Left, Ø5U8
      Right, Ø5U7
    Azygos, Ø5UØ
    Basilic
      Left, Ø5UC
      Right, Ø5UB
    Brachial
      Left, Ø5UA
      Right, Ø5U9
    Cephalic
      Left, Ø5UF
      Right, Ø5UD
    Colic, Ø6U7
    Common Iliac
      Left, Ø6UD
      Right, Ø6UC
    Esophageal, Ø6U3
    External Iliac
      Left, Ø6UG
      Right, Ø6UF
    External Jugular
      Left, Ø5UQ
      Right, Ø5UP
    Face
      Left, Ø5UV
      Right, Ø5UT
    Femoral
      Left, Ø6UN
      Right, Ø6UM
    Foot
      Left, Ø6UV
      Right, Ø6UT
    Gastric, Ø6U2
    Hand
      Left, Ø5UH
      Right, Ø5UG
    Hemiazygos, Ø5U1
    Hepatic, Ø6U4
    Hypogastric
      Left, Ø6UJ
      Right, Ø6UH
    Inferior Mesenteric, Ø6U6
    Innominate
      Left, Ø5U4
      Right, Ø5U3

Supplement — *continued*
  Vein — *continued*
    Internal Jugular
      Left, Ø5UN
      Right, Ø5UM
    Intracranial, Ø5UL
    Lower, Ø6UY
    Portal, Ø6U8
    Pulmonary
      Left, Ø2UT
      Right, Ø2US
    Renal
      Left, Ø6UB
      Right, Ø6U9
    Saphenous
      Left, Ø6UQ
      Right, Ø6UP
    Splenic, Ø6U1
    Subclavian
      Left, Ø5U6
      Right, Ø5U5
    Superior Mesenteric, Ø6U5
    Upper, Ø5UY
    Vertebral
      Left, Ø5US
      Right, Ø5UR
  Vena Cava
    Inferior, Ø6UØ
    Superior, Ø2UV
  Ventricle
    Left, Ø2UL
    Right, Ø2UK
  Vertebra
    Cervical, ØPU3
    Lumbar, ØQUØ
    Thoracic, ØPU4
  Vesicle
    Bilateral, ØVU3
    Left, ØVU2
    Right, ØVU1
  Vocal Cord
    Left, ØCUV
    Right, ØCUT
  Vulva, ØUUM
  Wrist Region
    Left, ØXUH
    Right, ØXUG

Supraclavicular (Virchow's) lymph node
  use Lymphatic, Left Neck
  use Lymphatic, Right Neck
Supraclavicular nerve *use* Cervical Plexus
Suprahyoid lymph node *use* Lymphatic, Head
Suprahyoid muscle
  use Neck Muscle, Left
  use Neck Muscle, Right
Suprainguinal lymph node *use* Lymphatic, Pelvis
Supraorbital vein
  use Face Vein, Left
  use Face Vein, Right
Suprarenal gland
  use Adrenal Gland
  use Adrenal Gland, Bilateral
  use Adrenal Gland, Left
  use Adrenal Gland, Right
Suprarenal plexus *use* Abdominal Sympathetic Nerve
Suprascapular nerve *use* Brachial Plexus
Supraspinatus fascia
  use Subcutaneous Tissue and Fascia, Left Upper Arm
  use Subcutaneous Tissue and Fascia, Right Upper Arm
Supraspinatus muscle
  use Shoulder Muscle, Left
  use Shoulder Muscle, Right
Supraspinous ligament
  use Lower Spine Bursa and Ligament
  use Upper Spine Bursa and Ligament
Suprasternal notch *use* Sternum
Supratrochlear lymph node
  use Lymphatic, Left Upper Extremity
  use Lymphatic, Right Upper Extremity
Sural artery
  use Popliteal Artery, Left
  use Popliteal Artery, Right
Suspension
  Bladder Neck *see* Reposition, Bladder Neck, ØTSC
  Kidney *see* Reposition, Urinary System, ØTS
  Urethra *see* Reposition, Urinary System, ØTS
  Urethrovesical *see* Reposition, Bladder Neck, ØTSC

▼ Subterms under main terms may continue to next column or page

Index

Suspension — Tissue Expander

Tissue Expander — *continued*
  Insertion of device in — *continued*
    Subcutaneous Tissue and Fascia — *continued*
      Foot — *continued*
        Right, ØJHQ
      Hand
        Left, ØJHK
        Right, ØJHJ
      Lower Arm
        Left, ØJHH
        Right, ØJHG
      Lower Leg
        Left, ØJHP
        Right, ØJHN
      Neck
        Left, ØJH5
        Right, ØJH4
      Pelvic Region, ØJHC
      Perineum, ØJHB
      Scalp, ØJHØ
      Upper Arm
        Left, ØJHF
        Right, ØJHD
      Upper Leg
        Left, ØJHM
        Right, ØJHL
  Removal of device from
    Breast
      Left, ØHPU
      Right, ØHPT
    Subcutaneous Tissue and Fascia
      Head and Neck, ØJPS
      Lower Extremity, ØJPW
      Trunk, ØJPT
      Upper Extremity, ØJPV
  Revision of device in
    Breast
      Left, ØHWU
      Right, ØHWT
    Subcutaneous Tissue and Fascia
      Head and Neck, ØJWS
      Lower Extremity, ØJWW
      Trunk, ØJWT
      Upper Extremity, ØJWV

Tissue expander (inflatable) (injectable)
  use Tissue Expander in Skin and Breast
  use Tissue Expander in Subcutaneous Tissue and Fascia

Tissue Plasminogen Activator (tPA) (r-tPA) *use* Other Thrombolytic

Titanium Sternal Fixation System (TSFS)
  use Internal Fixation Device, Rigid Plate in, ØPS
  use Internal Fixation Device, Rigid Plate in, ØPH

Tomographic (Tomo) Nuclear Medicine Imaging
  Abdomen, CW2Ø
  Abdomen and Chest, CW24
  Abdomen and Pelvis, CW21
  Anatomical Regions, Multiple, CW2YYZZ
  Bladder, Kidneys and Ureters, CT23
  Brain, CØ2Ø
  Breast, CH2YYZZ
    Bilateral, CH22
    Left, CH21
    Right, CH2Ø
  Bronchi and Lungs, CB22
  Central Nervous System, CØ2YYZZ
  Cerebrospinal Fluid, CØ25
  Chest, CW23
  Chest and Abdomen, CW24
  Chest and Neck, CW26
  Digestive System, CD2YYZZ
  Endocrine System, CG2YYZZ
  Extremity
    Lower, CW2D
      Bilateral, CP2F
      Left, CP2D
      Right, CP2C
    Upper, CW2M
      Bilateral, CP2B
      Left, CP29
      Right, CP28
  Gallbladder, CF24
  Gastrointestinal Tract, CD27
  Gland, Parathyroid, CG21
  Head and Neck, CW2B
  Heart, C22YYZZ
    Right and Left, C226
  Hepatobiliary System and Pancreas, CF2YYZZ

Tomographic (Tomo) Nuclear Medicine Imaging —
continued
  Kidneys, Ureters and Bladder, CT23
  Liver, CF25
  Liver and Spleen, CF26
  Lungs and Bronchi, CB22
  Lymphatics and Hematologic System, C72YYZZ
  Musculoskeletal System, Other, CP2YYZZ
  Myocardium, C22G
  Neck and Chest, CW26
  Neck and Head, CW2B
  Pancreas and Hepatobiliary System, CF2YYZZ
  Pelvic Region, CW2J
  Pelvis, CP26
  Pelvis and Abdomen, CW21
  Pelvis and Spine, CP27
  Respiratory System, CB2YYZZ
  Skin, CH2YYZZ
  Skull, CP21
  Skull and Cervical Spine, CP23
  Spine
    Cervical, CP22
    Cervical and Skull, CP23
    Lumbar, CP2H
    Thoracic, CP2G
    Thoracolumbar, CP2J
  Spine and Pelvis, CP27
  Spleen, C722
  Spleen and Liver, CF26
  Subcutaneous Tissue, CH2YYZZ
  Thorax, CP24
  Ureters, Kidneys and Bladder, CT23
  Urinary System, CT2YYZZ

Tomography, computerized *see* Computerized Tomography (CT Scan)

Tongue, base of *use* Pharynx

Tonometry, 4AØ7XBZ

Tonsillectomy
  see Excision, Mouth and Throat, ØCB
  see Resection, Mouth and Throat, ØCT

Tonsillotomy *see* Drainage, Mouth and Throat, ØC9

**Total Anomalous Pulmonary Venous Return (TAPVR)
repair**
  see Bypass, Atrium, Left, Ø217
  see Bypass, Vena Cava, Superior, Ø21V

Total artificial (replacement) heart *use* Synthetic Substitute

Total parenteral nutrition (TPN) *see* Introduction of Nutritional Substance

Trachectomy
  see Excision, Trachea, ØBB1
  see Resection, Trachea, ØBT1

Trachelectomy
  see Excision, Cervix, ØUBC
  see Resection, Cervix, ØUTC

Trachelopexy
  see Repair, Cervix, ØUQC
  see Reposition, Cervix, ØUSC

Tracheloplasty *see* Repair, Cervix, ØUQC

Trachelorrhaphy *see* Repair, Cervix, ØUQC

Trachelotomy *see* Drainage, Cervix, ØU9C

Tracheobronchial lymph node *use* Lymphatic, Thorax

Tracheoesophageal fistulization, ØB11ØD6

Tracheolysis *see* Release, Respiratory System, ØBN

Tracheoplasty
  see Repair, Respiratory System, ØBQ
  see Supplement, Respiratory System, ØBU

Tracheorrhaphy *see* Repair, Respiratory System, ØBQ

Tracheoscopy, ØBJ18ZZ

Tracheostomy *see* Bypass, Respiratory System, ØB1

Tracheostomy Device
  Bypass, Trachea, ØB11
  Change device in, Trachea, ØB21XFZ
  Removal of device from, Trachea, ØBP1
  Revision of device in, Trachea, ØBW1

Tracheostomy tube *use* Tracheostomy Device in Respiratory System

Tracheotomy *see* Drainage, Respiratory System, ØB9

Traction
  Abdominal Wall, 2W63X
  Arm
    Lower
      Left, 2W6DX
      Right, 2W6CX
    Upper
      Left, 2W6BX
      Right, 2W6AX
  Back, 2W65X

Traction — *continued*
  Chest Wall, 2W64X
  Extremity
    Lower
      Left, 2W6MX
      Right, 2W6LX
    Upper
      Left, 2W69X
      Right, 2W68X
  Face, 2W61X
  Finger
    Left, 2W6KX
    Right, 2W6JX
  Foot
    Left, 2W6TX
    Right, 2W6SX
  Hand
    Left, 2W6FX
    Right, 2W6EX
  Head, 2W6ØX
  Inguinal Region
    Left, 2W67X
    Right, 2W66X
  Leg
    Lower
      Left, 2W6RX
      Right, 2W6QX
    Upper
      Left, 2W6PX
      Right, 2W6NX
  Neck, 2W62X
  Thumb
    Left, 2W6HX
    Right, 2W6GX
  Toe
    Left, 2W6VX
    Right, 2W6UX

Tractotomy *see* Division, Central Nervous System and Cranial Nerves, ØØ8

Tragus
  use External Ear, Bilateral
  use External Ear, Left
  use External Ear, Right

Training, caregiver *see* Caregiver Training

**TRAM (transverse rectus abdominis myocutaneous)
flap reconstruction**
  Free *see* Replacement, Skin and Breast, ØHR
  Pedicled *see* Transfer, Muscles, ØKX

Transection *see* Division

Transfer
  Buccal Mucosa, ØCX4
  Bursa and Ligament
    Abdomen
      Left, ØMXJ
      Right, ØMXH
    Ankle
      Left, ØMXR
      Right, ØMXQ
    Elbow
      Left, ØMX4
      Right, ØMX3
    Foot
      Left, ØMXT
      Right, ØMXS
    Hand
      Left, ØMX8
      Right, ØMX7
    Head and Neck, ØMXØ
    Hip
      Left, ØMXM
      Right, ØMXL
    Knee
      Left, ØMXP
      Right, ØMXN
    Lower Extremity
      Left, ØMXW
      Right, ØMXV
    Perineum, ØMXK
    Rib(s), ØMXG
    Shoulder
      Left, ØMX2
      Right, ØMX1
    Spine
      Lower, ØMXD
      Upper, ØMXC
    Sternum, ØMXF
    Upper Extremity
      Left, ØMXB

Transfer — *continued*
  Bursa and Ligament — *continued*
    Upper Extremity — *continued*
      Right, ØMX9
    Wrist
      Left, ØMX6
      Right, ØMX5
  Finger
    Left, ØXXPØZM
    Right, ØXXNØZL
  Gingiva
    Lower, ØCX6
    Upper, ØCX5
  Intestine
    Large, ØDXE
    Small, ØDX8
  Lip
    Lower, ØCX1
    Upper, ØCXØ
  Muscle
    Abdomen
      Left, ØKXL
      Right, ØKXK
    Extraocular
      Left, Ø8XM
      Right, Ø8XL
    Facial, ØKX1
    Foot
      Left, ØKXW
      Right, ØKXV
    Hand
      Left, ØKXD
      Right, ØKXC
    Head, ØKXØ
    Hip
      Left, ØKXP
      Right, ØKXN
    Lower Arm and Wrist
      Left, ØKXB
      Right, ØKX9
    Lower Leg
      Left, ØKXT
      Right, ØKXS
    Neck
      Left, ØKX3
      Right, ØKX2
    Perineum, ØKXM
    Shoulder
      Left, ØKX6
      Right, ØKX5
    Thorax
      Left, ØKXJ
      Right, ØKXH
    Tongue, Palate, Pharynx, ØKX4
    Trunk
      Left, ØKXG
      Right, ØKXF
    Upper Arm
      Left, ØKX8
      Right, ØKX7
    Upper Leg
      Left, ØKXR
      Right, ØKXQ
  Nerve
    Abducens, ØØXL
    Accessory, ØØXR
    Acoustic, ØØXN
    Cervical, Ø1X1
    Facial, ØØXM
    Femoral, Ø1XD
    Glossopharyngeal, ØØXP
    Hypoglossal, ØØXS
    Lumbar, Ø1XB
    Median, Ø1X5
    Oculomotor, ØØXH
    Olfactory, ØØXF
    Optic, ØØXG
    Peroneal, Ø1XH
    Phrenic, Ø1X2
    Pudendal, Ø1XC
    Radial, Ø1X6
    Sciatic, Ø1XF
    Thoracic, Ø1X8
    Tibial, Ø1XG
    Trigeminal, ØØXK
    Trochlear, ØØXJ
    Ulnar, Ø1X4
    Vagus, ØØXQ
  Palate, Soft, ØCX3

Transfer — *continued*
  Prepuce, ØVXT
  Skin
    Abdomen, ØHX7XZZ
    Back, ØHX6XZZ
    Buttock, ØHX8XZZ
    Chest, ØHX5XZZ
    Ear
      Left, ØHX3XZZ
      Right, ØHX2XZZ
    Face, ØHX1XZZ
    Foot
      Left, ØHXNXZZ
      Right, ØHXMXZZ
    Hand
      Left, ØHXGXZZ
      Right, ØHXFXZZ
    Inguinal, ØHXAXZZ
    Lower Arm
      Left, ØHXEXZZ
      Right, ØHXDXZZ
    Lower Leg
      Left, ØHXLXZZ
      Right, ØHXKXZZ
    Neck, ØHX4XZZ
    Perineum, ØHX9XZZ
    Scalp, ØHXØXZZ
    Upper Arm
      Left, ØHXCXZZ
      Right, ØHXBXZZ
    Upper Leg
      Left, ØHXJXZZ
      Right, ØHXHXZZ
  Stomach, ØDX6
  Subcutaneous Tissue and Fascia
    Abdomen, ØJX8
    Back, ØJX7
    Buttock, ØJX9
    Chest, ØJX6
    Face, ØJX1
    Foot
      Left, ØJXR
      Right, ØJXQ
    Hand
      Left, ØJXK
      Right, ØJXJ
    Lower Arm
      Left, ØJXH
      Right, ØJXG
    Lower Leg
      Left, ØJXP
      Right, ØJXN
    Neck
      Left, ØJX5
      Right, ØJX4
    Pelvic Region, ØJXC
    Perineum, ØJXB
    Scalp, ØJXØ
    Upper Arm
      Left, ØJXF
      Right, ØJXD
    Upper Leg
      Left, ØJXM
      Right, ØJXL
  Tendon
    Abdomen
      Left, ØLXG
      Right, ØLXF
    Ankle
      Left, ØLXT
      Right, ØLXS
    Foot
      Left, ØLXW
      Right, ØLXV
    Hand
      Left, ØLX8
      Right, ØLX7
    Head and Neck, ØLXØ
    Hip
      Left, ØLXK
      Right, ØLXJ
    Knee
      Left, ØLXR
      Right, ØLXQ
    Lower Arm and Wrist
      Left, ØLX6
      Right, ØLX5
    Lower Leg
      Left, ØLXP

Transfer — *continued*
  Tendon — *continued*
    Lower Leg — *continued*
      Right, ØLXN
    Perineum, ØLXH
    Shoulder
      Left, ØLX2
      Right, ØLX1
    Thorax
      Left, ØLXD
      Right, ØLXC
    Trunk
      Left, ØLXB
      Right, ØLX9
    Upper Arm
      Left, ØLX4
      Right, ØLX3
    Upper Leg
      Left, ØLXM
      Right, ØLXL
  Tongue, ØCX7
Transfusion
  Artery
    Central
      Antihemophilic Factors, 3Ø26
      Blood
        Platelets, 3Ø26
        Red Cells, 3Ø26
          Frozen, 3Ø26
        White Cells, 3Ø26
        Whole, 3Ø26
      Bone Marrow, 3Ø26
      Factor IX, 3Ø26
      Fibrinogen, 3Ø26
      Globulin, 3Ø26
      Plasma
        Fresh, 3Ø26
        Frozen, 3Ø26
      Plasma Cryoprecipitate, 3Ø26
      Serum Albumin, 3Ø26
      Stem Cells
        Cord Blood, 3Ø26
        Hematopoietic, 3Ø26
    Peripheral
      Antihemophilic Factors, 3Ø25
      Blood
        Platelets, 3Ø25
        Red Cells, 3Ø25
          Frozen, 3Ø25
        White Cells, 3Ø25
        Whole, 3Ø25
      Bone Marrow, 3Ø25
      Factor IX, 3Ø25
      Fibrinogen, 3Ø25
      Globulin, 3Ø25
      Plasma
        Fresh, 3Ø25
        Frozen, 3Ø25
      Plasma Cryoprecipitate, 3Ø25
      Serum Albumin, 3Ø25
      Stem Cells
        Cord Blood, 3Ø25
        Hematopoietic, 3Ø25
  Products of Conception
    Antihemophilic Factors, 3Ø27
    Blood
      Platelets, 3Ø27
      Red Cells, 3Ø27
        Frozen, 3Ø27
      White Cells, 3Ø27
      Whole, 3Ø27
    Factor IX, 3Ø27
    Fibrinogen, 3Ø27
    Globulin, 3Ø27
    Plasma
      Fresh, 3Ø27
      Frozen, 3Ø27
    Plasma Cryoprecipitate, 3Ø27
    Serum Albumin, 3Ø27
  Vein
    4-Factor Prothrombin Complex Concentrate, 3Ø28ØB1
    Central
      Antihemophilic Factors, 3Ø24
      Blood
        Platelets, 3Ø24
        Red Cells, 3Ø24
          Frozen, 3Ø24
        White Cells, 3Ø24

▼ **Subterms under main terms may continue to next column or page**

Transfusion — *continued*
  Vein — *continued*
    Central — *continued*
      Blood — *continued*
        Whole, 3Ø24
      Bone Marrow, 3Ø24
      Factor IX, 3Ø24
      Fibrinogen, 3Ø24
      Globulin, 3Ø24
      Plasma
        Fresh, 3Ø24
        Frozen, 3Ø24
      Plasma Cryoprecipitate, 3Ø24
      Serum Albumin, 3Ø24
      Stem Cells
        Cord Blood, 3Ø24
        Embryonic, 3Ø24
        Hematopoietic, 3Ø24
    Peripheral
      Antihemophilic Factors, 3Ø23
      Blood
        Platelets, 3Ø23
        Red Cells, 3Ø23
          Frozen, 3Ø23
        White Cells, 3Ø23
        Whole, 3Ø23
      Bone Marrow, 3Ø23
      Factor IX, 3Ø23
      Fibrinogen, 3Ø23
      Globulin, 3Ø23
      Plasma
        Fresh, 3Ø23
        Frozen, 3Ø23
      Plasma Cryoprecipitate, 3Ø23
      Serum Albumin, 3Ø23
      Stem Cells
        Cord Blood, 3Ø23
        Embryonic, 3Ø23
        Hematopoietic, 3Ø23
Transplant *see* Transplantation
Transplantation
  Bone marrow *see* Transfusion, Circulatory, 3Ø2
  Esophagus, ØDY5ØZ
  Face, ØWY2ØZ
  Hand
    Left, ØXYKØZ
    Right, ØXYJØZ
  Heart, Ø2YAØZ
  Hematopoietic cell *see* Transfusion, Circulatory, 3Ø2
  Intestine
    Large, ØDYEØZ
    Small, ØDY8ØZ
  Kidney
    Left, ØTY1ØZ
    Right, ØTYØØZ
  Liver, ØFYØØZ
  Lung
    Bilateral, ØBYMØZ
    Left, ØBYLØZ
    Lower Lobe
      Left, ØBYJØZ
      Right, ØBYFØZ
    Middle Lobe, Right, ØBYDØZ
    Right, ØBYKØZ
    Upper Lobe
      Left, ØBYGØZ
      Right, ØBYCØZ
  Lung Lingula, ØBYHØZ
  Ovary
    Left, ØUY1ØZ
    Right, ØUYØØZ
  Pancreas, ØFYGØZ
  Products of Conception, 1ØYØ
  Spleen, Ø7YPØZ
  Stem cell *see* Transfusion, Circulatory, 3Ø2
  Stomach, ØDY6ØZ
  Thymus, Ø7YMØZ
  Uterus, ØUY9ØZ
Transposition
  see Bypass
  see Reposition
  see Transfer
Transversalis fascia *use* Subcutaneous Tissue and Fascia, Trunk
Transverse acetabular ligament
  use Hip Bursa and Ligament, Left
  use Hip Bursa and Ligament, Right

Transverse (cutaneous) cervical nerve *use* Cervical Plexus
Transverse facial artery
  use Temporal Artery, Left
  use Temporal Artery, Right
Transverse foramen *use* Cervical Vertebra
Transverse humeral ligament
  use Shoulder Bursa and Ligament, Left
  use Shoulder Bursa and Ligament, Right
Transverse ligament of atlas *use* Head and Neck Bursa and Ligament
Transverse process
  use Cervical Vertebra
  use Lumbar Vertebra
  use Thoracic Vertebra
Transverse Rectus Abdominis Myocutaneous Flap
  Replacement
    Bilateral, ØHRVØ76
    Left, ØHRUØ76
    Right, ØHRTØ76
  Transfer
    Left, ØKXL
    Right, ØKXK
Transverse scapular ligament
  use Shoulder Bursa and Ligament, Left
  use Shoulder Bursa and Ligament, Right
Transverse thoracis muscle
  use Thorax Muscle, Left
  use Thorax Muscle, Right
Transversospinalis muscle
  use Trunk Muscle, Left
  use Trunk Muscle, Right
Transversus abdominis muscle
  use Abdomen Muscle, Left
  use Abdomen Muscle, Right
Trapezium bone
  use Carpal, Left
  use Carpal, Right
Trapezius muscle
  use Trunk Muscle, Left
  use Trunk Muscle, Right
Trapezoid bone
  use Carpal, Left
  use Carpal, Right
Triceps brachii muscle
  use Upper Arm Muscle, Left
  use Upper Arm Muscle, Right
Tricuspid annulus *use* Tricuspid Valve
Trifacial nerve *use* Trigeminal Nerve
Trifecta™ Valve (aortic) *use* Zooplastic Tissue in Heart and Great Vessels
Trigone of bladder *use* Bladder
Trimming, excisional *see* Excision
Triquetral bone
  use Carpal, Left
  use Carpal, Right
Trochanteric bursa
  use Hip Bursa and Ligament, Left
  use Hip Bursa and Ligament, Right
TUMT (transurethral microwave thermotherapy of prostate), ØV5Ø7ZZ
TUNA (transurethral needle ablation of prostate), ØV5Ø7ZZ
Tunneled central venous catheter *use* Vascular Access Device, Tunneled in Subcutaneous Tissue and Fascia
Tunneled spinal (intrathecal) catheter *use* Infusion Device
Turbinectomy
  see Excision, Ear, Nose, Sinus, Ø9B
  see Resection, Ear, Nose, Sinus, Ø9T
Turbinoplasty
  see Repair, Ear, Nose, Sinus, Ø9Q
  see Replacement, Ear, Nose, Sinus, Ø9R
  see Supplement, Ear, Nose, Sinus, Ø9U
Turbinotomy
  see Division, Ear, Nose, Sinus, Ø98
  see Drainage, Ear, Nose, Sinus, Ø99
TURP (transurethral resection of prostate), ØVBØ7ZZ
  see Excision, Prostate, ØVBØ
  see Resection, Prostate, ØVTØ
Twelfth cranial nerve *use* Hypoglossal Nerve
Two lead pacemaker *use* Pacemaker, Dual Chamber in, ØJH
Tympanic cavity
  use Middle Ear, Left
  use Middle Ear, Right

Tympanic nerve *use* Glossopharyngeal Nerve
Tympanic part of temporal bone
  use Temporal Bone, Left
  use Temporal Bone, Right
Tympanogram *see* Hearing Assessment, Diagnostic Audiology, F13
Tympanoplasty
  see Repair, Ear, Nose, Sinus, Ø9Q
  see Replacement, Ear, Nose, Sinus, Ø9R
  see Supplement, Ear, Nose, Sinus, Ø9U
Tympanosympathectomy *see* Excision, Nerve, Head and Neck Sympathetic, Ø1BK
Tympanotomy *see* Drainage, Ear, Nose, Sinus, Ø99

U

Ulnar collateral carpal ligament
  use Wrist Bursa and Ligament, Left
  use Wrist Bursa and Ligament, Right
Ulnar collateral ligament
  use Elbow Bursa and Ligament, Left
  use Elbow Bursa and Ligament, Right
Ulnar notch
  use Radius, Left
  use Radius, Right
Ulnar vein
  use Brachial Vein, Left
  use Brachial Vein, Right
Ultrafiltration
  Hemodialysis *see* Performance, Urinary, 5A1D
  Therapeutic plasmapheresis *see* Pheresis, Circulatory, 6A55
Ultraflex™ Precision Colonic Stent System *use* Intraluminal Device
ULTRAPRO Hernia System (UHS) *use* Synthetic Substitute
ULTRAPRO Partially Absorbable Lightweight Mesh *use* Synthetic Substitute
ULTRAPRO Plug *use* Synthetic Substitute
Ultrasonic osteogenic stimulator
  use Bone Growth Stimulator in Head and Facial Bones
  use Bone Growth Stimulator in Lower Bones
  use Bone Growth Stimulator in Upper Bones
Ultrasonography
  Abdomen, BW4ØZZZ
  Abdomen and Pelvis, BW41ZZZ
  Abdominal Wall, BH49ZZZ
  Aorta
    Abdominal, Intravascular, B44ØZZ3
    Thoracic, Intravascular, B34ØZZ3
  Appendix, BD48ZZZ
  Artery
    Brachiocephalic-Subclavian, Right, Intravascular, B341ZZ3
    Celiac and Mesenteric, Intravascular, B44KZZ3
    Common Carotid
      Bilateral, Intravascular, B345ZZ3
      Left, Intravascular, B344ZZ3
      Right, Intravascular, B343ZZ3
    Coronary
      Multiple, B241YZZ
        Intravascular, B241ZZ3
        Transesophageal, B241ZZ4
      Single, B24ØYZZ
        Intravascular, B24ØZZ3
        Transesophageal, B24ØZZ4
    Femoral, Intravascular, B44LZZ3
    Inferior Mesenteric, Intravascular, B445ZZ3
    Internal Carotid
      Bilateral, Intravascular, B348ZZ3
      Left, Intravascular, B347ZZ3
      Right, Intravascular, B346ZZ3
    Intra-Abdominal, Other, Intravascular, B44BZZ3
    Intracranial, Intravascular, B34RZZ3
    Lower Extremity
      Bilateral, Intravascular, B44HZZ3
      Left, Intravascular, B44GZZ3
      Right, Intravascular, B44FZZ3
    Mesenteric and Celiac, Intravascular, B44KZZ3
    Ophthalmic, Intravascular, B34VZZ3
    Penile, Intravascular, B44NZZ3
    Pulmonary
      Left, Intravascular, B34TZZ3
      Right, Intravascular, B34SZZ3
    Renal
      Bilateral, Intravascular, B448ZZ3
      Left, Intravascular, B447ZZ3

Ultrasonography — *continued*
  Artery — *continued*
    Renal — *continued*
      Right, Intravascular, B446ZZ3
    Subclavian, Left, Intravascular, B342ZZ3
    Superior Mesenteric, Intravascular, B444ZZ3
    Upper Extremity
      Bilateral, Intravascular, B34KZZ3
      Left, Intravascular, B34JZZ3
      Right, Intravascular, B34HZZ3
  Bile Duct, BF40ZZZ
  Bile Duct and Gallbladder, BF43ZZZ
  Bladder, BT40ZZZ
    and Kidney, BT4JZZZ
  Brain, B040ZZZ
  Breast
    Bilateral, BH42ZZZ
    Left, BH41ZZZ
    Right, BH40ZZZ
  Chest Wall, BH4BZZZ
  Coccyx, BR4FZZZ
  Connective Tissue
    Lower Extremity, BL41ZZZ
    Upper Extremity, BL40ZZZ
  Duodenum, BD49ZZZ
  Elbow
    Left, Densitometry, BP4HZZ1
    Right, Densitometry, BP4GZZ1
  Esophagus, BD41ZZZ
  Extremity
    Lower, BH48ZZZ
    Upper, BH47ZZZ
  Eye
    Bilateral, B847ZZZ
    Left, B846ZZZ
    Right, B845ZZZ
  Fallopian Tube
    Bilateral, BU42
    Left, BU41
    Right, BU40
  Fetal Umbilical Cord, BY47ZZZ
  Fetus
    First Trimester, Multiple Gestation, BY4BZZZ
    Second Trimester, Multiple Gestation, BY4DZZZ
    Single
      First Trimester, BY49ZZZ
      Second Trimester, BY4CZZZ
      Third Trimester, BY4FZZZ
    Third Trimester, Multiple Gestation, BY4GZZZ
  Gallbladder, BF42ZZZ
  Gallbladder and Bile Duct, BF43ZZZ
  Gastrointestinal Tract, BD47ZZZ
  Gland
    Adrenal
      Bilateral, BG42ZZZ
      Left, BG41ZZZ
      Right, BG40ZZZ
    Parathyroid, BG43ZZZ
    Thyroid, BG44ZZZ
  Hand
    Left, Densitometry, BP4PZZ1
    Right, Densitometry, BP4NZZ1
  Head and Neck, BH4CZZZ
  Heart
    Left, B245YZZ
      Intravascular, B245ZZ3
      Transesophageal, B245ZZ4
    Pediatric, B24DYZZ
      Intravascular, B24DZZ3
      Transesophageal, B24DZZ4
    Right, B244YZZ
      Intravascular, B244ZZ3
      Transesophageal, B244ZZ4
    Right and Left, B246YZZ
      Intravascular, B246ZZ3
      Transesophageal, B246ZZ4
  Heart with Aorta, B24BYZZ
    Intravascular, B24BZZ3
    Transesophageal, B24BZZ4
  Hepatobiliary System, All, BF4CZZZ
  Hip
    Bilateral, BQ42ZZZ
    Left, BQ41ZZZ
    Right, BQ40ZZZ
  Kidney
    and Bladder, BT4JZZZ
    Bilateral, BT43ZZZ
    Left, BT42ZZZ
    Right, BT41ZZZ

Ultrasonography — *continued*
  Kidney — *continued*
    Transplant, BT49ZZZ
  Knee
    Bilateral, BQ49ZZZ
    Left, BQ48ZZZ
    Right, BQ47ZZZ
  Liver, BF45ZZZ
  Liver and Spleen, BF46ZZZ
  Mediastinum, BB4CZZZ
  Neck, BW4FZZZ
  Ovary
    Bilateral, BU45
    Left, BU44
    Right, BU43
  Ovary and Uterus, BU4C
  Pancreas, BF47ZZZ
  Pelvic Region, BW4GZZZ
  Pelvis and Abdomen, BW41ZZZ
  Penis, BV4BZZZ
  Pericardium, B24CYZZ
    Intravascular, B24CZZ3
    Transesophageal, B24CZZ4
  Placenta, BY48ZZZ
  Pleura, BB4BZZZ
  Prostate and Seminal Vesicle, BV49ZZZ
  Rectum, BD4CZZZ
  Sacrum, BR4FZZZ
  Scrotum, BV44ZZZ
  Seminal Vesicle and Prostate, BV49ZZZ
  Shoulder
    Left, Densitometry, BP49ZZ1
    Right, Densitometry, BP48ZZ1
  Spinal Cord, B04BZZZ
  Spine
    Cervical, BR40ZZZ
    Lumbar, BR49ZZZ
    Thoracic, BR47ZZZ
  Spleen and Liver, BF46ZZZ
  Stomach, BD42ZZZ
  Tendon
    Lower Extremity, BL43ZZZ
    Upper Extremity, BL42ZZZ
  Ureter
    Bilateral, BT48ZZZ
    Left, BT47ZZZ
    Right, BT46ZZZ
  Urethra, BT45ZZZ
  Uterus, BU46
  Uterus and Ovary, BU4C
  Vein
    Jugular
      Left, Intravascular, B544ZZ3
      Right, Intravascular, B543ZZ3
    Lower Extremity
      Bilateral, Intravascular, B54DZZ3
      Left, Intravascular, B54CZZ3
      Right, Intravascular, B54BZZ3
    Portal, Intravascular, B54TZZ3
    Renal
      Bilateral, Intravascular, B54LZZ3
      Left, Intravascular, B54KZZ3
      Right, Intravascular, B54JZZ3
    Spanchnic, Intravascular, B54TZZ3
    Subclavian
      Left, Intravascular, B547ZZ3
      Right, Intravascular, B546ZZ3
    Upper Extremity
      Bilateral, Intravascular, B54PZZ3
      Left, Intravascular, B54NZZ3
      Right, Intravascular, B54MZZ3
    Vena Cava
      Inferior, Intravascular, B549ZZ3
      Superior, Intravascular, B548ZZ3
    Wrist
      Left, Densitometry, BP4MZZ1
      Right, Densitometry, BP4LZZ1
Ultrasound bone healing system
  use Bone Growth Stimulator in Head and Facial Bones
  use Bone Growth Stimulator in Lower Bones
  use Bone Growth Stimulator in Upper Bones
Ultrasound Therapy
  Heart, 6A75
  No Qualifier, 6A75
  Vessels
    Head and Neck, 6A75
    Other, 6A75
    Peripheral, 6A75
Ultraviolet Light Therapy, Skin, 6A80

Umbilical artery
  use Internal Iliac Artery, Left
  use Internal Iliac Artery, Right
  use Lower Artery
Uniplanar external fixator
  use External Fixation Device, Monoplanar in, 0PH
  use External Fixation Device, Monoplanar in, 0PS
  use External Fixation Device, Monoplanar in, 0QH
  use External Fixation Device, Monoplanar in, 0QS
Upper GI series *see* Fluoroscopy, Gastrointestinal, Upper, BD1-5
Ureteral orifice
  use Ureter
  use Ureter, Left
  use Ureter, Right
  use Ureters, Bilateral
Ureterectomy
  see Excision, Urinary System, 0TB
  see Resection, Urinary System, 0TT
Ureterocolostomy *see* Bypass, Urinary System, 0T1
Ureterocystostomy *see* Bypass, Urinary System, 0T1
Ureteroenterostomy *see* Bypass, Urinary System, 0T1
Ureteroileostomy *see* Bypass, Urinary System, 0T1
Ureterolithotomy *see* Extirpation, Urinary System, 0TC
Ureterolysis *see* Release, Urinary System, 0TN
Ureteroneocystostomy
  see Bypass, Urinary System, 0T1
  see Reposition, Urinary System, 0TS
Ureteropelvic junction (UPJ)
  use Kidney Pelvis, Left
  use Kidney Pelvis, Right
Ureteropexy
  see Repair, Urinary System, 0TQ
  see Reposition, Urinary System, 0TS
Ureteroplasty
  see Repair, Urinary System, 0TQ
  see Replacement, Urinary System, 0TR
  see Supplement, Urinary System, 0TU
Ureteroplication *see* Restriction, Urinary System, 0TV
Ureteropyelography *see* Fluoroscopy, Urinary System, BT1
Ureterorrhaphy *see* Repair, Urinary System, 0TQ
Ureteroscopy, 0TJ98ZZ
Ureterostomy
  see Bypass, Urinary System, 0T1
  see Drainage, Urinary System, 0T9
Ureterotomy *see* Drainage, Urinary System, 0T9
Ureteroureterostomy *see* Bypass, Urinary System, 0T1
Ureterovesical orifice
  use Ureter
  use Ureter, Left
  use Ureter, Right
  use Ureters, Bilateral
Urethral catheterization, indwelling, 0T9B70Z
Urethrectomy
  see Excision, Urethra, 0TBD
  see Resection, Urethra, 0TTD
Urethrolithotomy *see* Extirpation, Urethra, 0TCD
Urethrolysis *see* Release, Urethra, 0TND
Urethropexy
  see Repair, Urethra, 0TQD
  see Reposition, Urethra, 0TSD
Urethroplasty
  see Repair, Urethra, 0TQD
  see Replacement, Urethra, 0TRD
  see Supplement, Urethra, 0TUD
Urethrorrhaphy *see* Repair, Urethra, 0TQD
Urethroscopy, 0TJD8ZZ
Urethrotomy *see* Drainage, Urethra, 0T9D
Uridine Triacetate, XW0DX82
Urinary incontinence stimulator lead *use* Stimulator Lead in Urinary System
Urography *see* Fluoroscopy, Urinary System, BT1
Ustekinumab *use* Other New Technology Therapeutic Substance
Uterine Artery
  use Internal Iliac Artery, Left
  use Internal Iliac Artery, Right
Uterine artery embolization (UAE) *see* Occlusion, Lower Arteries, 04L
Uterine cornu *use* Uterus
Uterine tube
  use Fallopian Tube, Left
  use Fallopian Tube, Right
Uterine vein
  use Hypogastric Vein, Left

Uterine vein — *continued*
  use Hypogastric Vein, Right
Uvulectomy
  see Excision, Uvula, ØCBN
  see Resection, Uvula, ØCTN
Uvulorrhaphy *see* Repair, Uvula, ØCQN
Uvulotomy *see* Drainage, Uvula, ØC9N

V

Vaccination *see* Introduction of Serum, Toxoid, and Vaccine
Vacuum extraction, obstetric, 10D07Z6
Vaginal artery
  use Internal Iliac Artery, Left
  use Internal Iliac Artery, Right
Vaginal pessary *use* Intraluminal Device, Pessary in Female Reproductive System
Vaginal vein
  use Hypogastric Vein, Left
  use Hypogastric Vein, Right
Vaginectomy
  see Excision, Vagina, ØUBG
  see Resection, Vagina, ØUTG
Vaginofixation
  see Repair, Vagina, ØUQG
  see Reposition, Vagina, ØUSG
Vaginoplasty
  see Repair, Vagina, ØUQG
  see Supplement, Vagina, ØUUG
Vaginorrhaphy *see* Repair, Vagina, ØUQG
Vaginoscopy, ØUJH8ZZ
Vaginotomy *see* Drainage, Female Reproductive System, ØU9
Vagotomy *see* Division, Nerve, Vagus, 008Q
Valiant Thoracic Stent Graft *use* Intraluminal Device
Valvotomy, valvulotomy
  see Division, Heart and Great Vessels, Ø28
  see Release, Heart and Great Vessels, Ø2N
Valvuloplasty
  see Repair, Heart and Great Vessels, Ø2Q
  see Replacement, Heart and Great Vessels, Ø2R
  see Supplement, Heart and Great Vessels, Ø2U
Valvuloplasty, Alfieri Stitch *see* Restriction, Valve, Mitral, Ø2VG
Vascular Access Device
  Totally Implantable
    Insertion of device in
      Abdomen, ØJH8
      Chest, ØJH6
      Lower Arm
        Left, ØJHH
        Right, ØJHG
      Lower Leg
        Left, ØJHP
        Right, ØJHN
      Upper Arm
        Left, ØJHF
        Right, ØJHD
      Upper Leg
        Left, ØJHM
        Right, ØJHL
    Removal of device from
      Lower Extremity, ØJPW
      Trunk, ØJPT
      Upper Extremity, ØJPV
    Revision of device in
      Lower Extremity, ØJWW
      Trunk, ØJWT
      Upper Extremity, ØJWV
  Tunneled
    Insertion of device in
      Abdomen, ØJH8
      Chest, ØJH6
      Lower Arm
        Left, ØJHH
        Right, ØJHG
      Lower Leg
        Left, ØJHP
        Right, ØJHN
      Upper Arm
        Left, ØJHF
        Right, ØJHD
      Upper Leg
        Left, ØJHM
        Right, ØJHL

Vascular Access Device — *continued*
  Tunneled — *continued*
    Removal of device from
      Lower Extremity, ØJPW
      Trunk, ØJPT
      Upper Extremity, ØJPV
    Revision of device in
      Lower Extremity, ØJWW
      Trunk, ØJWT
      Upper Extremity, ØJWV
Vasectomy *see* Excision, Male Reproductive System, ØVB
Vasography
  see Fluoroscopy, Male Reproductive System, BV1
  see Plain Radiography, Male Reproductive System, BVØ
Vasoligation *see* Occlusion, Male Reproductive System, ØVL
Vasorrhaphy *see* Repair, Male Reproductive System, ØVQ
Vasostomy *see* Bypass, Male Reproductive System, ØV1
Vasotomy
  With ligation *see* Occlusion, Male Reproductive System, ØVL
  Drainage *see* Drainage, Male Reproductive System, ØV9
Vasovasostomy *see* Repair, Male Reproductive System, ØVQ
Vastus intermedius muscle
  use Upper Leg Muscle, Left
  use Upper Leg Muscle, Right
Vastus lateralis muscle
  use Upper Leg Muscle, Left
  use Upper Leg Muscle, Right
Vastus medialis muscle
  use Upper Leg Muscle, Left
  use Upper Leg Muscle, Right
VCG (vectorcardiogram) *see* Measurement, Cardiac, 4A02
Vectra® Vascular Access Graft *use* Vascular Access Device, Tunneled in Subcutaneous Tissue and Fascia
Venectomy
  see Excision, Lower Veins, Ø6B
  see Excision, Upper Veins, Ø5B
Venography
  see Fluoroscopy, Veins, B51
  see Plain Radiography, Veins, B50
Venorrhaphy
  see Repair, Lower Veins, Ø6Q
  see Repair, Upper Veins, Ø5Q
Venotripsy
  see Occlusion, Lower Veins, Ø6L
  see Occlusion, Upper Veins, Ø5L
Ventricular fold *use* Larynx
Ventriculoatriostomy *see* Bypass, Central Nervous System and Cranial Nerves, 001
Ventriculocisternostomy *see* Bypass, Central Nervous System and Cranial Nerves, 001
Ventriculogram, cardiac
  Combined left and right heart *see* Fluoroscopy, Heart, Right and Left, B216
  Left ventricle *see* Fluoroscopy, Heart, Left, B215
  Right ventricle *see* Fluoroscopy, Heart, Right, B214
Ventriculopuncture, through previously implanted catheter, 8C01X6J
Ventriculoscopy, 00J04ZZ
Ventriculostomy
  External drainage *see* Drainage, Cerebral Ventricle, 0096
  Internal shunt *see* Bypass, Cerebral Ventricle, 0016
Ventriculovenostomy *see* Bypass, Cerebral Ventricle, 0016
Ventrio™ Hernia Patch *use* Synthetic Substitute
VEP (visual evoked potential), 4A07X0Z
Vermiform appendix *use* Appendix
Vermilion border
  use Lower Lip
  use Upper Lip
Versa *use* Pacemaker, Dual Chamber in, ØJH
Version, obstetric
  External, 10S0XZZ
  Internal, 10S07ZZ
Vertebral arch
  use Cervical Vertebra
  use Lumbar Vertebra
  use Thoracic Vertebra
Vertebral body
  use Cervical Vertebra
  use Lumbar Vertebra

Vertebral body — *continued*
  use Thoracic Vertebra
Vertebral canal *use* Spinal Canal
Vertebral foramen
  use Cervical Vertebra
  use Lumbar Vertebra
  use Thoracic Vertebra
Vertebral lamina
  use Cervical Vertebra
  use Lumbar Vertebra
  use Thoracic Vertebra
Vertebral pedicle
  use Cervical Vertebra
  use Lumbar Vertebra
  use Thoracic Vertebra
Vesical vein
  use Hypogastric Vein, Left
  use Hypogastric Vein, Right
Vesicotomy *see* Drainage, Urinary System, ØT9
Vesiculectomy
  see Excision, Male Reproductive System, ØVB
  see Resection, Male Reproductive System, ØVT
Vesiculogram, seminal *see* Plain Radiography, Male Reproductive System, BVØ
Vesiculotomy *see* Drainage, Male Reproductive System, ØV9
Vestibular Assessment, F15Z
Vestibular (Scarpa's) ganglion *use* Acoustic Nerve
Vestibular nerve *use* Acoustic Nerve
Vestibular Treatment, FØC
Vestibulocochlear nerve *use* Acoustic Nerve
VH-IVUS (virtual histology intravascular ultrasound) *see* Ultrasonography, Heart, B24
Virchow's (supraclavicular) lymph node
  use Lymphatic, Left Neck
  use Lymphatic, Right Neck
Virtuoso (II) (DR) (VR) *use* Defibrillator Generator in, ØJH
Vistogard(R) *use* Uridine Triacetate
Vitrectomy
  see Excision, Eye, Ø8B
  see Resection, Eye, Ø8T
Vitreous body
  use Vitreous, Left
  use Vitreous, Right
Viva (XT) (S) *use* Cardiac Resynchronization Defibrillator Pulse Generator in, ØJH
Vocal fold
  use Vocal Cord, Left
  use Vocal Cord, Right
Vocational
  Assessment *see* Activities of Daily Living Assessment, Rehabilitation, FØ2
  Retraining *see* Activities of Daily Living Treatment, Rehabilitation, FØ8
Volar (palmar) digital vein
  use Hand Vein, Left
  use Hand Vein, Right
Volar (palmar) metacarpal vein
  use Hand Vein, Left
  use Hand Vein, Right
Vomer bone *use* Nasal Septum
Vomer of nasal septum *use* Nasal Bone
Voraxaze *use* Glucarpidase
Vulvectomy
  see Excision, Female Reproductive System, ØUB
  see Resection, Female Reproductive System, ØUT
VYXEOS™ *use* Cytarabine and Daunorubicin Liposome Antineoplastic

W

WALLSTENT® Endoprosthesis *use* Intraluminal Device
Washing *see* Irrigation
Wedge resection, pulmonary *see* Excision, Respiratory System, ØBB
Window *see* Drainage
Wiring, dental, 2W31X9Z

X

Xact Carotid Stent System *use* Intraluminal Device
Xenograft *use* Zooplastic Tissue in Heart and Great Vessels
XIENCE Everolimus Eluting Coronary Stent System *use* Intraluminal Device, Drug-eluting in Heart and Great Vessels

 Subterms under main terms may continue to next column or page

Xiphoid process *use* Sternum
XLIF® System *use* Interbody Fusion Device in Lower Joints
X-ray *see* Plain Radiography
X-STOP® Spacer
    use Spinal Stabilization Device, Interspinous Process
       in, ØRH
    use Spinal Stabilization Device, Interspinous Process
       in, ØSH

Y

Yoga Therapy, 8EØZXY4

Z

Zenith AAA Endovascular Graft
    use Intraluminal Device

Zenith AAA Endovascular Graft — *continued*
    use Intraluminal Device, Branched or Fenestrated,
       One or Two Arteries in, Ø4V
    use Intraluminal Device, Branched or Fenestrated,
       Three or More Arteries in, Ø4V
Zenith Flex® AAA Endovascular Graft *use* Intraluminal
    Device
Zenith TX2® TAA Endovascular Graft *use* Intraluminal
    Device
Zenith® Renu™ AAA Ancillary Graft *use* Intraluminal
    Device
**Zilver® PTX® (paclitaxel) Drug-Eluting Peripheral
    Stent**
    use Intraluminal Device, Drug-eluting in Lower Arter-
       ies
    use Intraluminal Device, Drug-eluting in Upper Arter-
       ies
Zimmer® NexGen® LPS Mobile Bearing Knee *use* Syn-
    thetic Substitute

Zimmer® NexGen® LPS-Flex Mobile Knee *use* Synthetic
    Substitute
ZINPLAVA™ *use* Bezlotoxumab Monoclonal Antibody
Zonule of Zinn
    use Lens, Left
    use Lens, Right
**Zooplastic Tissue, Rapid Deployment Technique,
    Replacement**, X2RF
Zotarolimus-eluting Coronary Stent *use* Intraluminal
    Device, Drug-eluting in Heart and Great Vessels
Z-plasty, skin for scar contracture *see* Release, Skin and
    Breast, ØHN
Zygomatic process of frontal bone *use* Frontal Bone
Zygomatic process of temporal bone
    use Temporal Bone, Left
    use Temporal Bone, Right
Zygomaticus muscle *use* Facial Muscle
Zyvox *use* Oxazolidinones

 Subterms under main terms may continue to next column or page

ICD-10-PCS Tables

Central Nervous System and Cranial Nerves 001–00X

Character Meanings

This Character Meaning table is provided as a guide to assist the user in the identification of character members that may be found in this section of code tables. It **SHOULD NOT** be used to build a PCS code.

Operation–Character 3		Body Part–Character 4		Approach–Character 5		Device–Character 6		Qualifier–Character 7	
1	Bypass	0	Brain	0	Open	0	Drainage Device	0	Nasopharynx
2	Change	1	Cerebral Meninges	3	Percutaneous	2	Monitoring Device	1	Mastoid Sinus
5	Destruction	2	Dura Mater	4	Percutaneous Endoscopic	3	Infusion Device	2	Atrium
7	Dilation	3	Epidural Space, Intracranial	X	External	4	Radioactive Element, Cesium-131 Collagen Implant	3	Blood Vessel
8	Division	4	Subdural Space, Intracranial			7	Autologous Tissue Substitute	4	Pleural Cavity
9	Drainage	5	Subarachnoid Space, Intracranial			J	Synthetic Substitute	5	Intestine
B	Excision	6	Cerebral Ventricle			K	Nonautologous Tissue Substitute	6	Peritoneal Cavity
C	Extirpation	7	Cerebral Hemisphere			M	Neurostimulator Lead	7	Urinary Tract
D	Extraction	8	Basal Ganglia			Y	Other Device	8	Bone Marrow
F	Fragmentation	9	Thalamus			Z	No Device	9	Fallopian Tube
H	Insertion	A	Hypothalamus					B	Cerebral Cisterns
J	Inspection	B	Pons					F	Olfactory Nerve
K	Map	C	Cerebellum					G	Optic Nerve
N	Release	D	Medulla Oblongata					H	Oculomotor Nerve
P	Removal	E	Cranial Nerve					J	Trochlear Nerve
Q	Repair	F	Olfactory Nerve					K	Trigeminal Nerve
R	Replacement	G	Optic Nerve					L	Abducens Nerve
S	Reposition	H	Oculomotor Nerve					M	Facial Nerve
T	Resection	J	Trochlear Nerve					N	Acoustic Nerve
U	Supplement	K	Trigeminal Nerve					P	Glossopharyngeal Nerve
W	Revision	L	Abducens Nerve					Q	Vagus Nerve
X	Transfer	M	Facial Nerve					R	Accessory Nerve
		N	Acoustic Nerve					S	Hypoglossal Nerve
		P	Glossopharyngeal Nerve					X	Diagnostic
		Q	Vagus Nerve					Z	No Qualifier
		R	Accessory Nerve						
		S	Hypoglossal Nerve						
		T	Spinal Meninges						
		U	Spinal Canal						
		V	Spinal Cord						
		W	Cervical Spinal Cord						
		X	Thoracic Spinal Cord						
		Y	Lumbar Spinal Cord						

AHA Coding Clinic for table 001

2017, 4Q, 39-41	Dilation and bypass of cerebral ventricle
2015, 2Q, 9	Revision of ventriculoperitoneal (VP) shunt
2013, 2Q, 36	Insertion of ventriculoperitoneal shunt with laparoscopic assistance

AHA Coding Clinic for table 007

2017, 4Q, 39-41	Dilation and bypass of cerebral ventricle

AHA Coding Clinic for table 009

2017, 1Q, 50	Failed lumbar puncture
2015, 3Q, 10	Open evacuation of subdural hematoma
2015, 3Q, 11	Percutaneous drainage of subdural hematoma
2015, 3Q, 12	Subdural evacuation portal system (SEPS) placement
2015, 3Q, 12	Placement of ventriculostomy catheter via burr hole
2015, 2Q, 30	Drainage of syrinx
2015, 1Q, 31	Intrathecal chemotherapy
2014, 1Q, 8	Diagnostic lumbar tap
2014, 1Q, 8	Lumbar drainage port aspiration

AHA Coding Clinic for table 00B

2017, 3Q, 17	Resection of schwannoma and placement of DuraGen and Lorenz cranial plating system
2016, 2Q, 12	Resection of malignant neoplasm of infratemporal fossa
2016, 2Q, 18	Amygdalohippocampectomy
2014, 4Q, 34	Resection of brain malignancy with implantation of chemotherapeutic wafer
2014, 3Q, 24	Repair of lipomyelomeningocele and tethered cord

AHA Coding Clinic for table 00C

2017, 4Q, 48	New and revised body part values - Extirpation spinal canal
2016, 2Q, 29	Decompressive craniectomy with cryopreservation and storage of bone flap
2015, 3Q, 10	Open evacuation of subdural hematoma
2015, 3Q, 11	Percutaneous drainage of subdural hematoma
2015, 3Q, 13	Evacuation of intracerebral hematoma

AHA Coding Clinic for table 00D

2015, 3Q, 13	Nonexcisional debridement of cranial wound with removal and replacement of hardware

AHA Coding Clinic for table 00H

2017, 4Q, 30-31	Radiotherapeutic brain implant
2017, 3Q, 13	Implantation of bilateral neurostimulator electrodes
2014, 3Q, 19	End of life replacement of Baclofen pump

AHA Coding Clinic for table 00J

2017, 1Q, 50	Failed lumbar puncture

AHA Coding Clinic for table 00N

2017, 3Q, 10	Repair of Chiari malformation
2017, 2Q, 23	Decompression of spinal cord and placement of instrumentation
2016, 2Q, 29	Decompressive craniectomy with cryopreservation and storage of bone flap
2015, 2Q, 20	Cervical laminoplasty
2015, 2Q, 21	Multiple decompressive cervical laminectomies
2015, 2Q, 34	Decompressive laminectomy
2014, 3Q, 24	Repair of lipomyelomeningocele and tethered cord

AHA Coding Clinic for table 00P

2014, 3Q, 19	End of life replacement of Baclofen pump

AHA Coding Clinic for table 00Q

2014, 3Q, 7	Hemi-cranioplasty for repair of cranial defect
2013, 3Q, 25	Fracture of frontal bone with repair and coagulation for hemostasis

AHA Coding Clinic for table 00S

2014, 4Q, 35	Reimplantation of buccal nerve

AHA Coding Clinic for table 00U

2018, 1Q, 9	Craniectomy with DuraGaurd placement
2017, 4Q, 62	Added and revised device values - Nerve substitutes
2017, 3Q, 10	Repair of Chiari malformation
2017, 3Q, 17	Resection of schwannoma and placement of DuraGen and Lorenz cranial plating system
2015, 4Q, 39	Dural patch graft
2014, 3Q, 24	Repair of lipomyelomeningocele and tethered cord

Brain

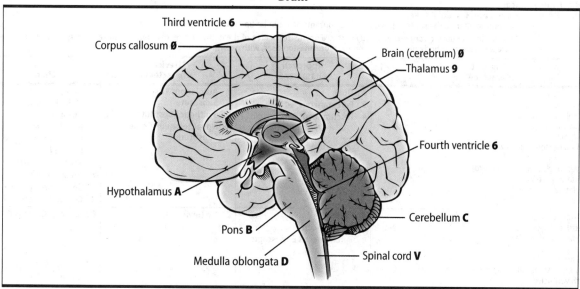

Cranial Nerves

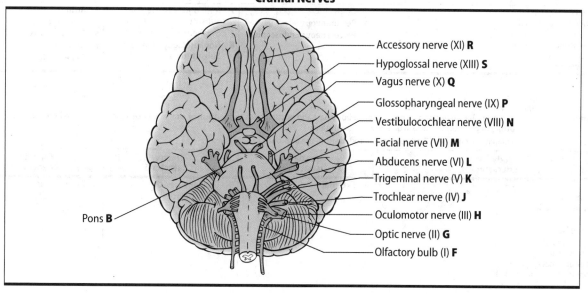

Ø Medical and Surgical
Ø Central Nervous System and Cranial Nerves
1 Bypass   Definition: Altering the route of passage of the contents of a tubular body part

Explanation: Rerouting contents of a body part to a downstream area of the normal route, to a similar route and body part, or to an abnormal route and dissimilar body part. Includes one or more anastomoses, with or without the use of a device.

Body Part Character 4	Approach Character 5	Device Character 6	Qualifier Character 7
6 Cerebral Ventricle Aqueduct of Sylvius Cerebral aqueduct (Sylvius) Choroid plexus Ependyma Foramen of Monro (intraventricular) Fourth ventricle Interventricular foramen (Monro) Left lateral ventricle Right lateral ventricle Third ventricle	**Ø** Open **3** Percutaneous **4** Percutaneous Endoscopic	**7** Autologous Tissue Substitute **J** Synthetic Substitute **K** Nonautologous Tissue Substitute	**Ø** Nasopharynx **1** Mastoid Sinus **2** Atrium **3** Blood Vessel **4** Pleural Cavity **5** Intestine **6** Peritoneal Cavity **7** Urinary Tract **8** Bone Marrow **B** Cerebral Cisterns
6 Cerebral Ventricle Aqueduct of Sylvius Cerebral aqueduct (Sylvius) Choroid plexus Ependyma Foramen of Monro (intraventricular) Fourth ventricle Interventricular foramen (Monro) Left lateral ventricle Right lateral ventricle Third ventricle	**Ø** Open **3** Percutaneous **4** Percutaneous Endoscopic	**Z** No Device	**B** Cerebral Cisterns
U Spinal Canal Epidural space, spinal Extradural space, spinal Subarachnoid space, spinal Subdural space, spinal Vertebral canal	**Ø** Open **3** Percutaneous **4** Percutaneous Endoscopic	**7** Autologous Tissue Substitute **J** Synthetic Substitute **K** Nonautologous Tissue Substitute	**2** Atrium **4** Pleural Cavity **6** Peritoneal Cavity **7** Urinary Tract **9** Fallopian Tube

Ø Medical and Surgical
Ø Central Nervous System and Cranial Nerves
2 Change   Definition: Taking out or off a device from a body part and putting back an identical or similar device in or on the same body part without cutting or puncturing the skin or a mucous membrane

Explanation: All CHANGE procedures are coded using the approach EXTERNAL

Body Part Character 4	Approach Character 5	Device Character 6	Qualifier Character 7
Ø Brain Cerebrum Corpus callosum Encephalon **E Cranial Nerve** **U Spinal Canal** Epidural space, spinal Extradural space, spinal Subarachnoid space, spinal Subdural space, spinal Vertebral canal	**X** External	**Ø** Drainage Device **Y** Other Device	**Z** No Qualifier

Non-OR   All body part, approach, device, and qualifier values

LC Limited Coverage   NC Noncovered   ⊞ Combination Member   HAC associated procedure   Combination Only   DRG Non-OR   Non-OR   New/Revised in GREEN

128   ICD-10-PCS 2019

Ø   **Medical and Surgical**
Ø   **Central Nervous System and Cranial Nerves**
5   **Destruction**   Definition: Physical eradication of all or a portion of a body part by the direct use of energy, force, or a destructive agent
                   Explanation: None of the body part is physically taken out

Body Part Character 4		Approach Character 5	Device Character 6	Qualifier Character 7

Ø Brain
  Cerebrum
  Corpus callosum
  Encephalon
1 Cerebral Meninges
  Arachnoid mater,
    intracranial
  Leptomeninges,
    intracranial
  Pia mater, intracranial
2 Dura Mater
  Diaphragma sellae
  Dura mater, intracranial
  Falx cerebri
  Tentorium cerebelli
6 Cerebral Ventricle
  Aqueduct of Sylvius
  Cerebral aqueduct (Sylvius)
  Choroid plexus
  Ependyma
  Foramen of Monro
    (intraventricular)
  Fourth ventricle
  Interventricular foramen
    (Monro)
  Left lateral ventricle
  Right lateral ventricle
  Third ventricle
7 Cerebral Hemisphere
  Frontal lobe
  Occipital lobe
  Parietal lobe
  Temporal lobe
8 Basal Ganglia
  Basal nuclei
  Claustrum
  Corpus striatum
  Globus pallidus
  Substantia nigra
  Subthalamic nucleus
9 Thalamus
  Epithalamus
  Geniculate nucleus
  Metathalamus
  Pulvinar
A Hypothalamus
  Mammillary body
B Pons
  Apneustic center
  Basis pontis
  Locus ceruleus
  Pneumotaxic center
  Pontine tegmentum
  Superior olivary nucleus
C Cerebellum
  Culmen
D Medulla Oblongata
  Myelencephalon
F Olfactory Nerve
  First cranial nerve
  Olfactory bulb
G Optic Nerve
  Optic chiasma
  Second cranial nerve
	H Oculomotor Nerve
	  Third cranial nerve
	J Trochlear Nerve
	  Fourth cranial nerve
	K Trigeminal Nerve
	  Fifth cranial nerve
	  Gasserian ganglion
	  Mandibular nerve
	  Maxillary nerve
	  Ophthalmic nerve
	  Trifacial nerve
	L Abducens Nerve
	  Sixth cranial nerve
	M Facial Nerve
	  Chorda tympani
	  Geniculate ganglion
	  Greater superficial petrosal
	    nerve
	  Nerve to the stapedius
	  Parotid plexus
	  Posterior auricular nerve
	  Seventh cranial nerve
	  Submandibular ganglion
	N Acoustic Nerve
	  Cochlear nerve
	  Eighth cranial nerve
	  Scarpa's (vestibular)
	    ganglion
	  Spiral ganglion
	  Vestibular (Scarpa's)
	    ganglion
	  Vestibular nerve
	  Vestibulocochlear nerve
	P Glossopharyngeal Nerve
	  Carotid sinus nerve
	  Ninth cranial nerve
	  Tympanic nerve
	Q Vagus Nerve
	  Anterior vagal trunk
	  Pharyngeal plexus
	  Pneumogastric nerve
	  Posterior vagal trunk
	  Pulmonary plexus
	  Recurrent laryngeal nerve
	  Superior laryngeal nerve
	  Tenth cranial nerve
	R Accessory Nerve
	  Eleventh cranial nerve
	S Hypoglossal Nerve
	  Twelfth cranial nerve
	T Spinal Meninges
	  Arachnoid mater, spinal
	  Denticulate (dentate)
	    ligament
	  Dura mater, spinal
	  Filum terminale
	  Leptomeninges, spinal
	  Pia mater, spinal
	W Cervical Spinal Cord
	X Thoracic Spinal Cord
	Y Lumbar Spinal Cord
	  Cauda equina
	  Conus medullaris
		Ø Open
		3 Percutaneous
		4 Percutaneous Endoscopic
			Z No Device	**Z No Qualifier**

Non-OR   Ø05[F,G,H,J,K,L,M,N,P,Q,R,S][Ø,3,4]ZZ

LC Limited Coverage   **NC** Noncovered   ⊞ Combination Member   HAC associated procedure   Combination Only   DRG Non-OR   Non-OR   New/Revised in GREEN

ICD-10-PCS 2019   129

Ø   **Medical and Surgical**
Ø   **Central Nervous System and Cranial Nerves**
7   **Dilation**   Definition: Expanding an orifice or the lumen of a tubular body part

                           Explanation: The orifice can be a natural orifice or an artificially created orifice. Accomplished by stretching a tubular body part using intraluminal pressure or by cutting part of the orifice or wall of the tubular body part.

Body Part Character 4	Approach Character 5	Device Character 6	Qualifier Character 7
6 Cerebral Ventricle Aqueduct of Sylvius Cerebral aqueduct (Sylvius) Choroid plexus Ependyma Foramen of Monro (intraventricular) Fourth ventricle Interventricular foramen (Monro) Left lateral ventricle Right lateral ventricle Third ventricle	**Ø** Open **3** Percutaneous **4** Percutaneous Endoscopic	**Z** No Device	**Z** No Qualifier

Ø   **Medical and Surgical**
Ø   **Central Nervous System and Cranial Nerves**
8   **Division**   Definition: Cutting into a body part, without draining fluids and/or gases from the body part, in order to separate or transect a body part

                           Explanation: All or a portion of the body part is separated into two or more portions

Body Part Character 4	Approach Character 5	Device Character 6	Qualifier Character 7
Ø Brain Cerebrum Corpus callosum Encephalon **7 Cerebral Hemisphere** Frontal lobe Occipital lobe Parietal lobe Temporal lobe **8 Basal Ganglia** Basal nuclei Claustrum Corpus striatum Globus pallidus Substantia nigra Subthalamic nucleus **F Olfactory Nerve** First cranial nerve Olfactory bulb **G Optic Nerve** Optic chiasma Second cranial nerve **H Oculomotor Nerve** Third cranial nerve **J Trochlear Nerve** Fourth cranial nerve **K Trigeminal Nerve** Fifth cranial nerve Gasserian ganglion Mandibular nerve Maxillary nerve Ophthalmic nerve Trifacial nerve **L Abducens Nerve** Sixth cranial nerve **M Facial Nerve** Chorda tympani Geniculate ganglion Greater superficial petrosal nerve Nerve to the stapedius Parotid plexus Posterior auricular nerve Seventh cranial nerve Submandibular ganglion **N Acoustic Nerve** Cochlear nerve Eighth cranial nerve Scarpa's (vestibular) ganglion Spiral ganglion Vestibular (Scarpa's) ganglion Vestibular nerve Vestibulocochlear nerve **P Glossopharyngeal Nerve** Carotid sinus nerve Ninth cranial nerve Tympanic nerve **Q Vagus Nerve** Anterior vagal trunk Pharyngeal plexus Pneumogastric nerve Posterior vagal trunk Pulmonary plexus Recurrent laryngeal nerve Superior laryngeal nerve Tenth cranial nerve **R Accessory Nerve** Eleventh cranial nerve **S Hypoglossal Nerve** Twelfth cranial nerve **W Cervical Spinal Cord** **X Thoracic Spinal Cord** **Y Lumbar Spinal Cord** Cauda equina Conus medullaris	**Ø** Open **3** Percutaneous **4** Percutaneous Endoscopic	**Z** No Device	**Z** No Qualifier

LC Limited Coverage   **NC** Noncovered   ⊞ Combination Member   HAC associated procedure   Combination Only   DRG Non-OR   Non-OR   New/Revised in GREEN

130   ICD-10-PCS 2019

007–008

0   **Medical and Surgical**
0   **Central Nervous System and Cranial Nerves**
9   **Drainage**   Definition: Taking or letting out fluids and/or gases from a body part

Explanation: The qualifier DIAGNOSTIC is used to identify drainage procedures that are biopsies

Body Part Character 4		Approach Character 5	Device Character 6	Qualifier Character 7

0 **Brain**
  Cerebrum
  Corpus callosum
  Encephalon
1 **Cerebral Meninges**
  Arachnoid mater,
    intracranial
  Leptomeninges,
    intracranial
  Pia mater, intracranial
2 **Dura Mater**
  Diaphragma sellae
  Dura mater, intracranial
  Falx cerebri
  Tentorium cerebelli
3 **Epidural Space,**
  Intracranial
  Extradural space,
    intracranial
4 **Subdural Space,**
  Intracranial
5 **Subarachnoid Space,**
  Intracranial
6 **Cerebral Ventricle**
  Aqueduct of Sylvius
  Cerebral aqueduct (Sylvius)
  Choroid plexus
  Ependyma
  Foramen of Monro
    (intraventricular)
  Fourth ventricle
  Interventricular foramen
    (Monro)
  Left lateral ventricle
  Right lateral ventricle
  Third ventricle
7 **Cerebral Hemisphere**
  Frontal lobe
  Occipital lobe
  Parietal lobe
  Temporal lobe
8 **Basal Ganglia**
  Basal nuclei
  Claustrum
  Corpus striatum
  Globus pallidus
  Substantia nigra
  Subthalamic nucleus
9 **Thalamus**
  Epithalamus
  Geniculate nucleus
  Metathalamus
  Pulvinar
A **Hypothalamus**
  Mammillary body
B **Pons**
  Apneustic center
  Basis pontis
  Locus ceruleus
  Pneumotaxic center
  Pontine tegmentum
  Superior olivary nucleus
C **Cerebellum**
  Culmen
D **Medulla Oblongata**
  Myelencephalon
F **Olfactory Nerve**
  First cranial nerve
  Olfactory bulb
	G **Optic Nerve**
	  Optic chiasma
	  Second cranial nerve
	H **Oculomotor Nerve**
	  Third cranial nerve
	J **Trochlear Nerve**
	  Fourth cranial nerve
	K **Trigeminal Nerve**
	  Fifth cranial nerve
	  Gasserian ganglion
	  Mandibular nerve
	  Maxillary nerve
	  Ophthalmic nerve
	  Trifacial nerve
	L **Abducens Nerve**
	  Sixth cranial nerve
	M **Facial Nerve**
	  Chorda tympani
	  Geniculate ganglion
	  Greater superficial petrosal
	    nerve
	  Nerve to the stapedius
	  Parotid plexus
	  Posterior auricular nerve
	  Seventh cranial nerve
	  Submandibular ganglion
	N **Acoustic Nerve**
	  Cochlear nerve
	  Eighth cranial nerve
	  Scarpa's (vestibular) ganglion
	  Spiral ganglion
	  Vestibular (Scarpa's) ganglion
	  Vestibular nerve
	  Vestibulocochlear nerve
	P **Glossopharyngeal Nerve**
	  Carotid sinus nerve
	  Ninth cranial nerve
	  Tympanic nerve
	Q **Vagus Nerve**
	  Anterior vagal trunk
	  Pharyngeal plexus
	  Pneumogastric nerve
	  Posterior vagal trunk
	  Pulmonary plexus
	  Recurrent laryngeal nerve
	  Superior laryngeal nerve
	  Tenth cranial nerve
	R **Accessory Nerve**
	  Eleventh cranial nerve
	S **Hypoglossal Nerve**
	  Twelfth cranial nerve
	T **Spinal Meninges**
	  Arachnoid mater, spinal
	  Denticulate (dentate)
	    ligament
	  Dura mater, spinal
	  Filum terminale
	  Leptomeninges, spinal
	  Pia mater, spinal
	U **Spinal Canal**
	  Epidural space, spinal
	  Extradural space, spinal
	  Subarachnoid space, spinal
	  Subdural space, spinal
	  Vertebral canal
	W **Cervical Spinal Cord**
	X **Thoracic Spinal Cord**
	Y **Lumbar Spinal Cord**
	  Cauda equina
	  Conus medullaris
		0 Open
		3 Percutaneous
		4 Percutaneous Endoscopic
			0 Drainage Device	**Z** No Qualifier

009 Continued on next page

Non-OR   009[T,W,X,Y]30Z
Non-OR   009U[3,4]0Z

Ø   **Medical and Surgical**   *009 Continued*
Ø   **Central Nervous System and Cranial Nerves**
9   **Drainage**   Definition: Taking or letting out fluids and/or gases from a body part
                   Explanation: The qualifier DIAGNOSTIC is used to identify drainage procedures that are biopsies

Body Part Character 4		Approach Character 5	Device Character 6	Qualifier Character 7

Ø Brain
  Cerebrum
  Corpus callosum
  Encephalon
1 Cerebral Meninges
  Arachnoid mater,
    intracranial
  Leptomeninges,
    intracranial
  Pia mater, intracranial
2 Dura Mater
  Diaphragma sellae
  Dura mater, intracranial
  Falx cerebri
  Tentorium cerebelli
3 Epidural Space,
  Intracranial
  Extradural space,
    intracranial
4 Subdural Space,
  Intracranial
5 Subarachnoid Space,
  Intracranial
6 Cerebral Ventricle
  Aqueduct of Sylvius
  Cerebral aqueduct (Sylvius)
  Choroid plexus
  Ependyma
  Foramen of Monro
    (intraventricular)
  Fourth ventricle
  Interventricular foramen
    (Monro)
  Left lateral ventricle
  Right lateral ventricle
  Third ventricle
7 Cerebral Hemisphere
  Frontal lobe
  Occipital lobe
  Parietal lobe
  Temporal lobe
8 Basal Ganglia
  Basal nuclei
  Claustrum
  Corpus striatum
  Globus pallidus
  Substantia nigra
  Subthalamic nucleus
9 Thalamus
  Epithalamus
  Geniculate nucleus
  Metathalamus
  Pulvinar
A Hypothalamus
  Mammillary body
B Pons
  Apneustic center
  Basis pontis
  Locus ceruleus
  Pneumotaxic center
  Pontine tegmentum
  Superior olivary nucleus
C Cerebellum
  Culmen
D Medulla Oblongata
  Myelencephalon
F Olfactory Nerve
  First cranial nerve
  Olfactory bulb
	G Optic Nerve
	  Optic chiasma
	  Second cranial nerve
	H Oculomotor Nerve
	  Third cranial nerve
	J Trochlear Nerve
	  Fourth cranial nerve
	K Trigeminal Nerve
	  Fifth cranial nerve
	  Gasserian ganglion
	  Mandibular nerve
	  Maxillary nerve
	  Ophthalmic nerve
	  Trifacial nerve
	L Abducens Nerve
	  Sixth cranial nerve
	M Facial Nerve
	  Chorda tympani
	  Geniculate ganglion
	  Greater superficial petrosal
	    nerve
	  Nerve to the stapedius
	  Parotid plexus
	  Posterior auricular nerve
	  Seventh cranial nerve
	  Submandibular ganglion
	N Acoustic Nerve
	  Cochlear nerve
	  Eighth cranial nerve
	  Scarpa's (vestibular) ganglion
	  Spiral ganglion
	  Vestibular (Scarpa's) ganglion
	  Vestibular nerve
	  Vestibulocochlear nerve
	P Glossopharyngeal Nerve
	  Carotid sinus nerve
	  Ninth cranial nerve
	  Tympanic nerve
	Q Vagus Nerve
	  Anterior vagal trunk
	  Pharyngeal plexus
	  Pneumogastric nerve
	  Posterior vagal trunk
	  Pulmonary plexus
	  Recurrent laryngeal nerve
	  Superior laryngeal nerve
	  Tenth cranial nerve
	R Accessory Nerve
	  Eleventh cranial nerve
	S Hypoglossal Nerve
	  Twelfth cranial nerve
	T Spinal Meninges
	  Arachnoid mater, spinal
	  Denticulate (dentate)
	    ligament
	  Dura mater, spinal
	  Filum terminale
	  Leptomeninges, spinal
	  Pia mater, spinal
	U Spinal Canal
	  Epidural space, spinal
	  Extradural space, spinal
	  Subarachnoid space, spinal
	  Subdural space, spinal
	  Vertebral canal
	W Cervical Spinal Cord
	X Thoracic Spinal Cord
	Y Lumbar Spinal Cord
	  Cauda equina
	  Conus medullaris
		Ø Open
		3 Percutaneous
		4 Percutaneous Endoscopic
			Z No Device	**X Diagnostic**
				Z No Qualifier

Non-OR   009[Ø,1,2,3,4,5,6,7,8,9,A,B,C,D,F,G,H,J,K,L,M,N,P,Q,R,S][3,4]ZX
Non-OR   009[T,W,X,Y]3Z[X,Z]
Non-OR   009U[3,4]Z[X,Z]

🔲 Limited Coverage   🔲 Noncovered   ⊞ Combination Member   HAC associated procedure   Combination Only   DRG Non-OR   Non-OR   New/Revised in GREEN

132   ICD-10-PCS 2019

0   **Medical and Surgical**
0   **Central Nervous System and Cranial Nerves**
B   **Excision**   Definition: Cutting out or off, without replacement, a portion of a body part

                     Explanation: The qualifier DIAGNOSTIC is used to identify excision procedures that are biopsies

Body Part Character 4		Approach Character 5	Device Character 6	Qualifier Character 7
0 Brain Cerebrum Corpus callosum Encephalon **1 Cerebral Meninges** Arachnoid mater, intracranial Leptomeninges, intracranial Pia mater, intracranial **2 Dura Mater** Diaphragma sellae Dura mater, intracranial Falx cerebri Tentorium cerebelli **6 Cerebral Ventricle** Aqueduct of Sylvius Cerebral aqueduct (Sylvius) Choroid plexus Ependyma Foramen of Monro (intraventricular) Fourth ventricle Interventricular foramen (Monro) Left lateral ventricle Right lateral ventricle Third ventricle **7 Cerebral Hemisphere** Frontal lobe Occipital lobe Parietal lobe Temporal lobe **8 Basal Ganglia** Basal nuclei Claustrum Corpus striatum Globus pallidus Substantia nigra Subthalamic nucleus **9 Thalamus** Epithalamus Geniculate nucleus Metathalamus Pulvinar **A Hypothalamus** Mammillary body **B Pons** Apneustic center Basis pontis Locus ceruleus Pneumotaxic center Pontine tegmentum Superior olivary nucleus **C Cerebellum** Culmen **D Medulla Oblongata** Myelencephalon **F Olfactory Nerve** First cranial nerve Olfactory bulb **G Optic Nerve** Optic chiasma Second cranial nerve	**H Oculomotor Nerve** Third cranial nerve **J Trochlear Nerve** Fourth cranial nerve **K Trigeminal Nerve** Fifth cranial nerve Gasserian ganglion Mandibular nerve Maxillary nerve Ophthalmic nerve Trifacial nerve **L Abducens Nerve** Sixth cranial nerve **M Facial Nerve** Chorda tympani Geniculate ganglion Greater superficial petrosal nerve Nerve to the stapedius Parotid plexus Posterior auricular nerve Seventh cranial nerve Submandibular ganglion **N Acoustic Nerve** Cochlear nerve Eighth cranial nerve Scarpa's (vestibular) ganglion Spiral ganglion Vestibular (Scarpa's) ganglion Vestibular nerve Vestibulocochlear nerve **P Glossopharyngeal Nerve** Carotid sinus nerve Ninth cranial nerve Tympanic nerve **Q Vagus Nerve** Anterior vagal trunk Pharyngeal plexus Pneumogastric nerve Posterior vagal trunk Pulmonary plexus Recurrent laryngeal nerve Superior laryngeal nerve Tenth cranial nerve **R Accessory Nerve** Eleventh cranial nerve **S Hypoglossal Nerve** Twelfth cranial nerve **T Spinal Meninges** Arachnoid mater, spinal Denticulate (dentate) ligament Dura mater, spinal Filum terminale Leptomeninges, spinal Pia mater, spinal **W Cervical Spinal Cord** **X Thoracic Spinal Cord** **Y Lumbar Spinal Cord** Cauda equina Conus medullaris	**0** Open **3** Percutaneous **4** Percutaneous Endoscopic	**Z** No Device	**X** Diagnostic **Z** No Qualifier

Non-OR   00B[0,1,2,6,7,8,9,A,B,C,D,F,G,H,J,K,L,M,N,P,Q,R,S][3,4]ZX

Central Nervous System and Cranial Nerves

0　**Medical and Surgical**
0　**Central Nervous System and Cranial Nerves**
C　**Extirpation**　　　Definition: Taking or cutting out solid matter from a body part

Explanation: The solid matter may be an abnormal byproduct of a biological function or a foreign body; it may be imbedded in a body part or in the lumen of a tubular body part. The solid matter may or may not have been previously broken into pieces.

Body Part Character 4		Approach Character 5	Device Character 6	Qualifier Character 7
0 **Brain**	G **Optic Nerve**	0 Open	Z No Device	Z No Qualifier
Cerebrum	Optic chiasma	3 Percutaneous		
Corpus callosum	Second cranial nerve	4 Percutaneous Endoscopic		
Encephalon	H **Oculomotor Nerve**			
1 **Cerebral Meninges**	Third cranial nerve			
Arachnoid mater, intracranial	J **Trochlear Nerve**			
Leptomeninges, intracranial	Fourth cranial nerve			
Pia mater, intracranial	K **Trigeminal Nerve**			
2 **Dura Mater**	Fifth cranial nerve			
Diaphragma sellae	Gasserian ganglion			
Dura mater, intracranial	Mandibular nerve			
Falx cerebri	Maxillary nerve			
Tentorium cerebelli	Ophthalmic nerve			
3 **Epidural Space, Intracranial**	Trifacial nerve			
Extradural space, intracranial	L **Abducens Nerve**			
	Sixth cranial nerve			
4 **Subdural Space, Intracranial**	M **Facial Nerve**			
5 **Subarachnoid Space, Intracranial**	Chorda tympani			
	Geniculate ganglion			
6 **Cerebral Ventricle**	Greater superficial petrosal nerve			
Aqueduct of Sylvius	Nerve to the stapedius			
Cerebral aqueduct (Sylvius)	Parotid plexus			
Choroid plexus	Posterior auricular nerve			
Ependyma	Seventh cranial nerve			
Foramen of Monro (intraventricular)	Submandibular ganglion			
Fourth ventricle	N **Acoustic Nerve**			
Interventricular foramen (Monro)	Cochlear nerve			
Left lateral ventricle	Eighth cranial nerve			
Right lateral ventricle	Scarpa's (vestibular) ganglion			
Third ventricle	Spiral ganglion			
7 **Cerebral Hemisphere**	Vestibular (Scarpa's) ganglion			
Frontal lobe	Vestibular nerve			
Occipital lobe	Vestibulocochlear nerve			
Parietal lobe	P **Glossopharyngeal Nerve**			
Temporal lobe	Carotid sinus nerve			
8 **Basal Ganglia**	Ninth cranial nerve			
Basal nuclei	Tympanic nerve			
Claustrum	Q **Vagus Nerve**			
Corpus striatum	Anterior vagal trunk			
Globus pallidus	Pharyngeal plexus			
Substantia nigra	Pneumogastric nerve			
Subthalamic nucleus	Posterior vagal trunk			
9 **Thalamus**	Pulmonary plexus			
Epithalamus	Recurrent laryngeal nerve			
Geniculate nucleus	Superior laryngeal nerve			
Metathalamus	Tenth cranial nerve			
Pulvinar	R **Accessory Nerve**			
A **Hypothalamus**	Eleventh cranial nerve			
Mammillary body	S **Hypoglossal Nerve**			
B **Pons**	Twelfth cranial nerve			
Apneustic center	T **Spinal Meninges**			
Basis pontis	Arachnoid mater, spinal			
Locus ceruleus	Denticulate (dentate) ligament			
Pneumotaxic center	Dura mater, spinal			
Pontine tegmentum	Filum terminale			
Superior olivary nucleus	Leptomeninges, spinal			
C **Cerebellum**	Pia mater, spinal			
Culmen	U **Spinal Canal**			
D **Medulla Oblongata**	W **Cervical Spinal Cord**			
Myelencephalon	X **Thoracic Spinal Cord**			
F **Olfactory Nerve**	Y **Lumbar Spinal Cord**			
First cranial nerve	Cauda equina			
Olfactory bulb	Conus medullaris			

0   Medical and Surgical
0   Central Nervous System and Cranial Nerves
D   Extraction   Definition: Pulling or stripping out or off all or a portion of a body part by the use of force

                    Explanation: The qualifier DIAGNOSTIC is used to identify extraction procedures that are biopsies

Body Part Character 4		Approach Character 5	Device Character 6	Qualifier Character 7
1 Cerebral Meninges Arachnoid mater, intracranial Leptomeninges, intracranial Pia mater, intracranial **2 Dura Mater** Diaphragma sellae Dura mater, intracranial Falx cerebri Tentorium cerebelli **F Olfactory Nerve** First cranial nerve Olfactory bulb **G Optic Nerve** Optic chiasma Second cranial nerve **H Oculomotor Nerve** Third cranial nerve **J Trochlear Nerve** Fourth cranial nerve **K Trigeminal Nerve** Fifth cranial nerve Gasserian ganglion Mandibular nerve Maxillary nerve Ophthalmic nerve Trifacial nerve **L Abducens Nerve** Sixth cranial nerve **M Facial Nerve** Chorda tympani Geniculate ganglion Greater superficial petrosal nerve Nerve to the stapedius Parotid plexus Posterior auricular nerve Seventh cranial nerve Submandibular ganglion	**N Acoustic Nerve** Cochlear nerve Eighth cranial nerve Scarpa's (vestibular) ganglion Spiral ganglion Vestibular (Scarpa's) ganglion Vestibular nerve Vestibulocochlear nerve **P Glossopharyngeal Nerve** Carotid sinus nerve Ninth cranial nerve Tympanic nerve **Q Vagus Nerve** Anterior vagal trunk Pharyngeal plexus Pneumogastric nerve Posterior vagal trunk Pulmonary plexus Recurrent laryngeal nerve Superior laryngeal nerve Tenth cranial nerve **R Accessory Nerve** Eleventh cranial nerve **S Hypoglossal Nerve** Twelfth cranial nerve **T Spinal Meninges** Arachnoid mater, spinal Denticulate (dentate) ligament Dura mater, spinal Filum terminale Leptomeninges, spinal Pia mater, spinal	**0 Open** **3 Percutaneous** **4 Percutaneous Endoscopic**	**Z No Device**	**Z No Qualifier**

0   Medical and Surgical
0   Central Nervous System and Cranial Nerves
F   Fragmentation   Definition: Breaking solid matter in a body part into pieces

                    Explanation: Physical force (e.g., manual, ultrasonic) applied directly or indirectly is used to break the solid matter into pieces. The solid matter may be an abnormal byproduct of a biological function or a foreign body. The pieces of solid matter are not taken out.

Body Part Character 4	Approach Character 5	Device Character 6	Qualifier Character 7
3 Epidural Space, Intracranial **NC** Extradural space, intracranial **4 Subdural Space, Intracranial** **NC** **5 Subarachnoid Space, Intracranial** **NC** **6 Cerebral Ventricle** **NC** Aqueduct of Sylvius Cerebral aqueduct (Sylvius) Choroid plexus Ependyma Foramen of Monro (intraventricular) Fourth ventricle Interventricular foramen (Monro) Left lateral ventricle Right lateral ventricle Third ventricle **U Spinal Canal** Epidural space, spinal Extradural space, spinal Subarachnoid space, spinal Subdural space, spinal Vertebral canal	**0 Open** **3 Percutaneous** **4 Percutaneous Endoscopic** **X External**	**Z No Device**	**Z No Qualifier**

Non-OR   00F[3,4,5,6]XZZ
NC   00F[3,4,5,6]XZZ

LC Limited Coverage   **NC** Noncovered   ⊞ Combination Member   HAC associated procedure   Combination Only   DRG Non-OR   Non-OR   New/Revised in GREEN

Central Nervous System and Cranial Nerves

Ø　**Medical and Surgical**
Ø　**Central Nervous System and Cranial Nerves**
H　**Insertion**　　Definition: Putting in a nonbiological appliance that monitors, assists, performs, or prevents a physiological function but does not physically take the place of a body part

Explanation: None

Body Part Character 4		Approach Character 5	Device Character 6	Qualifier Character 7
Ø **Brain** ⊞ Cerebrum Corpus callosum Encephalon		Ø Open	2 Monitoring Device 3 Infusion Device 4 Radioactive Element, 　Cesium-131 Collagen 　Implant M Neurostimulator Lead Y Other Device	Z No Qualifier
Ø **Brain** ⊞ Cerebrum Corpus callosum Encephalon		3 Percutaneous 4 Percutaneous Endoscopic	2 Monitoring Device 3 Infusion Device M Neurostimulator Lead Y Other Device	Z No Qualifier
6 **Cerebral Ventricle** ⊞ Aqueduct of Sylvius Cerebral aqueduct (Sylvius) Choroid plexus Ependyma Foramen of Monro 　(intraventricular) Fourth ventricle Interventricular 　foramen (Monro) Left lateral ventricle Right lateral ventricle Third ventricle	E **Cranial Nerve** ⊞ U **Spinal Canal** ⊞ 　Epidural space, spinal 　Extradural space, spinal 　Subarachnoid space, 　　spinal 　Subdural space, spinal 　Vertebral canal V **Spinal Cord** ⊞	Ø Open 3 Percutaneous 4 Percutaneous Endoscopic	2 Monitoring Device 3 Infusion Device M Neurostimulator Lead Y Other Device	Z No Qualifier

DRG Non-OR	ØØHØØ4Z	**See Appendix L for Procedure Combinations**
Non-OR	ØØH[E,U,V]32Z	⊞　ØØHØØMZ
Non-OR	ØØH[E,U][3,4]YZ	⊞　ØØHØ[3,4]MZ
Non-OR	ØØH[U,V][Ø,3,4]3Z	⊞　ØØH[6,E,U,V][Ø,3,4]MZ

Ø　**Medical and Surgical**
Ø　**Central Nervous System and Cranial Nerves**
J　**Inspection**　　Definition: Visually and/or manually exploring a body part

Explanation: Visual exploration may be performed with or without optical instrumentation. Manual exploration may be performed directly or through intervening body layers.

Body Part Character 4		Approach Character 5	Device Character 6	Qualifier Character 7
Ø **Brain** Cerebrum Corpus callosum Encephalon E **Cranial Nerve**	U **Spinal Canal** 　Epidural space, spinal 　Extradural space, spinal 　Subarachnoid space, spinal 　Subdural space, spinal 　Vertebral canal V **Spinal Cord**	Ø Open 3 Percutaneous 4 Percutaneous Endoscopic	Z No Device	Z No Qualifier

Non-OR	ØØJ[Ø,E,U,V]3ZZ

Ø　**Medical and Surgical**
Ø　**Central Nervous System and Cranial Nerves**
K　**Map**　　Definition: Locating the route of passage of electrical impulses and/or locating functional areas in a body part

Explanation: Applicable only to the cardiac conduction mechanism and the central nervous system

Body Part Character 4		Approach Character 5	Device Character 6	Qualifier Character 7
Ø **Brain** Cerebrum Corpus callosum Encephalon 7 **Cerebral Hemisphere** Frontal lobe Occipital lobe Parietal lobe Temporal lobe 8 **Basal Ganglia** Basal nuclei Claustrum Corpus striatum Globus pallidus Substantia nigra Subthalamic nucleus	9 **Thalamus** Epithalamus Geniculate nucleus Metathalamus Pulvinar A **Hypothalamus** Mammillary body B **Pons** Apneustic center Basis pontis Locus ceruleus Pneumotaxic center Pontine tegmentum Superior olivary nucleus C **Cerebellum** Culmen D **Medulla Oblongata** Myelencephalon	Ø Open 3 Percutaneous 4 Percutaneous Endoscopic	Z No Device	Z No Qualifier

ᴸᶜ Limited Coverage　ᴺᶜ Noncovered　⊞ Combination Member　HAC associated procedure　Combination Only　DRG Non-OR　Non-OR　New/Revised in GREEN

Ø　**Medical and Surgical**
Ø　**Central Nervous System and Cranial Nerves**
N　**Release**　　　Definition: Freeing a body part from an abnormal physical constraint by cutting or by the use of force
　　　　　　　　　　Explanation: Some of the restraining tissue may be taken out but none of the body part is taken out

Body Part Character 4		Approach Character 5	Device Character 6	Qualifier Character 7
Ø **Brain** 　Cerebrum 　Corpus callosum 　Encephalon 1 **Cerebral Meninges** 　Arachnoid mater, 　　intracranial 　Leptomeninges, 　　intracranial 　Pia mater, intracranial 2 **Dura Mater** 　Diaphragma sellae 　Dura mater, intracranial 　Falx cerebri 　Tentorium cerebelli 6 **Cerebral Ventricle** 　Aqueduct of Sylvius 　Cerebral aqueduct (Sylvius) 　Choroid plexus 　Ependyma 　Foramen of Monro 　　(intraventricular) 　Fourth ventricle 　Interventricular foramen 　　(Monro) 　Left lateral ventricle 　Right lateral ventricle 　Third ventricle 7 **Cerebral Hemisphere** 　Frontal lobe 　Occipital lobe 　Parietal lobe 　Temporal lobe 8 **Basal Ganglia** 　Basal nuclei 　Claustrum 　Corpus striatum 　Globus pallidus 　Substantia nigra 　Subthalamic nucleus 9 **Thalamus** 　Epithalamus 　Geniculate nucleus 　Metathalamus 　Pulvinar A **Hypothalamus** 　Mammillary body B **Pons** 　Apneustic center 　Basis pontis 　Locus ceruleus 　Pneumotaxic center 　Pontine tegmentum 　Superior olivary nucleus C **Cerebellum** 　Culmen D **Medulla Oblongata** 　Myelencephalon F **Olfactory Nerve** 　First cranial nerve 　Olfactory bulb G **Optic Nerve** 　Optic chiasma 　Second cranial nerve	H **Oculomotor Nerve** 　Third cranial nerve J **Trochlear Nerve** 　Fourth cranial nerve K **Trigeminal Nerve** 　Fifth cranial nerve 　Gasserian ganglion 　Mandibular nerve 　Maxillary nerve 　Ophthalmic nerve 　Trifacial nerve L **Abducens Nerve** 　Sixth cranial nerve M **Facial Nerve** 　Chorda tympani 　Geniculate ganglion 　Greater superficial petrosal 　　nerve 　Nerve to the stapedius 　Parotid plexus 　Posterior auricular nerve 　Seventh cranial nerve 　Submandibular ganglion N **Acoustic Nerve** 　Cochlear nerve 　Eighth cranial nerve 　Scarpa's (vestibular) 　　ganglion 　Spiral ganglion 　Vestibular (Scarpa's) 　　ganglion 　Vestibular nerve 　Vestibulocochlear nerve P **Glossopharyngeal Nerve** 　Carotid sinus nerve 　Ninth cranial nerve 　Tympanic nerve Q **Vagus Nerve** 　Anterior vagal trunk 　Pharyngeal plexus 　Pneumogastric nerve 　Posterior vagal trunk 　Pulmonary plexus 　Recurrent laryngeal nerve 　Superior laryngeal nerve 　Tenth cranial nerve R **Accessory Nerve** 　Eleventh cranial nerve S **Hypoglossal Nerve** 　Twelfth cranial nerve T **Spinal Meninges** 　Arachnoid mater, spinal 　Denticulate (dentate) 　　ligament 　Dura mater, spinal 　Filum terminale 　Leptomeninges, spinal 　Pia mater, spinal W **Cervical Spinal Cord** X **Thoracic Spinal Cord** Y **Lumbar Spinal Cord** 　Cauda equina 　Conus medullaris	Ø Open 3 Percutaneous 4 Percutaneous Endoscopic	Z No Device	Z No Qualifier

LC Limited Coverage　NC Noncovered　⊞ Combination Member　HAC associated procedure　Combination Only　DRG Non-OR　Non-OR　New/Revised in GREEN

ICD-10-PCS 2019　　　　　　　　　　　　　　　　　　　　　　　　　　　　　　　　　　　　　　137

Central Nervous System and Cranial Nerves

Ø   **Medical and Surgical**
Ø   **Central Nervous System and Cranial Nerves**
P   **Removal**   Definition: Taking out or off a device from a body part

Explanation: If a device is taken out and a similar device put in without cutting or puncturing the skin or mucous membrane, the procedure is coded to the root operation CHANGE. Otherwise, the procedure for taking out a device is coded to the root operation REMOVAL.

Body Part Character 4	Approach Character 5	Device Character 6	Qualifier Character 7
Ø **Brain** Cerebrum Corpus callosum Encephalon V **Spinal Cord**	Ø Open 3 Percutaneous 4 Percutaneous Endoscopic	Ø Drainage Device 2 Monitoring Device 3 Infusion Device 7 Autologous Tissue Substitute J Synthetic Substitute K Nonautologous Tissue Substitute M Neurostimulator Lead Y Other Device	Z No Qualifier
Ø **Brain** Cerebrum Corpus callosum Encephalon V **Spinal Cord**	X External	Ø Drainage Device 2 Monitoring Device 3 Infusion Device M Neurostimulator Lead	Z No Qualifier
6 **Cerebral Ventricle** Aqueduct of Sylvius Cerebral aqueduct (Sylvius) Choroid plexus Ependyma Foramen of Monro (intraventricular) Fourth ventricle Interventricular foramen (Monro) Left lateral ventricle Right lateral ventricle Third ventricle U **Spinal Canal** Epidural space, spinal Extradural space, spinal Subarachnoid space, spinal Subdural space, spinal Vertebral canal	Ø Open 3 Percutaneous 4 Percutaneous Endoscopic	Ø Drainage Device 2 Monitoring Device 3 Infusion Device J Synthetic Substitute M Neurostimulator Lead Y Other Device	Z No Qualifier
6 **Cerebral Ventricle** Aqueduct of Sylvius Cerebral aqueduct (Sylvius) Choroid plexus Ependyma Foramen of Monro (intraventricular) Fourth ventricle Interventricular foramen (Monro) Left lateral ventricle Right lateral ventricle Third ventricle U **Spinal Canal** Epidural space, spinal Extradural space, spinal Subarachnoid space, spinal Subdural space, spinal Vertebral canal	X External	Ø Drainage Device 2 Monitoring Device 3 Infusion Device M Neurostimulator Lead	Z No Qualifier
E **Cranial Nerve**	Ø Open 3 Percutaneous 4 Percutaneous Endoscopic	Ø Drainage Device 2 Monitoring Device 3 Infusion Device 7 Autologous Tissue Substitute M Neurostimulator Lead Y Other Device	Z No Qualifier
E **Cranial Nerve**	X External	Ø Drainage Device 2 Monitoring Device 3 Infusion Device M Neurostimulator Lead	Z No Qualifier

Non-OR   00P[0,V]3[0,2,3]Z
Non-OR   00P[0,V][3,4]YZ
Non-OR   00P[0,V]X[0,2,3,M]Z
Non-OR   00P[6,U]3[0,2,3]Z
Non-OR   00P[6,U][3,4]YZ
Non-OR   00P[6,U]X[0,2,3,M]Z
Non-OR   00PE3[0,2,3]Z
Non-OR   00PE[3,4]YZ
Non-OR   00PEX[0,2,3,M]Z

LC Limited Coverage   NC Noncovered   ⊞ Combination Member   HAC associated procedure   Combination Only   DRG Non-OR   Non-OR   New/Revised in GREEN

Ø Medical and Surgical
Ø Central Nervous System and Cranial Nerves
Q Repair   Definition: Restoring, to the extent possible, a body part to its normal anatomic structure and function

                 Explanation: Used only when the method to accomplish the repair is not one of the other root operations

Body Part Character 4		Approach Character 5	Device Character 6	Qualifier Character 7
Ø Brain Cerebrum Corpus callosum Encephalon **1 Cerebral Meninges** Arachnoid mater, intracranial Leptomeninges, intracranial Pia mater, intracranial **2 Dura Mater** Diaphragma sellae Dura mater, intracranial Falx cerebri Tentorium cerebelli **6 Cerebral Ventricle** Aqueduct of Sylvius Cerebral aqueduct (Sylvius) Choroid plexus Ependyma Foramen of Monro (intraventricular) Fourth ventricle Interventricular foramen (Monro) Left lateral ventricle Right lateral ventricle Third ventricle **7 Cerebral Hemisphere** Frontal lobe Occipital lobe Parietal lobe Temporal lobe **8 Basal Ganglia** Basal nuclei Claustrum Corpus striatum Globus pallidus Substantia nigra Subthalamic nucleus **9 Thalamus** Epithalamus Geniculate nucleus Metathalamus Pulvinar **A Hypothalamus** Mammillary body **B Pons** Apneustic center Basis pontis Locus ceruleus Pneumotaxic center Pontine tegmentum Superior olivary nucleus **C Cerebellum** Culmen **D Medulla Oblongata** Myelencephalon **F Olfactory Nerve** First cranial nerve Olfactory bulb **G Optic Nerve** Optic chiasma Second cranial nerve	**H Oculomotor Nerve** Third cranial nerve **J Trochlear Nerve** Fourth cranial nerve **K Trigeminal Nerve** Fifth cranial nerve Gasserian ganglion Mandibular nerve Maxillary nerve Ophthalmic nerve Trifacial nerve **L Abducens Nerve** Sixth cranial nerve **M Facial Nerve** Chorda tympani Geniculate ganglion Greater superficial petrosal nerve Nerve to the stapedius Parotid plexus Posterior auricular nerve Seventh cranial nerve Submandibular ganglion **N Acoustic Nerve** Cochlear nerve Eighth cranial nerve Scarpa's (vestibular) ganglion Spiral ganglion Vestibular (Scarpa's) ganglion Vestibular nerve Vestibulocochlear nerve **P Glossopharyngeal Nerve** Carotid sinus nerve Ninth cranial nerve Tympanic nerve **Q Vagus Nerve** Anterior vagal trunk Pharyngeal plexus Pneumogastric nerve Posterior vagal trunk Pulmonary plexus Recurrent laryngeal nerve Superior laryngeal nerve Tenth cranial nerve **R Accessory Nerve** Eleventh cranial nerve **S Hypoglossal Nerve** Twelfth cranial nerve **T Spinal Meninges** Arachnoid mater, spinal Denticulate (dentate) ligament Dura mater, spinal Filum terminale Leptomeninges, spinal Pia mater, spinal **W Cervical Spinal Cord** **X Thoracic Spinal Cord** **Y Lumbar Spinal Cord** Cauda equina Conus medullaris	**Ø Open** **3 Percutaneous** **4 Percutaneous Endoscopic**	**Z No Device**	**Z No Qualifier**

LC Limited Coverage   **NC** Noncovered   ⊞ Combination Member   HAC associated procedure   Combination Only   DRG Non-OR   Non-OR   New/Revised in GREEN

Central Nervous System and Cranial Nerves *(side tab)*

0 **Medical and Surgical**
0 **Central Nervous System and Cranial Nerves**
R **Replacement**   Definition: Putting in or on biological or synthetic material that physically takes the place and/or function of all or a portion of a body part

                            Explanation: The body part may have been taken out or replaced, or may be taken out, physically eradicated, or rendered nonfunctional during the REPLACEMENT procedure. A REMOVAL procedure is coded for taking out the device used in a previous replacement procedure.

Body Part Character 4		Approach Character 5	Device Character 6	Qualifier Character 7

1 Cerebral Meninges
  Arachnoid mater,
    intracranial
  Leptomeninges,
    intracranial
  Pia mater, intracranial
2 Dura Mater
  Diaphragma sellae
  Dura mater, intracranial
  Falx cerebri
  Tentorium cerebelli
6 Cerebral Ventricle
  Aqueduct of Sylvius
  Cerebral aqueduct (Sylvius)
  Choroid plexus
  Ependyma
  Foramen of Monro
    (intraventricular)
  Fourth ventricle
  Interventricular foramen
    (Monro)
  Left lateral ventricle
  Right lateral ventricle
  Third ventricle
F Olfactory Nerve
  First cranial nerve
  Olfactory bulb
G Optic Nerve
  Optic chiasma
  Second cranial nerve
H Oculomotor Nerve
  Third cranial nerve
J Trochlear Nerve
  Fourth cranial nerve
K Trigeminal Nerve
  Fifth cranial nerve
  Gasserian ganglion
  Mandibular nerve
  Maxillary nerve
  Ophthalmic nerve
  Trifacial nerve
L Abducens Nerve
  Sixth cranial nerve
	M Facial Nerve
	  Chorda tympani
	  Geniculate ganglion
	  Greater superficial petrosal
	    nerve
	  Nerve to the stapedius
	  Parotid plexus
	  Posterior auricular nerve
	  Seventh cranial nerve
	  Submandibular ganglion
	N Acoustic Nerve
	  Cochlear nerve
	  Eighth cranial nerve
	  Scarpa's (vestibular)
	    ganglion
	  Spiral ganglion
	  Vestibular (Scarpa's)
	    ganglion
	  Vestibular nerve
	  Vestibulocochlear nerve
	P Glossopharyngeal Nerve
	  Carotid sinus nerve
	  Ninth cranial nerve
	  Tympanic nerve
	Q Vagus Nerve
	  Anterior vagal trunk
	  Pharyngeal plexus
	  Pneumogastric nerve
	  Posterior vagal trunk
	  Pulmonary plexus
	  Recurrent laryngeal nerve
	  Superior laryngeal nerve
	  Tenth cranial nerve
	R Accessory Nerve
	  Eleventh cranial nerve
	S Hypoglossal Nerve
	  Twelfth cranial nerve
	T Spinal Meninges
	  Arachnoid mater, spinal
	  Denticulate (dentate)
	    ligament
	  Dura mater, spinal
	  Filum terminale
	  Leptomeninges, spinal
	  Pia mater, spinal
		0 Open
		4 Percutaneous Endoscopic
			7 Autologous Tissue
			  Substitute
			J Synthetic Substitute
			K Nonautologous Tissue
			  Substitute
				Z No Qualifier

0   Medical and Surgical
0   Central Nervous System and Cranial Nerves
S   Reposition   Definition: Moving to its normal location, or other suitable location, all or a portion of a body part

Explanation: The body part is moved to a new location from an abnormal location, or from a normal location where it is not functioning correctly. The body part may or may not be cut out or off to be moved to the new location.

Body Part Character 4		Approach Character 5	Device Character 6	Qualifier Character 7

F   Olfactory Nerve
   First cranial nerve
   Olfactory bulb
G   Optic Nerve
   Optic chiasma
   Second cranial nerve
H   Oculomotor Nerve
   Third cranial nerve
J   Trochlear Nerve
   Fourth cranial nerve
K   Trigeminal Nerve
   Fifth cranial nerve
   Gasserian ganglion
   Mandibular nerve
   Maxillary nerve
   Ophthalmic nerve
   Trifacial nerve
L   Abducens Nerve
   Sixth cranial nerve
M   Facial Nerve
   Chorda tympani
   Geniculate ganglion
   Greater superficial petrosal
      nerve
   Nerve to the stapedius
   Parotid plexus
   Posterior auricular nerve
   Seventh cranial nerve
   Submandibular ganglion
	N Acoustic Nerve
	   Cochlear nerve
	   Eighth cranial nerve
	   Scarpa's (vestibular)
	      ganglion
	   Spiral ganglion
	   Vestibular (Scarpa's)
	      ganglion
	   Vestibular nerve
	   Vestibulocochlear nerve
	P Glossopharyngeal Nerve
	   Carotid sinus nerve
	   Ninth cranial nerve
	   Tympanic nerve
	Q Vagus Nerve
	   Anterior vagal trunk
	   Pharyngeal plexus
	   Pneumogastric nerve
	   Posterior vagal trunk
	   Pulmonary plexus
	   Recurrent laryngeal nerve
	   Superior laryngeal nerve
	   Tenth cranial nerve
	R Accessory Nerve
	   Eleventh cranial nerve
	S Hypoglossal Nerve
	   Twelfth cranial nerve
	W Cervical Spinal Cord
	X Thoracic Spinal Cord
	Y Lumbar Spinal Cord
	   Cauda equina
	   Conus medullaris
		0 Open
		3 Percutaneous
		4 Percutaneous Endoscopic
			Z No Device	**Z No Qualifier**

0   Medical and Surgical
0   Central Nervous System and Cranial Nerves
T   Resection   Definition: Cutting out or off, without replacement, all of a body part

Explanation: None

Body Part Character 4	Approach Character 5	Device Character 6	Qualifier Character 7

7   Cerebral Hemisphere
   Frontal lobe
   Occipital lobe
   Parietal lobe
   Temporal lobe
	0 Open
	3 Percutaneous
	4 Percutaneous Endoscopic
		Z No Device	**Z No Qualifier**

Ø   **Medical and Surgical**
Ø   **Central Nervous System and Cranial Nerves**
U   **Supplement**   Definition: Putting in or on biological or synthetic material that physically reinforces and/or augments the function of a portion of a body part
          Explanation: The biological material is non-living, or is living and from the same individual. The body part may have been previously replaced, and the SUPPLEMENT procedure is performed to physically reinforce and/or augment the function of the replaced body part.

Body Part — Character 4	Approach — Character 5	Device — Character 6	Qualifier — Character 7
1 Cerebral Meninges Arachnoid mater, intracranial; Leptomeninges, intracranial; Pia mater, intracranial **2 Dura Mater** Diaphragma sellae; Dura mater, intracranial; Falx cerebri; Tentorium cerebelli **6 Cerebral Ventricle** Aqueduct of Sylvius; Cerebral aqueduct (Sylvius); Choroid plexus; Ependyma; Foramen of Monro (intraventricular); Fourth ventricle; Interventricular foramen (Monro); Left lateral ventricle; Right lateral ventricle; Third ventricle **F Olfactory Nerve** First cranial nerve; Olfactory bulb **G Optic Nerve** Optic chiasma; Second cranial nerve **H Oculomotor Nerve** Third cranial nerve **J Trochlear Nerve** Fourth cranial nerve **K Trigeminal Nerve** Fifth cranial nerve; Gasserian ganglion; Mandibular nerve; Maxillary nerve; Ophthalmic nerve; Trifacial nerve **L Abducens Nerve** Sixth cranial nerve **M Facial Nerve** Chorda tympani; Geniculate ganglion; Greater superficial petrosal nerve; Nerve to the stapedius; Parotid plexus; Posterior auricular nerve; Seventh cranial nerve; Submandibular ganglion **N Acoustic Nerve** Cochlear nerve; Eighth cranial nerve; Scarpa's (vestibular) ganglion; Spiral ganglion; Vestibular (Scarpa's) ganglion; Vestibular nerve; Vestibulocochlear nerve **P Glossopharyngeal Nerve** Carotid sinus nerve; Ninth cranial nerve; Tympanic nerve **Q Vagus Nerve** Anterior vagal trunk; Pharyngeal plexus; Pneumogastric nerve; Posterior vagal trunk; Pulmonary plexus; Recurrent laryngeal nerve; Superior laryngeal nerve; Tenth cranial nerve **R Accessory Nerve** Eleventh cranial nerve **S Hypoglossal Nerve** Twelfth cranial nerve **T Spinal Meninges** Arachnoid mater, spinal; Denticulate (dentate) ligament; Dura mater, spinal; Filum terminale; Leptomeninges, spinal; Pia mater, spinal	**Ø** Open **3** Percutaneous **4** Percutaneous Endoscopic	**7** Autologous Tissue Substitute **J** Synthetic Substitute **K** Nonautologous Tissue Substitute	**Z** No Qualifier

Ø Medical and Surgical
Ø Central Nervous System and Cranial Nerves
W Revision   Definition: Correcting, to the extent possible, a portion of a malfunctioning device or the position of a displaced device

              Explanation: Revision can include correcting a malfunctioning or displaced device by taking out or putting in components of the device such as a screw or pin

Body Part Character 4	Approach Character 5	Device Character 6	Qualifier Character 7

Ø Brain
  Cerebrum
  Corpus callosum
  Encephalon
V Spinal Cord
	Ø Open
	3 Percutaneous
	4 Percutaneous Endoscopic
		Ø Drainage Device
		2 Monitoring Device
		3 Infusion Device
		7 Autologous Tissue
		    Substitute
		J Synthetic Substitute
		K Nonautologous Tissue
		    Substitute
		M Neurostimulator Lead
		Y Other Device
			Z No Qualifier

Ø Brain
  Cerebrum
  Corpus callosum
  Encephalon
V Spinal Cord
	X External	**Ø** Drainage Device
		2 Monitoring Device
		3 Infusion Device
		7 Autologous Tissue
		    Substitute
		J Synthetic Substitute
		K Nonautologous Tissue
		    Substitute
		M Neurostimulator Lead
			Z No Qualifier

6 Cerebral Ventricle
  Aqueduct of Sylvius
  Cerebral aqueduct (Sylvius)
  Choroid plexus
  Ependyma
  Foramen of Monro (intraventricular)
  Fourth ventricle
  Interventricular foramen (Monro)
  Left lateral ventricle
  Right lateral ventricle
  Third ventricle
U Spinal Canal
  Epidural space, spinal
  Extradural space, spinal
  Subarachnoid space, spinal
  Subdural space, spinal
  Vertebral canal
	Ø Open
	3 Percutaneous
	4 Percutaneous Endoscopic
		Ø Drainage Device
		2 Monitoring Device
		3 Infusion Device
		J Synthetic Substitute
		M Neurostimulator Lead
		Y Other Device
			Z No Qualifier

6 Cerebral Ventricle
  Aqueduct of Sylvius
  Cerebral aqueduct (Sylvius)
  Choroid plexus
  Ependyma
  Foramen of Monro (intraventricular)
  Fourth ventricle
  Interventricular foramen (Monro)
  Left lateral ventricle
  Right lateral ventricle
  Third ventricle
U Spinal Canal
  Epidural space, spinal
  Extradural space, spinal
  Subarachnoid space, spinal
  Subdural space, spinal
  Vertebral canal
	X External	**Ø** Drainage Device
		2 Monitoring Device
		3 Infusion Device
		J Synthetic Substitute
		M Neurostimulator Lead
			Z No Qualifier

E Cranial Nerve	**Ø** Open **3** Percutaneous **4** Percutaneous Endoscopic	**Ø** Drainage Device **2** Monitoring Device **3** Infusion Device **7** Autologous Tissue Substitute **M** Neurostimulator Lead **Y** Other Device	**Z** No Qualifier
E Cranial Nerve	**X** External	**Ø** Drainage Device **2** Monitoring Device **3** Infusion Device **7** Autologous Tissue Substitute **M** Neurostimulator Lead	**Z** No Qualifier

Non-OR   Ø0W[Ø,V][3,4]YZ
Non-OR   Ø0W[Ø,V]X[Ø,2,3,7,J,K,M]Z
Non-OR   Ø0W[6,U][3,4]YZ
Non-OR   Ø0W[6,U]X[Ø,2,3,J,M]Z
Non-OR   Ø0WE[3,4]YZ
Non-OR   Ø0WEX[Ø,2,3,7,M]Z

LC Limited Coverage   NC Noncovered   ⊞ Combination Member   HAC associated procedure   Combination Only   DRG Non-OR   Non-OR   New/Revised in GREEN

Central Nervous System and Cranial Nerves

Ø   **Medical and Surgical**
Ø   **Central Nervous System and Cranial Nerves**
X   **Transfer**   Definition: Moving, without taking out, all or a portion of a body part to another location to take over the function of all or a portion of a body part
                       Explanation: The body part transferred remains connected to its vascular and nervous supply

Body Part Character 4	Approach Character 5	Device Character 6	Qualifier Character 7

F **Olfactory Nerve**
   First cranial nerve
   Olfactory bulb
G **Optic Nerve**
   Optic chiasma
   Second cranial nerve
H **Oculomotor Nerve**
   Third cranial nerve
J **Trochlear Nerve**
   Fourth cranial nerve
K **Trigeminal Nerve**
   Fifth cranial nerve
   Gasserian ganglion
   Mandibular nerve
   Maxillary nerve
   Ophthalmic nerve
   Trifacial nerve
L **Abducens Nerve**
   Sixth cranial nerve
M **Facial Nerve**
   Chorda tympani
   Geniculate ganglion
   Greater superficial petrosal nerve
   Nerve to the stapedius
   Parotid plexus
   Posterior auricular nerve
   Seventh cranial nerve
   Submandibular ganglion
N **Acoustic Nerve**
   Cochlear nerve
   Eighth cranial nerve
   Scarpa's (vestibular) ganglion
   Spiral ganglion
   Vestibular (Scarpa's) ganglion
   Vestibular nerve
   Vestibulocochlear nerve
P **Glossopharyngeal Nerve**
   Carotid sinus nerve
   Ninth cranial nerve
   Tympanic nerve
Q **Vagus Nerve**
   Anterior vagal trunk
   Pharyngeal plexus
   Pneumogastric nerve
   Posterior vagal trunk
   Pulmonary plexus
   Recurrent laryngeal nerve
   Superior laryngeal nerve
   Tenth cranial nerve
R **Accessory Nerve**
   Eleventh cranial nerve
S **Hypoglossal Nerve**
   Twelfth cranial nerve
	Ø Open
	4 Percutaneous Endoscopic
		Z No Device	**F** Olfactory Nerve
			G Optic Nerve
			H Oculomotor Nerve
			J Trochlear Nerve
			K Trigeminal Nerve
			L Abducens Nerve
			M Facial Nerve
			N Acoustic Nerve
			P Glossopharyngeal Nerve
			Q Vagus Nerve
			R Accessory Nerve
			S Hypoglossal Nerve

LC Limited Coverage   **NC** Noncovered   ⊞ Combination Member   HAC associated procedure   Combination Only   DRG Non-OR   Non-OR   New/Revised in GREEN

144   ICD-10-PCS 2019

Peripheral Nervous System Ø12–Ø1X

Character Meanings

This Character Meaning table is provided as a guide to assist the user in the identification of character members that may be found in this section of code tables. It **SHOULD NOT** be used to build a PCS code.

Operation–Character 3	Body Part–Character 4	Approach–Character 5	Device–Character 6	Qualifier–Character 7
2 Change	Ø Cervical Plexus	Ø Open	Ø Drainage Device	1 Cervical Nerve
5 Destruction	1 Cervical Nerve	3 Percutaneous	2 Monitoring Device	2 Phrenic Nerve
8 Division	2 Phrenic Nerve	4 Percutaneous Endoscopic	7 Autologous Tissue Substitute	4 Ulnar Nerve
9 Drainage	3 Brachial Plexus	X External	M Neurostimulator Lead	5 Median Nerve
B Excision	4 Ulnar Nerve		Y Other Device	6 Radial Nerve
C Extirpation	5 Median Nerve		Z No Device	8 Thoracic Nerve
D Extraction	6 Radial Nerve			B Lumbar Nerve
H Insertion	8 Thoracic Nerve			C Perineal Nerve
J Inspection	9 Lumbar Plexus			D Femoral Nerve
N Release	A Lumbosacral Plexus			F Sciatic Nerve
P Removal	B Lumbar Nerve			G Tibial Nerve
Q Repair	C Pudendal Nerve			H Peroneal Nerve
R Replacement	D Femoral Nerve			X Diagnostic
S Reposition	F Sciatic Nerve			Z No Qualifier
U Supplement	G Tibial Nerve			
W Revision	H Peroneal Nerve			
X Transfer	K Head and Neck Sympathetic Nerve			
	L Thoracic Sympathetic Nerve			
	M Abdominal Sympathetic Nerve			
	N Lumbar Sympathetic Nerve			
	P Sacral Sympathetic Nerve			
	Q Sacral Plexus			
	R Sacral Nerve			
	Y Peripheral Nerve			

AHA Coding Clinic for table Ø1B
2018, 2Q, 22   Excision of synovial cyst
2017, 2Q, 19   Thoracic outlet decompression with sympathectomy

AHA Coding Clinic for table Ø1N
2018, 2Q, 22   Excision of synovial cyst
2017, 2Q, 19   Thoracic outlet decompression with sympathectomy
2016, 2Q, 16   Decompressive laminectomy/foraminotomy and lumbar discectomy
2016, 2Q, 17   Removal of longitudinal ligament to decompress cervical nerve root
2016, 2Q, 23   Thoracic outlet syndrome and release of brachial plexus
2015, 2Q, 34   Decompressive laminectomy
2014, 3Q, 33   Radial fracture treatment with open reduction internal fixation, and release of carpal ligament

AHA Coding Clinic for table Ø1U
2017, 4Q, 62   Added and revised device values - Nerve substitutes

Median and Ulnar Nerves

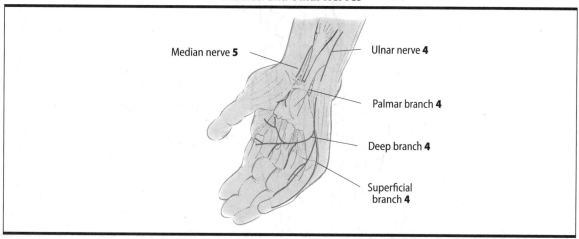

Median nerve **5**

Ulnar nerve **4**

Palmar branch **4**

Deep branch **4**

Superficial branch **4**

Peripheral Nervous System

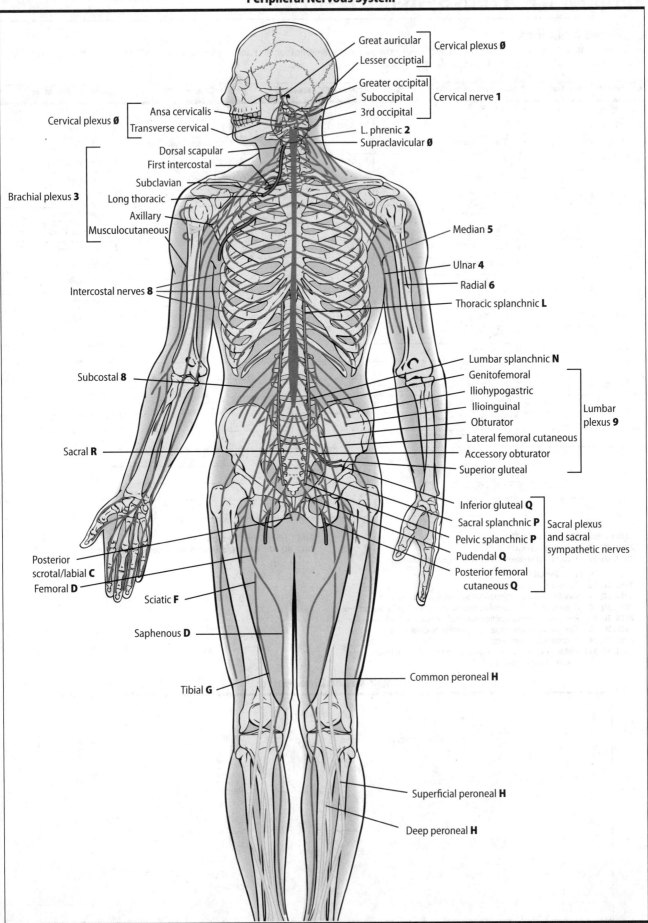

Great auricular — Cervical plexus Ø
Lesser occiptial

Greater occipital
Suboccipital — Cervical nerve 1
3rd occipital

Ansa cervicalis — L. phrenic 2
Cervical plexus Ø — Supraclavicular Ø
Transverse cervical

Dorsal scapular
First intercostal
Subclavian
Brachial plexus 3 — Long thoracic
Axillary
Musculocutaneous

Median 5

Ulnar 4
Radial 6
Thoracic splanchnic L

Intercostal nerves 8

Lumbar splanchnic N
Genitofemoral
Iliohypogastric
Ilioinguinal
Subcostal 8 — Obturator — Lumbar plexus 9
Lateral femoral cutaneous
Accessory obturator
Sacral R — Superior gluteal

Inferior gluteal Q
Sacral splanchnic P — Sacral plexus and sacral sympathetic nerves
Pelvic splanchnic P
Pudendal Q
Posterior — Posterior femoral cutaneous Q
scrotal/labial C
Femoral D
Sciatic F

Saphenous D

Common peroneal H

Tibial G

Superficial peroneal H

Deep peroneal H

Ø   Medical and Surgical
1   Peripheral Nervous System
2   Change   Definition: Taking out or off a device from a body part and putting back an identical or similar device in or on the same body part without cutting or puncturing the skin or a mucous membrane

                     Explanation: All CHANGE procedures are coded using the approach EXTERNAL

Body Part Character 4	Approach Character 5	Device Character 6	Qualifier Character 7
Y Peripheral Nerve	**X** External	**Ø** Drainage Device **Y** Other Device	**Z** No Qualifier

    Non-OR   All body part, approach, device, and qualifier values

---

Ø   Medical and Surgical
1   Peripheral Nervous System
5   Destruction   Definition: Physical eradication of all or a portion of a body part by the direct use of energy, force, or a destructive agent

                     Explanation: None of the body part is physically taken out

Body Part Character 4	Approach Character 5	Device Character 6	Qualifier Character 7

Ø Cervical Plexus
    Ansa cervicalis
    Cutaneous (transverse) cervical nerve
    Great auricular nerve
    Lesser occipital nerve
    Supraclavicular nerve
    Transverse (cutaneous) cervical nerve
1 Cervical Nerve
    Greater occipital nerve
    Spinal nerve, cervical
    Suboccipital nerve
    Third occipital nerve
2 Phrenic Nerve
    Accessory phrenic nerve
3 Brachial Plexus
    Axillary nerve
    Dorsal scapular nerve
    First intercostal nerve
    Long thoracic nerve
    Musculocutaneous nerve
    Subclavius nerve
    Suprascapular nerve
4 Ulnar Nerve
    Cubital nerve
5 Median Nerve
    Anterior interosseous nerve
    Palmar cutaneous nerve
6 Radial Nerve
    Dorsal digital nerve
    Musculospiral nerve
    Palmar cutaneous nerve
    Posterior interosseous nerve
8 Thoracic Nerve
    Intercostal nerve
    Intercostobrachial nerve
    Spinal nerve, thoracic
    Subcostal nerve
9 Lumbar Plexus
    Accessory obturator nerve
    Genitofemoral nerve
    Iliohypogastric nerve
    Ilioinguinal nerve
    Lateral femoral cutaneous nerve
    Obturator nerve
    Superior gluteal nerve
A Lumbosacral Plexus
B Lumbar Nerve
    Lumbosacral trunk
    Spinal nerve, lumbar
    Superior clunic (cluneal) nerve
C Pudendal Nerve
    Posterior labial nerve
    Posterior scrotal nerve
D Femoral Nerve
    Anterior crural nerve
    Saphenous nerve
F Sciatic Nerve
    Ischiatic nerve
G Tibial Nerve
    Lateral plantar nerve
    Medial plantar nerve
    Medial popliteal nerve
    Medial sural cutaneous nerve
 	
H Peroneal Nerve
    Common fibular nerve
    Common peroneal nerve
    External popliteal nerve
    Lateral sural cutaneous nerve
K Head and Neck Sympathetic Nerve
    Cavernous plexus
    Cervical ganglion
    Ciliary ganglion
    Internal carotid plexus
    Otic ganglion
    Pterygopalatine (sphenopalatine)
      ganglion
    Sphenopalatine (pterygopalatine)
      ganglion
    Stellate ganglion
    Submandibular ganglion
    Submaxillary ganglion
L Thoracic Sympathetic Nerve
    Cardiac plexus
    Esophageal plexus
    Greater splanchnic nerve
    Inferior cardiac nerve
    Least splanchnic nerve
    Lesser splanchnic nerve
    Middle cardiac nerve
    Pulmonary plexus
    Superior cardiac nerve
    Thoracic aortic plexus
    Thoracic ganglion
M Abdominal Sympathetic Nerve
    Abdominal aortic plexus
    Auerbach's (myenteric) plexus
    Celiac (solar) plexus
    Celiac ganglion
    Gastric plexus
    Hepatic plexus
    Inferior hypogastric plexus
    Inferior mesenteric ganglion
    Inferior mesenteric plexus
    Meissner's (submucous) plexus
    Myenteric (Auerbach's) plexus
    Pancreatic plexus
    Pelvic splanchnic nerve
    Renal plexus
    Solar (celiac) plexus
    Splenic plexus
    Submucous (Meissner's) plexus
    Superior hypogastric plexus
    Superior mesenteric ganglion
    Superior mesenteric plexus
    Suprarenal plexus
N Lumbar Sympathetic Nerve
    Lumbar ganglion
    Lumbar splanchnic nerve
P Sacral Sympathetic Nerve
    Ganglion impar (ganglion of
      Walther)
    Pelvic splanchnic nerve
    Sacral ganglion
    Sacral splanchnic nerve
Q Sacral Plexus
    Inferior gluteal nerve
    Posterior femoral cutaneous nerve
    Pudendal nerve
R Sacral Nerve
    Spinal nerve, sacral
	Ø Open
	3 Percutaneous
	4 Percutaneous
	     Endoscopic
		Z No Device	**Z** No Qualifier

    Non-OR   Ø15[Ø,2,3,4,5,6,9,A,C,D,F,G,H,Q][Ø,3,4]ZZ   **Non-OR**   Ø15[1,8,B,R]3ZZ

LC Limited Coverage   **NC** Noncovered   ⊞ Combination Member   HAC associated procedure   Combination Only   DRG Non-OR   Non-OR   New/Revised in GREEN

Peripheral Nervous System

Ø   Medical and Surgical
1   Peripheral Nervous System
8   Division   Definition: Cutting into a body part, without draining fluids and/or gases from the body part, in order to separate or transect a body part
                      Explanation: All or a portion of the body part is separated into two or more portions

Body Part Character 4		Approach Character 5	Device Character 6	Qualifier Character 7

Ø Cervical Plexus
Ansa cervicalis
Cutaneous (transverse) cervical
   nerve
Great auricular nerve
Lesser occipital nerve
Supraclavicular nerve
Transverse (cutaneous) cervical
   nerve
1 Cervical Nerve
Greater occipital nerve
Spinal nerve, cervical
Suboccipital nerve
Third occipital nerve
2 Phrenic Nerve
Accessory phrenic nerve
3 Brachial Plexus
Axillary nerve
Dorsal scapular nerve
First intercostal nerve
Long thoracic nerve
Musculocutaneous nerve
Subclavius nerve
Suprascapular nerve
4 Ulnar Nerve
Cubital nerve
5 Median Nerve
Anterior interosseous nerve
Palmar cutaneous nerve
6 Radial Nerve
Dorsal digital nerve
Musculospiral nerve
Palmar cutaneous nerve
Posterior interosseous nerve
8 Thoracic Nerve
Intercostal nerve
Intercostobrachial nerve
Spinal nerve, thoracic
Subcostal nerve
9 Lumbar Plexus
Accessory obturator nerve
Genitofemoral nerve
Iliohypogastric nerve
Ilioinguinal nerve
Lateral femoral cutaneous
   nerve
Obturator nerve
Superior gluteal nerve
A Lumbosacral Plexus
B Lumbar Nerve
Lumbosacral trunk
Spinal nerve, lumbar
Superior clunic (cluneal) nerve
C Pudendal Nerve
Posterior labial nerve
Posterior scrotal nerve
D Femoral Nerve
Anterior crural nerve
Saphenous nerve
F Sciatic Nerve
Ischiatic nerve
	G Tibial Nerve
	Lateral plantar nerve
	Medial plantar nerve
	Medial popliteal nerve
	Medial sural cutaneous nerve
	H Peroneal Nerve
	Common fibular nerve
	Common peroneal nerve
	External popliteal nerve
	Lateral sural cutaneous nerve
	K Head and Neck Sympathetic
	Nerve
	Cavernous plexus
	Cervical ganglion
	Ciliary ganglion
	Internal carotid plexus
	Otic ganglion
	Pterygopalatine
	   (sphenopalatine) ganglion
	Sphenopalatine
	   (pterygopalatine) ganglion
	Stellate ganglion
	Submandibular ganglion
	Submaxillary ganglion
	L Thoracic Sympathetic Nerve
	Cardiac plexus
	Esophageal plexus
	Greater splanchnic nerve
	Inferior cardiac nerve
	Least splanchnic nerve
	Lesser splanchnic nerve
	Middle cardiac nerve
	Pulmonary plexus
	Superior cardiac nerve
	Thoracic aortic plexus
	Thoracic ganglion
	M Abdominal Sympathetic
	Nerve
	Abdominal aortic plexus
	Auerbach's (myenteric) plexus
	Celiac (solar) plexus
	Celiac ganglion
	Gastric plexus
	Hepatic plexus
	Inferior hypogastric plexus
	Inferior mesenteric ganglion
	Inferior mesenteric plexus
	Meissner's (submucous) plexus
	Myenteric (Auerbach's) plexus
	Pancreatic plexus
	Pelvic splanchnic nerve
	Renal plexus
	Solar (celiac) plexus
	Splenic plexus
	Submucous (Meissner's) plexus
	Superior hypogastric plexus
	Superior mesenteric ganglion
	Superior mesenteric plexus
	Suprarenal plexus
	N Lumbar Sympathetic Nerve
	Lumbar ganglion
	Lumbar splanchnic nerve
	P Sacral Sympathetic Nerve
	Ganglion impar (ganglion of
	   Walther)
	Pelvic splanchnic nerve
	Sacral ganglion
	Sacral splanchnic nerve
	Q Sacral Plexus
	Inferior gluteal nerve
	Posterior femoral cutaneous
	   nerve
	Pudendal nerve
	R Sacral Nerve
	Spinal nerve, sacral
		Ø Open
		3 Percutaneous
		4 Percutaneous Endoscopic
			Z No Device	**Z No Qualifier**

LC Limited Coverage   NC Noncovered   ⊞ Combination Member   HAC associated procedure   Combination Only   DRG Non-OR   Non-OR   New/Revised in GREEN

148   ICD-10-PCS 2019

Ø   **Medical and Surgical**
1   **Peripheral Nervous System**
9   **Drainage**   Definition: Taking or letting out fluids and/or gases from a body part
                  Explanation: The qualifier DIAGNOSTIC is used to identify drainage procedures that are biopsies

Body Part Character 4		Approach Character 5	Device Character 6	Qualifier Character 7

Ø Cervical Plexus
  Ansa cervicalis
  Cutaneous (transverse) cervical
    nerve
  Great auricular nerve
  Lesser occipital nerve
  Supraclavicular nerve
  Transverse (cutaneous) cervical
    nerve
1 Cervical Nerve
  Greater occipital nerve
  Spinal nerve, cervical
  Suboccipital nerve
  Third occipital nerve
2 Phrenic Nerve
  Accessory phrenic nerve
3 Brachial Plexus
  Axillary nerve
  Dorsal scapular nerve
  First intercostal nerve
  Long thoracic nerve
  Musculocutaneous nerve
  Subclavius nerve
  Suprascapular nerve
4 Ulnar Nerve
  Cubital nerve
5 Median Nerve
  Anterior interosseous nerve
  Palmar cutaneous nerve
6 Radial Nerve
  Dorsal digital nerve
  Musculospiral nerve
  Palmar cutaneous nerve
  Posterior interosseous nerve
8 Thoracic Nerve
  Intercostal nerve
  Intercostobrachial nerve
  Spinal nerve, thoracic
  Subcostal nerve
9 Lumbar Plexus
  Accessory obturator nerve
  Genitofemoral nerve
  Iliohypogastric nerve
  Ilioinguinal nerve
  Lateral femoral cutaneous
    nerve
  Obturator nerve
  Superior gluteal nerve
A Lumbosacral Plexus
B Lumbar Nerve
  Lumbosacral trunk
  Spinal nerve, lumbar
  Superior clunic (cluneal) nerve
C Pudendal Nerve
  Posterior labial nerve
  Posterior scrotal nerve
D Femoral Nerve
  Anterior crural nerve
  Saphenous nerve
F Sciatic Nerve
  Ischiatic nerve
G Tibial Nerve
  Lateral plantar nerve
  Medial plantar nerve
  Medial popliteal nerve
  Medial sural cutaneous nerve
	H Peroneal Nerve
	  Common fibular nerve
	  Common peroneal nerve
	  External popliteal nerve
	  Lateral sural cutaneous nerve
	**K Head and Neck Sympathetic
	   Nerve**
	  Cavernous plexus
	  Cervical ganglion
	  Ciliary ganglion
	  Internal carotid plexus
	  Otic ganglion
	  Pterygopalatine
	    (sphenopalatine) ganglion
	  Sphenopalatine
	    (pterygopalatine) ganglion
	  Stellate ganglion
	  Submandibular ganglion
	  Submaxillary ganglion
	L Thoracic Sympathetic Nerve
	  Cardiac plexus
	  Esophageal plexus
	  Greater splanchnic nerve
	  Inferior cardiac nerve
	  Least splanchnic nerve
	  Lesser splanchnic nerve
	  Middle cardiac nerve
	  Pulmonary plexus
	  Superior cardiac nerve
	  Thoracic aortic plexus
	  Thoracic ganglion
	**M Abdominal Sympathetic
	   Nerve**
	  Abdominal aortic plexus
	  Auerbach's (myenteric) plexus
	  Celiac (solar) plexus
	  Celiac ganglion
	  Gastric plexus
	  Hepatic plexus
	  Inferior hypogastric plexus
	  Inferior mesenteric ganglion
	  Inferior mesenteric plexus
	  Meissner's (submucous) plexus
	  Myenteric (Auerbach's) plexus
	  Pancreatic plexus
	  Pelvic splanchnic nerve
	  Renal plexus
	  Solar (celiac) plexus
	  Splenic plexus
	  Submucous (Meissner's) plexus
	  Superior hypogastric plexus
	  Superior mesenteric ganglion
	  Superior mesenteric plexus
	  Suprarenal plexus
	N Lumbar Sympathetic Nerve
	  Lumbar ganglion
	  Lumbar splanchnic nerve
	P Sacral Sympathetic Nerve
	  Ganglion impar (ganglion of
	    Walther)
	  Pelvic splanchnic nerve
	  Sacral ganglion
	  Sacral splanchnic nerve
	Q Sacral Plexus
	  Inferior gluteal nerve
	  Posterior femoral cutaneous
	    nerve
	  Pudendal nerve
	R Sacral Nerve
	  Spinal nerve, sacral
		Ø Open
		3 Percutaneous
		4 Percutaneous Endoscopic
			Ø Drainage Device	**Z No Qualifier**

Ø19 Continued on next page

Non-OR   Ø19[Ø,1,2,3,4,5,6,8,9,A,B,C,D,F,G,H,K,L,M,N,P,Q,R]3ØZ

LC Limited Coverage   **NC** Noncovered   ⊞ Combination Member   HAC associated procedure   Combination Only   DRG Non-OR   Non-OR   New/Revised in GREEN
ICD-10-PCS 2019   **149**

Ø19–Ø19

Ø19 Continued

Ø   Medical and Surgical
1   Peripheral Nervous System
9   Drainage   Definition: Taking or letting out fluids and/or gases from a body part
              Explanation: The qualifier DIAGNOSTIC is used to identify drainage procedures that are biopsies

Body Part Character 4		Approach Character 5	Device Character 6	Qualifier Character 7

Ø   Cervical Plexus
Ansa cervicalis
Cutaneous (transverse) cervical
  nerve
Great auricular nerve
Lesser occipital nerve
Supraclavicular nerve
Transverse (cutaneous) cervical
  nerve
1   Cervical Nerve
Greater occipital nerve
Spinal nerve, cervical
Suboccipital nerve
Third occipital nerve
2   Phrenic Nerve
Accessory phrenic nerve
3   Brachial Plexus
Axillary nerve
Dorsal scapular nerve
First intercostal nerve
Long thoracic nerve
Musculocutaneous nerve
Subclavius nerve
Suprascapular nerve
4   Ulnar Nerve
Cubital nerve
5   Median Nerve
Anterior interosseous nerve
Palmar cutaneous nerve
6   Radial Nerve
Dorsal digital nerve
Musculospiral nerve
Palmar cutaneous nerve
Posterior interosseous nerve
8   Thoracic Nerve
Intercostal nerve
Intercostobrachial nerve
Spinal nerve, thoracic
Subcostal nerve
9   Lumbar Plexus
Accessory obturator nerve
Genitofemoral nerve
Iliohypogastric nerve
Ilioinguinal nerve
Lateral femoral cutaneous
  nerve
Obturator nerve
Superior gluteal nerve
A   Lumbosacral Plexus
B   Lumbar Nerve
Lumbosacral trunk
Spinal nerve, lumbar
Superior clunic (cluneal) nerve
C   Pudendal Nerve
Posterior labial nerve
Posterior scrotal nerve
D   Femoral Nerve
Anterior crural nerve
Saphenous nerve
F   Sciatic Nerve
Ischiatic nerve
G   Tibial Nerve
Lateral plantar nerve
Medial plantar nerve
Medial popliteal nerve
Medial sural cutaneous nerve
	H Peroneal Nerve
	Common fibular nerve
	Common peroneal nerve
	External popliteal nerve
	Lateral sural cutaneous nerve
	**K Head and Neck Sympathetic
	   Nerve**
	Cavernous plexus
	Cervical ganglion
	Ciliary ganglion
	Internal carotid plexus
	Otic ganglion
	Pterygopalatine
	  (sphenopalatine) ganglion
	Sphenopalatine
	  (pterygopalatine) ganglion
	Stellate ganglion
	Submandibular ganglion
	Submaxillary ganglion
	L Thoracic Sympathetic Nerve
	Cardiac plexus
	Esophageal plexus
	Greater splanchnic nerve
	Inferior cardiac nerve
	Least splanchnic nerve
	Lesser splanchnic nerve
	Middle cardiac nerve
	Pulmonary plexus
	Superior cardiac nerve
	Thoracic aortic plexus
	Thoracic ganglion
	**M Abdominal Sympathetic
	   Nerve**
	Abdominal aortic plexus
	Auerbach's (myenteric) plexus
	Celiac (solar) plexus
	Celiac ganglion
	Gastric plexus
	Hepatic plexus
	Inferior hypogastric plexus
	Inferior mesenteric ganglion
	Inferior mesenteric plexus
	Meissner's (submucous) plexus
	Myenteric (Auerbach's) plexus
	Pancreatic plexus
	Pelvic splanchnic nerve
	Renal plexus
	Solar (celiac) plexus
	Splenic plexus
	Submucous (Meissner's) plexus
	Superior hypogastric plexus
	Superior mesenteric ganglion
	Superior mesenteric plexus
	Suprarenal plexus
	N Lumbar Sympathetic Nerve
	Lumbar ganglion
	Lumbar splanchnic nerve
	P Sacral Sympathetic Nerve
	Ganglion impar (ganglion of
	  Walther)
	Pelvic splanchnic nerve
	Sacral ganglion
	Sacral splanchnic nerve
	Q Sacral Plexus
	Inferior gluteal nerve
	Posterior femoral cutaneous
	  nerve
	Pudendal nerve
	R Sacral Nerve
	Spinal nerve, sacral
		Ø Open
		3 Percutaneous
		4 Percutaneous Endoscopic
			Z No Device	**X Diagnostic**
				Z No Qualifier

Non-OR	Ø19[Ø,1,2,3,4,5,6,8,9,A,B,C,D,F,G,H,Q,R][3,4]ZX
Non-OR	Ø19[Ø,1,2,3,4,5,6,8,9,A,B,C,D,F,G,H,K,L,M,N,P,Q,R]3ZZ

Ø   Medical and Surgical
1   Peripheral Nervous System
B   Excision   Definition: Cutting out or off, without replacement, a portion of a body part
           Explanation: The qualifier DIAGNOSTIC is used to identify excision procedures that are biopsies

Body Part Character 4		Approach Character 5	Device Character 6	Qualifier Character 7
Ø **Cervical Plexus** Ansa cervicalis Cutaneous (transverse) cervical nerve Great auricular nerve Lesser occipital nerve Supraclavicular nerve Transverse (cutaneous) cervical nerve 1 **Cervical Nerve** Greater occipital nerve Spinal nerve, cervical Suboccipital nerve Third occipital nerve 2 **Phrenic Nerve** Accessory phrenic nerve 3 **Brachial Plexus** Axillary nerve Dorsal scapular nerve First intercostal nerve Long thoracic nerve Musculocutaneous nerve Subclavius nerve Suprascapular nerve 4 **Ulnar Nerve** Cubital nerve 5 **Median Nerve** Anterior interosseous nerve Palmar cutaneous nerve 6 **Radial Nerve** Dorsal digital nerve Musculospiral nerve Palmar cutaneous nerve Posterior interosseous nerve 8 **Thoracic Nerve** Intercostal nerve Intercostobrachial nerve Spinal nerve, thoracic Subcostal nerve 9 **Lumbar Plexus** Accessory obturator nerve Genitofemoral nerve Iliohypogastric nerve Ilioinguinal nerve Lateral femoral cutaneous nerve Obturator nerve Superior gluteal nerve A **Lumbosacral Plexus** B **Lumbar Nerve** Lumbosacral trunk Spinal nerve, lumbar Superior clunic (cluneal) nerve C **Pudendal Nerve** Posterior labial nerve Posterior scrotal nerve D **Femoral Nerve** Anterior crural nerve Saphenous nerve F **Sciatic Nerve** Ischiatic nerve G **Tibial Nerve** Lateral plantar nerve Medial plantar nerve Medial popliteal nerve Medial sural cutaneous nerve	H **Peroneal Nerve** Common fibular nerve Common peroneal nerve External popliteal nerve Lateral sural cutaneous nerve K **Head and Neck Sympathetic Nerve** Cavernous plexus Cervical ganglion Ciliary ganglion Internal carotid plexus Otic ganglion Pterygopalatine (sphenopalatine) ganglion Sphenopalatine (pterygopalatine) ganglion Stellate ganglion Submandibular ganglion Submaxillary ganglion L **Thoracic Sympathetic Nerve** Cardiac plexus Esophageal plexus Greater splanchnic nerve Inferior cardiac nerve Least splanchnic nerve Lesser splanchnic nerve Middle cardiac nerve Pulmonary plexus Superior cardiac nerve Thoracic aortic plexus Thoracic ganglion M **Abdominal Sympathetic Nerve** Abdominal aortic plexus Auerbach's (myenteric) plexus Celiac (solar) plexus Celiac ganglion Gastric plexus Hepatic plexus Inferior hypogastric plexus Inferior mesenteric ganglion Inferior mesenteric plexus Meissner's (submucous) plexus Myenteric (Auerbach's) plexus Pancreatic plexus Pelvic splanchnic nerve Renal plexus Solar (celiac) plexus Splenic plexus Submucous (Meissner's) plexus Superior hypogastric plexus Superior mesenteric ganglion Superior mesenteric plexus Suprarenal plexus N **Lumbar Sympathetic Nerve** Lumbar ganglion Lumbar splanchnic nerve P **Sacral Sympathetic Nerve** Ganglion impar (ganglion of Walther) Pelvic splanchnic nerve Sacral ganglion Sacral splanchnic nerve Q **Sacral Plexus** Inferior gluteal nerve Posterior femoral cutaneous nerve Pudendal nerve R **Sacral Nerve** Spinal nerve, sacral	Ø Open 3 Percutaneous 4 Percutaneous Endoscopic	Z No Device	X Diagnostic Z No Qualifier

Non-OR   01B[Ø,1,2,3,4,5,6,8,9,A,B,C,D,F,G,H,Q,R][3,4]ZX

LC Limited Coverage   NC Noncovered   ⊞ Combination Member   HAC associated procedure   Combination Only   DRG Non-OR   Non-OR   New/Revised in GREEN

Peripheral Nervous System

Ø   Medical and Surgical
1   Peripheral Nervous System
C   Extirpation   Definition: Taking or cutting out solid matter from a body part

Explanation: The solid matter may be an abnormal byproduct of a biological function or a foreign body; it may be imbedded in a body part or in the lumen of a tubular body part. The solid matter may or may not have been previously broken into pieces. .

Body Part Character 4		Approach Character 5	Device Character 6	Qualifier Character 7

Ø Cervical Plexus
  Ansa cervicalis
  Cutaneous (transverse) cervical
    nerve
  Great auricular nerve
  Lesser occipital nerve
  Supraclavicular nerve
  Transverse (cutaneous) cervical
    nerve
1 Cervical Nerve
  Greater occipital nerve
  Spinal nerve, cervical
  Suboccipital nerve
  Third occipital nerve
2 Phrenic Nerve
  Accessory phrenic nerve
3 Brachial Plexus
  Axillary nerve
  Dorsal scapular nerve
  First intercostal nerve
  Long thoracic nerve
  Musculocutaneous nerve
  Subclavius nerve
  Suprascapular nerve
4 Ulnar Nerve
  Cubital nerve
5 Median Nerve
  Anterior interosseous nerve
  Palmar cutaneous nerve
6 Radial Nerve
  Dorsal digital nerve
  Musculospiral nerve
  Palmar cutaneous nerve
  Posterior interosseous nerve
8 Thoracic Nerve
  Intercostal nerve
  Intercostobrachial nerve
  Spinal nerve, thoracic
  Subcostal nerve
9 Lumbar Plexus
  Accessory obturator nerve
  Genitofemoral nerve
  Iliohypogastric nerve
  Ilioinguinal nerve
  Lateral femoral cutaneous
    nerve
  Obturator nerve
  Superior gluteal nerve
A Lumbosacral Plexus
B Lumbar Nerve
  Lumbosacral trunk
  Spinal nerve, lumbar
  Superior clunic (cluneal) nerve
C Pudendal Nerve
  Posterior labial nerve
  Posterior scrotal nerve
D Femoral Nerve
  Anterior crural nerve
  Saphenous nerve
F Sciatic Nerve
  Ischiatic nerve
G Tibial Nerve
  Lateral plantar nerve
  Medial plantar nerve
  Medial popliteal nerve
  Medial sural cutaneous nerve
	H Peroneal Nerve
	  Common fibular nerve
	  Common peroneal nerve
	  External popliteal nerve
	  Lateral sural cutaneous nerve
	K Head and Neck Sympathetic
	  Nerve
	  Cavernous plexus
	  Cervical ganglion
	  Ciliary ganglion
	  Internal carotid plexus
	  Otic ganglion
	  Pterygopalatine
	    (sphenopalatine) ganglion
	  Sphenopalatine
	    (pterygopalatine) ganglion
	  Stellate ganglion
	  Submandibular ganglion
	  Submaxillary ganglion
	L Thoracic Sympathetic Nerve
	  Cardiac plexus
	  Esophageal plexus
	  Greater splanchnic nerve
	  Inferior cardiac nerve
	  Least splanchnic nerve
	  Lesser splanchnic nerve
	  Middle cardiac nerve
	  Pulmonary plexus
	  Superior cardiac nerve
	  Thoracic aortic plexus
	  Thoracic ganglion
	M Abdominal Sympathetic
	  Nerve
	  Abdominal aortic plexus
	  Auerbach's (myenteric) plexus
	  Celiac (solar) plexus
	  Celiac ganglion
	  Gastric plexus
	  Hepatic plexus
	  Inferior hypogastric plexus
	  Inferior mesenteric ganglion
	  Inferior mesenteric plexus
	  Meissner's (submucous) plexus
	  Myenteric (Auerbach's) plexus
	  Pancreatic plexus
	  Pelvic splanchnic nerve
	  Renal plexus
	  Solar (celiac) plexus
	  Splenic plexus
	  Submucous (Meissner's) plexus
	  Superior hypogastric plexus
	  Superior mesenteric ganglion
	  Superior mesenteric plexus
	  Suprarenal plexus
	N Lumbar Sympathetic Nerve
	  Lumbar ganglion
	  Lumbar splanchnic nerve
	P Sacral Sympathetic Nerve
	  Ganglion impar (ganglion of
	    Walther)
	  Pelvic splanchnic nerve
	  Sacral ganglion
	  Sacral splanchnic nerve
	Q Sacral Plexus
	  Inferior gluteal nerve
	  Posterior femoral cutaneous
	    nerve
	  Pudendal nerve
	R Sacral Nerve
	  Spinal nerve, sacral
		Ø Open
		3 Percutaneous
		4 Percutaneous Endoscopic
			Z No Device	**Z No Qualifier**

LC Limited Coverage   NC Noncovered   ⊞ Combination Member   HAC associated procedure   Combination Only   DRG Non-OR   Non-OR   New/Revised in GREEN

152   ICD-10-PCS 2019

01C-01C

0   Medical and Surgical
1   Peripheral Nervous System
D   Extraction   Definition: Pulling or stripping out or off all or a portion of a body part by the use of force
               Explanation: The qualifier DIAGNOSTIC is used to identify extraction procedures that are biopsies

Body Part Character 4		Approach Character 5	Device Character 6	Qualifier Character 7

0 Cervical Plexus
Ansa cervicalis
Cutaneous (transverse) cervical
   nerve
Great auricular nerve
Lesser occipital nerve
Supraclavicular nerve
Transverse (cutaneous) cervical
   nerve
1 Cervical Nerve
Greater occipital nerve
Spinal nerve, cervical
Suboccipital nerve
Third occipital nerve
2 Phrenic Nerve
Accessory phrenic nerve
3 Brachial Plexus
Axillary nerve
Dorsal scapular nerve
First intercostal nerve
Long thoracic nerve
Musculocutaneous nerve
Subclavius nerve
Suprascapular nerve
4 Ulnar Nerve
Cubital nerve
5 Median Nerve
Anterior interosseous nerve
Palmar cutaneous nerve
6 Radial Nerve
Dorsal digital nerve
Musculospiral nerve
Palmar cutaneous nerve
Posterior interosseous nerve
8 Thoracic Nerve
Intercostal nerve
Intercostobrachial nerve
Spinal nerve, thoracic
Subcostal nerve
9 Lumbar Plexus
Accessory obturator nerve
Genitofemoral nerve
Iliohypogastric nerve
Ilioinguinal nerve
Lateral femoral cutaneous nerve
Obturator nerve
Superior gluteal nerve
A Lumbosacral Plexus
B Lumbar Nerve
Lumbosacral trunk
Spinal nerve, lumbar
Superior clunic (cluneal) nerve
C Pudendal Nerve]
Posterior labial nerve
Posterior scrotal nerve
D Femoral Nerve
Anterior crural nerve
Saphenous nerve
F Sciatic Nerve
Ischiatic nerve
G Tibial Nerve
Lateral plantar nerve
Medial plantar nerve
Medial popliteal nerve
Medial sural cutaneous nerve
	H Peroneal Nerve
	Common fibular nerve
	Common peroneal nerve
	External popliteal nerve
	Lateral sural cutaneous nerve
	**K Head and Neck Sympathetic
	Nerve**
	Cavernous plexus
	Cervical ganglion
	Ciliary ganglion
	Internal carotid plexus
	Otic ganglion
	Pterygopalatine
	   (sphenopalatine) ganglion
	Sphenopalatine
	   (pterygopalatine) ganglion
	Stellate ganglion
	Submandibular ganglion
	Submaxillary ganglion
	L Thoracic Sympathetic Nerve
	Cardiac plexus
	Esophageal plexus
	Greater splanchnic nerve
	Inferior cardiac nerve
	Least splanchnic nerve
	Lesser splanchnic nerve
	Middle cardiac nerve
	Pulmonary plexus
	Superior cardiac nerve
	Thoracic aortic plexus
	Thoracic ganglion
	M Abdominal Sympathetic Nerve
	Abdominal aortic plexus
	Auerbach's (myenteric) plexus
	Celiac (solar) plexus
	Celiac ganglion
	Gastric plexus
	Hepatic plexus
	Inferior hypogastric plexus
	Inferior mesenteric ganglion
	Inferior mesenteric plexus
	Meissner's (submucous) plexus
	Myenteric (Auerbach's) plexus
	Pancreatic plexus
	Pelvic splanchnic nerve
	Renal plexus
	Solar (celiac) plexus
	Splenic plexus
	Submucous (Meissner's) plexus
	Superior hypogastric plexus
	Superior mesenteric ganglion
	Superior mesenteric plexus
	Suprarenal plexus
	N Lumbar Sympathetic Nerve
	Lumbar ganglion
	Lumbar splanchnic nerve
	P Sacral Sympathetic Nerve
	Ganglion impar (ganglion of
	   Walther)
	Pelvic splanchnic nerve
	Sacral ganglion
	Sacral splanchnic nerve
	Q Sacral Plexus
	Inferior gluteal nerve
	Posterior femoral cutaneous
	   nerve
	Pudendal nerve
	R Sacral Nerve
	Spinal nerve, sacral
		0 Open
		3 Percutaneous
		4 Percutaneous Endoscopic
			Z No Device	**Z No Qualifier**

LC Limited Coverage   NC Noncovered   ⊞ Combination Member   HAC associated procedure   Combination Only   DRG Non-OR   Non-OR   New/Revised in GREEN

ICD-10-PCS 2019   153

Ø   **Medical and Surgical**
1   **Peripheral Nervous System**
H   **Insertion**   Definition: Putting in a nonbiological appliance that monitors, assists, performs, or prevents a physiological function but does not physically take the place of a body part

                    Explanation: None

Body Part Character 4		Approach Character 5	Device Character 6	Qualifier Character 7
Y Peripheral Nerve	⊞	Ø Open 3 Percutaneous 4 Percutaneous Endoscopic	2 Monitoring Device M Neurostimulator Lead Y Other Device	Z No Qualifier

Non-OR   Ø1HY[3,4]YZ

                                            See Appendix L for Procedure Combinations
                                            ⊞   Ø1HY[Ø,3,4]MZ

Ø   **Medical and Surgical**
1   **Peripheral Nervous System**
J   **Inspection**   Definition: Visually and/or manually exploring a body part

                    Explanation: Visual exploration may be performed with or without optical instrumentation. Manual exploration may be performed directly or through intervening body layers.

Body Part Character 4	Approach Character 5	Device Character 6	Qualifier Character 7
Y Peripheral Nerve	Ø Open 3 Percutaneous 4 Percutaneous Endoscopic	Z No Device	Z No Qualifier

Non-OR   Ø1JY3ZZ

Peripheral Nervous System

Ø   **Medical and Surgical**
1   **Peripheral Nervous System**
N   **Release**   Definition: Freeing a body part from an abnormal physical constraint by cutting or by the use of force
                    Explanation: Some of the restraining tissue may be taken out but none of the body part is taken out

Body Part Character 4		Approach Character 5	Device Character 6	Qualifier Character 7

Ø Cervical Plexus
Ansa cervicalis
Cutaneous (transverse) cervical
   nerve
Great auricular nerve
Lesser occipital nerve
Supraclavicular nerve
Transverse (cutaneous) cervical
   nerve
1 Cervical Nerve
Greater occipital nerve
Spinal nerve, cervical
Suboccipital nerve
Third occipital nerve
2 Phrenic Nerve
Accessory phrenic nerve
3 Brachial Plexus
Axillary nerve
Dorsal scapular nerve
First intercostal nerve
Long thoracic nerve
Musculocutaneous nerve
Subclavius nerve
Suprascapular nerve
4 Ulnar Nerve
Cubital nerve
5 Median Nerve
Anterior interosseous nerve
Palmar cutaneous nerve
6 Radial Nerve
Dorsal digital nerve
Musculospiral nerve
Palmar cutaneous nerve
Posterior interosseous nerve
8 Thoracic Nerve
Intercostal nerve
Intercostobrachial nerve
Spinal nerve, thoracic
Subcostal nerve
9 Lumbar Plexus
Accessory obturator nerve
Genitofemoral nerve
Iliohypogastric nerve
Ilioinguinal nerve
Lateral femoral cutaneous nerve
Obturator nerve
Superior gluteal nerve
A Lumbosacral Plexus
B Lumbar Nerve
Lumbosacral trunk
Spinal nerve, lumbar
Superior clunic (cluneal) nerve
C Pudendal Nerve
Posterior labial nerve
Posterior scrotal nerve
D Femoral Nerve
Anterior crural nerve
Saphenous nerve
F Sciatic Nerve
Ischiatic nerve
G Tibial Nerve
Lateral plantar nerve
Medial plantar nerve
Medial popliteal nerve
Medial sural cutaneous nerve
	H Peroneal Nerve
	Common fibular nerve
	Common peroneal nerve
	External popliteal nerve
	Lateral sural cutaneous nerve
	K Head and Neck Sympathetic Nerve
	Cavernous plexus
	Cervical ganglion
	Ciliary ganglion
	Internal carotid plexus
	Otic ganglion
	Pterygopalatine
	   (sphenopalatine) ganglion
	Sphenopalatine
	   (pterygopalatine) ganglion
	Stellate ganglion
	Submandibular ganglion
	Submaxillary ganglion
	L Thoracic Sympathetic Nerve
	Cardiac plexus
	Esophageal plexus
	Greater splanchnic nerve
	Inferior cardiac nerve
	Least splanchnic nerve
	Lesser splanchnic nerve
	Middle cardiac nerve
	Pulmonary plexus
	Superior cardiac nerve
	Thoracic aortic plexus
	Thoracic ganglion
	M Abdominal Sympathetic Nerve
	Abdominal aortic plexus
	Auerbach's (myenteric) plexus
	Celiac (solar) plexus
	Celiac ganglion
	Gastric plexus
	Hepatic plexus
	Inferior hypogastric plexus
	Inferior mesenteric ganglion
	Inferior mesenteric plexus
	Meissner's (submucous) plexus
	Myenteric (Auerbach's) plexus
	Pancreatic plexus
	Pelvic splanchnic nerve
	Renal plexus
	Solar (celiac) plexus
	Splenic plexus
	Submucous (Meissner's) plexus
	Superior hypogastric plexus
	Superior mesenteric ganglion
	Superior mesenteric plexus
	Suprarenal plexus
	N Lumbar Sympathetic Nerve
	Lumbar ganglion
	Lumbar splanchnic nerve
	P Sacral Sympathetic Nerve
	Ganglion impar (ganglion of
	   Walther)
	Pelvic splanchnic nerve
	Sacral ganglion
	Sacral splanchnic nerve
	Q Sacral Plexus
	Inferior gluteal nerve
	Posterior femoral cutaneous
	   nerve
	Pudendal nerve
	R Sacral Nerve
	Spinal nerve, sacral
		Ø Open
		3 Percutaneous
		4 Percutaneous Endoscopic
			Z No Device	**Z No Qualifier**

Peripheral Nervous System *(left margin)*

Ø   Medical and Surgical
1   Peripheral Nervous System
P   Removal   Definition: Taking out or off a device from a body part

Explanation: If a device is taken out and a similar device put in without cutting or puncturing the skin or mucous membrane, the procedure is coded to the root operation CHANGE. Otherwise, the procedure for taking out a device is coded to the root operation REMOVAL.

Body Part Character 4	Approach Character 5	Device Character 6	Qualifier Character 7
Y Peripheral Nerve	Ø Open 3 Percutaneous 4 Percutaneous Endoscopic	Ø Drainage Device 2 Monitoring Device 7 Autologous Tissue Substitute M Neurostimulator Lead Y Other Device	Z No Qualifier
Y Peripheral Nerve	X External	Ø Drainage Device 2 Monitoring Device M Neurostimulator Lead	Z No Qualifier

Non-OR	Ø1PY3[Ø,2]Z
Non-OR	Ø1PY[3,4]YZ
Non-OR	Ø1PYX[Ø,2,M]Z

01P–01P *(left margin)*

🔲 Limited Coverage   🔲 Noncovered   ⊞ Combination Member   HAC associated procedure   Combination Only   DRG Non-OR   Non-OR   New/Revised in GREEN

156   ICD-10-PCS 2019

0   **Medical and Surgical**
1   **Peripheral Nervous System**
Q   **Repair**   Definition: Restoring, to the extent possible, a body part to its normal anatomic structure and function
                        Explanation: Used only when the method to accomplish the repair is not one of the other root operations

Body Part Character 4		Approach Character 5	Device Character 6	Qualifier Character 7

0 Cervical Plexus
  Ansa cervicalis
  Cutaneous (transverse) cervical
    nerve
  Great auricular nerve
  Lesser occipital nerve
  Supraclavicular nerve
  Transverse (cutaneous) cervical
    nerve
1 Cervical Nerve
  Greater occipital nerve
  Spinal nerve, cervical
  Suboccipital nerve
  Third occipital nerve
2 Phrenic Nerve
  Accessory phrenic nerve
3 Brachial Plexus
  Axillary nerve
  Dorsal scapular nerve
  First intercostal nerve
  Long thoracic nerve
  Musculocutaneous nerve
  Subclavius nerve
  Suprascapular nerve
4 Ulnar Nerve
  Cubital nerve
5 Median Nerve
  Anterior interosseous nerve
  Palmar cutaneous nerve
6 Radial Nerve
  Dorsal digital nerve
  Musculospiral nerve
  Palmar cutaneous nerve
  Posterior interosseous nerve
8 Thoracic Nerve
  Intercostal nerve
  Intercostobrachial nerve
  Spinal nerve, thoracic
  Subcostal nerve
9 Lumbar Plexus
  Accessory obturator nerve
  Genitofemoral nerve
  Iliohypogastric nerve
  Ilioinguinal nerve
  Lateral femoral cutaneous
    nerve
  Obturator nerve
  Superior gluteal nerve
A Lumbosacral Plexus
B Lumbar Nerve
  Lumbosacral trunk
  Spinal nerve, lumbar
  Superior clunic (cluneal) nerve
C Pudendal Nerve
  Posterior labial nerve
  Posterior scrotal nerve
D Femoral Nerve
  Anterior crural nerve
  Saphenous nerve
F Sciatic Nerve
  Ischiatic nerve
G Tibial Nerve
  Lateral plantar nerve
  Medial plantar nerve
  Medial popliteal nerve
  Medial sural cutaneous nerve
	H Peroneal Nerve
	  Common fibular nerve
	  Common peroneal nerve
	  External popliteal nerve
	  Lateral sural cutaneous nerve
	K Head and Neck Sympathetic
	  Nerve
	  Cavernous plexus
	  Cervical ganglion
	  Ciliary ganglion
	  Internal carotid plexus
	  Otic ganglion
	  Pterygopalatine
	    (sphenopalatine) ganglion
	  Sphenopalatine
	    (pterygopalatine) ganglion
	  Stellate ganglion
	  Submandibular ganglion
	  Submaxillary ganglion
	L Thoracic Sympathetic Nerve
	  Cardiac plexus
	  Esophageal plexus
	  Greater splanchnic nerve
	  Inferior cardiac nerve
	  Least splanchnic nerve
	  Lesser splanchnic nerve
	  Middle cardiac nerve
	  Pulmonary plexus
	  Superior cardiac nerve
	  Thoracic aortic plexus
	  Thoracic ganglion
	M Abdominal Sympathetic
	  Nerve
	  Abdominal aortic plexus
	  Auerbach's (myenteric) plexus
	  Celiac (solar) plexus
	  Celiac ganglion
	  Gastric plexus
	  Hepatic plexus
	  Inferior hypogastric plexus
	  Inferior mesenteric ganglion
	  Inferior mesenteric plexus
	  Meissner's (submucous) plexus
	  Myenteric (Auerbach's) plexus
	  Pancreatic plexus
	  Pelvic splanchnic nerve
	  Renal plexus
	  Solar (celiac) plexus
	  Splenic plexus
	  Submucous (Meissner's) plexus
	  Superior hypogastric plexus
	  Superior mesenteric ganglion
	  Superior mesenteric plexus
	  Suprarenal plexus
	N Lumbar Sympathetic Nerve
	  Lumbar ganglion
	  Lumbar splanchnic nerve
	P Sacral Sympathetic Nerve
	  Ganglion impar (ganglion of
	    Walther)
	  Pelvic splanchnic nerve
	  Sacral ganglion
	  Sacral splanchnic nerve
	Q Sacral Plexus
	  Inferior gluteal nerve
	  Posterior femoral cutaneous
	    nerve
	  Pudendal nerve
	R Sacral Nerve
	  Spinal nerve, sacral
		0 Open
		3 Percutaneous
		4 Percutaneous Endoscopic
			Z No Device	**Z No Qualifier**

LC Limited Coverage   **NC** Noncovered   ⊞ Combination Member   HAC associated procedure   Combination Only   DRG Non-OR   Non-OR   New/Revised in GREEN

ICD-10-PCS 2019   157

01Q-01Q

Peripheral Nervous System

0   **Medical and Surgical**
1   **Peripheral Nervous System**
R   **Replacement**   Definition: Putting in or on biological or synthetic material that physically takes the place and/or function of all or a portion of a body part
                         Explanation: The body part may have been taken out or replaced, or may be taken out, physically eradicated, or rendered nonfunctional during the REPLACEMENT procedure. A REMOVAL procedure is coded for taking out the device used in a previous replacement procedure.

Body Part Character 4	Approach Character 5	Device Character 6	Qualifier Character 7

1   **Cervical Nerve**
    Greater occipital nerve
    Spinal nerve, cervical
    Suboccipital nerve
    Third occipital nerve
2   **Phrenic Nerve**
    Accessory phrenic nerve
4   **Ulnar Nerve**
    Cubital nerve
5   **Median Nerve**
    Anterior interosseous nerve
    Palmar cutaneous nerve
6   **Radial Nerve**
    Dorsal digital nerve
    Musculospiral nerve
    Palmar cutaneous nerve
    Posterior interosseous nerve
8   **Thoracic Nerve**
    Intercostal nerve
    Intercostobrachial nerve
    Spinal nerve, thoracic
    Subcostal nerve
B   **Lumbar Nerve**
    Lumbosacral trunk
    Spinal nerve, lumbar
    Superior clunic (cluneal) nerve
C   **Pudendal Nerve**
    Posterior labial nerve
    Posterior scrotal nerve
D   **Femoral Nerve**
    Anterior crural nerve
    Saphenous nerve
F   **Sciatic Nerve**
    Ischiatic nerve
G   **Tibial Nerve**
    Lateral plantar nerve
    Medial plantar nerve
    Medial popliteal nerve
    Medial sural cutaneous nerve
H   **Peroneal Nerve**
    Common fibular nerve
    Common peroneal nerve
    External popliteal nerve
    Lateral sural cutaneous nerve
R   **Sacral Nerve**
    Spinal nerve, sacral
	0 Open
	4 Percutaneous Endoscopic
		7 Autologous Tissue Substitute
		J Synthetic Substitute
		K Nonautologous Tissue Substitute
			Z No Qualifier

0   Medical and Surgical
1   Peripheral Nervous System
S   Reposition   Definition: Moving to its normal location, or other suitable location, all or a portion of a body part

Explanation: The body part is moved to a new location from an abnormal location, or from a normal location where it is not functioning correctly. The body part may or may not be cut out or off to be moved to the new location.

Body Part Character 4	Approach Character 5	Device Character 6	Qualifier Character 7

0 Cervical Plexus
  Ansa cervicalis
  Cutaneous (transverse) cervical nerve
  Great auricular nerve
  Lesser occipital nerve
  Supraclavicular nerve
  Transverse (cutaneous) cervical nerve
1 Cervical Nerve
  Greater occipital nerve
  Spinal nerve, cervical
  Suboccipital nerve
  Third occipital nerve
2 Phrenic Nerve
  Accessory phrenic nerve
3 Brachial Plexus
  Axillary nerve
  Dorsal scapular nerve
  First intercostal nerve
  Long thoracic nerve
  Musculocutaneous nerve
  Subclavius nerve
  Suprascapular nerve
4 Ulnar Nerve
  Cubital nerve
5 Median Nerve
  Anterior interosseous nerve
  Palmar cutaneous nerve
6 Radial Nerve
  Dorsal digital nerve
  Musculospiral nerve
  Palmar cutaneous nerve
  Posterior interosseous nerve
8 Thoracic Nerve
  Intercostal nerve
  Intercostobrachial nerve
  Spinal nerve, thoracic
  Subcostal nerve
9 Lumbar Plexus
  Accessory obturator nerve
  Genitofemoral nerve
  Iliohypogastric nerve
  Ilioinguinal nerve
  Lateral femoral cutaneous nerve
  Obturator nerve
  Superior gluteal nerve
A Lumbosacral Plexus
B Lumbar Nerve
  Lumbosacral trunk
  Spinal nerve, lumbar
  Superior clunic (cluneal) nerve
C Pudendal Nerve
  Posterior labial nerve
  Posterior scrotal nerve
D Femoral Nerve
  Anterior crural nerve
  Saphenous nerve
F Sciatic Nerve
  Ischiatic nerve
G Tibial Nerve
  Lateral plantar nerve
  Medial plantar nerve
  Medial popliteal nerve
  Medial sural cutaneous nerve
H Peroneal Nerve
  Common fibular nerve
  Common peroneal nerve
  External popliteal nerve
  Lateral sural cutaneous nerve
Q Sacral Plexus
  Inferior gluteal nerve
  Posterior femoral cutaneous nerve
  Pudendal nerve
R Sacral Nerve
  Spinal nerve, sacral
	0 Open
	3 Percutaneous
	4 Percutaneous Endoscopic
		Z No Device	**Z No Qualifier**

LC Limited Coverage   NC Noncovered   ⊞ Combination Member   HAC associated procedure   Combination Only   DRG Non-OR   Non-OR   New/Revised in GREEN

ICD-10-PCS 2019   159

0   Medical and Surgical
1   Peripheral Nervous System
U   Supplement   Definition: Putting in or on biological or synthetic material that physically reinforces and/or augments the function of a portion of a body part

Explanation: The biological material is non-living, or is living and from the same individual. The body part may have been previously replaced, and the SUPPLEMENT procedure is performed to physically reinforce and/or augment the function of the replaced body part.

Body Part Character 4	Approach Character 5	Device Character 6	Qualifier Character 7

1 Cervical Nerve
  Greater occipital nerve
  Spinal nerve, cervical
  Suboccipital nerve
  Third occipital nerve
2 Phrenic Nerve
  Accessory phrenic nerve
4 Ulnar Nerve
  Cubital nerve
5 Median Nerve
  Anterior interosseous nerve
  Palmar cutaneous nerve
6 Radial Nerve
  Dorsal digital nerve
  Musculospiral nerve
  Palmar cutaneous nerve
  Posterior interosseous nerve
8 Thoracic Nerve
  Intercostal nerve
  Intercostobrachial nerve
  Spinal nerve, thoracic
  Subcostal nerve
B Lumbar Nerve
  Lumbosacral trunk
  Spinal nerve, lumbar
  Superior clunic (cluneal) nerve
C Pudendal Nerve
  Posterior labial nerve
  Posterior scrotal nerve
D Femoral Nerve
  Anterior crural nerve
  Saphenous nerve
F Sciatic Nerve
  Ischiatic nerve
G Tibial Nerve
  Lateral plantar nerve
  Medial plantar nerve
  Medial popliteal nerve
  Medial sural cutaneous nerve
H Peroneal Nerve
  Common fibular nerve
  Common peroneal nerve
  External popliteal nerve
  Lateral sural cutaneous nerve
R Sacral Nerve
  Spinal nerve, sacral
	0 Open
	3 Percutaneous
	4 Percutaneous Endoscopic
		7 Autologous Tissue Substitute
		J Synthetic Substitute
		K Nonautologous Tissue Substitute
			Z No Qualifier

0   Medical and Surgical
1   Peripheral Nervous System
W   Revision   Definition: Correcting, to the extent possible, a portion of a malfunctioning device or the position of a displaced device

Explanation: Revision can include correcting a malfunctioning or displaced device by taking out or putting in components of the device such as a screw or pin

Body Part Character 4	Approach Character 5	Device Character 6	Qualifier Character 7
Y Peripheral Nerve	**0 Open** **3 Percutaneous** **4 Percutaneous Endoscopic**	**0 Drainage Device** **2 Monitoring Device** **7 Autologous Tissue Substitute** **M Neurostimulator Lead** **Y Other Device**	**Z No Qualifier**
Y Peripheral Nerve	**X External**	**0 Drainage Device** **2 Monitoring Device** **7 Autologous Tissue Substitute** **M Neurostimulator Lead**	**Z No Qualifier**

Non-OR   01WY[3,4]YZ
Non-OR   01WYX[0,2,7,M]Z

LC Limited Coverage   NC Noncovered   ⊞ Combination Member   HAC associated procedure   Combination Only   DRG Non-OR   Non-OR   New/Revised in GREEN

160   ICD-10-PCS 2019

0   Medical and Surgical
1   Peripheral Nervous System
X   Transfer   Definition: Moving, without taking out, all or a portion of a body part to another location to take over the function of all or a portion of a body part
                      Explanation: The body part transferred remains connected to its vascular and nervous supply

Body Part Character 4	Approach Character 5	Device Character 6	Qualifier Character 7

1   Cervical Nerve
    Greater occipital nerve
    Spinal nerve, cervical
    Suboccipital nerve
    Third occipital nerve
2   Phrenic Nerve
    Accessory phrenic nerve
	0 Open
	4 Percutaneous Endoscopic
		Z No Device	**1 Cervical Nerve**
			2 Phrenic Nerve

4   Ulnar Nerve
    Cubital nerve
5   Median Nerve
    Anterior interosseous nerve
    Palmar cutaneous nerve
6   Radial Nerve
    Dorsal digital nerve
    Musculospiral nerve
    Palmar cutaneous nerve
    Posterior interosseous nerve
	0 Open
	4 Percutaneous Endoscopic
		Z No Device	**4 Ulnar Nerve**
			5 Median Nerve
			6 Radial Nerve

8   Thoracic Nerve
    Intercostal nerve
    Intercostobrachial nerve
    Spinal nerve, thoracic
    Subcostal nerve
	0 Open
	4 Percutaneous Endoscopic
		Z No Device	**8 Thoracic Nerve**

B   Lumbar Nerve
    Lumbosacral trunk
    Spinal nerve, lumbar
    Superior clunic (cluneal) nerve
C   Pudendal Nerve
    Posterior labial nerve
    Posterior scrotal nerve
	0 Open
	4 Percutaneous Endoscopic
		Z No Device	**B Lumbar Nerve**
			C Perineal Nerve

D   Femoral Nerve
    Anterior crural nerve
    Saphenous nerve
F   Sciatic Nerve
    Ischiatic nerve
G   Tibial Nerve
    Lateral plantar nerve
    Medial plantar nerve
    Medial popliteal nerve
    Medial sural cutaneous nerve
H   Peroneal Nerve
    Common fibular nerve
    Common peroneal nerve
    External popliteal nerve
    Lateral sural cutaneous nerve
	0 Open
	4 Percutaneous Endoscopic
		Z No Device	**D Femoral Nerve**
			F Sciatic Nerve
			G Tibial Nerve
			H Peroneal Nerve

Heart and Great Vessels Ø21–Ø2Y

Character Meanings

This Character Meaning table is provided as a guide to assist the user in the identification of character members that may be found in this section of code tables. It **SHOULD NOT** be used to build a PCS code.

Operation–Character 3	Body Part–Character 4	Approach–Character 5	Device–Character 6	Qualifier–Character 7
1 Bypass	Ø Coronary Artery, One Artery	Ø Open	Ø Monitoring Device, Pressure Sensor	Ø Allogeneic
4 Creation	1 Coronary Artery, Two Arteries	3 Percutaneous	2 Monitoring Device	1 Syngeneic
5 Destruction	2 Coronary Artery, Three Arteries	4 Percutaneous Endoscopic	3 Infusion Device	2 Zooplastic OR Common Atrioventricular Valve
7 Dilation	3 Coronary Artery, Four or More Arteries	X External	4 Intraluminal Device, Drug-eluting	3 Coronary Artery
8 Division	4 Coronary Vein		5 Intraluminal Device, Drug-eluting, Two	4 Coronary Vein
B Excision	5 Atrial Septum		6 Intraluminal Device, Drug-eluting, Three	5 Coronary Circulation
C Extirpation	6 Atrium, Right		7 Intraluminal Device, Drug-eluting, Four or More OR Autologous Tissue Substitute	6 Bifurcation
F Fragmentation	7 Atrium, Left		8 Zooplastic Tissue	7 Atrium, Left
H Insertion	8 Conduction Mechanism		9 Autologous Venous Tissue	8 Internal Mammary, Right
J Inspection	9 Chordae Tendineae		A Autologous Arterial Tissue	9 Internal Mammary, Left
K Map	A Heart		C Extraluminal Device	A Innominate Artery
L Occlusion	B Heart, Right		D Intraluminal Device	B Subclavian
N Release	C Heart, Left		E Intraluminal Device, Two OR Intraluminal Device, Branched or Fenestrated, One or Two Arteries	C Thoracic Artery
P Removal	D Papillary Muscle		F Intraluminal Device, Three OR Intraluminal Device, Branched or Fenestrated, Three or More Arteries	D Carotid
Q Repair	F Aortic Valve		G Intraluminal Device, Four or More	E Atrioventricular Valve, Left
R Replacement	G Mitral Valve		J Synthetic Substitute OR Cardiac Lead, Pacemaker	F Abdominal Artery
S Reposition	H Pulmonary Valve		K Nonautologous Tissue Substitute OR Cardiac Lead, Defibrillator	G Atrioventricular Valve, Right OR Axillary Artery
T Resection	J Tricuspid Valve		M Cardiac Lead	H Transapical OR Brachial Artery
U Supplement	K Ventricle, Right		N Intracardiac Pacemaker	J Truncal Valve OR Temporary OR Intraoperative
V Restriction	L Ventricle, Left		Q Implantable Heart Assist System	K Left Atrial Appendage
W Revision	M Ventricular Septum		R Short-term External Heart Assist System	P Pulmonary Trunk
Y Transplantation	N Pericardium		T Intraluminal Device, Radioactive	Q Pulmonary Artery, Right
	P Pulmonary Trunk		Y Other Device	R Pulmonary Artery, Left
	Q Pulmonary Artery, Right		Z No Device	S Pulmonary Vein, Right OR Biventricular
	R Pulmonary Artery, Left			T Pulmonary Vein, Left OR Ductus Arteriosus

Continued on next page

Continued from previous page

Operation–Character 3	Body Part–Character 4	Approach–Character 5	Device–Character 6	Qualifier–Character 7
	S Pulmonary Vein, Right			U Pulmonary Vein, Confluence
	T Pulmonary Vein, Left			V Lower Extremity Artery
	V Superior Vena Cava			W Aorta
	W Thoracic Aorta, Descending			X Diagnostic
	X Thoracic Aorta, Ascending/ Arch			Z No Qualifier
	Y Great Vessel			

AHA Coding Clinic for table 021

2017, 4Q, 56	Added approach values - Percutaneous heart valve procedures
2017, 1Q, 19	Norwood Sano procedure
2016, 4Q, 80-81	Thoracic aorta, ascending/arch and descending
2016, 4Q, 82-83	Coronary artery, number of arteries
2016, 4Q, 102-109	Correction of congenital heart defects
2016, 4Q, 144	Repair of atrial septal defect and anomalous pulmonary venous return
2016, 4Q, 145	Modified Warden procedure for repair of septal defect and right partial anomalous pulmonary venous return
2016, 1Q, 27	Aortocoronary bypass graft utilizing Y-graft
2015, 4Q, 22, 24	Congenital heart corrective procedures
2015, 3Q, 16	Revision of previous truncus arteriosus surgery with ventricle to pulmonary artery conduit
2014, 3Q, 3	Blalock-Taussig shunt procedure
2014, 3Q, 8	Coronary artery bypass graft utilizing internal mammary as pedicle graft
2014, 3Q, 20	MAZE procedure performed with coronary artery bypass graft
2014, 3Q, 29	Fontan completion procedure stage II
2014, 3Q, 30	Creation of conduit from right ventricle to pulmonary artery
2014, 1Q, 10	Repair of thoracic aortic aneurysm & coronary artery bypass graft
2013, 2Q, 37	Coronary artery release performed during coronary artery bypass graft

AHA Coding Clinic for table 024

2016, 4Q, 101	Root operation Creation
2016, 4Q, 102-109	Correction of congenital heart defects

AHA Coding Clinic for table 025

2016, 4Q, 80-81	Thoracic aorta, ascending/arch and descending
2016, 3Q, 43-44	Peri-pulmonary catheter ablation
2016, 3Q, 44-45	Maze procedure
2016, 2Q, 17	Photodynamic therapy for treatment of malignant mesothelioma
2014, 4Q, 47	Catheter ablation of peripulmonary veins
2014, 3Q, 19	Ablation of ventricular tachycardia with Impella® support
2014, 3Q, 20	MAZE procedure performed with coronary artery bypass graft
2013, 2Q, 38	Catheter ablation to treat atrial fibrillation

AHA Coding Clinic for table 027

2018, 2Q, 24	Coronary artery bifurcation
2017, 4Q, 32-33	Corrective surgery of left ventricular outflow tract obstruction
2016, 4Q, 80-81	Thoracic aorta, ascending/arch and descending
2016, 4Q, 82-83	Coronary artery, number of arteries
2016, 4Q, 84-85	Coronary Artery, number of stents
2016, 4Q, 86-88	Coronary and peripheral artery bifurcation
2016, 1Q, 16	Pulmonary valvotomy and dilation of annulus
2015, 4Q, 13	New Section X codes—New Technology procedures
2015, 3Q, 9	Failed attempt to treat coronary artery occlusion
2015, 3Q, 10	Coronary angioplasty with unsuccessful stent insertion
2015, 3Q, 16	Revision of previous truncus arteriosus surgery with ventricle to pulmonary artery conduit
2015, 2Q, 3-5	Coronary artery intervention site
2014, 2Q, 4	Coronary angioplasty of bypassed vessel

AHA Coding Clinic for table 02B

2017, 1Q, 38	Mitral valve repair and chordae tendineae transfer
2016, 4Q, 80-81	Thoracic aorta, ascending/arch and descending
2015, 2Q, 23	Annuloplasty ring

AHA Coding Clinic for table 02C

2018, 2Q, 24	Coronary artery bifurcation
2017, 2Q, 23	Thrombectomy via Fogarty catheter
2016, 4Q, 80-81	Thoracic aorta, ascending/arch and descending
2016, 4Q, 82-83	Coronary artery, number of arteries
2016, 4Q, 86-87	Coronary and peripheral artery bifurcation
2016, 2Q, 24	Repair/decalcification of mitral valve
2016, 2Q, 25	Aortic valve surgery with excision of calcium deposits

AHA Coding Clinic for table 02H

2018, 2Q, 3-5	Intra-aortic balloon pump
2018, 1Q, 19	Pacing lead attached to automatic implantable cardioverter defibrillator
2017, 4Q, 42-45	Insertion of external heart assist devices
2017, 4Q, 63-64	Added and revised device values - Vascular access reservoir
2017, 4Q, 104	Placement of Watchman ™ left atrial appendage device
2017, 3Q, 11	Placement of peripherally inserted central catheter using 3CG ECG technology
2017, 2Q, 24	Tunneled catheter versus totally implantable catheter
2017, 2Q, 26	Exchange of tunneled catheter
2017, 1Q, 10-11	External heart assist device
2016, 4Q, 80-81	Thoracic aorta, ascending/arch and descending
2016, 4Q, 95	Intracardiac pacemaker
2016, 4Q, 137-138	Heart assist device systems
2016, 2Q, 15	Removal and replacement of tunneled internal jugular catheter
2015, 4Q, 14	New Section X codes—New Technology procedures
2015, 4Q, 26-31	Vascular access devices
2015, 3Q, 35	Swan Ganz catheterization
2015, 2Q, 31	Leadless pacemaker insertion
2015, 2Q, 33	Totally implantable central venous access device (Port-a-Cath)
2013, 3Q, 18	Placement of peripherally inserted central catheter (PICC)

AHA Coding Clinic for table 02J

2015, 3Q, 9	Failed attempt to treat coronary artery occlusion

AHA Coding Clinic for table 02L

2017, 4Q, 31	Resuscitative endovascular balloon occlusion of the aorta
2017, 4Q, 33-34	Occlusion/ligation of pulmonary trunk & right pulmonary artery
2016, 4Q, 102-109	Correction of congenital heart defects
2016, 2Q, 26	Embolization of pulmonary arteriovenous fistula
2015, 4Q, 23	Congenital heart corrective procedures
2014, 3Q, 20	MAZE procedure performed with coronary artery bypass graft

AHA Coding Clinic for table 02N

2017, 4Q, 35	Release of myocardial bridge
2016, 4Q, 80-81	Thoracic aorta, ascending/arch and descending
2014, 3Q, 16	Repair of Tetralogy of Fallot

AHA Coding Clinic for table 02P

2018, 2Q, 3-5	Intra-aortic balloon pump
2017, 4Q, 42-45	Insertion of external heart assist devices
2017, 4Q, 104	Placement of Watchman ™ left atrial appendage device
2017, 3Q, 18	Intra-aortic balloon pump removal
2017, 2Q, 24	Tunneled catheter versus totally implantable catheter
2017, 2Q, 26	Exchange of tunneled catheter
2017, 1Q, 11	External heart assist device
2017, 1Q, 13	SynCardia total artificial heart
2016, 4Q, 95-96	Intracardiac pacemaker
2016, 4Q, 137-139	Heart assist device systems
2016, 3Q, 19	Nonoperative removal of peripherally inserted central catheter
2016, 2Q, 15	Removal and replacement of tunneled internal jugular catheter
2015, 4Q, 31	Vascular access devices
2015, 3Q, 33	Approach values for repositioning and removal of cardiac lead

AHA Coding Clinic for table 02Q

2018, 1Q, 12	Percutaneous balloon valvuloplasty & cardiac catheterization with ventriculogram
2017, 1Q, 18	Sutureless repair of pulmonary vein stenosis
2016, 4Q, 80-81	Thoracic aorta, ascending/arch and descending
2016, 4Q, 82-83	Coronary artery, number of arteries
2016, 4Q, 101	Root operation Creation
2016, 4Q, 102-109	Correction of congenital heart defects
2015, 4Q, 23	Congenital heart corrective procedures
2015, 3Q, 16	Vascular ring surgery and double aortic arch
2015, 2Q, 23	Annuloplasty ring
2013, 3Q, 26	Transcatheter replacement of heart valve (TAVR) with measurements

AHA Coding Clinic for table 02R

2018, 1Q, 12	Percutaneous balloon valvuloplasty & cardiac catheterization with ventriculogram
2017, 4Q, 55-56	Added approach values - Percutaneous heart valve procedures
2017, 1Q, 13	SynCardia total artificial heart
2016, 4Q, 80-81	Thoracic aorta, ascending/arch and descending
2016, 3Q, 32	Transcatheter tricuspid valve replacement
2014, 1Q, 10	Repair of thoracic aortic aneurysm & coronary artery bypass graft

AHA Coding Clinic for table 02S

2016, 4Q, 80-81	Thoracic aorta, ascending/arch and descending
2016, 4Q, 82-83	Coronary artery, number of arteries
2016, 4Q, 102-109	Correction of congenital heart defects
2015, 4Q, 23	Congenital heart corrective procedures

AHA Coding Clinic for table 02U

2018, 1Q, 12	Percutaneous balloon valvuloplasty & cardiac catheterization with ventriculogram
2017, 4Q, 36	Alfieri stitch procedure
2017, 3Q, 7	Senning procedure (arterial switch)
2017, 1Q, 19	Norwood Sano procedure
2016, 4Q, 80-81	Thoracic aorta, ascending/arch and descending
2016, 4Q, 101	Root operation Creation
2016, 4Q, 102-109	Correction of congenital heart defects
2016, 2Q, 23	Repair of tetralogy of Fallot with autologous pericardial patch graft
2016, 2Q, 26	Aortic valve replacement with aortic root enlargement
2015, 4Q, 22-24	Congenital heart corrective procedures
2015, 3Q, 16	Revision of previous truncus arteriosus surgery with ventricle to pulmonary artery conduit
2015, 2Q, 23	Annuloplasty ring
2014, 3Q, 16	Repair of Tetralogy of Fallot

AHA Coding Clinic for table 02V

2017, 4Q, 35-36	Alfieri stitch procedure
2016, 4Q, 80-81	Thoracic aorta, ascending/arch and descending
2016, 4Q, 89-92	Branched and fenestrated endograft repair of aneurysms

AHA Coding Clinic for table 02W

2018, 1Q, 17	Repositioning of Impella short-term external heart assist device
2017, 4Q, 42-45	Insertion of external heart assist devices
2017, 4Q, 55-56	Added approach values - Percutaneous heart valve procedures
2016, 4Q, 85	Coronary Artery, number of stents
2016, 4Q, 95-96	Intracardiac pacemaker
2015, 3Q, 32	Approach values for repositioning and removal of cardiac lead
2014, 3Q, 31	Closure of paravalvular leak using Amplatzer® vascular plug

AHA Coding Clinic for table 02Y

2013, 3Q, 18	Heart transplant surgery

Coronary Arteries

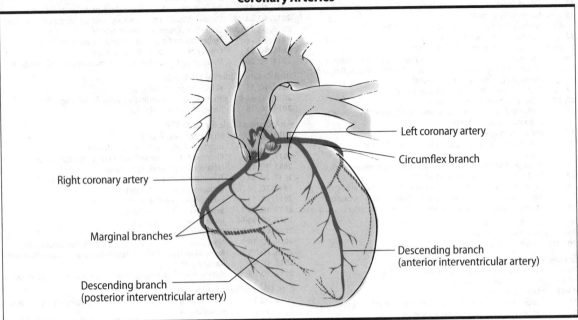

- Left coronary artery
- Circumflex branch
- Right coronary artery
- Marginal branches
- Descending branch (anterior interventricular artery)
- Descending branch (posterior interventricular artery)

Heart Anatomy

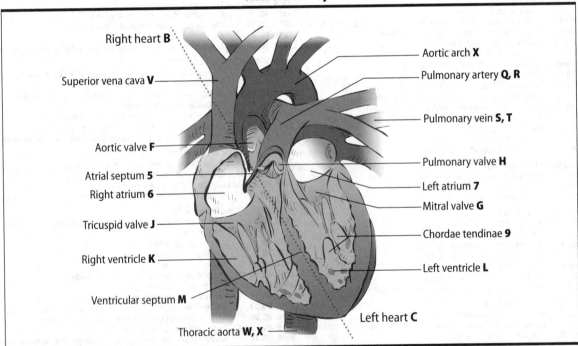

- Right heart **B**
- Superior vena cava **V**
- Aortic valve **F**
- Atrial septum **5**
- Right atrium **6**
- Tricuspid valve **J**
- Right ventricle **K**
- Ventricular septum **M**
- Thoracic aorta **W, X**
- Aortic arch **X**
- Pulmonary artery **Q, R**
- Pulmonary vein **S, T**
- Pulmonary valve **H**
- Left atrium **7**
- Mitral valve **G**
- Chordae tendinae **9**
- Left ventricle **L**
- Left heart **C**

Ø   Medical and Surgical
2   Heart and Great Vessels
1   Bypass   Definition: Altering the route of passage of the contents of a tubular body part

Explanation: Rerouting contents of a body part to a downstream area of the normal route, to a similar route and body part, or to an abnormal route and dissimilar body part. Includes one or more anastomoses, with or without the use of a device.

Body Part Character 4	Approach Character 5	Device Character 6	Qualifier Character 7
Ø Coronary Artery, One Artery 1 Coronary Artery, Two Arteries 2 Coronary Artery, Three Arteries 3 Coronary Artery, Four or More Arteries	Ø Open	8 Zooplastic Tissue 9 Autologous Venous Tissue A Autologous Arterial Tissue J Synthetic Substitute K Nonautologous Tissue Substitute	3 Coronary Artery 8 Internal Mammary, Right 9 Internal Mammary, Left C Thoracic Artery F Abdominal Artery W Aorta
Ø Coronary Artery, One Artery 1 Coronary Artery, Two Arteries 2 Coronary Artery, Three Arteries 3 Coronary Artery, Four or More Arteries	Ø Open	Z No Device	3 Coronary Artery 8 Internal Mammary, Right 9 Internal Mammary, Left C Thoracic Artery F Abdominal Artery
Ø Coronary Artery, One Artery 1 Coronary Artery, Two Arteries 2 Coronary Artery, Three Arteries 3 Coronary Artery, Four or More Arteries	3 Percutaneous	4 Intraluminal Device, Drug-eluting D Intraluminal Device	4 Coronary Vein
Ø Coronary Artery, One Artery 1 Coronary Artery, Two Arteries 2 Coronary Artery, Three Arteries 3 Coronary Artery, Four or More Arteries	4 Percutaneous Endoscopic	4 Intraluminal Device, Drug-eluting D Intraluminal Device	4 Coronary Vein
Ø Coronary Artery, One Artery 1 Coronary Artery, Two Arteries 2 Coronary Artery, Three Arteries 3 Coronary Artery, Four or More Arteries	4 Percutaneous Endoscopic	8 Zooplastic Tissue 9 Autologous Venous Tissue A Autologous Arterial Tissue J Synthetic Substitute K Nonautologous Tissue Substitute	3 Coronary Artery 8 Internal Mammary, Right 9 Internal Mammary, Left C Thoracic Artery F Abdominal Artery W Aorta
Ø Coronary Artery, One Artery 1 Coronary Artery, Two Arteries 2 Coronary Artery, Three Arteries 3 Coronary Artery, Four or More Arteries	4 Percutaneous Endoscopic	Z No Device	3 Coronary Artery 8 Internal Mammary, Right 9 Internal Mammary, Left C Thoracic Artery F Abdominal Artery

6 Atrium, Right
   Atrium dextrum cordis
   Right auricular appendix
   Sinus venosus
	Ø Open
	4 Percutaneous Endoscopic
		8 Zooplastic Tissue
		9 Autologous Venous Tissue
		A Autologous Arterial Tissue
		J Synthetic Substitute
		K Nonautologous Tissue Substitute
			P Pulmonary Trunk
			Q Pulmonary Artery, Right
			R Pulmonary Artery, Left

6 Atrium, Right
   Atrium dextrum cordis
   Right auricular appendix
   Sinus venosus
	Ø Open
	4 Percutaneous Endoscopic
		Z No Device	7 Atrium, Left
			P Pulmonary Trunk
			Q Pulmonary Artery, Right
			R Pulmonary Artery, Left

6 Atrium, Right
   Atrium dextrum cordis
   Right auricular appendix
   Sinus venosus
	3 Percutaneous	Z No Device	7 Atrium, Left

7 Atrium, Left
   Atrium pulmonale
   Left auricular appendix
V Superior Vena Cava
   Precava
	Ø Open
	4 Percutaneous Endoscopic
		8 Zooplastic Tissue
		9 Autologous Venous Tissue
		A Autologous Arterial Tissue
		J Synthetic Substitute
		K Nonautologous Tissue Substitute
		Z No Device
			P Pulmonary Trunk
			Q Pulmonary Artery, Right
			R Pulmonary Artery, Left
			S Pulmonary Vein, Right
			T Pulmonary Vein, Left
			U Pulmonary Vein, Confluence

K Ventricle, Right Conus arteriosus L Ventricle, Left	Ø Open 4 Percutaneous Endoscopic	8 Zooplastic Tissue 9 Autologous Venous Tissue A Autologous Arterial Tissue J Synthetic Substitute K Nonautologous Tissue Substitute	P Pulmonary Trunk Q Pulmonary Artery, Right R Pulmonary Artery, Left

Ø21 Continued on next page

HAC	Ø21[Ø,1,2,3]Ø[8,9,A,J,K][3,8,9,C,F,W] when reported with SDx J98.51 or J98.59
HAC	Ø21[Ø,1,2,3]ØZ[3,8,9,C,F] when reported with SDx J98.51 or J98.59
HAC	Ø21[Ø,1,2,3]4[8,9,A,J,K][3,8,9,C,F,W] when reported with SDx J98.51 or J98.59
HAC	Ø21[Ø,1,2,3]4Z[3,8,9,C,F] when reported with SDx J98.51 or J98.59=

🄻🄲 Limited Coverage   🄽🄲 Noncovered   ⊞ Combination Member   HAC associated procedure   Combination Only   DRG Non-OR   Non-OR   New/Revised in GREEN

ICD-10-PCS 2019   167

Ø21–Ø21

Heart and Great Vessels

Ø Medical and Surgical
2 Heart and Great Vessels
1 Bypass   Definition: Altering the route of passage of the contents of a tubular body part

Explanation: Rerouting contents of a body part to a downstream area of the normal route, to a similar route and body part, or to an abnormal route and dissimilar body part. Includes one or more anastomoses, with or without the use of a device.

Body Part Character 4	Approach Character 5	Device Character 6	Qualifier Character 7
K Ventricle, Right Conus arteriosus **L** Ventricle, Left	**Ø** Open **4** Percutaneous Endoscopic	**Z** No Device	**5** Coronary Circulation **8** Internal Mammary, Right **9** Internal Mammary, Left **C** Thoracic Artery **F** Abdominal Artery **P** Pulmonary Trunk **Q** Pulmonary Artery, Right **R** Pulmonary Artery, Left **W** Aorta
P Pulmonary Trunk **Q** Pulmonary Artery, Right **R** Pulmonary Artery, Left Arterial canal (duct) Botallo's duct Pulmoaortic canal	**Ø** Open **4** Percutaneous Endoscopic	**8** Zooplastic Tissue **9** Autologous Venous Tissue **A** Autologous Arterial Tissue **J** Synthetic Substitute **K** Nonautologous Tissue Substitute **Z** No Device	**A** Innominate Artery **B** Subclavian **D** Carotid
W Thoracic Aorta, Descending	**Ø** Open	**8** Zooplastic Tissue **9** Autologous Venous Tissue **A** Autologous Arterial Tissue **J** Synthetic Substitute **K** Nonautologous Tissue Substitute	**B** Subclavian **D** Carotid **F** Abdominal Artery **G** Axillary Artery **H** Brachial Artery **P** Pulmonary Trunk **Q** Pulmonary Artery, Right **R** Pulmonary Artery, Left **V** Lower Extremity Artery
W Thoracic Aorta, Descending	**Ø** Open	**Z** No Device	**B** Subclavian **D** Carotid **P** Pulmonary Trunk **Q** Pulmonary Artery, Right **R** Pulmonary Artery, Left
W Thoracic Aorta, Descending	**4** Percutaneous Endoscopic	**8** Zooplastic Tissue **9** Autologous Venous Tissue **A** Autologous Arterial Tissue **J** Synthetic Substitute **K** Nonautologous Tissue Substitute **Z** No Device	**B** Subclavian **D** Carotid **P** Pulmonary Trunk **Q** Pulmonary Artery, Right **R** Pulmonary Artery, Left
X Thoracic Aorta, Ascending/Arch Aortic arch Ascending aorta	**Ø** Open **4** Percutaneous Endoscopic	**8** Zooplastic Tissue **9** Autologous Venous Tissue **A** Autologous Arterial Tissue **J** Synthetic Substitute **K** Nonautologous Tissue Substitute **Z** No Device	**B** Subclavian **D** Carotid **P** Pulmonary Trunk **Q** Pulmonary Artery, Right **R** Pulmonary Artery, Left

Ø Medical and Surgical
2 Heart and Great Vessels
4 Creation   Definition: Putting in or on biological or synthetic material to form a new body part that to the extent possible replicates the anatomic structure or function of an absent body part

Explanation: Used for gender reassignment surgery and corrective procedures in individuals with congenital anomalies

Body Part Character 4	Approach Character 5	Device Character 6	Qualifier Character 7
F Aortic Valve Aortic annulus	**Ø** Open	**7** Autologous Tissue **8** Zooplastic Tissue **J** Synthetic Substitute **K** Nonautologous Tissue Substitute	**J** Truncal Valve
G Mitral Valve Bicuspid valve Left atrioventricular valve Mitral annulus **J** Tricuspid Valve Right atrioventricular valve Tricuspid annulus	**Ø** Open	**7** Autologous Tissue **8** Zooplastic Tissue **J** Synthetic Substitute **K** Nonautologous Tissue Substitute	**2** Common Atrioventricular Valve

LC Limited Coverage   **NC** Noncovered   ⊞ Combination Member   HAC associated procedure   Combination Only   DRG Non-OR   Non-OR   New/Revised in GREEN

168   ICD-10-PCS 2019

Ø Medical and Surgical
2 Heart and Great Vessels
5 Destruction   Definition: Physical eradication of all or a portion of a body part by the direct use of energy, force, or a destructive agent
                     Explanation: None of the body part is physically taken out

Body Part Character 4	Approach Character 5	Device Character 6	Qualifier Character 7

4 Coronary Vein
5 Atrial Septum
     Interatrial septum
6 Atrium, Right
     Atrium dextrum cordis
     Right auricular appendix
     Sinus venosus
8 Conduction Mechanism
     Atrioventricular node
     Bundle of His
     Bundle of Kent
     Sinoatrial node
9 Chordae Tendineae
D Papillary Muscle
F Aortic Valve
     Aortic annulus
G Mitral Valve
     Bicuspid valve
     Left atrioventricular valve
     Mitral annulus
H Pulmonary Valve
     Pulmonary annulus
     Pulmonic valve
J Tricuspid Valve
     Right atrioventricular valve
     Tricuspid annulus
K Ventricle, Right
     Conus arteriosus
L Ventricle, Left
M Ventricular Septum
     Interventricular septum
N Pericardium
P Pulmonary Trunk
Q Pulmonary Artery, Right
R Pulmonary Artery, Left
     Arterial canal (duct)
     Botallo's duct
     Pulmoaortic canal
S Pulmonary Vein, Right
     Right inferior pulmonary vein
     Right superior pulmonary vein
T Pulmonary Vein, Left
     Left inferior pulmonary vein
     Left superior pulmonary vein
V Superior Vena Cava
     Precava
W Thoracic Aorta, Descending
X Thoracic Aorta, Ascending/Arch
     Aortic arch
     Ascending aorta
	Ø Open
	3 Percutaneous
	4 Percutaneous Endoscopic
		Z No Device	Z No Qualifier

7 Atrium, Left
     Atrium pulmonale
     Left auricular appendix
	Ø Open
	3 Percutaneous
	4 Percutaneous Endoscopic
		Z No Device	K Left Atrial Appendage
			Z No Qualifier

DRG Non-OR   Ø257[Ø,3,4]ZK

Heart and Great Vessels

Ø   Medical and Surgical
2   Heart and Great Vessels
7   Dilation   Definition: Expanding an orifice or the lumen of a tubular body part

Explanation: The orifice can be a natural orifice or an artificially created orifice. Accomplished by stretching a tubular body part using intraluminal pressure or by cutting part of the orifice or wall of the tubular body part.

Body Part Character 4	Approach Character 5	Device Character 6	Qualifier Character 7
Ø Coronary Artery, One Artery 1 Coronary Artery, Two Arteries 2 Coronary Artery, Three Arteries 3 Coronary Artery, Four or More Arteries	Ø Open 3 Percutaneous 4 Percutaneous Endoscopic	4 Intraluminal Device, Drug-eluting 5 Intraluminal Device, Drug-eluting, Two 6 Intraluminal Device, Drug-eluting, Three 7 Intraluminal Device, Drug-eluting, Four or More D Intraluminal Device E Intraluminal Device, Two F Intraluminal Device, Three G Intraluminal Device, Four or More T Intraluminal Device, Radioactive Z No Device	6 Bifurcation Z No Qualifier

F Aortic Valve
    Aortic annulus
G Mitral Valve
    Bicuspid valve
    Left atrioventricular valve
    Mitral annulus
H Pulmonary Valve
    Pulmonary annulus
    Pulmonic valve
J Tricuspid Valve
    Right atrioventricular valve
    Tricuspid annulus
K Ventricle, Right
    Conus arteriosus
L Ventricle, Left
P Pulmonary Trunk
Q Pulmonary Artery, Right
S Pulmonary Vein, Right
    Right inferior pulmonary vein
    Right superior pulmonary vein
T Pulmonary Vein, Left
    Left inferior pulmonary vein
    Left superior pulmonary vein
V Superior Vena Cava
    Precava
W Thoracic Aorta, Descending
X Thoracic Aorta, Ascending/Arch
    Aortic arch
    Ascending aorta
	Ø Open
	3 Percutaneous
	4 Percutaneous Endoscopic
		4 Intraluminal Device, Drug-eluting
		D Intraluminal Device
		Z No Device
			Z No Qualifier

R Pulmonary Artery, Left
    Arterial canal (duct)
    Botallo's duct
    Pulmoaortic canal
	Ø Open
	3 Percutaneous
	4 Percutaneous Endoscopic
		4 Intraluminal Device, Drug-eluting
		D Intraluminal Device
		Z No Device
			T Ductus Arteriosus
			Z No Qualifier

Ø   Medical and Surgical
2   Heart and Great Vessels
8   Division   Definition: Cutting into a body part, without draining fluids and/or gases from the body part, in order to separate or transect a body part

Explanation: All or a portion of the body part is separated into two or more portions.

Body Part Character 4	Approach Character 5	Device Character 6	Qualifier Character 7

8 Conduction Mechanism
    Atrioventricular node
    Bundle of His
    Bundle of Kent
    Sinoatrial node
9 Chordae Tendineae
D Papillary Muscle
	Ø Open
	3 Percutaneous
	4 Percutaneous Endoscopic
		Z No Device	Z No Qualifier

LC Limited Coverage   NC Noncovered   ⊞ Combination Member   HAC associated procedure   Combination Only   DRG Non-OR   Non-OR   New/Revised in GREEN

170   ICD-10-PCS 2019

Ø   Medical and Surgical
2   Heart and Great Vessels
B   Excision   Definition: Cutting out or off, without replacement, a portion of a body part

Explanation: The qualifier DIAGNOSTIC is used to identify excision procedures that are biopsies

Body Part Character 4	Approach Character 5	Device Character 6	Qualifier Character 7

4   Coronary Vein
5   Atrial Septum
       Interatrial septum
6   Atrium, Right
       Atrium dextrum cordis
       Right auricular appendix
       Sinus venosus
8   Conduction Mechanism
       Atrioventricular node
       Bundle of His
       Bundle of Kent
       Sinoatrial node
9   Chordae Tendineae
D   Papillary Muscle
F   Aortic Valve
       Aortic annulus
G   Mitral Valve
       Bicuspid valve
       Left atrioventricular valve
       Mitral annulus
H   Pulmonary Valve
       Pulmonary annulus
       Pulmonic valve
J   Tricuspid Valve
       Right atrioventricular valve
       Tricuspid annulus
K   Ventricle, Right   NC
       Conus arteriosus
L   Ventricle, Left   NC
M   Ventricular Septum
       Interventricular septum
N   Pericardium
P   Pulmonary Trunk
Q   Pulmonary Artery, Right
R   Pulmonary Artery, Left
       Arterial canal (duct)
       Botallo's duct
       Pulmoaortic canal
S   Pulmonary Vein, Right
       Right inferior pulmonary vein
       Right superior pulmonary vein
T   Pulmonary Vein, Left
       Left inferior pulmonary vein
       Left superior pulmonary vein
V   Superior Vena Cava
       Precava
W   Thoracic Aorta, Descending
X   Thoracic Aorta, Ascending/Arch
       Aortic arch
       Ascending aorta
	Ø Open
	3 Percutaneous
	4 Percutaneous Endoscopic
		Z No Device	**X Diagnostic**
			Z No Qualifier

7   Atrium, Left
       Atrium pulmonale
       Left auricular appendix
	Ø Open
	3 Percutaneous
	4 Percutaneous Endoscopic
		Z No Device	**K Left Atrial Appendage**
			X Diagnostic
			Z No Qualifier

DRG Non-OR	Ø2B7[Ø,3,4]ZK
Non-OR	Ø2B[4,5,6,8,9,D,F,G,H,J,K,L,M][Ø,3,4]ZX
NC	Ø2B[K,L][Ø,3,4]ZZ

LC Limited Coverage   NC Noncovered   ⊞ Combination Member   HAC associated procedure   Combination Only   DRG Non-OR   Non-OR   New/Revised in GREEN

Heart and Great Vessels

0   **Medical and Surgical**
2   **Heart and Great Vessels**
C   **Extirpation**   Definition: Taking or cutting out solid matter from a body part

Explanation: The solid matter may be an abnormal byproduct of a biological function or a foreign body; it may be imbedded in a body part or in the lumen of a tubular body part. The solid matter may or may not have been previously broken into pieces.

Body Part Character 4	Approach Character 5	Device Character 6	Qualifier Character 7
0 Coronary Artery, One Artery **1** Coronary Artery, Two Arteries **2** Coronary Artery, Three Arteries **3** Coronary Artery, Four or More Arteries	**0** Open **3** Percutaneous **4** Percutaneous Endoscopic	**Z** No Device	**6** Bifurcation **Z** No Qualifier

4 Coronary Vein
5 Atrial Septum
   Interatrial septum
6 Atrium, Right
   Atrium dextrum cordis
   Right auricular appendix
   Sinus venosus
7 Atrium, Left
   Atrium pulmonale
   Left auricular appendix
8 Conduction Mechanism
   Atrioventricular node
   Bundle of His
   Bundle of Kent
   Sinoatrial node
9 Chordae Tendineae
D Papillary Muscle
F Aortic Valve
   Aortic annulus
G Mitral Valve
   Bicuspid valve
   Left atrioventricular valve
   Mitral annulus
H Pulmonary Valve
   Pulmonary annulus
   Pulmonic valve
J Tricuspid Valve
   Right atrioventricular valve
   Tricuspid annulus
K Ventricle, Right
   Conus arteriosus
L Ventricle, Left
M Ventricular Septum
   Interventricular septum
N Pericardium
P Pulmonary Trunk
Q Pulmonary Artery, Right
R Pulmonary Artery, Left
   Arterial canal (duct)
   Botallo's duct
   Pulmoaortic canal
S Pulmonary Vein, Right
   Right inferior pulmonary vein
   Right superior pulmonary vein
T Pulmonary Vein, Left
   Left inferior pulmonary vein
   Left superior pulmonary vein
V Superior Vena Cava
   Precava
W Thoracic Aorta, Descending
X Thoracic Aorta, Ascending/Arch
   Aortic arch
   Ascending aorta
	0 Open
	3 Percutaneous
	4 Percutaneous Endoscopic
		Z No Device	**Z** No Qualifier

0   **Medical and Surgical**
2   **Heart and Great Vessels**
F   **Fragmentation**   Definition: Breaking solid matter in a body part into pieces

Explanation: Physical force (e.g., manual, ultrasonic) applied directly or indirectly is used to break the solid matter into pieces. The solid matter may be an abnormal byproduct of a biological function or a foreign body. The pieces of solid matter are not taken out.

Body Part Character 4	Approach Character 5	Device Character 6	Qualifier Character 7
N Pericardium NC	**0** Open **3** Percutaneous **4** Percutaneous Endoscopic **X** External	**Z** No Device	**Z** No Qualifier

Non-OR   02FNXZZ
NC   02FNXZZ

LC Limited Coverage   NC Noncovered   ⊞ Combination Member   HAC associated procedure   Combination Only   DRG Non-OR   Non-OR   New/Revised in GREEN

172   ICD-10-PCS 2019

0   Medical and Surgical
2   Heart and Great Vessels
H   Insertion   Definition: Putting in a nonbiological appliance that monitors, assists, performs, or prevents a physiological function but does not physically take the place of a body part
                    Explanation: None

Body Part — Character 4	Approach — Character 5	Device — Character 6	Qualifier — Character 7

4   Coronary Vein ⊞
6   Atrium, Right ⊞
    Atrium dextrum cordis
    Right auricular appendix
    Sinus venosus
7   Atrium, Left ⊞
    Atrium pulmonale
    Left auricular appendix
K   Ventricle, Right ⊞
    Conus arteriosus
L   Ventricle, Left ⊞
	0 Open
	3 Percutaneous
	4 Percutaneous Endoscopic
		0 Monitoring Device, Pressure Sensor
		2 Monitoring Device
		3 Infusion Device
		D Intraluminal Device
		J Cardiac Lead, Pacemaker
		K Cardiac Lead, Defibrillator
		M Cardiac Lead
		N Intracardiac Pacemaker
		Y Other Device
			Z No Qualifier

A Heart LC NC	0 Open 3 Percutaneous 4 Percutaneous Endoscopic	Q Implantable Heart Assist System Y Other Device	Z No Qualifier
A Heart ⊞	0 Open 3 Percutaneous 4 Percutaneous Endoscopic	R Short-term External Heart Assist System	J Intraoperative S Biventricular Z No Qualifier
N Pericardium ⊞	0 Open 3 Percutaneous 4 Percutaneous Endoscopic	0 Monitoring Device, Pressure Sensor 2 Monitoring Device J Cardiac Lead, Pacemaker K Cardiac Lead, Defibrillator M Cardiac Lead Y Other Device	Z No Qualifier

P   Pulmonary Trunk
Q   Pulmonary Artery, Right
R   Pulmonary Artery, Left
    Arterial canal (duct)
    Botallo's duct
    Pulmoaortic canal
S   Pulmonary Vein, Right
    Right inferior pulmonary vein
    Right superior pulmonary vein
T   Pulmonary Vein, Left
    Left inferior pulmonary vein
    Left superior pulmonary vein
V   Superior Vena Cava
    Precava
W   Thoracic Aorta, Descending
	0 Open
	3 Percutaneous
	4 Percutaneous Endoscopic
		0 Monitoring Device, Pressure Sensor
		2 Monitoring Device
		3 Infusion Device
		D Intraluminal Device
		Y Other Device
			Z No Qualifier

X   Thoracic Aorta, Ascending/Arch
    Aortic arch
    Ascending aorta
	0 Open
	3 Percutaneous
	4 Percutaneous Endoscopic
		0 Monitoring Device, Pressure Sensor
		2 Monitoring Device
		3 Infusion Device
		D Intraluminal Device
			Z No Qualifier

DRG Non-OR	02H[4,6,7][0,4][J,M]Z	
DRG Non-OR	02H[6,7]3JZ	
DRG Non-OR	02H[K,L][0,3,4][J,M]Z	
DRG Non-OR	02HK32Z	
Non-OR	02H[4,6,7,L]3[2,3]Z	
Non-OR	02H[6,7]3MZ	
Non-OR	02HK3[0,3]Z	
Non-OR	02HN32Z	
Non-OR	02HP[0,3,4][0,2,3]Z	
Non-OR	02H[Q,R][0,3,4][2,3]Z	
Non-OR	02H[S,T,V,W][0,3,4]3Z	
Non-OR	02H[S,T,V,W]32Z	
Non-OR	02HW[0,3]0Z	
Non-OR	02HX[0,3,4][0,3]Z	

HAC   02H43[J,K,M]Z when reported with SDx K68.11 or T81.4XXA or T82.6XXA or T82.7XXA
HAC   02H[6,K]33Z when reported with SDx J95.811
HAC   02H[6,7]3[J,M]Z when reported with SDx K68.11 or T81.4XXA or T82.6XXA or T82.7XXA
HAC   02H[K,L]3JZ when reported with SDx K68.11 or T81.4XXA or T82.6XXA or T82.7XXA
HAC   02HN[0,3,4][J,M]Z when reported with SDx K68.11 or T81.4XXA or T82.6XXA or T82.7XXA
HAC   02H[S,T,V][3,4]3Z when reported with SDx J95.811
LC   02HA0QZ
NC   02HA[3,4]QZ

See Appendix L for Procedure Combinations
⊞   02H[4,6,7,K,L][0,3,4]KZ
⊞   02H43[J,M]Z
⊞   02HA[0,4]R[S,Z]
⊞   02HA3RS
⊞   02HN[0,3,4][J,K,M]Z

LC Limited Coverage   NC Noncovered   ⊞ Combination Member   HAC associated procedure   Combination Only   DRG Non-OR   Non-OR   New/Revised in GREEN
ICD-10-PCS 2019   173

02H–02H

Ø   Medical and Surgical
2   Heart and Great Vessels
J   Inspection   Definition: Visually and/or manually exploring a body part

Explanation: Visual exploration may be performed with or without optical instrumentation. Manual exploration may be performed directly or through intervening body layers.

Body Part Character 4	Approach Character 5	Device Character 6	Qualifier Character 7
A Heart Y Great Vessel	Ø Open 3 Percutaneous 4 Percutaneous Endoscopic	Z No Device	Z No Qualifier

Non-OR   Ø2J[A,Y]3ZZ

Ø   Medical and Surgical
2   Heart and Great Vessels
K   Map   Definition: Locating the route of passage of electrical impulses and/or locating functional areas in a body part

Explanation: Applicable only to the cardiac conduction mechanism and the central nervous system

Body Part Character 4	Approach Character 5	Device Character 6	Qualifier Character 7

8   Conduction Mechanism
    Atrioventricular node
    Bundle of His
    Bundle of Kent
    Sinoatrial node
	Ø Open
	3 Percutaneous
	4 Percutaneous Endoscopic
		Z No Device	Z No Qualifier

DRG Non-OR   Ø2K8[Ø,3,4]ZZ

Ø   Medical and Surgical
2   Heart and Great Vessels
L   Occlusion   Definition: Completely closing an orifice or the lumen of a tubular body part

Explanation: The orifice can be a natural orifice or an artificially created orifice

Body Part Character 4	Approach Character 5	Device Character 6	Qualifier Character 7

7   Atrium, Left
    Atrium pulmonale
    Left auricular appendix
	Ø Open
	3 Percutaneous
	4 Percutaneous Endoscopic
		C Extraluminal Device
		D Intraluminal Device
		Z No Device
			K Left Atrial Appendage

H   Pulmonary Valve
    Pulmonary annulus
    Pulmonic valve
P   Pulmonary Trunk
Q   Pulmonary Artery, Right
S   Pulmonary Vein, Right
    Right inferior pulmonary vein
    Right superior pulmonary vein
T   Pulmonary Vein, Left
    Left inferior pulmonary vein
    Left superior pulmonary vein
V   Superior Vena Cava
    Precava
	Ø Open
	3 Percutaneous
	4 Percutaneous Endoscopic
		C Extraluminal Device
		D Intraluminal Device
		Z No Device
			Z No Qualifier

R   Pulmonary Artery, Left
    Arterial canal (duct)
    Botallo's duct
    Pulmoaortic canal
	Ø Open
	3 Percutaneous
	4 Percutaneous Endoscopic
		C Extraluminal Device
		D Intraluminal Device
		Z No Device
			T Ductus Arteriosus
			Z No Qualifier

W Thoracic Aorta, Descending	3 Percutaneous	D Intraluminal Device	J Temporary

DRG Non-OR   Ø2L7[Ø,3,4][C,D,Z]K

LC Limited Coverage   **NC** Noncovered   ⊞ Combination Member   HAC associated procedure   Combination Only   DRG Non-OR   Non-OR   New/Revised in GREEN

174   ICD-10-PCS 2019

0   **Medical and Surgical**
2   **Heart and Great Vessels**
N   **Release**   Definition: Freeing a body part from an abnormal physical constraint by cutting or by the use of force
                         Explanation: Some of the restraining tissue may be taken out but none of the body part is taken out

Body Part Character 4	Approach Character 5	Device Character 6	Qualifier Character 7

0 **Coronary Artery, One Artery**
1 **Coronary Artery, Two Arteries**
2 **Coronary Artery, Three Arteries**
3 **Coronary Artery, Four or More Arteries**
4 **Coronary Vein**
5 **Atrial Septum**
    Interatrial septum
6 **Atrium, Right**
    Atrium dextrum cordis
    Right auricular appendix
    Sinus venosus
7 **Atrium, Left**
    Atrium pulmonale
    Left auricular appendix
8 **Conduction Mechanism**
    Atrioventricular node
    Bundle of His
    Bundle of Kent
    Sinoatrial node
9 **Chordae Tendineae**
D **Papillary Muscle**
F **Aortic Valve**
    Aortic annulus
G **Mitral Valve**
    Bicuspid valve
    Left atrioventricular valve
    Mitral annulus
H **Pulmonary Valve**
    Pulmonary annulus
    Pulmonic valve
J **Tricuspid Valve**
    Right atrioventricular valve
    Tricuspid annulus
K **Ventricle, Right**
    Conus arteriosus
L **Ventricle, Left**
M **Ventricular Septum**
    Interventricular septum
N **Pericardium**
P **Pulmonary Trunk**
Q **Pulmonary Artery, Right**
R **Pulmonary Artery, Left**
    Arterial canal (duct)
    Botallo's duct
    Pulmoaortic canal
S **Pulmonary Vein, Right**
    Right inferior pulmonary vein
    Right superior pulmonary vein
T **Pulmonary Vein, Left**
    Left inferior pulmonary vein
    Left superior pulmonary vein
V **Superior Vena Cava**
    Precava
W **Thoracic Aorta, Descending**
X **Thoracic Aorta, Ascending/Arch**
    Aortic arch
    Ascending aorta
	0 Open
	3 Percutaneous
	4 Percutaneous Endoscopic
		Z No Device	**Z** No Qualifier

LC Limited Coverage   **NC** Noncovered   ⊞ Combination Member   HAC associated procedure   Combination Only   DRG Non-OR   Non-OR   New/Revised in GREEN

ICD-10-PCS 2019   175

02N–02N

Heart and Great Vessels

Ø   **Medical and Surgical**
2   **Heart and Great Vessels**
P   **Removal**   Definition: Taking out or off a device from a body part

Explanation: If a device is taken out and a similar device put in without cutting or puncturing the skin or mucous membrane, the procedure is coded to the root operation CHANGE. Otherwise, the procedure for taking out a device is coded to the root operation REMOVAL.

Body Part Character 4	Approach Character 5	Device Character 6	Qualifier Character 7
A Heart	**Ø** Open **3** Percutaneous **4** Percutaneous Endoscopic	**2** Monitoring Device **3** Infusion Device **7** Autologous Tissue Substitute **8** Zooplastic Tissue **C** Extraluminal Device **D** Intraluminal Device **J** Synthetic Substitute **K** Nonautologous Tissue Substitute **M** Cardiac Lead **N** Intracardiac Pacemaker **Q** Implantable Heart Assist System **Y** Other Device	**Z** No Qualifier
A Heart ⊞	**Ø** Open **3** Percutaneous **4** Percutaneous Endoscopic	**R** Short-term External Heart Assist System	**S** Biventricular **Z** No Qualifier
A Heart	**X** External	**2** Monitoring Device **3** Infusion Device **D** Intraluminal Device **M** Cardiac Lead	**Z** No Qualifier
Y Great Vessel	**Ø** Open **3** Percutaneous **4** Percutaneous Endoscopic	**2** Monitoring Device **3** Infusion Device **7** Autologous Tissue Substitute **8** Zooplastic Tissue **C** Extraluminal Device **D** Intraluminal Device **J** Synthetic Substitute **K** Nonautologous Tissue Substitute **Y** Other Device	**Z** No Qualifier
Y Great Vessel	**X** External	**2** Monitoring Device **3** Infusion Device **D** Intraluminal Device	**Z** No Qualifier

Non-OR	Ø2PA3[2,3,D]Z
Non-OR	Ø2PA[3,4]YZ
Non-OR	Ø2PAX[2,3,D,M]Z
Non-OR	Ø2PY3[2,3,D]Z
Non-OR	Ø2PY[3,4]YZ
Non-OR	Ø2PYX[2,3,D]Z
HAC	Ø2PA[Ø,3,4]MZ when reported with SDx K68.11 or T81.4XXA or T82.6XXA or T82.7XXA
HAC	Ø2PAXMZ when reported with SDx K68.11 or T81.4XXA or T82.6XXA or T82.7XXA

See Appendix L for Procedure Combinations
⊞   Ø2PA[Ø,3,4]RZ

LC Limited Coverage   NC Noncovered   ⊞ Combination Member   HAC associated procedure   Combination Only   DRG Non-OR   Non-OR   New/Revised in GREEN

176   ICD-10-PCS 2019

0   **Medical and Surgical**
2   **Heart and Great Vessels**
Q   **Repair**   Definition: Restoring, to the extent possible, a body part to its normal anatomic structure and function
                    Explanation: Used only when the method to accomplish the repair is not one of the other root operations

Body Part Character 4	Approach Character 5	Device Character 6	Qualifier Character 7

0 **Coronary Artery, One Artery**
1 **Coronary Artery, Two Arteries**
2 **Coronary Artery, Three Arteries**
3 **Coronary Artery, Four or More
    Arteries**
4 **Coronary Vein**
5 **Atrial Septum**
    Interatrial septum
6 **Atrium, Right**
    Atrium dextrum cordis
    Right auricular appendix
    Sinus venosus
7 **Atrium, Left**
    Atrium pulmonale
    Left auricular appendix
8 **Conduction Mechanism**
    Atrioventricular node
    Bundle of His
    Bundle of Kent
    Sinoatrial node
9 **Chordae Tendineae**
A **Heart**
B **Heart, Right**
    Right coronary sulcus
C **Heart, Left**
    Left coronary sulcus
    Obtuse margin
D **Papillary Muscle**
H **Pulmonary Valve**
    Pulmonary annulus
    Pulmonic valve
K **Ventricle, Right**
    Conus arteriosus
L **Ventricle, Left**
M **Ventricular Septum**
    Interventricular septum
N **Pericardium**
P **Pulmonary Trunk**
Q **Pulmonary Artery, Right**
R **Pulmonary Artery, Left**
    Arterial canal (duct)
    Botallo's duct
    Pulmoaortic canal
S **Pulmonary Vein, Right**
    Right inferior pulmonary vein
    Right superior pulmonary vein
T **Pulmonary Vein, Left**
    Left inferior pulmonary vein
    Left superior pulmonary vein
V **Superior Vena Cava**
    Precava
W **Thoracic Aorta, Descending**
X **Thoracic Aorta, Ascending/Arch**
    Aortic arch
    Ascending aorta
	0 **Open**
	3 **Percutaneous**
	4 **Percutaneous Endoscopic**
		Z **No Device**	**Z** **No Qualifier**

F **Aortic Valve** Aortic annulus	**0** **Open** **3** **Percutaneous** **4** **Percutaneous Endoscopic**	**Z** **No Device**	**J** **Truncal Valve** **Z** **No Qualifier**

G **Mitral Valve**
    Bicuspid valve
    Left atrioventricular valve
    Mitral annulus
	0 **Open**
	3 **Percutaneous**
	4 **Percutaneous Endoscopic**
		Z **No Device**	**E** **Atrioventricular Valve, Left**
			Z **No Qualifier**

J **Tricuspid Valve**
    Right atrioventricular valve
    Tricuspid annulus
	0 **Open**
	3 **Percutaneous**
	4 **Percutaneous Endoscopic**
		Z **No Device**	**G** **Atrioventricular Valve, Right**
			Z **No Qualifier**

Heart and Great Vessels *(side tab)*

0   **Medical and Surgical**
2   **Heart and Great Vessels**
R   **Replacement**   Definition: Putting in or on biological or synthetic material that physically takes the place and/or function of all or a portion of a body part
                         Explanation: The body part may have been taken out or replaced, or may be taken out, physically eradicated, or rendered nonfunctional during the REPLACEMENT procedure. A REMOVAL procedure is coded for taking out the device used in a previous replacement procedure.

Body Part Character 4	Approach Character 5	Device Character 6	Qualifier Character 7

5   **Atrial Septum**
    Interatrial septum
6   **Atrium, Right**
    Atrium dextrum cordis
    Right auricular appendix
    Sinus venosus
7   **Atrium, Left**
    Atrium pulmonale
    Left auricular appendix
9   **Chordae Tendineae**
D   **Papillary Muscle**
K   **Ventricle, Right**   ⊞ LC NC
    Conus arteriosus
L   **Ventricle, Left**   ⊞ LC NC
M   **Ventricular Septum**
    Interventricular septum
N   **Pericardium**
P   **Pulmonary Trunk**
Q   **Pulmonary Artery, Right**
R   **Pulmonary Artery, Left**
    Arterial canal (duct)
    Botallo's duct
    Pulmoaortic canal
S   **Pulmonary Vein, Right**
    Right inferior pulmonary vein
    Right superior pulmonary vein
T   **Pulmonary Vein, Left**
    Left inferior pulmonary vein
    Left superior pulmonary vein
V   **Superior Vena Cava**
    Precava
W   **Thoracic Aorta, Descending**
X   **Thoracic Aorta, Ascending/Arch**
    Aortic arch
    Ascending aorta
	0 Open
	4 Percutaneous Endoscopic
		7 Autologous Tissue Substitute
		8 Zooplastic Tissue
		J Synthetic Substitute
		K Nonautologous Tissue Substitute
			Z No Qualifier

F   **Aortic Valve**
    Aortic annulus
G   **Mitral Valve**
    Bicuspid valve
    Left atrioventricular valve
    Mitral annulus
H   **Pulmonary Valve**
    Pulmonary annulus
    Pulmonic valve
J   **Tricuspid Valve**
    Right atrioventricular valve
    Tricuspid annulus
	0 Open
	4 Percutaneous Endoscopic
		7 Autologous Tissue Substitute
		8 Zooplastic Tissue
		J Synthetic Substitute
		K Nonautologous Tissue Substitute
			Z No Qualifier

F   **Aortic Valve**
    Aortic annulus
G   **Mitral Valve**
    Bicuspid valve
    Left atrioventricular valve
    Mitral annulus
H   **Pulmonary Valve**
    Pulmonary annulus
    Pulmonic valve
J   **Tricuspid Valve**
    Right atrioventricular valve
    Tricuspid annulus
	3 Percutaneous	**7** Autologous Tissue Substitute
		8 Zooplastic Tissue
		J Synthetic Substitute
		K Nonautologous Tissue Substitute
			H Transapical
			Z No Qualifier

LC	02RK0JZ with 02RL0JZ with diagnosis code Z00.6
NC	02RK0JZ with 02RL0JZ without diagnosis code Z00.6

See Appendix L for Procedure Combinations
⊞   02R[K,L]0JZ

0 Medical and Surgical
2 Heart and Great Vessels
S Reposition   Definition: Moving to its normal location, or other suitable location, all or a portion of a body part

       Explanation: The body part is moved to a new location from an abnormal location, or from a normal location where it is not functioning correctly. The body part may or may not be cut out or off to be moved to the new location.

Body Part Character 4	Approach Character 5	Device Character 6	Qualifier Character 7

0 Coronary Artery, One Artery
1 Coronary Artery, Two Arteries
P Pulmonary Trunk
Q Pulmonary Artery, Right
R Pulmonary Artery, Left
   Arterial canal (duct)
   Botallo's duct
   Pulmoaortic canal
S Pulmonary Vein, Right
   Right inferior pulmonary vein
   Right superior pulmonary vein
T Pulmonary Vein, Left
   Left inferior pulmonary vein
   Left superior pulmonary vein
V Superior Vena Cava
   Precava
W Thoracic Aorta, Descending
X Thoracic Aorta, Ascending/Arch
   Aortic arch
   Ascending aorta
	0 Open	**Z** No Device	**Z** No Qualifier

0 Medical and Surgical
2 Heart and Great Vessels
T Resection   Definition: Cutting out or off, without replacement, all of a body part

       Explanation: None

Body Part Character 4	Approach Character 5	Device Character 6	Qualifier Character 7

5 Atrial Septum
   Interatrial septum
8 Conduction Mechanism
   Atrioventricular node
   Bundle of His
   Bundle of Kent
   Sinoatrial node
9 Chordae Tendineae
D Papillary Muscle
H Pulmonary Valve
   Pulmonary annulus
   Pulmonic valve
M Ventricular Septum
   Interventricular septum
N Pericardium
	0 Open
	3 Percutaneous
	4 Percutaneous Endoscopic
		Z No Device	**Z** No Qualifier

LC Limited Coverage   NC Noncovered   ⊞ Combination Member   HAC associated procedure   Combination Only   DRG Non-OR   Non-OR   New/Revised in GREEN

ICD-10-PCS 2019   179

Heart and Great Vessels

Ø   **Medical and Surgical**
2   **Heart and Great Vessels**
U   **Supplement**   Definition: Putting in or on biological or synthetic material that physically reinforces and/or augments the function of a portion of a body part
         Explanation: The biological material is non-living, or is living and from the same individual. The body part may have been previously replaced, and the SUPPLEMENT procedure is performed to physically reinforce and/or augment the function of the replaced body part.

Body Part Character 4	Approach Character 5	Device Character 6	Qualifier Character 7

5 Atrial Septum
  Interatrial septum
6 Atrium, Right
  Atrium dextrum cordis
  Right auricular appendix
  Sinus venosus
7 Atrium, Left
  Atrium pulmonale
  Left auricular appendix
9 Chordae Tendineae
A Heart
D Papillary Muscle
H Pulmonary Valve
  Pulmonary annulus
  Pulmonic valve
K Ventricle, Right
  Conus arteriosus
L Ventricle, Left
M Ventricular Septum
  Interventricular septum
N Pericardium
P Pulmonary Trunk
Q Pulmonary Artery, Right
R Pulmonary Artery, Left
  Arterial canal (duct)
  Botallo's duct
  Pulmoaortic canal
S Pulmonary Vein, Right
  Right inferior pulmonary vein
  Right superior pulmonary vein
T Pulmonary Vein, Left
  Left inferior pulmonary vein
  Left superior pulmonary vein
V Superior Vena Cava
  Precava
W Thoracic Aorta, Descending
X Thoracic Aorta, Ascending/Arch
  Aortic arch
  Ascending aorta
	Ø Open
	3 Percutaneous
	4 Percutaneous Endoscopic
		7 Autologous Tissue Substitute
		8 Zooplastic Tissue
		J Synthetic Substitute
		K Nonautologous Tissue Substitute
			Z No Qualifier

F Aortic Valve Aortic annulus	Ø Open 3 Percutaneous 4 Percutaneous Endoscopic	7 Autologous Tissue Substitute 8 Zooplastic Tissue J Synthetic Substitute K Nonautologous Tissue Substitute	J Truncal Valve Z No Qualifier

G Mitral Valve
  Bicuspid valve
  Left atrioventricular valve
  Mitral annulus
	Ø Open
	3 Percutaneous
	4 Percutaneous Endoscopic
		7 Autologous Tissue Substitute
		8 Zooplastic Tissue
		J Synthetic Substitute
		K Nonautologous Tissue Substitute
			E Atrioventricular Valve, Left
			Z No Qualifier

J Tricuspid Valve
  Right atrioventricular valve
  Tricuspid annulus
	Ø Open
	3 Percutaneous
	4 Percutaneous Endoscopic
		7 Autologous Tissue Substitute
		8 Zooplastic Tissue
		J Synthetic Substitute
		K Nonautologous Tissue Substitute
			G Atrioventricular Valve, Right
			Z No Qualifier

DRG Non-OR   02U7[3,4]JZ

LC Limited Coverage   **NC** Noncovered   ⊞ Combination Member   HAC associated procedure   Combination Only   DRG Non-OR   Non-OR   New/Revised in GREEN

Ø   Medical and Surgical
2   Heart and Great Vessels
V   Restriction   Definition: Partially closing an orifice or the lumen of a tubular body part
                          Explanation: The orifice can be a natural orifice or an artificially created orifice

Body Part Character 4	Approach Character 5	Device Character 6	Qualifier Character 7
A Heart	Ø Open 3 Percutaneous 4 Percutaneous Endoscopic	C Extraluminal Device Z No Device	Z No Qualifier

G   Mitral Valve
      Bicuspid valve
      Left atrioventricular valve
      Mitral annulus
	Ø Open
	3 Percutaneous
	4 Percutaneous Endoscopic
		Z No Device	Z No Qualifier

P   Pulmonary Trunk
Q   Pulmonary Artery, Right
S   Pulmonary Vein, Right
      Right inferior pulmonary vein
      Right superior pulmonary vein
T   Pulmonary Vein, Left
      Left inferior pulmonary vein
      Left superior pulmonary vein
V   Superior Vena Cava
      Precava
	Ø Open
	3 Percutaneous
	4 Percutaneous Endoscopic
		C Extraluminal Device
		D Intraluminal Device
		Z No Device
			Z No Qualifier

R   Pulmonary Artery, Left
      Arterial canal (duct)
      Botallo's duct
      Pulmoaortic canal
	Ø Open
	3 Percutaneous
	4 Percutaneous Endoscopic
		C Extraluminal Device
		D Intraluminal Device
		Z No Device
			T Ductus Arteriosus
			Z No Qualifier

W   Thoracic Aorta, Descending
X   Thoracic Aorta, Ascending/Arch
      Aortic arch
      Ascending aorta
	Ø Open
	3 Percutaneous
	4 Percutaneous Endoscopic
		C Extraluminal Device
		D Intraluminal Device
		E Intraluminal Device, Branched or
		     Fenestrated, One or Two Arteries
		F Intraluminal Device, Branched or
		     Fenestrated, Three or More Arteries
		Z No Device
			Z No Qualifier

Heart and Great Vessels

Ø   **Medical and Surgical**
2   **Heart and Great Vessels**
W   **Revision**   Definition: Correcting, to the extent possible, a portion of a malfunctioning device or the position of a displaced device
                     Explanation: Revision can include correcting a malfunctioning or displaced device by taking out or putting in components of the device such as a screw or pin

Body Part Character 4	Approach Character 5	Device Character 6	Qualifier Character 7

5   **Atrial Septum**
     Interatrial septum
M   **Ventricular Septum**
     Interventricular septum
	Ø Open
	4 Percutaneous Endoscopic
		J Synthetic Substitute	Z No Qualifier

A **Heart** ⊞ LC NC	Ø Open 3 Percutaneous 4 Percutaneous Endoscopic	2 Monitoring Device 3 Infusion Device 7 Autologous Tissue Substitute 8 Zooplastic Tissue C Extraluminal Device D Intraluminal Device J Synthetic Substitute K Nonautologous Tissue Substitute M Cardiac Lead N Intracardiac Pacemaker Q Implantable Heart Assist System Y Other Device	Z No Qualifier
A Heart ⊞	Ø Open 3 Percutaneous 4 Percutaneous Endoscopic	R Short-term External Heart Assist System	S Biventricular Z No Qualifier
A Heart	X External	2 Monitoring Device 3 Infusion Device 7 Autologous Tissue Substitute 8 Zooplastic Tissue C Extraluminal Device D Intraluminal Device J Synthetic Substitute K Nonautologous Tissue Substitute M Cardiac Lead N Intracardiac Pacemaker Q Implantable Heart Assist System	Z No Qualifier
A Heart	X External	R Short-term External Heart Assist System	S Biventricular Z No Qualifier

F   **Aortic Valve**
     Aortic annulus
G   **Mitral Valve**
     Bicuspid valve
     Left atrioventricular valve
     Mitral annulus
H   **Pulmonary Valve**
     Pulmonary annulus
     Pulmonic valve
J   **Tricuspid Valve**
     Right atrioventricular valve
     Tricuspid annulus
	Ø Open
	3 Percutaneous
	4 Percutaneous Endoscopic
		7 Autologous Tissue Substitute
		8 Zooplastic Tissue
		J Synthetic Substitute
		K Nonautologous Tissue Substitute
			Z No Qualifier

Y **Great Vessel**	Ø Open 3 Percutaneous 4 Percutaneous Endoscopic	2 Monitoring Device 3 Infusion Device 7 Autologous Tissue Substitute 8 Zooplastic Tissue C Extraluminal Device D Intraluminal Device J Synthetic Substitute K Nonautologous Tissue Substitute Y Other Device	Z No Qualifier
Y **Great Vessel**	X External	2 Monitoring Device 3 Infusion Device 7 Autologous Tissue Substitute 8 Zooplastic Tissue C Extraluminal Device D Intraluminal Device J Synthetic Substitute K Nonautologous Tissue Substitute	Z No Qualifier

Non-OR 02WA3[2,3,D]Z	**HAC** 02WA[Ø,3,4]MZ when reported with SDx K68.11 or T81.4XXA	
Non-OR 02WA[3,4]YZ	or T82.6XXA or T82.7XXA	
Non-OR 02WAX[2,3,7,8,C,D,J,K,M,N,Q]Z	**LC** 02WAØ[J,Q]Z	
Non-OR 02WAXRZ	**NC** 02WA[3,4]QZ	
Non-OR 02WY3[2,3,D]Z		
Non-OR 02WY[3,4]YZ	**See Appendix L for Procedure Combinations**	
Non-OR 02WYX[2,3,7,8,C,D,J,K]Z	⊞ 02WA[Ø,3,4]QZ	
	⊞ 02WA[Ø,3,4]RZ	

LC Limited Coverage   **NC** Noncovered   ⊞ Combination Member   HAC associated procedure   Combination Only   DRG Non-OR   Non-OR   New/Revised in GREEN

Ø Medical and Surgical
2 Heart and Great Vessels
Y Transplantation   Definition: Putting in or on all or a portion of a living body part taken from another individual or animal to physically take the place and/or function of all or a portion of a similar body part

                       Explanation: The native body part may or may not be taken out, and the transplanted body part may take over all or a portion of its function

Body Part Character 4	Approach Character 5	Device Character 6	Qualifier Character 7
A Heart LC	Ø Open	Z No Device	Ø Allogeneic 1 Syngeneic 2 Zooplastic

     LC   Ø2YAØZ[Ø,1,2]

Upper Arteries Ø31–Ø3W

Character Meanings

This Character Meaning table is provided as a guide to assist the user in the identification of character members that may be found in this section of code tables. It **SHOULD NOT** be used to build a PCS code.

Operation–Character 3	Body Part–Character 4	Approach–Character 5	Device–Character 6	Qualifier–Character 7
1 Bypass	Ø Internal Mammary Artery, Right	Ø Open	Ø Drainage Device	Ø Upper Arm Artery, Right
5 Destruction	1 Internal Mammary Artery, Left	3 Percutaneous	2 Monitoring Device	1 Upper Arm Artery, Left OR Drug-Coated Balloon
7 Dilation	2 Innominate Artery	4 Percutaneous Endoscopic	3 Infusion Device	2 Upper Arm Artery, Bilateral
9 Drainage	3 Subclavian Artery, Right	X External	4 Intraluminal Device, Drug-eluting	3 Lower Arm Artery, Right
B Excision	4 Subclavian Artery, Left		5 Intraluminal Device, Drug-eluting, Two	4 Lower Arm Artery, Left
C Extirpation	5 Axillary Artery, Right		6 Intraluminal Device, Drug-eluting, Three	5 Lower Arm Artery, Bilateral
H Insertion	6 Axillary Artery, Left		7 Intraluminal Device, Drug-eluting, Four or More OR Autologous Tissue Substitute	6 Upper Leg Artery, Right OR Bifurcation
J Inspection	7 Brachial Artery, Right		9 Autologous Venous Tissue	7 Upper Leg Artery, Left OR Stent Retriever
L Occlusion	8 Brachial Artery, Left		A Autologous Arterial Tissue	8 Upper Leg Artery, Bilateral
N Release	9 Ulnar Artery, Right		B Intraluminal Device, Bioactive	9 Lower Leg Artery, Right
P Removal	A Ulnar Artery, Left		C Extraluminal Device	B Lower Leg Artery, Left
Q Repair	B Radial Artery, Right		D Intraluminal Device	C Lower Leg Artery, Bilateral
R Replacement	C Radial Artery, Left		E Intraluminal Device, Two	D Upper Arm Vein
S Reposition	D Hand Artery, Right		F Intraluminal Device, Three	F Lower Arm Vein
U Supplement	F Hand Artery, Left		G Intraluminal Device, Four or More	G Intracranial Artery
V Restriction	G Intracranial Artery		J Synthetic Substitute	J Extracranial Artery, Right
W Revision	H Common Carotid Artery, Right		K Nonautologous Tissue Substitute	K Extracranial Artery, Left
	J Common Carotid Artery, Left		M Stimulator Lead	M Pulmonary Artery, Right
	K Internal Carotid Artery, Right		Y Other Device	N Pulmonary Artery, Left
	L Internal Carotid Artery, Left		Z No Device	T Abdominal Artery
	M External Carotid Artery, Right			V Superior Vena Cava
	N External Carotid Artery, Left			X Diagnostic
	P Vertebral Artery, Right			Y Upper Artery
	Q Vertebral Artery, Left			Z No Qualifier
	R Face Artery			
	S Temporal Artery, Right			
	T Temporal Artery, Left			
	U Thyroid Artery, Right			
	V Thyroid Artery, Left			
	Y Upper Artery			

AHA Coding Clinic for table Ø31

2017, 4Q, 64-65	New qualifier values - Left to right carotid bypass
2017, 2Q, 22	Carotid artery to subclavian artery transposition
2017, 1Q, 31	Left to right common carotid artery bypass
2016, 3Q, 37	Insertion of arteriovenous graft using HeRO device
2016, 3Q, 39	Revision of arteriovenous graft
2013, 4Q, 125	Stage II cephalic vein transposition (superficialization) of arteriovenous fistula
2013, 1Q, 27	Creation of radial artery fistula

AHA Coding Clinic for table Ø37

2018, 2Q, 24	Coronary artery bifurcation
2016, 4Q, 86	Peripheral artery, number of stents
2016, 4Q, 86-87	Coronary and peripheral artery bifurcation
2015, 1Q, 32	Deployment of stent for herniated/migrated coil in basilar artery

AHA Coding Clinic for table Ø3B

2016, 2Q, 12	Resection of malignant neoplasm of infratemporal fossa

AHA Coding Clinic for table Ø3C

2018, 2Q, 24	Coronary artery bifurcation
2017, 4Q, 64-65	New qualifier values - Left to right carotid bypass
2017, 2Q, 23	Thrombectomy via Fogarty catheter
2016, 4Q, 86-87	Coronary and peripheral artery bifurcation
2016, 2Q, 11	Carotid endarterectomy with patch angioplasty
2015, 1Q, 29	Discontinued carotid endarterectomy

AHA Coding Clinic for table Ø3H

2016, 2Q, 32	Arterial catheter placement

AHA Coding Clinic for table Ø3J

2015, 1Q, 29	Discontinued carotid endarterectomy

AHA Coding Clinic for table Ø3L

2016, 2Q, 30	Clipping (occlusion) of cerebral artery, decompressive craniectomy and storage of bone flap in abdominal wall
2014, 4Q, 20	Control of epistaxis
2014, 4Q, 37	Endovascular embolization of arteriovenous malformation using Onyx-18 liquid

AHA Coding Clinic for table Ø3Q

2017, 1Q, 31	Left to right common carotid artery bypass

AHA Coding Clinic for table Ø3S

2017, 2Q, 22	Carotid artery to subclavian artery transposition
2015, 3Q, 27	Moyamoya disease and hemispheric pial synagiosis with craniotomy

AHA Coding Clinic for table Ø3U

2016, 2Q, 11	Carotid endarterectomy with patch angioplasty

AHA Coding Clinic for table Ø3V

2016, 1Q, 19	Embolization of superior hypophyseal aneurysm using stent-assisted coil

AHA Coding Clinic for table Ø3W

2016, 3Q, 39	Revision of arteriovenous graft
2015, 1Q, 32	Deployment of stent for herniated/migrated coil in basilar artery

Upper Arteries

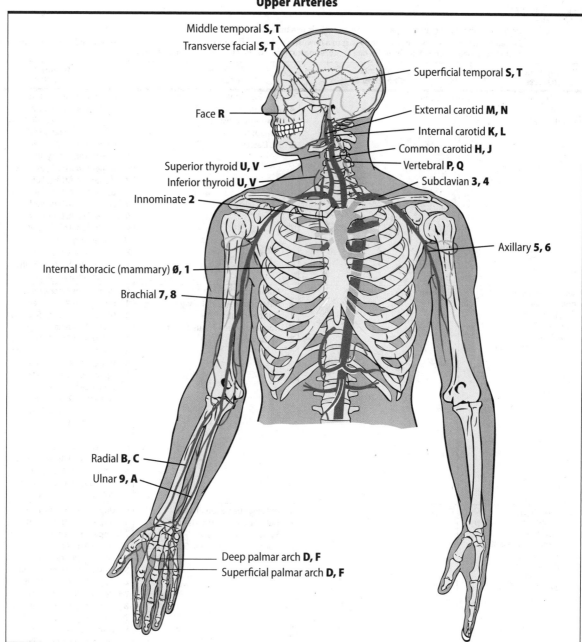

Middle temporal **S, T**
Transverse facial **S, T**
Superficial temporal **S, T**
Face **R**
External carotid **M, N**
Internal carotid **K, L**
Common carotid **H, J**
Superior thyroid **U, V**
Vertebral **P, Q**
Inferior thyroid **U, V**
Subclavian **3, 4**
Innominate **2**
Axillary **5, 6**
Internal thoracic (mammary) **Ø, 1**
Brachial **7, 8**
Radial **B, C**
Ulnar **9, A**
Deep palmar arch **D, F**
Superficial palmar arch **D, F**

Head and Neck Arteries

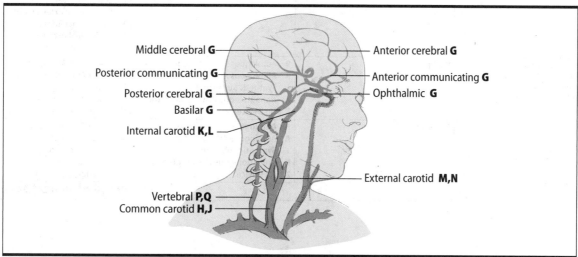

Middle cerebral **G**
Anterior cerebral **G**
Posterior communicating **G**
Anterior communicating **G**
Posterior cerebral **G**
Ophthalmic **G**
Basilar **G**
Internal carotid **K,L**
External carotid **M,N**
Vertebral **P,Q**
Common carotid **H,J**

Upper Arteries

Ø   **Medical and Surgical**
3   **Upper Arteries**
1   **Bypass**   Definition: Altering the route of passage of the contents of a tubular body part

Explanation: Rerouting contents of a body part to a downstream area of the normal route, to a similar route and body part, or to an abnormal route and dissimilar body part. Includes one or more anastomoses, with or without the use of a device.

Body Part Character 4	Approach Character 5	Device Character 6	Qualifier Character 7
2 Innominate Artery Brachiocephalic artery Brachiocephalic trunk	Ø Open	9 Autologous Venous Tissue A Autologous Arterial Tissue J Synthetic Substitute K Nonautologous Tissue Substitute Z No Device	Ø Upper Arm Artery, Right 1 Upper Arm Artery, Left 2 Upper Arm Artery, Bilateral 3 Lower Arm Artery, Right 4 Lower Arm Artery, Left 5 Lower Arm Artery, Bilateral 6 Upper Leg Artery, Right 7 Upper Leg Artery, Left 8 Upper Leg Artery, Bilateral 9 Lower Leg Artery, Right B Lower Leg Artery, Left C Lower Leg Artery, Bilateral D Upper Arm Vein F Lower Arm Vein J Extracranial Artery, Right K Extracranial Artery, Left
3 Subclavian Artery, Right Costocervical trunk Dorsal scapular artery Internal thoracic artery **4 Subclavian Artery, Left** *See 3 Subclavian Artery, Right*	Ø Open	9 Autologous Venous Tissue A Autologous Arterial Tissue J Synthetic Substitute K Nonautologous Tissue Substitute Z No Device	Ø Upper Arm Artery, Right 1 Upper Arm Artery, Left 2 Upper Arm Artery, Bilateral 3 Lower Arm Artery, Right 4 Lower Arm Artery, Left 5 Lower Arm Artery, Bilateral 6 Upper Leg Artery, Right 7 Upper Leg Artery, Left 8 Upper Leg Artery, Bilateral 9 Lower Leg Artery, Right B Lower Leg Artery, Left C Lower Leg Artery, Bilateral D Upper Arm Vein F Lower Arm Vein J Extracranial Artery, Right K Extracranial Artery, Left M Pulmonary Artery, Right N Pulmonary Artery, Left
5 Axillary Artery, Right Anterior circumflex humeral artery Lateral thoracic artery Posterior circumflex humeral artery Subscapular artery Superior thoracic artery Thoracoacromial artery **6 Axillary Artery, Left** *See 5 Axillary Artery, Right*	Ø Open	9 Autologous Venous Tissue A Autologous Arterial Tissue J Synthetic Substitute K Nonautologous Tissue Substitute Z No Device	Ø Upper Arm Artery, Right 1 Upper Arm Artery, Left 2 Upper Arm Artery, Bilateral 3 Lower Arm Artery, Right 4 Lower Arm Artery, Left 5 Lower Arm Artery, Bilateral 6 Upper Leg Artery, Right 7 Upper Leg Artery, Left 8 Upper Leg Artery, Bilateral 9 Lower Leg Artery, Right B Lower Leg Artery, Left C Lower Leg Artery, Bilateral D Upper Arm Vein F Lower Arm Vein J Extracranial Artery, Right K Extracranial Artery, Left T Abdominal Artery V Superior Vena Cava
7 Brachial Artery, Right Inferior ulnar collateral artery Profunda brachii Superior ulnar collateral artery	Ø Open	9 Autologous Venous Tissue A Autologous Arterial Tissue J Synthetic Substitute K Nonautologous Tissue Substitute Z No Device	Ø Upper Arm Artery, Right 3 Lower Arm Artery, Right D Upper Arm Vein F Lower Arm Vein V Superior Vena Cava
8 Brachial Artery, Left Inferior ulnar collateral artery Profunda brachii Superior ulnar collateral artery	Ø Open	9 Autologous Venous Tissue A Autologous Arterial Tissue J Synthetic Substitute K Nonautologous Tissue Substitute Z No Device	1 Upper Arm Artery, Left 4 Lower Arm Artery, Left D Upper Arm Vein F Lower Arm Vein V Superior Vena Cava

Ø31 Continued on next page

LC Limited Coverage   NC Noncovered   ⊞ Combination Member   HAC associated procedure   Combination Only   DRG Non-OR   Non-OR   New/Revised in GREEN

188   ICD-10-PCS 2019

Ø   Medical and Surgical
3   Upper Arteries
1   Bypass

031 Continued

Definition: Altering the route of passage of the contents of a tubular body part

Explanation: Rerouting contents of a body part to a downstream area of the normal route, to a similar route and body part, or to an abnormal route and dissimilar body part. Includes one or more anastomoses, with or without the use of a device.

Body Part Character 4	Approach Character 5	Device Character 6	Qualifier Character 7
9 Ulnar Artery, Right Anterior ulnar recurrent artery Common interosseous artery Posterior ulnar recurrent artery **B Radial Artery, Right** Radial recurrent artery	**Ø Open**	**9 Autologous Venous Tissue** **A Autologous Arterial Tissue** **J Synthetic Substitute** **K Nonautologous Tissue Substitute** **Z No Device**	**3 Lower Arm Artery, Right** **F Lower Arm Vein**
A Ulnar Artery, Left Anterior ulnar recurrent artery Common interosseous artery Posterior ulnar recurrent artery **C Radial Artery, Left** Radial recurrent artery	**Ø Open**	**9 Autologous Venous Tissue** **A Autologous Arterial Tissue** **J Synthetic Substitute** **K Nonautologous Tissue Substitute** **Z No Device**	**4 Lower Arm Artery, Left** **F Lower Arm Vein**

G   Intracranial Artery
Anterior cerebral artery
Anterior choroidal artery
Anterior communicating artery
Basilar artery
Circle of Willis
Internal carotid artery, intracranial
    portion
Middle cerebral artery
Ophthalmic artery
Posterior cerebral artery
Posterior communicating artery
Posterior inferior cerebellar artery
    (PICA)
S   Temporal Artery, Right
Middle temporal artery
Superficial temporal artery
Transverse facial artery
T   Temporal Artery, Left
See S Temporal Artery, Right
	Ø Open	**9 Autologous Venous Tissue**
		A Autologous Arterial Tissue
		J Synthetic Substitute
		K Nonautologous Tissue Substitute
		Z No Device
			G Intracranial Artery

H Common Carotid Artery, Right **J Common Carotid Artery, Left**	**Ø Open**	**9 Autologous Venous Tissue** **A Autologous Arterial Tissue** **J Synthetic Substitute** **K Nonautologous Tissue Substitute** **Z No Device**	**G Intracranial Artery** **J Extracranial Artery, Right** **K Extracranial Artery, Left** **Y Upper Artery**
K Internal Carotid Artery, Right Caroticotympanic artery Carotid sinus **L Internal Carotid Artery, Left** Caroticotympanic artery Carotid sinus **M External Carotid Artery, Right** Ascending pharyngeal artery Internal maxillary artery Lingual artery Maxillary artery Occipital artery Posterior auricular artery Superior thyroid artery **N External Carotid Artery, Left** Ascending pharyngeal artery Internal maxillary artery Lingual artery Maxillary artery Occipital artery Posterior auricular artery Superior thyroid artery	**Ø Open**	**9 Autologous Venous Tissue** **A Autologous Arterial Tissue** **J Synthetic Substitute** **K Nonautologous Tissue Substitute** **Z No Device**	**J Extracranial Artery, Right** **K Extracranial Artery, Left**

LC Limited Coverage   NC Noncovered   ⊞ Combination Member   HAC associated procedure   Combination Only   DRG Non-OR   Non-OR   New/Revised in GREEN

ICD-10-PCS 2019   189

031–031

Ø   **Medical and Surgical**
3   **Upper Arteries**
5   **Destruction**   Definition: Physical eradication of all or a portion of a body part by the direct use of energy, force, or a destructive agent

                       Explanation: None of the body part is physically taken out

Body Part Character 4		Approach Character 5	Device Character 6	Qualifier Character 7
Ø Internal Mammary Artery, Right Anterior intercostal artery Internal thoracic artery Musculophrenic artery Pericardiophrenic artery Superior epigastric artery **1 Internal Mammary Artery, Left** *See Ø Internal Mammary Artery, Right* **2 Innominate Artery** Brachiocephalic artery Brachiocephalic trunk **3 Subclavian Artery, Right** Costocervical trunk Dorsal scapular artery Internal thoracic artery **4 Subclavian Artery, Left** *See 3 Subclavian Artery, Right* **5 Axillary Artery, Right** Anterior circumflex humeral artery Lateral thoracic artery Posterior circumflex humeral artery Subscapular artery Superior thoracic artery Thoracoacromial artery **6 Axillary Artery, Left** *See 5 Axillary Artery, Right* **7 Brachial Artery, Right** Inferior ulnar collateral artery Profunda brachii Superior ulnar collateral artery **8 Brachial Artery, Left** *See 7 Brachial Artery, Right* **9 Ulnar Artery, Right** Anterior ulnar recurrent artery Common interosseous artery Posterior ulnar recurrent artery **A Ulnar Artery, Left** *See 9 Ulnar Artery, Right* **B Radial Artery, Right** Radial recurrent artery **C Radial Artery, Left** *See B Radial Artery, Right* **D Hand Artery, Right** Deep palmar arch Princeps pollicis artery Radialis indicis Superficial palmar arch **F Hand Artery, Left** *See D Hand Artery, Right* **G Intracranial Artery** Anterior cerebral artery Anterior choroidal artery Anterior communicating artery Basilar artery Circle of Willis Internal carotid artery, intracranial portion Middle cerebral artery Ophthalmic artery Posterior cerebral artery Posterior communicating artery Posterior inferior cerebellar artery (PICA)	**H Common Carotid Artery, Right** **J Common Carotid Artery, Left** **K Internal Carotid Artery, Right** Caroticotympanic artery Carotid sinus **L Internal Carotid Artery, Left** *See K Internal Carotid Artery, Right* **M External Carotid Artery, Right** Ascending pharyngeal artery Internal maxillary artery Lingual artery Maxillary artery Occipital artery Posterior auricular artery Superior thyroid artery **N External Carotid Artery, Left** *See M External Carotid Artery, Right* **P Vertebral Artery, Right** Anterior spinal artery Posterior spinal artery **Q Vertebral Artery, Left** *See P Vertebral Artery, Right* **R Face Artery** Angular artery Ascending palatine artery External maxillary artery Facial artery Inferior labial artery Submental artery Superior labial artery **S Temporal Artery, Right** Middle temporal artery Superficial temporal artery Transverse facial artery **T Temporal Artery, Left** *See S Temporal Artery, Right* **U Thyroid Artery, Right** Cricothyroid artery Hyoid artery Sternocleidomastoid artery Superior laryngeal artery Superior thyroid artery Thyrocervical trunk **V Thyroid Artery, Left** *See U Thyroid Artery, Right* **Y Upper Artery** Aortic intercostal artery Bronchial artery Esophageal artery Subcostal artery	**Ø Open** **3 Percutaneous** **4 Percutaneous Endoscopic**	**Z No Device**	**Z No Qualifier**

LC Limited Coverage   **NC** Noncovered   ⊞ Combination Member   HAC associated procedure   Combination Only   DRG Non-OR   Non-OR   New/Revised in GREEN

190   ICD-10-PCS 2019

Ø   Medical and Surgical
3   Upper Arteries
7   Dilation   Definition: Expanding an orifice or the lumen of a tubular body part

Explanation: The orifice can be a natural orifice or an artificially created orifice. Accomplished by stretching a tubular body part using intraluminal pressure or by cutting part of the orifice or wall of the tubular body part.

Body Part Character 4		Approach Character 5	Device Character 6	Qualifier Character 7

Ø Internal Mammary Artery, Right
    Anterior intercostal artery
    Internal thoracic artery
    Musculophrenic artery
    Pericardiophrenic artery
    Superior epigastric artery
1 Internal Mammary Artery, Left
    See Ø Internal Mammary Artery, Right
2 Innominate Artery
    Brachiocephalic artery
    Brachiocephalic trunk
3 Subclavian Artery, Right
    Costocervical trunk
    Dorsal scapular artery
    Internal thoracic artery
4 Subclavian Artery, Left
    See 3 Subclavian Artery, Right
5 Axillary Artery, Right
    Anterior circumflex humeral artery
    Lateral thoracic artery
    Posterior circumflex humeral artery
    Subscapular artery
    Superior thoracic artery
    Thoracoacromial artery
	6 Axillary Artery, Left
	    See 5 Axillary Artery, Right
	7 Brachial Artery, Right
	    Inferior ulnar collateral artery
	    Profunda brachii
	    Superior ulnar collateral artery
	8 Brachial Artery, Left
	    See 7 Brachial Artery, Right
	9 Ulnar Artery, Right
	    Anterior ulnar recurrent artery
	    Common interosseous artery
	    Posterior ulnar recurrent artery
	A Ulnar Artery, Left
	    See 9 Ulnar Artery, Right
	B Radial Artery, Right
	    Radial recurrent artery
	C Radial Artery, Left
	    See B Radial Artery, Right
		Ø Open
		3 Percutaneous
		4 Percutaneous Endoscopic
			4 Intraluminal Device, Drug-eluting
			5 Intraluminal Device, Drug-eluting, Two
			6 Intraluminal Device, Drug-eluting, Three
			7 Intraluminal Device, Drug-eluting, Four or More
			E Intraluminal Device, Two
			F Intraluminal Device, Three
			G Intraluminal Device, Four or More
				6 Bifurcation
				Z No Qualifier

Ø Internal Mammary Artery, Right
    Anterior intercostal artery
    Internal thoracic artery
    Musculophrenic artery
    Pericardiophrenic artery
    Superior epigastric artery
1 Internal Mammary Artery, Left
    See Ø Internal Mammary Artery, Right
2 Innominate Artery
    Brachiocephalic artery
    Brachiocephalic trunk
3 Subclavian Artery, Right
    Costocervical trunk
    Dorsal scapular artery
    Internal thoracic artery
4 Subclavian Artery, Left
    See 3 Subclavian Artery, Right
5 Axillary Artery, Right
    Anterior circumflex humeral artery
    Lateral thoracic artery
    Posterior circumflex humeral artery
    Subscapular artery
    Superior thoracic artery
    Thoracoacromial artery
	6 Axillary Artery, Left
	    See 5 Axillary Artery, Right
	7 Brachial Artery, Right
	    Inferior ulnar collateral artery
	    Profunda brachii
	    Superior ulnar collateral artery
	8 Brachial Artery, Left
	    See 7 Brachial Artery, Right
	9 Ulnar Artery, Right
	    Anterior ulnar recurrent artery
	    Common interosseous artery
	    Posterior ulnar recurrent artery
	A Ulnar Artery, Left
	    See 9 Ulnar Artery, Right
	B Radial Artery, Right
	    Radial recurrent artery
	C Radial Artery, Left
	    See B Radial Artery, Right
		Ø Open
		3 Percutaneous
		4 Percutaneous Endoscopic
			D Intraluminal Device
			Z No Device
				1 Drug-Coated Balloon
				6 Bifurcation
				Z No Qualifier

037 Continued on next page

Upper Arteries

0	Medical and Surgical	*037 Continued*
3	Upper Arteries	
7	Dilation	

Definition: Expanding an orifice or the lumen of a tubular body part

Explanation: The orifice can be a natural orifice or an artificially created orifice. Accomplished by stretching a tubular body part using intraluminal pressure or by cutting part of the orifice or wall of the tubular body part.

Body Part Character 4		Approach Character 5	Device Character 6	Qualifier Character 7
D Hand Artery, Right Deep palmar arch Princeps pollicis artery Radialis indicis Superficial palmar arch **F** Hand Artery, Left *See D Hand Artery, Right* **G** Intracranial Artery **NC** Anterior cerebral artery Anterior choroidal artery Anterior communicating artery Basilar artery Circle of Willis Internal carotid artery, intracranial portion Middle cerebral artery Ophthalmic artery Posterior cerebral artery Posterior communicating artery Posterior inferior cerebellar artery (PICA) **H** Common Carotid Artery, Right **J** Common Carotid Artery, Left **K** Internal Carotid Artery, Right Caroticotympanic artery Carotid sinus **L** Internal Carotid Artery, Left *See K Internal Carotid Artery, Right* **M** External Carotid Artery, Right Ascending pharyngeal artery Internal maxillary artery Lingual artery Maxillary artery Occipital artery Posterior auricular artery Superior thyroid artery	**N** External Carotid Artery, Left *See M External Carotid Artery, Right* **P** Vertebral Artery, Right Anterior spinal artery Posterior spinal artery **Q** Vertebral Artery, Left *See P Vertebral Artery, Right* **R** Face Artery Angular artery Ascending palatine artery External maxillary artery Facial artery Inferior labial artery Submental artery Superior labial artery **S** Temporal Artery, Right Middle temporal artery Superficial temporal artery Transverse facial artery **T** Temporal Artery, Left *See S Temporal Artery, Right* **U** Thyroid Artery, Right Cricothyroid artery Hyoid artery Sternocleidomastoid artery Superior laryngeal artery Superior thyroid artery Thyrocervical trunk **V** Thyroid Artery, Left *See U Thyroid Artery, Right* **Y** Upper Artery Aortic intercostal artery Bronchial artery Esophageal artery Subcostal artery	**0** Open **3** Percutaneous **4** Percutaneous Endoscopic	**4** Intraluminal Device, Drug-eluting **5** Intraluminal Device, Drug-eluting, Two **6** Intraluminal Device, Drug-eluting, Three **7** Intraluminal Device, Drug-eluting, Four or More **D** Intraluminal Device **E** Intraluminal Device, Two **F** Intraluminal Device, Three **G** Intraluminal Device, Four or More **Z** No Device	**6** Bifurcation **Z** No Qualifier

NC   037G[3,4]Z[6,Z]

LC Limited Coverage   **NC** Noncovered   ⊞ Combination Member   HAC associated procedure   Combination Only   DRG Non-OR   Non-OR   New/Revised in GREEN

192   ICD-10-PCS 2019

Ø   **Medical and Surgical**
3   **Upper Arteries**
9   **Drainage**   Definition: Taking or letting out fluids and/or gases from a body part
                   Explanation: The qualifier DIAGNOSTIC is used to identify drainage procedures that are biopsies

Body Part Character 4		Approach Character 5	Device Character 6	Qualifier Character 7
Ø Internal Mammary Artery, Right Anterior intercostal artery Internal thoracic artery Musculophrenic artery Pericardiophrenic artery Superior epigastric artery **1 Internal Mammary Artery, Left** *See Ø Internal Mammary Artery, Right above* **2 Innominate Artery** Brachiocephalic artery Brachiocephalic trunk **3 Subclavian Artery, Right** Costocervical trunk Dorsal scapular artery Internal thoracic artery **4 Subclavian Artery, Left** *See 3 Subclavian Artery, Right* **5 Axillary Artery, Right** Anterior circumflex humeral artery Lateral thoracic artery Posterior circumflex humeral artery Subscapular artery Superior thoracic artery Thoracoacromial artery **6 Axillary Artery, Left** *See 5 Axillary Artery, Right* **7 Brachial Artery, Right** Inferior ulnar collateral artery Profunda brachii Superior ulnar collateral artery **8 Brachial Artery, Left** *See 7 Brachial Artery, Right* **9 Ulnar Artery, Right** Anterior ulnar recurrent artery Common interosseous artery Posterior ulnar recurrent artery **A Ulnar Artery, Left** *See 9 Ulnar Artery, Right* **B Radial Artery, Right** Radial recurrent artery **C Radial Artery, Left** *See B Radial Artery, Right* **D Hand Artery, Right** Deep palmar arch Princeps pollicis artery Radialis indicis Superficial palmar arch **F Hand Artery, Left** *See D Hand Artery, Right* **G Intracranial Artery** Anterior cerebral artery Anterior choroidal artery Anterior communicating artery Basilar artery Circle of Willis Internal carotid artery, intracranial portion Middle cerebral artery Ophthalmic artery Posterior cerebral artery Posterior communicating artery Posterior inferior cerebellar artery (PICA)	**H Common Carotid Artery, Right** **J Common Carotid Artery, Left** **K Internal Carotid Artery, Right** Caroticotympanic artery Carotid sinus **L Internal Carotid Artery, Left** *See K Internal Carotid Artery, Right* **M External Carotid Artery, Right** Ascending pharyngeal artery Internal maxillary artery Lingual artery Maxillary artery Occipital artery Posterior auricular artery Superior thyroid artery **N External Carotid Artery, Left** *See M External Carotid Artery, Right* **P Vertebral Artery, Right** Anterior spinal artery Posterior spinal artery **Q Vertebral Artery, Left** *See P Vertebral Artery, Right* **R Face Artery** Angular artery Ascending palatine artery External maxillary artery Facial artery Inferior labial artery Submental artery Superior labial artery **S Temporal Artery, Right** Middle temporal artery Superficial temporal artery Transverse facial artery **T Temporal Artery, Left** *See S Temporal Artery, Right* **U Thyroid Artery, Right** Cricothyroid artery Hyoid artery Sternocleidomastoid artery Superior laryngeal artery Superior thyroid artery Thyrocervical trunk **V Thyroid Artery, Left** *See U Thyroid Artery, Right* **Y Upper Artery** Aortic intercostal artery Bronchial artery Esophageal artery Subcostal artery	**Ø Open** **3 Percutaneous** **4 Percutaneous Endoscopic**	**Ø Drainage Device**	**Z No Qualifier**

Ø39 Continued on next page

Non-OR   Ø39[Ø,1,2,3,4,5,6,7,8,9,A,B,C,D,F,G,H,J,K,L,M,N,P,Q,R,S,T,U,V,Y][Ø,3,4]ØZ

0   Medical and Surgical   *039 Continued*
3   Upper Arteries
9   Drainage   Definition: Taking or letting out fluids and/or gases from a body part
                          Explanation: The qualifier DIAGNOSTIC is used to identify drainage procedures that are biopsies

Body Part Character 4		Approach Character 5	Device Character 6	Qualifier Character 7

0 Internal Mammary Artery, Right
  Anterior intercostal artery
  Internal thoracic artery
  Musculophrenic artery
  Pericardiophrenic artery
  Superior epigastric artery
1 Internal Mammary Artery, Left
  See 0 Internal Mammary Artery, Right
2 Innominate Artery
  Brachiocephalic artery
  Brachiocephalic trunk
3 Subclavian Artery, Right
  Costocervical trunk
  Dorsal scapular artery
  Internal thoracic artery
4 Subclavian Artery, Left
  See 3 Subclavian Artery, Right
5 Axillary Artery, Right
  Anterior circumflex humeral
    artery
  Lateral thoracic artery
  Posterior circumflex humeral
    artery
  Subscapular artery
  Superior thoracic artery
  Thoracoacromial artery
6 Axillary Artery, Left
  See 5 Axillary Artery, Right
7 Brachial Artery, Right
  Inferior ulnar collateral artery
  Profunda brachii
  Superior ulnar collateral artery
8 Brachial Artery, Left
  See 7 Brachial Artery, Right
9 Ulnar Artery, Right
  Anterior ulnar recurrent artery
  Common interosseous artery
  Posterior ulnar recurrent artery
A Ulnar Artery, Left
  See 9 Ulnar Artery, Right
B Radial Artery, Right
  Radial recurrent artery
C Radial Artery, Left
  See B Radial Artery, Right
D Hand Artery, Right
  Deep palmar arch
  Princeps pollicis artery
  Radialis indicis
  Superficial palmar arch
F Hand Artery, Left
  See D Hand Artery, Right
G Intracranial Artery
  Anterior cerebral artery
  Anterior choroidal artery
  Anterior communicating artery
  Basilar artery
  Circle of Willis
  Internal carotid artery,
    intracranial portion
  Middle cerebral artery
  Ophthalmic artery
  Posterior cerebral artery
  Posterior communicating artery
  Posterior inferior cerebellar
    artery (PICA)
	H Common Carotid Artery, Right
	J Common Carotid Artery, Left
	K Internal Carotid Artery, Right
	  Caroticotympanic artery
	  Carotid sinus
	L Internal Carotid Artery, Left
	  See K Internal Carotid Artery, Right
	M External Carotid Artery, Right
	  Ascending pharyngeal artery
	  Internal maxillary artery
	  Lingual artery
	  Maxillary artery
	  Occipital artery
	  Posterior auricular artery
	  Superior thyroid artery
	N External Carotid Artery, Left
	  See M External Carotid Artery, Right
	P Vertebral Artery, Right
	  Anterior spinal artery
	  Posterior spinal artery
	Q Vertebral Artery, Left
	  See P Vertebral Artery, Right
	R Face Artery
	  Angular artery
	  Ascending palatine artery
	  External maxillary artery
	  Facial artery
	  Inferior labial artery
	  Submental artery
	  Superior labial artery
	S Temporal Artery, Right
	  Middle temporal artery
	  Superficial temporal artery
	  Transverse facial artery
	T Temporal Artery, Left
	  See S Temporal Artery, Right
	U Thyroid Artery, Right
	  Cricothyroid artery
	  Hyoid artery
	  Sternocleidomastoid artery
	  Superior laryngeal artery
	  Superior thyroid artery
	  Thyrocervical trunk
	V Thyroid Artery, Left
	  See U Thyroid Artery, Right
	Y Upper Artery
	  Aortic intercostal artery
	  Bronchial artery
	  Esophageal artery
	  Subcostal artery
		0 Open
		3 Percutaneous
		4 Percutaneous Endoscopic
			Z No Device	**X Diagnostic**
				Z No Qualifier

Non-OR   039[0,1,2,3,4,5,6,7,8,9,A,B,C,D,F,G,H,J,K,L,M,N,P,Q,R,S,T,U,V,Y]3ZX
Non-OR   039[0,1,2,3,4,5,6,7,8,9,A,B,C,D,F,G,H,J,K,L,M,N,P,Q,R,S,T,U,V,Y][0,3,4]ZZ

0   Medical and Surgical
3   Upper Arteries
B   Excision   Definition: Cutting out or off, without replacement, a portion of a body part
                  Explanation: The qualifier DIAGNOSTIC is used to identify excision procedures that are biopsies

Body Part Character 4		Approach Character 5	Device Character 6	Qualifier Character 7
0 Internal Mammary Artery, Right Anterior intercostal artery Internal thoracic artery Musculophrenic artery Pericardiophrenic artery Superior epigastric artery **1 Internal Mammary Artery, Left** *See 0 Internal Mammary Artery, Right* **2 Innominate Artery** Brachiocephalic artery Brachiocephalic trunk **3 Subclavian Artery, Right** Costocervical trunk Dorsal scapular artery Internal thoracic artery **4 Subclavian Artery, Left** *See 3 Subclavian Artery, Right* **5 Axillary Artery, Right** Anterior circumflex humeral artery Lateral thoracic artery Posterior circumflex humeral artery Subscapular artery Superior thoracic artery Thoracoacromial artery **6 Axillary Artery, Left** *See 5 Axillary Artery, Right* **7 Brachial Artery, Right** Inferior ulnar collateral artery Profunda brachii Superior ulnar collateral artery **8 Brachial Artery, Left** *See 7 Brachial Artery, Right* **9 Ulnar Artery, Right** Anterior ulnar recurrent artery Common interosseous artery Posterior ulnar recurrent artery **A Ulnar Artery, Left** *See 9 Ulnar Artery, Right* **B Radial Artery, Right** Radial recurrent artery **C Radial Artery, Left** *See B Radial Artery, Right* **D Hand Artery, Right** Deep palmar arch Princeps pollicis artery Radialis indicis Superficial palmar arch **F Hand Artery, Left** *See D Hand Artery, Right* **G Intracranial Artery** Anterior cerebral artery Anterior choroidal artery Anterior communicating artery Basilar artery Circle of Willis Internal carotid artery, intracranial portion Middle cerebral artery Ophthalmic artery Posterior cerebral artery Posterior communicating artery Posterior inferior cerebellar artery (PICA)	**H Common Carotid Artery, Right** **J Common Carotid Artery, Left** **K Internal Carotid Artery, Right** Caroticotympanic artery Carotid sinus **L Internal Carotid Artery, Left** *See K Internal Carotid Artery, Right* **M External Carotid Artery, Right** Ascending pharyngeal artery Internal maxillary artery Lingual artery Maxillary artery Occipital artery Posterior auricular artery Superior thyroid artery **N External Carotid Artery, Left** *See M External Carotid Artery, Right* **P Vertebral Artery, Right** Anterior spinal artery Posterior spinal artery **Q Vertebral Artery, Left** *See P Vertebral Artery, Right* **R Face Artery** Angular artery Ascending palatine artery External maxillary artery Facial artery Inferior labial artery Submental artery Superior labial artery **S Temporal Artery, Right** Middle temporal artery Superficial temporal artery Transverse facial artery **T Temporal Artery, Left** *See S Temporal Artery, Right* **U Thyroid Artery, Right** Cricothyroid artery Hyoid artery Sternocleidomastoid artery Superior laryngeal artery Superior thyroid artery Thyrocervical trunk **V Thyroid Artery, Left** *See U Thyroid Artery, Right* **Y Upper Artery** Aortic intercostal artery Bronchial artery Esophageal artery Subcostal artery	**0 Open** **3 Percutaneous** **4 Percutaneous Endoscopic**	**Z No Device**	**X Diagnostic** **Z No Qualifier**

LC Limited Coverage   **NC** Noncovered   ⊞ Combination Member   HAC associated procedure   Combination Only   DRG Non-OR   Non-OR   New/Revised in GREEN

ICD-10-PCS 2019   195

03B–03B

Ø   Medical and Surgical
3   Upper Arteries
C   Extirpation   Definition: Taking or cutting out solid matter from a body part

Explanation: The solid matter may be an abnormal byproduct of a biological function or a foreign body; it may be imbedded in a body part or in the lumen of a tubular body part. The solid matter may or may not have been previously broken into pieces.

Body Part Character 4		Approach Character 5	Device Character 6	Qualifier Character 7

Ø Internal Mammary Artery, Right
  Anterior intercostal artery
  Internal thoracic artery
  Musculophrenic artery
  Pericardiophrenic artery
  Superior epigastric artery
1 Internal Mammary Artery, Left
  See Ø Internal Mammary Artery, Right
2 Innominate Artery
  Brachiocephalic artery
  Brachiocephalic trunk
3 Subclavian Artery, Right
  Costocervical trunk
  Dorsal scapular artery
  Internal thoracic artery
4 Subclavian Artery, Left
  See 3 Subclavian Artery, Right
5 Axillary Artery, Right
  Anterior circumflex humeral artery
  Lateral thoracic artery
  Posterior circumflex humeral artery
  Subscapular artery
  Superior thoracic artery
  Thoracoacromial artery
6 Axillary Artery, Left
  See 5 Axillary Artery, Right
7 Brachial Artery, Right
  Inferior ulnar collateral artery
  Profunda brachii
  Superior ulnar collateral artery
8 Brachial Artery, Left
  See 7 Brachial Artery, Right
9 Ulnar Artery, Right
  Anterior ulnar recurrent artery
  Common interosseous artery
  Posterior ulnar recurrent artery
	A Ulnar Artery, Left
	  See 9 Ulnar Artery, Right
	B Radial Artery, Right
	  Radial recurrent artery
	C Radial Artery, Left
	  See B Radial Artery, Right
	D Hand Artery, Right
	  Deep palmar arch
	  Princeps pollicis artery
	  Radialis indicis
	  Superficial palmar arch
	F Hand Artery, Left
	  See D Hand Artery, Right
	R Face Artery
	  Angular artery
	  Ascending palatine artery
	  External maxillary artery
	  Facial artery
	  Inferior labial artery
	  Submental artery
	  Superior labial artery
	S Temporal Artery, Right
	  Middle temporal artery
	  Superficial temporal artery
	  Transverse facial artery
	T Temporal Artery, Left
	  See S Temporal Artery, Right
	U Thyroid Artery, Right
	  Cricothyroid artery
	  Hyoid artery
	  Sternocleidomastoid artery
	  Superior laryngeal artery
	  Superior thyroid artery
	  Thyrocervical trunk
	V Thyroid Artery, Left
	  See U Thyroid Artery, Right
	Y Upper Artery
	  Aortic intercostal artery
	  Bronchial artery
	  Esophageal artery
	  Subcostal artery
		Ø Open
		3 Percutaneous
		4 Percutaneous Endoscopic
			Z No Device	**6** Bifurcation
				Z No Qualifier

G Intracranial Artery
  Anterior cerebral artery
  Anterior choroidal artery
  Anterior communicating artery
  Basilar artery
  Circle of Willis
  Internal carotid artery, intracranial portion
  Middle cerebral artery
  Ophthalmic artery
  Posterior cerebral artery
  Posterior communicating artery
  Posterior inferior cerebellar artery (PICA)
H Common Carotid Artery, Right
J Common Carotid Artery, Left
K Internal Carotid Artery, Right
  Caroticotympanic artery
  Carotid sinus
	L Internal Carotid Artery, Left
	  See K Internal Carotid Artery, Right
	M External Carotid Artery, Right
	  Ascending pharyngeal artery
	  Internal maxillary artery
	  Lingual artery
	  Maxillary artery
	  Occipital artery
	  Posterior auricular artery
	  Superior thyroid artery
	N External Carotid Artery, Left
	  See M External Carotid Artery, Right
	P Vertebral Artery, Right
	  Anterior spinal artery
	  Posterior spinal artery
	Q Vertebral Artery, Left
	  See P Vertebral Artery, Right
		Ø Open
		4 Percutaneous Endoscopic
			Z No Device	**6** Bifurcation
				Z No Qualifier

Ø3C Continued on next page

0   Medical and Surgical
3   Upper Arteries
C   Extirpation   Definition: Taking or cutting out solid matter from a body part

03C Continued

Explanation: The solid matter may be an abnormal byproduct of a biological function or a foreign body; it may be imbedded in a body part or in the lumen of a tubular body part. The solid matter may or may not have been previously broken into pieces.

Body Part Character 4		Approach Character 5	Device Character 6	Qualifier Character 7

G Intracranial Artery
    Anterior cerebral artery
    Anterior choroidal artery
    Anterior communicating
      artery
    Basilar artery
    Circle of Willis
    Internal carotid artery,
      intracranial portion
    Middle cerebral artery
    Ophthalmic artery
    Posterior cerebral artery
    Posterior communicating
      artery
    Posterior inferior cerebellar
      artery (PICA)
H Common Carotid Artery,
    Right
J Common Carotid Artery, Left
K Internal Carotid Artery, Right
    Caroticotympanic artery
    Carotid sinus
	L Internal Carotid Artery, Left
	    See K Internal Carotid Artery,
	    Right
	M External Carotid Artery, Right
	    Ascending pharyngeal artery
	    Internal maxillary artery
	    Lingual artery
	    Maxillary artery
	    Occipital artery
	    Posterior auricular artery
	    Superior thyroid artery
	N External Carotid Artery, Left
	    See M External Carotid Artery,
	    Right
	P Vertebral Artery, Right
	    Anterior spinal artery
	    Posterior spinal artery
	Q Vertebral Artery, Left
	    See P Vertebral Artery, Right
		3 Percutaneous	**Z** No Device	**6** Bifurcation
				7 Stent Retriever
				Z No Qualifier

LC Limited Coverage   NC Noncovered   ⊞ Combination Member   HAC associated procedure   Combination Only   DRG Non-OR   Non-OR   New/Revised in GREEN

ICD-10-PCS 2019   197

03C–03C

0   **Medical and Surgical**
3   **Upper Arteries**
H   **Insertion**   Definition: Putting in a nonbiological appliance that monitors, assists, performs, or prevents a physiological function but does not physically take the place of a body part
                 Explanation: None

Body Part Character 4		Approach Character 5	Device Character 6	Qualifier Character 7

0 **Internal Mammary Artery, Right**
  Anterior intercostal artery
  Internal thoracic artery
  Musculophrenic artery
  Pericardiophrenic artery
  Superior epigastric artery
1 **Internal Mammary Artery, Left**
  See 0 Internal Mammary Artery, Right
2 **Innominate Artery**
  Brachiocephalic artery
  Brachiocephalic trunk
3 **Subclavian Artery, Right**
  Costocervical trunk
  Dorsal scapular artery
  Internal thoracic artery
4 **Subclavian Artery, Left**
  See 3 Subclavian Artery, Right
5 **Axillary Artery, Right**
  Anterior circumflex humeral artery
  Lateral thoracic artery
  Posterior circumflex humeral artery
  Subscapular artery
  Superior thoracic artery
  Thoracoacromial artery
6 **Axillary Artery, Left**
  See 5 Axillary Artery, Right
7 **Brachial Artery, Right**
  Inferior ulnar collateral artery
  Profunda brachii
  Superior ulnar collateral artery
8 **Brachial Artery, Left**
  See 7 Brachial Artery, Right
9 **Ulnar Artery, Right**
  Anterior ulnar recurrent artery
  Common interosseous artery
  Posterior ulnar recurrent artery
A **Ulnar Artery, Left**
  See 9 Ulnar Artery, Right
B **Radial Artery, Right**
  Radial recurrent artery
C **Radial Artery, Left**
  See B Radial Artery, Right
D **Hand Artery, Right**
  Deep palmar arch
  Princeps pollicis artery
  Radialis indicis
  Superficial palmar arch
F **Hand Artery, Left**
  See D Hand Artery, Right
	G **Intracranial Artery**
	  Anterior cerebral artery
	  Anterior choroidal artery
	  Anterior communicating artery
	  Basilar artery
	  Circle of Willis
	  Internal carotid artery, intracranial portion
	  Middle cerebral artery
	  Ophthalmic artery
	  Posterior cerebral artery
	  Posterior communicating artery
	  Posterior inferior cerebellar artery (PICA)
	H **Common Carotid Artery, Right**
	J **Common Carotid Artery, Left**
	M **External Carotid Artery, Right**
	  Ascending pharyngeal artery
	  Internal maxillary artery
	  Lingual artery
	  Maxillary artery
	  Occipital artery
	  Posterior auricular artery
	  Superior thyroid artery
	N **External Carotid Artery, Left**
	  See M External Carotid Artery, Right
	P **Vertebral Artery, Right**
	  Anterior spinal artery
	  Posterior spinal artery
	Q **Vertebral Artery, Left**
	  See P Vertebral Artery, Right
	R **Face Artery**
	  Angular artery
	  Ascending palatine artery
	  External maxillary artery
	  Facial artery
	  Inferior labial artery
	  Submental artery
	  Superior labial artery
	S **Temporal Artery, Right**
	  Middle temporal artery
	  Superficial temporal artery
	  Transverse facial artery
	T **Temporal Artery, Left**
	  See S Temporal Artery, Right
	U **Thyroid Artery, Right**
	  Cricothyroid artery
	  Hyoid artery
	  Sternocleidomastoid artery
	  Superior laryngeal artery
	  Superior thyroid artery
	  Thyrocervical trunk
	V **Thyroid Artery, Left**
	  See U Thyroid Artery, Right
		0 Open
		3 Percutaneous
		4 Percutaneous Endoscopic
			3 Infusion Device
			D Intraluminal Device
				Z No Qualifier

K **Internal Carotid Artery, Right**
  Caroticotympanic artery
  Carotid sinus
L **Internal Carotid Artery, Left**
  See K Internal Carotid Artery, Right
		0 Open
		3 Percutaneous
		4 Percutaneous Endoscope
			3 Infusion Device
			D Intraluminal Device
			M Stimulator Lead
				Z No Qualifier

Y **Upper Artery**
  Aortic intercostal artery
  Bronchial artery
  Esophageal artery
  Subcostal artery
		0 Open
		3 Percutaneous
		4 Percutaneous Endoscopic
			2 Monitoring Device
			3 Infusion Device
			D Intraluminal Device
			Y Other Device
				Z No Qualifier

Non-OR	03H[0,1,2,3,4,5,6,7,8,9,A,B,C,D,F,G,H,J,M,N,P,Q,R,S,T,U,V][0,3,4]3Z	
Non-OR	03H[K,L][0,3,4]3Z	
Non-OR	03HY[0,3,4]3Z	
Non-OR	03HY32Z	
Non-OR	03HY[3,4]YZ	

LC Limited Coverage   **NC** Noncovered   ⊞ Combination Member   HAC associated procedure   Combination Only   DRG Non-OR   Non-OR   New/Revised in GREEN

198   ICD-10-PCS 2019

Ø   Medical and Surgical
3   Upper Arteries
J   Inspection   Definition: Visually and/or manually exploring a body part

Explanation: Visual exploration may be performed with or without optical instrumentation. Manual exploration may be performed directly or through intervening body layers.

Body Part Character 4	Approach Character 5	Device Character 6	Qualifier Character 7

Y   **Upper Artery**
    Aortic intercostal artery
    Bronchial artery
    Esophageal artery
    Subcostal artery
	Ø Open
	3 Percutaneous
	4 Percutaneous Endoscopic
	X External
		Z No Device	**Z** No Qualifier

Non-OR   Ø3JY[3,4,X]ZZ

0 Medical and Surgical
3 Upper Arteries
L Occlusion   Definition: Completely closing an orifice or the lumen of a tubular body part
            Explanation: The orifice can be a natural orifice or an artificially created orifice

Body Part Character 4		Approach Character 5	Device Character 6	Qualifier Character 7
0 Internal Mammary Artery, Right Anterior intercostal artery Internal thoracic artery Musculophrenic artery Pericardiophrenic artery Superior epigastric artery **1 Internal Mammary Artery, Left** *See 0 Internal Mammary Artery, Left* **2 Innominate Artery** Brachiocephalic artery Brachiocephalic trunk **3 Subclavian Artery, Right** Costocervical trunk Dorsal scapular artery Internal thoracic artery **4 Subclavian Artery, Left** *See 3 Subclavian Artery, Right* **5 Axillary Artery, Right** Anterior circumflex humeral artery Lateral thoracic artery Posterior circumflex humeral artery Subscapular artery Superior thoracic artery Thoracoacromial artery **6 Axillary Artery, Left** *See 5 Axillary Artery, Right* **7 Brachial Artery, Right** Inferior ulnar collateral artery Profunda brachii Superior ulnar collateral artery **8 Brachial Artery, Left** *See 7 Brachial Artery, Right* **9 Ulnar Artery, Right** Anterior ulnar recurrent artery Common interosseous artery Posterior ulnar recurrent artery	**A Ulnar Artery, Left** *See 9 Ulnar Artery, Right* **B Radial Artery, Right** Radial recurrent artery **C Radial Artery, Left** *See B Radial Artery, Right* **D Hand Artery, Right** Deep palmar arch Princeps pollicis artery Radialis indicis Superficial palmar arch **F Hand Artery, Left** *See D Hand Artery, Right* **R Face Artery** Angular artery Ascending palatine artery External maxillary artery Facial artery Inferior labial artery Submental artery Superior labial artery **S Temporal Artery, Right** Middle temporal artery Superficial temporal artery Transverse facial artery **T Temporal Artery, Left** *See S Temporal Artery, Right* **U Thyroid Artery, Right** Cricothyroid artery Hyoid artery Sternocleidomastoid artery Superior laryngeal artery Superior thyroid artery Thyrocervical trunk **V Thyroid Artery, Left** *See U Thyroid Artery, Right* **Y Upper Artery** Aortic intercostal artery Bronchial artery Esophageal artery Subcostal artery	**0 Open** **3 Percutaneous** **4 Percutaneous Endoscopic**	**C Extraluminal Device** **D Intraluminal Device** **Z No Device**	**Z No Qualifier**
G Intracranial Artery Anterior cerebral artery Anterior choroidal artery Anterior communicating artery Basilar artery Circle of Willis Internal carotid artery, intracranial portion Middle cerebral artery Ophthalmic artery Posterior cerebral artery Posterior communicating artery Posterior inferior cerebellar artery (PICA) **H Common Carotid Artery, Right** **J Common Carotid Artery, Left** **K Internal Carotid Artery, Right** Caroticotympanic artery Carotid sinus	**L Internal Carotid Artery, Left** *See K Internal Carotid Artery, Right* **M External Carotid Artery, Right** Ascending pharyngeal artery Internal maxillary artery Lingual artery Maxillary artery Occipital artery Posterior auricular artery Superior thyroid artery **N External Carotid Artery, Left** *See M External Carotid Artery, Right* **P Vertebral Artery, Right** Anterior spinal artery Posterior spinal artery **Q Vertebral Artery, Left** *See P Vertebral Artery, Right*	**0 Open** **3 Percutaneous** **4 Percutaneous Endoscopic**	**B Intraluminal Device, Bioactive** **C Extraluminal Device** **D Intraluminal Device** **Z No Device**	**Z No Qualifier**

0   **Medical and Surgical**
3   **Upper Arteries**
N   **Release**

Definition: Freeing a body part from an abnormal physical constraint by cutting or by the use of force
Explanation: Some of the restraining tissue may be taken out but none of the body part is taken out

Body Part Character 4		Approach Character 5	Device Character 6	Qualifier Character 7
0 **Internal Mammary Artery, Right** Anterior intercostal artery Internal thoracic artery Musculophrenic artery Pericardiophrenic artery Superior epigastric artery **1** **Internal Mammary Artery, Left** *See 0 Internal Mammary Artery, Right* **2** **Innominate Artery** Brachiocephalic artery Brachiocephalic trunk **3** **Subclavian Artery, Right** Costocervical trunk Dorsal scapular artery Internal thoracic artery **4** **Subclavian Artery, Left** *See 3 Subclavian Artery, Right* **5** **Axillary Artery, Right** Anterior circumflex humeral artery Lateral thoracic artery Posterior circumflex humeral artery Subscapular artery Superior thoracic artery Thoracoacromial artery **6** **Axillary Artery, Left** *See 5 Axillary Artery, Right* **7** **Brachial Artery, Right** Inferior ulnar collateral artery Profunda brachii Superior ulnar collateral artery **8** **Brachial Artery, Left** *See 7 Brachial Artery, Right* **9** **Ulnar Artery, Right** Anterior ulnar recurrent artery Common interosseous artery Posterior ulnar recurrent artery **A** **Ulnar Artery, Left** *See 9 Ulnar Artery, Right* **B** **Radial Artery, Right** Radial recurrent artery **C** **Radial Artery, Left** *See B Radial Artery, Right* **D** **Hand Artery, Right** Deep palmar arch Princeps pollicis artery Radialis indicis Superficial palmar arch **F** **Hand Artery, Left** *See D Hand Artery, Right* **G** **Intracranial Artery** Anterior cerebral artery Anterior choroidal artery Anterior communicating artery Basilar artery Circle of Willis Internal carotid artery, intracranial portion Middle cerebral artery Ophthalmic artery Posterior cerebral artery Posterior communicating artery Posterior inferior cerebellar artery (PICA)	**H** **Common Carotid Artery, Right** **J** **Common Carotid Artery, Left** **K** **Internal Carotid Artery, Right** Caroticotympanic artery Carotid sinus **L** **Internal Carotid Artery, Left** *See K Internal Carotid Artery, Right* **M** **External Carotid Artery, Right** Ascending pharyngeal artery Internal maxillary artery Lingual artery Maxillary artery Occipital artery Posterior auricular artery Superior thyroid artery **N** **External Carotid Artery, Left** *See M External Carotid Artery, Right* **P** **Vertebral Artery, Right** Anterior spinal artery Posterior spinal artery **Q** **Vertebral Artery, Left** *See P Vertebral Artery, Right* **R** **Face Artery** Angular artery Ascending palatine artery External maxillary artery Facial artery Inferior labial artery Submental artery Superior labial artery **S** **Temporal Artery, Right** Middle temporal artery Superficial temporal artery Transverse facial artery **T** **Temporal Artery, Left** *See S Temporal Artery, Right* **U** **Thyroid Artery, Right** Cricothyroid artery Hyoid artery Sternocleidomastoid artery Superior laryngeal artery Superior thyroid artery Thyrocervical trunk **V** **Thyroid Artery, Left** *See U Thyroid Artery, Right* **Y** **Upper Artery** Aortic intercostal artery Bronchial artery Esophageal artery Subcostal artery	**0** Open **3** Percutaneous **4** Percutaneous Endoscopic	**Z** No Device	**Z** No Qualifier

Ø　Medical and Surgical
3　Upper Arteries
P　Removal　　Definition: Taking out or off a device from a body part

Explanation: If a device is taken out and a similar device put in without cutting or puncturing the skin or mucous membrane, the procedure is coded to the root operation CHANGE. Otherwise, the procedure for taking out a device is coded to the root operation REMOVAL.

Body Part Character 4	Approach Character 5	Device Character 6	Qualifier Character 7
Y　Upper Artery 　　Aortic intercostal artery 　　Bronchial artery 　　Esophageal artery 　　Subcostal artery	**Ø　Open** **3　Percutaneous** **4　Percutaneous Endoscopic**	**Ø　Drainage Device** **2　Monitoring Device** **3　Infusion Device** **7　Autologous Tissue Substitute** **C　Extraluminal Device** **D　Intraluminal Device** **J　Synthetic Substitute** **K　Nonautologous Tissue Substitute** **M　Stimulator Lead** **Y　Other Device**	**Z　No Qualifier**
Y　Upper Artery 　　Aortic intercostal artery 　　Bronchial artery 　　Esophageal artery 　　Subcostal artery	**X　External**	**Ø　Drainage Device** **2　Monitoring Device** **3　Infusion Device** **D　Intraluminal Device** **M　Stimulator Lead**	**Z　No Qualifier**

Non-OR　Ø3PY3[Ø,2,3,D]Z
Non-OR　Ø3PY[3,4]YZ
Non-OR　Ø3PYX[Ø,2,3,D,M]Z

Upper Arteries

0   **Medical and Surgical**
3   **Upper Arteries**
Q   **Repair**   Definition: Restoring, to the extent possible, a body part to its normal anatomic structure and function
                 Explanation: Used only when the method to accomplish the repair is not one of the other root operations

Body Part Character 4		Approach Character 5	Device Character 6	Qualifier Character 7
0 **Internal Mammary Artery, Right** Anterior intercostal artery Internal thoracic artery Musculophrenic artery Pericardiophrenic artery Superior epigastric artery **1** **Internal Mammary Artery, Left** *See 0 Internal Mammary Artery, Right* **2** **Innominate Artery** Brachiocephalic artery Brachiocephalic trunk **3** **Subclavian Artery, Right** Costocervical trunk Dorsal scapular artery Internal thoracic artery **4** **Subclavian Artery, Left** *See 3 Subclavian Artery, Right* **5** **Axillary Artery, Right** Anterior circumflex humeral artery Lateral thoracic artery Posterior circumflex humeral artery Subscapular artery Superior thoracic artery Thoracoacromial artery **6** **Axillary Artery, Left** *See 5 Axillary Artery, Right* **7** **Brachial Artery, Right** Inferior ulnar collateral artery Profunda brachii Superior ulnar collateral artery **8** **Brachial Artery, Left** *See 7 Brachial Artery, Right* **9** **Ulnar Artery, Right** Anterior ulnar recurrent artery Common interosseous artery Posterior ulnar recurrent artery **A** **Ulnar Artery, Left** *See 9 Ulnar Artery, Right* **B** **Radial Artery, Right** Radial recurrent artery **C** **Radial Artery, Left** *See B Radial Artery, Right* **D** **Hand Artery, Right** Deep palmar arch Princeps pollicis artery Radialis indicis Superficial palmar arch **F** **Hand Artery, Left** *See D Hand Artery, Right* **G** **Intracranial Artery** Anterior cerebral artery Anterior choroidal artery Anterior communicating artery Basilar artery Circle of Willis Internal carotid artery, intracranial portion Middle cerebral artery Ophthalmic artery Posterior cerebral artery Posterior communicating artery Posterior inferior cerebellar artery (PICA)	**H** **Common Carotid Artery, Right** **J** **Common Carotid Artery, Left** **K** **Internal Carotid Artery, Right** Caroticotympanic artery Carotid sinus **L** **Internal Carotid Artery, Left** *See K Internal Carotid Artery, Right* **M** **External Carotid Artery, Right** Ascending pharyngeal artery Internal maxillary artery Lingual artery Maxillary artery Occipital artery Posterior auricular artery Superior thyroid artery **N** **External Carotid Artery, Left** *See M External Carotid Artery, Right* **P** **Vertebral Artery, Right** Anterior spinal artery Posterior spinal artery **Q** **Vertebral Artery, Left** *See P Vertebral Artery, Right* **R** **Face Artery** Angular artery Ascending palatine artery External maxillary artery Facial artery Inferior labial artery Submental artery Superior labial artery **S** **Temporal Artery, Right** Middle temporal artery Superficial temporal artery Transverse facial artery **T** **Temporal Artery, Left** *See S Temporal Artery, Right* **U** **Thyroid Artery, Right** Cricothyroid artery Hyoid artery Sternocleidomastoid artery Superior laryngeal artery Superior thyroid artery Thyrocervical trunk **V** **Thyroid Artery, Left** *See U Thyroid Artery, Right* **Y** **Upper Artery** Aortic intercostal artery Bronchial artery Esophageal artery Subcostal artery	**0** Open **3** Percutaneous **4** Percutaneous Endoscopic	**Z** No Device	**Z** No Qualifier

LC Limited Coverage   **NC** Noncovered   ⊞ Combination Member   HAC associated procedure   Combination Only   DRG Non-OR   Non-OR   New/Revised in GREEN

ICD-10-PCS 2019   **203**

03Q–03Q

Ø   Medical and Surgical
3   Upper Arteries
R   Replacement   Definition: Putting in or on biological or synthetic material that physically takes the place and/or function of all or a portion of a body part
Explanation: The body part may have been taken out or replaced, or may be taken out, physically eradicated, or rendered nonfunctional during the REPLACEMENT procedure. A REMOVAL procedure is coded for taking out the device used in a previous replacement procedure.

Body Part Character 4		Approach Character 5	Device Character 6	Qualifier Character 7

Ø Internal Mammary Artery, Right
Anterior intercostal artery
Internal thoracic artery
Musculophrenic artery
Pericardiophrenic artery
Superior epigastric artery
1 Internal Mammary Artery, Left
See Ø Internal Mammary Artery, Right
2 Innominate Artery
Brachiocephalic artery
Brachiocephalic trunk
3 Subclavian Artery, Right
Costocervical trunk
Dorsal scapular artery
Internal thoracic artery
4 Subclavian Artery, Left
See 3 Subclavian Artery, Right
5 Axillary Artery, Right
Anterior circumflex humeral
   artery
Lateral thoracic artery
Posterior circumflex humeral
   artery
Subscapular artery
Superior thoracic artery
Thoracoacromial artery
6 Axillary Artery, Left
See 5 Axillary Artery, Right
7 Brachial Artery, Right
Inferior ulnar collateral artery
Profunda brachii
Superior ulnar collateral artery
8 Brachial Artery, Left
See 7 Brachial Artery, Right
9 Ulnar Artery, Right
Anterior ulnar recurrent artery
Common interosseous artery
Posterior ulnar recurrent
   artery
A Ulnar Artery, Left
See 9 Ulnar Artery, Right
B Radial Artery, Right
Radial recurrent artery
C Radial Artery, Left
See B Radial Artery, Right
D Hand Artery, Right
Deep palmar arch
Princeps pollicis artery
Radialis indicis
Superficial palmar arch
F Hand Artery, Left
See D Hand Artery, Right
G Intracranial Artery
Anterior cerebral artery
Anterior choroidal artery
Anterior communicating
   artery
Basilar artery
Circle of Willis
Internal carotid artery,
   intracranial portion
Middle cerebral artery
Ophthalmic artery
Posterior cerebral artery
Posterior communicating artery
Posterior inferior cerebellar
   artery (PICA)
	H Common Carotid Artery, Right
	J Common Carotid Artery, Left
	K Internal Carotid Artery, Right
	Caroticotympanic artery
	Carotid sinus
	L Internal Carotid Artery, Left
	See K Internal Carotid Artery, Right
	M External Carotid Artery, Right
	Ascending pharyngeal artery
	Internal maxillary artery
	Lingual artery
	Maxillary artery
	Occipital artery
	Posterior auricular artery
	Superior thyroid artery
	N External Carotid Artery, Left
	See M External Carotid Artery, Right
	P Vertebral Artery, Right
	Anterior spinal artery
	Posterior spinal artery
	Q Vertebral Artery, Left
	See P Vertebral Artery, Right
	R Face Artery
	Angular artery
	Ascending palatine artery
	External maxillary artery
	Facial artery
	Inferior labial artery
	Submental artery
	Superior labial artery
	S Temporal Artery, Right
	Middle temporal artery
	Superficial temporal artery
	Transverse facial artery
	T Temporal Artery, Left
	See S Temporal Artery, Right
	U Thyroid Artery, Right
	Cricothyroid artery
	Hyoid artery
	Sternocleidomastoid artery
	Superior laryngeal artery
	Superior thyroid artery
	Thyrocervical trunk
	V Thyroid Artery, Left
	See U Thyroid Artery, Right
	Y Upper Artery
	Aortic intercostal artery
	Bronchial artery
	Esophageal artery
	Subcostal artery
		Ø Open
		4 Percutaneous Endoscopic
			7 Autologous Tissue Substitute
			J Synthetic Substitute
			K Nonautologous Tissue Substitute
				Z No Qualifier

LC Limited Coverage   NC Noncovered   ⊞ Combination Member   HAC associated procedure   Combination Only   DRG Non-OR   Non-OR   New/Revised in GREEN

0　Medical and Surgical
3　Upper Arteries
S　Reposition

Definition: Moving to its normal location, or other suitable location, all or a portion of a body part

Explanation: The body part is moved to a new location from an abnormal location, or from a normal location where it is not functioning correctly. The body part may or may not be cut out or off to be moved to the new location.

Body Part Character 4		Approach Character 5	Device Character 6	Qualifier Character 7
0 Internal Mammary Artery, Right Anterior intercostal artery Internal thoracic artery Musculophrenic artery Pericardiophrenic artery Superior epigastric artery **1 Internal Mammary Artery, Left** *See 0 Internal Mammary Artery, Right* **2 Innominate Artery** Brachiocephalic artery Brachiocephalic trunk **3 Subclavian Artery, Right** Costocervical trunk Dorsal scapular artery Internal thoracic artery **4 Subclavian Artery, Left** *See 3 Subclavian Artery, Right* **5 Axillary Artery, Right** Anterior circumflex humeral artery Lateral thoracic artery Posterior circumflex humeral artery Subscapular artery Superior thoracic artery Thoracoacromial artery **6 Axillary Artery, Left** *See 5 Axillary Artery, Right* **7 Brachial Artery, Right** Inferior ulnar collateral artery Profunda brachii Superior ulnar collateral artery **8 Brachial Artery, Left** *See 7 Brachial Artery, Right* **9 Ulnar Artery, Right** Anterior ulnar recurrent artery Common interosseous artery Posterior ulnar recurrent artery **A Ulnar Artery, Left** *See 9 Ulnar Artery, Right* **B Radial Artery, Right** Radial recurrent artery **C Radial Artery, Left** *See B Radial Artery, Right* **D Hand Artery, Right** Deep palmar arch Princeps pollicis artery Radialis indicis Superficial palmar arch **F Hand Artery, Left** *See D Hand Artery, Right* **G Intracranial Artery** Anterior cerebral artery Anterior choroidal artery Anterior communicating artery Basilar artery Circle of Willis Internal carotid artery, intracranial portion Middle cerebral artery Ophthalmic artery Posterior cerebral artery Posterior communicating artery Posterior inferior cerebellar artery (PICA)	**H Common Carotid Artery, Right** **J Common Carotid Artery, Left** **K Internal Carotid Artery, Right** Caroticotympanic artery Carotid sinus **L Internal Carotid Artery, Left** *See K Internal Carotid Artery, Right* **M External Carotid Artery, Right** Ascending pharyngeal artery Internal maxillary artery Lingual artery Maxillary artery Occipital artery Posterior auricular artery Superior thyroid artery **N External Carotid Artery, Left** *See M External Carotid Artery, Right* **P Vertebral Artery, Right** Anterior spinal artery Posterior spinal artery **Q Vertebral Artery, Left** *See P Vertebral Artery, Right* **R Face Artery** Angular artery Ascending palatine artery External maxillary artery Facial artery Inferior labial artery Submental artery Superior labial artery **S Temporal Artery, Right** Middle temporal artery Superficial temporal artery Transverse facial artery **T Temporal Artery, Left** *See S Temporal Artery, Right* **U Thyroid Artery, Right** Cricothyroid artery Hyoid artery Sternocleidomastoid artery Superior laryngeal artery Superior thyroid artery Thyrocervical trunk **V Thyroid Artery, Left** *See U Thyroid Artery, Right* **Y Upper Artery** Aortic intercostal artery Bronchial artery Esophageal artery Subcostal artery	**0 Open** **3 Percutaneous** **4 Percutaneous Endoscopic**	**Z No Device**	**Z No Qualifier**

LC Limited Coverage　　NC Noncovered　　⊞ Combination Member　　HAC associated procedure　　Combination Only　　DRG Non-OR　　Non-OR　　New/Revised in GREEN

ICD-10-PCS 2019　　　　　　　　　　　　　　　　　　　　　　　　　　　　　　　　　　　　205

Upper Arteries

Ø **Medical and Surgical**
3 **Upper Arteries**
U **Supplement**

Definition: Putting in or on biological or synthetic material that physically reinforces and/or augments the function of a portion of a body part

Explanation: The biological material is non-living, or is living and from the same individual. The body part may have been previously replaced, and the SUPPLEMENT procedure is performed to physically reinforce and/or augment the function of the replaced body part.

Body Part — Character 4		Approach — Character 5	Device — Character 6	Qualifier — Character 7
Ø Internal Mammary Artery, Right Anterior intercostal artery Internal thoracic artery Musculophrenic artery Pericardiophrenic artery Superior epigastric artery **1** Internal Mammary Artery, Left *See Ø Internal Mammary Artery, Right* **2** Innominate Artery Brachiocephalic artery Brachiocephalic trunk **3** Subclavian Artery, Right Costocervical trunk Dorsal scapular artery Internal thoracic artery **4** Subclavian Artery, Left *See 3 Subclavian Artery, Right* **5** Axillary Artery, Right Anterior circumflex humeral artery Lateral thoracic artery Posterior circumflex humeral artery Subscapular artery Superior thoracic artery Thoracoacromial artery **6** Axillary Artery, Left *See 5 Axillary Artery, Right* **7** Brachial Artery, Right Inferior ulnar collateral artery Profunda brachii Superior ulnar collateral artery **8** Brachial Artery, Left *See 7 Brachial Artery, Right* **9** Ulnar Artery, Right Anterior ulnar recurrent artery Common interosseous artery Posterior ulnar recurrent artery **A** Ulnar Artery, Left *See 9 Ulnar Artery, Right* **B** Radial Artery, Right Radial recurrent artery **C** Radial Artery, Left *See B Radial Artery, Right* **D** Hand Artery, Right Deep palmar arch Princeps pollicis artery Radialis indicis Superficial palmar arch **F** Hand Artery, Left *See D Hand Artery, Right* **G** Intracranial Artery Anterior cerebral artery Anterior choroidal artery Anterior communicating artery Basilar artery Circle of Willis Internal carotid artery, intracranial portion Middle cerebral artery Ophthalmic artery Posterior cerebral artery Posterior communicating artery Posterior inferior cerebellar artery (PICA)	**H** Common Carotid Artery, Right **J** Common Carotid Artery, Left **K** Internal Carotid Artery, Right Caroticotympanic artery Carotid sinus **L** Internal Carotid Artery, Left *See K Internal Carotid Artery, Right* **M** External Carotid Artery, Right Ascending pharyngeal artery Internal maxillary artery Lingual artery Maxillary artery Occipital artery Posterior auricular artery Superior thyroid artery **N** External Carotid Artery, Left *See M External Carotid Artery, Right* **P** Vertebral Artery, Right Anterior spinal artery Posterior spinal artery **Q** Vertebral Artery, Left *See P Vertebral Artery, Right* **R** Face Artery Angular artery Ascending palatine artery External maxillary artery Facial artery Inferior labial artery Submental artery Superior labial artery **S** Temporal Artery, Right Middle temporal artery Superficial temporal artery Transverse facial artery **T** Temporal Artery, Left *See S Temporal Artery, Right* **U** Thyroid Artery, Right Cricothyroid artery Hyoid artery Sternocleidomastoid artery Superior laryngeal artery Superior thyroid artery Thyrocervical trunk **V** Thyroid Artery, Left *See U Thyroid Artery, Right* **Y** Upper Artery Aortic intercostal artery Bronchial artery Esophageal artery Subcostal artery	**Ø** Open **3** Percutaneous **4** Percutaneous Endoscopic	**7** Autologous Tissue Substitute **J** Synthetic Substitute **K** Nonautologous Tissue Substitute	**Z** No Qualifier

LC Limited Coverage   NC Noncovered   ⊞ Combination Member   HAC associated procedure   Combination Only   DRG Non-OR   Non-OR   New/Revised in GREEN

206   ICD-10-PCS 2019

Ø   Medical and Surgical
3   Upper Arteries
V   Restriction   Definition: Partially closing an orifice or the lumen of a tubular body part
                  Explanation: The orifice can be a natural orifice or an artificially created orifice

Body Part Character 4		Approach Character 5	Device Character 6	Qualifier Character 7
Ø Internal Mammary Artery, Right Anterior intercostal artery Internal thoracic artery Musculophrenic artery Pericardiophrenic artery Superior epigastric artery **1 Internal Mammary Artery, Left** *See Ø Internal Mammary Artery, Right* **2 Innominate Artery** Brachiocephalic artery Brachiocephalic trunk **3 Subclavian Artery, Right** Costocervical trunk Dorsal scapular artery Internal thoracic artery **4 Subclavian Artery, Left** *See 3 Subclavian Artery, Right* **5 Axillary Artery, Right** Anterior circumflex humeral artery Lateral thoracic artery Posterior circumflex humeral artery Subscapular artery Superior thoracic artery Thoracoacromial artery **6 Axillary Artery, Left** *See 5 Axillary Artery, Right* **7 Brachial Artery, Right** Inferior ulnar collateral artery Profunda brachii Superior ulnar collateral artery **8 Brachial Artery, Left** *See 7 Brachial Artery, Right* **9 Ulnar Artery, Right** Anterior ulnar recurrent artery Common interosseous artery Posterior ulnar recurrent artery **A Ulnar Artery, Left** *See 9 Ulnar Artery, Right*	**B Radial Artery, Right** Radial recurrent artery **C Radial Artery, Left** *See B Radial Artery, Right* **D Hand Artery, Right** Deep palmar arch Princeps pollicis artery Radialis indicis Superficial palmar arch **F Hand Artery, Left** *See D Hand Artery, Right* **R Face Artery** Angular artery Ascending palatine artery External maxillary artery Facial artery Inferior labial artery Submental artery Superior labial artery **S Temporal Artery, Right** Middle temporal artery Superficial temporal artery Transverse facial artery **T Temporal Artery, Left** *See S Temporal Artery, Right* **U Thyroid Artery, Right** Cricothyroid artery Hyoid artery Sternocleidomastoid artery Superior laryngeal artery Superior thyroid artery Thyrocervical trunk **V Thyroid Artery, Left** *See U Thyroid Artery, Right* **Y Upper Artery** Aortic intercostal artery Bronchial artery Esophageal artery Subcostal artery	**Ø Open** **3 Percutaneous** **4 Percutaneous Endoscopic**	**C Extraluminal Device** **D Intraluminal Device** **Z No Device**	**Z No Qualifier**
G Intracranial Artery Anterior cerebral artery Anterior choroidal artery Anterior communicating artery Basilar artery Circle of Willis Internal carotid artery, intracranial portion Middle cerebral artery Ophthalmic artery Posterior cerebral artery Posterior communicating artery Posterior inferior cerebellar artery (PICA) **H Common Carotid Artery, Right** **J Common Carotid Artery, Left** **K Internal Carotid Artery, Right** Caroticotympanic artery Carotid sinus	**L Internal Carotid Artery, Left** *See K Internal Carotid Artery, Right* **M External Carotid Artery, Right** Ascending pharyngeal artery Internal maxillary artery Lingual artery Maxillary artery Occipital artery Posterior auricular artery Superior thyroid artery **N External Carotid Artery, Left** *See M External Carotid Artery, Right* **P Vertebral Artery, Right** Anterior spinal artery Posterior spinal artery **Q Vertebral Artery, Left** *See P Vertebral Artery, Right*	**Ø Open** **3 Percutaneous** **4 Percutaneous Endoscopic**	**B Intraluminal Device, Bioactive** **C Extraluminal Device** **D Intraluminal Device** **Z No Device**	**Z No Qualifier**

LC Limited Coverage   **NC** Noncovered   ⊞ Combination Member   HAC associated procedure   Combination Only   DRG Non-OR   Non-OR   New/Revised in GREEN

ICD-10-PCS 2019   **207**

Ø   Medical and Surgical
3   Upper Arteries
W   Revision

Definition: Correcting, to the extent possible, a portion of a malfunctioning device or the position of a displaced device

Explanation: Revision can include correcting a malfunctioning or displaced device by taking out or putting in components of the device such as a screw or pin

Body Part Character 4	Approach Character 5	Device Character 6	Qualifier Character 7
Y **Upper Artery** Aortic intercostal artery Bronchial artery Esophageal artery Subcostal artery	**Ø** Open **3** Percutaneous **4** Percutaneous Endoscopic	**Ø** Drainage Device **2** Monitoring Device **3** Infusion Device **7** Autologous Tissue Substitute **C** Extraluminal Device **D** Intraluminal Device **J** Synthetic Substitute **K** Nonautologous Tissue Substitute **M** Stimulator Lead **Y** Other Device	**Z** No Qualifier
Y **Upper Artery** Aortic intercostal artery Bronchial artery Esophageal artery Subcostal artery	**X** External	**Ø** Drainage Device **2** Monitoring Device **3** Infusion Device **7** Autologous Tissue Substitute **C** Extraluminal Device **D** Intraluminal Device **J** Synthetic Substitute **K** Nonautologous Tissue Substitute **M** Stimulator Lead	**Z** No Qualifier

Non-OR   03WY3[0,2,3,D]Z
Non-OR   03WY[3,4]YZ
Non-OR   03WYX[0,2,3,7,C,D,J,K,M]Z

LC Limited Coverage   NC Noncovered   ⊞ Combination Member   HAC associated procedure   Combination Only   DRG Non-OR   Non-OR   New/Revised in GREEN

208   ICD-10-PCS 2019

Lower Arteries Ø41–Ø4W

Character Meanings

This Character Meaning table is provided as a guide to assist the user in the identification of character members that may be found in this section of code tables. It **SHOULD NOT** be used to build a PCS code.

Operation–Character 3	Body Part–Character 4	Approach–Character 5	Device–Character 6	Qualifier–Character 7
1 Bypass	Ø Abdominal Aorta	Ø Open	Ø Drainage Device	Ø Abdominal Aorta
5 Destruction	1 Celiac Artery	3 Percutaneous	1 Radioactive Element	1 Celiac Artery OR Drug-Coated Balloon
7 Dilation	2 Gastric Artery	4 Percutaneous Endoscopic	2 Monitoring Device	2 Mesenteric Artery
9 Drainage	3 Hepatic Artery	X External	3 Infusion Device	3 Renal Artery, Right
B Excision	4 Splenic Artery		4 Intraluminal Device, Drug-eluting	4 Renal Artery, Left
C Extirpation	5 Superior Mesenteric Artery		5 Intraluminal Device, Drug-eluting, Two	5 Renal Artery, Bilateral
H Insertion	6 Colic Artery, Right		6 Intraluminal Device, Drug-eluting, Three	6 Common Iliac Artery, Right OR Bifurcation
J Inspection	7 Colic Artery, Left		7 Intraluminal Device, Drug-eluting, Four or More OR Autologous Tissue Substitute	7 Common Iliac Artery, Left
L Occlusion	8 Colic Artery, Middle		9 Autologous Venous Tissue	8 Common Iliac Arteries, Bilateral
N Release	9 Renal Artery, Right		A Autologous Arterial Tissue	9 Internal Iliac Artery, Right
P Removal	A Renal Artery, Left		C Extraluminal Device	B Internal Iliac Artery, Left
Q Repair	B Inferior Mesenteric Artery		D Intraluminal Device	C Internal Iliac Arteries, Bilateral
R Replacement	C Common Iliac Artery, Right		E Intraluminal Device, Two OR Intraluminal Device, Branched or Fenestrated, One or Two Arteries	D External Iliac Artery, Right
S Reposition	D Common Iliac Artery, Left		F Intraluminal Device, Three OR Intraluminal Device, Branched or Fenestrated, Three or More Arteries	F External Iliac Artery, Left
U Supplement	E Internal Iliac Artery, Right		G Intraluminal Device, Four or More	G External Iliac Arteries, Bilateral
V Restriction	F Internal Iliac Artery, Left		J Synthetic Substitute	H Femoral Artery, Right
W Revision	H External Iliac Artery, Right		K Nonautologous Tissue Substitute	J Femoral Artery, Left OR Temporary
	J External Iliac Artery, Left		Y Other Device	K Femoral Arteries, Bilateral
	K Femoral Artery, Right		Z No Device	L Popliteal Artery
	L Femoral Artery, Left			M Peroneal Artery
	M Popliteal Artery, Right			N Posterior Tibial Artery
	N Popliteal Artery, Left			P Foot Artery
	P Anterior Tibial Artery, Right			Q Lower Extremity Artery
	Q Anterior Tibial Artery, Left			R Lower Artery
	R Posterior Tibial Artery, Right			S Lower Extremity Vein
	S Posterior Tibial Artery, Left			T Uterine Artery, Right
	T Peroneal Artery, Right			U Uterine Artery, Left
	U Peroneal Artery, Left			X Diagnostic
	V Foot Artery, Right			Z No Qualifier
	W Foot Artery, Left			
	Y Lower Artery			

AHA Coding Clinic for table Ø41

2017, 4Q, 46-47	New and revised body part values - Bypass hepatic artery to renal artery
2017, 3Q, 5	Femoral artery to posterior tibial artery bypass using autologous and synthetic grafts
2017, 3Q, 16	Abdominal aortic debranching with bypass of external iliac artery to bilateral renal arteries and superior mesenteric artery
2017, 1Q, 32	Peroneal artery to dorsalis pedis artery bypass using saphenous vein graft
2016, 2Q, 18	Femoral-tibial artery bypass and saphenous vein graft
2015, 3Q, 28	Bilateral renal artery bypass

AHA Coding Clinic for table Ø47

2018, 2Q, 24	Coronary artery bifurcation
2016, 4Q, 86	Peripheral artery, number of stents
2016, 4Q, 86-88	Coronary and peripheral artery bifurcation
2016, 3Q, 39	Infrarenal abdominal aortic aneurysm repair with iliac graft extension
2015, 4Q, 4-7, 15	Drug-coated balloon angioplasty in peripheral vessels
2015, 3Q, 9	Aborted endovascular stenting of superficial femoral artery

AHA Coding Clinic for table Ø4C

2018, 2Q, 24	Coronary artery bifurcation
2017, 2Q, 23	Thrombectomy via Fogarty catheter
2016, 4Q, 86-88	Coronary and peripheral artery bifurcation
2016, 1Q, 31	Iliofemoral endarterectomy with patch repair
2015, 1Q, 29	Discontinued carotid endarterectomy
2015, 1Q, 36	Percutaneous mechanical thrombectomy of femoropopliteal bypass graft

AHA Coding Clinic for table Ø4H

2017, 1Q, 30	Insertion of umbilical artery catheter

AHA Coding Clinic for table Ø4L

2018, 2Q, 18	Transverse rectus abdominis myocutaneous (TRAM) delay
2017, 4Q, 31	Resuscitative endovascular balloon occlusion of the aorta
2015, 2Q, 27	Uterine artery embolization using Gelfoam
2014, 3Q, 26	Coil embolization of gastroduodenal artery with chemoembolization of hepatic artery
2014, 1Q, 24	Endovascular embolization for gastrointestinal bleeding

AHA Coding Clinic for table Ø4N

2015, 2Q, 28	Release and replacement of celiac artery

AHA Coding Clinic for table Ø4Q

2014, 1Q, 21	Repair of femoral artery pseudoaneurysm

AHA Coding Clinic for table Ø4R

2015, 2Q, 28	Release and replacement of celiac artery

AHA Coding Clinic for table Ø4U

2016, 2Q, 18	Femoral-tibial artery bypass and saphenous vein graft
2016, 1Q, 31	Iliofemoral endarterectomy with patch repair
2014, 4Q, 37	Bovine patch arterioplasty
2014, 1Q, 22	Repair of pseudoaneurysm of femoral-popliteal bypass graft

AHA Coding Clinic for table Ø4V

2018, 2Q, 24	Coronary artery bifurcation
2016, 4Q, 86-87	Coronary and peripheral artery bifurcation
2016, 4Q, 89-93	Branched and fenestrated endograft repair of aneurysms
2016, 3Q, 39	Infrarenal abdominal aortic aneurysm repair with iliac graft extension
2014, 1Q, 9	Endovascular repair of abdominal aortic aneurysm

AHA Coding Clinic for table Ø4W

2015, 1Q, 36	Revision of femoropopliteal bypass graft
2014, 1Q, 9	Endovascular repair of endoleak
2014, 1Q, 22	Repair of pseudoaneurysm of femoral-popliteal bypass graft

Lower Arteries

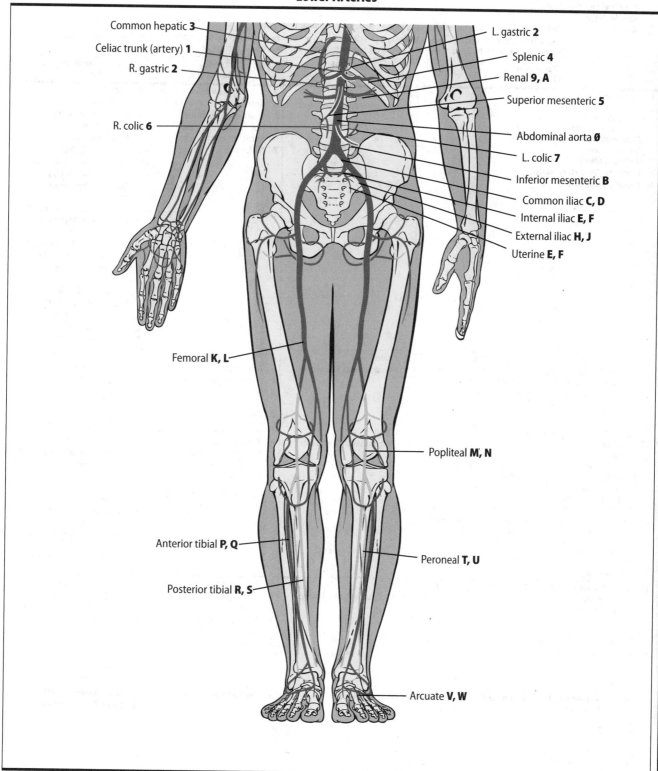

Common hepatic **3**
Celiac trunk (artery) **1**
R. gastric **2**
R. colic **6**

L. gastric **2**
Splenic **4**
Renal **9, A**
Superior mesenteric **5**
Abdominal aorta **Ø**
L. colic **7**
Inferior mesenteric **B**
Common iliac **C, D**
Internal iliac **E, F**
External iliac **H, J**
Uterine **E, F**

Femoral **K, L**

Popliteal **M, N**

Anterior tibial **P, Q**

Peroneal **T, U**

Posterior tibial **R, S**

Arcuate **V, W**

Lower Arteries *(left margin)*

Ø Medical and Surgical
4 Lower Arteries
1 Bypass

Definition: Altering the route of passage of the contents of a tubular body part

Explanation: Rerouting contents of a body part to a downstream area of the normal route, to a similar route and body part, or to an abnormal route and dissimilar body part. Includes one or more anastomoses, with or without the use of a device.

Body Part Character 4	Approach Character 5	Device Character 6	Qualifier Character 7
Ø Abdominal Aorta Inferior phrenic artery Lumbar artery Median sacral artery Middle suprarenal artery Ovarian artery Testicular artery **C Common Iliac Artery, Right** **D Common Iliac Artery, Left**	**Ø Open** **4 Percutaneous Endoscopic**	**9 Autologous Venous Tissue** **A Autologous Arterial Tissue** **J Synthetic Substitute** **K Nonautologous Tissue Substitute** **Z No Device**	**Ø Abdominal Aorta** **1 Celiac Artery** **2 Mesenteric Artery** **3 Renal Artery, Right** **4 Renal Artery, Left** **5 Renal Artery, Bilateral** **6 Common Iliac Artery, Right** **7 Common Iliac Artery, Left** **8 Common Iliac Arteries, Bilateral** **9 Internal Iliac Artery, Right** **B Internal Iliac Artery, Left** **C Internal Iliac Arteries, Bilateral** **D External Iliac Artery, Right** **F External Iliac Artery, Left** **G External Iliac Arteries, Bilateral** **H Femoral Artery, Right** **J Femoral Artery, Left** **K Femoral Arteries, Bilateral** **Q Lower Extremity Artery** **R Lower Artery**
3 Hepatic Artery Common hepatic artery Gastroduodenal artery Hepatic artery proper **4 Splenic Artery** Left gastroepiploic artery Pancreatic artery Short gastric artery	**Ø Open** **4 Percutaneous Endoscopic**	**9 Autologous Venous Tissue** **A Autologous Arterial Tissue** **J Synthetic Substitute** **K Nonautologous Tissue Substitute** **Z No Device**	**3 Renal Artery, Right** **4 Renal Artery, Left** **5 Renal Artery, Bilateral**
E Internal Iliac Artery, Right Deferential artery Hypogastric artery Iliolumbar artery Inferior gluteal artery Inferior vesical artery Internal pudendal artery Lateral sacral artery Middle rectal artery Obturator artery Superior gluteal artery Umbilical artery Uterine artery Vaginal artery **F Internal Iliac Artery, Left** *See E Internal Iliac Artery, Right* **H External Iliac Artery, Right** Deep circumflex iliac artery Inferior epigastric artery **J External Iliac Artery, Left** *See H External Iliac Artery, Right*	**Ø Open** **4 Percutaneous Endoscopic**	**9 Autologous Venous Tissue** **A Autologous Arterial Tissue** **J Synthetic Substitute** **K Nonautologous Tissue Substitute** **Z No Device**	**9 Internal Iliac Artery, Right** **B Internal Iliac Artery, Left** **C Internal Iliac Arteries, Bilateral** **D External Iliac Artery, Right** **F External Iliac Artery, Left** **G External Iliac Arteries, Bilateral** **H Femoral Artery, Right** **J Femoral Artery, Left** **K Femoral Arteries, Bilateral** **P Foot Artery** **Q Lower Extremity Artery**
K Femoral Artery, Right Circumflex iliac artery Deep femoral artery Descending genicular artery External pudendal artery Superficial epigastric artery **L Femoral Artery, Left** *See K Femoral Artery, Right*	**Ø Open** **4 Percutaneous Endoscopic**	**9 Autologous Venous Tissue** **A Autologous Arterial Tissue** **J Synthetic Substitute** **K Nonautologous Tissue Substitute** **Z No Device**	**H Femoral Artery, Right** **J Femoral Artery, Left** **K Femoral Arteries, Bilateral** **L Popliteal Artery** **M Peroneal Artery** **N Posterior Tibial Artery** **P Foot Artery** **Q Lower Extremity Artery** **S Lower Extremity Vein**
K Femoral Artery, Right Circumflex iliac artery Deep femoral artery Descending genicular artery External pudendal artery Superficial epigastric artery **L Femoral Artery, Left** *See K Femoral Artery, Right*	**3 Percutaneous**	**J Synthetic Substitute**	**Q Lower Extremity Artery** **S Lower Extremity Vein**
M Popliteal Artery, Right Inferior genicular artery Middle genicular artery Superior genicular artery Sural artery **N Popliteal Artery, Left** *See M Popliteal Artery, Right*	**Ø Open** **4 Percutaneous Endoscopic**	**9 Autologous Venous Tissue** **A Autologous Arterial Tissue** **J Synthetic Substitute** **K Nonautologous Tissue Substitute** **Z No Device**	**L Popliteal Artery** **M Peroneal Artery** **P Foot Artery** **Q Lower Extremity Artery** **S Lower Extremity Vein**

Ø41 Continued on next page

LC Limited Coverage   NC Noncovered   ⊞ Combination Member   HAC associated procedure   Combination Only   DRG Non-OR   Non-OR   New/Revised in GREEN

Ø   Medical and Surgical
4   Lower Arteries
1   Bypass

041 Continued

Definition: Altering the route of passage of the contents of a tubular body part

Explanation: Rerouting contents of a body part to a downstream area of the normal route, to a similar route and body part, or to an abnormal route and dissimilar body part. Includes one or more anastomoses, with or without the use of a device.

Body Part Character 4		Approach Character 5	Device Character 6	Qualifier Character 7
M Popliteal Artery, Right Inferior genicular artery Middle genicular artery Superior genicular artery Sural artery	**N** Popliteal Artery, Left *See M Popliteal Artery, Right*	**3** Percutaneous	**J** Synthetic Substitute	**Q** Lower Extremity Artery **S** Lower Extremity Vein
P Anterior Tibial Artery, Right Anterior lateral malleolar artery Anterior medial malleolar artery Anterior tibial recurrent artery Dorsalis pedis artery Posterior tibial recurrent artery	**Q** Anterior Tibial Artery, Left *See P Anterior Tibial Artery, Right* **R** Posterior Tibial Artery, Right **S** Posterior Tibial Artery, Left	**Ø** Open **3** Percutaneous **4** Percutaneous Endoscopic	**J** Synthetic Substitute	**Q** Lower Extremity Artery **S** Lower Extremity Vein
T Peroneal Artery, Right Fibular artery **U** Peroneal Artery, Left *See T Peroneal Artery, Right*	**V** Foot Artery, Right Arcuate artery Dorsal metatarsal artery Lateral plantar artery Lateral tarsal artery Medial plantar artery **W** Foot Artery, Left *See V Foot Artery, Right*	**Ø** Open **4** Percutaneous Endoscopic	**9** Autologous Venous Tissue **A** Autologous Arterial Tissue **J** Synthetic Substitute **K** Nonautologous Tissue Substitute **Z** No Device	**P** Foot Artery **Q** Lower Extremity Artery **S** Lower Extremity Vein
T Peroneal Artery, Right Fibular artery **U** Peroneal Artery, Left *See T Peroneal Artery, Right*	**V** Foot Artery, Right Arcuate artery Dorsal metatarsal artery Lateral plantar artery Lateral tarsal artery Medial plantar artery **W** Foot Artery, Left *See V Foot Artery, Right*	**3** Percutaneous	**J** Synthetic Substitute	**Q** Lower Extremity Artery **S** Lower Extremity Vein

LC Limited Coverage **NC** Noncovered ⊞ Combination Member HAC associated procedure Combination Only DRG Non-OR Non-OR New/Revised in GREEN

ICD-10-PCS 2019

213

041–041

Lower Arteries

Ø   **Medical and Surgical**
4   **Lower Arteries**
5   **Destruction**   Definition: Physical eradication of all or a portion of a body part by the direct use of energy, force, or a destructive agent
                          Explanation: None of the body part is physically taken out

Body Part Character 4		Approach Character 5	Device Character 6	Qualifier Character 7

Ø **Abdominal Aorta**
  Inferior phrenic artery
  Lumbar artery
  Median sacral artery
  Middle suprarenal artery
  Ovarian artery
  Testicular artery
1 **Celiac Artery**
  Celiac trunk
2 **Gastric Artery**
  Left gastric artery
  Right gastric artery
3 **Hepatic Artery**
  Common hepatic artery
  Gastroduodenal artery
  Hepatic artery proper
4 **Splenic Artery**
  Left gastroepiploic artery
  Pancreatic artery
  Short gastric artery
5 **Superior Mesenteric Artery**
  Ileal artery
  Ileocolic artery
  Inferior pancreaticoduodenal
    artery
  Jejunal artery
6 **Colic Artery, Right**
7 **Colic Artery, Left**
8 **Colic Artery, Middle**
9 **Renal Artery, Right**
  Inferior suprarenal artery
  Renal segmental artery
A **Renal Artery, Left**
  See 9 Renal Artery, Right
B **Inferior Mesenteric Artery**
  Sigmoid artery
  Superior rectal artery
C **Common Iliac Artery, Right**
D **Common Iliac Artery, Left**
E **Internal Iliac Artery, Right**
  Deferential artery
  Hypogastric artery
  Iliolumbar artery
  Inferior gluteal artery
  Inferior vesical artery
  Internal pudendal artery
  Lateral sacral artery
  Middle rectal artery
  Obturator artery
  Superior gluteal artery
  Umbilical artery
  Uterine artery
  Vaginal artery
	F **Internal Iliac Artery, Left**
	  See E Internal Iliac Artery, Right
	H **External Iliac Artery, Right**
	  Deep circumflex iliac artery
	  Inferior epigastric artery
	J **External Iliac Artery, Left**
	  See H External Iliac Artery, Right
	K **Femoral Artery, Right**
	  Circumflex iliac artery
	  Deep femoral artery
	  Descending genicular artery
	  External pudendal artery
	  Superficial epigastric artery
	L **Femoral Artery, Left**
	  See K Femoral Artery, Right
	M **Popliteal Artery, Right**
	  Inferior genicular artery
	  Middle genicular artery
	  Superior genicular artery
	  Sural artery
	N **Popliteal Artery, Left**
	  See M Popliteal Artery, Right
	P **Anterior Tibial Artery, Right**
	  Anterior lateral malleolar
	    artery
	  Anterior medial malleolar
	    artery
	  Anterior tibial recurrent artery
	  Dorsalis pedis artery
	  Posterior tibial recurrent artery
	Q **Anterior Tibial Artery, Left**
	  *See P Anterior Tibial Artery,
	    Right*
	R **Posterior Tibial Artery, Right**
	S **Posterior Tibial Artery, Left**
	T **Peroneal Artery, Right**
	  Fibular artery
	U **Peroneal Artery, Left**
	  See T Peroneal Artery, Right
	V **Foot Artery, Right**
	  Arcuate artery
	  Dorsal metatarsal artery
	  Lateral plantar artery
	  Lateral tarsal artery
	  Medial plantar artery
	W **Foot Artery, Left**
	  See V Foot Artery, Right
	Y **Lower Artery**
	  Umbilical artery
		Ø Open
		3 Percutaneous
		4 Percutaneous Endoscopic
			Z No Device	**Z** No Qualifier

LC Limited Coverage   **NC** Noncovered   ⊞ Combination Member   HAC associated procedure   Combination Only   DRG Non-OR   Non-OR   New/Revised in GREEN

214   ICD-10-PCS 2019

Ø   Medical and Surgical
4   Lower Arteries
7   Dilation   Definition: Expanding an orifice or the lumen of a tubular body part

Explanation: The orifice can be a natural orifice or an artificially created orifice. Accomplished by stretching a tubular body part using intraluminal pressure or by cutting part of the orifice or wall of the tubular body part.

Body Part Character 4		Approach Character 5	Device Character 6	Qualifier Character 7

Ø Abdominal Aorta
Inferior phrenic artery
Lumbar artery
Median sacral artery
Middle suprarenal artery
Ovarian artery
Testicular artery
1 Celiac Artery
Celiac trunk
2 Gastric Artery
Left gastric artery
Right gastric artery
3 Hepatic Artery
Common hepatic artery
Gastroduodenal artery
Hepatic artery proper
4 Splenic Artery
Left gastroepiploic artery
Pancreatic artery
Short gastric artery
5 Superior Mesenteric Artery
Ileal artery
Ileocolic artery
Inferior pancreaticoduodenal
    artery
Jejunal artery
6 Colic Artery, Right
7 Colic Artery, Left
8 Colic Artery, Middle
9 Renal Artery, Right
Inferior suprarenal artery
Renal segmental artery
A Renal Artery, Left
See 9 Renal Artery, Right
B Inferior Mesenteric Artery
Sigmoid artery
Superior rectal artery
C Common Iliac Artery, Right
D Common Iliac Artery, Left
E Internal Iliac Artery, Right
Deferential artery
Hypogastric artery
Iliolumbar artery
Inferior gluteal artery
Inferior vesical artery
Internal pudendal artery
Lateral sacral artery
Middle rectal artery
Obturator artery
Superior gluteal artery
Umbilical artery
Uterine artery
Vaginal artery
	F Internal Iliac Artery, Left
	See E Internal Iliac Artery, Right
	H External Iliac Artery, Right
	Deep circumflex iliac artery
	Inferior epigastric artery
	J External Iliac Artery, Left
	See H External Iliac Artery, Right
	K Femoral Artery, Right
	Circumflex iliac artery
	Deep femoral artery
	Descending genicular artery
	External pudendal artery
	Superficial epigastric artery
	L Femoral Artery, Left
	See K Femoral Artery, Right
	M Popliteal Artery, Right
	Inferior genicular artery
	Middle genicular artery
	Superior genicular artery
	Sural artery
	N Popliteal Artery, Left
	See M Popliteal Artery, Right
	P Anterior Tibial Artery, Right
	Anterior lateral malleolar
	    artery
	Anterior medial malleolar
	    artery
	Anterior tibial recurrent artery
	Dorsalis pedis artery
	Posterior tibial recurrent artery
	Q Anterior Tibial Artery, Left
	*See P Anterior Tibial Artery,
	    Right*
	R Posterior Tibial Artery, Right
	S Posterior Tibial Artery, Left
	T Peroneal Artery, Right
	Fibular artery
	U Peroneal Artery, Left
	See T Peroneal Artery, Right
	V Foot Artery, Right
	Arcuate artery
	Dorsal metatarsal artery
	Lateral plantar artery
	Lateral tarsal artery
	Medial plantar artery
	W Foot Artery, Left
	See V Foot Artery, Right
	Y Lower Artery
	Umbilical artery
		Ø Open
		3 Percutaneous
		4 Percutaneous Endoscopic
			**4 Intraluminal Device,
			    Drug-eluting**
			D Intraluminal Device
			Z No Device
				1 Drug-Coated Balloon
				6 Bifurcation
				Z No Qualifier

Ø47 Continued on next page

LC Limited Coverage   **NC** Noncovered   ⊞ Combination Member   HAC associated procedure   Combination Only   DRG Non-OR   Non-OR   New/Revised in GREEN

ICD-10-PCS 2019   215

047–047

Lower Arteries

Ø47 Continued

Ø   Medical and Surgical
4   Lower Arteries
7   Dilation   Definition: Expanding an orifice or the lumen of a tubular body part

Explanation: The orifice can be a natural orifice or an artificially created orifice. Accomplished by stretching a tubular body part using intraluminal pressure or by cutting part of the orifice or wall of the tubular body part.

Body Part Character 4		Approach Character 5	Device Character 6	Qualifier Character 7

Ø Abdominal Aorta
Inferior phrenic artery
Lumbar artery
Median sacral artery
Middle suprarenal artery
Ovarian artery
Testicular artery
1 Celiac Artery
Celiac trunk
2 Gastric Artery
Left gastric artery
Right gastric artery
3 Hepatic Artery
Common hepatic artery
Gastroduodenal artery
Hepatic artery proper
4 Splenic Artery
Left gastroepiploic artery
Pancreatic artery
Short gastric artery
5 Superior Mesenteric Artery
Ileal artery
Ileocolic artery
Inferior pancreaticoduodenal
   artery
Jejunal artery
6 Colic Artery, Right
7 Colic Artery, Left
8 Colic Artery, Middle
9 Renal Artery, Right
Inferior suprarenal artery
Renal segmental artery
A Renal Artery, Left
See 9 Renal Artery, Right
B Inferior Mesenteric Artery
Sigmoid artery
Superior rectal artery
C Common Iliac Artery, Right
D Common Iliac Artery, Left
E Internal Iliac Artery, Right
Deferential artery
Hypogastric artery
Iliolumbar artery
Inferior gluteal artery
Inferior vesical artery
Internal pudendal artery
Lateral sacral artery
Middle rectal artery
Obturator artery
Superior gluteal artery
Umbilical artery
Uterine artery
Vaginal artery
	F Internal Iliac Artery, Left
	See E Internal Iliac Artery, Right
	H External Iliac Artery, Right
	Deep circumflex iliac artery
	Inferior epigastric artery
	J External Iliac Artery, Left
	See H External Iliac Artery, Right
	K Femoral Artery, Right
	Circumflex iliac artery
	Deep femoral artery
	Descending genicular artery
	External pudendal artery
	Superficial epigastric artery
	L Femoral Artery, Left
	See K Femoral Artery, Right
	M Popliteal Artery, Right
	Inferior genicular artery
	Middle genicular artery
	Superior genicular artery
	Sural artery
	N Popliteal Artery, Left
	See M Popliteal Artery, Right
	P Anterior Tibial Artery, Right
	Anterior lateral malleolar
	   artery
	Anterior medial malleolar
	   artery
	Anterior tibial recurrent artery
	Dorsalis pedis artery
	Posterior tibial recurrent artery
	Q Anterior Tibial Artery, Left
	See P Anterior Tibial Artery,
	* Right*
	R Posterior Tibial Artery, Right
	S Posterior Tibial Artery, Left
	T Peroneal Artery, Right
	Fibular artery
	U Peroneal Artery, Left
	See T Peroneal Artery, Right
	V Foot Artery, Right
	Arcuate artery
	Dorsal metatarsal artery
	Lateral plantar artery
	Lateral tarsal artery
	Medial plantar artery
	W Foot Artery, Left
	See V Foot Artery, Right
	Y Lower Artery
	Umbilical artery
		Ø Open
		3 Percutaneous
		4 Percutaneous Endoscopic
			5 Intraluminal Device, Drug-eluting, Two
			6 Intraluminal Device, Drug-eluting, Three
			7 Intraluminal Device, Drug-eluting, Four or More
			E Intraluminal Device, Two
			F Intraluminal Device, Three
			G Intraluminal Device, Four or More
				6 Bifurcation
				Z No Qualifier

LC Limited Coverage   **NC** Noncovered   ⊞ Combination Member   HAC associated procedure   Combination Only   DRG Non-OR   Non-OR   New/Revised in GREEN

216   ICD-10-PCS 2019

Ø   Medical and Surgical
4   Lower Arteries
9   Drainage   Definition: Taking or letting out fluids and/or gases from a body part
                 Explanation: The qualifier DIAGNOSTIC is used to identify drainage procedures that are biopsies

Body Part Character 4		Approach Character 5	Device Character 6	Qualifier Character 7
Ø Abdominal Aorta	**F Internal Iliac Artery, Left**	**Ø Open**	**Ø Drainage Device**	**Z No Qualifier**
Inferior phrenic artery	*See E Internal Iliac Artery, Right*	**3 Percutaneous**		
Lumbar artery	**H External Iliac Artery, Right**	**4 Percutaneous Endoscopic**		
Median sacral artery	Deep circumflex iliac artery			
Middle suprarenal artery	Inferior epigastric artery			
Ovarian artery	**J External Iliac Artery, Left**			
Testicular artery	*See H External Iliac Artery, Right*			
1 Celiac Artery	**K Femoral Artery, Right**			
Celiac trunk	Circumflex iliac artery			
2 Gastric Artery	Deep femoral artery			
Left gastric artery	Descending genicular artery			
Right gastric artery	External pudendal artery			
3 Hepatic Artery	Superficial epigastric artery			
Common hepatic artery	**L Femoral Artery, Left**			
Gastroduodenal artery	*See K Femoral Artery, Right*			
Hepatic artery proper	**M Popliteal Artery, Right**			
4 Splenic Artery	Inferior genicular artery			
Left gastroepiploic artery	Middle genicular artery			
Pancreatic artery	Superior genicular artery			
Short gastric artery	Sural artery			
5 Superior Mesenteric Artery	**N Popliteal Artery, Left**			
Ileal artery	*See M Popliteal Artery, Right*			
Ileocolic artery	**P Anterior Tibial Artery, Right**			
Inferior pancreaticoduodenal artery	Anterior lateral malleolar artery			
Jejunal artery	Anterior medial malleolar artery			
6 Colic Artery, Right	Anterior tibial recurrent artery			
7 Colic Artery, Left	Dorsalis pedis artery			
8 Colic Artery, Middle	Posterior tibial recurrent artery			
9 Renal Artery, Right	**Q Anterior Tibial Artery, Left**			
Inferior suprarenal artery	*See P Anterior Tibial Artery, Right*			
Renal segmental artery	**R Posterior Tibial Artery, Right**			
A Renal Artery, Left	**S Posterior Tibial Artery, Left**			
See 9 Renal Artery, Right	**T Peroneal Artery, Right**			
B Inferior Mesenteric Artery	Fibular artery			
Sigmoid artery	**U Peroneal Artery, Left**			
Superior rectal artery	*See T Peroneal Artery, Right*			
C Common Iliac Artery, Right	**V Foot Artery, Right**			
D Common Iliac Artery, Left	Arcuate artery			
E Internal Iliac Artery, Right	Dorsal metatarsal artery			
Deferential artery	Lateral plantar artery			
Hypogastric artery	Lateral tarsal artery			
Iliolumbar artery	Medial plantar artery			
Inferior gluteal artery	**W Foot Artery, Left**			
Inferior vesical artery	*See V Foot Artery, Right*			
Internal pudendal artery	**Y Lower Artery**			
Lateral sacral artery	Umbilical artery			
Middle rectal artery				
Obturator artery				
Superior gluteal artery				
Umbilical artery				
Uterine artery				
Vaginal artery				

049 Continued on next page

Non-OR   049[Ø,1,2,3,4,5,6,7,8,9,A,B,C,D,E,F,H,J,K,L,M,N,P,Q,R,S,T,U,V,W,Y][Ø,3,4]ØZ

LC Limited Coverage   NC Noncovered   ⊞ Combination Member   HAC associated procedure   Combination Only   DRG Non-OR   Non-OR   New/Revised in GREEN
ICD-10-PCS 2019   217

049–049

0 **Medical and Surgical**
4 **Lower Arteries**
9 **Drainage**   Definition: Taking or letting out fluids and/or gases from a body part
                            Explanation: The qualifier DIAGNOSTIC is used to identify drainage procedures that are biopsies

Body Part Character 4		Approach Character 5	Device Character 6	Qualifier Character 7

0 Abdominal Aorta
Inferior phrenic artery
Lumbar artery
Median sacral artery
Middle suprarenal artery
Ovarian artery
Testicular artery
1 **Celiac Artery**
Celiac trunk
2 **Gastric Artery**
Left gastric artery
Right gastric artery
3 **Hepatic Artery**
Common hepatic artery
Gastroduodenal artery
Hepatic artery proper
4 **Splenic Artery**
Left gastroepiploic artery
Pancreatic artery
Short gastric artery
5 **Superior Mesenteric Artery**
Ileal artery
Ileocolic artery
Inferior pancreaticoduodenal
  artery
Jejunal artery
6 **Colic Artery, Right**
7 **Colic Artery, Left**
8 **Colic Artery, Middle**
9 **Renal Artery, Right**
Inferior suprarenal artery
Renal segmental artery
A **Renal Artery, Left**
See 9 Renal Artery, Right
B **Inferior Mesenteric Artery**
Sigmoid artery
Superior rectal artery
C **Common Iliac Artery, Right**
D **Common Iliac Artery, Left**
E **Internal Iliac Artery, Right**
Deferential artery
Hypogastric artery
Iliolumbar artery
Inferior gluteal artery
Inferior vesical artery
Internal pudendal artery
Lateral sacral artery
Middle rectal artery
Obturator artery
Superior gluteal artery
Umbilical artery
Uterine artery
Vaginal artery
	F **Internal Iliac Artery, Left**
	See E Internal Iliac Artery, Right
	H **External Iliac Artery, Right**
	Deep circumflex iliac artery
	Inferior epigastric artery
	J **External Iliac Artery, Left**
	See H External Iliac Artery, Right
	K **Femoral Artery, Right**
	Circumflex iliac artery
	Deep femoral artery
	Descending genicular artery
	External pudendal artery
	Superficial epigastric artery
	L **Femoral Artery, Left**
	See K Femoral Artery, Right
	M **Popliteal Artery, Right**
	Inferior genicular artery
	Middle genicular artery
	Superior genicular artery
	Sural artery
	N **Popliteal Artery, Left**
	See M Popliteal Artery, Right
	P **Anterior Tibial Artery, Right**
	Anterior lateral malleolar
	  artery
	Anterior medial malleolar
	  artery
	Anterior tibial recurrent artery
	Dorsalis pedis artery
	Posterior tibial recurrent artery
	Q **Anterior Tibial Artery, Left**
	*See P Anterior Tibial Artery,
	  Right*
	R **Posterior Tibial Artery, Right**
	S **Posterior Tibial Artery, Left**
	T **Peroneal Artery, Right**
	Fibular artery
	U **Peroneal Artery, Left**
	See T Peroneal Artery, Right
	V **Foot Artery, Right**
	Arcuate artery
	Dorsal metatarsal artery
	Lateral plantar artery
	Lateral tarsal artery
	Medial plantar artery
	W **Foot Artery, Left**
	See V Foot Artery, Right
	Y **Lower Artery**
	Umbilical artery
		0 Open
		3 Percutaneous
		4 Percutaneous Endoscopic
			Z No Device	**X** Diagnostic
				Z No Qualifier

Non-OR 049[0,1,2,3,4,5,6,7,8,9,A,B,C,D,E,F,H,J,K,L,M,N,P,Q,R,S,T,U,V,W,Y]3ZX
Non-OR 049[0,1,2,3,4,5,6,7,8,9,A,B,C,D,E,F,H,J,K,L,M,N,P,Q,R,S,T,U,V,W,Y][0,3,4]ZZ

Ø   Medical and Surgical
4   Lower Arteries
B   Excision

Definition: Cutting out or off, without replacement, a portion of a body part

Explanation: The qualifier DIAGNOSTIC is used to identify excision procedures that are biopsies

Body Part Character 4		Approach Character 5	Device Character 6	Qualifier Character 7
Ø Abdominal Aorta Inferior phrenic artery Lumbar artery Median sacral artery Middle suprarenal artery Ovarian artery Testicular artery **1 Celiac Artery** Celiac trunk **2 Gastric Artery** Left gastric artery Right gastric artery **3 Hepatic Artery** Common hepatic artery Gastroduodenal artery Hepatic artery proper **4 Splenic Artery** Left gastroepiploic artery Pancreatic artery Short gastric artery **5 Superior Mesenteric Artery** Ileal artery Ileocolic artery Inferior pancreaticoduodenal artery Jejunal artery **6 Colic Artery, Right** **7 Colic Artery, Left** **8 Colic Artery, Middle** **9 Renal Artery, Right** Inferior suprarenal artery Renal segmental artery **A Renal Artery, Left** *See 9 Renal Artery, Right* **B Inferior Mesenteric Artery** Sigmoid artery Superior rectal artery **C Common Iliac Artery, Right** **D Common Iliac Artery, Left** **E Internal Iliac Artery, Right** Deferential artery Hypogastric artery Iliolumbar artery Inferior gluteal artery Inferior vesical artery Internal pudendal artery Lateral sacral artery Middle rectal artery Obturator artery Superior gluteal artery Umbilical artery Uterine artery Vaginal artery	**F Internal Iliac Artery, Left** *See E Internal Iliac Artery, Right* **H External Iliac Artery, Right** Deep circumflex iliac artery Inferior epigastric artery **J External Iliac Artery, Left** *See H External Iliac Artery, Right* **K Femoral Artery, Right** Circumflex iliac artery Deep femoral artery Descending genicular artery External pudendal artery Superficial epigastric artery **L Femoral Artery, Left** *See K Femoral Artery, Right* **M Popliteal Artery, Right** Inferior genicular artery Middle genicular artery Superior genicular artery Sural artery **N Popliteal Artery, Left** *See M Popliteal Artery, Right* **P Anterior Tibial Artery, Right** Anterior lateral malleolar artery Anterior medial malleolar artery Anterior tibial recurrent artery Dorsalis pedis artery Posterior tibial recurrent artery **Q Anterior Tibial Artery, Left** *See P Anterior Tibial Artery, Right* **R Posterior Tibial Artery, Right** **S Posterior Tibial Artery, Left** **T Peroneal Artery, Right** Fibular artery **U Peroneal Artery, Left** *See T Peroneal Artery, Right* **V Foot Artery, Right** Arcuate artery Dorsal metatarsal artery Lateral plantar artery Lateral tarsal artery Medial plantar artery **W Foot Artery, Left** *See V Foot Artery, Right* **Y Lower Artery** Umbilical artery	**Ø Open** **3 Percutaneous** **4 Percutaneous Endoscopic**	**Z No Device**	**X Diagnostic** **Z No Qualifier**

■ Limited Coverage   ■ Noncovered   ⊞ Combination Member   HAC associated procedure   Combination Only   DRG Non-OR   Non-OR   New/Revised in GREEN

ICD-10-PCS 2019   219

04B–04B

Lower Arteries

04C–04C

0 **Medical and Surgical**
4 **Lower Arteries**
C **Extirpation**　　Definition: Taking or cutting out solid matter from a body part

Explanation: The solid matter may be an abnormal byproduct of a biological function or a foreign body; it may be imbedded in a body part or in the lumen of a tubular body part. The solid matter may or may not have been previously broken into pieces.

Body Part Character 4		Approach Character 5	Device Character 6	Qualifier Character 7
0 **Abdominal Aorta** 　Inferior phrenic artery 　Lumbar artery 　Median sacral artery 　Middle suprarenal artery 　Ovarian artery 　Testicular artery **1** **Celiac Artery** 　Celiac trunk **2** **Gastric Artery** 　Left gastric artery 　Right gastric artery **3** **Hepatic Artery** 　Common hepatic artery 　Gastroduodenal artery 　Hepatic artery proper **4** **Splenic Artery** 　Left gastroepiploic artery 　Pancreatic artery 　Short gastric artery **5** **Superior Mesenteric Artery** 　Ileal artery 　Ileocolic artery 　Inferior pancreaticoduodenal 　　artery 　Jejunal artery **6** **Colic Artery, Right** **7** **Colic Artery, Left** **8** **Colic Artery, Middle** **9** **Renal Artery, Right** 　Inferior suprarenal artery 　Renal segmental artery **A** **Renal Artery, Left** 　*See 9 Renal Artery, Right* **B** **Inferior Mesenteric Artery** 　Sigmoid artery 　Superior rectal artery **C** **Common Iliac Artery, Right** **D** **Common Iliac Artery, Left** **E** **Internal Iliac Artery, Right** 　Deferential artery 　Hypogastric artery 　Iliolumbar artery 　Inferior gluteal artery 　Inferior vesical artery 　Internal pudendal artery 　Lateral sacral artery 　Middle rectal artery 　Obturator artery 　Superior gluteal artery 　Umbilical artery 　Uterine artery 　Vaginal artery	**F** **Internal Iliac Artery, Left** 　*See E Internal Iliac Artery, Right* **H** **External Iliac Artery, Right** 　Deep circumflex iliac artery 　Inferior epigastric artery **J** **External Iliac Artery, Left** 　*See H External Iliac Artery, Right* **K** **Femoral Artery, Right** 　Circumflex iliac artery 　Deep femoral artery 　Descending genicular artery 　External pudendal artery 　Superficial epigastric artery **L** **Femoral Artery, Left** 　*See K Femoral Artery, Right* **M** **Popliteal Artery, Right** 　Inferior genicular artery 　Middle genicular artery 　Superior genicular artery 　Sural artery **N** **Popliteal Artery, Left** 　*See M Popliteal Artery, Right* **P** **Anterior Tibial Artery, Right** 　Anterior lateral malleolar artery 　Anterior medial malleolar artery 　Anterior tibial recurrent artery 　Dorsalis pedis artery 　Posterior tibial recurrent artery **Q** **Anterior Tibial Artery, Left** 　*See P Anterior Tibial Artery, 　　Right* **R** **Posterior Tibial Artery, Right** **S** **Posterior Tibial Artery, Left** **T** **Peroneal Artery, Right** 　Fibular artery **U** **Peroneal Artery, Left** 　*See T Peroneal Artery, Right* **V** **Foot Artery, Right** 　Arcuate artery 　Dorsal metatarsal artery 　Lateral plantar artery 　Lateral tarsal artery 　Medial plantar artery **W** **Foot Artery, Left** 　*See V Foot Artery, Right* **Y** **Lower Artery** 　Umbilical artery	**0** Open **3** Percutaneous **4** Percutaneous Endoscopic	**Z** No Device	**6** Bifurcation **Z** No Qualifier

LC Limited Coverage　NC Noncovered　⊞ Combination Member　HAC associated procedure　Combination Only　DRG Non-OR　Non-OR　New/Revised in GREEN

220　　　　　　　　　　　　　　　　　　　　　　　　　　　　　　　　　　　　　　ICD-10-PCS 2019

Ø Medical and Surgical
4 Lower Arteries
H Insertion   Definition: Putting in a nonbiological appliance that monitors, assists, performs, or prevents a physiological function but does not physically take the place of a body part
               Explanation: None

Body Part Character 4		Approach Character 5	Device Character 6	Qualifier Character 7
Ø Abdominal Aorta Inferior phrenic artery Lumbar artery Median sacral artery Middle suprarenal artery Ovarian artery Testicular artery		**Ø** Open **3** Percutaneous **4** Percutaneous Endoscopic	**2** Monitoring Device **3** Infusion Device **D** Intraluminal Device	**Z** No Qualifier
1 Celiac Artery Celiac trunk **2 Gastric Artery** Left gastric artery Right gastric artery **3 Hepatic Artery** Common hepatic artery Gastroduodenal artery Hepatic artery proper **4 Splenic Artery** Left gastroepiploic artery Pancreatic artery Short gastric artery **5 Superior Mesenteric Artery** Ileal artery Ileocolic artery Inferior pancreaticoduodenal artery Jejunal artery **6 Colic Artery, Right** **7 Colic Artery, Left** **8 Colic Artery, Middle** **9 Renal Artery, Right** Inferior suprarenal artery Renal segmental artery **A Renal Artery, Left** *See 9 Renal Artery, Right* **B Inferior Mesenteric Artery** Sigmoid artery Superior rectal artery **C Common Iliac Artery, Right** **D Common Iliac Artery, Left** **E Internal Iliac Artery, Right** Deferential artery Hypogastric artery Iliolumbar artery Inferior gluteal artery Inferior vesical artery Internal pudendal artery Lateral sacral artery Middle rectal artery Obturator artery Superior gluteal artery Umbilical artery Uterine artery Vaginal artery	**F Internal Iliac Artery, Left** *See E Internal Iliac Artery, Right* **H External Iliac Artery, Right** Deep circumflex iliac artery Inferior epigastric artery **J External Iliac Artery, Left** *See H External Iliac Artery, Right* **K Femoral Artery, Right** Circumflex iliac artery Deep femoral artery Descending genicular artery External pudendal artery Superficial epigastric artery **L Femoral Artery, Left** *See K Femoral Artery, Right* **M Popliteal Artery, Right** Inferior genicular artery Middle genicular artery Superior genicular artery Sural artery **N Popliteal Artery, Left** *See M Popliteal Artery, Right* **P Anterior Tibial Artery, Right** Anterior lateral malleolar artery Anterior medial malleolar artery Anterior tibial recurrent artery Dorsalis pedis artery Posterior tibial recurrent artery **Q Anterior Tibial Artery, Left** *See P Anterior Tibial Artery, Right* **R Posterior Tibial Artery, Right** **S Posterior Tibial Artery, Left** **T Peroneal Artery, Right** Fibular artery **U Peroneal Artery, Left** *See T Peroneal Artery, Right* **V Foot Artery, Right** Arcuate artery Dorsal metatarsal artery Lateral plantar artery Lateral tarsal artery Medial plantar artery **W Foot Artery, Left** *See V Foot Artery, Right*	**Ø** Open **3** Percutaneous **4** Percutaneous Endoscopic	**3** Infusion Device **D** Intraluminal Device	**Z** No Qualifier
Y Lower Artery Umbilical artery		**Ø** Open **3** Percutaneous **4** Percutaneous Endoscopic	**2** Monitoring Device **3** Infusion Device **D** Intraluminal Device **Y** Other Device	**Z** No Qualifier

Non-OR   04HØ[Ø,3,4][2,3]Z
Non-OR   04H[1,2,3,4,5,6,7,8,9,A,B,C,D,E,F,H,J,K,L,M,N,P,Q,R,S,T,U,V,W][Ø,3,4]3Z
Non-OR   04HY32Z
Non-OR   04HY[Ø,3,4]3Z
Non-OR   04HY[3,4]YZ

LC Limited Coverage   NC Noncovered   ⊞ Combination Member   HAC associated procedure   Combination Only   DRG Non-OR   Non-OR   New/Revised in GREEN
ICD-10-PCS 2019   221

04H–04H

Ø   Medical and Surgical
4   Lower Arteries
J   Inspection   Definition: Visually and/or manually exploring a body part

Explanation: Visual exploration may be performed with or without optical instrumentation. Manual exploration may be performed directly or through intervening body layers.

Body Part Character 4	Approach Character 5	Device Character 6	Qualifier Character 7
Y Lower Artery Umbilical artery	**Ø Open** **3 Percutaneous** **4 Percutaneous Endoscopic** **X External**	**Z No Device**	**Z No Qualifier**

Non-OR   Ø4JY[3,4,X]ZZ

Ø   Medical and Surgical
4   Lower Arteries
L   Occlusion   Definition: Completely closing an orifice or the lumen of a tubular body part

Explanation: The orifice can be a natural orifice or an artificially created orifice

Body Part Character 4	Approach Character 5	Device Character 6	Qualifier Character 7
Ø Abdominal Aorta Inferior phrenic artery Lumbar artery Median sacral artery Middle suprarenal artery Ovarian artery Testicular artery	**Ø Open** **4 Percutaneous Endoscopic**	**C Extraluminal Device** **D Intraluminal Device** **Z No Device**	**Z No Qualifier**
Ø Abdominal Aorta Inferior phrenic artery Lumbar artery Median sacral artery Middle suprarenal artery Ovarian artery Testicular artery	**3 Percutaneous**	**C Extraluminal Device** **Z No Device**	**Z No Qualifier**
Ø Abdominal Aorta Inferior phrenic artery Lumbar artery Median sacral artery Middle suprarenal artery Ovarian artery Testicular artery	**3 Percutaneous**	**D Intraluminal Device**	**J Temporary** **Z No Qualifier**

Ø4L Continued on next page

Ø   **Medical and Surgical**   *Ø4L Continued*
4   **Lower Arteries**
L   **Occlusion**   Definition: Completely closing an orifice or the lumen of a tubular body part
                     Explanation: The orifice can be a natural orifice or an artificially created orifice

Body Part Character 4		Approach Character 5	Device Character 6	Qualifier Character 7

1 Celiac Artery
Celiac trunk
2 Gastric Artery
Left gastric artery
Right gastric artery
3 Hepatic Artery
Common hepatic artery
Gastroduodenal artery
Hepatic artery proper
4 Splenic Artery
Left gastroepiploic artery
Pancreatic artery
Short gastric artery
5 Superior Mesenteric Artery
Ileal artery
Ileocolic artery
Inferior pancreaticoduodenal
   artery
Jejunal artery
6 Colic Artery, Right
7 Colic Artery, Left
8 Colic Artery, Middle
9 Renal Artery, Right
Inferior suprarenal artery
Renal segmental artery
A Renal Artery, Left
See 9 Renal Artery, Right
B Inferior Mesenteric Artery
Sigmoid artery
Superior rectal artery
C Common Iliac Artery, Right
D Common Iliac Artery, Left
H External Iliac Artery, Right
Deep circumflex iliac artery
Inferior epigastric artery
J External Iliac Artery, Left
See H External Iliac Artery, Right
	K Femoral Artery, Right
	Circumflex iliac artery
	Deep femoral artery
	Descending genicular artery
	External pudendal artery
	Superficial epigastric artery
	L Femoral Artery, Left
	See K Femoral Artery, Right
	M Popliteal Artery, Right
	Inferior genicular artery
	Middle genicular artery
	Superior genicular artery
	Sural artery
	N Popliteal Artery, Left
	See M Popliteal Artery, Right
	P Anterior Tibial Artery, Right
	Anterior lateral malleolar
	   artery
	Anterior medial malleolar
	   artery
	Anterior tibial recurrent artery
	Dorsalis pedis artery
	Posterior tibial recurrent artery
	Q Anterior Tibial Artery, Left
	See P Anterior Tibial Artery,
	* Right*
	R Posterior Tibial Artery, Right
	S Posterior Tibial Artery, Left
	T Peroneal Artery, Right
	Fibular artery
	U Peroneal Artery, Left
	See T Peroneal Artery, Right
	V Foot Artery, Right
	Arcuate artery
	Dorsal metatarsal artery
	Lateral plantar artery
	Lateral tarsal artery
	Medial plantar artery
	W Foot Artery, Left
	See V Foot Artery, Right
	Y Lower Artery
	Umbilical artery
		Ø Open
		3 Percutaneous
		4 Percutaneous Endoscopic
			C Extraluminal Device
			D Intraluminal Device
			Z No Device
				Z No Qualifier

E Internal Iliac Artery, Right Deferential artery Hypogastric artery Iliolumbar artery Inferior gluteal artery Inferior vesical artery Internal pudendal artery Lateral sacral artery Middle rectal artery Obturator artery Superior gluteal artery Umbilical artery Uterine artery Vaginal artery		**Ø Open** **3 Percutaneous** **4 Percutaneous Endoscopic**	**C Extraluminal Device** **D Intraluminal Device** **Z No Device**	**T Uterine Artery, Right** ♀ **Z No Qualifier**
F Internal Iliac Artery, Left Deferential artery Hypogastric artery Iliolumbar artery Inferior gluteal artery Inferior vesical artery Internal pudendal artery Lateral sacral artery Middle rectal artery Obturator artery Superior gluteal artery Umbilical artery Uterine Artery Vaginal artery		**Ø Open** **3 Percutaneous** **4 Percutaneous Endoscopic**	**C Extraluminal Device** **D Intraluminal Device** **Z No Device**	**U Uterine Artery, Left** ♀ **Z No Qualifier**

Non-OR   Ø4L23DZ
♀   Ø4LE[Ø,3,4][C,D,Z]T
♀   Ø4LF[Ø,3,4][C,D,Z]U

LC Limited Coverage   NC Noncovered   ⊞ Combination Member   HAC associated procedure   Combination Only   DRG Non-OR   Non-OR   New/Revised in GREEN
ICD-10-PCS 2019   223

Ø4L–Ø4L

Lower Arteries

Ø **Medical and Surgical**
4 **Lower Arteries**
N **Release**   Definition: Freeing a body part from an abnormal physical constraint by cutting or by the use of force
              Explanation: Some of the restraining tissue may be taken out but none of the body part is taken out

Body Part Character 4	Approach Character 5	Device Character 6	Qualifier Character 7

Ø **Abdominal Aorta**
  Inferior phrenic artery
  Lumbar artery
  Median sacral artery
  Middle suprarenal artery
  Ovarian artery
  Testicular artery
1 **Celiac Artery**
  Celiac trunk
2 **Gastric Artery**
  Left gastric artery
  Right gastric artery
3 **Hepatic Artery**
  Common hepatic artery
  Gastroduodenal artery
  Hepatic artery proper
4 **Splenic Artery**
  Left gastroepiploic artery
  Pancreatic artery
  Short gastric artery
5 **Superior Mesenteric Artery**
  Ileal artery
  Ileocolic artery
  Inferior pancreaticoduodenal artery
  Jejunal artery
6 **Colic Artery, Right**
7 **Colic Artery, Left**
8 **Colic Artery, Middle**
9 **Renal Artery, Right**
  Inferior suprarenal artery
  Renal segmental artery
A **Renal Artery, Left**
  See 9 Renal Artery, Right
B **Inferior Mesenteric Artery**
  Sigmoid artery
  Superior rectal artery
C **Common Iliac Artery, Right**
D **Common Iliac Artery, Left**
E **Internal Iliac Artery, Right**
  Deferential artery
  Hypogastric artery
  Iliolumbar artery
  Inferior gluteal artery
  Inferior vesical artery
  Internal pudendal artery
  Lateral sacral artery
  Middle rectal artery
  Obturator artery
  Superior gluteal artery
  Umbilical artery
  Uterine artery
  Vaginal artery
	F **Internal Iliac Artery, Left**
	  See E Internal Iliac Artery, Right
	H **External Iliac Artery, Right**
	  Deep circumflex iliac artery
	  Inferior epigastric artery
	J **External Iliac Artery, Left**
	  See H External Iliac Artery, Right
	K **Femoral Artery, Right**
	  Circumflex iliac artery
	  Deep femoral artery
	  Descending genicular artery
	  External pudendal artery
	  Superficial epigastric artery
	L **Femoral Artery, Left**
	  See K Femoral Artery, Right
	M **Popliteal Artery, Right**
	  Inferior genicular artery
	  Middle genicular artery
	  Superior genicular artery
	  Sural artery
	N **Popliteal Artery, Left**
	  See M Popliteal Artery, Right
	P **Anterior Tibial Artery, Right**
	  Anterior lateral malleolar artery
	  Anterior medial malleolar artery
	  Anterior tibial recurrent artery
	  Dorsalis pedis artery
	  Posterior tibial recurrent artery
	Q **Anterior Tibial Artery, Left**
	  See P Anterior Tibial Artery, Right
	R **Posterior Tibial Artery, Right**
	S **Posterior Tibial Artery, Left**
	T **Peroneal Artery, Right**
	  Fibular artery
	U **Peroneal Artery, Left**
	  See T Peroneal Artery, Right
	V **Foot Artery, Right**
	  Arcuate artery
	  Dorsal metatarsal artery
	  Lateral plantar artery
	  Lateral tarsal artery
	  Medial plantar artery
	W **Foot Artery, Left**
	  See V Foot Artery, Right
	Y **Lower Artery**
	  Umbilical artery
		Ø **Open**
		3 **Percutaneous**
		4 **Percutaneous Endoscopic**
			Z **No Device**	Z **No Qualifier**

LC Limited Coverage   NC Noncovered   ⊞ Combination Member   HAC associated procedure   Combination Only   DRG Non-OR   Non-OR   New/Revised in GREEN

224   ICD-10-PCS 2019

0   **Medical and Surgical**
4   **Lower Arteries**
P   **Removal**   Definition: Taking out or off a device from a body part

                       Explanation: If a device is taken out and a similar device put in without cutting or puncturing the skin or mucous membrane, the procedure is coded to the root operation CHANGE. Otherwise, the procedure for taking out a device is coded to the root operation REMOVAL.

Body Part Character 4	Approach Character 5	Device Character 6	Qualifier Character 7

Y **Lower Artery**
    Umbilical artery
	0 Open
	3 Percutaneous
	4 Percutaneous Endoscopic
		0 Drainage Device
		2 Monitoring Device
		3 Infusion Device
		7 Autologous Tissue
		    Substitute
		C Extraluminal Device
		D Intraluminal Device
		J Synthetic Substitute
		K Nonautologous Tissue
		    Substitute
		Y Other Device
			Z No Qualifier

Y **Lower Artery** Umbilical artery	**X** External	**0** Drainage Device **1** Radioactive Element **2** Monitoring Device **3** Infusion Device **D** Intraluminal Device	**Z** No Qualifier

Non-OR   04PY3[0,2,3,D]Z
Non-OR   04PY[3,4]YZ
Non-OR   04PYX[0,1,2,3,D]Z

Lower Arteries

0 Medical and Surgical
4 Lower Arteries
Q Repair Definition: Restoring, to the extent possible, a body part to its normal anatomic structure and function

Explanation: Used only when the method to accomplish the repair is not one of the other root operations

Body Part Character 4		Approach Character 5	Device Character 6	Qualifier Character 7
0 Abdominal Aorta	**F Internal Iliac Artery, Left**	**0 Open**	**Z No Device**	**Z No Qualifier**
Inferior phrenic artery	*See E Internal Iliac Artery, Right*	**3 Percutaneous**		
Lumbar artery	**H External Iliac Artery, Right**	**4 Percutaneous Endoscopic**		
Median sacral artery	Deep circumflex iliac artery			
Middle suprarenal artery	Inferior epigastric artery			
Ovarian artery	**J External Iliac Artery, Left**			
Testicular artery	*See H External Iliac Artery, Right*			
1 Celiac Artery	**K Femoral Artery, Right**			
Celiac trunk	Circumflex iliac artery			
2 Gastric Artery	Deep femoral artery			
Left gastric artery	Descending genicular artery			
Right gastric artery	External pudendal artery			
3 Hepatic Artery	Superficial epigastric artery			
Common hepatic artery	**L Femoral Artery, Left**			
Gastroduodenal artery	*See K Femoral Artery, Right*			
Hepatic artery proper	**M Popliteal Artery, Right**			
4 Splenic Artery	Inferior genicular artery			
Left gastroepiploic artery	Middle genicular artery			
Pancreatic artery	Superior genicular artery			
Short gastric artery	Sural artery			
5 Superior Mesenteric Artery	**N Popliteal Artery, Left**			
Ileal artery	*See M Popliteal Artery, Right*			
Ileocolic artery	**P Anterior Tibial Artery, Right**			
Inferior pancreaticoduodenal artery	Anterior lateral malleolar artery			
Jejunal artery	Anterior medial malleolar artery			
6 Colic Artery, Right	Anterior tibial recurrent artery			
7 Colic Artery, Left	Dorsalis pedis artery			
8 Colic Artery, Middle	Posterior tibial recurrent artery			
9 Renal Artery, Right	**Q Anterior Tibial Artery, Left**			
Inferior suprarenal artery	*See P Anterior Tibial Artery, Right*			
Renal segmental artery	**R Posterior Tibial Artery, Right**			
A Renal Artery, Left	**S Posterior Tibial Artery, Left**			
See 9 Renal Artery, Right	**T Peroneal Artery, Right**			
B Inferior Mesenteric Artery	Fibular artery			
Sigmoid artery	**U Peroneal Artery, Left**			
Superior rectal artery	*See T Peroneal Artery, Right*			
C Common Iliac Artery, Right	**V Foot Artery, Right**			
D Common Iliac Artery, Left	Arcuate artery			
E Internal Iliac Artery, Right	Dorsal metatarsal artery			
Deferential artery	Lateral plantar artery			
Hypogastric artery	Lateral tarsal artery			
Iliolumbar artery	Medial plantar artery			
Inferior gluteal artery	**W Foot Artery, Left**			
Inferior vesical artery	*See V Foot Artery, Right*			
Internal pudendal artery	**Y Lower Artery**			
Lateral sacral artery	Umbilical artery			
Middle rectal artery				
Obturator artery				
Superior gluteal artery				
Umbilical artery				
Uterine artery				
Vaginal artery				

LC Limited Coverage NC Noncovered ⊞ Combination Member HAC associated procedure Combination Only DRG Non-OR Non-OR New/Revised in GREEN

226 ICD-10-PCS 2019

Lower Arteries

Ø   **Medical and Surgical**
4   **Lower Arteries**
R   **Replacement**   Definition: Putting in or on biological or synthetic material that physically takes the place and/or function of all or a portion of a body part
          Explanation: The body part may have been taken out or replaced, or may be taken out, physically eradicated, or rendered nonfunctional during the REPLACEMENT procedure. A REMOVAL procedure is coded for taking out the device used in a previous replacement procedure.

Body Part Character 4		Approach Character 5	Device Character 6	Qualifier Character 7

Ø Abdominal Aorta
  Inferior phrenic artery
  Lumbar artery
  Median sacral artery
  Middle suprarenal artery
  Ovarian artery
  Testicular artery
1 Celiac Artery
  Celiac trunk
2 Gastric Artery
  Left gastric artery
  Right gastric artery
3 Hepatic Artery
  Common hepatic artery
  Gastroduodenal artery
  Hepatic artery proper
4 Splenic Artery
  Left gastroepiploic artery
  Pancreatic artery
  Short gastric artery
5 Superior Mesenteric Artery
  Ileal artery
  Ileocolic artery
  Inferior pancreaticoduodenal
    artery
  Jejunal artery
6 Colic Artery, Right
7 Colic Artery, Left
8 Colic Artery, Middle
9 Renal Artery, Right
  Inferior suprarenal artery
  Renal segmental artery
A Renal Artery, Left
  See 9 Renal Artery, Right
B Inferior Mesenteric Artery
  Sigmoid artery
  Superior rectal artery
C Common Iliac Artery, Right
D Common Iliac Artery, Left
E Internal Iliac Artery, Right
  Deferential artery
  Hypogastric artery
  Iliolumbar artery
  Inferior gluteal artery
  Inferior vesical artery
  Internal pudendal artery
  Lateral sacral artery
  Middle rectal artery
  Obturator artery
  Superior gluteal artery
  Umbilical artery
  Uterine artery
  Vaginal artery
	F Internal Iliac Artery, Left
	  See E Internal Iliac Artery, Right
	H External Iliac Artery, Right
	  Deep circumflex iliac artery
	  Inferior epigastric artery
	J External Iliac Artery, Left
	  See H External Iliac Artery, Right
	K Femoral Artery, Right
	  Circumflex iliac artery
	  Deep femoral artery
	  Descending genicular artery
	  External pudendal artery
	  Superficial epigastric artery
	L Femoral Artery, Left
	  See K Femoral Artery, Right
	M Popliteal Artery, Right
	  Inferior genicular artery
	  Middle genicular artery
	  Superior genicular artery
	  Sural artery
	N Popliteal Artery, Left
	  See M Popliteal Artery, Right
	P Anterior Tibial Artery, Right
	  Anterior lateral malleolar
	    artery
	  Anterior medial malleolar
	    artery
	  Anterior tibial recurrent artery
	  Dorsalis pedis artery
	  Posterior tibial recurrent artery
	Q Anterior Tibial Artery, Left
	  See P Anterior Tibial Artery,
	    Right
	R Posterior Tibial Artery, Right
	S Posterior Tibial Artery, Left
	T Peroneal Artery, Right
	  Fibular artery
	U Peroneal Artery, Left
	  See T Peroneal Artery, Right
	V Foot Artery, Right
	  Arcuate artery
	  Dorsal metatarsal artery
	  Lateral plantar artery
	  Lateral tarsal artery
	  Medial plantar artery
	W Foot Artery, Left
	  See V Foot Artery, Right
	Y Lower Artery
	  Umbilical artery
		Ø Open
		4 Percutaneous Endoscopic
			7 Autologous Tissue
			  Substitute
			J Synthetic Substitute
			K Nonautologous Tissue
			  Substitute
				Z No Qualifier

🔵 Limited Coverage   🔵 Noncovered   ✚ Combination Member   HAC associated procedure   Combination Only   DRG Non-OR   Non-OR   New/Revised in GREEN

ICD-10-PCS 2019   227

Ø   **Medical and Surgical**
4   **Lower Arteries**
S   **Reposition**   Definition: Moving to its normal location, or other suitable location, all or a portion of a body part

Explanation: The body part is moved to a new location from an abnormal location, or from a normal location where it is not functioning correctly. The body part may or may not be cut out or off to be moved to the new location.

Body Part Character 4	Approach Character 5	Device Character 6	Qualifier Character 7

Ø   **Abdominal Aorta**
   Inferior phrenic artery
   Lumbar artery
   Median sacral artery
   Middle suprarenal artery
   Ovarian artery
   Testicular artery
1   **Celiac Artery**
   Celiac trunk
2   **Gastric Artery**
   Left gastric artery
   Right gastric artery
3   **Hepatic Artery**
   Common hepatic artery
   Gastroduodenal artery
   Hepatic artery proper
4   **Splenic Artery**
   Left gastroepiploic artery
   Pancreatic artery
   Short gastric artery
5   **Superior Mesenteric Artery**
   Ileal artery
   Ileocolic artery
   Inferior pancreaticoduodenal
      artery
   Jejunal artery
6   **Colic Artery, Right**
7   **Colic Artery, Left**
8   **Colic Artery, Middle**
9   **Renal Artery, Right**
   Inferior suprarenal artery
   Renal segmental artery
A   **Renal Artery, Left**
   See 9 Renal Artery, Right
B   **Inferior Mesenteric Artery**
   Sigmoid artery
   Superior rectal artery
C   **Common Iliac Artery, Right**
D   **Common Iliac Artery, Left**
E   **Internal Iliac Artery, Right**
   Deferential artery
   Hypogastric artery
   Iliolumbar artery
   Inferior gluteal artery
   Inferior vesical artery
   Internal pudendal artery
   Lateral sacral artery
   Middle rectal artery
   Obturator artery
   Superior gluteal artery
   Umbilical artery
   Uterine artery
   Vaginal artery
	Ø **Open**
	3 **Percutaneous**
	4 **Percutaneous Endoscopic**
		Z **No Device**	**Z** **No Qualifier**

F   **Internal Iliac Artery, Left**
   See E Internal Iliac Artery, Right
H   **External Iliac Artery, Right**
   Deep circumflex iliac artery
   Inferior epigastric artery
J   **External Iliac Artery, Left**
   See H External Iliac Artery, Right
K   **Femoral Artery, Right**
   Circumflex iliac artery
   Deep femoral artery
   Descending genicular artery
   External pudendal artery
   Superficial epigastric artery
L   **Femoral Artery, Left**
   See K Femoral Artery, Right
M   **Popliteal Artery, Right**
   Inferior genicular artery
   Middle genicular artery
   Superior genicular artery
   Sural artery
N   **Popliteal Artery, Left**
   See M Popliteal Artery, Right
P   **Anterior Tibial Artery, Right**
   Anterior lateral malleolar
      artery
   Anterior medial malleolar
      artery
   Anterior tibial recurrent artery
   Dorsalis pedis artery
   Posterior tibial recurrent artery
Q   **Anterior Tibial Artery, Left**
   See P Anterior Tibial Artery,
    Right
R   **Posterior Tibial Artery, Right**
S   **Posterior Tibial Artery, Left**
T   **Peroneal Artery, Right**
   Fibular artery
U   **Peroneal Artery, Left**
   See T Peroneal Artery, Right
V   **Foot Artery, Right**
   Arcuate artery
   Dorsal metatarsal artery
   Lateral plantar artery
   Lateral tarsal artery
   Medial plantar artery
W   **Foot Artery, Left**
   See V Foot Artery, Right
Y   **Lower Artery**
   Umbilical artery			

LC Limited Coverage   **NC** Noncovered   ⊞ Combination Member   HAC associated procedure   Combination Only   DRG Non-OR   Non-OR   New/Revised in GREEN

228   ICD-10-PCS 2019

0   **Medical and Surgical**
4   **Lower Arteries**
U   **Supplement**   Definition: Putting in or on biological or synthetic material that physically reinforces and/or augments the function of a portion of a body part
                   Explanation: The biological material is non-living, or is living and from the same individual. The body part may have been previously replaced, and the SUPPLEMENT procedure is performed to physically reinforce and/or augment the function of the replaced body part.

Body Part Character 4		Approach Character 5	Device Character 6	Qualifier Character 7

0 Abdominal Aorta
   Inferior phrenic artery
   Lumbar artery
   Median sacral artery
   Middle suprarenal artery
   Ovarian artery
   Testicular artery
1 Celiac Artery
   Celiac trunk
2 Gastric Artery
   Left gastric artery
   Right gastric artery
3 Hepatic Artery
   Common hepatic artery
   Gastroduodenal artery
   Hepatic artery proper
4 Splenic Artery
   Left gastroepiploic artery
   Pancreatic artery
   Short gastric artery
5 Superior Mesenteric Artery
   Ileal artery
   Ileocolic artery
   Inferior pancreaticoduodenal
     artery
   Jejunal artery
6 Colic Artery, Right
7 Colic Artery, Left
8 Colic Artery, Middle
9 Renal Artery, Right
   Inferior suprarenal artery
   Renal segmental artery
A Renal Artery, Left
   See 9 Renal Artery, Right
B Inferior Mesenteric Artery
   Sigmoid artery
   Superior rectal artery
C Common Iliac Artery, Right
D Common Iliac Artery, Left
E Internal Iliac Artery, Right
   Deferential artery
   Hypogastric artery
   Iliolumbar artery
   Inferior gluteal artery
   Inferior vesical artery
   Internal pudendal artery
   Lateral sacral artery
   Middle rectal artery
   Obturator artery
   Superior gluteal artery
   Umbilical artery
   Uterine artery
   Vaginal artery
	F Internal Iliac Artery, Left
	   See E Internal Iliac Artery, Right
	H External Iliac Artery, Right
	   Deep circumflex iliac artery
	   Inferior epigastric artery
	J External Iliac Artery, Left
	   See H External Iliac Artery, Right
	K Femoral Artery, Right
	   Circumflex iliac artery
	   Deep femoral artery
	   Descending genicular artery
	   External pudendal artery
	   Superficial epigastric artery
	L Femoral Artery, Left
	   See K Femoral Artery, Right
	M Popliteal Artery, Right
	   Inferior genicular artery
	   Middle genicular artery
	   Superior genicular artery
	   Sural artery
	N Popliteal Artery, Left
	   See M Popliteal Artery, Right
	P Anterior Tibial Artery, Right
	   Anterior lateral malleolar
	     artery
	   Anterior medial malleolar
	     artery
	   Anterior tibial recurrent artery
	   Dorsalis pedis artery
	   Posterior tibial recurrent artery
	Q Anterior Tibial Artery, Left
	   See P Anterior Tibial Artery,
	     Right
	R Posterior Tibial Artery, Right
	S Posterior Tibial Artery, Left
	T Peroneal Artery, Right
	   Fibular artery
	U Peroneal Artery, Left
	   See T Peroneal Artery, Right
	V Foot Artery, Right
	   Arcuate artery
	   Dorsal metatarsal artery
	   Lateral plantar artery
	   Lateral tarsal artery
	   Medial plantar artery
	W Foot Artery, Left
	   See V Foot Artery, Right
	Y Lower Artery
	   Umbilical artery
		0 Open
		3 Percutaneous
		4 Percutaneous Endoscopic
			7 Autologous Tissue
			   Substitute
			J Synthetic Substitute
			K Nonautologous Tissue
			   Substitute
				Z No Qualifier

LC Limited Coverage   NC Noncovered   ⊞ Combination Member   HAC associated procedure   Combination Only   DRG Non-OR   Non-OR   New/Revised in GREEN

ICD-10-PCS 2019   229

04U–04U

Lower Arteries

0   **Medical and Surgical**
4   **Lower Arteries**
V   **Restriction**   Definition: Partially closing an orifice or the lumen of a tubular body part
                         Explanation: The orifice can be a natural orifice or an artificially created orifice

Body Part Character 4		Approach Character 5	Device Character 6	Qualifier Character 7

0 **Abdominal Aorta**
   Inferior phrenic artery
   Lumbar artery
   Median sacral artery
   Middle suprarenal artery
   Ovarian artery
   Testicular artery
		0 Open
		3 Percutaneous
		4 Percutaneous Endoscopic
			C Extraluminal Device
			E Intraluminal Device, Branched or Fenestrated, One or Two Arteries
			F Intraluminal Device, Branched or Fenestrated, Three or More Arteries
			Z No Device
				6 Bifurcation
				Z No Qualifier

0 **Abdominal Aorta**
   Inferior phrenic artery
   Lumbar artery
   Median sacral artery
   Middle suprarenal artery
   Ovarian artery
   Testicular artery
		0 Open
		3 Percutaneous
		4 Percutaneous Endoscopic
			D Intraluminal Device	**6** Bifurcation
				J Temporary
				Z No Qualifier

1 **Celiac Artery**
   Celiac trunk
2 **Gastric Artery**
   Left gastric artery
   Right gastric artery
3 **Hepatic Artery**
   Common hepatic artery
   Gastroduodenal artery
   Hepatic artery proper
4 **Splenic Artery**
   Left gastroepiploic artery
   Pancreatic artery
   Short gastric artery
5 **Superior Mesenteric Artery**
   Ileal artery
   Ileocolic artery
   Inferior pancreaticoduodenal artery
   Jejunal artery
6 **Colic Artery, Right**
7 **Colic Artery, Left**
8 **Colic Artery, Middle**
9 **Renal Artery, Right**
   Inferior suprarenal artery
   Renal segmental artery
A **Renal Artery, Left**
   See 9 Renal Artery, Right
B **Inferior Mesenteric Artery**
   Sigmoid artery
   Superior rectal artery
E **Internal Iliac Artery, Right**
   Deferential artery
   Hypogastric artery
   Iliolumbar artery
   Inferior gluteal artery
   Inferior vesical artery
   Internal pudendal artery
   Lateral sacral artery
   Middle rectal artery
   Obturator artery
   Superior gluteal artery
   Umbilical artery
   Uterine artery
   Vaginal artery
F **Internal Iliac Artery, Left**
   See E Internal Iliac Artery, Right
	H **External Iliac Artery, Right**
	   Deep circumflex iliac artery
	   Inferior epigastric artery
	J **External Iliac Artery, Left**
	   See H External Iliac Artery, Right
	K **Femoral Artery, Right**
	   Circumflex iliac artery
	   Deep femoral artery
	   Descending genicular artery
	   External pudendal artery
	   Superficial epigastric artery
	L **Femoral Artery, Left**
	   See K Femoral Artery, Right
	M **Popliteal Artery, Right**
	   Inferior genicular artery
	   Middle genicular artery
	   Superior genicular artery
	   Sural artery
	N **Popliteal Artery, Left**
	   See M Popliteal Artery, Right
	P **Anterior Tibial Artery, Right**
	   Anterior lateral malleolar artery
	   Anterior medial malleolar artery
	   Anterior tibial recurrent artery
	   Dorsalis pedis artery
	   Posterior tibial recurrent artery
	Q **Anterior Tibial Artery, Left**
	   See P Anterior Tibial Artery, Right
	R **Posterior Tibial Artery, Right**
	S **Posterior Tibial Artery, Left**
	T **Peroneal Artery, Right**
	   Fibular artery
	U **Peroneal Artery, Left**
	   See T Peroneal Artery, Right
	V **Foot Artery, Right**
	   Arcuate artery
	   Dorsal metatarsal artery
	   Lateral plantar artery
	   Lateral tarsal artery
	   Medial plantar artery
	W **Foot Artery, Left**
	   See V Foot Artery, Right
	Y **Lower Artery**
	   Umbilical artery
		0 Open
		3 Percutaneous
		4 Percutaneous Endoscopic
			C Extraluminal Device
			D Intraluminal Device
			Z No Device
				Z No Qualifier

C **Common Iliac Artery, Right** **D** **Common Iliac Artery, Left**		**0** Open **3** Percutaneous **4** Percutaneous Endoscopic	**C** Extraluminal Device **D** Intraluminal Device **E** Intraluminal Device, Branched or Fenestrated, One or Two Arteries **Z** No Device	**Z** No Qualifier

LC Limited Coverage   NC Noncovered   ⊞ Combination Member   HAC associated procedure   Combination Only   DRG Non-OR   Non-OR   New/Revised in GREEN

230   ICD-10-PCS 2019

0   **Medical and Surgical**
4   **Lower Arteries**
W   **Revision**   Definition: Correcting, to the extent possible, a portion of a malfunctioning device or the position of a displaced device

Explanation: Revision can include correcting a malfunctioning or displaced device by taking out or putting in components of the device such as a screw or pin

Body Part Character 4	Approach Character 5	Device Character 6	Qualifier Character 7
Y **Lower Artery** Umbilical artery	**0** Open **3** Percutaneous **4** Percutaneous Endoscopic	**0** Drainage Device **2** Monitoring Device **3** Infusion Device **7** Autologous Tissue Substitute **C** Extraluminal Device **D** Intraluminal Device **J** Synthetic Substitute **K** Nonautologous Tissue Substitute **Y** Other Device	**Z** No Qualifier
Y **Lower Artery** Umbilical artery	**X** External	**0** Drainage Device **2** Monitoring Device **3** Infusion Device **7** Autologous Tissue Substitute **C** Extraluminal Device **D** Intraluminal Device **J** Synthetic Substitute **K** Nonautologous Tissue Substitute	**Z** No Qualifier

Non-OR   04WY3[0,2,3,D]Z
Non-OR   04WY[3,4]YZ
Non-OR   04WYX[0,2,3,7,C,D,J,K]Z

LC Limited Coverage **NC** Noncovered ⊞ Combination Member HAC associated procedure Combination Only DRG Non-OR Non-OR New/Revised in GREEN

Upper Veins Ø51–Ø5W

Character Meanings

This Character Meaning table is provided as a guide to assist the user in the identification of character members that may be found in this section of code tables. It **SHOULD NOT** be used to build a PCS code.

Operation–Character 3		Body Part–Character 4		Approach–Character 5		Device–Character 6		Qualifier–Character 7	
1	Bypass	Ø	Azygos Vein	Ø	Open	Ø	Drainage Device	1	Drug-Coated Balloon
5	Destruction	1	Hemiazygos Vein	3	Percutaneous	2	Monitoring Device	X	Diagnostic
7	Dilation	3	Innominate Vein, Right	4	Percutaneous Endoscopic	3	Infusion Device	Y	Upper Vein
9	Drainage	4	Innominate Vein, Left	X	External	7	Autologous Tissue Substitute	Z	No Qualifier
B	Excision	5	Subclavian Vein, Right			9	Autologous Venous Tissue		
C	Extirpation	6	Subclavian Vein, Left			A	Autologous Arterial Tissue		
D	Extraction	7	Axillary Vein, Right			C	Extraluminal Device		
H	Insertion	8	Axillary Vein, Left			D	Intraluminal Device		
J	Inspection	9	Brachial Vein, Right			J	Synthetic Substitute		
L	Occlusion	A	Brachial Vein, Left			K	Nonautologous Tissue Substitute		
N	Release	B	Basilic Vein, Right			M	Neurostimulator Lead		
P	Removal	C	Basilic Vein, Left			Y	Other Device		
Q	Repair	D	Cephalic Vein, Right			Z	No Device		
R	Replacement	F	Cephalic Vein, Left						
S	Reposition	G	Hand Vein, Right						
U	Supplement	H	Hand Vein, Left						
V	Restriction	L	Intracranial Vein						
W	Revision	M	Internal Jugular Vein, Right						
		N	Internal Jugular Vein, Left						
		P	External Jugular Vein, Right						
		Q	External Jugular Vein, Left						
		R	Vertebral Vein, Right						
		S	Vertebral Vein, Left						
		T	Face Vein, Right						
		V	Face Vein, Left						
		Y	Upper Vein						

AHA Coding Clinic for table Ø51
2017, 3Q, 15   Bypass of innominate vein to atrial appendage

AHA Coding Clinic for table Ø5B
2016, 2Q, 12   Resection of malignant neoplasm of infratemporal fossa

AHA Coding Clinic for table Ø5H
2016, 4Q, 97-98   Phrenic neurostimulator

AHA Coding Clinic for table Ø5P
2016, 4Q, 97-98   Phrenic neurostimulator

AHA Coding Clinic for table Ø5Q
2017, 3Q, 15   Bypass of innominate vein to atrial appendage

AHA Coding Clinic for table Ø5S
2013, 4Q, 125   Stage II cephalic vein transposition (superficialization) of arteriovenous fistula

AHA Coding Clinic for table Ø5W
2016, 4Q, 97-98   Phrenic neurostimulator

Head and Neck Veins

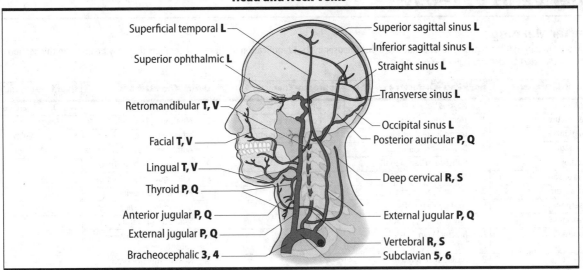

Superficial temporal **L**
Superior ophthalmic **L**
Retromandibular **T, V**
Facial **T, V**
Lingual **T, V**
Thyroid **P, Q**
Anterior jugular **P, Q**
External jugular **P, Q**
Bracheocephalic **3, 4**

Superior sagittal sinus **L**
Inferior sagittal sinus **L**
Straight sinus **L**
Transverse sinus **L**
Occipital sinus **L**
Posterior auricular **P, Q**
Deep cervical **R, S**
External jugular **P, Q**
Vertebral **R, S**
Subclavian **5, 6**

Upper Veins

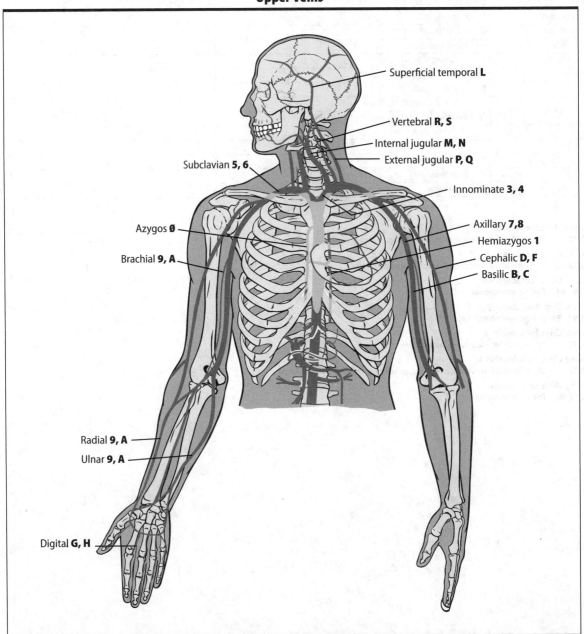

Superficial temporal **L**
Vertebral **R, S**
Internal jugular **M, N**
External jugular **P, Q**
Subclavian **5, 6**
Innominate **3, 4**
Azygos **Ø**
Axillary **7,8**
Hemiazygos **1**
Brachial **9, A**
Cephalic **D, F**
Basilic **B, C**
Radial **9, A**
Ulnar **9, A**
Digital **G, H**

Ø   **Medical and Surgical**
5   **Upper Veins**
1   **Bypass**   Definition: Altering the route of passage of the contents of a tubular body part

                     Explanation: Rerouting contents of a body part to a downstream area of the normal route, to a similar route and body part, or to an abnormal route and dissimilar body part. Includes one or more anastomoses, with or without the use of a device.

Body Part Character 4		Approach Character 5	Device Character 6	Qualifier Character 7
Ø Azygos Vein Right ascending lumbar vein Right subcostal vein **1** Hemiazygos Vein Left ascending lumbar vein Left subcostal vein **3** Innominate Vein, Right Brachiocephalic vein Inferior thyroid vein **4** Innominate Vein, Left *See 3 Innominate Vein, Right* **5** Subclavian Vein, Right **6** Subclavian Vein, Left **7** Axillary Vein, Right **8** Axillary Vein, Left **9** Brachial Vein, Right Radial vein Ulnar vein **A** Brachial Vein, Left *See 9 Brachial Vein, Right* **B** Basilic Vein, Right Median antebrachial vein Median cubital vein **C** Basilic Vein, Left *See B Basilic Vein, Right* **D** Cephalic Vein, Right Accessory cephalic vein **F** Cephalic Vein, Left *See D Cephalic Vein, Right* **G** Hand Vein, Right Dorsal metacarpal vein Palmar (volar) digital vein Palmar (volar) metacarpal vein Superficial palmar venous arch Volar (palmar) digital vein Volar (palmar) metacarpal vein	**H** Hand Vein, Left *See G Hand Vein, Right* **L** Intracranial Vein Anterior cerebral vein Basal (internal) cerebral vein Dural venous sinus Great cerebral vein Inferior cerebellar vein Inferior cerebral vein Internal (basal) cerebral vein Middle cerebral vein Ophthalmic vein Superior cerebellar vein Superior cerebral vein **M** Internal Jugular Vein, Right **N** Internal Jugular Vein, Left **P** External Jugular Vein, Right Posterior auricular vein **Q** External Jugular Vein, Left *See P External Jugular Vein, Right* **R** Vertebral Vein, Right Deep cervical vein Suboccipital venous plexus **S** Vertebral Vein, Left *See R Vertebral Vein, Right* **T** Face Vein, Right Angular vein Anterior facial vein Common facial vein Deep facial vein Frontal vein Posterior facial (retromandibular) vein Supraorbital vein **V** Face Vein, Left *See T Face Vein, Right*	**Ø** Open **4** Percutaneous Endoscopic	**7** Autologous Tissue Substitute **9** Autologous Venous Tissue **A** Autologous Arterial Tissue **J** Synthetic Substitute **K** Nonautologous Tissue Substitute **Z** No Device	**Y** Upper Vein

LC Limited Coverage   NC Noncovered   ⊞ Combination Member   HAC associated procedure   Combination Only   DRG Non-OR   Non-OR   New/Revised in GREEN

ICD-10-PCS 2019   235

Ø51–Ø51

Ø   Medical and Surgical
5   Upper Veins
5   Destruction   Definition: Physical eradication of all or a portion of a body part by the direct use of energy, force, or a destructive agent
                 Explanation: None of the body part is physically taken out

Body Part Character 4		Approach Character 5	Device Character 6	Qualifier Character 7

Ø Azygos Vein
  Right ascending lumbar vein
  Right subcostal vein
1 Hemiazygos Vein
  Left ascending lumbar vein
  Left subcostal vein
3 Innominate Vein, Right
  Brachiocephalic vein
  Inferior thyroid vein
4 Innominate Vein, Left
  See 3 Innominate Vein, Right
5 Subclavian Vein, Right
6 Subclavian Vein, Left
7 Axillary Vein, Right
8 Axillary Vein, Left
9 Brachial Vein, Right
  Radial vein
  Ulnar vein
A Brachial Vein, Left
  See 9 Brachial Vein, Right
B Basilic Vein, Right
  Median antebrachial vein
  Median cubital vein
C Basilic Vein, Left
  See B Basilic Vein, Right
D Cephalic Vein, Right
  Accessory cephalic vein
F Cephalic Vein, Left
  See D Cephalic Vein, Right
G Hand Vein, Right
  Dorsal metacarpal vein
  Palmar (volar) digital vein
  Palmar (volar) metacarpal vein
  Superficial palmar venous arch
  Volar (palmar) digital vein
  Volar (palmar) metacarpal vein
	H Hand Vein, Left
	  See G Hand Vein, Right
	L Intracranial Vein
	  Anterior cerebral vein
	  Basal (internal) cerebral vein
	  Dural venous sinus
	  Great cerebral vein
	  Inferior cerebellar vein
	  Inferior cerebral vein
	  Internal (basal) cerebral vein
	  Middle cerebral vein
	  Ophthalmic vein
	  Superior cerebellar vein
	  Superior cerebral vein
	M Internal Jugular Vein, Right
	N Internal Jugular Vein, Left
	P External Jugular Vein, Right
	  Posterior auricular vein
	Q External Jugular Vein, Left
	  See P External Jugular Vein,
	    Right
	R Vertebral Vein, Right
	  Deep cervical vein
	  Suboccipital venous plexus
	S Vertebral Vein, Left
	  See R Vertebral Vein, Right
	T Face Vein, Right
	  Angular vein
	  Anterior facial vein
	  Common facial vein
	  Deep facial vein
	  Frontal vein
	  Posterior facial
	    (retromandibular) vein
	  Supraorbital vein
	V Face Vein, Left
	  See T Face Vein, Right
	Y Upper Vein
		Ø Open
		3 Percutaneous
		4 Percutaneous Endoscopic
			Z No Device	**Z No Qualifier**

LC Limited Coverage   NC Noncovered   ⊞ Combination Member   HAC associated procedure   Combination Only   DRG Non-OR   Non-OR   New/Revised in GREEN

236   ICD-10-PCS 2019

Ø   **Medical and Surgical**
5   **Upper Veins**
7   **Dilation**   Definition: Expanding an orifice or the lumen of a tubular body part

Explanation: The orifice can be a natural orifice or an artificially created orifice. Accomplished by stretching a tubular body part using intraluminal pressure or by cutting part of the orifice or wall of the tubular body part.

Body Part Character 4		Approach Character 5	Device Character 6	Qualifier Character 7

Ø **Azygos Vein**
  Right ascending lumbar vein
  Right subcostal vein
1 **Hemiazygos Vein**
  Left ascending lumbar vein
  Left subcostal vein
G **Hand Vein, Right**
  Dorsal metacarpal vein
  Palmar (volar) digital vein
  Palmar (volar) metacarpal vein
  Superficial palmar venous arch
  Volar (palmar) digital vein
  Volar (palmar) metacarpal vein
H **Hand Vein, Left**
  See G Hand Vein, Right
L **Intracranial Vein** NC
  Anterior cerebral vein
  Basal (internal) cerebral vein
  Dural venous sinus
  Great cerebral vein
  Inferior cerebellar vein
  Inferior cerebral vein
  Internal (basal) cerebral vein
  Middle cerebral vein
  Ophthalmic vein
  Superior cerebellar vein
  Superior cerebral vein
	M **Internal Jugular Vein, Right**
	N **Internal Jugular Vein, Left**
	P **External Jugular Vein, Right**
	  Posterior auricular vein
	Q **External Jugular Vein, Left**
	  See P External Jugular Vein,
	    Right
	R **Vertebral Vein, Right**
	  Deep cervical vein
	  Suboccipital venous plexus
	S **Vertebral Vein, Left**
	  See R Vertebral Vein, Right
	T **Face Vein, Right**
	  Angular vein
	  Anterior facial vein
	  Common facial vein
	  Deep facial vein
	  Frontal vein
	  Posterior facial
	    (retromandibular) vein
	  Supraorbital vein
	V **Face Vein, Left**
	  See T Face Vein, Right
	Y **Upper Vein**
		Ø Open
		3 Percutaneous
		4 Percutaneous Endoscopic
			D Intraluminal Device
			Z No Device
				Z No Qualifier

3 **Innominate Vein, Right**
  Brachiocephalic vein
  Inferior thyroid vein
4 **Innominate Vein, Left**
  See 3 Innominate Vein, Right
5 **Subclavian Vein, Right**
6 **Subclavian Vein, Left**
7 **Axillary Vein, Right**
8 **Axillary Vein, Left**
9 **Brachial Vein, Right**
  Radial vein
  Ulnar vein
	A **Brachial Vein, Left**
	  See 9 Brachial Vein, Right
	B **Basilic Vein, Right**
	  Median antebrachial vein
	  Median cubital vein
	C **Basilic Vein, Left**
	  See B Basilic Vein, Right
	D **Cephalic Vein, Right**
	  Accessory cephalic vein
	F **Cephalic Vein, Left**
	  See D Cephalic Vein, Right
		Ø Open
		3 Percutaneous
		4 Percutaneous Endoscopic
			D Intraluminal Device
			Z No Device
				1 Drug-Coated Balloon
				Z No Qualifier

NC   Ø57L[3,4]ZZ

LC Limited Coverage   NC Noncovered   ⊞ Combination Member   HAC associated procedure   Combination Only   DRG Non-OR   Non-OR   New/Revised in GREEN
ICD-10-PCS 2019   237

Ø57–Ø57

Ø   Medical and Surgical
5   Upper Veins
9   Drainage   Definition: Taking or letting out fluids and/or gases from a body part
                   Explanation: The qualifier DIAGNOSTIC is used to identify drainage procedures that are biopsies

Body Part Character 4		Approach Character 5	Device Character 6	Qualifier Character 7

Ø Azygos Vein
   Right ascending lumbar vein
   Right subcostal vein
1 Hemiazygos Vein
   Left ascending lumbar vein
   Left subcostal vein
3 Innominate Vein, Right
   Brachiocephalic vein
   Inferior thyroid vein
4 Innominate Vein, Left
   See 3 Innominate Vein, Right
5 Subclavian Vein, Right
6 Subclavian Vein, Left
7 Axillary Vein, Right
8 Axillary Vein, Left
9 Brachial Vein, Right
   Radial vein
   Ulnar vein
A Brachial Vein, Left
   See 9 Brachial Vein, Right
B Basilic Vein, Right
   Median antebrachial vein
   Median cubital vein
C Basilic Vein, Left
   See B Basilic Vein, Right
D Cephalic Vein, Right
   Accessory cephalic vein
F Cephalic Vein, Left
   See D Cephalic Vein, Right
G Hand Vein, Right
   Dorsal metacarpal vein
   Palmar (volar) digital vein
   Palmar (volar) metacarpal vein
   Superficial palmar venous arch
   Volar (palmar) digital vein
   Volar (palmar) metacarpal vein
	H Hand Vein, Left
	   See G Hand Vein, Right
	L Intracranial Vein
	   Anterior cerebral vein
	   Basal (internal) cerebral vein
	   Dural venous sinus
	   Great cerebral vein
	   Inferior cerebellar vein
	   Inferior cerebral vein
	   Internal (basal) cerebral vein
	   Middle cerebral vein
	   Ophthalmic vein
	   Superior cerebellar vein
	   Superior cerebral vein
	M Internal Jugular Vein, Right
	N Internal Jugular Vein, Left
	P External Jugular Vein, Right
	   Posterior auricular vein
	Q External Jugular Vein, Left
	   See P External Jugular Vein, Right
	R Vertebral Vein, Right
	   Deep cervical vein
	   Suboccipital venous plexus
	S Vertebral Vein, Left
	   See R Vertebral Vein, Right
	T Face Vein, Right
	   Angular vein
	   Anterior facial vein
	   Common facial vein
	   Deep facial vein
	   Frontal vein
	   Posterior facial
	     (retromandibular) vein
	   Supraorbital vein
	V Face Vein, Left
	   See T Face Vein, Right
	Y Upper Vein
		Ø Open
		3 Percutaneous
		4 Percutaneous Endoscopic
			Ø Drainage Device	Z No Qualifier

Ø Azygos Vein
   Right ascending lumbar vein
   Right subcostal vein
1 Hemiazygos Vein
   Left ascending lumbar vein
   Left subcostal vein
3 Innominate Vein, Right
   Brachiocephalic vein
   Inferior thyroid vein
4 Innominate Vein, Left
   See 3 Innominate Vein, Right
5 Subclavian Vein, Right
6 Subclavian Vein, Left
7 Axillary Vein, Right
8 Axillary Vein, Left
9 Brachial Vein, Right
   Radial vein
   Ulnar vein
A Brachial Vein, Left
   See 9 Brachial Vein, Right
B Basilic Vein, Right
   Median antebrachial vein
   Median cubital vein
C Basilic Vein, Left
   See B Basilic Vein, Right
D Cephalic Vein, Right
   Accessory cephalic vein
F Cephalic Vein, Left
   See D Cephalic Vein, Right
G Hand Vein, Right
   Dorsal metacarpal vein
   Palmar (volar) digital vein
   Palmar (volar) metacarpal vein
   Superficial palmar venous arch
   Volar (palmar) digital vein
   Volar (palmar) metacarpal vein
	H Hand Vein, Left
	   See G Hand Vein, Right
	L Intracranial Vein
	   Anterior cerebral vein
	   Basal (internal) cerebral vein
	   Dural venous sinus
	   Great cerebral vein
	   Inferior cerebellar vein
	   Inferior cerebral vein
	   Internal (basal) cerebral vein
	   Middle cerebral vein
	   Ophthalmic vein
	   Superior cerebellar vein
	   Superior cerebral vein
	M Internal Jugular Vein, Right
	N Internal Jugular Vein, Left
	P External Jugular Vein, Right
	   Posterior auricular vein
	Q External Jugular Vein, Left
	   See P External Jugular Vein, Right
	R Vertebral Vein, Right
	   Deep cervical vein
	   Suboccipital venous plexus
	S Vertebral Vein, Left
	   See R Vertebral Vein, Right
	T Face Vein, Right
	   Angular vein
	   Anterior facial vein
	   Common facial vein
	   Deep facial vein
	   Frontal vein
	   Posterior facial
	     (retromandibular) vein
	   Supraorbital vein
	V Face Vein, Left
	   See T Face Vein, Right
	Y Upper Vein
		Ø Open
		3 Percutaneous
		4 Percutaneous Endoscopic
			Z No Device	X Diagnostic
				Z No Qualifier

Non-OR   Ø59[Ø,1,3,4,5,6,7,8,9,A,B,C,D,F,G,H,L,M,N,P,Q,R,S,T,V,Y][Ø,3,4]ØZ
Non-OR   Ø59[Ø,1,3,4,5,6,7,8,9,A,B,C,D,F,G,H,L,M,N,P,Q,R,S,T,V,Y]3ZX
Non-OR   Ø59[Ø,1,3,4,5,6,7,8,9,A,B,C,D,F,G,H,L,M,N,P,Q,R,S,T,V,Y][Ø,3,4]ZZ

LC Limited Coverage   NC Noncovered   ⊞ Combination Member   HAC associated procedure   Combination Only   DRG Non-OR   Non-OR   New/Revised in GREEN

238   ICD-10-PCS 2019

0   Medical and Surgical
5   Upper Veins
B   Excision   Definition: Cutting out or off, without replacement, a portion of a body part

                    Explanation: The qualifier DIAGNOSTIC is used to identify excision procedures that are biopsies

Body Part Character 4		Approach Character 5	Device Character 6	Qualifier Character 7
0 Azygos Vein Right ascending lumbar vein Right subcostal vein **1 Hemiazygos Vein** Left ascending lumbar vein Left subcostal vein **3 Innominate Vein, Right** Brachiocephalic vein Inferior thyroid vein **4 Innominate Vein, Left** *See 3 Innominate Vein, Right* **5 Subclavian Vein, Right** **6 Subclavian Vein, Left** **7 Axillary Vein, Right** **8 Axillary Vein, Left** **9 Brachial Vein, Right** Radial vein Ulnar vein **A Brachial Vein, Left** *See 9 Brachial Vein, Right* **B Basilic Vein, Right** Median antebrachial vein Median cubital vein **C Basilic Vein, Left** *See B Basilic Vein, Right* **D Cephalic Vein, Right** Accessory cephalic vein **F Cephalic Vein, Left** *See D Cephalic Vein, Right* **G Hand Vein, Right** Dorsal metacarpal vein Palmar (volar) digital vein Palmar (volar) metacarpal vein Superficial palmar venous arch Volar (palmar) digital vein Volar (palmar) metacarpal vein	**H Hand Vein, Left** *See G Hand Vein, Right* **L Intracranial Vein** Anterior cerebral vein Basal (internal) cerebral vein Dural venous sinus Great cerebral vein Inferior cerebellar vein Inferior cerebral vein Internal (basal) cerebral vein Middle cerebral vein Ophthalmic vein Superior cerebellar vein Superior cerebral vein **M Internal Jugular Vein, Right** **N Internal Jugular Vein, Left** **P External Jugular Vein, Right** Posterior auricular vein **Q External Jugular Vein, Left** *See P External Jugular Vein, Right* **R Vertebral Vein, Right** Deep cervical vein Suboccipital venous plexus **S Vertebral Vein, Left** *See R Vertebral Vein, Right* **T Face Vein, Right** Angular vein Anterior facial vein Common facial vein Deep facial vein Frontal vein Posterior facial (retromandibular) vein Supraorbital vein **V Face Vein, Left** *See T Face Vein, Right* **Y Upper Vein**	**0 Open** **3 Percutaneous** **4 Percutaneous Endoscopic**	**Z No Device**	**X Diagnostic** **Z No Qualifier**

0 Medical and Surgical
5 Upper Veins
C Extirpation

Definition: Taking or cutting out solid matter from a body part

Explanation: The solid matter may be an abnormal byproduct of a biological function or a foreign body; it may be imbedded in a body part or in the lumen of a tubular body part. The solid matter may or may not have been previously broken into pieces.

Body Part — Character 4	Approach — Character 5	Device — Character 6	Qualifier — Character 7

0 Azygos Vein
  Right ascending lumbar vein
  Right subcostal vein
1 Hemiazygos Vein
  Left ascending lumbar vein
  Left subcostal vein
3 Innominate Vein, Right
  Brachiocephalic vein
  Inferior thyroid vein
4 Innominate Vein, Left
  See 3 Innominate Vein, Right
5 Subclavian Vein, Right
6 Subclavian Vein, Left
7 Axillary Vein, Right
8 Axillary Vein, Left
9 Brachial Vein, Right
  Radial vein
  Ulnar vein
A Brachial Vein, Left
  See 9 Brachial Vein, Right
B Basilic Vein, Right
  Median antebrachial vein
  Median cubital vein
C Basilic Vein, Left
  See B Basilic Vein, Right
D Cephalic Vein, Right
  Accessory cephalic vein
F Cephalic Vein, Left
  See D Cephalic Vein, Right
G Hand Vein, Right
  Dorsal metacarpal vein
  Palmar (volar) digital vein
  Palmar (volar) metacarpal vein
  Superficial palmar venous arch
  Volar (palmar) digital vein
  Volar (palmar) metacarpal vein
H Hand Vein, Left
  See G Hand Vein, Right
L Intracranial Vein
  Anterior cerebral vein
  Basal (internal) cerebral vein
  Dural venous sinus
  Great cerebral vein
  Inferior cerebellar vein
  Inferior cerebral vein
  Internal (basal) cerebral vein
  Middle cerebral vein
  Ophthalmic vein
  Superior cerebellar vein
  Superior cerebral vein
M Internal Jugular Vein, Right
N Internal Jugular Vein, Left
P External Jugular Vein, Right
  Posterior auricular vein
Q External Jugular Vein, Left
  See P External Jugular Vein, Right
R Vertebral Vein, Right
  Deep cervical vein
  Suboccipital venous plexus
S Vertebral Vein, Left
  See R Vertebral Vein, Right
T Face Vein, Right
  Angular vein
  Anterior facial vein
  Common facial vein
  Deep facial vein
  Frontal vein
  Posterior facial (retromandibular) vein
  Supraorbital vein
V Face Vein, Left
  See T Face Vein, Right
Y Upper Vein
	0 Open
	3 Percutaneous
	4 Percutaneous Endoscopic
		Z No Device	Z No Qualifier

0 Medical and Surgical
5 Upper Veins
D Extraction

Definition: Pulling or stripping out or off all or a portion of a body part by the use of force

Explanation: The qualifier DIAGNOSTIC is used to identify extraction procedures that are biopsies

Body Part — Character 4	Approach — Character 5	Device — Character 6	Qualifier — Character 7

9 Brachial Vein, Right
  Radial vein
  Ulnar vein
A Brachial Vein, Left
  See 9 Brachial Vein, Right
B Basilic Vein, Right
  Median antebrachial vein
  Median cubital vein
C Basilic Vein, Left
  See B Basilic Vein, Right
D Cephalic Vein, Right
  Accessory cephalic vein
F Cephalic Vein, Left
  See D Cephalic Vein, Right
G Hand Vein, Right
  Dorsal metacarpal vein
  Palmar (volar) digital vein
  Palmar (volar) metacarpal vein
  Superficial palmar venous arch
  Volar (palmar) digital vein
  Volar (palmar) metacarpal vein
H Hand Vein, Left
  See G Hand Vein, Right
Y Upper Vein
	0 Open
	3 Percutaneous
		Z No Device	Z No Qualifier

0   Medical and Surgical
5   Upper Veins
H   Insertion   Definition: Putting in a nonbiological appliance that monitors, assists, performs, or prevents a physiological function but does not physically take the place of a body part
                 Explanation: None

Body Part Character 4		Approach Character 5	Device Character 6	Qualifier Character 7

0   Azygos Vein ⊞
    Right ascending lumbar vein
    Right subcostal vein
		0 Open
		3 Percutaneous
		4 Percutaneous Endoscopic
			2 Monitoring Device
			3 Infusion Device
			D Intraluminal Device
			M Neurostimulator Lead
				Z No Qualifier

1   Hemiazygos Vein
    Left ascending lumbar vein
    Left subcostal vein
5   Subclavian Vein, Right
6   Subclavian Vein, Left
7   Axillary Vein, Right
8   Axillary Vein, Left
9   Brachial Vein, Right
    Radial vein
    Ulnar vein
A   Brachial Vein, Left
    See 9 Brachial Vein, Right
B   Basilic Vein, Right
    Median antebrachial vein
    Median cubital vein
C   Basilic Vein, Left
    See B Basilic Vein, Right
D   Cephalic Vein, Right
    Accessory cephalic vein
F   Cephalic Vein, Left
    See D Cephalic Vein, Right
G   Hand Vein, Right
    Dorsal metacarpal vein
    Palmar (volar) digital vein
    Palmar (volar) metacarpal vein
    Superficial palmar venous arch
    Volar (palmar) digital vein
    Volar (palmar) metacarpal vein
H   Hand Vein, Left
    See G Hand Vein, Right
	L Intracranial Vein
	    Anterior cerebral vein
	    Basal (internal) cerebral vein
	    Dural venous sinus
	    Great cerebral vein
	    Inferior cerebellar vein
	    Inferior cerebral vein
	    Internal (basal) cerebral vein
	    Middle cerebral vein
	    Ophthalmic vein
	    Superior cerebellar vein
	    Superior cerebral vein
	M Internal Jugular Vein, Right
	N Internal Jugular Vein, Left
	P External Jugular Vein, Right
	    Posterior auricular vein
	Q External Jugular Vein, Left
	    See P External Jugular Vein, Right
	R Vertebral Vein, Right
	    Deep cervical vein
	    Suboccipital venous plexus
	S Vertebral Vein, Left
	    See R Vertebral Vein, Right
	T Face Vein, Right
	    Angular vein
	    Anterior facial vein
	    Common facial vein
	    Deep facial vein
	    Frontal vein
	    Posterior facial (retromandibular) vein
	    Supraorbital vein
	V Face Vein, Left
	    See T Face Vein, Right
		0 Open
		3 Percutaneous
		4 Percutaneous Endoscopic
			3 Infusion Device
			D Intraluminal Device
				Z No Qualifier

3   Innominate Vein, Right ⊞
    Brachiocephalic vein
    Inferior thyroid vein
4   Innominate Vein, Left ⊞
    See 3 Innominate Vein, Right
		0 Open
		3 Percutaneous
		4 Percutaneous Endoscopic
			3 Infusion Device
			D Intraluminal Device
			M Neurostimulator Lead
				Z No Qualifier

Y Upper Vein		**0 Open** **3 Percutaneous** **4 Percutaneous Endoscopic**	**2 Monitoring Device** **3 Infusion Device** **D Intraluminal Device** **Y Other Device**	**Z No Qualifier**

Non-OR	05H0[0,3,4]3Z	
Non-OR	05H[1,5,6,7,8,9,A,B,C,D,F,G,H,L,M,N,P,Q,R,S,T,V][0,3,4]3Z	
Non-OR	05H[3,4][0,3,4]3Z	
Non-OR	05HY[0,3,4]3Z	
Non-OR	05HY32Z	
Non-OR	05HY[3,4]YZ	
HAC	05H0[3,4]3Z when reported with SDx J95.811	
HAC	05H[1,5,6][3,4]3Z when reported with SDx J95.811	
HAC	05H[M,N,P,Q]33Z when reported with SDx J95.811	
HAC	05H[3,4][3,4]3Z when reported with SDx J95.811	

See Appendix L for Procedure Combinations
    ⊞   05H0[0,3,4]MZ
    ⊞   05H[3,4][0,3,4]MZ

0   Medical and Surgical
5   Upper Veins
J   Inspection   Definition: Visually and/or manually exploring a body part
                     Explanation: Visual exploration may be performed with or without optical instrumentation. Manual exploration may be performed directly or through intervening body layers.

Body Part Character 4	Approach Character 5	Device Character 6	Qualifier Character 7
Y Upper Vein	**0 Open** **3 Percutaneous** **4 Percutaneous Endoscopic** **X External**	**Z No Device**	**Z No Qualifier**

Non-OR   05JY[3,X]ZZ

⊡ Limited Coverage   ⊠ Noncovered   ⊞ Combination Member   HAC associated procedure   Combination Only   DRG Non-OR   Non-OR   New/Revised in GREEN

Ø   Medical and Surgical
5   Upper Veins
L   Occlusion   Definition: Completely closing an orifice or the lumen of a tubular body part
                      Explanation: The orifice can be a natural orifice or an artificially created orifice

Body Part Character 4		Approach Character 5	Device Character 6	Qualifier Character 7

Ø Azygos Vein
   Right ascending lumbar vein
   Right subcostal vein
1 Hemiazygos Vein
   Left ascending lumbar vein
   Left subcostal vein
3 Innominate Vein, Right
   Brachiocephalic vein
   Inferior thyroid vein
4 Innominate Vein, Left
   See 3 Innominate Vein, Right
5 Subclavian Vein, Right
6 Subclavian Vein, Left
7 Axillary Vein, Right
8 Axillary Vein, Left
9 Brachial Vein, Right
   Radial vein
   Ulnar vein
A Brachial Vein, Left
   See 9 Brachial Vein, Right
B Basilic Vein, Right
   Median antebrachial vein
   Median cubital vein
C Basilic Vein, Left
   See B Basilic Vein, Right
D Cephalic Vein, Right
   Accessory cephalic vein
F Cephalic Vein, Left
   See D Cephalic Vein, Right
G Hand Vein, Right
   Dorsal metacarpal vein
   Palmar (volar) digital vein
   Palmar (volar) metacarpal vein
   Superficial palmar venous arch
   Volar (palmar) digital vein
   Volar (palmar) metacarpal vein
	H Hand Vein, Left
	   See G Hand Vein, Right
	L Intracranial Vein
	   Anterior cerebral vein
	   Basal (internal) cerebral vein
	   Dural venous sinus
	   Great cerebral vein
	   Inferior cerebellar vein
	   Inferior cerebral vein
	   Internal (basal) cerebral vein
	   Middle cerebral vein
	   Ophthalmic vein
	   Superior cerebellar vein
	   Superior cerebral vein
	M Internal Jugular Vein, Right
	N Internal Jugular Vein, Left
	P External Jugular Vein, Right
	   Posterior auricular vein
	Q External Jugular Vein, Left
	   See P External Jugular Vein,
	     Right
	R Vertebral Vein, Right
	   Deep cervical vein
	   Suboccipital venous plexus
	S Vertebral Vein, Left
	   See R Vertebral Vein, Right
	T Face Vein, Right
	   Angular vein
	   Anterior facial vein
	   Common facial vein
	   Deep facial vein
	   Frontal vein
	   Posterior facial
	     (retromandibular) vein
	   Supraorbital vein
	V Face Vein, Left
	   See T Face Vein, Right
	Y Upper Vein
		Ø Open
		3 Percutaneous
		4 Percutaneous Endoscopic
			C Extraluminal Device
			D Intraluminal Device
			Z No Device
				Z No Qualifier

Ø   Medical and Surgical
5   Upper Veins
N   Release   Definition: Freeing a body part from an abnormal physical constraint by cutting or by the use of force
                         Explanation: Some of the restraining tissue may be taken out but none of the body part is taken out

Body Part Character 4		Approach Character 5	Device Character 6	Qualifier Character 7

Ø **Azygos Vein**
  Right ascending lumbar vein
  Right subcostal vein
1 **Hemiazygos Vein**
  Left ascending lumbar vein
  Left subcostal vein
3 **Innominate Vein, Right**
  Brachiocephalic vein
  Inferior thyroid vein
4 **Innominate Vein, Left**
  See 3 Innominate Vein, Right
5 **Subclavian Vein, Right**
6 **Subclavian Vein, Left**
7 **Axillary Vein, Right**
8 **Axillary Vein, Left**
9 **Brachial Vein, Right**
  Radial vein
  Ulnar vein
A **Brachial Vein, Left**
  See 9 Brachial Vein, Right
B **Basilic Vein, Right**
  Median antebrachial vein
  Median cubital vein
C **Basilic Vein, Left**
  See B Basilic Vein, Right
D **Cephalic Vein, Right**
  Accessory cephalic vein
F **Cephalic Vein, Left**
  See D Cephalic Vein, Right
G **Hand Vein, Right**
  Dorsal metacarpal vein
  Palmar (volar) digital vein
  Palmar (volar) metacarpal vein
  Superficial palmar venous arch
  Volar (palmar) digital vein
  Volar (palmar) metacarpal vein
	H **Hand Vein, Left**
	  See G Hand Vein, Right
	L **Intracranial Vein**
	  Anterior cerebral vein
	  Basal (internal) cerebral vein
	  Dural venous sinus
	  Great cerebral vein
	  Inferior cerebellar vein
	  Inferior cerebral vein
	  Internal (basal) cerebral vein
	  Middle cerebral vein
	  Ophthalmic vein
	  Superior cerebellar vein
	  Superior cerebral vein
	M **Internal Jugular Vein, Right**
	N **Internal Jugular Vein, Left**
	P **External Jugular Vein, Right**
	  Posterior auricular vein
	Q **External Jugular Vein, Left**
	  See P External Jugular Vein,
	    Right
	R **Vertebral Vein, Right**
	  Deep cervical vein
	  Suboccipital venous plexus
	S **Vertebral Vein, Left**
	  See R Vertebral Vein, Right
	T **Face Vein, Right**
	  Angular vein
	  Anterior facial vein
	  Common facial vein
	  Deep facial vein
	  Frontal vein
	  Posterior facial
	    (retromandibular) vein
	  Supraorbital vein
	V **Face Vein, Left**
	  See T Face Vein, Right
	Y **Upper Vein**
		Ø Open
		3 Percutaneous
		4 Percutaneous Endoscopic
			Z No Device	**Z** No Qualifier

LC Limited Coverage   NC Noncovered   ⊞ Combination Member   HAC associated procedure   Combination Only   DRG Non-OR   Non-OR   New/Revised in GREEN

Ø   Medical and Surgical
5   Upper Veins
P   Removal   Definition: Taking out or off a device from a body part

Explanation: If a device is taken out and a similar device put in without cutting or puncturing the skin or mucous membrane, the procedure is coded to the root operation CHANGE. Otherwise, the procedure for taking out a device is coded to the root operation REMOVAL.

Body Part Character 4	Approach Character 5	Device Character 6	Qualifier Character 7
Ø Azygos Vein Right ascending lumbar vein Right subcostal vein	**Ø** Open **3** Percutaneous **4** Percutaneous Endoscopic **X** External	**2** Monitoring Device **M** Neurostimulator Lead	**Z** No Qualifier
3 Innominate Vein, Right Brachiocephalic vein Inferior thyroid vein **4 Innominate Vein, Left** *See 3 Innominate Vein, Right*	**Ø** Open **3** Percutaneous **4** Percutaneous Endoscopic **X** External	**M** Neurostimulator Lead	**Z** No Qualifier
Y Upper Vein	**Ø** Open **3** Percutaneous **4** Percutaneous Endoscopic	**Ø** Drainage Device **2** Monitoring Device **3** Infusion Device **7** Autologous Tissue Substitute **C** Extraluminal Device **D** Intraluminal Device **J** Synthetic Substitute **K** Nonautologous Tissue Substitute **Y** Other Device	**Z** No Qualifier
Y Upper Vein	**X** External	**Ø** Drainage Device **2** Monitoring Device **3** Infusion Device **D** Intraluminal Device	**Z** No Qualifier

Non-OR   Ø5PØ[Ø,3,4,X]2Z
Non-OR   Ø5PY3[Ø,2,3]Z
Non-OR   Ø5PY[3,4]YZ
Non-OR   Ø5PYX[Ø,2,3,D]Z

LC Limited Coverage   NC Noncovered   ⊞ Combination Member   HAC associated procedure   Combination Only   DRG Non-OR   Non-OR   New/Revised in GREEN

244   ICD-10-PCS 2019

0   **Medical and Surgical**
5   **Upper Veins**
Q   **Repair**   Definition: Restoring, to the extent possible, a body part to its normal anatomic structure and function

Explanation: Used only when the method to accomplish the repair is not one of the other root operations

Body Part Character 4		Approach Character 5	Device Character 6	Qualifier Character 7

0 **Azygos Vein**
   Right ascending lumbar vein
   Right subcostal vein
1 **Hemiazygos Vein**
   Left ascending lumbar vein
   Left subcostal vein
3 **Innominate Vein, Right**
   Brachiocephalic vein
   Inferior thyroid vein
4 **Innominate Vein, Left**
   See 3 Innominate Vein, Right
5 **Subclavian Vein, Right**
6 **Subclavian Vein, Left**
7 **Axillary Vein, Right**
8 **Axillary Vein, Left**
9 **Brachial Vein, Right**
   Radial vein
   Ulnar vein
A **Brachial Vein, Left**
   See 9 Brachial Vein, Right
B **Basilic Vein, Right**
   Median antebrachial vein
   Median cubital vein
C **Basilic Vein, Left**
   See B Basilic Vein, Right
D **Cephalic Vein, Right**
   Accessory cephalic vein
F **Cephalic Vein, Left**
   See D Cephalic Vein, Right
G **Hand Vein, Right**
   Dorsal metacarpal vein
   Palmar (volar) digital vein
   Palmar (volar) metacarpal vein
   Superficial palmar venous arch
   Volar (palmar) digital vein
   Volar (palmar) metacarpal vein
	H **Hand Vein, Left**
	   See G Hand Vein, Right
	L **Intracranial Vein**
	   Anterior cerebral vein
	   Basal (internal) cerebral vein
	   Dural venous sinus
	   Great cerebral vein
	   Inferior cerebellar vein
	   Inferior cerebral vein
	   Internal (basal) cerebral vein
	   Middle cerebral vein
	   Ophthalmic vein
	   Superior cerebellar vein
	   Superior cerebral vein
	M **Internal Jugular Vein, Right**
	N **Internal Jugular Vein, Left**
	P **External Jugular Vein, Right**
	   Posterior auricular vein
	Q **External Jugular Vein, Left**
	   See P External Jugular Vein,
	     Right
	R **Vertebral Vein, Right**
	   Deep cervical vein
	   Suboccipital venous plexus
	S **Vertebral Vein, Left**
	   See R Vertebral Vein, Right
	T **Face Vein, Right**
	   Angular vein
	   Anterior facial vein
	   Common facial vein
	   Deep facial vein
	   Frontal vein
	   Posterior facial
	     (retromandibular) vein
	   Supraorbital vein
	V **Face Vein, Left**
	   See T Face Vein, Right
	Y **Upper Vein**
		0 Open
		3 Percutaneous
		4 Percutaneous Endoscopic
			Z No Device	**Z** No Qualifier

Ø **Medical and Surgical**
5 **Upper Veins**
R **Replacement**   Definition: Putting in or on biological or synthetic material that physically takes the place and/or function of all or a portion of a body part
    Explanation: The body part may have been taken out or replaced, or may be taken out, physically eradicated, or rendered nonfunctional during the REPLACEMENT procedure. A REMOVAL procedure is coded for taking out the device used in a previous replacement procedure.

Body Part Character 4		Approach Character 5	Device Character 6	Qualifier Character 7

Ø **Azygos Vein**
    Right ascending lumbar vein
    Right subcostal vein
1 **Hemiazygos Vein**
    Left ascending lumbar vein
    Left subcostal vein
3 **Innominate Vein, Right**
    Brachiocephalic vein
    Inferior thyroid vein
4 **Innominate Vein, Left**
    See 3 Innominate Vein, Right
5 **Subclavian Vein, Right**
6 **Subclavian Vein, Left**
7 **Axillary Vein, Right**
8 **Axillary Vein, Left**
9 **Brachial Vein, Right**
    Radial vein
    Ulnar vein
A **Brachial Vein, Left**
    See 9 Brachial Vein, Right
B **Basilic Vein, Right**
    Median antebrachial vein
    Median cubital vein
C **Basilic Vein, Left**
    See B Basilic Vein, Right
D **Cephalic Vein, Right**
    Accessory cephalic vein
F **Cephalic Vein, Left**
    See D Cephalic Vein, Right
G **Hand Vein, Right**
    Dorsal metacarpal vein
    Palmar (volar) digital vein
    Palmar (volar) metacarpal vein
    Superficial palmar venous arch
    Volar (palmar) digital vein
    Volar (palmar) metacarpal vein
	H **Hand Vein, Left**
	    See G Hand Vein, Right
	L **Intracranial Vein**
	    Anterior cerebral vein
	    Basal (internal) cerebral vein
	    Dural venous sinus
	    Great cerebral vein
	    Inferior cerebellar vein
	    Inferior cerebral vein
	    Internal (basal) cerebral vein
	    Middle cerebral vein
	    Ophthalmic vein
	    Superior cerebellar vein
	    Superior cerebral vein
	M **Internal Jugular Vein, Right**
	N **Internal Jugular Vein, Left**
	P **External Jugular Vein, Right**
	    Posterior auricular vein
	Q **External Jugular Vein, Left**
	    See P External Jugular Vein,
	    Right
	R **Vertebral Vein, Right**
	    Deep cervical vein
	    Suboccipital venous plexus
	S **Vertebral Vein, Left**
	    See R Vertebral Vein, Right
	T **Face Vein, Right**
	    Angular vein
	    Anterior facial vein
	    Common facial vein
	    Deep facial vein
	    Frontal vein
	    Posterior facial
	       (retromandibular) vein
	    Supraorbital vein
	V **Face Vein, Left**
	    See T Face Vein, Right
	Y **Upper Vein**
		Ø **Open**
		4 **Percutaneous Endoscopic**
			7 **Autologous Tissue**
			    Substitute
			J **Synthetic Substitute**
			K **Nonautologous Tissue**
			    Substitute
				Z **No Qualifier**

LC Limited Coverage   **NC** Noncovered   ⊞ Combination Member   HAC associated procedure   Combination Only   DRG Non-OR   Non-OR   New/Revised in GREEN

246   ICD-10-PCS 2019

0   **Medical and Surgical**
5   **Upper Veins**
S   **Reposition**   Definition: Moving to its normal location, or other suitable location, all or a portion of a body part

                 Explanation: The body part is moved to a new location from an abnormal location, or from a normal location where it is not functioning correctly. The body part may or may not be cut out or off to be moved to the new location.

Body Part Character 4		Approach Character 5	Device Character 6	Qualifier Character 7

0   **Azygos Vein**
    Right ascending lumbar vein
    Right subcostal vein
1   **Hemiazygos Vein**
    Left ascending lumbar vein
    Left subcostal vein
3   **Innominate Vein, Right**
    Brachiocephalic vein
    Inferior thyroid vein
4   **Innominate Vein, Left**
    See 3 Innominate Vein, Right
5   **Subclavian Vein, Right**
6   **Subclavian Vein, Left**
7   **Axillary Vein, Right**
8   **Axillary Vein, Left**
9   **Brachial Vein, Right**
    Radial vein
    Ulnar vein
A   **Brachial Vein, Left**
    See 9 Brachial Vein, Right
B   **Basilic Vein, Right**
    Median antebrachial vein
    Median cubital vein
C   **Basilic Vein, Left**
    See B Basilic Vein, Right
D   **Cephalic Vein, Right**
    Accessory cephalic vein
F   **Cephalic Vein, Left**
    See D Cephalic Vein, Right
G   **Hand Vein, Right**
    Dorsal metacarpal vein
    Palmar (volar) digital vein
    Palmar (volar) metacarpal vein
    Superficial palmar venous arch
    Volar (palmar) digital vein
    Volar (palmar) metacarpal vein
	H **Hand Vein, Left**
	    See G Hand Vein, Right
	L **Intracranial Vein**
	    Anterior cerebral vein
	    Basal (internal) cerebral vein
	    Dural venous sinus
	    Great cerebral vein
	    Inferior cerebellar vein
	    Inferior cerebral vein
	    Internal (basal) cerebral vein
	    Middle cerebral vein
	    Ophthalmic vein
	    Superior cerebellar vein
	    Superior cerebral vein
	M **Internal Jugular Vein, Right**
	N **Internal Jugular Vein, Left**
	P **External Jugular Vein, Right**
	    Posterior auricular vein
	Q **External Jugular Vein, Left**
	    See P External Jugular Vein,
	        Right
	R **Vertebral Vein, Right**
	    Deep cervical vein
	    Suboccipital venous plexus
	S **Vertebral Vein, Left**
	    See R Vertebral Vein, Right
	T **Face Vein, Right**
	    Angular vein
	    Anterior facial vein
	    Common facial vein
	    Deep facial vein
	    Frontal vein
	    Posterior facial
	        (retromandibular) vein
	    Supraorbital vein
	V **Face Vein, Left**
	    See T Face Vein, Right
	Y **Upper Vein**
		0 Open
		3 Percutaneous
		4 Percutaneous Endoscopic
			Z No Device	**Z** No Qualifier

Ø   Medical and Surgical
5   Upper Veins
U   Supplement   Definition: Putting in or on biological or synthetic material that physically reinforces and/or augments the function of a portion of a body part
Explanation: The biological material is non-living, or is living and from the same individual. The body part may have been previously replaced, and the SUPPLEMENT procedure is performed to physically reinforce and/or augment the function of the replaced body part.

Body Part Character 4		Approach Character 5	Device Character 6	Qualifier Character 7

Ø Azygos Vein
Right ascending lumbar vein
Right subcostal vein
1 Hemiazygos Vein
Left ascending lumbar vein
Left subcostal vein
3 Innominate Vein, Right
Brachiocephalic vein
Inferior thyroid vein
4 Innominate Vein, Left
See 3 Innominate Vein, Right
5 Subclavian Vein, Right
6 Subclavian Vein, Left
7 Axillary Vein, Right
8 Axillary Vein, Left
9 Brachial Vein, Right
Radial vein
Ulnar vein
A Brachial Vein, Left
See 9 Brachial Vein, Right
B Basilic Vein, Right
Median antebrachial vein
Median cubital vein
C Basilic Vein, Left
See B Basilic Vein, Right
D Cephalic Vein, Right
Accessory cephalic vein
F Cephalic Vein, Left
See D Cephalic Vein, Right
G Hand Vein, Right
Dorsal metacarpal vein
Palmar (volar) digital vein
Palmar (volar) metacarpal vein
Superficial palmar venous arch
Volar (palmar) digital vein
Volar (palmar) metacarpal vein
	H Hand Vein, Left
	See G Hand Vein, Right
	L Intracranial Vein
	Anterior cerebral vein
	Basal (internal) cerebral vein
	Dural venous sinus
	Great cerebral vein
	Inferior cerebellar vein
	Inferior cerebral vein
	Internal (basal) cerebral vein
	Middle cerebral vein
	Ophthalmic vein
	Superior cerebellar vein
	Superior cerebral vein
	M Internal Jugular Vein, Right
	N Internal Jugular Vein, Left
	P External Jugular Vein, Right
	Posterior auricular vein
	Q External Jugular Vein, Left
	See P External Jugular Vein, Right
	R Vertebral Vein, Right
	Deep cervical vein
	Suboccipital venous plexus
	S Vertebral Vein, Left
	See R Vertebral Vein, Right
	T Face Vein, Right
	Angular vein
	Anterior facial vein
	Common facial vein
	Deep facial vein
	Frontal vein
	Posterior facial
	    (retromandibular) vein
	Supraorbital vein
	V Face Vein, Left
	See T Face Vein, Right
	Y Upper Vein
		Ø Open
		3 Percutaneous
		4 Percutaneous Endoscopic
			7 Autologous Tissue
			   Substitute
			J Synthetic Substitute
			K Nonautologous Tissue
			   Substitute
				Z No Qualifier

LC Limited Coverage   NC Noncovered   ⊞ Combination Member   HAC associated procedure   Combination Only   DRG Non-OR   Non-OR   New/Revised in GREEN

Ø   Medical and Surgical
5   Upper Veins
V   Restriction   Definition: Partially closing an orifice or the lumen of a tubular body part
                         Explanation: The orifice can be a natural orifice or an artificially created orifice

Body Part Character 4		Approach Character 5	Device Character 6	Qualifier Character 7

Ø   Azygos Vein
    Right ascending lumbar vein
    Right subcostal vein
1   Hemiazygos Vein
    Left ascending lumbar vein
    Left subcostal vein
3   Innominate Vein, Right
    Brachiocephalic vein
    Inferior thyroid vein
4   Innominate Vein, Left
    See 3 Innominate Vein, Right
5   Subclavian Vein, Right
6   Subclavian Vein, Left
7   Axillary Vein, Right
8   Axillary Vein, Left
9   Brachial Vein, Right
    Radial vein
    Ulnar vein
A   Brachial Vein, Left
    See 9 Brachial Vein, Right
B   Basilic Vein, Right
    Median antebrachial vein
    Median cubital vein
C   Basilic Vein, Left
    See B Basilic Vein, Right
D   Cephalic Vein, Right
    Accessory cephalic vein
F   Cephalic Vein, Left
    See D Cephalic Vein, Right
G   Hand Vein, Right
    Dorsal metacarpal vein
    Palmar (volar) digital vein
    Palmar (volar) metacarpal vein
    Superficial palmar venous arch
    Volar (palmar) digital vein
    Volar (palmar) metacarpal vein
	H Hand Vein, Left
	    See G Hand Vein, Right
	L Intracranial Vein
	    Anterior cerebral vein
	    Basal (internal) cerebral vein
	    Dural venous sinus
	    Great cerebral vein
	    Inferior cerebellar vein
	    Inferior cerebral vein
	    Internal (basal) cerebral vein
	    Middle cerebral vein
	    Ophthalmic vein
	    Superior cerebellar vein
	    Superior cerebral vein
	M Internal Jugular Vein, Right
	N Internal Jugular Vein, Left
	P External Jugular Vein, Right
	    Posterior auricular vein
	Q External Jugular Vein, Left
	    See P External Jugular Vein,
	       Right
	R Vertebral Vein, Right
	    Deep cervical vein
	    Suboccipital venous plexus
	S Vertebral Vein, Left
	    See R Vertebral Vein, Right
	T Face Vein, Right
	    Angular vein
	    Anterior facial vein
	    Common facial vein
	    Deep facial vein
	    Frontal vein
	    Posterior facial
	       (retromandibular) vein
	    Supraorbital vein
	V Face Vein, Left
	    See T Face Vein, Right
	Y Upper Vein
		Ø Open
		3 Percutaneous
		4 Percutaneous Endoscopic
			C Extraluminal Device
			D Intraluminal Device
			Z No Device
				Z No Qualifier

Upper Veins

Ø   Medical and Surgical
5   Upper Veins
W   Revision   Definition: Correcting, to the extent possible, a portion of a malfunctioning device or the position of a displaced device
                           Explanation: Revision can include correcting a malfunctioning or displaced device by taking out or putting in components of the device such as a screw or pin

Body Part Character 4	Approach Character 5	Device Character 6	Qualifier Character 7

Ø Azygos Vein
    Right ascending lumbar vein
    Right subcostal vein
	Ø Open
	3 Percutaneous
	4 Percutaneous Endoscopic
	X External
		2 Monitoring Device
		M Neurostimulator Lead
			Z No Qualifier

3 Innominate Vein, Right
    Brachiocephalic vein
    Inferior thyroid vein
4 Innominate Vein, Left
    See 3 Innominate Vein, Right
	Ø Open
	3 Percutaneous
	4 Percutaneous Endoscopic
	X External
		M Neurostimulator Lead	**Z** No Qualifier

Y Upper Vein	**Ø** Open **3** Percutaneous **4** Percutaneous Endoscopic	**Ø** Drainage Device **2** Monitoring Device **3** Infusion Device **7** Autologous Tissue Substitute **C** Extraluminal Device **D** Intraluminal Device **J** Synthetic Substitute **K** Nonautologous Tissue Substitute **Y** Other Device	**Z** No Qualifier
Y Upper Vein	**X** External	**Ø** Drainage Device **2** Monitoring Device **3** Infusion Device **7** Autologous Tissue Substitute **C** Extraluminal Device **D** Intraluminal Device **J** Synthetic Substitute **K** Nonautologous Tissue Substitute	**Z** No Qualifier

Non-OR	Ø5WØXMZ
Non-OR	Ø5W[3,4]XMZ
Non-OR	Ø5WY3[Ø,2,3,D]Z
Non-OR	Ø5WY[3,4]YZ
Non-OR	Ø5WYX[Ø,2,3,7,C,D,J,K]Z

Lower Veins Ø61–Ø6W

Character Meanings

This Character Meaning table is provided as a guide to assist the user in the identification of character members that may be found in this section of code tables. It **SHOULD NOT** be used to build a PCS code.

Operation–Character 3		Body Part–Character 4		Approach–Character 5		Device–Character 6		Qualifier–Character 7	
1	Bypass	Ø	Inferior Vena Cava	Ø	Open	Ø	Drainage Device	4	Hepatic Vein
5	Destruction	1	Splenic Vein	3	Percutaneous	2	Monitoring Device	5	Superior Mesenteric Vein
7	Dilation	2	Gastric Vein	4	Percutaneous Endoscopic	3	Infusion Device	6	Inferior Mesenteric Vein
9	Drainage	3	Esophageal Vein	7	Via Natural or Artificial Opening	7	Autologous Tissue Substitute	9	Renal Vein, Right
B	Excision	4	Hepatic Vein	8	Via Natural or Artificial Opening Endoscopic	9	Autologous Venous Tissue	B	Renal Vein, Left
C	Extirpation	5	Superior Mesenteric Vein	X	External	A	Autologous Arterial Tissue	C	Hemorrhoidal Plexus
D	Extraction	6	Inferior Mesenteric Vein			C	Extraluminal Device	P	Pulmonary Trunk
H	Insertion	7	Colic Vein			D	Intraluminal Device	Q	Pulmonary Artery, Right
J	Inspection	8	Portal Vein			J	Synthetic Substitute	R	Pulmonary Artery, Left
L	Occlusion	9	Renal Vein, Right			K	Nonautologous Tissue Substitute	T	Via Umbilical Vein
N	Release	B	Renal Vein, Left			Y	Other Device	X	Diagnostic
P	Removal	C	Common Iliac Vein, Right			Z	No Device	Y	Lower Vein
Q	Repair	D	Common Iliac Vein, Left					Z	No Qualifier
R	Replacement	F	External Iliac Vein, Right						
S	Reposition	G	External Iliac Vein, Left						
U	Supplement	H	Hypogastric Vein, Right						
V	Restriction	J	Hypogastric Vein, Left						
W	Revision	M	Femoral Vein, Right						
		N	Femoral Vein, Left						
		P	Saphenous Vein, Right						
		Q	Saphenous Vein, Left						
		T	Foot Vein, Right						
		V	Foot Vein, Left						
		Y	Lower Vein						

AHA Coding Clinic for table Ø61

| 2017, 4Q, 36-38 | Fontan completion procedure |
| 2017, 4Q, 66-67 | New qualifier values - Portal to hepatic shunt |

AHA Coding Clinic for table Ø6B

2017, 3Q, 5	Femoral artery to posterior tibial artery bypass using autologous and synthetic grafts
2017, 1Q, 31	Left to right common carotid artery bypass
2017, 1Q, 32	Peroneal artery to dorsalis pedis artery bypass using saphenous vein graft
2016, 1Q, 31	Femoral to peroneal artery bypass with in-situ saphenous vein graft and lysis of valves
2016, 2Q, 18	Femoral-tibial artery bypass and saphenous vein graft
2016, 1Q, 27	Aortocoronary bypass graft utilizing Y-graft
2014, 3Q, 8	Excision of saphenous vein for coronary artery bypass graft
2014, 3Q, 20	MAZE procedure performed with coronary artery bypass graft
2014, 1Q, 10	Repair of thoracic aortic aneurysm & coronary artery bypass graft

AHA Coding Clinic for table Ø6H

2017, 3Q, 11	Placement of peripherally inserted central catheter using 3CG ECG technology
2017, 1Q, 31	Umbilical vein catheterization
2017, 1Q, 31	Central catheter placement in femoral vein
2013, 3Q, 18	Heart transplant surgery

AHA Coding Clinic for table Ø6L

2018, 2Q, 18	Transverse rectus abdominis myocutaneous (TRAM) delay
2017, 4Q, 57-58	Added approach values - Transorifice esophageal vein banding
2013, 4Q, 112	Endoscopic banding of esophageal varices

AHA Coding Clinic for table Ø6V

| 2018, 1Q, 10 | Revision of transjugular intrahepatic portosystemic shunt |

AHA Coding Clinic for table Ø6W

| 2018, 1Q, 10 | Revision of transjugular intrahepatic portosystemic shunt |
| 2014, 3Q, 25 | Revision of transjugular intrahepatic portosystemic shunt (TIPS) |

Lower Veins

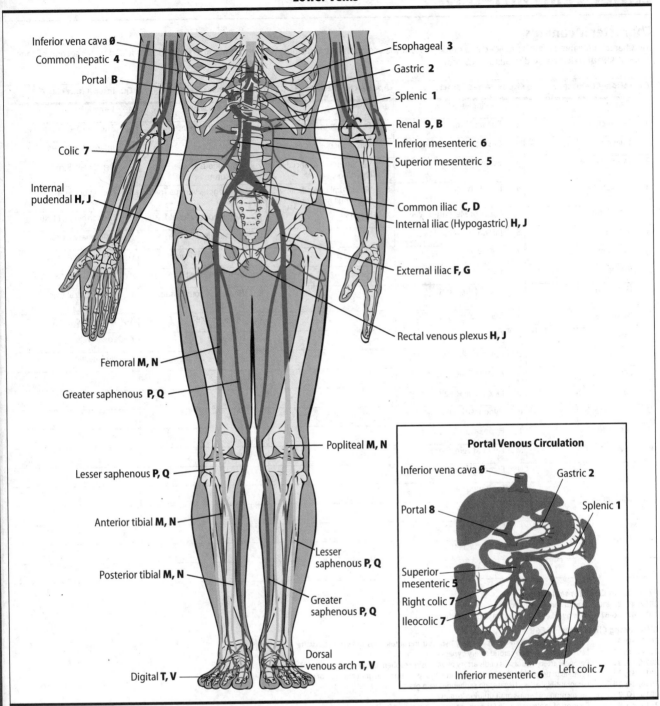

Inferior vena cava **Ø**
Common hepatic **4**
Portal **B**
Colic **7**
Internal pudendal **H, J**
Femoral **M, N**
Greater saphenous **P, Q**
Lesser saphenous **P, Q**
Anterior tibial **M, N**
Posterior tibial **M, N**
Digital **T, V**

Esophageal **3**
Gastric **2**
Splenic **1**
Renal **9, B**
Inferior mesenteric **6**
Superior mesenteric **5**
Common iliac **C, D**
Internal iliac (Hypogastric) **H, J**
External iliac **F, G**
Rectal venous plexus **H, J**
Popliteal **M, N**
Lesser saphenous **P, Q**
Greater saphenous **P, Q**
Dorsal venous arch **T, V**

Portal Venous Circulation

Inferior vena cava **Ø**
Portal **8**
Superior mesenteric **5**
Right colic **7**
Ileocolic **7**
Gastric **2**
Splenic **1**
Inferior mesenteric **6**
Left colic **7**

Ø Medical and Surgical
6 Lower Veins
1 Bypass

Definition: Altering the route of passage of the contents of a tubular body part

Explanation: Rerouting contents of a body part to a downstream area of the normal route, to a similar route and body part, or to an abnormal route and dissimilar body part. Includes one or more anastomoses, with or without the use of a device.

Body Part Character 4		Approach Character 5	Device Character 6	Qualifier Character 7
Ø Inferior Vena Cava Postcava Right inferior phrenic vein Right ovarian vein Right second lumbar vein Right suprarenal vein Right testicular vein		**Ø** Open **4** Percutaneous Endoscopic	**7** Autologous Tissue Substitute **9** Autologous Venous Tissue **A** Autologous Arterial Tissue **J** Synthetic Substitute **K** Nonautologous Tissue Substitute **Z** No Device	**5** Superior Mesenteric Vein **6** Inferior Mesenteric Vein **P** Pulmonary Trunk **Q** Pulmonary Artery, Right **R** Pulmonary Artery, Left **Y** Lower Vein
1 Splenic Vein Left gastroepiploic vein Pancreatic vein		**Ø** Open **4** Percutaneous Endoscopic	**7** Autologous Tissue Substitute **9** Autologous Venous Tissue **A** Autologous Arterial Tissue **J** Synthetic Substitute **K** Nonautologous Tissue Substitute **Z** No Device	**9** Renal Vein, Right **B** Renal Vein, Left **Y** Lower Vein
2 Gastric Vein **3 Esophageal Vein** **4 Hepatic Vein** **5 Superior Mesenteric Vein** Right gastroepiploic vein **6 Inferior Mesenteric Vein** Sigmoid vein Superior rectal vein **7 Colic Vein** Ileocolic vein Left colic vein Middle colic vein Right colic vein **9 Renal Vein, Right** **B Renal Vein, Left** Left inferior phrenic vein Left ovarian vein Left second lumbar vein Left suprarenal vein Left testicular vein **C Common Iliac Vein, Right** **D Common Iliac Vein, Left** **F External Iliac Vein, Right** **G External Iliac Vein, Left** **H Hypogastric Vein, Right** Gluteal vein Internal iliac vein Internal pudendal vein Lateral sacral vein Middle hemorrhoidal vein Obturator vein Uterine vein Vaginal vein Vesical vein	**J Hypogastric Vein, Left** *See H Hypogastric Vein, Right* **M Femoral Vein, Right** Deep femoral (profunda femoris) vein Popliteal vein Profunda femoris (deep femoral) vein **N Femoral Vein, Left** *See M Femoral Vein, Right* **P Saphenous Vein, Right** External pudendal vein Great(er) saphenous vein Lesser saphenous vein Small saphenous vein Superficial circumflex iliac vein Superficial epigastric vein **Q Saphenous Vein, Left** *See P Saphenous Vein, Right* **T Foot Vein, Right** Common digital vein Dorsal metatarsal vein Dorsal venous arch Plantar digital vein Plantar metatarsal vein Plantar venous arch **V Foot Vein, Left** *See T Foot Vein, Right*	**Ø** Open **4** Percutaneous Endoscopic	**7** Autologous Tissue Substitute **9** Autologous Venous Tissue **A** Autologous Arterial Tissue **J** Synthetic Substitute **K** Nonautologous Tissue Substitute **Z** No Device	**Y** Lower Vein
8 Portal Vein Hepatic portal vein		**Ø** Open	**7** Autologous Tissue Substitute **9** Autologous Venous Tissue **A** Autologous Arterial Tissue **J** Synthetic Substitute **K** Nonautologous Tissue Substitute **Z** No Device	**9** Renal Vein, Right **B** Renal Vein, Left **Y** Lower Vein
8 Portal Vein Hepatic portal vein		**3** Percutaneous	**J** Synthetic Substitute	**4** Hepatic Vein **Y** Lower Vein
8 Portal Vein Hepatic portal vein		**4** Percutaneous Endoscopic	**7** Autologous Tissue Substitute **9** Autologous Venous Tissue **A** Autologous Arterial Tissue **K** Nonautologous Tissue Substitute **Z** No Device	**9** Renal Vein, Right **B** Renal Vein, Left **Y** Lower Vein
8 Portal Vein Hepatic portal vein		**4** Percutaneous Endoscopic	**J** Synthetic Substitute	**4** Hepatic Vein **9** Renal Vein, Right **B** Renal Vein, Left **Y** Lower Vein

0   Medical and Surgical
6   Lower Veins
5   Destruction   Definition: Physical eradication of all or a portion of a body part by the direct use of energy, force, or a destructive agent
                       Explanation: None of the body part is physically taken out

Body Part Character 4	Approach Character 5	Device Character 6	Qualifier Character 7
0 Inferior Vena Cava Postcava Right inferior phrenic vein Right ovarian vein Right second lumbar vein Right suprarenal vein Right testicular vein **1 Splenic Vein** Left gastroepiploic vein Pancreatic vein **2 Gastric Vein** **3 Esophageal Vein** **4 Hepatic Vein** **5 Superior Mesenteric Vein** Right gastroepiploic vein **6 Inferior Mesenteric Vein** Sigmoid vein Superior rectal vein **7 Colic Vein** Ileocolic vein Left colic vein Middle colic vein Right colic vein **8 Portal Vein** Hepatic portal vein **9 Renal Vein, Right** **B Renal Vein, Left** Left inferior phrenic vein Left ovarian vein Left second lumbar vein Left suprarenal vein Left testicular vein **C Common Iliac Vein, Right** **D Common Iliac Vein, Left** **F External Iliac Vein, Right** **G External Iliac Vein, Left** **H Hypogastric Vein, Right** Gluteal vein Internal iliac vein Internal pudendal vein Lateral sacral vein Middle hemorrhoidal vein Obturator vein Uterine vein Vaginal vein Vesical vein **J Hypogastric Vein, Left** *See H Hypogastric Vein, Right* **M Femoral Vein, Right** Deep femoral (profunda femoris) vein Popliteal vein Profunda femoris (deep femoral) vein **N Femoral Vein, Left** *See M Femoral Vein, Right* **P Saphenous Vein, Right** External pudendal vein Great(er) saphenous vein Lesser saphenous vein Small saphenous vein Superficial circumflex iliac vein Superficial epigastric vein **Q Saphenous Vein, Left** *See P Saphenous Vein, Right* **T Foot Vein, Right** Common digital vein Dorsal metatarsal vein Dorsal venous arch Plantar digital vein Plantar metatarsal vein Plantar venous arch **V Foot Vein, Left** *See T Foot Vein, Right*	**0** Open **3** Percutaneous **4** Percutaneous Endoscopic	**Z** No Device	**Z** No Qualifier
Y Lower Vein	**0** Open **3** Percutaneous **4** Percutaneous Endoscopic	**Z** No Device	**C** Hemorrhoidal Plexus **Z** No Qualifier

LC Limited Coverage   NC Noncovered   ⊞ Combination Member   HAC associated procedure   Combination Only   DRG Non-OR   Non-OR   New/Revised in GREEN

254   ICD-10-PCS 2019

065–065

0   Medical and Surgical
6   Lower Veins
7   Dilation   Definition: Expanding an orifice or the lumen of a tubular body part

Explanation: The orifice can be a natural orifice or an artificially created orifice. Accomplished by stretching a tubular body part using intraluminal pressure or by cutting part of the orifice or wall of the tubular body part.

Body Part Character 4	Approach Character 5	Device Character 6	Qualifier Character 7
0 Inferior Vena Cava Postcava Right inferior phrenic vein Right ovarian vein Right second lumbar vein Right suprarenal vein Right testicular vein	**0** Open **3** Percutaneous **4** Percutaneous Endoscopic	**D** Intraluminal Device **Z** No Device	**Z** No Qualifier
1 Splenic Vein Left gastroepiploic vein Pancreatic vein			
2 Gastric Vein			
3 Esophageal Vein			
4 Hepatic Vein			
5 Superior Mesenteric Vein Right gastroepiploic vein			
6 Inferior Mesenteric Vein Sigmoid vein Superior rectal vein			
7 Colic Vein Ileocolic vein Left colic vein Middle colic vein Right colic vein			
8 Portal Vein Hepatic portal vein			
9 Renal Vein, Right			
B Renal Vein, Left Left inferior phrenic vein Left ovarian vein Left second lumbar vein Left suprarenal vein Left testicular vein			
C Common Iliac Vein, Right			
D Common Iliac Vein, Left			
F External Iliac Vein, Right			
G External Iliac Vein, Left			
H Hypogastric Vein, Right Gluteal vein Internal iliac vein Internal pudendal vein Lateral sacral vein Middle hemorrhoidal vein Obturator vein Uterine vein Vaginal vein Vesical vein			
J Hypogastric Vein, Left *See H Hypogastric Vein, Right*			
M Femoral Vein, Right Deep femoral (profunda femoris) vein Popliteal vein Profunda femoris (deep femoral) vein			
N Femoral Vein, Left *See M Femoral Vein, Right*			
P Saphenous Vein, Right External pudendal vein Great(er) saphenous vein Lesser saphenous vein Small saphenous vein Superficial circumflex iliac vein Superficial epigastric vein			
Q Saphenous Vein, Left *See P Saphenous Vein, Right*			
T Foot Vein, Right Common digital vein Dorsal metatarsal vein Dorsal venous arch Plantar digital vein Plantar metatarsal vein Plantar venous arch			
V Foot Vein, Left *See T Foot Vein, Right*			
Y Lower Vein			

Ø   Medical and Surgical
6   Lower Veins
9   Drainage   Definition: Taking or letting out fluids and/or gases from a body part

Explanation: The qualifier DIAGNOSTIC is used to identify drainage procedures that are biopsies

Body Part Character 4		Approach Character 5	Device Character 6	Qualifier Character 7

Ø Inferior Vena Cava
 Postcava
 Right inferior phrenic vein
 Right ovarian vein
 Right second lumbar vein
 Right suprarenal vein
 Right testicular vein
 1 Splenic Vein
 Left gastroepiploic vein
 Pancreatic vein
 2 Gastric Vein
 3 Esophageal Vein
 4 Hepatic Vein
 5 Superior Mesenteric Vein
 Right gastroepiploic vein
 6 Inferior Mesenteric Vein
 Sigmoid vein
 Superior rectal vein
 7 Colic Vein
 Ileocolic vein
 Left colic vein
 Middle colic vein
 Right colic vein
 8 Portal Vein
 Hepatic portal vein
 9 Renal Vein, Right
 B Renal Vein, Left
 Left inferior phrenic vein
 Left ovarian vein
 Left second lumbar vein
 Left suprarenal vein
 Left testicular vein
 C Common Iliac Vein, Right
 D Common Iliac Vein, Left
 F External Iliac Vein, Right
 G External Iliac Vein, Left
	H Hypogastric Vein, Right
	 Gluteal vein
	 Internal iliac vein
	 Internal pudendal vein
	 Lateral sacral vein
	 Middle hemorrhoidal vein
	 Obturator vein
	 Uterine vein
	 Vaginal vein
	 Vesical vein
	 J Hypogastric Vein, Left
	 See H Hypogastric Vein, Right
	 M Femoral Vein, Right
	 Deep femoral (profunda
	  femoris) vein
	 Popliteal vein
	 Profunda femoris (deep
	  femoral) vein
	 N Femoral Vein, Left
	 See M Femoral Vein, Right
	 P Saphenous Vein, Right
	 External pudendal vein
	 Great(er) saphenous vein
	 Lesser saphenous vein
	 Small saphenous vein
	 Superficial circumflex iliac vein
	 Superficial epigastric vein
	 Q Saphenous Vein, Left
	 See P Saphenous Vein, Right
	 T Foot Vein, Right
	 Common digital vein
	 Dorsal metatarsal vein
	 Dorsal venous arch
	 Plantar digital vein
	 Plantar metatarsal vein
	 Plantar venous arch
	 V Foot Vein, Left
	 See T Foot Vein, Right
	 Y Lower Vein
		Ø Open
		 3 Percutaneous
		 4 Percutaneous Endoscopic
			Ø Drainage Device	**Z No Qualifier**

Ø69 Continued on next page

Non-OR	Ø69[Ø,1,2,4,5,6,7,8,9,B,C,D,F,G,H,J,M,N,P,Q,T,V,Y][Ø,3,4]ØZ
Non-OR	Ø69330Z

LC Limited Coverage   **NC** Noncovered   ⊞ Combination Member   HAC associated procedure   Combination Only   DRG Non-OR   Non-OR   New/Revised in GREEN

256   ICD-10-PCS 2019

Ø69–Ø69

Ø   Medical and Surgical
6   Lower Veins
069 Continued
9   Drainage   Definition: Taking or letting out fluids and/or gases from a body part

Explanation: The qualifier DIAGNOSTIC is used to identify drainage procedures that are biopsies

Body Part Character 4		Approach Character 5	Device Character 6	Qualifier Character 7

Ø   Inferior Vena Cava
    Postcava
    Right inferior phrenic vein
    Right ovarian vein
    Right second lumbar vein
    Right suprarenal vein
    Right testicular vein
1   Splenic Vein
    Left gastroepiploic vein
    Pancreatic vein
2   Gastric Vein
3   Esophageal Vein
4   Hepatic Vein
5   Superior Mesenteric Vein
    Right gastroepiploic vein
6   Inferior Mesenteric Vein
    Sigmoid vein
    Superior rectal vein
7   Colic Vein
    Ileocolic vein
    Left colic vein
    Middle colic vein
    Right colic vein
8   Portal Vein
    Hepatic portal vein
9   Renal Vein, Right
B   Renal Vein, Left
    Left inferior phrenic vein
    Left ovarian vein
    Left second lumbar vein
    Left suprarenal vein
    Left testicular vein
C   Common Iliac Vein, Right
D   Common Iliac Vein, Left
F   External Iliac Vein, Right
G   External Iliac Vein, Left
	H Hypogastric Vein, Right
	    Gluteal vein
	    Internal iliac vein
	    Internal pudendal vein
	    Lateral sacral vein
	    Middle hemorrhoidal vein
	    Obturator vein
	    Uterine vein
	    Vaginal vein
	    Vesical vein
	J Hypogastric Vein, Left
	    See H Hypogastric Vein, Right
	M Femoral Vein, Right
	    Deep femoral (profunda
	      femoris) vein
	    Popliteal vein
	    Profunda femoris (deep
	      femoral) vein
	N Femoral Vein, Left
	    See M Femoral Vein, Right
	P Saphenous Vein, Right
	    External pudendal vein
	    Great(er) saphenous vein
	    Lesser saphenous vein
	    Small saphenous vein
	    Superficial circumflex iliac vein
	    Superficial epigastric vein
	Q Saphenous Vein, Left
	    See P Saphenous Vein, Right
	T Foot Vein, Right
	    Common digital vein
	    Dorsal metatarsal vein
	    Dorsal venous arch
	    Plantar digital vein
	    Plantar metatarsal vein
	    Plantar venous arch
	V Foot Vein, Left
	    See T Foot Vein, Right
	Y Lower Vein
		Ø Open
		3 Percutaneous
		4 Percutaneous Endoscopic
			Z No Device	**X Diagnostic**
				Z No Qualifier

Non-OR   069[Ø,1,2,3,4,5,6,7,8,9,B,C,D,F,G,H,J,M,N,P,Q,T,V,Y]3ZX
Non-OR   069[Ø,1,2,4,5,6,7,8,9,B,C,D,F,G,H,J,M,N,P,Q,T,V,Y][Ø,3,4]ZZ
Non-OR   06933ZZ

Lower Veins

Ø   **Medical and Surgical**
6   **Lower Veins**
B   **Excision**   Definition: Cutting out or off, without replacement, a portion of a body part

Explanation: The qualifier DIAGNOSTIC is used to identify excision procedures that are biopsies

Body Part Character 4		Approach Character 5	Device Character 6	Qualifier Character 7
Ø **Inferior Vena Cava** Postcava Right inferior phrenic vein Right ovarian vein Right second lumbar vein Right suprarenal vein Right testicular vein **1** **Splenic Vein** Left gastroepiploic vein Pancreatic vein **2** **Gastric Vein** **3** **Esophageal Vein** **4** **Hepatic Vein** **5** **Superior Mesenteric Vein** Right gastroepiploic vein **6** **Inferior Mesenteric Vein** Sigmoid vein Superior rectal vein **7** **Colic Vein** Ileocolic vein Left colic vein Middle colic vein Right colic vein **8** **Portal Vein** Hepatic portal vein **9** **Renal Vein, Right** **B** **Renal Vein, Left** Left inferior phrenic vein Left ovarian vein Left second lumbar vein Left suprarenal vein Left testicular vein **C** **Common Iliac Vein, Right** **D** **Common Iliac Vein, Left** **F** **External Iliac Vein, Right** **G** **External Iliac Vein, Left**	**H** **Hypogastric Vein, Right** Gluteal vein Internal iliac vein Internal pudendal vein Lateral sacral vein Middle hemorrhoidal vein Obturator vein Uterine vein Vaginal vein Vesical vein **J** **Hypogastric Vein, Left** *See H Hypogastric Vein, Right* **M** **Femoral Vein, Right** Deep femoral (profunda femoris) vein Popliteal vein Profunda femoris (deep femoral) vein **N** **Femoral Vein, Left** *See M Femoral Vein, Right* **P** **Saphenous Vein, Right** External pudendal vein Great(er) saphenous vein Lesser saphenous vein Small saphenous vein Superficial circumflex iliac vein Superficial epigastric vein **Q** **Saphenous Vein, Left** *See P Saphenous Vein, Right* **T** **Foot Vein, Right** Common digital vein Dorsal metatarsal vein Dorsal venous arch Plantar digital vein Plantar metatarsal vein Plantar venous arch **V** **Foot Vein, Left** *See T Foot Vein, Right*	**Ø** Open **3** Percutaneous **4** Percutaneous Endoscopic	**Z** No Device	**X** Diagnostic **Z** No Qualifier
Y Lower Vein		**Ø** Open **3** Percutaneous **4** Percutaneous Endoscopic	**Z** No Device	**C** Hemorrhoidal Plexus **X** Diagnostic **Z** No Qualifier

LC Limited Coverage   NC Noncovered   ⊞ Combination Member   HAC associated procedure   Combination Only   DRG Non-OR   Non-OR   New/Revised in GREEN

258   ICD-10-PCS 2019

Ø   Medical and Surgical
6   Lower Veins
C   Extirpation   Definition: Taking or cutting out solid matter from a body part

Explanation: The solid matter may be an abnormal byproduct of a biological function or a foreign body; it may be imbedded in a body part or in the lumen of a tubular body part. The solid matter may or may not have been previously broken into pieces.

Body Part Character 4		Approach Character 5	Device Character 6	Qualifier Character 7

Ø Inferior Vena Cava
Postcava
Right inferior phrenic vein
Right ovarian vein
Right second lumbar vein
Right suprarenal vein
Right testicular vein
1 Splenic Vein
Left gastroepiploic vein
Pancreatic vein
2 Gastric Vein
3 Esophageal Vein
4 Hepatic Vein
5 Superior Mesenteric Vein
Right gastroepiploic vein
6 Inferior Mesenteric Vein
Sigmoid vein
Superior rectal vein
7 Colic Vein
Ileocolic vein
Left colic vein
Middle colic vein
Right colic vein
8 Portal Vein
Hepatic portal vein
9 Renal Vein, Right
B Renal Vein, Left
Left inferior phrenic vein
Left ovarian vein
Left second lumbar vein
Left suprarenal vein
Left testicular vein
C Common Iliac Vein, Right
D Common Iliac Vein, Left
F External Iliac Vein, Right
G External Iliac Vein, Left
	H Hypogastric Vein, Right
	Gluteal vein
	Internal iliac vein
	Internal pudendal vein
	Lateral sacral vein
	Middle hemorrhoidal vein
	Obturator vein
	Uterine vein
	Vaginal vein
	Vesical vein
	J Hypogastric Vein, Left
	See H Hypogastric Vein, Right
	M Femoral Vein, Right
	Deep femoral (profunda
	  femoris) vein
	Popliteal vein
	Profunda femoris (deep
	  femoral) vein
	N Femoral Vein, Left
	See M Femoral Vein, Right
	P Saphenous Vein, Right
	External pudendal vein
	Great(er) saphenous vein
	Lesser saphenous vein
	Small saphenous vein
	Superficial circumflex iliac vein
	Superficial epigastric vein
	Q Saphenous Vein, Left
	See P Saphenous Vein, Right
	T Foot Vein, Right
	Common digital vein
	Dorsal metatarsal vein
	Dorsal venous arch
	Plantar digital vein
	Plantar metatarsal vein
	Plantar venous arch
	V Foot Vein, Left
	See T Foot Vein, Right
	Y Lower Vein
		Ø Open
		3 Percutaneous
		4 Percutaneous Endoscopic
			Z No Device	**Z No Qualifier**

Ø   Medical and Surgical
6   Lower Veins
D   Extraction   Definition: Pulling or stripping out or off all or a portion of a body part by the use of force

Explanation: The qualifier DIAGNOSTIC is used to identify extraction procedures that are biopsies

Body Part Character 4		Approach Character 5	Device Character 6	Qualifier Character 7

M Femoral Vein, Right
Deep femoral (profunda
  femoris) vein
Popliteal vein
Profunda femoris (deep
  femoral) vein
N Femoral Vein, Left
See M Femoral Vein, Right
P Saphenous Vein, Right
External pudendal vein
Great(er) saphenous vein
Lesser saphenous vein
Small saphenous vein
Superficial circumflex iliac vein
Superficial epigastric vein
Q Saphenous Vein, Left
See P Saphenous Vein, Right
	T Foot Vein, Right
	Common digital vein
	Dorsal metatarsal vein
	Dorsal venous arch
	Plantar digital vein
	Plantar metatarsal vein
	Plantar venous arch
	V Foot Vein, Left
	See T Foot Vein, Right
	Y Lower Vein
		Ø Open
		3 Percutaneous
		4 Percutaneous Endoscopic
			Z No Device	**Z No Qualifier**

LC Limited Coverage   NC Noncovered   ⊞ Combination Member   HAC associated procedure   Combination Only   DRG Non-OR   Non-OR   New/Revised in GREEN

ICD-10-PCS 2019

259

06C–06D

0   Medical and Surgical
6   Lower Veins
H   Insertion   Definition: Putting in a nonbiological appliance that monitors, assists, performs, or prevents a physiological function but does not physically take the place of a body part

Explanation: None

Body Part Character 4		Approach Character 5	Device Character 6	Qualifier Character 7
0 Inferior Vena Cava Postcava Right inferior phrenic vein Right ovarian vein Right second lumbar vein Right suprarenal vein Right testicular vein		0 Open 3 Percutaneous	3 Infusion Device	T Via Umbilical Vein Z No Qualifier
0 Inferior Vena Cava Postcava Right inferior phrenic vein Right ovarian vein Right second lumbar vein Right suprarenal vein Right testicular vein		0 Open 3 Percutaneous	D Intraluminal Device	Z No Qualifier
0 Inferior Vena Cava Postcava Right inferior phrenic vein Right ovarian vein Right second lumbar vein Right suprarenal vein Right testicular vein		4 Percutaneous Endoscopic	3 Infusion Device D Intraluminal Device	Z No Qualifier
1 Splenic Vein 　Left gastroepiploic vein 　Pancreatic vein **2 Gastric Vein** **3 Esophageal Vein** **4 Hepatic Vein** **5 Superior Mesenteric Vein** 　Right gastroepiploic vein **6 Inferior Mesenteric Vein** 　Sigmoid vein 　Superior rectal vein **7 Colic Vein** 　Ileocolic vein 　Left colic vein 　Middle colic vein 　Right colic vein **8 Portal Vein** 　Hepatic portal vein **9 Renal Vein, Right** **B Renal Vein, Left** 　Left inferior phrenic vein 　Left ovarian vein 　Left second lumbar vein 　Left suprarenal vein 　Left testicular vein **C Common Iliac Vein, Right** **D Common Iliac Vein, Left** **F External Iliac Vein, Right** **G External Iliac Vein, Left**	**H Hypogastric Vein, Right** 　Gluteal vein 　Internal iliac vein 　Internal pudendal vein 　Lateral sacral vein 　Middle hemorrhoidal vein 　Obturator vein 　Uterine vein 　Vaginal vein 　Vesical vein **J Hypogastric Vein, Left** 　*See H Hypogastric Vein, Right* **M Femoral Vein, Right** 　Deep femoral (profunda 　　femoris) vein 　Popliteal vein 　Profunda femoris (deep 　　femoral) vein **N Femoral Vein, Left** 　*See M Femoral Vein, Right* **P Saphenous Vein, Right** 　External pudendal vein 　Great(er) saphenous vein 　Lesser saphenous vein 　Small saphenous vein 　Superficial circumflex iliac vein 　Superficial epigastric vein **Q Saphenous Vein, Left** 　*See P Saphenous Vein, Right* **T Foot Vein, Right** 　Common digital vein 　Dorsal metatarsal vein 　Dorsal venous arch 　Plantar digital vein 　Plantar metatarsal vein 　Plantar venous arch **V Foot Vein, Left** 　*See T Foot Vein, Right*	0 Open 3 Percutaneous 4 Percutaneous Endoscopic	3 Infusion Device D Intraluminal Device	Z No Qualifier
Y Lower Vein		0 Open 3 Percutaneous 4 Percutaneous Endoscopic	2 Monitoring Device 3 Infusion Device D Intraluminal Device Y Other Device	Z No Qualifier

Non-OR	06H0[0,3]3[T,Z]
Non-OR	06H03DZ
Non-OR	06H043Z
Non-OR	06H[1,2,3,4,5,6,7,8,9,B,C,D,F,G,H,J,M,N,P,Q,T,V][0,3,4]3Z
Non-OR	06HY[0,3,4]3Z
Non-OR	06HY32Z
Non-OR	06HY[3,4]YZ

LG Limited Coverage   NC Noncovered   ⊞ Combination Member   HAC associated procedure   Combination Only   DRG Non-OR   Non-OR   New/Revised in GREEN

0   **Medical and Surgical**
6   **Lower Veins**
J   **Inspection**   Definition: Visually and/or manually exploring a body part

Explanation: Visual exploration may be performed with or without optical instrumentation. Manual exploration may be performed directly or through intervening body layers.

Body Part Character 4	Approach Character 5	Device Character 6	Qualifier Character 7
Y Lower Vein	0 Open 3 Percutaneous 4 Percutaneous Endoscopic X External	Z No Device	Z No Qualifier

Non-OR   06JY[3,X]ZZ

---

0   **Medical and Surgical**
6   **Lower Veins**
L   **Occlusion**   Definition: Completely closing an orifice or the lumen of a tubular body part

Explanation: The orifice can be a natural orifice or an artificially created orifice

Body Part Character 4	Approach Character 5	Device Character 6	Qualifier Character 7

0 **Inferior Vena Cava**
   Postcava
   Right inferior phrenic vein
   Right ovarian vein
   Right second lumbar vein
   Right suprarenal vein
   Right testicular vein
1 **Splenic Vein**
   Left gastroepiploic vein
   Pancreatic vein
2 **Gastric Vein**
4 **Hepatic Vein**
5 **Superior Mesenteric Vein**
   Right gastroepiploic vein
6 **Inferior Mesenteric Vein**
   Sigmoid vein
   Superior rectal vein
7 **Colic Vein**
   Ileocolic vein
   Left colic vein
   Middle colic vein
   Right colic vein
8 **Portal Vein**
   Hepatic portal vein
9 **Renal Vein, Right**
B **Renal Vein, Left**
   Left inferior phrenic vein
   Left ovarian vein
   Left second lumbar vein
   Left suprarenal vein
   Left testicular vein
C **Common Iliac Vein, Right**
D **Common Iliac Vein, Left**
F **External Iliac Vein, Right**
G **External Iliac Vein, Left**
 	
H **Hypogastric Vein, Right**
   Gluteal vein
   Internal iliac vein
   Internal pudendal vein
   Lateral sacral vein
   Middle hemorrhoidal vein
   Obturator vein
   Uterine vein
   Vaginal vein
   Vesical vein
J **Hypogastric Vein, Left**
   See H Hypogastric Vein, Right
M **Femoral Vein, Right**
   Deep femoral (profunda
     femoris) vein
   Popliteal vein
   Profunda femoris (deep
     femoral) vein
N **Femoral Vein, Left**
   See M Femoral Vein, Right
P **Saphenous Vein, Right**
   External pudendal vein
   Great(er) saphenous vein
   Lesser saphenous vein
   Small saphenous vein
   Superficial circumflex iliac vein
   Superficial epigastric vein
Q **Saphenous Vein, Left**
   See P Saphenous Vein, Right
T **Foot Vein, Right**
   Common digital vein
   Dorsal metatarsal vein
   Dorsal venous arch
   Plantar digital vein
   Plantar metatarsal vein
   Plantar venous arch
V **Foot Vein, Left**
   See T Foot Vein, Right
	0 Open
	3 Percutaneous
	4 Percutaneous Endoscopic
		C Extraluminal Device
		D Intraluminal Device
		Z No Device
			Z No Qualifier

3 **Esophageal Vein**	0 Open
	3 Percutaneous
	4 Percutaneous Endoscopic
	7 Via Natural or Artificial
	   Opening
	8 Via Natural or Artificial
	   Opening Endoscopic
		C Extraluminal Device
		D Intraluminal Device
		Z No Device
			Z No Qualifier

Y **Lower Vein**	0 Open 3 Percutaneous 4 Percutaneous Endoscopic	C Extraluminal Device D Intraluminal Device Z No Device	C Hemorrhoidal Plexus Z No Qualifier

Non-OR   06L3[3,4,7,8][C,D,Z]Z

LC Limited Coverage   NC Noncovered   ⊞ Combination Member   HAC associated procedure   Combination Only   DRG Non-OR   Non-OR   New/Revised in GREEN

ICD-10-PCS 2019   261

06J–06L

Lower Veins

0   **Medical and Surgical**
6   **Lower Veins**
N   **Release**

Definition: Freeing a body part from an abnormal physical constraint by cutting or by the use of force

Explanation: Some of the restraining tissue may be taken out but none of the body part is taken out

Body Part Character 4		Approach Character 5	Device Character 6	Qualifier Character 7
0 Inferior Vena Cava Postcava Right inferior phrenic vein Right ovarian vein Right second lumbar vein Right suprarenal vein Right testicular vein **1** Splenic Vein Left gastroepiploic vein Pancreatic vein **2** Gastric Vein **3** Esophageal Vein **4** Hepatic Vein **5** Superior Mesenteric Vein Right gastroepiploic vein **6** Inferior Mesenteric Vein Sigmoid vein Superior rectal vein **7** Colic Vein Ileocolic vein Left colic vein Middle colic vein Right colic vein **8** Portal Vein Hepatic portal vein **9** Renal Vein, Right **B** Renal Vein, Left Left inferior phrenic vein Left ovarian vein Left second lumbar vein Left suprarenal vein Left testicular vein **C** Common Iliac Vein, Right **D** Common Iliac Vein, Left **F** External Iliac Vein, Right **G** External Iliac Vein, Left	**H** Hypogastric Vein, Right Gluteal vein Internal iliac vein Internal pudendal vein Lateral sacral vein Middle hemorrhoidal vein Obturator vein Uterine vein Vaginal vein Vesical vein **J** Hypogastric Vein, Left *See H Hypogastric Vein, Right* **M** Femoral Vein, Right Deep femoral (profunda femoris) vein Popliteal vein Profunda femoris (deep femoral) vein **N** Femoral Vein, Left *See M Femoral Vein, Right* **P** Saphenous Vein, Right External pudendal vein Great(er) saphenous vein Lesser saphenous vein Small saphenous vein Superficial circumflex iliac vein Superficial epigastric vein **Q** Saphenous Vein, Left *See P Saphenous Vein, Right* **T** Foot Vein, Right Common digital vein Dorsal metatarsal vein Dorsal venous arch Plantar digital vein Plantar metatarsal vein Plantar venous arch **V** Foot Vein, Left *See T Foot Vein, Right* **Y** Lower Vein	**0** Open **3** Percutaneous **4** Percutaneous Endoscopic	**Z** No Device	**Z** No Qualifier

0   **Medical and Surgical**
6   **Lower Veins**
P   **Removal**

Definition: Taking out or off a device from a body part

Explanation: If a device is taken out and a similar device put in without cutting or puncturing the skin or mucous membrane, the procedure is coded to the root operation CHANGE. Otherwise, the procedure for taking out a device is coded to the root operation REMOVAL.

Body Part Character 4	Approach Character 5	Device Character 6	Qualifier Character 7
Y Lower Vein	**0** Open **3** Percutaneous **4** Percutaneous Endoscopic	**0** Drainage Device **2** Monitoring Device **3** Infusion Device **7** Autologous Tissue Substitute **C** Extraluminal Device **D** Intraluminal Device **J** Synthetic Substitute **K** Nonautologous Tissue Substitute **Y** Other Device	**Z** No Qualifier
Y Lower Vein	**X** External	**0** Drainage Device **2** Monitoring Device **3** Infusion Device **D** Intraluminal Device	**Z** No Qualifier

Non-OR	06PY3[0,2,3]Z
Non-OR	06PY[3,4]YZ
Non-OR	06PYX[0,2,3,D]Z

LC Limited Coverage   NC Noncovered   ⊞ Combination Member   HAC associated procedure   Combination Only   DRG Non-OR   Non-OR   New/Revised in GREEN

262   ICD-10-PCS 2019

0   **Medical and Surgical**
6   **Lower Veins**
Q   **Repair**   Definition: Restoring, to the extent possible, a body part to its normal anatomic structure and function
                          Explanation: Used only when the method to accomplish the repair is not one of the other root operations

Body Part Character 4	Approach Character 5	Device Character 6	Qualifier Character 7

0 **Inferior Vena Cava**
   Postcava
   Right inferior phrenic vein
   Right ovarian vein
   Right second lumbar vein
   Right suprarenal vein
   Right testicular vein
1 **Splenic Vein**
   Left gastroepiploic vein
   Pancreatic vein
2 **Gastric Vein**
3 **Esophageal Vein**
4 **Hepatic Vein**
5 **Superior Mesenteric Vein**
   Right gastroepiploic vein
6 **Inferior Mesenteric Vein**
   Sigmoid vein
   Superior rectal vein
7 **Colic Vein**
   Ileocolic vein
   Left colic vein
   Middle colic vein
   Right colic vein
8 **Portal Vein**
   Hepatic portal vein
9 **Renal Vein, Right**
B **Renal Vein, Left**
   Left inferior phrenic vein
   Left ovarian vein
   Left second lumbar vein
   Left suprarenal vein
   Left testicular vein
C **Common Iliac Vein, Right**
D **Common Iliac Vein, Left**
F **External Iliac Vein, Right**
G **External Iliac Vein, Left**
H **Hypogastric Vein, Right**
   Gluteal vein
   Internal iliac vein
   Internal pudendal vein
   Lateral sacral vein
   Middle hemorrhoidal vein
   Obturator vein
   Uterine vein
   Vaginal vein
   Vesical vein
J **Hypogastric Vein, Left**
   See H Hypogastric Vein, Right
M **Femoral Vein, Right**
   Deep femoral (profunda femoris) vein
   Popliteal vein
   Profunda femoris (deep femoral) vein
N **Femoral Vein, Left**
   See M Femoral Vein, Right
P **Saphenous Vein, Right**
   External pudendal vein
   Great(er) saphenous vein
   Lesser saphenous vein
   Small saphenous vein
   Superficial circumflex iliac vein
   Superficial epigastric vein
Q **Saphenous Vein, Left**
   See P Saphenous Vein, Right
T **Foot Vein, Right**
   Common digital vein
   Dorsal metatarsal vein
   Dorsal venous arch
   Plantar digital vein
   Plantar metatarsal vein
   Plantar venous arch
V **Foot Vein, Left**
   See T Foot Vein, Right
Y **Lower Vein**
	0 Open
	3 Percutaneous
	4 Percutaneous Endoscopic
		Z No Device	**Z** No Qualifier

LC Limited Coverage   **NC** Noncovered   ⊞ Combination Member   HAC associated procedure   Combination Only   DRG Non-OR   Non-OR   New/Revised in GREEN

ICD-10-PCS 2019   **263**

06Q–06Q

Ø   Medical and Surgical
6   Lower Veins
R   Replacement   Definition: Putting in or on biological or synthetic material that physically takes the place and/or function of all or a portion of a body part
                                 Explanation: The body part may have been taken out or replaced, or may be taken out, physically eradicated, or rendered nonfunctional during
                                 the REPLACEMENT procedure. A REMOVAL procedure is coded for taking out the device used in a previous replacement procedure.

Body Part Character 4	Approach Character 5	Device Character 6	Qualifier Character 7
Ø Inferior Vena Cava Postcava Right inferior phrenic vein Right ovarian vein Right second lumbar vein Right suprarenal vein Right testicular vein	**Ø Open** **4 Percutaneous Endoscopic**	**7 Autologous Tissue Substitute** **J Synthetic Substitute** **K Nonautologous Tissue Substitute**	**Z No Qualifier**
1 Splenic Vein Left gastroepiploic vein Pancreatic vein			
2 Gastric Vein			
3 Esophageal Vein			
4 Hepatic Vein			
5 Superior Mesenteric Vein Right gastroepiploic vein			
6 Inferior Mesenteric Vein Sigmoid vein Superior rectal vein			
7 Colic Vein Ileocolic vein Left colic vein Middle colic vein Right colic vein			
8 Portal Vein Hepatic portal vein			
9 Renal Vein, Right			
B Renal Vein, Left Left inferior phrenic vein Left ovarian vein Left second lumbar vein Left suprarenal vein Left testicular vein			
C Common Iliac Vein, Right			
D Common Iliac Vein, Left			
F External Iliac Vein, Right			
G External Iliac Vein, Left			
H Hypogastric Vein, Right Gluteal vein Internal iliac vein Internal pudendal vein Lateral sacral vein Middle hemorrhoidal vein Obturator vein Uterine vein Vaginal vein Vesical vein			
J Hypogastric Vein, Left *See H Hypogastric Vein, Right*			
M Femoral Vein, Right Deep femoral (profunda femoris) vein Popliteal vein Profunda femoris (deep femoral) vein			
N Femoral Vein, Left *See M Femoral Vein, Right*			
P Saphenous Vein, Right External pudendal vein Great(er) saphenous vein Lesser saphenous vein Small saphenous vein Superficial circumflex iliac vein Superficial epigastric vein			
Q Saphenous Vein, Left *See P Saphenous Vein, Right*			
T Foot Vein, Right Common digital vein Dorsal metatarsal vein Dorsal venous arch Plantar digital vein Plantar metatarsal vein Plantar venous arch			
V Foot Vein, Left *See T Foot Vein, Right*			
Y Lower Vein			

Ø **Medical and Surgical**
6 **Lower Veins**
S **Reposition** Definition: Moving to its normal location, or other suitable location, all or a portion of a body part
Explanation: The body part is moved to a new location from an abnormal location, or from a normal location where it is not functioning correctly. The body part may or may not be cut out or off to be moved to the new location.

Body Part Character 4	Approach Character 5	Device Character 6	Qualifier Character 7
Ø Inferior Vena Cava Postcava Right inferior phrenic vein Right ovarian vein Right second lumbar vein Right suprarenal vein Right testicular vein	**Ø** Open **3** Percutaneous **4** Percutaneous Endoscopic	**Z** No Device	**Z** No Qualifier
1 Splenic Vein Left gastroepiploic vein Pancreatic vein			
2 Gastric Vein			
3 Esophageal Vein			
4 Hepatic Vein			
5 Superior Mesenteric Vein Right gastroepiploic vein			
6 Inferior Mesenteric Vein Sigmoid vein Superior rectal vein			
7 Colic Vein Ileocolic vein Left colic vein Middle colic vein Right colic vein			
8 Portal Vein Hepatic portal vein			
9 Renal Vein, Right			
B Renal Vein, Left Left inferior phrenic vein Left ovarian vein Left second lumbar vein Left suprarenal vein Left testicular vein			
C Common Iliac Vein, Right			
D Common Iliac Vein, Left			
F External Iliac Vein, Right			
G External Iliac Vein, Left			
H Hypogastric Vein, Right Gluteal vein Internal iliac vein Internal pudendal vein Lateral sacral vein Middle hemorrhoidal vein Obturator vein Uterine vein Vaginal vein Vesical vein			
J Hypogastric Vein, Left *See H Hypogastric Vein, Right*			
M Femoral Vein, Right Deep femoral (profunda femoris) vein Popliteal vein Profunda femoris (deep femoral) vein			
N Femoral Vein, Left *See M Femoral Vein, Right*			
P Saphenous Vein, Right External pudendal vein Great(er) saphenous vein Lesser saphenous vein Small saphenous vein Superficial circumflex iliac vein Superficial epigastric vein			
Q Saphenous Vein, Left *See P Saphenous Vein, Right*			
T Foot Vein, Right Common digital vein Dorsal metatarsal vein Dorsal venous arch Plantar digital vein Plantar metatarsal vein Plantar venous arch			
V Foot Vein, Left *See T Foot Vein, Right*			
Y Lower Vein			

Ø   Medical and Surgical
6   Lower Veins
U   Supplement   Definition: Putting in or on biological or synthetic material that physically reinforces and/or augments the function of a portion of a body part
                  Explanation: The biological material is non-living, or is living and from the same individual. The body part may have been previously replaced, and the SUPPLEMENT procedure is performed to physically reinforce and/or augment the function of the replaced body part.

Body Part Character 4	Approach Character 5	Device Character 6	Qualifier Character 7

Ø Inferior Vena Cava
   Postcava
   Right inferior phrenic vein
   Right ovarian vein
   Right second lumbar vein
   Right suprarenal vein
   Right testicular vein
1 Splenic Vein
   Left gastroepiploic vein
   Pancreatic vein
2 Gastric Vein
3 Esophageal Vein
4 Hepatic Vein
5 Superior Mesenteric Vein
   Right gastroepiploic vein
6 Inferior Mesenteric Vein
   Sigmoid vein
   Superior rectal vein
7 Colic Vein
   Ileocolic vein
   Left colic vein
   Middle colic vein
   Right colic vein
8 Portal Vein
   Hepatic portal vein
9 Renal Vein, Right
B Renal Vein, Left
   Left inferior phrenic vein
   Left ovarian vein
   Left second lumbar vein
   Left suprarenal vein
   Left testicular vein
C Common Iliac Vein, Right
D Common Iliac Vein, Left
F External Iliac Vein, Right
G External Iliac Vein, Left
H Hypogastric Vein, Right
   Gluteal vein
   Internal iliac vein
   Internal pudendal vein
   Lateral sacral vein
   Middle hemorrhoidal vein
   Obturator vein
   Uterine vein
   Vaginal vein
   Vesical vein
J Hypogastric Vein, Left
   See H Hypogastric Vein, Right
M Femoral Vein, Right
   Deep femoral (profunda femoris) vein
   Popliteal vein
   Profunda femoris (deep femoral) vein
N Femoral Vein, Left
   See M Femoral Vein, Right
P Saphenous Vein, Right
   External pudendal vein
   Great(er) saphenous vein
   Lesser saphenous vein
   Small saphenous vein
   Superficial circumflex iliac vein
   Superficial epigastric vein
Q Saphenous Vein, Left
   See P Saphenous Vein, Right
T Foot Vein, Right
   Common digital vein
   Dorsal metatarsal vein
   Dorsal venous arch
   Plantar digital vein
   Plantar metatarsal vein
   Plantar venous arch
V Foot Vein, Left
   See T Foot Vein, Right
Y Lower Vein
	Ø Open
	3 Percutaneous
	4 Percutaneous Endoscopic
		7 Autologous Tissue Substitute
		J Synthetic Substitute
		K Nonautologous Tissue Substitute
			Z No Qualifier

LC Limited Coverage   NC Noncovered   ⊞ Combination Member   HAC associated procedure   Combination Only   DRG Non-OR   Non-OR   New/Revised in GREEN

266   ICD-10-PCS 2019

06U–06U

0   Medical and Surgical
6   Lower Veins
V   Restriction   Definition: Partially closing an orifice or the lumen of a tubular body part
                      Explanation: The orifice can be a natural orifice or an artificially created orifice

Body Part Character 4	Approach Character 5	Device Character 6	Qualifier Character 7
0 **Inferior Vena Cava** Postcava Right inferior phrenic vein Right ovarian vein Right second lumbar vein Right suprarenal vein Right testicular vein **1** **Splenic Vein** Left gastroepiploic vein Pancreatic vein **2** **Gastric Vein** **3** **Esophageal Vein** **4** **Hepatic Vein** **5** **Superior Mesenteric Vein** Right gastroepiploic vein **6** **Inferior Mesenteric Vein** Sigmoid vein Superior rectal vein **7** **Colic Vein** Ileocolic vein Left colic vein Middle colic vein Right colic vein **8** **Portal Vein** Hepatic portal vein **9** **Renal Vein, Right** **B** **Renal Vein, Left** Left inferior phrenic vein Left ovarian vein Left second lumbar vein Left suprarenal vein Left testicular vein **C** **Common Iliac Vein, Right** **D** **Common Iliac Vein, Left** **F** **External Iliac Vein, Right** **G** **External Iliac Vein, Left** **H** **Hypogastric Vein, Right** Gluteal vein Internal iliac vein Internal pudendal vein Lateral sacral vein Middle hemorrhoidal vein Obturator vein Uterine vein Vaginal vein Vesical vein **J** **Hypogastric Vein, Left** *See H Hypogastric Vein, Right* **M** **Femoral Vein, Right** Deep femoral (profunda femoris) vein Popliteal vein Profunda femoris (deep femoral) vein **N** **Femoral Vein, Left** *See M Femoral Vein, Right* **P** **Saphenous Vein, Right** External pudendal vein Great(er) saphenous vein Lesser saphenous vein Small saphenous vein Superficial circumflex iliac vein Superficial epigastric vein **Q** **Saphenous Vein, Left** *See P Saphenous Vein, Right* **T** **Foot Vein, Right** Common digital vein Dorsal metatarsal vein Dorsal venous arch Plantar digital vein Plantar metatarsal vein Plantar venous arch **V** **Foot Vein, Left** *See T Foot Vein, Right* **Y** **Lower Vein**	**0** Open **3** Percutaneous **4** Percutaneous Endoscopic	**C** Extraluminal Device **D** Intraluminal Device **Z** No Device	**Z** No Qualifier

LC Limited Coverage   **NC** Noncovered   ⊞ Combination Member   HAC associated procedure   Combination Only   DRG Non-OR   Non-OR   New/Revised in GREEN
ICD-10-PCS 2019   267

06V–06V

0   Medical and Surgical
6   Lower Veins
W   Revision

Definition: Correcting, to the extent possible, a portion of a malfunctioning device or the position of a displaced device

Explanation: Revision can include correcting a malfunctioning or displaced device by taking out or putting in components of the device such as a screw or pin

Body Part Character 4	Approach Character 5	Device Character 6	Qualifier Character 7
Y Lower Vein	0 Open 3 Percutaneous 4 Percutaneous Endoscopic	0 Drainage Device 2 Monitoring Device 3 Infusion Device 7 Autologous Tissue Substitute C Extraluminal Device D Intraluminal Device J Synthetic Substitute K Nonautologous Tissue Substitute Y Other Device	Z No Qualifier
Y Lower Vein	X External	0 Drainage Device 2 Monitoring Device 3 Infusion Device 7 Autologous Tissue Substitute C Extraluminal Device D Intraluminal Device J Synthetic Substitute K Nonautologous Tissue Substitute	Z No Qualifier

Non-OR   06WY3[0,2,3,D]Z
Non-OR   06WY[3,4]YZ
Non-OR   06WYX[0,2,3,7,C,D,J,K]Z

LC Limited Coverage   NC Noncovered   ⊞ Combination Member   HAC associated procedure   Combination Only   DRG Non-OR   Non-OR   New/Revised in GREEN

268   ICD-10-PCS 2019

Lymphatic and Hemic Systems Ø72–Ø7Y

Character Meanings*

This Character Meaning table is provided as a guide to assist the user in the identification of character members that may be found in this section of code tables. It **SHOULD NOT** be used to build a PCS code.

Operation–Character 3		Body Part–Character 4		Approach–Character 5		Device–Character 6		Qualifier–Character 7	
2	Change	Ø	Lymphatic, Head	Ø	Open	Ø	Drainage Device	Ø	Allogeneic
5	Destruction	1	Lymphatic, Right Neck	3	Percutaneous	3	Infusion Device	1	Syngeneic
9	Drainage	2	Lymphatic, Left Neck	4	Percutaneous Endoscopic	7	Autologous Tissue Substitute	2	Zooplastic
B	Excision	3	Lymphatic, Right Upper Extremity	8	Via Natural or Artificial Opening Endoscopic	C	Extraluminal Device	X	Diagnostic
C	Extirpation	4	Lymphatic, Left Upper Extremity	X	External	D	Intraluminal Device	Z	No Qualifier
D	Extraction	5	Lymphatic, Right Axillary			J	Synthetic Substitute		
H	Insertion	6	Lymphatic, Left Axillary			K	Nonautologous Tissue Substitute		
J	Inspection	7	Lymphatic, Thorax			Y	Other Device		
L	Occlusion	8	Lymphatic, Internal Mammary, Right			Z	No Device		
N	Release	9	Lymphatic, Internal Mammary, Left						
P	Removal	B	Lymphatic, Mesenteric						
Q	Repair	C	Lymphatic, Pelvis						
S	Reposition	D	Lymphatic, Aortic						
T	Resection	F	Lymphatic, Right Lower Extremity						
U	Supplement	G	Lymphatic, Left Lower Extremity						
V	Restriction	H	Lymphatic, Right Inguinal						
W	Revision	J	Lymphatic, Left Inguinal						
Y	Transplantation	K	Thoracic Duct						
		L	Cisterna Chyli						
		M	Thymus						
		N	Lymphatic						
		P	Spleen						
		Q	Bone Marrow, Sternum						
		R	Bone Marrow, Iliac						
		S	Bone Marrow, Vertebral						
		T	Bone Marrow						

* Includes lymph vessels and lymph nodes.

AHA Coding Clinic for table Ø79
2017, 1Q, 34	Lymphovenous bypass following mastectomy
2014, 1Q, 26	Transbronchial needle aspiration lymph node biopsy
2013, 4Q, 111	Transbronchial needle aspiration lymph node biopsy

AHA Coding Clinic for table Ø7B
2018, 1Q, 22	Resection of lymph node chains
2016, 1Q, 30	Axillary lymph node resection with modified radical mastectomy
2014, 3Q, 10	Selective excision of paratracheal lymph nodes
2014, 1Q, 20	Fiducial marker placement
2014, 1Q, 26	Transbronchial endoscopic lymph node aspiration biopsy

AHA Coding Clinic for table Ø7D
| 2013, 4Q, 111 | Root operation for bone marrow biopsy |

AHA Coding Clinic for table Ø7Q
| 2017, 1Q, 34 | Lymphovenous bypass following mastectomy |

AHA Coding Clinic for table Ø7T
2018, 1Q, 22	Resection of lymph node chains
2016, 2Q, 12	Resection of malignant neoplasm of infratemporal fossa
2016, 1Q, 30	Axillary lymph node resection with modified radical mastectomy
2015, 4Q, 13	New Section X codes—New Technology procedures
2014, 3Q, 9	Radical resection of level I lymph nodes
2014, 3Q, 16	Repair of Tetralogy of Fallot

Lymphatic System

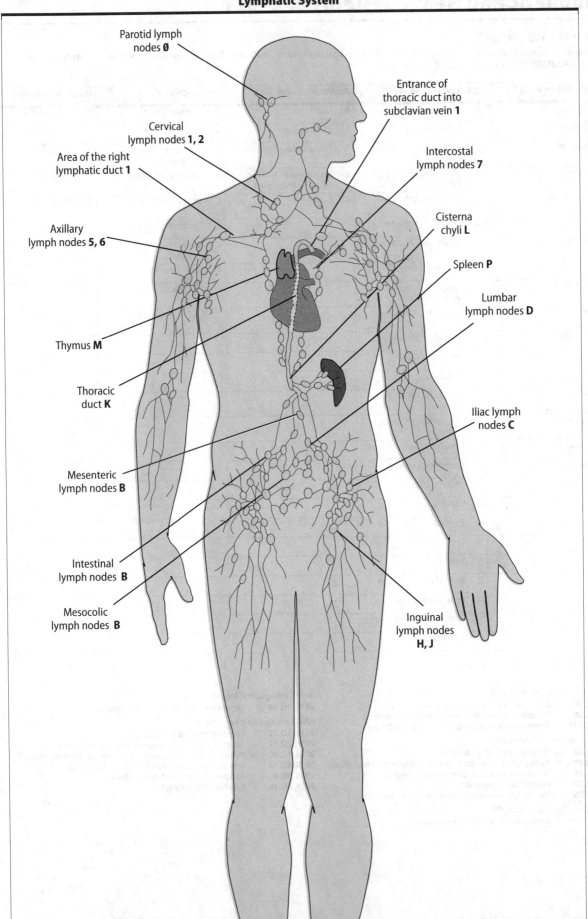

Parotid lymph nodes Ø

Cervical lymph nodes 1, 2

Area of the right lymphatic duct 1

Axillary lymph nodes 5, 6

Thymus M

Thoracic duct K

Mesenteric lymph nodes B

Intestinal lymph nodes B

Mesocolic lymph nodes B

Entrance of thoracic duct into subclavian vein 1

Intercostal lymph nodes 7

Cisterna chyli L

Spleen P

Lumbar lymph nodes D

Iliac lymph nodes C

Inguinal lymph nodes H, J

Ø   Medical and Surgical
7   Lymphatic and Hemic Systems
2   Change   Definition: Taking out or off a device from a body part and putting back an identical or similar device in or on the same body part without cutting or puncturing the skin or a mucous membrane

          Explanation: All CHANGE procedures are coded using the approach EXTERNAL

Body Part Character 4		Approach Character 5	Device Character 6	Qualifier Character 7

K Thoracic Duct
   Left jugular trunk
   Left subclavian trunk
L Cisterna Chyli
   Intestinal lymphatic trunk
   Lumbar lymphatic trunk
	M Thymus
	   Thymus gland
	N Lymphatic
	P Spleen
	   Accessory spleen
	T Bone Marrow
		X External	**Ø** Drainage Device
			Y Other Device
				Z No Qualifier

Non-OR   All body part, approach, device, and qualifier values

Ø   Medical and Surgical
7   Lymphatic and Hemic Systems
5   Destruction   Definition: Physical eradication of all or a portion of a body part by the direct use of energy, force, or a destructive agent

          Explanation: None of the body part is physically taken out

Body Part Character 4		Approach Character 5	Device Character 6	Qualifier Character 7

Ø Lymphatic, Head
   Buccinator lymph node
   Infraauricular lymph node
   Infraparotid lymph node
   Parotid lymph node
   Preauricular lymph node
   Submandibular lymph node
   Submaxillary lymph node
   Submental lymph node
   Subparotid lymph node
   Suprahyoid lymph node
1 Lymphatic, Right Neck
   Cervical lymph node
   Jugular lymph node
   Mastoid (postauricular) lymph node
   Occipital lymph node
   Postauricular (mastoid) lymph node
   Retropharyngeal lymph node
   Right jugular trunk
   Right lymphatic duct
   Right subclavian trunk
   Supraclavicular (Virchow's) lymph node
   Virchow's (supraclavicular) lymph node
2 Lymphatic, Left Neck
   Cervical lymph node
   Jugular lymph node
   Mastoid (postauricular) lymph node
   Occipital lymph node
   Postauricular (mastoid) lymph node
   Retropharyngeal lymph node
   Supraclavicular (Virchow's) lymph node
   Virchow's (supraclavicular) lymph node
3 Lymphatic, Right Upper Extremity
   Cubital lymph node
   Deltopectoral (infraclavicular) lymph
     node
   Epitrochlear lymph node
   Infraclavicular (deltopectoral) lymph
     node
   Supratrochlear lymph node
4 Lymphatic, Left Upper Extremity
   See 3 Lymphatic, Right Upper Extremity
5 Lymphatic, Right Axillary
   Anterior (pectoral) lymph node
   Apical (subclavicular) lymph node
   Brachial (lateral) lymph node
   Central axillary lymph node
   Lateral (brachial) lymph node
   Pectoral (anterior) lymph node
   Posterior (subscapular) lymph node
   Subclavicular (apical) lymph node
   Subscapular (posterior) lymph node
	6 Lymphatic, Left Axillary
	   See 5 Lymphatic, Right Axillary
	7 Lymphatic, Thorax
	   Intercostal lymph node
	   Mediastinal lymph node
	   Parasternal lymph node
	   Paratracheal lymph node
	   Tracheobronchial lymph node
	8 Lymphatic, Internal Mammary, Right
	9 Lymphatic, Internal Mammary, Left
	B Lymphatic, Mesenteric
	   Inferior mesenteric lymph node
	   Pararectal lymph node
	   Superior mesenteric lymph node
	C Lymphatic, Pelvis
	   Common iliac (subaortic) lymph node
	   Gluteal lymph node
	   Iliac lymph node
	   Inferior epigastric lymph node
	   Obturator lymph node
	   Sacral lymph node
	   Subaortic (common iliac) lymph node
	   Suprainguinal lymph node
	D Lymphatic, Aortic
	   Celiac lymph node
	   Gastric lymph node
	   Hepatic lymph node
	   Lumbar lymph node
	   Pancreaticosplenic lymph node
	   Paraaortic lymph node
	   Retroperitoneal lymph node
	F Lymphatic, Right Lower Extremity
	   Femoral lymph node
	   Popliteal lymph node
	G Lymphatic, Left Lower Extremity
	   See F Lymphatic, Right Lower Extremity
	H Lymphatic, Right Inguinal
	J Lymphatic, Left Inguinal
	K Thoracic Duct
	   Left jugular trunk
	   Left subclavian trunk
	L Cisterna Chyli
	   Intestinal lymphatic trunk
	   Lumbar lymphatic trunk
	M Thymus
	   Thymus gland
	P Spleen
	   Accessory spleen
		Ø Open
		3 Percutaneous
		4 Percutaneous
		   Endoscopic
			Z No Device	**Z** No Qualifier

LC Limited Coverage   **NC** Noncovered   ⊞ Combination Member   HAC associated procedure   Combination Only   DRG Non-OR   Non-OR   New/Revised in GREEN

ICD-10-PCS 2019   271

Ø   Medical and Surgical
7   Lymphatic and Hemic Systems
9   Drainage   Definition: Taking or letting out fluids and/or gases from a body part
                 Explanation: The qualifier DIAGNOSTIC is used to identify drainage procedures that are biopsies

Body Part Character 4		Approach Character 5	Device Character 6	Qualifier Character 7

Ø Lymphatic, Head
  Buccinator lymph node
  Infraauricular lymph node
  Infraparotid lymph node
  Parotid lymph node
  Preauricular lymph node
  Submandibular lymph node
  Submaxillary lymph node
  Submental lymph node
  Subparotid lymph node
  Suprahyoid lymph node
1 Lymphatic, Right Neck
  Cervical lymph node
  Jugular lymph node
  Mastoid (postauricular) lymph node
  Occipital lymph node
  Postauricular (mastoid) lymph node
  Retropharyngeal lymph node
  Right jugular trunk
  Right lymphatic duct
  Right subclavian trunk
  Supraclavicular (Virchow's) lymph
    node
  Virchow's (supraclavicular) lymph
    node
2 Lymphatic, Left Neck
  Cervical lymph node
  Jugular lymph node
  Mastoid (postauricular) lymph node
  Occipital lymph node
  Postauricular (mastoid) lymph node
  Retropharyngeal lymph node
  Supraclavicular (Virchow's) lymph
    node
  Virchow's (supraclavicular) lymph
    node
3 Lymphatic, Right Upper Extremity
  Cubital lymph node
  Deltopectoral (infraclavicular) lymph
    node
  Epitrochlear lymph node
  Infraclavicular (deltopectoral) lymph
    node
  Supratrochlear lymph node
4 Lymphatic, Left Upper Extremity
  See 3 Lymphatic, Right Upper Extremity
5 Lymphatic, Right Axillary
  Anterior (pectoral) lymph node
  Apical (subclavicular) lymph node
  Brachial (lateral) lymph node
  Central axillary lymph node
  Lateral (brachial) lymph node
  Pectoral (anterior) lymph node
  Posterior (subscapular) lymph node
  Subclavicular (apical) lymph node
  Subscapular (posterior) lymph node
	6 Lymphatic, Left Axillary
	  See 5 Lymphatic, Right Axillary
	7 Lymphatic, Thorax
	  Intercostal lymph node
	  Mediastinal lymph node
	  Parasternal lymph node
	  Paratracheal lymph node
	  Tracheobronchial lymph node
	8 Lymphatic, Internal Mammary, Right
	9 Lymphatic, Internal Mammary, Left
	B Lymphatic, Mesenteric
	  Inferior mesenteric lymph node
	  Pararectal lymph node
	  Superior mesenteric lymph node
	C Lymphatic, Pelvis
	  Common iliac (subaortic) lymph node
	  Gluteal lymph node
	  Iliac lymph node
	  Inferior epigastric lymph node
	  Obturator lymph node
	  Sacral lymph node
	  Subaortic (common iliac) lymph node
	  Suprainguinal lymph node
	D Lymphatic, Aortic
	  Celiac lymph node
	  Gastric lymph node
	  Hepatic lymph node
	  Lumbar lymph node
	  Pancreaticosplenic lymph node
	  Paraaortic lymph node
	  Retroperitoneal lymph node
	F Lymphatic, Right Lower Extremity
	  Femoral lymph node
	  Popliteal lymph node
	G Lymphatic, Left Lower Extremity
	  See F Lymphatic, Right Lower Extremity
	H Lymphatic, Right Inguinal
	J Lymphatic, Left Inguinal
	K Thoracic Duct
	  Left jugular trunk
	  Left subclavian trunk
	L Cisterna Chyli
	  Intestinal lymphatic trunk
	  Lumbar lymphatic trunk
		Ø Open
		3 Percutaneous
		4 Percutaneous
		  Endoscopic
		8 Via Natural or
		  Artificial Opening
		  Endoscopic
			Ø Drainage Device	**Z No Qualifier**

Ø79 Continued on next page

Non-OR	Ø79[Ø,1,2,3,4,5,6,7,8,9,B,C,D,F,G,H,J,K,L][3,8]ØZ

LC Limited Coverage   NC Noncovered   ⊞ Combination Member   HAC associated procedure   Combination Only   DRG Non-OR   Non-OR   New/Revised in GREEN

272   ICD-10-PCS 2019

Ø   Medical and Surgical
7   Lymphatic and Hemic Systems   *079 Continued*
9   Drainage   Definition: Taking or letting out fluids and/or gases from a body part
                       Explanation: The qualifier DIAGNOSTIC is used to identify drainage procedures that are biopsies

Body Part Character 4		Approach Character 5	Device Character 6	Qualifier Character 7

Ø Lymphatic, Head
Buccinator lymph node
Infraauricular lymph node
Infraparotid lymph node
Parotid lymph node
Preauricular lymph node
Submandibular lymph node
Submaxillary lymph node
Submental lymph node
Subparotid lymph node
Suprahyoid lymph node
1 Lymphatic, Right Neck
Cervical lymph node
Jugular lymph node
Mastoid (postauricular) lymph node
Occipital lymph node
Postauricular (mastoid) lymph node
Retropharyngeal lymph node
Right jugular trunk
Right lymphatic duct
Right subclavian trunk
Supraclavicular (Virchow's) lymph
   node
Virchow's (supraclavicular) lymph
   node
2 Lymphatic, Left Neck
Cervical lymph node
Jugular lymph node
Mastoid (postauricular) lymph node
Occipital lymph node
Postauricular (mastoid) lymph node
Retropharyngeal lymph node
Supraclavicular (Virchow's) lymph
   node
Virchow's (supraclavicular) lymph
   node
3 Lymphatic, Right Upper Extremity
Cubital lymph node
Deltopectoral (infraclavicular) lymph
   node
Epitrochlear lymph node
Infraclavicular (deltopectoral) lymph
   node
Supratrochlear lymph node
4 Lymphatic, Left Upper Extremity
See 3 Lymphatic, Right Upper Extremity
5 Lymphatic, Right Axillary
Anterior (pectoral) lymph node
Apical (subclavicular) lymph node
Brachial (lateral) lymph node
Central axillary lymph node
Lateral (brachial) lymph node
Pectoral (anterior) lymph node
Posterior (subscapular) lymph node
Subclavicular (apical) lymph node
Subscapular (posterior) lymph node
	6 Lymphatic, Left Axillary
	See 5 Lymphatic, Right Axillary
	7 Lymphatic, Thorax
	Intercostal lymph node
	Mediastinal lymph node
	Parasternal lymph node
	Paratracheal lymph node
	Tracheobronchial lymph node
	8 Lymphatic, Internal Mammary, Right
	9 Lymphatic, Internal Mammary, Left
	B Lymphatic, Mesenteric
	Inferior mesenteric lymph node
	Pararectal lymph node
	Superior mesenteric lymph node
	C Lymphatic, Pelvis
	Common iliac (subaortic) lymph node
	Gluteal lymph node
	Iliac lymph node
	Inferior epigastric lymph node
	Obturator lymph node
	Sacral lymph node
	Subaortic (common iliac) lymph node
	Suprainguinal lymph node
	D Lymphatic, Aortic
	Celiac lymph node
	Gastric lymph node
	Hepatic lymph node
	Lumbar lymph node
	Pancreaticosplenic lymph node
	Paraaortic lymph node
	Retroperitoneal lymph node
	F Lymphatic, Right Lower Extremity
	Femoral lymph node
	Popliteal lymph node
	G Lymphatic, Left Lower Extremity
	See F Lymphatic, Right Lower Extremity
	H Lymphatic, Right Inguinal
	J Lymphatic, Left Inguinal
	K Thoracic Duct
	Left jugular trunk
	Left subclavian trunk
	L Cisterna Chyli
	Intestinal lymphatic trunk
	Lumbar lymphatic trunk
		Ø Open
		3 Percutaneous
		4 Percutaneous Endoscopic
		8 Via Natural or Artificial Opening Endoscopic
			Z No Device	**X Diagnostic**
				Z No Qualifier

M Thymus Thymus gland **P Spleen** Accessory spleen **T Bone Marrow**		**Ø Open** **3 Percutaneous** **4 Percutaneous Endoscopic**	**Ø Drainage Device**	**Z No Qualifier**
M Thymus Thymus gland **P Spleen** Accessory spleen **T Bone Marrow**		**Ø Open** **3 Percutaneous** **4 Percutaneous Endoscopic**	**Z No Device**	**X Diagnostic** **Z No Qualifier**

Non-OR	079[Ø,1,2,3,4,5,6,7,8,9,B,C,D,F,G,H,J,K,L]8ZX
Non-OR	079[Ø,1,2,3,4,5,6,7,8,9,B,C,D,F,G,H,J,K,L][3,8]ZZ
Non-OR	079M3ØZ
Non-OR	079P[3,4]ØZ
Non-OR	079T[Ø,3,4]ØZ
Non-OR	079M3ZZ
Non-OR	079P[3,4]Z[X,Z]
Non-OR	079T[Ø,3,4]Z[X,Z]

Ø   Medical and Surgical
7   Lymphatic and Hemic Systems
B   Excision   Definition: Cutting out or off, without replacement, a portion of a body part
                           Explanation: The qualifier DIAGNOSTIC is used to identify excision procedures that are biopsies

Body Part Character 4		Approach Character 5	Device Character 6	Qualifier Character 7

Ø Lymphatic, Head
Buccinator lymph node
Infraauricular lymph node
Infraparotid lymph node
Parotid lymph node
Preauricular lymph node
Submandibular lymph node
Submaxillary lymph node
Submental lymph node
Subparotid lymph node
Suprahyoid lymph node
1 Lymphatic, Right Neck
Cervical lymph node
Jugular lymph node
Mastoid (postauricular) lymph node
Occipital lymph node
Postauricular (mastoid) lymph node
Retropharyngeal lymph node
Right jugular trunk
Right lymphatic duct
Right subclavian trunk
Supraclavicular (Virchow's) lymph
   node
Virchow's (supraclavicular) lymph
   node
2 Lymphatic, Left Neck
Cervical lymph node
Jugular lymph node
Mastoid (postauricular) lymph node
Occipital lymph node
Postauricular (mastoid) lymph node
Retropharyngeal lymph node
Supraclavicular (Virchow's) lymph
   node
Virchow's (supraclavicular) lymph
   node
3 Lymphatic, Right Upper Extremity
Cubital lymph node
Deltopectoral (infraclavicular) lymph
   node
Epitrochlear lymph node
Infraclavicular (deltopectoral) lymph
   node
Supratrochlear lymph node
4 Lymphatic, Left Upper Extremity
See 3 Lymphatic, Right Upper Extremity
5 Lymphatic, Right Axillary
Anterior (pectoral) lymph node
Apical (subclavicular) lymph node
Brachial (lateral) lymph node
Central axillary lymph node
Lateral (brachial) lymph node
Pectoral (anterior) lymph node
Posterior (subscapular) lymph node
Subclavicular (apical) lymph node
Subscapular (posterior) lymph node
	6 Lymphatic, Left Axillary
	See 5 Lymphatic, Right Axillary
	7 Lymphatic, Thorax
	Intercostal lymph node
	Mediastinal lymph node
	Parasternal lymph node
	Paratracheal lymph node
	Tracheobronchial lymph node
	8 Lymphatic, Internal Mammary, Right
	9 Lymphatic, Internal Mammary, Left
	B Lymphatic, Mesenteric
	Inferior mesenteric lymph node
	Pararectal lymph node
	Superior mesenteric lymph node
	C Lymphatic, Pelvis
	Common iliac (subaortic) lymph node
	Gluteal lymph node
	Iliac lymph node
	Inferior epigastric lymph node
	Obturator lymph node
	Sacral lymph node
	Subaortic (common iliac) lymph node
	Suprainguinal lymph node
	D Lymphatic, Aortic
	Celiac lymph node
	Gastric lymph node
	Hepatic lymph node
	Lumbar lymph node
	Pancreaticosplenic lymph node
	Paraaortic lymph node
	Retroperitoneal lymph node
	F Lymphatic, Right Lower Extremity
	Femoral lymph node
	Popliteal lymph node
	G Lymphatic, Left Lower Extremity
	See F Lymphatic, Right Lower Extremity
	H Lymphatic, Right Inguinal ⊞
	J Lymphatic, Left Inguinal ⊞
	K Thoracic Duct
	Left jugular trunk
	Left subclavian trunk
	L Cisterna Chyli
	Intestinal lymphatic trunk
	Lumbar lymphatic trunk
	M Thymus
	Thymus gland
	P Spleen
	Accessory spleen
		Ø Open
		3 Percutaneous
		4 Percutaneous
		   Endoscopic
			Z No Device	**X Diagnostic**
				Z No Qualifier

Non-OR   Ø7BP[3,4]ZX

See Appendix L for Procedure Combinations
   ⊞   Ø7B[H,J][Ø,4]ZZ

LC Limited Coverage   NC Noncovered   ⊞ Combination Member   HAC associated procedure   Combination Only   DRG Non-OR   Non-OR   New/Revised in GREEN

274   ICD-10-PCS 2019

0   Medical and Surgical
7   Lymphatic and Hemic Systems
C   Extirpation   Definition: Taking or cutting out solid matter from a body part

Explanation: The solid matter may be an abnormal byproduct of a biological function or a foreign body; it may be imbedded in a body part or in the lumen of a tubular body part. The solid matter may or may not have been previously broken into pieces.

Body Part Character 4		Approach Character 5	Device Character 6	Qualifier Character 7
0 Lymphatic, Head Buccinator lymph node Infraauricular lymph node Infraparotid lymph node Parotid lymph node Preauricular lymph node Submandibular lymph node Submaxillary lymph node Submental lymph node Subparotid lymph node Suprahyoid lymph node **1 Lymphatic, Right Neck** Cervical lymph node Jugular lymph node Mastoid (postauricular) lymph node Occipital lymph node Postauricular (mastoid) lymph node Retropharyngeal lymph node Right jugular trunk Right lymphatic duct Right subclavian trunk Supraclavicular (Virchow's) lymph node Virchow's (supraclavicular) lymph node **2 Lymphatic, Left Neck** Cervical lymph node Jugular lymph node Mastoid (postauricular) lymph node Occipital lymph node Postauricular (mastoid) lymph node Retropharyngeal lymph node Supraclavicular (Virchow's) lymph node Virchow's (supraclavicular) lymph node **3 Lymphatic, Right Upper Extremity** Cubital lymph node Deltopectoral (infraclavicular) lymph node Epitrochlear lymph node Infraclavicular (deltopectoral) lymph node Supratrochlear lymph node **4 Lymphatic, Left Upper Extremity** *See 3 Lymphatic, Right Upper Extremity* **5 Lymphatic, Right Axillary** Anterior (pectoral) lymph node Apical (subclavicular) lymph node Brachial (lateral) lymph node Central axillary lymph node Lateral (brachial) lymph node Pectoral (anterior) lymph node Posterior (subscapular) lymph node Subclavicular (apical) lymph node Subscapular (posterior) lymph node	**6 Lymphatic, Left Axillary** *See 5 Lymphatic, Right Axillary* **7 Lymphatic, Thorax** Intercostal lymph node Mediastinal lymph node Parasternal lymph node Paratracheal lymph node Tracheobronchial lymph node **8 Lymphatic, Internal Mammary, Right** **9 Lymphatic, Internal Mammary, Left** **B Lymphatic, Mesenteric** Inferior mesenteric lymph node Pararectal lymph node Superior mesenteric lymph node **C Lymphatic, Pelvis** Common iliac (subaortic) lymph node Gluteal lymph node Iliac lymph node Inferior epigastric lymph node Obturator lymph node Sacral lymph node Subaortic (common iliac) lymph node Suprainguinal lymph node **D Lymphatic, Aortic** Celiac lymph node Gastric lymph node Hepatic lymph node Lumbar lymph node Pancreaticosplenic lymph node Paraaortic lymph node Retroperitoneal lymph node **F Lymphatic, Right Lower Extremity** Femoral lymph node Popliteal lymph node **G Lymphatic, Left Lower Extremity** *See F Lymphatic, Right Lower Extremity* **H Lymphatic, Right Inguinal** **J Lymphatic, Left Inguinal** **K Thoracic Duct** Left jugular trunk Left subclavian trunk **L Cisterna Chyli** Intestinal lymphatic trunk Lumbar lymphatic trunk **M Thymus** Thymus gland **P Spleen** Accessory spleen	**0 Open** **3 Percutaneous** **4 Percutaneous Endoscopic**	**Z No Device**	**Z No Qualifier**

Non-OR   07CP[3,4]ZZ

LC Limited Coverage   NC Noncovered   ⊞ Combination Member   HAC associated procedure   Combination Only   DRG Non-OR   Non-OR   New/Revised in GREEN

ICD-10-PCS 2019   275

Lymphatic and Hemic Systems (side tab)

0   Medical and Surgical
7   Lymphatic and Hemic Systems
D   Extraction   Definition: Pulling or stripping out or off all or a portion of a body part by the use of force
                      Explanation: The qualifier DIAGNOSTIC is used to identify extraction procedures that are biopsies

Body Part Character 4		Approach Character 5	Device Character 6	Qualifier Character 7

0 Lymphatic, Head
  Buccinator lymph node
  Infraauricular lymph node
  Infraparotid lymph node
  Parotid lymph node
  Preauricular lymph node
  Submandibular lymph node
  Submaxillary lymph node
  Submental lymph node
  Subparotid lymph node
  Suprahyoid lymph node
1 Lymphatic, Right Neck
  Cervical lymph node
  Jugular lymph node
  Mastoid (postauricular) lymph node
  Occipital lymph node
  Postauricular (mastoid) lymph node
  Retropharyngeal lymph node
  Right jugular trunk
  Right lymphatic duct
  Right subclavian trunk
  Supraclavicular (Virchow's) lymph node
  Virchow's (supraclavicular) lymph node
2 Lymphatic, Left Neck
  Cervical lymph node
  Jugular lymph node
  Mastoid (postauricular) lymph node
  Occipital lymph node
  Postauricular (mastoid) lymph node
  Retropharyngeal lymph node
  Supraclavicular (Virchow's) lymph node
  Virchow's (supraclavicular) lymph node
3 Lymphatic, Right Upper Extremity
  Cubital lymph node
  Deltopectoral (infraclavicular) lymph node
  Epitrochlear lymph node
  Infraclavicular (deltopectoral) lymph node
  Supratrochlear lymph node
4 Lymphatic, Left Upper Extremity
  See 3 Lymphatic, Right Upper Extremity
5 Lymphatic, Right Axillary
  Anterior (pectoral) lymph node
  Apical (subclavicular) lymph node
  Brachial (lateral) lymph node
  Central axillary lymph node
  Lateral (brachial) lymph node
  Pectoral (anterior) lymph node
  Posterior (subscapular) lymph node
  Subclavicular (apical) lymph node
  Subscapular (posterior) lymph node
	6 Lymphatic, Left Axillary
	  See 5 Lymphatic, Right Axillary
	7 Lymphatic, Thorax
	  Intercostal lymph node
	  Mediastinal lymph node
	  Parasternal lymph node
	  Paratracheal lymph node
	  Tracheobronchial lymph node
	8 Lymphatic, Internal Mammary, Right
	9 Lymphatic, Internal Mammary, Left
	B Lymphatic, Mesenteric
	  Inferior mesenteric lymph node
	  Pararectal lymph node
	  Superior mesenteric lymph node
	C Lymphatic, Pelvis
	  Common iliac (subaortic) lymph node
	  Gluteal lymph node
	  Iliac lymph node
	  Inferior epigastric lymph node
	  Obturator lymph node
	  Sacral lymph node
	  Subaortic (common iliac) lymph node
	  Suprainguinal lymph node
	D Lymphatic, Aortic
	  Celiac lymph node
	  Gastric lymph node
	  Hepatic lymph node
	  Lumbar lymph node
	  Pancreaticosplenic lymph node
	  Paraaortic lymph node
	  Retroperitoneal lymph node
	F Lymphatic, Right Lower Extremity
	  Femoral lymph node
	  Popliteal lymph node
	G Lymphatic, Left Lower Extremity
	  See F Lymphatic, Right Lower Extremity
	H Lymphatic, Right Inguinal
	J Lymphatic, Left Inguinal
	K Thoracic Duct
	  Left jugular trunk
	  Left subclavian trunk
	L Cisterna Chyli
	  Intestinal lymphatic trunk
	  Lumbar lymphatic trunk
		3 Percutaneous
		4 Percutaneous Endoscopic
		8 Via Natural or Artificial Opening Endoscopic
			Z No Device	**X** Diagnostic

M Thymus
  Thymus gland
P Spleen
  Accessory spleen
		3 Percutaneous
		4 Percutaneous Endoscopic
			Z No Device	**X** Diagnostic

Q Bone Marrow, Sternum **R** Bone Marrow, Iliac **S** Bone Marrow, Vertebral		**0** Open **3** Percutaneous	**Z** No Device	**X** Diagnostic **Z** No Qualifier

Non-OR   All body part, approach, device, and qualifier values

LC Limited Coverage   **NC** Noncovered   ⊞ Combination Member   HAC associated procedure   Combination Only   DRG Non-OR   Non-OR   New/Revised in GREEN

276   ICD-10-PCS 2019

07D–07D (side tab)

Ø   Medical and Surgical
7   Lymphatic and Hemic Systems
H   Insertion   Definition: Putting in a nonbiological appliance that monitors, assists, performs, or prevents a physiological function but does not physically take the place of a body part

               Explanation: None

Body Part Character 4	Approach Character 5	Device Character 6	Qualifier Character 7

K Thoracic Duct
   Left jugular trunk
   Left subclavian trunk
L Cisterna Chyli
   Intestinal lymphatic trunk
   Lumbar lymphatic trunk
M Thymus
   Thymus gland
N Lymphatic
P Spleen
   Accessory spleen
	Ø Open
	3 Percutaneous
	4 Percutaneous Endoscopic
		3 Infusion Device
		Y Other Device
			Z No Qualifier

Non-OR   07H[K,L,M,N,P][Ø,3,4]3Z
Non-OR   07H[K,L,M]3YZ
Non-OR   07H[N,P][3,4]YZ

Ø   Medical and Surgical
7   Lymphatic and Hemic Systems
J   Inspection   Definition: Visually and/or manually exploring a body part

               Explanation: Visual exploration may be performed with or without optical instrumentation. Manual exploration may be performed directly or through intervening body layers.

Body Part Character 4	Approach Character 5	Device Character 6	Qualifier Character 7

K Thoracic Duct
   Left jugular trunk
   Left subclavian trunk
L Cisterna Chyli
   Intestinal lymphatic trunk
   Lumbar lymphatic trunk
M Thymus
   Thymus gland
T Bone Marrow
	Ø Open
	3 Percutaneous
	4 Percutaneous Endoscopic
		Z No Device	**Z** No Qualifier

N Lymphatic	**Ø** Open **3** Percutaneous **4** Percutaneous Endoscopic **8** Via Natural or Artificial Opening Endoscopic **X** External	**Z** No Device	**Z** No Qualifier
P Spleen Accessory spleen	**Ø** Open **3** Percutaneous **4** Percutaneous Endoscopic **X** External	**Z** No Device	**Z** No Qualifier

Non-OR   07J[K,L,M]3ZZ
Non-OR   07JT[Ø,3,4]ZZ
Non-OR   07JN[3,8,X]ZZ
Non-OR   07JP[3,4,X]ZZ

LC Limited Coverage   NC Noncovered   ⊞ Combination Member   HAC associated procedure   Combination Only   DRG Non-OR   Non-OR   New/Revised in GREEN

Lymphatic and Hemic Systems

Ø   Medical and Surgical
7   Lymphatic and Hemic Systems
L   Occlusion   Definition: Completely closing an orifice or the lumen of a tubular body part
                            Explanation: The orifice can be a natural orifice or an artificially created orifice

Body Part Character 4		Approach Character 5	Device Character 6	Qualifier Character 7
Ø Lymphatic, Head	**6 Lymphatic, Left Axillary**	**Ø** Open	**C** Extraluminal Device	**Z** No Qualifier
Buccinator lymph node	*See 5 Lymphatic, Right Axillary*	**3** Percutaneous	**D** Intraluminal Device	
Infraauricular lymph node	**7 Lymphatic, Thorax**	**4** Percutaneous	**Z** No Device	
Infraparotid lymph node	Intercostal lymph node	Endoscopic		
Parotid lymph node	Mediastinal lymph node			
Preauricular lymph node	Parasternal lymph node			
Submandibular lymph node	Paratracheal lymph node			
Submaxillary lymph node	Tracheobronchial lymph node			
Submental lymph node	**8 Lymphatic, Internal Mammary, Right**			
Subparotid lymph node	**9 Lymphatic, Internal Mammary, Left**			
Suprahyoid lymph node	**B Lymphatic, Mesenteric**			
1 Lymphatic, Right Neck	Inferior mesenteric lymph node			
Cervical lymph node	Pararectal lymph node			
Jugular lymph node	Superior mesenteric lymph node			
Mastoid (postauricular) lymph node	**C Lymphatic, Pelvis**			
Occipital lymph node	Common iliac (subaortic) lymph node			
Postauricular (mastoid) lymph node	Gluteal lymph node			
Retropharyngeal lymph node	Iliac lymph node			
Right jugular trunk	Inferior epigastric lymph node			
Right lymphatic duct	Obturator lymph node			
Right subclavian trunk	Sacral lymph node			
Supraclavicular (Virchow's) lymph node	Subaortic (common iliac) lymph node			
Virchow's (supraclavicular) lymph node	Suprainguinal lymph node			
2 Lymphatic, Left Neck	**D Lymphatic, Aortic**			
Cervical lymph node	Celiac lymph node			
Jugular lymph node	Gastric lymph node			
Mastoid (postauricular) lymph node	Hepatic lymph node			
Occipital lymph node	Lumbar lymph node			
Postauricular (mastoid) lymph node	Pancreaticosplenic lymph node			
Retropharyngeal lymph node	Paraaortic lymph node			
Supraclavicular (Virchow's) lymph node	Retroperitoneal lymph node			
Virchow's (supraclavicular) lymph node	**F Lymphatic, Right Lower Extremity**			
3 Lymphatic, Right Upper Extremity	Femoral lymph node			
Cubital lymph node	Popliteal lymph node			
Deltopectoral (infraclavicular) lymph node	**G Lymphatic, Left Lower Extremity**			
Epitrochlear lymph node	*See F Lymphatic, Right Lower Extremity*			
Infraclavicular (deltopectoral) lymph node	**H Lymphatic, Right Inguinal**			
Supratrochlear lymph node	**J Lymphatic, Left Inguinal**			
4 Lymphatic, Left Upper Extremity	**K Thoracic Duct**			
See 3 Lymphatic, Right Upper Extremity	Left jugular trunk			
5 Lymphatic, Right Axillary	Left subclavian trunk			
Anterior (pectoral) lymph node	**L Cisterna Chyli**			
Apical (subclavicular) lymph node	Intestinal lymphatic trunk			
Brachial (lateral) lymph node	Lumbar lymphatic trunk			
Central axillary lymph node				
Lateral (brachial) lymph node				
Pectoral (anterior) lymph node				
Posterior (subscapular) lymph node				
Subclavicular (apical) lymph node				
Subscapular (posterior) lymph node				

0   Medical and Surgical
7   Lymphatic and Hemic Systems
N   Release   Definition: Freeing a body part from an abnormal physical constraint by cutting or by the use of force
                     Explanation: Some of the restraining tissue may be taken out but none of the body part is taken out

Body Part Character 4		Approach Character 5	Device Character 6	Qualifier Character 7
0 Lymphatic, Head Buccinator lymph node Infraauricular lymph node Infraparotid lymph node Parotid lymph node Preauricular lymph node Submandibular lymph node Submaxillary lymph node Submental lymph node Subparotid lymph node Suprahyoid lymph node **1 Lymphatic, Right Neck** Cervical lymph node Jugular lymph node Mastoid (postauricular) lymph node Occipital lymph node Postauricular (mastoid) lymph node Retropharyngeal lymph node Right jugular trunk Right lymphatic duct Right subclavian trunk Supraclavicular (Virchow's) lymph node Virchow's (supraclavicular) lymph node **2 Lymphatic, Left Neck** Cervical lymph node Jugular lymph node Mastoid (postauricular) lymph node Occipital lymph node Postauricular (mastoid) lymph node Retropharyngeal lymph node Supraclavicular (Virchow's) lymph node Virchow's (supraclavicular) lymph node **3 Lymphatic, Right Upper Extremity** Cubital lymph node Deltopectoral (infraclavicular) lymph node Epitrochlear lymph node Infraclavicular (deltopectoral) lymph node Supratrochlear lymph node **4 Lymphatic, Left Upper Extremity** *See 3 Lymphatic, Right Upper Extremity* **5 Lymphatic, Right Axillary** Anterior (pectoral) lymph node Apical (subclavicular) lymph node Brachial (lateral) lymph node Central axillary lymph node Lateral (brachial) lymph node Pectoral (anterior) lymph node Posterior (subscapular) lymph node Subclavicular (apical) lymph node Subscapular (posterior) lymph node	**6 Lymphatic, Left Axillary** *See 5 Lymphatic, Right Axillary* **7 Lymphatic, Thorax** Intercostal lymph node Mediastinal lymph node Parasternal lymph node Paratracheal lymph node Tracheobronchial lymph node **8 Lymphatic, Internal Mammary, Right** **9 Lymphatic, Internal Mammary, Left** **B Lymphatic, Mesenteric** Inferior mesenteric lymph node Pararectal lymph node Superior mesenteric lymph node **C Lymphatic, Pelvis** Common iliac (subaortic) lymph node Gluteal lymph node Iliac lymph node Inferior epigastric lymph node Obturator lymph node Sacral lymph node Subaortic (common iliac) lymph node Suprainguinal lymph node **D Lymphatic, Aortic** Celiac lymph node Gastric lymph node Hepatic lymph node Lumbar lymph node Pancreaticosplenic lymph node Paraaortic lymph node Retroperitoneal lymph node **F Lymphatic, Right Lower Extremity** Femoral lymph node Popliteal lymph node **G Lymphatic, Left Lower Extremity** *See F Lymphatic, Right Lower Extremity* **H Lymphatic, Right Inguinal** **J Lymphatic, Left Inguinal** **K Thoracic Duct** Left jugular trunk Left subclavian trunk **L Cisterna Chyli** Intestinal lymphatic trunk Lumbar lymphatic trunk **M Thymus** Thymus gland **P Spleen** Accessory spleen	**0 Open** **3 Percutaneous** **4 Percutaneous Endoscopic**	**Z No Device**	**Z No Qualifier**

LC Limited Coverage   **NC** Noncovered   ⊞ Combination Member   HAC associated procedure   Combination Only   DRG Non-OR   Non-OR   New/Revised in GREEN

ICD-10-PCS 2019   279

0 Medical and Surgical
7 Lymphatic and Hemic Systems
P Removal Definition: Taking out or off a device from a body part

Explanation: If a device is taken out and a similar device put in without cutting or puncturing the skin or mucous membrane, the procedure is coded to the root operation CHANGE. Otherwise, the procedure for taking out a device is coded to the root operation REMOVAL.

Body Part Character 4	Approach Character 5	Device Character 6	Qualifier Character 7
K Thoracic Duct Left jugular trunk Left subclavian trunk L Cisterna Chyli Intestinal lymphatic trunk Lumbar lymphatic trunk N Lymphatic	0 Open 3 Percutaneous 4 Percutaneous Endoscopic	0 Drainage Device 3 Infusion Device 7 Autologous Tissue Substitute C Extraluminal Device D Intraluminal Device J Synthetic Substitute K Nonautologous Tissue Substitute Y Other Device	Z No Qualifier
K Thoracic Duct Left jugular trunk Left subclavian trunk L Cisterna Chyli Intestinal lymphatic trunk Lumbar lymphatic trunk N Lymphatic	X External	0 Drainage Device 3 Infusion Device D Intraluminal Device	Z No Qualifier
M Thymus Thymus gland P Spleen Accessory spleen	0 Open 3 Percutaneous 4 Percutaneous Endoscopic	0 Drainage Device 3 Infusion Device Y Other Device	Z No Qualifier
M Thymus Thymus gland P Spleen Accessory spleen	X External	0 Drainage Device 3 Infusion Device	Z No Qualifier
T Bone Marrow	0 Open 3 Percutaneous 4 Percutaneous Endoscopic X External	0 Drainage Device	Z No Qualifier

Non-OR	07P[K,L,N][3,4]YZ
Non-OR	07P[K,L,N]X[0,3,D]Z
Non-OR	07P[M,P][3,4]YZ
Non-OR	07P[M,P]X[0,3]Z
Non-OR	07PT[0,3,4,X]0Z

LC Limited Coverage NC Noncovered ⊞ Combination Member HAC associated procedure Combination Only DRG Non-OR Non-OR New/Revised in GREEN

280 ICD-10-PCS 2019

0   **Medical and Surgical**
7   **Lymphatic and Hemic Systems**
Q   **Repair**   Definition: Restoring, to the extent possible, a body part to its normal anatomic structure and function
                     Explanation: Used only when the method to accomplish the repair is not one of the other root operations

Body Part Character 4		Approach Character 5	Device Character 6	Qualifier Character 7

0   **Lymphatic, Head**
    Buccinator lymph node
    Infraauricular lymph node
    Infraparotid lymph node
    Parotid lymph node
    Preauricular lymph node
    Submandibular lymph node
    Submaxillary lymph node
    Submental lymph node
    Subparotid lymph node
    Suprahyoid lymph node
1   **Lymphatic, Right Neck**
    Cervical lymph node
    Jugular lymph node
    Mastoid (postauricular) lymph node
    Occipital lymph node
    Postauricular (mastoid) lymph node
    Retropharyngeal lymph node
    Right jugular trunk
    Right lymphatic duct
    Right subclavian trunk
    Supraclavicular (Virchow's) lymph
       node
    Virchow's (supraclavicular) lymph
       node
2   **Lymphatic, Left Neck**
    Cervical lymph node
    Jugular lymph node
    Mastoid (postauricular) lymph node
    Occipital lymph node
    Postauricular (mastoid) lymph node
    Retropharyngeal lymph node
    Supraclavicular (Virchow's) lymph
       node
    Virchow's (supraclavicular) lymph
       node
3   **Lymphatic, Right Upper Extremity**
    Cubital lymph node
    Deltopectoral (infraclavicular) lymph
       node
    Epitrochlear lymph node
    Infraclavicular (deltopectoral) lymph
       node
    Supratrochlear lymph node
4   **Lymphatic, Left Upper Extremity**
    See 3 Lymphatic, Right Upper Extremity
5   **Lymphatic, Right Axillary**
    Anterior (pectoral) lymph node
    Apical (subclavicular) lymph node
    Brachial (lateral) lymph node
    Central axillary lymph node
    Lateral (brachial) lymph node
    Pectoral (anterior) lymph node
    Posterior (subscapular) lymph node
    Subclavicular (apical) lymph node
    Subscapular (posterior) lymph node
	6 **Lymphatic, Left Axillary**
	    See 5 Lymphatic, Right Axillary
	7 **Lymphatic, Thorax**
	    Intercostal lymph node
	    Mediastinal lymph node
	    Parasternal lymph node
	    Paratracheal lymph node
	    Tracheobronchial lymph node
	8 **Lymphatic, Internal Mammary, Right**
	9 **Lymphatic, Internal Mammary, Left**
	B **Lymphatic, Mesenteric**
	    Inferior mesenteric lymph node
	    Pararectal lymph node
	    Superior mesenteric lymph node
	C **Lymphatic, Pelvis**
	    Common iliac (subaortic) lymph node
	    Gluteal lymph node
	    Iliac lymph node
	    Inferior epigastric lymph node
	    Obturator lymph node
	    Sacral lymph node
	    Subaortic (common iliac) lymph node
	    Suprainguinal lymph node
	D **Lymphatic, Aortic**
	    Celiac lymph node
	    Gastric lymph node
	    Hepatic lymph node
	    Lumbar lymph node
	    Pancreaticosplenic lymph node
	    Paraaortic lymph node
	    Retroperitoneal lymph node
	F **Lymphatic, Right Lower Extremity**
	    Femoral lymph node
	    Popliteal lymph node
	G **Lymphatic, Left Lower Extremity**
	    See F Lymphatic, Right Lower Extremity
	H **Lymphatic, Right Inguinal**
	J **Lymphatic, Left Inguinal**
	K **Thoracic Duct**
	    Left jugular trunk
	    Left subclavian trunk
	L **Cisterna Chyli**
	    Intestinal lymphatic trunk
	    Lumbar lymphatic trunk
		0 Open
		3 Percutaneous
		4 Percutaneous
		    Endoscopic
		8 Via Natural or
		    Artificial Opening
		    Endoscopic
			Z No Device	**Z** No Qualifier

M   **Thymus**
    Thymus gland
P   **Spleen**
    Accessory spleen
		0 Open
		3 Percutaneous
		4 Percutaneous
		    Endoscopic
			Z No Device	**Z** No Qualifier

Lymphatic and Hemic Systems

Ø Medical and Surgical
7 Lymphatic and Hemic Systems
S Reposition   Definition: Moving to its normal location, or other suitable location, all or a portion of a body part

Explanation: The body part is moved to a new location from an abnormal location, or from a normal location where it is not functioning correctly. The body part may or may not be cut out or off to be moved to the new location.

Body Part Character 4	Approach Character 5	Device Character 6	Qualifier Character 7
M Thymus Thymus gland **P Spleen** Accessory spleen	Ø Open	Z No Device	Z No Qualifier

Ø Medical and Surgical
7 Lymphatic and Hemic Systems
T Resection   Definition: Cutting out or off, without replacement, all of a body part

Explanation: None

Body Part Character 4	Approach Character 5	Device Character 6	Qualifier Character 7
Ø Lymphatic, Head Buccinator lymph node Infraauricular lymph node Infraparotid lymph node Parotid lymph node Preauricular lymph node Submandibular lymph node Submaxillary lymph node Submental lymph node Subparotid lymph node Suprahyoid lymph node **1 Lymphatic, Right Neck** Cervical lymph node Jugular lymph node Mastoid (postauricular) lymph node Occipital lymph node Postauricular (mastoid) lymph node Retropharyngeal lymph node Right jugular trunk Right lymphatic duct Right subclavian trunk Supraclavicular (Virchow's) lymph node Virchow's (supraclavicular) lymph node **2 Lymphatic, Left Neck** Cervical lymph node Jugular lymph node Mastoid (postauricular) lymph node Occipital lymph node Postauricular (mastoid) lymph node Retropharyngeal lymph node Supraclavicular (Virchow's) lymph node Virchow's (supraclavicular) lymph node **3 Lymphatic, Right Upper Extremity** Cubital lymph node Deltopectoral (infraclavicular) lymph node Epitrochlear lymph node Infraclavicular (deltopectoral) lymph node Supratrochlear lymph node **4 Lymphatic, Left Upper Extremity** See 3 Lymphatic, Right Upper Extremity **5 Lymphatic, Right Axillary** ⊞ Anterior (pectoral) lymph node Apical (subclavicular) lymph node Brachial (lateral) lymph node Central axillary lymph node Lateral (brachial) lymph node Pectoral (anterior) lymph node Posterior (subscapular) lymph node Subclavicular (apical) lymph node Subscapular (posterior) lymph node **6 Lymphatic, Left Axillary** ⊞ See 5 Lymphatic, Right Axillary **7 Lymphatic, Thorax** ⊞ Intercostal lymph node Mediastinal lymph node Parasternal lymph node Paratracheal lymph node Tracheobronchial lymph node **8 Lymphatic, Internal Mammary, Right** ⊞ **9 Lymphatic, Internal Mammary, Left** ⊞ **B Lymphatic, Mesenteric** Inferior mesenteric lymph node Pararectal lymph node Superior mesenteric lymph node **C Lymphatic, Pelvis** Common iliac (subaortic) lymph node Gluteal lymph node Iliac lymph node Inferior epigastric lymph node Obturator lymph node Sacral lymph node Subaortic (common iliac) lymph node Suprainguinal lymph node **D Lymphatic, Aortic** Celiac lymph node Gastric lymph node Hepatic lymph node Lumbar lymph node Pancreaticosplenic lymph node Paraaortic lymph node Retroperitoneal lymph node **F Lymphatic, Right Lower Extremity** Femoral lymph node Popliteal lymph node **G Lymphatic, Left Lower Extremity** See F Lymphatic, Right Lower Extremity **H Lymphatic, Right Inguinal** **J Lymphatic, Left Inguinal** **K Thoracic Duct** Left jugular trunk Left subclavian trunk **L Cisterna Chyli** Intestinal lymphatic trunk Lumbar lymphatic trunk **M Thymus** Thymus gland **P Spleen** Accessory spleen	Ø Open 4 Percutaneous Endoscopic	Z No Device	Z No Qualifier

See Appendix L for Procedure Combinations
⊞   Ø7T[5,6,7,8,9]ØZZ

Ø   **Medical and Surgical**
7   **Lymphatic and Hemic Systems**
U   **Supplement**   Definition: Putting in or on biological or synthetic material that physically reinforces and/or augments the function of a portion of a body part
                Explanation: The biological material is non-living, or is living and from the same individual. The body part may have been previously replaced, and the SUPPLEMENT procedure is performed to physically reinforce and/or augment the function of the replaced body part.

Body Part Character 4		Approach Character 5	Device Character 6	Qualifier Character 7

Ø Lymphatic, Head
  Buccinator lymph node
  Infraauricular lymph node
  Infraparotid lymph node
  Parotid lymph node
  Preauricular lymph node
  Submandibular lymph node
  Submaxillary lymph node
  Submental lymph node
  Subparotid lymph node
  Suprahyoid lymph node
 	
1 Lymphatic, Right Neck
  Cervical lymph node
  Jugular lymph node
  Mastoid (postauricular) lymph node
  Occipital lymph node
  Postauricular (mastoid) lymph node
  Retropharyngeal lymph node
  Right jugular trunk
  Right lymphatic duct
  Right subclavian trunk
  Supraclavicular (Virchow's) lymph
    node
  Virchow's (supraclavicular) lymph
    node
 	
2 Lymphatic, Left Neck
  Cervical lymph node
  Jugular lymph node
  Mastoid (postauricular) lymph node
  Occipital lymph node
  Postauricular (mastoid) lymph node
  Retropharyngeal lymph node
  Supraclavicular (Virchow's) lymph
    node
  Virchow's (supraclavicular) lymph
    node
 	
3 Lymphatic, Right Upper Extremity
  Cubital lymph node
  Deltopectoral (infraclavicular) lymph
    node
  Epitrochlear lymph node
  Infraclavicular (deltopectoral) lymph
    node
  Supratrochlear lymph node
 	
4 Lymphatic, Left Upper Extremity
  See 3 Lymphatic, Right Upper Extremity
 	
5 Lymphatic, Right Axillary
  Anterior (pectoral) lymph node
  Apical (subclavicular) lymph node
  Brachial (lateral) lymph node
  Central axillary lymph node
  Lateral (brachial) lymph node
  Pectoral (anterior) lymph node
  Posterior (subscapular) lymph node
  Subclavicular (apical) lymph node
  Subscapular (posterior) lymph node
	6 Lymphatic, Left Axillary
	  See 5 Lymphatic, Right Axillary
	
	7 Lymphatic, Thorax
	  Intercostal lymph node
	  Mediastinal lymph node
	  Parasternal lymph node
	  Paratracheal lymph node
	  Tracheobronchial lymph node
	
	8 Lymphatic, Internal Mammary, Right
	9 Lymphatic, Internal Mammary, Left
	B Lymphatic, Mesenteric
	  Inferior mesenteric lymph node
	  Pararectal lymph node
	  Superior mesenteric lymph node
	
	C Lymphatic, Pelvis
	  Common iliac (subaortic) lymph node
	  Gluteal lymph node
	  Iliac lymph node
	  Inferior epigastric lymph node
	  Obturator lymph node
	  Sacral lymph node
	  Subaortic (common iliac) lymph node
	  Suprainguinal lymph node
	
	D Lymphatic, Aortic
	  Celiac lymph node
	  Gastric lymph node
	  Hepatic lymph node
	  Lumbar lymph node
	  Pancreaticosplenic lymph node
	  Paraaortic lymph node
	  Retroperitoneal lymph node
	
	F Lymphatic, Right Lower Extremity
	  Femoral lymph node
	  Popliteal lymph node
	
	G Lymphatic, Left Lower Extremity
	  See F Lymphatic, Right Lower Extremity
	H Lymphatic, Right Inguinal
	J Lymphatic, Left Inguinal
	K Thoracic Duct
	  Left jugular trunk
	  Left subclavian trunk
	
	L Cisterna Chyli
	  Intestinal lymphatic trunk
	  Lumbar lymphatic trunk
		Ø Open
		4 Percutaneous Endoscopic
			7 Autologous Tissue Substitute
			J Synthetic Substitute
			K Nonautologous Tissue Substitute
				Z No Qualifier

0 Medical and Surgical
7 Lymphatic and Hemic Systems
V Restriction   Definition: Partially closing an orifice or the lumen of a tubular body part
                        Explanation: The orifice can be a natural orifice or an artificially created orifice

Body Part Character 4		Approach Character 5	Device Character 6	Qualifier Character 7
0 Lymphatic, Head	**6 Lymphatic, Left Axillary**	**0** Open	**C** Extraluminal Device	**Z** No Qualifier
Buccinator lymph node	*See 5 Lymphatic, Right Axillary*	**3** Percutaneous	**D** Intraluminal Device	
Infraauricular lymph node	**7 Lymphatic, Thorax**	**4** Percutaneous	**Z** No Device	
Infraparotid lymph node	Intercostal lymph node	Endoscopic		
Parotid lymph node	Mediastinal lymph node			
Preauricular lymph node	Parasternal lymph node			
Submandibular lymph node	Paratracheal lymph node			
Submaxillary lymph node	Tracheobronchial lymph node			
Submental lymph node	**8 Lymphatic, Internal Mammary, Right**			
Subparotid lymph node	**9 Lymphatic, Internal Mammary, Left**			
Suprahyoid lymph node	**B Lymphatic, Mesenteric**			
1 Lymphatic, Right Neck	Inferior mesenteric lymph node			
Cervical lymph node	Pararectal lymph node			
Jugular lymph node	Superior mesenteric lymph node			
Mastoid (postauricular) lymph node	**C Lymphatic, Pelvis**			
Occipital lymph node	Common iliac (subaortic) lymph node			
Postauricular (mastoid) lymph node	Gluteal lymph node			
Retropharyngeal lymph node	Iliac lymph node			
Right jugular trunk	Inferior epigastric lymph node			
Right lymphatic duct	Obturator lymph node			
Right subclavian trunk	Sacral lymph node			
Supraclavicular (Virchow's) lymph node	Subaortic (common iliac) lymph node			
Virchow's (supraclavicular) lymph node	Suprainguinal lymph node			
2 Lymphatic, Left Neck	**D Lymphatic, Aortic**			
Cervical lymph node	Celiac lymph node			
Jugular lymph node	Gastric lymph node			
Mastoid (postauricular) lymph node	Hepatic lymph node			
Occipital lymph node	Lumbar lymph node			
Postauricular (mastoid) lymph node	Pancreaticosplenic lymph node			
Retropharyngeal lymph node	Paraaortic lymph node			
Supraclavicular (Virchow's) lymph node	Retroperitoneal lymph node			
Virchow's (supraclavicular) lymph node	**F Lymphatic, Right Lower Extremity**			
3 Lymphatic, Right Upper Extremity	Femoral lymph node			
Cubital lymph node	Popliteal lymph node			
Deltopectoral (infraclavicular) lymph node	**G Lymphatic, Left Lower Extremity**			
Epitrochlear lymph node	*See F Lymphatic, Right Lower Extremity*			
Infraclavicular (deltopectoral) lymph node	**H Lymphatic, Right Inguinal**			
Supratrochlear lymph node	**J Lymphatic, Left Inguinal**			
4 Lymphatic, Left Upper Extremity	**K Thoracic Duct**			
See 3 Lymphatic, Right Upper Extremity	Left jugular trunk			
5 Lymphatic, Right Axillary	Left subclavian trunk			
Anterior (pectoral) lymph node	**L Cisterna Chyli**			
Apical (subclavicular) lymph node	Intestinal lymphatic trunk			
Brachial (lateral) lymph node	Lumbar lymphatic trunk			
Central axillary lymph node				
Lateral (brachial) lymph node				
Pectoral (anterior) lymph node				
Posterior (subscapular) lymph node				
Subclavicular (apical) lymph node				
Subscapular (posterior) lymph node				

Ø   **Medical and Surgical**
7   **Lymphatic and Hemic Systems**
W   **Revision**   Definition: Correcting, to the extent possible, a portion of a malfunctioning device or the position of a displaced device
                      Explanation: Revision can include correcting a malfunctioning or displaced device by taking out or putting in components of the device such as a screw or pin

Body Part Character 4	Approach Character 5	Device Character 6	Qualifier Character 7

K Thoracic Duct
   Left jugular trunk
   Left subclavian trunk
L Cisterna Chyli
   Intestinal lymphatic trunk
   Lumbar lymphatic trunk
N Lymphatic
	Ø Open
	3 Percutaneous
	4 Percutaneous Endoscopic
		Ø Drainage Device
		3 Infusion Device
		7 Autologous Tissue
		   Substitute
		C Extraluminal Device
		D Intraluminal Device
		J Synthetic Substitute
		K Nonautologous Tissue
		   Substitute
		Y Other Device
			Z No Qualifier

K Thoracic Duct
   Left jugular trunk
   Left subclavian trunk
L Cisterna Chyli
   Intestinal lymphatic trunk
   Lumbar lymphatic trunk
N Lymphatic
	X External	**Ø** Drainage Device
		3 Infusion Device
		7 Autologous Tissue
		   Substitute
		C Extraluminal Device
		D Intraluminal Device
		J Synthetic Substitute
		K Nonautologous Tissue
		   Substitute
			Z No Qualifier

M Thymus
   Thymus gland
P Spleen
   Accessory spleen
	Ø Open
	3 Percutaneous
	4 Percutaneous Endoscopic
		Ø Drainage Device
		3 Infusion Device
		Y Other Device
			Z No Qualifier

M Thymus
   Thymus gland
P Spleen
   Accessory spleen
	X External	**Ø** Drainage Device
		3 Infusion Device
			Z No Qualifier

T Bone Marrow	**Ø** Open **3** Percutaneous **4** Percutaneous Endoscopic **X** External	**Ø** Drainage Device	**Z** No Qualifier

Non-OR   Ø7W[K,L,N][3,4]YZ
Non-OR   Ø7W[K,L,N]X[Ø,3,7,C,D,J,K]Z
Non-OR   Ø7W[M,P][3,4]YZ
Non-OR   Ø7W[M,P]X[Ø,3]Z
Non-OR   Ø7WT[Ø,3,4,X]ØZ

Ø   **Medical and Surgical**
7   **Lymphatic and Hemic Systems**
Y   **Transplantation**   Definition: Putting in or on all or a portion of a living body part taken from another individual or animal to physically take the place and/or function of all or a portion of a similar body part
                        Explanation: The native body part may or may not be taken out, and the transplanted body part may take over all or a portion of its function

Body Part Character 4	Approach Character 5	Device Character 6	Qualifier Character 7

M Thymus
   Thymus gland
P Spleen
   Accessory spleen
	Ø Open	**Z** No Device	**Ø** Allogeneic
			1 Syngeneic
			2 Zooplastic

Eye Ø8Ø–Ø8X

Character Meanings

This Character Meaning table is provided as a guide to assist the user in the identification of character members that may be found in this section of code tables. It **SHOULD NOT** be used to build a PCS code.

Operation–Character 3	Body Part–Character 4	Approach–Character 5	Device–Character 6	Qualifier–Character 7
Ø Alteration	Ø Eye, Right	Ø Open	Ø Drainage Device OR Synthetic Substitute, Intraocular Telescope	3 Nasal Cavity
1 Bypass	1 Eye, Left	3 Percutaneous	1 Radioactive Element	4 Sclera
2 Change	2 Anterior Chamber, Right	7 Via Natural or Artificial Opening	3 Infusion Device	X Diagnostic
5 Destruction	3 Anterior Chamber, Left	8 Via Natural or Artificial Opening Endoscopic	5 Epiretinal Visual Prosthesis	Z No Qualifier
7 Dilation	4 Vitreous, Right	X External	7 Autologous Tissue Substitute	
9 Drainage	5 Vitreous, Left		C Extraluminal Device	
B Excision	6 Sclera, Right		D Intraluminal Device	
C Extirpation	7 Sclera, Left		J Synthetic Substitute	
D Extraction	8 Cornea, Right		K Nonautologous Tissue Substitute	
F Fragmentation	9 Cornea, Left		Y Other Device	
H Insertion	A Choroid, Right		Z No Device	
J Inspection	B Choroid, Left			
L Occlusion	C Iris, Right			
M Reattachment	D Iris, Left			
N Release	E Retina, Right			
P Removal	F Retina, Left			
Q Repair	G Retinal Vessel, Right			
R Replacement	H Retinal Vessel, Left			
S Reposition	J Lens, Right			
T Resection	K Lens, Left			
U Supplement	L Extraocular Muscle, Right			
V Restriction	M Extraocular Muscle, Left			
W Revision	N Upper Eyelid, Right			
X Transfer	P Upper Eyelid, Left			
	Q Lower Eyelid, Right			
	R Lower Eyelid, Left			
	S Conjunctiva, Right			
	T Conjunctiva, Left			
	V Lacrimal Gland, Right			
	W Lacrimal Gland, Left			
	X Lacrimal Duct, Right			
	Y Lacrimal Duct, Left			

AHA Coding Clinic for table Ø89
2016, 2Q, 21   Laser trabeculoplasty

AHA Coding Clinic for table Ø8B
2014, 4Q, 35   Vitrectomy with air/fluid exchange
2014, 4Q, 36   Pars plans vitrectomy without mention of instillation of oil, air or fluid

AHA Coding Clinic for table Ø8J
2015, 1Q, 35   Attempted removal of foreign body from cornea

AHA Coding Clinic for table Ø8N
2015, 2Q, 24   Penetrating keratoplasty and anterior segment reconstruction

AHA Coding Clinic for table Ø8R
2015, 2Q, 24   Penetrating keratoplasty and anterior segment reconstruction
2015, 2Q, 25   Penetrating keratoplasty and placement of viscoelastic eye with paracentesis

AHA Coding Clinic for table Ø8T
2015, 2Q, 12   Orbital exenteration

AHA Coding Clinic for table Ø8U
2014, 3Q, 31   Corneal amniotic membrane transplantation

Eye

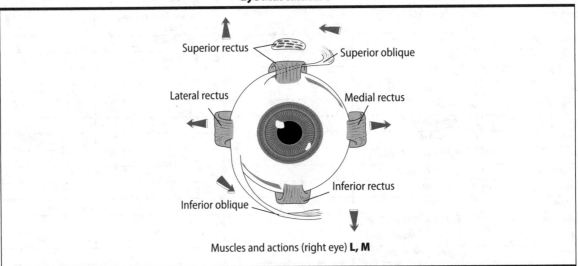

Sclera **6, 7**

Cornea **8, 9**

Iris **C, D**

Anterior chamber **2, 3**

Posterior chamber **Ø, 1**

Ciliary body **Ø, 1**

Conjunctiva **S, T**

Choroid (uvea) **A, B**

Vitreous body **4, 5**

Lens **J, K**

Optic disk **E, F**

Fovea **E, F**

Retina **E, F**

Eye Musculature

Superior rectus

Superior oblique

Lateral rectus

Medial rectus

Inferior oblique

Inferior rectus

Muscles and actions (right eye) **L, M**

Lacrimal System

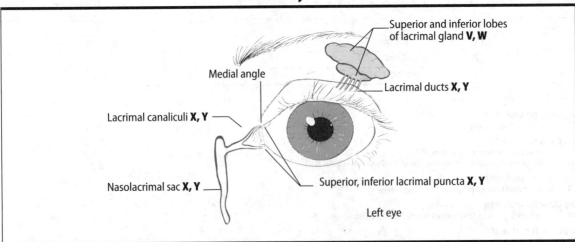

Superior and inferior lobes of lacrimal gland **V, W**

Medial angle

Lacrimal ducts **X, Y**

Lacrimal canaliculi **X, Y**

Nasolacrimal sac **X, Y**

Superior, inferior lacrimal puncta **X, Y**

Left eye

Ø   Medical and Surgical
8   Eye
Ø   Alteration   Definition: Modifying the anatomic structure of a body part without affecting the function of the body part

Explanation: Principal purpose is to improve appearance

Body Part Character 4	Approach Character 5	Device Character 6	Qualifier Character 7
N Upper Eyelid, Right Lateral canthus Levator palpebrae superioris muscle Orbicularis oculi muscle Superior tarsal plate **P** Upper Eyelid, Left *See N Upper Eyelid, Right* **Q** Lower Eyelid, Right Inferior tarsal plate Medial canthus **R** Lower Eyelid, Left *See Q Lower Eyelid, Right*	**Ø** Open **3** Percutaneous **X** External	**7** Autologous Tissue Substitute **J** Synthetic Substitute **K** Nonautologous Tissue Substitute **Z** No Device	**Z** No Qualifier

Non-OR   All body part, approach, device, and qualifier values

---

Ø   Medical and Surgical
8   Eye
1   Bypass   Definition: Altering the route of passage of the contents of a tubular body part

Explanation: Rerouting contents of a body part to a downstream area of the normal route, to a similar route and body part, or to an abnormal route and dissimilar body part. Includes one or more anastomoses, with or without the use of a device.

Body Part Character 4	Approach Character 5	Device Character 6	Qualifier Character 7
2 Anterior Chamber, Right Aqueous humour **3** Anterior Chamber, Left *See 2 Anterior Chamber, Right*	**3** Percutaneous	**J** Synthetic Substitute **K** Nonautologous Tissue Substitute **Z** No Device	**4** Sclera
X Lacrimal Duct, Right Lacrimal canaliculus Lacrimal punctum Lacrimal sac Nasolacrimal duct **Y** Lacrimal Duct, Left *See X Lacrimal Duct, Right*	**Ø** Open **3** Percutaneous	**J** Synthetic Substitute **K** Nonautologous Tissue Substitute **Z** No Device	**3** Nasal Cavity

---

Ø   Medical and Surgical
8   Eye
2   Change   Definition: Taking out or off a device from a body part and putting back an identical or similar device in or on the same body part without cutting or puncturing the skin or a mucous membrane

Explanation: All CHANGE procedures are coded using the approach EXTERNAL

Body Part Character 4	Approach Character 5	Device Character 6	Qualifier Character 7
Ø Eye, Right Ciliary body Posterior chamber **1** Eye, Left *See Ø Eye, Right*	**X** External	**Ø** Drainage Device **Y** Other Device	**Z** No Qualifier

Non-OR   All body part, approach, device, and qualifier values

---

LC Limited Coverage   NC Noncovered   ⊞ Combination Member   HAC associated procedure   Combination Only   DRG Non-OR   Non-OR   New/Revised in GREEN

ICD-10-PCS 2019   289

Ø   Medical and Surgical
8   Eye
5   Destruction   Definition: Physical eradication of all or a portion of a body part by the direct use of energy, force, or a destructive agent
Explanation: None of the body part is physically taken out

Body Part Character 4		Approach Character 5	Device Character 6	Qualifier Character 7

Ø Eye, Right
   Ciliary body
   Posterior chamber
1 Eye, Left
   See Ø Eye, Right
6 Sclera, Right
7 Sclera, Left
	8 Cornea, Right
	9 Cornea, Left
	S Conjunctiva, Right
	   Plica semilunaris
	T Conjunctiva, Left
	   See S Conjunctiva, Right
		X External	**Z** No Device	**Z** No Qualifier

2 Anterior Chamber, Right
   Aqueous humour
3 Anterior Chamber, Left
   See 2 Anterior Chamber, Right
4 Vitreous, Right
   Vitreous body
5 Vitreous, Left
   See 4 Vitreous, Right
C Iris, Right
D Iris, Left
	E Retina, Right
	   Fovea
	   Macula
	   Optic disc
	F Retina, Left
	   See E Retina, Right
	G Retinal Vessel, Right
	H Retinal Vessel, Left
	J Lens, Right
	   Zonule of Zinn
	K Lens, Left
	   See J Lens, Right
		3 Percutaneous	**Z** No Device	**Z** No Qualifier

A Choroid, Right
B Choroid, Left
L Extraocular Muscle, Right
   Inferior oblique muscle
   Inferior rectus muscle
   Lateral rectus muscle
   Medial rectus muscle
   Superior oblique muscle
   Superior rectus muscle
	M Extraocular Muscle, Left
	   See L Extraocular Muscle, Right
	V Lacrimal Gland, Right
	W Lacrimal Gland, Left
		Ø Open
		3 Percutaneous
			Z No Device	**Z** No Qualifier

N Upper Eyelid, Right
   Lateral canthus
   Levator palpebrae superioris
      muscle
   Orbicularis oculi muscle
   Superior tarsal plate
P Upper Eyelid, Left
   See N Upper Eyelid, Right
	Q Lower Eyelid, Right
	   Inferior tarsal plate
	   Medial canthus
	R Lower Eyelid, Left
	   See Q Lower Eyelid, Right
		Ø Open
		3 Percutaneous
		X External
			Z No Device	**Z** No Qualifier

X Lacrimal Duct, Right
   Lacrimal canaliculus
   Lacrimal punctum
   Lacrimal sac
   Nasolacrimal duct
	Y Lacrimal Duct, Left
	   See X Lacrimal Duct, Right
		Ø Open
		3 Percutaneous
		7 Via Natural or Artificial
		   Opening
		8 Via Natural or Artificial
		   Opening Endoscopic
			Z No Device	**Z** No Qualifier

Non-OR   Ø85[E,F]3ZZ

Ø   Medical and Surgical
8   Eye
7   Dilation   Definition: Expanding an orifice or the lumen of a tubular body part
Explanation: The orifice can be a natural orifice or an artificially created orifice. Accomplished by stretching a tubular body part using intraluminal pressure or by cutting part of the orifice or wall of the tubular body part.

Body Part Character 4	Approach Character 5	Device Character 6	Qualifier Character 7

X Lacrimal Duct, Right
   Lacrimal canaliculus
   Lacrimal punctum
   Lacrimal sac
   Nasolacrimal duct
Y Lacrimal Duct, Left
   See X Lacrimal Duct, Right
	Ø Open
	3 Percutaneous
	7 Via Natural or Artificial
	   Opening
	8 Via Natural or Artificial
	   Opening Endoscopic
		D Intraluminal Device
		Z No Device
			Z No Qualifier

Ø   **Medical and Surgical**
8   **Eye**
9   **Drainage**   Definition: Taking or letting out fluids and/or gases from a body part
                       Explanation: The qualifier DIAGNOSTIC is used to identify drainage procedures that are biopsies

Body Part Character 4		Approach Character 5	Device Character 6	Qualifier Character 7

Ø   **Eye, Right**
   Ciliary body
   Posterior chamber
1   **Eye, Left**
   See Ø Eye, Right
6   **Sclera, Right**
7   **Sclera, Left**
	8 **Cornea, Right**
	9 **Cornea, Left**
	S **Conjunctiva, Right**
	   Plica semilunaris
	T **Conjunctiva, Left**
	   See S Conjunctiva, Right
		X External	**Ø** Drainage Device	**Z** No Qualifier

Ø   **Eye, Right**
   Ciliary body
   Posterior chamber
1   **Eye, Left**
   See Ø Eye, Right
6   **Sclera, Right**
7   **Sclera, Left**
	8 **Cornea, Right**
	9 **Cornea, Left**
	S **Conjunctiva, Right**
	   Plica semilunaris
	T **Conjunctiva, Left**
	   See S Conjunctiva, Right
		X External	**Z** No Device	**X** Diagnostic
				Z No Qualifier

2   **Anterior Chamber, Right**
   Aqueous humour
3   **Anterior Chamber, Left**
   See 2 Anterior Chamber, Right
4   **Vitreous, Right**
   Vitreous body
5   **Vitreous, Left**
   See 4 Vitreous, Right
C   Iris, Right
D   Iris, Left
	E Retina, Right
	   Fovea
	   Macula
	   Optic disc
	F Retina, Left
	   See E Retina, Right
	G Retinal Vessel, Right
	H Retinal Vessel, Left
	J Lens, Right
	   Zonule of Zinn
	K Lens, Left
	   See J Lens, Right
		3 Percutaneous	**Ø** Drainage Device	**Z** No Qualifier

2   **Anterior Chamber, Right**
   Aqueous humour
3   **Anterior Chamber, Left**
   See 2 Anterior Chamber, Right
4   **Vitreous, Right**
   Vitreous body
5   **Vitreous, Left**
   See 4 Vitreous, Right
C   Iris, Right
D   Iris, Left
	E Retina, Right
	   Fovea
	   Macula
	   Optic disc
	F Retina, Left
	   See E Retina, Right
	G Retinal Vessel, Right
	H Retinal Vessel, Left
	J Lens, Right
	   Zonule of Zinn
	K Lens, Left
	   See J Lens, Right
		3 Percutaneous	**Z** No Device	**X** Diagnostic
				Z No Qualifier

A   Choroid, Right
B   Choroid, Left
L   Extraocular Muscle, Right
   Inferior oblique muscle
   Inferior rectus muscle
   Lateral rectus muscle
   Medial rectus muscle
   Superior oblique muscle
   Superior rectus muscle
	M Extraocular Muscle, Left
	   See L Extraocular Muscle, Right
	V Lacrimal Gland, Right
	W Lacrimal Gland, Left
		Ø Open
		3 Percutaneous
			Ø Drainage Device	**Z** No Qualifier

A   Choroid, Right
B   Choroid, Left
L   Extraocular Muscle, Right
   Inferior oblique muscle
   Inferior rectus muscle
   Lateral rectus muscle
   Medial rectus muscle
   Superior oblique muscle
   Superior rectus muscle
	M Extraocular Muscle, Left
	   See L Extraocular Muscle, Right
	V Lacrimal Gland, Right
	W Lacrimal Gland, Left
		Ø Open
		3 Percutaneous
			Z No Device	**X** Diagnostic
				Z No Qualifier

N   **Upper Eyelid, Right**
   Lateral canthus
   Levator palpebrae superioris
     muscle
   Orbicularis oculi muscle
   Superior tarsal plate
P   **Upper Eyelid, Left**
   See N Upper Eyelid, Right
	Q **Lower Eyelid, Right**
	   Inferior tarsal plate
	   Medial canthus
	R **Lower Eyelid, Left**
	   See Q Lower Eyelid, Right
		Ø Open
		3 Percutaneous
		X External
			Ø Drainage Device	**Z** No Qualifier

Ø89 Continued on next page

Non-OR	Ø89[Ø,1,6,7,8,9,S,T]XZ[X,Z]
Non-OR	Ø89[N,P,Q,R][Ø,3,X]ØZ

LC Limited Coverage   **NC** Noncovered   ⊞ Combination Member   HAC associated procedure   Combination Only   DRG Non-OR   Non-OR   New/Revised in GREEN

ICD-10-PCS 2019   291

Ø89–Ø89

0   Medical and Surgical
8   Eye

9   Drainage   Definition: Taking or letting out fluids and/or gases from a body part
Explanation: The qualifier DIAGNOSTIC is used to identify drainage procedures that are biopsies

Body Part Character 4		Approach Character 5	Device Character 6	Qualifier Character 7

N Upper Eyelid, Right
   Lateral canthus
   Levator palpebrae superioris
     muscle
   Orbicularis oculi muscle
   Superior tarsal plate
P Upper Eyelid, Left
   See N Upper Eyelid, Right
	Q Lower Eyelid, Right
	   Inferior tarsal plate
	   Medial canthus
	R Lower Eyelid, Left
	   See Q Lower Eyelid, Right
		0 Open
		3 Percutaneous
		X External
			Z No Device	X Diagnostic
				Z No Qualifier

X Lacrimal Duct, Right
   Lacrimal canaliculus
   Lacrimal punctum
   Lacrimal sac
   Nasolacrimal duct
	Y Lacrimal Duct, Left
	   See X Lacrimal Duct, Right
		0 Open
		3 Percutaneous
		7 Via Natural or Artificial
		   Opening
		8 Via Natural or Artificial
		   Opening Endoscopic
			0 Drainage Device	Z No Qualifier

X Lacrimal Duct, Right
   Lacrimal canaliculus
   Lacrimal punctum
   Lacrimal sac
   Nasolacrimal duct
	Y Lacrimal Duct, Left
	   See X Lacrimal Duct, Right
		0 Open
		3 Percutaneous
		7 Via Natural or Artificial
		   Opening
		8 Via Natural or Artificial
		   Opening Endoscopic
			Z No Device	X Diagnostic
				Z No Qualifier

Non-OR   089[N,P,Q,R]0ZZ
Non-OR   089[N,P,Q,R][3,X]Z[X,Z]

0   Medical and Surgical
8   Eye
B   Excision   Definition: Cutting out or off, without replacement, a portion of a body part
Explanation: The qualifier DIAGNOSTIC is used to identify excision procedures that are biopsies

Body Part Character 4		Approach Character 5	Device Character 6	Qualifier Character 7

0 Eye, Right
   Ciliary body
   Posterior chamber
1 Eye, Left
   See 0 Eye, Right
N Upper Eyelid, Right
   Lateral canthus
   Levator palpebrae superioris
     muscle
   Orbicularis oculi muscle
   Superior tarsal plate
	P Upper Eyelid, Left
	   See N Upper Eyelid, Right
	Q Lower Eyelid, Right
	   Inferior tarsal plate
	   Medial canthus
	R Lower Eyelid, Left
	   See Q Lower Eyelid, Right
		0 Open
		3 Percutaneous
		X External
			Z No Device	X Diagnostic
				Z No Qualifier

4 Vitreous, Right
   Vitreous body
5 Vitreous, Left
   See 4 Vitreous, Right
C Iris, Right
D Iris, Left
E Retina, Right
   Fovea
   Macula
   Optic disc
	F Retina, Left
	   See E Retina, Right
	J Lens, Right
	   Zonule of Zinn
	K Lens, Left
	   See J Lens, Right
		3 Percutaneous	Z No Device	X Diagnostic
				Z No Qualifier

6 Sclera, Right
7 Sclera, Left
8 Cornea, Right
9 Cornea, Left
	S Conjunctiva, Right
	   Plica semilunaris
	T Conjunctiva, Left
	   See S Conjunctiva, Right
		X External	Z No Device	X Diagnostic
				Z No Qualifier

A Choroid, Right
B Choroid, Left
L Extraocular Muscle, Right
   Inferior oblique muscle
   Inferior rectus muscle
   Lateral rectus muscle
   Medial rectus muscle
   Superior oblique muscle
   Superior rectus muscle
	M Extraocular Muscle, Left
	   See L Extraocular Muscle, Right
	V Lacrimal Gland, Right
	W Lacrimal Gland, Left
		0 Open
		3 Percutaneous
			Z No Device	X Diagnostic
				Z No Qualifier

X Lacrimal Duct, Right
   Lacrimal canaliculus
   Lacrimal punctum
   Lacrimal sac
   Nasolacrimal duct
	Y Lacrimal Duct, Left
	   See X Lacrimal Duct, Right
		0 Open
		3 Percutaneous
		7 Via Natural or Artificial
		   Opening
		8 Via Natural or Artificial
		   Opening Endoscopic
			Z No Device	X Diagnostic
				Z No Qualifier

LC Limited Coverage   NC Noncovered   ⊞ Combination Member   HAC associated procedure   Combination Only   DRG Non-OR   Non-OR   New/Revised in GREEN

292   ICD-10-PCS 2019

089–08B

0   **Medical and Surgical**
8   **Eye**
C   **Extirpation**   Definition: Taking or cutting out solid matter from a body part

Explanation: The solid matter may be an abnormal byproduct of a biological function or a foreign body; it may be imbedded in a body part or in the lumen of a tubular body part. The solid matter may or may not have been previously broken into pieces.

Body Part Character 4	Approach Character 5	Device Character 6	Qualifier Character 7

0   **Eye, Right**
    Ciliary body
    Posterior chamber
1   **Eye, Left**
    See 0 Eye, Right
6   **Sclera, Right**
7   **Sclera, Left**
8   **Cornea, Right**
9   **Cornea, Left**
S   **Conjunctiva, Right**
    Plica semilunaris
T   **Conjunctiva, Left**
    See S Conjunctiva, Right
	X External	**Z** No Device	**Z** No Qualifier

2   **Anterior Chamber, Right**
    Aqueous humour
3   **Anterior Chamber, Left**
    See 2 Anterior Chamber, Right
4   **Vitreous, Right**
    Vitreous body
5   **Vitreous, Left**
    See 4 Vitreous, Right
C   **Iris, Right**
D   **Iris, Left**
E   **Retina, Right**
    Fovea
    Macula
    Optic disc
F   **Retina, Left**
    See E Retina, Right
G   **Retinal Vessel, Right**
H   **Retinal Vessel, Left**
J   **Lens, Right**
    Zonule of Zinn
K   **Lens, Left**
    See J Lens, Right
	3 Percutaneous
	X External
		Z No Device	**Z** No Qualifier

A   **Choroid, Right**
B   **Choroid, Left**
L   **Extraocular Muscle, Right**
    Inferior oblique muscle
    Inferior rectus muscle
    Lateral rectus muscle
    Medial rectus muscle
    Superior oblique muscle
    Superior rectus muscle
M   **Extraocular Muscle, Left**
    See L Extraocular Muscle, Right
N   **Upper Eyelid, Right**
    Lateral canthus
    Levator palpebrae superioris muscle
    Orbicularis oculi muscle
    Superior tarsal plate
P   **Upper Eyelid, Left**
    See N Upper Eyelid, Right
Q   **Lower Eyelid, Right**
    Inferior tarsal plate
    Medial canthus
R   **Lower Eyelid, Left**
    See Q Lower Eyelid, Right
V   **Lacrimal Gland, Right**
W   **Lacrimal Gland, Left**
	0 Open
	3 Percutaneous
	X External
		Z No Device	**Z** No Qualifier

X   **Lacrimal Duct, Right**
    Lacrimal canaliculus
    Lacrimal punctum
    Lacrimal sac
    Nasolacrimal duct
Y   **Lacrimal Duct, Left**
    See X Lacrimal Duct, Right
	0 Open
	3 Percutaneous
	7 Via Natural or Artificial Opening
	8 Via Natural or Artificial Opening
	     Endoscopic
		Z No Device	**Z** No Qualifier

Non-OR   08C[0,1,6,7,S,T]XZZ
Non-OR   08C[2,3]XZZ
Non-OR   08C[N,P,Q,R][0,3,X]ZZ

LC Limited Coverage   **NC** Noncovered   ⊞ Combination Member   HAC associated procedure   Combination Only   DRG Non-OR   Non-OR   New/Revised in GREEN

Ø **Medical and Surgical**
8 **Eye**
D **Extraction**   Definition: Pulling or stripping out or off all or a portion of a body part by the use of force
Explanation: The qualifier DIAGNOSTIC is used to identify extraction procedures that are biopsies

Body Part Character 4	Approach Character 5	Device Character 6	Qualifier Character 7
8 Cornea, Right 9 Cornea, Left	X External	Z No Device	X Diagnostic Z No Qualifier

J Lens, Right
  Zonule of Zinn
K Lens, Left
  See J Lens, Right
	3 Percutaneous	Z No Device	Z No Qualifier

Ø **Medical and Surgical**
8 **Eye**
F **Fragmentation**   Definition: Breaking solid matter in a body part into pieces
Explanation: Physical force (e.g., manual, ultrasonic) applied directly or indirectly is used to break the solid matter into pieces. The solid matter may be an abnormal byproduct of a biological function or a foreign body. The pieces of solid matter are not taken out.

Body Part Character 4	Approach Character 5	Device Character 6	Qualifier Character 7

4 Vitreous, Right NC
  Vitreous body
5 Vitreous, Left NC
  See 4 Vitreous, Right
	3 Percutaneous
	X External
		Z No Device	Z No Qualifier

Non-OR   Ø8F[4,5]XZZ
NC   Ø8F[4,5]XZZ

Ø **Medical and Surgical**
8 **Eye**
H **Insertion**   Definition: Putting in a nonbiological appliance that monitors, assists, performs, or prevents a physiological function but does not physically take the place of a body part
Explanation: None

Body Part Character 4	Approach Character 5	Device Character 6	Qualifier Character 7

Ø Eye, Right
  Ciliary body
  Posterior chamber
1 Eye, Left
  See Ø Eye, Right
	Ø Open	5 Epiretinal Visual Prosthesis
		Y Other Device
			Z No Qualifier

Ø Eye, Right
  Ciliary body
  Posterior chamber
1 Eye, Left
  See Ø Eye, Right
	3 Percutaneous	1 Radioactive Element
		3 Infusion Device
		Y Other Device
			Z No Qualifier

Ø Eye, Right
  Ciliary body
  Posterior chamber
1 Eye, Left
  See Ø Eye, Right
	7 Via Natural or Artificial Opening
	8 Via Natural or Artificial Opening Endoscopic
		Y Other Device	Z No Qualifier

Ø Eye, Right
  Ciliary body
  Posterior chamber
1 Eye, Left
  See Ø Eye, Right
	X External	1 Radioactive Element
		3 Infusion Device
			Z No Qualifier

Non-OR   Ø8H[Ø,1]3YZ
Non-OR   Ø8H[Ø,1][7,8]YZ

0   **Medical and Surgical**
8   **Eye**
J   **Inspection**   Definition: Visually and/or manually exploring a body part

Explanation: Visual exploration may be performed with or without optical instrumentation. Manual exploration may be performed directly or through intervening body layers.

Body Part Character 4	Approach Character 5	Device Character 6	Qualifier Character 7

0 Eye, Right
  Ciliary body
  Posterior chamber
1 Eye, Left
  See 0 Eye, Right
J Lens, Right
  Zonule of Zinn
K Lens, Left
  See J Lens, Right
	X External	**Z** No Device	**Z** No Qualifier

L Extraocular Muscle, Right
  Inferior oblique muscle
  Inferior rectus muscle
  Lateral rectus muscle
  Medial rectus muscle
  Superior oblique muscle
  Superior rectus muscle
M Extraocular Muscle, Left
  See L Extraocular Muscle, Right
	0 Open
	X External
		Z No Device	**Z** No Qualifier

Non-OR   08J[0,1,J,K]XZZ
Non-OR   08J[L,M]XZZ

0   **Medical and Surgical**
8   **Eye**
L   **Occlusion**   Definition: Completely closing an orifice or the lumen of a tubular body part

Explanation: The orifice can be a natural orifice or an artificially created orifice

Body Part Character 4	Approach Character 5	Device Character 6	Qualifier Character 7

X Lacrimal Duct, Right
  Lacrimal canaliculus
  Lacrimal punctum
  Lacrimal sac
  Nasolacrimal duct
Y Lacrimal Duct, Left
  See X Lacrimal Duct, Right
	0 Open
	3 Percutaneous
		C Extraluminal Device
		D Intraluminal Device
		Z No Device
			Z No Qualifier

X Lacrimal Duct, Right
  Lacrimal canaliculus
  Lacrimal punctum
  Lacrimal sac
  Nasolacrimal duct
Y Lacrimal Duct, Left
  See X Lacrimal Duct, Right
	7 Via Natural or Artificial Opening
	8 Via Natural or Artificial Opening Endoscopic
		D Intraluminal Device
		Z No Device
			Z No Qualifier

0   **Medical and Surgical**
8   **Eye**
M   **Reattachment**   Definition: Putting back in or on all or a portion of a separated body part to its normal location or other suitable location

Explanation: Vascular circulation and nervous pathways may or may not be reestablished

Body Part Character 4	Approach Character 5	Device Character 6	Qualifier Character 7

N Upper Eyelid, Right
  Lateral canthus
  Levator palpebrae superioris muscle
  Orbicularis oculi muscle
  Superior tarsal plate
P Upper Eyelid, Left
  See N Upper Eyelid, Right
Q Lower Eyelid, Right
  Inferior tarsal plate
  Medial canthus
R Lower Eyelid, Left
  See Q Lower Eyelid, Right
	X External	**Z** No Device	**Z** No Qualifier

0 Medical and Surgical
8 Eye
N Release

Definition: Freeing a body part from an abnormal physical constraint by cutting or by the use of force
Explanation: Some of the restraining tissue may be taken out but none of the body part is taken out

Body Part Character 4	Approach Character 5	Device Character 6	Qualifier Character 7

0 Eye, Right
  Ciliary body
  Posterior chamber
1 Eye, Left
  See 0 Eye, Right
6 Sclera, Right
7 Sclera, Left
8 Cornea, Right
9 Cornea, Left
S Conjunctiva, Right
  Plica semilunaris
T Conjunctiva, Left
  See S Conjunctiva, Right
	X External	**Z** No Device	**Z** No Qualifier

2 Anterior Chamber, Right
  Aqueous humour
3 Anterior Chamber, Left
  See 2 Anterior Chamber, Right
4 Vitreous, Right
  Vitreous body
5 Vitreous, Left
  See 4 Vitreous, Right
C Iris, Right
D Iris, Left
E Retina, Right
  Fovea
  Macula
  Optic disc
F Retina, Left
  See E Retina, Right
G Retinal Vessel, Right
H Retinal Vessel, Left
J Lens, Right
  Zonule of Zinn
K Lens, Left
  See J Lens, Right
	3 Percutaneous	**Z** No Device	**Z** No Qualifier

A Choroid, Right
B Choroid, Left
L Extraocular Muscle, Right
  Inferior oblique muscle
  Inferior rectus muscle
  Lateral rectus muscle
  Medial rectus muscle
  Superior oblique muscle
  Superior rectus muscle
M Extraocular Muscle, Left
  See L Extraocular Muscle, Right
V Lacrimal Gland, Right
W Lacrimal Gland, Left
	0 Open
	3 Percutaneous
		Z No Device	**Z** No Qualifier

N Upper Eyelid, Right
  Lateral canthus
  Levator palpebrae superioris muscle
  Orbicularis oculi muscle
  Superior tarsal plate
P Upper Eyelid, Left
  See N Upper Eyelid, Right
Q Lower Eyelid, Right
  Inferior tarsal plate
  Medial canthus
R Lower Eyelid, Left
  See Q Lower Eyelid, Right
	0 Open
	3 Percutaneous
	X External
		Z No Device	**Z** No Qualifier

X Lacrimal Duct, Right
  Lacrimal canaliculus
  Lacrimal punctum
  Lacrimal sac
  Nasolacrimal duct
Y Lacrimal Duct, Left
  See X Lacrimal Duct, Right
	0 Open
	3 Percutaneous
	7 Via Natural or Artificial Opening
	8 Via Natural or Artificial Opening Endoscopic
		Z No Device	**Z** No Qualifier

LC Limited Coverage NC Noncovered ⊞ Combination Member HAC associated procedure Combination Only DRG Non-OR Non-OR New/Revised in GREEN

296 ICD-10-PCS 2019

0   **Medical and Surgical**
8   **Eye**
P   **Removal**   Definition: Taking out or off a device from a body part

Explanation: If a device is taken out and a similar device put in without cutting or puncturing the skin or mucous membrane, the procedure is coded to the root operation CHANGE. Otherwise, the procedure for taking out a device is coded to the root operation REMOVAL.

Body Part Character 4	Approach Character 5	Device Character 6	Qualifier Character 7

0 Eye, Right
   Ciliary body
   Posterior chamber
1 Eye, Left
   See 0 Eye, Right
	0 Open
	3 Percutaneous
	7 Via Natural or Artificial Opening
	8 Via Natural or Artificial Opening
	    Endoscopic
		0 Drainage Device
		1 Radioactive Element
		3 Infusion Device
		7 Autologous Tissue Substitute
		C Extraluminal Device
		D Intraluminal Device
		J Synthetic Substitute
		K Nonautologous Tissue Substitute
		Y Other Device
			Z No Qualifier

0 Eye, Right
   Ciliary body
   Posterior chamber
1 Eye, Left
   See 0 Eye, Right
	X External	**0** Drainage Device
		1 Radioactive Element
		3 Infusion Device
		7 Autologous Tissue Substitute
		C Extraluminal Device
		D Intraluminal Device
		J Synthetic Substitute
		K Nonautologous Tissue Substitute
			Z No Qualifier

J Lens, Right
   Zonule of Zinn
K Lens, Left
   See J Lens, Right
	3 Percutaneous	**J** Synthetic Substitute
		Y Other Device
			Z No Qualifier

L Extraocular Muscle, Right
   Inferior oblique muscle
   Inferior rectus muscle
   Lateral rectus muscle
   Medial rectus muscle
   Superior oblique muscle
   Superior rectus muscle
M Extraocular Muscle, Left
   See L Extraocular Muscle, Right
	0 Open
	3 Percutaneous
		0 Drainage Device
		7 Autologous Tissue Substitute
		J Synthetic Substitute
		K Nonautologous Tissue Substitute
		Y Other Device
			Z No Qualifier

Non-OR   08P[0,1]3YZ
Non-OR   08P[0,1][7,8][0,3,D,Y]Z
Non-OR   08P[0,1]X[0,1,3,C,D,J]Z
Non-OR   08P[J,K]3YZ
Non-OR   08P[L,M]3YZ

LC Limited Coverage   NC Noncovered   ⊞ Combination Member   HAC associated procedure   Combination Only   DRG Non-OR   Non-OR   New/Revised in GREEN
ICD-10-PCS 2019   297

08P–08P

Ø   Medical and Surgical
8   Eye
Q   Repair   Definition: Restoring, to the extent possible, a body part to its normal anatomic structure and function
                          Explanation: Used only when the method to accomplish the repair is not one of the other root operations

Body Part Character 4	Approach Character 5	Device Character 6	Qualifier Character 7

Ø Eye, Right
   Ciliary body
   Posterior chamber
1 Eye, Left
   See Ø Eye, Right
6 Sclera, Right
7 Sclera, Left
8 Cornea, Right   NC
9 Cornea, Left   NC
S Conjunctiva, Right
   Plica semilunaris
T Conjunctiva, Left
   See S Conjunctiva, Right
	X External	**Z No Device**	**Z No Qualifier**

2 Anterior Chamber, Right
   Aqueous humour
3 Anterior Chamber, Left
   See 2 Anterior Chamber, Right
4 Vitreous, Right
   Vitreous body
5 Vitreous, Left
   See 4 Vitreous, Right
C Iris, Right
D Iris, Left
E Retina, Right
   Fovea
   Macula
   Optic disc
F Retina, Left
   See E Retina, Right
G Retinal Vessel, Right
H Retinal Vessel, Left
J Lens, Right
   Zonule of Zinn
K Lens, Left
   See J Lens, Right
	3 Percutaneous	**Z No Device**	**Z No Qualifier**

A Choroid, Right
B Choroid, Left
L Extraocular Muscle, Right
   Inferior oblique muscle
   Inferior rectus muscle
   Lateral rectus muscle
   Medial rectus muscle
   Superior oblique muscle
   Superior rectus muscle
M Extraocular Muscle, Left
   See L Extraocular Muscle, Right
V Lacrimal Gland, Right
W Lacrimal Gland, Left
	Ø Open
	3 Percutaneous
		Z No Device	**Z No Qualifier**

N Upper Eyelid, Right
   Lateral canthus
   Levator palpebrae superioris muscle
   Orbicularis oculi muscle
   Superior tarsal plate
P Upper Eyelid, Left
   See N Upper Eyelid, Right
Q Lower Eyelid, Right
   Inferior tarsal plate
   Medial canthus
R Lower Eyelid, Left
   See Q Lower Eyelid, Right
	Ø Open
	3 Percutaneous
	X External
		Z No Device	**Z No Qualifier**

X Lacrimal Duct, Right
   Lacrimal canaliculus
   Lacrimal punctum
   Lacrimal sac
   Nasolacrimal duct
Y Lacrimal Duct, Left
   See X Lacrimal Duct, Right
	Ø Open
	3 Percutaneous
	7 Via Natural or Artificial Opening
	**8 Via Natural or Artificial Opening
	   Endoscopic**
		Z No Device	**Z No Qualifier**

Non-OR	Ø8Q[N,P,Q,R][Ø,3,X]ZZ
NC	Ø8Q[8,9]XZZ

LC Limited Coverage   NC Noncovered   ⊞ Combination Member   HAC associated procedure   Combination Only   DRG Non-OR   Non-OR   New/Revised in GREEN

298   ICD-10-PCS 2019

Ø   Medical and Surgical
8   Eye
R   Replacement   Definition: Putting in or on biological or synthetic material that physically takes the place and/or function of all or a portion of a body part

Explanation: The body part may have been taken out or replaced, or may be taken out, physically eradicated, or rendered nonfunctional during the REPLACEMENT procedure. A REMOVAL procedure is coded for taking out the device used in a previous replacement procedure.

Body Part Character 4	Approach Character 5	Device Character 6	Qualifier Character 7

Ø Eye, Right
  Ciliary body
  Posterior chamber
1 Eye, Left
  See Ø Eye, Right
A Choroid, Right
B Choroid, Left
	Ø Open
	3 Percutaneous
		7 Autologous Tissue Substitute
		J Synthetic Substitute
		K Nonautologous Tissue Substitute
			Z No Qualifier

4 Vitreous, Right
  Vitreous body
5 Vitreous, Left
  See 4 Vitreous, Right
C Iris, Right
D Iris, Left
G Retinal Vessel, Right
H Retinal Vessel, Left
	3 Percutaneous	7 Autologous Tissue Substitute
		J Synthetic Substitute
		K Nonautologous Tissue Substitute
			Z No Qualifier

6 Sclera, Right
7 Sclera, Left
S Conjunctiva, Right
  Plica semilunaris
T Conjunctiva, Left
  See S Conjunctiva, Right
	X External	7 Autologous Tissue Substitute
		J Synthetic Substitute
		K Nonautologous Tissue Substitute
			Z No Qualifier

8 Cornea, Right 9 Cornea, Left	3 Percutaneous X External	7 Autologous Tissue Substitute J Synthetic Substitute K Nonautologous Tissue Substitute	Z No Qualifier

J Lens, Right
  Zonule of Zinn
K Lens, Left
  See J Lens, Right
	3 Percutaneous	Ø Synthetic Substitute, Intraocular Telescope
		7 Autologous Tissue Substitute
		J Synthetic Substitute
		K Nonautologous Tissue Substitute
			Z No Qualifier

N Upper Eyelid, Right
  Lateral canthus
  Levator palpebrae superioris muscle
  Orbicularis oculi muscle
  Superior tarsal plate
P Upper Eyelid, Left
  See N Upper Eyelid, Right
Q Lower Eyelid, Right
  Inferior tarsal plate
  Medial canthus
R Lower Eyelid, Left
  See Q Lower Eyelid, Right
	Ø Open
	3 Percutaneous
	X External
		7 Autologous Tissue Substitute
		J Synthetic Substitute
		K Nonautologous Tissue Substitute
			Z No Qualifier

X Lacrimal Duct, Right
  Lacrimal canaliculus
  Lacrimal punctum
  Lacrimal sac
  Nasolacrimal duct
Y Lacrimal Duct, Left
  See X Lacrimal Duct, Right
	Ø Open
	3 Percutaneous
	7 Via Natural or Artificial Opening
	8 Via Natural or Artificial Opening Endoscopic
		7 Autologous Tissue Substitute
		J Synthetic Substitute
		K Nonautologous Tissue Substitute
			Z No Qualifier

LC Limited Coverage   NC Noncovered   ⊞ Combination Member   HAC associated procedure   Combination Only   DRG Non-OR   Non-OR   New/Revised in GREEN

ICD-10-PCS 2019   299

Ø8R-Ø8R

0   Medical and Surgical
8   Eye
S   Reposition   Definition: Moving to its normal location, or other suitable location, all or a portion of a body part

Explanation: The body part is moved to a new location from an abnormal location, or from a normal location where it is not functioning correctly. The body part may or may not be cut out or off to be moved to the new location.

Body Part Character 4	Approach Character 5	Device Character 6	Qualifier Character 7

C Iris, Right
D Iris, Left
G Retinal Vessel, Right
H Retinal Vessel, Left
J Lens, Right
   Zonule of Zinn
K Lens, Left
   See J Lens, Right
	3 Percutaneous	**Z** No Device	**Z** No Qualifier

L Extraocular Muscle, Right
   Inferior oblique muscle
   Inferior rectus muscle
   Lateral rectus muscle
   Medial rectus muscle
   Superior oblique muscle
   Superior rectus muscle
M Extraocular Muscle, Left
   See L Extraocular Muscle, Right
V Lacrimal Gland, Right
W Lacrimal Gland, Left
	0 Open
	3 Percutaneous
		Z No Device	**Z** No Qualifier

N Upper Eyelid, Right
   Lateral canthus
   Levator palpebrae superioris muscle
   Orbicularis oculi muscle
   Superior tarsal plate
P Upper Eyelid, Left
   See N Upper Eyelid, Right
Q Lower Eyelid, Right
   Inferior tarsal plate
   Medial canthus
R Lower Eyelid, Left
   See Q Lower Eyelid, Right
	0 Open
	3 Percutaneous
	X External
		Z No Device	**Z** No Qualifier

X Lacrimal Duct, Right
   Lacrimal canaliculus
   Lacrimal punctum
   Lacrimal sac
   Nasolacrimal duct
Y Lacrimal Duct, Left
   See X Lacrimal Duct, Right
	0 Open
	3 Percutaneous
	7 Via Natural or Artificial Opening
	8 Via Natural or Artificial Opening Endoscopic
		Z No Device	**Z** No Qualifier

LC Limited Coverage   NC Noncovered   ⊞ Combination Member   HAC associated procedure   Combination Only   DRG Non-OR   Non-OR   New/Revised in GREEN

300   ICD-10-PCS 2019

Ø   **Medical and Surgical**
8   **Eye**
T   **Resection**   Definition: Cutting out or off, without replacement, all of a body part
                      Explanation: None

Body Part Character 4	Approach Character 5	Device Character 6	Qualifier Character 7

Ø **Eye, Right**
   Ciliary body
   Posterior chamber
1 **Eye, Left**
   See Ø Eye, Right
8 **Cornea, Right**
9 **Cornea, Left**
	X External	**Z** No Device	**Z** No Qualifier

4 **Vitreous, Right**
   Vitreous body
5 **Vitreous, Left**
   See 4 Vitreous, Right
C **Iris, Right**
D **Iris, Left**
J **Lens, Right**
   Zonule of Zinn
K **Lens, Left**
   See J Lens, Right
	3 Percutaneous	**Z** No Device	**Z** No Qualifier

L **Extraocular Muscle, Right**
   Inferior oblique muscle
   Inferior rectus muscle
   Lateral rectus muscle
   Medial rectus muscle
   Superior oblique muscle
   Superior rectus muscle
M **Extraocular Muscle, Left**
   See L Extraocular Muscle, Right
V **Lacrimal Gland, Right**
W **Lacrimal Gland, Left**
	Ø Open
	3 Percutaneous
		Z No Device	**Z** No Qualifier

N **Upper Eyelid, Right**
   Lateral canthus
   Levator palpebrae superioris muscle
   Orbicularis oculi muscle
   Superior tarsal plate
P **Upper Eyelid, Left**
   See N Upper Eyelid, Right
Q **Lower Eyelid, Right**
   Inferior tarsal plate
   Medial canthus
R **Lower Eyelid, Left**
   See Q Lower Eyelid, Right
	Ø Open
	X External
		Z No Device	**Z** No Qualifier

X **Lacrimal Duct, Right**
   Lacrimal canaliculus
   Lacrimal punctum
   Lacrimal sac
   Nasolacrimal duct
Y **Lacrimal Duct, Left**
   See X Lacrimal Duct, Right
	Ø Open
	3 Percutaneous
	7 Via Natural or Artificial Opening
	8 Via Natural or Artificial Opening Endoscopic
		Z No Device	**Z** No Qualifier

0   Medical and Surgical
8   Eye
U   Supplement   Definition: Putting in or on biological or synthetic material that physically reinforces and/or augments the function of a portion of a body part
Explanation: The biological material is non-living, or is living and from the same individual. The body part may have been previously replaced, and the SUPPLEMENT procedure is performed to physically reinforce and/or augment the function of the replaced body part.

Body Part Character 4	Approach Character 5	Device Character 6	Qualifier Character 7

0 Eye, Right
  Ciliary body
  Posterior chamber
1 Eye, Left
  See 0 Eye, Right
C Iris, Right
D Iris, Left
E Retina, Right
  Fovea
  Macula
  Optic disc
F Retina, Left
  See E Retina, Right
G Retinal Vessel, Right
H Retinal Vessel, Left
L Extraocular Muscle, Right
  Inferior oblique muscle
  Inferior rectus muscle
  Lateral rectus muscle
  Medial rectus muscle
  Superior oblique muscle
  Superior rectus muscle
M Extraocular Muscle, Left
  See L Extraocular Muscle, Right
	0 Open
	3 Percutaneous
		7 Autologous Tissue Substitute
		J Synthetic Substitute
		K Nonautologous Tissue Substitute
			Z No Qualifier

8 Cornea, Right   **NC**
9 Cornea, Left   **NC**
N Upper Eyelid, Right
  Lateral canthus
  Levator palpebrae superioris muscle
  Orbicularis oculi muscle
  Superior tarsal plate
P Upper Eyelid, Left
  See N Upper Eyelid, Right
Q Lower Eyelid, Right
  Inferior tarsal plate
  Medial canthus
R Lower Eyelid, Left
  See Q Lower Eyelid, Right
	0 Open
	3 Percutaneous
	X External
		7 Autologous Tissue Substitute
		J Synthetic Substitute
		K Nonautologous Tissue Substitute
			Z No Qualifier

X Lacrimal Duct, Right
  Lacrimal canaliculus
  Lacrimal punctum
  Lacrimal sac
  Nasolacrimal duct
Y Lacrimal Duct, Left
  See X Lacrimal Duct, Right
	0 Open
	3 Percutaneous
	7 Via Natural or Artificial Opening
	8 Via Natural or Artificial Opening Endoscopic
		7 Autologous Tissue Substitute
		J Synthetic Substitute
		K Nonautologous Tissue Substitute
			Z No Qualifier

NC 08U[8,9][0,3,X]KZ

0   Medical and Surgical
8   Eye
V   Restriction   Definition: Partially closing an orifice or the lumen of a tubular body part
Explanation: The orifice can be a natural orifice or an artificially created orifice

Body Part Character 4	Approach Character 5	Device Character 6	Qualifier Character 7

X Lacrimal Duct, Right
  Lacrimal canaliculus
  Lacrimal punctum
  Lacrimal sac
  Nasolacrimal duct
Y Lacrimal Duct, Left
  See X Lacrimal Duct, Right
	0 Open
	3 Percutaneous
		C Extraluminal Device
		D Intraluminal Device
		Z No Device
			Z No Qualifier

X Lacrimal Duct, Right
  Lacrimal canaliculus
  Lacrimal punctum
  Lacrimal sac
  Nasolacrimal duct
Y Lacrimal Duct, Left
  See X Lacrimal Duct, Right
	7 Via Natural or Artificial Opening
	8 Via Natural or Artificial Opening Endoscopic
		D Intraluminal Device
		Z No Device
			Z No Qualifier

LC Limited Coverage   **NC** Noncovered   ⊞ Combination Member   HAC associated procedure   Combination Only   DRG Non-OR   Non-OR   New/Revised in GREEN
302   ICD-10-PCS 2019

08U–08V

0 Medical and Surgical
8 Eye
W Revision

Definition: Correcting, to the extent possible, a portion of a malfunctioning device or the position of a displaced device

Explanation: Revision can include correcting a malfunctioning or displaced device by taking out or putting in components of the device such as a screw or pin

Body Part Character 4	Approach Character 5	Device Character 6	Qualifier Character 7

0 Eye, Right
   Ciliary body
   Posterior chamber
1 Eye, Left
   See 0 Eye, Right
	0 Open
	3 Percutaneous
	7 Via Natural or Artificial Opening
	8 Via Natural or Artificial Opening
	   Endoscopic
		0 Drainage Device
		3 Infusion Device
		7 Autologous Tissue Substitute
		C Extraluminal Device
		D Intraluminal Device
		J Synthetic Substitute
		K Nonautologous Tissue Substitute
		Y Other Device
			Z No Qualifier

0 Eye, Right
   Ciliary body
   Posterior chamber
1 Eye, Left
   See 0 Eye, Right
	X External	0 Drainage Device
		3 Infusion Device
		7 Autologous Tissue Substitute
		C Extraluminal Device
		D Intraluminal Device
		J Synthetic Substitute
		K Nonautologous Tissue Substitute
			Z No Qualifier

J Lens, Right
   Zonule of Zinn
K Lens, Left
   See J Lens, Right
	3 Percutaneous	J Synthetic Substitute
		Y Other Device
			Z No Qualifier

J Lens, Right
   Zonule of Zinn
K Lens, Left
   See J Lens, Right
	X External	J Synthetic Substitute	Z No Qualifier

L Extraocular Muscle, Right
   Inferior oblique muscle
   Inferior rectus muscle
   Lateral rectus muscle
   Medial rectus muscle
   Superior oblique muscle
   Superior rectus muscle
M Extraocular Muscle, Left
   See L Extraocular Muscle, Right
	0 Open
	3 Percutaneous
		0 Drainage Device
		7 Autologous Tissue Substitute
		J Synthetic Substitute
		K Nonautologous Tissue Substitute
		Y Other Device
			Z No Qualifier

Non-OR	08W[0,1][3,7,8]YZ
Non-OR	08W[0,1]X[0,3,7,C,D,J,K]Z
Non-OR	08W[J,K]3YZ
Non-OR	08W[J,K]XJZ
Non-OR	08W[L,M]3YZ

0 Medical and Surgical
8 Eye
X Transfer

Definition: Moving, without taking out, all or a portion of a body part to another location to take over the function of all or a portion of a body part

Explanation: The body part transferred remains connected to its vascular and nervous supply

Body Part Character 4	Approach Character 5	Device Character 6	Qualifier Character 7

L Extraocular Muscle, Right
   Inferior oblique muscle
   Inferior rectus muscle
   Lateral rectus muscle
   Medial rectus muscle
   Superior oblique muscle
   Superior rectus muscle
M Extraocular Muscle, Left
   See L Extraocular Muscle, Right
	0 Open
	3 Percutaneous
		Z No Device	Z No Qualifier

Ear, Nose, Sinus Ø9Ø–Ø9W

Character Meanings*

This Character Meaning table is provided as a guide to assist the user in the identification of character members that may be found in this section of code tables. It **SHOULD NOT** be used to build a PCS code.

Operation–Character 3		Body Part–Character 4		Approach–Character 5		Device–Character 6		Qualifier–Character 7	
Ø	Alteration	Ø	External Ear, Right	Ø	Open	Ø	Drainage Device	Ø	Endolymphatic
1	Bypass	1	External Ear, Left	3	Percutaneous	4	Hearing Device, Bone Conduction	X	Diagnostic
2	Change	2	External Ear, Bilateral	4	Percutaneous Endoscopic	5	Hearing Device, Single Channel Cochlear Prosthesis	Z	No Qualifier
3	Control	3	External Auditory Canal, Right	7	Via Natural or Artificial Opening	6	Hearing Device, Multiple Channel Cochlear Prosthesis		
5	Destruction	4	External Auditory Canal, Left	8	Via Natural or Artificial Opening Endoscopic	7	Autologous Tissue Substitute		
7	Dilation	5	Middle Ear, Right	X	External	B	Intraluminal Device, Airway		
8	Division	6	Middle Ear, Left			D	Intraluminal Device		
9	Drainage	7	Tympanic Membrane, Right			J	Synthetic Substitute		
B	Excision	8	Tympanic Membrane, Left			K	Nonautologous Tissue Substitute		
C	Extirpation	9	Auditory Ossicle, Right			S	Hearing Device		
D	Extraction	A	Auditory Ossicle, Left			Y	Other Device		
H	Insertion	B	Mastoid Sinus, Right			Z	No Device		
J	Inspection	C	Mastoid Sinus, Left						
M	Reattachment	D	Inner Ear, Right						
N	Release	E	Inner Ear, Left						
P	Removal	F	Eustachian Tube, Right						
Q	Repair	G	Eustachian Tube, Left						
R	Replacement	H	Ear, Right						
S	Reposition	J	Ear, Left						
T	Resection	K	Nasal Mucosa and Soft Tissue						
U	Supplement	L	Nasal Turbinate						
W	Revision	M	Nasal Septum						
		N	Nasopharynx						
		P	Accessory Sinus						
		Q	Maxillary Sinus, Right						
		R	Maxillary Sinus, Left						
		S	Frontal Sinus, Right						
		T	Frontal Sinus, Left						
		U	Ethmoid Sinus, Right						
		V	Ethmoid Sinus, Left						
		W	Sphenoid Sinus, Right						
		X	Sphenoid Sinus, Left						
		Y	Sinus						

* Includes sinus ducts.

AHA Coding Clinic for table Ø95
2018, 1Q, 19   Control of epistaxis via silver nitrate cauterization

AHA Coding Clinic for table Ø9Q
2018, 1Q, 19   Control of epistaxis via silver nitrate cauterization
2017, 4Q, 106   Control of bleeding of external naris using suture
2014, 4Q, 20   Control of epistaxis
2014, 3Q, 22   Transsphenoidal removal of pituitary tumor and fat graft placement
2013, 4Q, 114   Balloon sinuplasty

Ear Anatomy

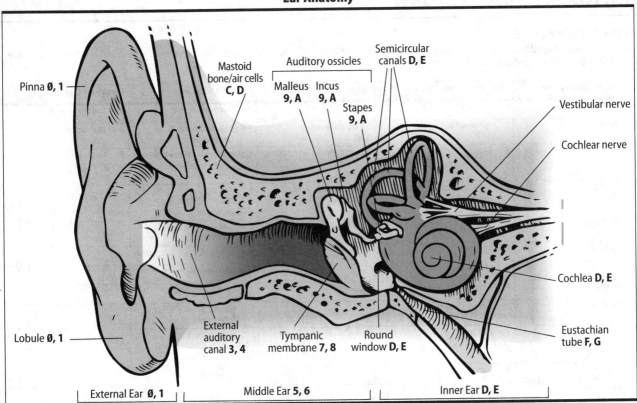

Pinna Ø, 1

Mastoid bone/air cells C, D

Auditory ossicles

Malleus 9, A

Incus 9, A

Stapes 9, A

Semicircular canals D, E

Vestibular nerve

Cochlear nerve

Cochlea D, E

Eustachian tube F, G

Round window D, E

Tympanic membrane 7, 8

External auditory canal 3, 4

Lobule Ø, 1

External Ear Ø, 1   Middle Ear 5, 6   Inner Ear D, E

Nasal Turbinates

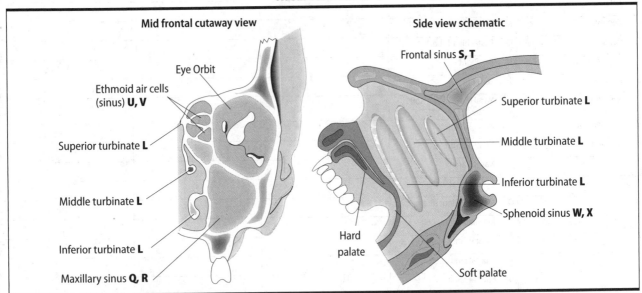

Mid frontal cutaway view

Side view schematic

Eye Orbit

Ethmoid air cells (sinus) U, V

Superior turbinate L

Middle turbinate L

Inferior turbinate L

Maxillary sinus Q, R

Frontal sinus S, T

Superior turbinate L

Middle turbinate L

Inferior turbinate L

Sphenoid sinus W, X

Hard palate

Soft palate

Paranasal Sinuses

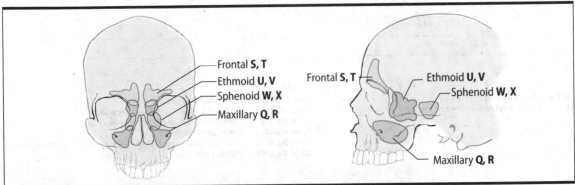

Frontal S, T
Ethmoid U, V
Sphenoid W, X
Maxillary Q, R

Frontal S, T

Ethmoid U, V

Sphenoid W, X

Maxillary Q, R

Ø　Medical and Surgical
9　Ear, Nose, Sinus
Ø　Alteration　Definition: Modifying the anatomic structure of a body part without affecting the function of the body part
　　　　　　　　　Explanation: Principal purpose is to improve appearance

Body Part Character 4		Approach Character 5	Device Character 6	Qualifier Character 7
Ø **External Ear, Right** Antihelix Antitragus Auricle Earlobe Helix Pinna Tragus **1** **External Ear, Left** *See Ø External Ear, Right*	**2** **External Ear, Bilateral** *See Ø External Ear, Right* **K** **Nasal Mucosa and Soft Tissue** Columella External naris Greater alar cartilage Internal naris Lateral nasal cartilage Lesser alar cartilage Nasal cavity Nostril	**Ø** Open **3** Percutaneous **4** Percutaneous Endoscopic **X** External	**7** Autologous Tissue Substitute **J** Synthetic Substitute **K** Nonautologous Tissue Substitute **Z** No Device	**Z** No Qualifier

Ø　Medical and Surgical
9　Ear, Nose, Sinus
1　Bypass　Definition: Altering the route of passage of the contents of a tubular body part
　　　　　　　Explanation: Rerouting contents of a body part to a downstream area of the normal route, to a similar route and body part, or to an abnormal route and dissimilar body part. Includes one or more anastomoses, with or without the use of a device.

Body Part Character 4	Approach Character 5	Device Character 6	Qualifier Character 7
D **Inner Ear, Right** Bony labyrinth Bony vestibule Cochlea Round window Semicircular canal **E** **Inner Ear, Left** *See D Inner Ear, Right*	**Ø** Open	**7** Autologous Tissue Substitute **J** Synthetic Substitute **K** Nonautologous Tissue Substitute **Z** No Device	**Ø** Endolymphatic

Ø　Medical and Surgical
9　Ear, Nose, Sinus
2　Change　Definition: Taking out or off a device from a body part and putting back an identical or similar device in or on the same body part without cutting or puncturing the skin or a mucous membrane
　　　　　　　Explanation: ALL CHANGE procedures are coded using the approach EXTERNAL

Body Part Character 4	Approach Character 5	Device Character 6	Qualifier Character 7
H **Ear, Right** **J** **Ear, Left** **K** **Nasal Mucosa and Soft Tissue** Columella External naris Greater alar cartilage Internal naris Lateral nasal cartilage Lesser alar cartilage Nasal cavity Nostril **Y** **Sinus**	**X** External	**Ø** Drainage Device **Y** Other Device	**Z** No Qualifier

Non-OR　All body part, approach, device, and qualifier values

Ø　Medical and Surgical
9　Ear, Nose, Sinus
3　Control　Definition: Stopping, or attempting to stop, postprocedural or other acute bleeding
　　　　　　　Explanation: The site of the bleeding is coded as an anatomical region and not to a specific body part

Body Part Character 4	Approach Character 5	Device Character 6	Qualifier Character 7
K **Nasal Mucosa and Soft Tissue** Columella External naris Greater alar cartilage Internal naris Lateral nasal cartilage Lesser alar cartilage Nasal cavity Nostril	**7** Via Natural or Artificial Opening **8** Via Natural or Artificial Opening Endoscopic	**Z** No Device	**Z** No Qualifier

Ear, Nose, Sinus *(side margin)*

Ø   **Medical and Surgical**
9   **Ear, Nose, Sinus**
5   **Destruction**   Definition: Physical eradication of all or a portion of a body part by the direct use of energy, force, or a destructive agent
                   Explanation: None of the body part is physically taken out

Body Part Character 4		Approach Character 5	Device Character 6	Qualifier Character 7
Ø External Ear, Right Antihelix Antitragus Auricle Earlobe Helix Pinna Tragus	**1 External Ear, Left** *See Ø External Ear, Right*	**Ø** Open **3** Percutaneous **4** Percutaneous Endoscopic **X** External	**Z** No Device	**Z** No Qualifier
3 External Auditory Canal, Right External auditory meatus	**4 External Auditory Canal, Left** *See 3 External Auditory Canal, Right*	**Ø** Open **3** Percutaneous **4** Percutaneous Endoscopic **7** Via Natural or Artificial Opening **8** Via Natural or Artificial Opening Endoscopic **X** External	**Z** No Device	**Z** No Qualifier
5 Middle Ear, Right Oval window Tympanic cavity **6 Middle Ear, Left** *See 5 Middle Ear, Right* **9 Auditory Ossicle, Right** Incus Malleus Stapes **A Auditory Ossicle, Left** *See 9 Auditory Ossicle, Right*	**D Inner Ear, Right** Bony labyrinth Bony vestibule Cochlea Round window Semicircular canal **E Inner Ear, Left** *See D Inner Ear, Right*	**Ø** Open **8** Via Natural or Artificial Opening Endoscopic	**Z** No Device	**Z** No Qualifier
7 Tympanic Membrane, Right Pars flaccida **8 Tympanic Membrane, Left** *See 7 Tympanic Membrane, Right* **F Eustachian Tube, Right** Auditory tube Pharyngotympanic tube **G Eustachian Tube, Left** *See F Eustachian Tube, Right*	**L Nasal Turbinate** Inferior turbinate Middle turbinate Nasal concha Superior turbinate **N Nasopharynx** Choana Fossa of Rosenmuller Pharyngeal recess Rhinopharynx	**Ø** Open **3** Percutaneous **4** Percutaneous Endoscopic **7** Via Natural or Artificial Opening **8** Via Natural or Artificial Opening Endoscopic	**Z** No Device	**Z** No Qualifier
B Mastoid Sinus, Right Mastoid air cells **C Mastoid Sinus, Left** *See B Mastoid Sinus, Right* **M Nasal Septum** Quadrangular cartilage Septal cartilage Vomer bone **P Accessory Sinus** **Q Maxillary Sinus, Right** Antrum of Highmore	**R Maxillary Sinus, Left** *See Q Maxillary Sinus, Right* **S Frontal Sinus, Right** **T Frontal Sinus, Left** **U Ethmoid Sinus, Right** Ethmoidal air cell **V Ethmoid Sinus, Left** *See U Ethmoid Sinus, Right* **W Sphenoid Sinus, Right** **X Sphenoid Sinus, Left**	**Ø** Open **3** Percutaneous **4** Percutaneous Endoscopic **8** Via Natural or Artificial Opening Endoscopic	**Z** No Device	**Z** No Qualifier
K Nasal Mucosa and Soft Tissue Columella External naris Greater alar cartilage Internal naris Lateral nasal cartilage Lesser alar cartilage Nasal cavity Nostril		**Ø** Open **3** Percutaneous **4** Percutaneous Endoscopic **8** Via Natural or Artificial Opening Endoscopic **X** External	**Z** No Device	**Z** No Qualifier

Non-OR   Ø95[Ø,1][Ø,3,4,X]ZZ
Non-OR   Ø95[3,4][Ø,3,4,7,8,X]ZZ
Non-OR   Ø95[F,G][Ø,3,4,7,8]ZZ
Non-OR   Ø95M[Ø,3,4,8]ZZ
Non-OR   Ø95K[Ø,3,4,8,X]ZZ

LC Limited Coverage   NC Noncovered   ⊞ Combination Member   HAC associated procedure   Combination Only   DRG Non-OR   Non-OR   New/Revised in GREEN

308   ICD-10-PCS 2019

095–095 *(side margin)*

Ø Medical and Surgical
9 Ear, Nose, Sinus
7 Dilation   Definition: Expanding an orifice or the lumen of a tubular body part

Explanation: The orifice can be a natural orifice or an artificially created orifice. Accomplished by stretching a tubular body part using intraluminal pressure or by cutting part of the orifice or wall of the tubular body part.

Body Part Character 4	Approach Character 5	Device Character 6	Qualifier Character 7
F Eustachian Tube, Right Auditory tube Pharyngotympanic tube G Eustachian Tube, Left *See F Eustachian Tube, Right*	Ø Open 7 Via Natural or Artificial Opening 8 Via Natural or Artificial Opening Endoscopic	D Intraluminal Device Z No Device	Z No Qualifier
F Eustachian Tube, Right Auditory tube Pharyngotympanic tube G Eustachian Tube, Left *See F Eustachian Tube, Right*	3 Percutaneous 4 Percutaneous Endoscopic	Z No Device	Z No Qualifier

Non-OR All body part, approach, device, and qualifier values

Ø Medical and Surgical
9 Ear, Nose, Sinus
8 Division   Definition: Cutting into a body part, without draining fluids and/or gases from the body part, in order to separate or transect a body part

Explanation: All or a portion of the body part is separated into two or more portions

Body Part Character 4	Approach Character 5	Device Character 6	Qualifier Character 7
L Nasal Turbinate Inferior turbinate Middle turbinate Nasal concha Superior turbinate	Ø Open 3 Percutaneous 4 Percutaneous Endoscopic 7 Via Natural or Artificial Opening 8 Via Natural or Artificial Opening Endoscopic	Z No Device	Z No Qualifier

Ear, Nose, Sinus

Ø   **Medical and Surgical**
9   **Ear, Nose, Sinus**
9   **Drainage**   Definition: Taking or letting out fluids and/or gases from a body part
                  Explanation: The qualifier DIAGNOSTIC is used to identify drainage procedures that are biopsies

Body Part Character 4		Approach Character 5	Device Character 6	Qualifier Character 7
Ø External Ear, Right Antihelix Antitragus Auricle Earlobe Helix Pinna Tragus	**1 External Ear, Left** *See Ø External Ear, Right*	**Ø** Open **3** Percutaneous **4** Percutaneous Endoscopic **X** External	**Ø** Drainage Device	**Z** No Qualifier
Ø External Ear, Right Antihelix Antitragus Auricle Earlobe Helix Pinna Tragus	**1 External Ear, Left** *See Ø External Ear, Right*	**Ø** Open **3** Percutaneous **4** Percutaneous Endoscopic **X** External	**Z** No Device	**X** Diagnostic **Z** No Qualifier
3 External Auditory Canal, Right External auditory meatus **4 External Auditory Canal, Left** *See 3 External Auditory Canal, Right*	**K Nasal Mucosa and Soft Tissue** Columella External naris Greater alar cartilage Internal naris Lateral nasal cartilage Lesser alar cartilage Nasal cavity Nostril	**Ø** Open **3** Percutaneous **4** Percutaneous Endoscopic **7** Via Natural or Artificial Opening **8** Via Natural or Artificial Opening Endoscopic **X** External	**Ø** Drainage Device	**Z** No Qualifier
3 External Auditory Canal, Right External auditory meatus **4 External Auditory Canal, Left** *See 3 External Auditory Canal, Right*	**K Nasal Mucosa and Soft Tissue** Columella External naris Greater alar cartilage Internal naris Lateral nasal cartilage Lesser alar cartilage Nasal cavity Nostril	**Ø** Open **3** Percutaneous **4** Percutaneous Endoscopic **7** Via Natural or Artificial Opening **8** Via Natural or Artificial Opening Endoscopic **X** External	**Z** No Device	**X** Diagnostic **Z** No Qualifier
5 Middle Ear, Right Oval window Tympanic cavity **6 Middle Ear, Left** *See 5 Middle Ear, Right* **9 Auditory Ossicle, Right** Incus Malleus Stapes	**A Auditory Ossicle, Left** *See 9 Auditory Ossicle, Right* **D Inner Ear, Right** Bony labyrinth Bony vestibule Cochlea Round window Semicircular canal **E Inner Ear, Left** *See D Inner Ear, Right*	**Ø** Open **7** Via Natural or Artificial Opening **8** Via Natural or Artificial Opening Endoscopic	**Ø** Drainage Device	**Z** No Qualifier
5 Middle Ear, Right Oval window Tympanic cavity **6 Middle Ear, Left** *See 5 Middle Ear, Right* **9 Auditory Ossicle, Right** Incus Malleus Stapes	**A Auditory Ossicle, Left** *See 9 Auditory Ossicle, Right* **D Inner Ear, Right** Bony labyrinth Bony vestibule Cochlea Round window Semicircular canal **E Inner Ear, Left** *See D Inner Ear, Right*	**Ø** Open **7** Via Natural or Artificial Opening **8** Via Natural or Artificial Opening Endoscopic	**Z** No Device	**X** Diagnostic **Z** No Qualifier

Ø99 Continued on next page

Non-OR	Ø99[Ø,1][Ø,3,4,X]ØZ
Non-OR	Ø99[Ø,1][Ø,3,4,X]Z[X,Z]
Non-OR	Ø99[3,4,K][Ø,3,4,7,8,X]ØZ
Non-OR	Ø99[3,4,K][Ø,3,4,7,8,X]Z[X,Z]
Non-OR	Ø99558ØZ
Non-OR	Ø99[6,9,A,D,E][7,8]ØZ
Non-OR	Ø99[5,6]ØZZ
Non-OR	Ø99[5,6,9,A,D,E][7,8]Z[X,Z]

LC Limited Coverage **NC** Noncovered ⊞ Combination Member HAC associated procedure Combination Only DRG Non-OR Non-OR New/Revised in GREEN

310   ICD-10-PCS 2019

Ø99–Ø99

Ø   Medical and Surgical   *Ø99 Continued*
9   Ear, Nose, Sinus
9   Drainage   Definition: Taking or letting out fluids and/or gases from a body part
                          Explanation: The qualifier DIAGNOSTIC is used to identify drainage procedures that are biopsies

Body Part Character 4		Approach Character 5	Device Character 6	Qualifier Character 7

7 Tympanic Membrane, Right
   Pars flaccida
8 Tympanic Membrane, Left
   See 7 Tympanic Membrane,
   Right
B Mastoid Sinus, Right
   Mastoid air cells
C Mastoid Sinus, Left
   See B Mastoid Sinus, Right
F Eustachian Tube, Right
   Auditory tube
   Pharyngotympanic tube
G Eustachian Tube, Left
   See F Eustachian Tube, Right
L Nasal Turbinate
   Inferior turbinate
   Middle turbinate
   Nasal concha
   Superior turbinate
M Nasal Septum
   Quadrangular cartilage
   Septal cartilage
   Vomer bone
	N Nasopharynx
	   Choana
	   Fossa of Rosenmuller
	   Pharyngeal recess
	   Rhinopharynx
	P Accessory Sinus
	Q Maxillary Sinus, Right
	   Antrum of Highmore
	R Maxillary Sinus, Left
	   See Q Maxillary Sinus, Right
	S Frontal Sinus, Right
	T Frontal Sinus, Left
	U Ethmoid Sinus, Right
	   Ethmoidal air cell
	V Ethmoid Sinus, Left
	   See U Ethmoid Sinus, Right
	W Sphenoid Sinus, Right
	X Sphenoid Sinus, Left
		Ø Open
		3 Percutaneous
		4 Percutaneous Endoscopic
		7 Via Natural or Artificial
		   Opening
		8 Via Natural or Artificial
		   Opening Endoscopic
			Ø Drainage Device	**Z** No Qualifier

7 Tympanic Membrane, Right
   Pars flaccida
8 Tympanic Membrane, Left
   See 7 Tympanic Membrane,
   Right
B Mastoid Sinus, Right
   Mastoid air cells
C Mastoid Sinus, Left
   See B Mastoid Sinus, Right
F Eustachian Tube, Right
   Auditory tube
   Pharyngotympanic tube
G Eustachian Tube, Left
   See F Eustachian Tube, Right
L Nasal Turbinate
   Inferior turbinate
   Middle turbinate
   Nasal concha
   Superior turbinate
M Nasal Septum
   Quadrangular cartilage
   Septal cartilage
   Vomer bone
	N Nasopharynx
	   Choana
	   Fossa of Rosenmuller
	   Pharyngeal recess
	   Rhinopharynx
	P Accessory Sinus
	Q Maxillary Sinus, Right
	   Antrum of Highmore
	R Maxillary Sinus, Left
	   See Q Maxillary Sinus, Right
	S Frontal Sinus, Right
	T Frontal Sinus, Left
	U Ethmoid Sinus, Right
	   Ethmoidal air cell
	V Ethmoid Sinus, Left
	   See U Ethmoid Sinus, Right
	W Sphenoid Sinus, Right
	X Sphenoid Sinus, Left
		Ø Open
		3 Percutaneous
		4 Percutaneous Endoscopic
		7 Via Natural or Artificial
		   Opening
		8 Via Natural or Artificial
		   Opening Endoscopic
			Z No Device	**X** Diagnostic
				Z No Qualifier

Non-OR	Ø99[B,C][3,7,8]ØZ
Non-OR	Ø99[F,G,L,M][Ø,3,4,7,8]ØZ
Non-OR	Ø99N3ØZ
Non-OR	Ø99[P,Q,R,S,T,U,V,W,X][3,4,7,8]ØZ
Non-OR	Ø99[7,8][Ø,3,4,7,8]ZZ
Non-OR	Ø99[7,8][7,8]ZX
Non-OR	Ø99[B,C]3ZZ
Non-OR	Ø99[B,C][7,8]Z[X,Z]
Non-OR	Ø99[F,G][Ø,3,4,7,8]ZZ
Non-OR	Ø99[F,G][7,8]ZX
Non-OR	Ø99[L,M][Ø,3,4,7,8]Z[X,Z]
Non-OR	Ø99N[Ø,3,4,7,8]ZX
Non-OR	Ø99N3ZZ
Non-OR	Ø99[P,Q,R,S,T,U,V,W,X][3,4,7,8]Z[X,Z]

Ear, Nose, Sinus *(side margin)*

0   **Medical and Surgical**
9   **Ear, Nose, Sinus**
B   **Excision**   Definition: Cutting out or off, without replacement, a portion of a body part
            Explanation: The qualifier DIAGNOSTIC is used to identify excision procedures that are biopsies

Body Part — Character 4		Approach — Character 5	Device — Character 6	Qualifier — Character 7
0 External Ear, Right Antihelix Antitragus Auricle Earlobe Helix Pinna Tragus	**1** External Ear, Left *See 0 External Ear, Right*	**0** Open **3** Percutaneous **4** Percutaneous Endoscopic **X** External	**Z** No Device	**X** Diagnostic **Z** No Qualifier
3 External Auditory Canal, Right External auditory meatus	**4** External Auditory Canal, Left *See 3 External Auditory Canal, Right*	**0** Open **3** Percutaneous **4** Percutaneous Endoscopic **7** Via Natural or Artificial Opening **8** Via Natural or Artificial Opening Endoscopic **X** External	**Z** No Device	**X** Diagnostic **Z** No Qualifier
5 Middle Ear, Right Oval window Tympanic cavity **6** Middle Ear, Left *See 5 Middle Ear, Right* **9** Auditory Ossicle, Right Incus Malleus Stapes	**A** Auditory Ossicle, Left *See 9 Auditory Ossicle, Right* **D** Inner Ear, Right Bony labyrinth Bony vestibule Cochlea Round window Semicircular canal **E** Inner Ear, Left *See D Inner Ear, Right*	**0** Open **8** Via Natural or Artificial Opening Endoscopic	**Z** No Device	**X** Diagnostic **Z** No Qualifier
7 Tympanic Membrane, Right Pars flaccida **8** Tympanic Membrane, Left *See 7 Tympanic Membrane, Right* **F** Eustachian Tube, Right Auditory tube Pharyngotympanic tube **G** Eustachian Tube, Left *See F Eustachian Tube, Right*	**L** Nasal Turbinate Inferior turbinate Middle turbinate Nasal concha Superior turbinate **N** Nasopharynx Choana Fossa of Rosenmuller Pharyngeal recess Rhinopharynx	**0** Open **3** Percutaneous **4** Percutaneous Endoscopic **7** Via Natural or Artificial Opening **8** Via Natural or Artificial Opening Endoscopic	**Z** No Device	**X** Diagnostic **Z** No Qualifier
B Mastoid Sinus, Right Mastoid air cells **C** Mastoid Sinus, Left *See B Mastoid Sinus, Right* **M** Nasal Septum Quadrangular cartilage Septal cartilage Vomer bone **P** Accessory Sinus **Q** Maxillary Sinus, Right Antrum of Highmore	**R** Maxillary Sinus, Left *See Q Maxillary Sinus, Right* **S** Frontal Sinus, Right **T** Frontal Sinus, Left **U** Ethmoid Sinus, Right Ethmoidal air cell **V** Ethmoid Sinus, Left *See U Ethmoid Sinus, Right* **W** Sphenoid Sinus, Right **X** Sphenoid Sinus, Left	**0** Open **3** Percutaneous **4** Percutaneous Endoscopic **8** Via Natural or Artificial Opening Endoscopic	**Z** No Device	**X** Diagnostic **Z** No Qualifier
K Nasal Mucosa and Soft Tissue Columella External naris Greater alar cartilage Internal naris Lateral nasal cartilage Lesser alar cartilage Nasal cavity Nostril		**0** Open **3** Percutaneous **4** Percutaneous Endoscopic **8** Via Natural or Artificial Opening Endoscopic **X** External	**Z** No Device	**X** Diagnostic **Z** No Qualifier

Non-OR   09B[0,1][0,3,4,X]Z[X,Z]
Non-OR   09B[3,4][0,3,4,7,8,X]Z[X,Z]
Non-OR   09B[F,G,L,N][0,3,4,7,8]Z[X,Z]
Non-OR   09BM[0,3,4,8]ZX
Non-OR   09B[P,Q,R,S,T,U,V,W,X][3,4,8]ZX
Non-OR   09BK8Z[X,Z]

0   **Medical and Surgical**
9   **Ear, Nose, Sinus**
C   **Extirpation**   Definition: Taking or cutting out solid matter from a body part

Explanation: The solid matter may be an abnormal byproduct of a biological function or a foreign body; it may be imbedded in a body part or in the lumen of a tubular body part. The solid matter may or may not have been previously broken into pieces.

Body Part Character 4		Approach Character 5	Device Character 6	Qualifier Character 7

0 External Ear, Right
  Antihelix
  Antitragus
  Auricle
  Earlobe
  Helix
  Pinna
  Tragus
	1 External Ear, Left
	  See 0 External Ear, Right
		0 Open
		3 Percutaneous
		4 Percutaneous Endoscopic
		X External
			Z No Device	**Z** No Qualifier

3 External Auditory Canal,
  Right
  External auditory meatus
	4 External Auditory Canal, Left
	  *See 3 External Auditory Canal,
	  Right*
		0 Open
		3 Percutaneous
		4 Percutaneous Endoscopic
		7 Via Natural or Artificial
		  Opening
		8 Via Natural or Artificial
		  Opening Endoscopic
		X External
			Z No Device	**Z** No Qualifier

5 Middle Ear, Right
  Oval window
  Tympanic cavity
6 Middle Ear, Left
  See 5 Middle Ear, Right
9 Auditory Ossicle, Right
  Incus
  Malleus
  Stapes
	A Auditory Ossicle, Left
	  See 9 Auditory Ossicle, Right
	D Inner Ear, Right
	  Bony labyrinth
	  Bony vestibule
	  Cochlea
	  Round window
	  Semicircular canal
	E Inner Ear, Left
	  See D Inner Ear, Right
		0 Open
		8 Via Natural or Artificial
		  Opening Endoscopic
			Z No Device	**Z** No Qualifier

7 Tympanic Membrane, Right
  Pars flaccida
8 Tympanic Membrane, Left
  *See 7 Tympanic Membrane,
  Right*
F Eustachian Tube, Right
  Auditory tube
  Pharyngotympanic tube
G Eustachian Tube, Left
  See F Eustachian Tube, Right
	L Nasal Turbinate
	  Inferior turbinate
	  Middle turbinate
	  Nasal concha
	  Superior turbinate
	N Nasopharynx
	  Choana
	  Fossa of Rosenmuller
	  Pharyngeal recess
	  Rhinopharynx
		0 Open
		3 Percutaneous
		4 Percutaneous Endoscopic
		7 Via Natural or Artificial
		  Opening
		8 Via Natural or Artificial
		  Opening Endoscopic
			Z No Device	**Z** No Qualifier

B Mastoid Sinus, Right
  Mastoid air cells
C Mastoid Sinus, Left
  See B Mastoid Sinus, Right
M Nasal Septum
  Quadrangular cartilage
  Septal cartilage
  Vomer bone
P Accessory Sinus
Q Maxillary Sinus, Right
  Antrum of Highmore
	R Maxillary Sinus, Left
	  See Q Maxillary Sinus, Right
	S Frontal Sinus, Right
	T Frontal Sinus, Left
	U Ethmoid Sinus, Right
	  Ethmoidal air cell
	V Ethmoid Sinus, Left
	  See U Ethmoid Sinus, Right
	W Sphenoid Sinus, Right
	X Sphenoid Sinus, Left
		0 Open
		3 Percutaneous
		4 Percutaneous Endoscopic
		8 Via Natural or Artificial
		  Opening Endoscopic
			Z No Device	**Z** No Qualifier

K Nasal Mucosa and Soft Tissue
  Columella
  External naris
  Greater alar cartilage
  Internal naris
  Lateral nasal cartilage
  Lesser alar cartilage
  Nasal cavity
  Nostril
		0 Open
		3 Percutaneous
		4 Percutaneous Endoscopic
		8 Via Natural or Artificial
		  Opening Endoscopic
		X External
			Z No Device	**Z** No Qualifier

Non-OR   09C[0,1][0,3,4,X]ZZ
Non-OR   09C[3,4][0,3,4,7,8,X]ZZ
Non-OR   09C[7,8,F,G,L][0,3,4,7,8]ZZ
Non-OR   09CM[0,3,4,8]ZZ
Non-OR   09CK8ZZ

LC Limited Coverage   **NC** Noncovered   ⊞ Combination Member   HAC associated procedure   Combination Only   DRG Non-OR   Non-OR   New/Revised in GREEN

ICD-10-PCS 2019   313

Ø   Medical and Surgical
9   Ear, Nose, Sinus
D   Extraction   Definition: Pulling or stripping out or off all or a portion of a body part by the use of force
Explanation: The qualifier DIAGNOSTIC is used to identify extraction procedures that are biopsies

Body Part Character 4	Approach Character 5	Device Character 6	Qualifier Character 7
7 Tympanic Membrane, Right Pars flaccida **8** Tympanic Membrane, Left *See 7 Tympanic Membrane, Right* **L** Nasal Turbinate Inferior turbinate Middle turbinate Nasal concha Superior turbinate	**Ø** Open **3** Percutaneous **4** Percutaneous Endoscopic **7** Via Natural or Artificial Opening **8** Via Natural or Artificial Opening Endoscopic	**Z** No Device	**Z** No Qualifier
9 Auditory Ossicle, Right Incus Malleus Stapes **A** Auditory Ossicle, Left *See 9 Auditory Ossicle, Right*	**Ø** Open	**Z** No Device	**Z** No Qualifier
B Mastoid Sinus, Right Mastoid air cells **C** Mastoid Sinus, Left *See B Mastoid Sinus, Right* **M** Nasal Septum Quadrangular cartilage Septal cartilage Vomer bone **P** Accessory Sinus **Q** Maxillary Sinus, Right Antrum of Highmore **R** Maxillary Sinus, Left *See Q Maxillary Sinus, Right* **S** Frontal Sinus, Right **T** Frontal Sinus, Left **U** Ethmoid Sinus, Right Ethmoidal air cell **V** Ethmoid Sinus, Left *See U Ethmoid Sinus, Right* **W** Sphenoid Sinus, Right **X** Sphenoid Sinus, Left	**Ø** Open **3** Percutaneous **4** Percutaneous Endoscopic	**Z** No Device	**Z** No Qualifier

Ø   Medical and Surgical
9   Ear, Nose, Sinus
H   Insertion   Definition: Putting in a nonbiological appliance that monitors, assists, performs, or prevents a physiological function but does not physically
take the place of a body part
Explanation: None

Body Part Character 4	Approach Character 5	Device Character 6	Qualifier Character 7
D Inner Ear, Right Bony labyrinth Bony vestibule Cochlea Round window Semicircular canal **E** Inner Ear, Left *See D Inner Ear, Right*	**Ø** Open **3** Percutaneous **4** Percutaneous Endoscopic	**4** Hearing Device, Bone Conduction **5** Hearing Device, Single Channel Cochlear Prosthesis **6** Hearing Device, Multiple Channel Cochlear Prosthesis **S** Hearing Device	**Z** No Qualifier
H Ear, Right **J** Ear, Left **K** Nasal Mucosa and Soft Tissue Columella External naris Greater alar cartilage Internal naris Lateral nasal cartilage Lesser alar cartilage Nasal cavity Nostril **Y** Sinus	**Ø** Open **3** Percutaneous **4** Percutaneous Endoscopic **7** Via Natural or Artificial Opening **8** Via Natural or Artificial Opening Endoscopic	**Y** Other Device	**Z** No Qualifier
N Nasopharynx Choana Fossa of Rosenmuller Pharyngeal recess Rhinopharynx	**7** Via Natural or Artificial Opening **8** Via Natural or Artificial Opening Endoscopic	**B** Intraluminal Device, Airway	**Z** No Qualifier

Non-OR   09H[H,J][3,4,7,8]YZ
Non-OR   09H[K,Y][0,3,4,7,8]YZ
Non-OR   09HN[7,8]BZ

Ø   Medical and Surgical
9   Ear, Nose, Sinus
J   Inspection   Definition: Visually and/or manually exploring a body part

Explanation: Visual exploration may be performed with or without optical instrumentation. Manual exploration may be performed directly or through intervening body layers.

Body Part Character 4	Approach Character 5	Device Character 6	Qualifier Character 7
7 Tympanic Membrane, Right Pars flaccida **8 Tympanic Membrane, Left** *See 7 Tympanic Membrane, Right* **H Ear, Right** **J Ear, Left**	**Ø** Open **3** Percutaneous **4** Percutaneous Endoscopic **7** Via Natural or Artificial Opening **8** Via Natural or Artificial Opening Endoscopic **X** External	**Z** No Device	**Z** No Qualifier
D Inner Ear, Right Bony labyrinth Bony vestibule Cochlea Round window Semicircular canal **E Inner Ear, Left** *See D Inner Ear, Right* **K Nasal Mucosa and Soft Tissue** Columella External naris Greater alar cartilage Internal naris Lateral nasal cartilage Lesser alar cartilage Nasal cavity Nostril **Y Sinus**	**Ø** Open **3** Percutaneous **4** Percutaneous Endoscopic **8** Via Natural or Artificial Opening Endoscopic **X** External	**Z** No Device	**Z** No Qualifier

Non-OR   Ø9J[7,8][3,7,8,X]ZZ
Non-OR   Ø9J[H,J][Ø,3,4,7,8,X]ZZ
Non-OR   Ø9J[D,E][3,8,X]ZZ
Non-OR   Ø9J[K,Y][Ø,3,4,8,X]ZZ

Ø   Medical and Surgical
9   Ear, Nose, Sinus
M   Reattachment   Definition: Putting back in or on all or a portion of a separated body part to its normal location or other suitable location

Explanation: Vascular circulation and nervous pathways may or may not be reestablished

Body Part Character 4	Approach Character 5	Device Character 6	Qualifier Character 7
Ø External Ear, Right Antihelix Antitragus Auricle Earlobe Helix Pinna Tragus **1 External Ear, Left** *See Ø External Ear, Right* **K Nasal Mucosa and Soft Tissue** Columella External naris Greater alar cartilage Internal naris Lateral nasal cartilage Lesser alar cartilage Nasal cavity Nostril	**X** External	**Z** No Device	**Z** No Qualifier

Ear, Nose, Sinus

0   Medical and Surgical
9   Ear, Nose, Sinus
N   Release   Definition: Freeing a body part from an abnormal physical constraint by cutting or by the use of force
                 Explanation: Some of the restraining tissue may be taken out but none of the body part is taken out

Body Part — Character 4		Approach — Character 5	Device — Character 6	Qualifier — Character 7
0 External Ear, Right Antihelix Antitragus Auricle Earlobe Helix Pinna Tragus	**1 External Ear, Left** *See 0 External Ear, Right*	**0** Open **3** Percutaneous **4** Percutaneous Endoscopic **X** External	**Z** No Device	**Z** No Qualifier
3 External Auditory Canal, Right External auditory meatus	**4 External Auditory Canal, Left** *See 3 External Auditory Canal, Right*	**0** Open **3** Percutaneous **4** Percutaneous Endoscopic **7** Via Natural or Artificial Opening **8** Via Natural or Artificial Opening Endoscopic **X** External	**Z** No Device	**Z** No Qualifier
5 Middle Ear, Right Oval window Tympanic cavity **6 Middle Ear, Left** *See 5 Middle Ear, Right* **9 Auditory Ossicle, Right** Incus Malleus Stapes	**A Auditory Ossicle, Left** *See 9 Auditory Ossicle, Right* **D Inner Ear, Right** Bony labyrinth Bony vestibule Cochlea Round window Semicircular canal **E Inner Ear, Left** *See D Inner Ear, Right*	**0** Open **8** Via Natural or Artificial Opening Endoscopic	**Z** No Device	**Z** No Qualifier
7 Tympanic Membrane, Right Pars flaccida **8 Tympanic Membrane, Left** *See 7 Tympanic Membrane, Right* **F Eustachian Tube, Right** Auditory tube Pharyngotympanic tube **G Eustachian Tube, Left** *See F Eustachian Tube, Right*	**L Nasal Turbinate** Inferior turbinate Middle turbinate Nasal concha Superior turbinate **N Nasopharynx** Choana Fossa of Rosenmuller Pharyngeal recess Rhinopharynx	**0** Open **3** Percutaneous **4** Percutaneous Endoscopic **7** Via Natural or Artificial Opening **8** Via Natural or Artificial Opening Endoscopic	**Z** No Device	**Z** No Qualifier
B Mastoid Sinus, Right Mastoid air cells **C Mastoid Sinus, Left** *See B Mastoid Sinus, Right* **M Nasal Septum** Quadrangular cartilage Septal cartilage Vomer bone **P Accessory Sinus** **Q Maxillary Sinus, Right** Antrum of Highmore	**R Maxillary Sinus, Left** *See Q Maxillary Sinus, Right* **S Frontal Sinus, Right** **T Frontal Sinus, Left** **U Ethmoid Sinus, Right** Ethmoidal air cell **V Ethmoid Sinus, Left** *See U Ethmoid Sinus, Right* **W Sphenoid Sinus, Right** **X Sphenoid Sinus, Left**	**0** Open **3** Percutaneous **4** Percutaneous Endoscopic **8** Via Natural or Artificial Opening Endoscopic	**Z** No Device	**Z** No Qualifier
K Nasal Mucosa and Soft Tissue Columella External naris Greater alar cartilage Internal naris Lateral nasal cartilage Lesser alar cartilage Nasal cavity Nostril		**0** Open **3** Percutaneous **4** Percutaneous Endoscopic **8** Via Natural or Artificial Opening Endoscopic **X** External	**Z** No Device	**Z** No Qualifier

Non-OR   09N[0,1]XZZ
Non-OR   09N[3,4]XZZ
Non-OR   09N[F,G,L][0,3,4,7,8]ZZ
Non-OR   09NM[0,3,4,8]ZZ
Non-OR   09NK[0,3,4,8,X]ZZ

Ø   Medical and Surgical
9   Ear, Nose, Sinus
P   Removal   Definition: Taking out or off a device from a body part

Explanation: If a device is taken out and a similar device put in without cutting or puncturing the skin or mucous membrane, the procedure is coded to the root operation CHANGE. Otherwise, the procedure for taking out a device is coded to the root operation REMOVAL.

Body Part Character 4	Approach Character 5	Device Character 6	Qualifier Character 7
7 Tympanic Membrane, Right Pars flaccida **8 Tympanic Membrane, Left** *See 7 Tympanic Membrane, Right*	**Ø Open** **7 Via Natural or Artificial Opening** **8 Via Natural or Artificial Opening Endoscopic** **X External**	**Ø Drainage Device**	**Z No Qualifier**
D Inner Ear, Right Bony labyrinth Bony vestibule Cochlea Round window Semicircular canal **E Inner Ear, Left** *See D Inner Ear, Right*	**Ø Open** **7 Via Natural or Artificial Opening** **8 Via Natural or Artificial Opening Endoscopic**	**S Hearing Device**	**Z No Qualifier**
H Ear, Right **J Ear, Left** **K Nasal Mucosa and Soft Tissue** Columella External naris Greater alar cartilage Internal naris Lateral nasal cartilage Lesser alar cartilage Nasal cavity Nostril	**Ø Open** **3 Percutaneous** **4 Percutaneous Endoscopic** **7 Via Natural or Artificial Opening** **8 Via Natural or Artificial Opening Endoscopic**	**Ø Drainage Device** **7 Autologous Tissue Substitute** **D Intraluminal Device** **J Synthetic Substitute** **K Nonautologous Tissue Substitute** **Y Other Device**	**Z No Qualifier**
H Ear, Right **J Ear, Left** **K Nasal Mucosa and Soft Tissue** Columella External naris Greater alar cartilage Internal naris Lateral nasal cartilage Lesser alar cartilage Nasal cavity Nostril	**X External**	**Ø Drainage Device** **7 Autologous Tissue Substitute** **D Intraluminal Device** **J Synthetic Substitute** **K Nonautologous Tissue Substitute**	**Z No Qualifier**
Y Sinus	**Ø Open** **3 Percutaneous** **4 Percutaneous Endoscopic**	**Ø Drainage Device** **Y Other Device**	**Z No Qualifier**
Y Sinus	**7 Via Natural or Artificial Opening** **8 Via Natural or Artificial Opening Endoscopic**	**Y Other Device**	**Z No Qualifier**
Y Sinus	**X External**	**Ø Drainage Device**	**Z No Qualifier**

Non-OR   09P[7,8][0,7,8,X]0Z
Non-OR   09P[H,J][3,4][0,J,K,Y]Z
Non-OR   09P[H,J][7,8][0,D,Y]Z
Non-OR   09PK[0,3,4,7,8][0,7,D,J,K,Y]Z
Non-OR   09P[H,J]X[0,7,D,J,K]Z
Non-OR   09PKX[0,7,D,J,K]Z
Non-OR   09PY[3,4]YZ
Non-OR   09PY[7,8]YZ
Non-OR   09PYX0Z

LC Limited Coverage   NC Noncovered   ⊞ Combination Member   HAC associated procedure   Combination Only   DRG Non-OR   Non-OR   New/Revised in GREEN

0 Medical and Surgical
9 Ear, Nose, Sinus
Q Repair

Definition: Restoring, to the extent possible, a body part to its normal anatomic structure and function
Explanation: Used only when the method to accomplish the repair is not one of the other root operations

Body Part Character 4	Approach Character 5	Device Character 6	Qualifier Character 7
0 External Ear, Right Antihelix Antitragus Auricle Earlobe Helix Pinna Tragus **1** External Ear, Left See 0 External Ear, Right **2** External Ear, Bilateral See 0 External Ear, Right	**0** Open **3** Percutaneous **4** Percutaneous Endoscopic **X** External	**Z** No Device	**Z** No Qualifier
3 External Auditory Canal, Right External auditory meatus **4** External Auditory Canal, Left See 3 External Auditory Canal, Right **F** Eustachian Tube, Right Auditory tube Pharyngotympanic tube **G** Eustachian Tube, Left See F Eustachian Tube, Right	**0** Open **3** Percutaneous **4** Percutaneous Endoscopic **7** Via Natural or Artificial Opening **8** Via Natural or Artificial Opening Endoscopic **X** External	**Z** No Device	**Z** No Qualifier
5 Middle Ear, Right Oval window Tympanic cavity **6** Middle Ear, Left See 5 Middle Ear, Right **9** Auditory Ossicle, Right Incus Malleus Stapes **A** Auditory Ossicle, Left See 9 Auditory Ossicle, Right **D** Inner Ear, Right Bony labyrinth Bony vestibule Cochlea Round window Semicircular canal **E** Inner Ear, Left See D Inner Ear, Right	**0** Open **8** Via Natural or Artificial Opening Endoscopic	**Z** No Device	**Z** No Qualifier
7 Tympanic Membrane, Right Pars flaccida **8** Tympanic Membrane, Left See 7 Tympanic Membrane, Right **L** Nasal Turbinate Inferior turbinate Middle turbinate Nasal concha Superior turbinate **N** Nasopharynx Choana Fossa of Rosenmuller Pharyngeal recess Rhinopharynx	**0** Open **3** Percutaneous **4** Percutaneous Endoscopic **7** Via Natural or Artificial Opening **8** Via Natural or Artificial Opening Endoscopic	**Z** No Device	**Z** No Qualifier
B Mastoid Sinus, Right Mastoid air cells **C** Mastoid Sinus, Left See B Mastoid Sinus, Right **M** Nasal Septum Quadrangular cartilage Septal cartilage Vomer bone **P** Accessory Sinus **Q** Maxillary Sinus, Right Antrum of Highmore **R** Maxillary Sinus, Left See Q Maxillary Sinus, Right **S** Frontal Sinus, Right **T** Frontal Sinus, Left **U** Ethmoid Sinus, Right Ethmoidal air cell **V** Ethmoid Sinus, Left See U Ethmoid Sinus, Right **W** Sphenoid Sinus, Right **X** Sphenoid Sinus, Left	**0** Open **3** Percutaneous **4** Percutaneous Endoscopic **8** Via Natural or Artificial Opening Endoscopic	**Z** No Device	**Z** No Qualifier
K Nasal Mucosa and Soft Tissue Columella External naris Greater alar cartilage Internal naris Lateral nasal cartilage Lesser alar cartilage Nasal cavity Nostril	**0** Open **3** Percutaneous **4** Percutaneous Endoscopic **8** Via Natural or Artificial Opening Endoscopic **X** External	**Z** No Device	**Z** No Qualifier

Non-OR 09Q[0,1,2]XZZ
Non-OR 09Q[3,4]XZZ
Non-OR 09Q[F,G][0,3,4,7,8,X]ZZ
Non-OR 09QKXZZ

Ear, Nose, Sinus

Ø   **Medical and Surgical**
9   **Ear, Nose, Sinus**
R   **Replacement**   Definition: Putting in or on biological or synthetic material that physically takes the place and/or function of all or a portion of a body part
                         Explanation: The body part may have been taken out or replaced, or may be taken out, physically eradicated, or rendered nonfunctional during
                         the REPLACEMENT procedure. A REMOVAL procedure is coded for taking out the device used in a previous replacement procedure.

Body Part Character 4	Approach Character 5	Device Character 6	Qualifier Character 7

Ø   **External Ear, Right**
    Antihelix
    Antitragus
    Auricle
    Earlobe
    Helix
    Pinna
    Tragus
1   **External Ear, Left**
    See Ø External Ear, Right
2   **External Ear, Bilateral**
    See Ø External Ear, Right
K   **Nasal Mucosa and Soft Tissue**
    Columella
    External naris
    Greater alar cartilage
    Internal naris
    Lateral nasal cartilage
    Lesser alar cartilage
    Nasal cavity
    Nostril
	Ø Open
	X External
		7 Autologous Tissue Substitute
		J Synthetic Substitute
		K Nonautologous Tissue Substitute
			Z No Qualifier

5   **Middle Ear, Right**
    Oval window
    Tympanic cavity
6   **Middle Ear, Left**
    See 5 Middle Ear, Right
9   **Auditory Ossicle, Right**
    Incus
    Malleus
    Stapes
A   **Auditory Ossicle, Left**
    See 9 Auditory Ossicle, Right
D   **Inner Ear, Right**
    Bony labyrinth
    Bony vestibule
    Cochlea
    Round window
    Semicircular canal
E   **Inner Ear, Left**
    See D Inner Ear, Right
	Ø Open	7 Autologous Tissue Substitute
		J Synthetic Substitute
		K Nonautologous Tissue Substitute
			Z No Qualifier

7   **Tympanic Membrane, Right**
    Pars flaccida
8   **Tympanic Membrane, Left**
    See 7 Tympanic Membrane, Right
N   **Nasopharynx**
    Choana
    Fossa of Rosenmuller
    Pharyngeal recess
    Rhinopharynx
	Ø Open
	7 Via Natural or Artificial Opening
	8 Via Natural or Artificial Opening
	    Endoscopic
		7 Autologous Tissue Substitute
		J Synthetic Substitute
		K Nonautologous Tissue Substitute
			Z No Qualifier

L   **Nasal Turbinate**
    Inferior turbinate
    Middle turbinate
    Nasal concha
    Superior turbinate
	Ø Open
	3 Percutaneous
	4 Percutaneous Endoscopic
	7 Via Natural or Artificial Opening
	8 Via Natural or Artificial Opening
	    Endoscopic
		7 Autologous Tissue Substitute
		J Synthetic Substitute
		K Nonautologous Tissue Substitute
			Z No Qualifier

M   **Nasal Septum**
    Quadrangular cartilage
    Septal cartilage
    Vomer bone
	Ø Open
	3 Percutaneous
	4 Percutaneous Endoscopic
		7 Autologous Tissue Substitute
		J Synthetic Substitute
		K Nonautologous Tissue Substitute
			Z No Qualifier

Ø **Medical and Surgical**
9 **Ear, Nose, Sinus**
S **Reposition**   Definition: Moving to its normal location, or other suitable location, all or a portion of a body part
        Explanation: The body part is moved to a new location from an abnormal location, or from a normal location where it is not functioning correctly. The body part may or may not be cut out or off to be moved to the new location.

Body Part Character 4	Approach Character 5	Device Character 6	Qualifier Character 7

Ø **External Ear, Right**
   Antihelix
   Antitragus
   Auricle
   Earlobe
   Helix
   Pinna
   Tragus
1 **External Ear, Left**
   See Ø External Ear, Right
2 **External Ear, Bilateral**
   See Ø External Ear, Right
K **Nasal Mucosa and Soft Tissue**
   Columella
   External naris
   Greater alar cartilage
   Internal naris
   Lateral nasal cartilage
   Lesser alar cartilage
   Nasal cavity
   Nostril
	Ø Open
	4 Percutaneous Endoscopic
	X External
		Z No Device	Z No Qualifier

7 **Tympanic Membrane, Right**
   Pars flaccida
8 **Tympanic Membrane, Left**
   See 7 Tympanic Membrane, Right
F **Eustachian Tube, Right**
   Auditory tube
   Pharyngotympanic tube
G **Eustachian Tube, Left**
   See F Eustachian Tube, Right
L **Nasal Turbinate**
   Inferior turbinate
   Middle turbinate
   Nasal concha
   Superior turbinate
	Ø Open
	4 Percutaneous Endoscopic
	7 Via Natural or Artificial Opening
	8 Via Natural or Artificial Opening
	   Endoscopic
		Z No Device	Z No Qualifier

9 **Auditory Ossicle, Right**
   Incus
   Malleus
   Stapes
A **Auditory Ossicle, Left**
   See 9 Auditory Ossicle, Right
M **Nasal Septum**
   Quadrangular cartilage
   Septal cartilage
   Vomer bone
	Ø Open
	4 Percutaneous Endoscopic
		Z No Device	Z No Qualifier

Non-OR   09S[F,G][Ø,4,7,8]ZZ

0   Medical and Surgical
9   Ear, Nose, Sinus
T   Resection   Definition: Cutting out or off, without replacement, all of a body part
                 Explanation: None

Body Part Character 4		Approach Character 5	Device Character 6	Qualifier Character 7
0 External Ear, Right Antihelix Antitragus Auricle Earlobe Helix Pinna Tragus	**1 External Ear, Left** *See 0 External Ear, Right*	**0 Open** **4 Percutaneous Endoscopic** **X External**	**Z No Device**	**Z No Qualifier**
5 Middle Ear, Right Oval window Tympanic cavity **6 Middle Ear, Left** *See 5 Middle Ear, Right* **9 Auditory Ossicle, Right** Incus Malleus Stapes	**A Auditory Ossicle, Left** *See 9 Auditory Ossicle, Right* **D Inner Ear, Right** Bony labyrinth Bony vestibule Cochlea Round window Semicircular canal **E Inner Ear, Left** *See D Inner Ear, Right*	**0 Open** **8 Via Natural or Artificial Opening Endoscopic**	**Z No Device**	**Z No Qualifier**
7 Tympanic Membrane, Right Pars flaccida **8 Tympanic Membrane, Left** *See 7 Tympanic Membrane, Right* **F Eustachian Tube, Right** Auditory tube Pharyngotympanic tube **G Eustachian Tube, Left** *See F Eustachian Tube, Right*	**L Nasal Turbinate** Inferior turbinate Middle turbinate Nasal concha Superior turbinate **N Nasopharynx** Choana Fossa of Rosenmuller Pharyngeal recess Rhinopharynx	**0 Open** **4 Percutaneous Endoscopic** **7 Via Natural or Artificial Opening** **8 Via Natural or Artificial Opening Endoscopic**	**Z No Device**	**Z No Qualifier**
B Mastoid Sinus, Right Mastoid air cells **C Mastoid Sinus, Left** *See B Mastoid Sinus, Right* **M Nasal Septum** Quadrangular cartilage Septal cartilage Vomer bone **P Accessory Sinus** **Q Maxillary Sinus, Right** Antrum of Highmore	**R Maxillary Sinus, Left** *See Q Maxillary Sinus, Right* **S Frontal Sinus, Right** **T Frontal Sinus, Left** **U Ethmoid Sinus, Right** Ethmoidal air cell **V Ethmoid Sinus, Left** *See U Ethmoid Sinus, Right* **W Sphenoid Sinus, Right** **X Sphenoid Sinus, Left**	**0 Open** **4 Percutaneous Endoscopic** **8 Via Natural or Artificial Opening Endoscopic**	**Z No Device**	**Z No Qualifier**
K Nasal Mucosa and Soft Tissue Columella External naris Greater alar cartilage Internal naris Lateral nasal cartilage Lesser alar cartilage Nasal cavity Nostril		**0 Open** **4 Percutaneous Endoscopic** **8 Via Natural or Artificial Opening Endoscopic** **X External**	**Z No Device**	**Z No Qualifier**

Non-OR   09T[F,G][0,4,7,8]ZZ

LC Limited Coverage   NC Noncovered   ⊞ Combination Member   HAC associated procedure   Combination Only   DRG Non-OR   Non-OR   New/Revised in GREEN
ICD-10-PCS 2019   321

09T–09T

Ø Medical and Surgical
9 Ear, Nose, Sinus
U Supplement   Definition: Putting in or on biological or synthetic material that physically reinforces and/or augments the function of a portion of a body part
    Explanation: The biological material is non-living, or is living and from the same individual. The body part may have been previously replaced, and the SUPPLEMENT procedure is performed to physically reinforce and/or augment the function of the replaced body part.

Body Part Character 4	Approach Character 5	Device Character 6	Qualifier Character 7
Ø External Ear, Right Antihelix Antitragus Auricle Earlobe Helix Pinna Tragus **1 External Ear, Left** *See Ø External Ear, Right* **2 External Ear, Bilateral** *See Ø External Ear, Right*	Ø Open X External	7 Autologous Tissue Substitute J Synthetic Substitute K Nonautologous Tissue Substitute	Z No Qualifier
5 Middle Ear, Right Oval window Tympanic cavity **6 Middle Ear, Left** *See 5 Middle Ear, Right* **9 Auditory Ossicle, Right** Incus Malleus Stapes **A Auditory Ossicle, Left** *See 9 Auditory Ossicle, Right* **D Inner Ear, Right** Bony labyrinth Bony vestibule Cochlea Round window Semicircular canal **E Inner Ear, Left** *See D Inner Ear, Right*	Ø Open 8 Via Natural or Artificial Opening Endoscopic	7 Autologous Tissue Substitute J Synthetic Substitute K Nonautologous Tissue Substitute	Z No Qualifier
7 Tympanic Membrane, Right Pars flaccida **8 Tympanic Membrane, Left** *See 7 Tympanic Membrane, Right* **N Nasopharynx** Choana Fossa of Rosenmuller Pharyngeal recess Rhinopharynx	Ø Open 7 Via Natural or Artificial Opening 8 Via Natural or Artificial Opening Endoscopic	7 Autologous Tissue Substitute J Synthetic Substitute K Nonautologous Tissue Substitute	Z No Qualifier
K Nasal Mucosa and Soft Tissue Columella External naris Greater alar cartilage Internal naris Lateral nasal cartilage Lesser alar cartilage Nasal cavity Nostril	Ø Open 8 Via Natural or Artificial Opening Endoscopic X External	7 Autologous Tissue Substitute J Synthetic Substitute K Nonautologous Tissue Substitute	Z No Qualifier
L Nasal Turbinate Inferior turbinate Middle turbinate Nasal concha Superior turbinate	Ø Open 3 Percutaneous 4 Percutaneous Endoscopic 7 Via Natural or Artificial Opening 8 Via Natural or Artificial Opening Endoscopic	7 Autologous Tissue Substitute J Synthetic Substitute K Nonautologous Tissue Substitute	Z No Qualifier
M Nasal Septum Quadrangular cartilage Septal cartilage Vomer bone	Ø Open 3 Percutaneous 4 Percutaneous Endoscopic 8 Via Natural or Artificial Opening Endoscopic	7 Autologous Tissue Substitute J Synthetic Substitute K Nonautologous Tissue Substitute	Z No Qualifier

Ø **Medical and Surgical**
9 **Ear, Nose, Sinus**
W **Revision** Definition: Correcting, to the extent possible, a portion of a malfunctioning device or the position of a displaced device
Explanation: Revision can include correcting a malfunctioning or displaced device by taking out or putting in components of the device such as a screw or pin

Body Part Character 4	Approach Character 5	Device Character 6	Qualifier Character 7
7 Tympanic Membrane, Right Pars flaccida 8 Tympanic Membrane, Left See 7 Tympanic Membrane, Right 9 Auditory Ossicle, Right Incus Malleus Stapes A Auditory Ossicle, Left See 9 Auditory Ossicle, Right	Ø Open 7 Via Natural or Artificial Opening 8 Via Natural or Artificial Opening Endoscopic	7 Autologous Tissue Substitute J Synthetic Substitute K Nonautologous Tissue Substitute	Z No Qualifier
D Inner Ear, Right Bony labyrinth Bony vestibule Cochlea Round window Semicircular canal E Inner Ear, Left See D Inner Ear, Right	Ø Open 7 Via Natural or Artificial Opening 8 Via Natural or Artificial Opening Endoscopic	S Hearing Device	Z No Qualifier
H Ear, Right J Ear, Left K Nasal Mucosa and Soft Tissue Columella External naris Greater alar cartilage Internal naris Lateral nasal cartilage Lesser alar cartilage Nasal cavity Nostril	Ø Open 3 Percutaneous 4 Percutaneous Endoscopic 7 Via Natural or Artificial Opening 8 Via Natural or Artificial Opening Endoscopic	Ø Drainage Device 7 Autologous Tissue Substitute D Intraluminal Device J Synthetic Substitute K Nonautologous Tissue Substitute Y Other Device	Z No Qualifier
H Ear, Right J Ear, Left K Nasal Mucosa and Soft Tissue Columella External naris Greater alar cartilage Internal naris Lateral nasal cartilage Lesser alar cartilage Nasal cavity Nostril	X External	Ø Drainage Device 7 Autologous Tissue Substitute D Intraluminal Device J Synthetic Substitute K Nonautologous Tissue Substitute	Z No Qualifier
Y Sinus	Ø Open 3 Percutaneous 4 Percutaneous Endoscopic	Ø Drainage Device Y Other Device	Z No Qualifier
Y Sinus	7 Via Natural or Artificial Opening 8 Via Natural or Artificial Opening Endoscopic	Y Other Device	Z No Qualifier
Y Sinus	X External	Ø Drainage Device	Z No Qualifier

Non-OR 09W[H,J][3,4][J,K,Y]Z
Non-OR 09W[H,J][7,8][D,Y]Z
Non-OR 09WK[Ø,3,4,7,8][Ø,7,D,J,K,Y]Z
Non-OR 09W[H,J,K]X[Ø,7,D,J,K]Z
Non-OR 09WY[3,4]YZ
Non-OR 09WY[7,8]YZ
Non-OR 09WYXØZ

Respiratory System ØB1–ØBY

Character Meanings

This Character Meaning table is provided as a guide to assist the user in the identification of character members that may be found in this section of code tables. It **SHOULD NOT** be used to build a PCS code.

Operation–Character 3	Body Part–Character 4	Approach–Character 5	Device–Character 6	Qualifier–Character 7
1 Bypass	Ø Tracheobronchial Tree	Ø Open	Ø Drainage Device	Ø Allogeneic
2 Change	1 Trachea	3 Percutaneous	1 Radioactive Element	1 Syngeneic
5 Destruction	2 Carina	4 Percutaneous Endoscopic	2 Monitoring Device	2 Zooplastic
7 Dilation	3 Main Bronchus, Right	7 Via Natural or Artificial Opening	3 Infusion Device	4 Cutaneous
9 Drainage	4 Upper Lobe Bronchus, Right	8 Via Natural or Artificial Opening Endoscopic	7 Autologous Tissue Substitute	6 Esophagus
B Excision	5 Middle Lobe Bronchus, Right	X External	C Extraluminal Device	X Diagnostic
C Extirpation	6 Lower Lobe Bronchus, Right		D Intraluminal Device	Z No Qualifier
D Extraction	7 Main Bronchus, Left		E Intraluminal Device, Endotracheal Airway	
F Fragmentation	8 Upper Lobe Bronchus, Left		F Tracheostomy Device	
H Insertion	9 Lingula Bronchus		G Intraluminal Device, Endobronchial Valve	
J Inspection	B Lower Lobe Bronchus, Left		J Synthetic Substitute	
L Occlusion	C Upper Lung Lobe, Right		K Nonautologous Tissue Substitute	
M Reattachment	D Middle Lung Lobe, Right		M Diaphragmatic Pacemaker Lead	
N Release	F Lower Lung Lobe, Right		Y Other Device	
P Removal	G Upper Lung Lobe, Left		Z No Device	
Q Repair	H Lung Lingula			
R Replacement	J Lower Lung Lobe, Left			
S Reposition	K Lung, Right			
T Resection	L Lung, Left			
U Supplement	M Lungs, Bilateral			
V Restriction	N Pleura, Right			
W Revision	P Pleura, Left			
Y Transplantation	Q Pleura			
	T Diaphragm			

AHA Coding Clinic for table ØB5
2016, 2Q, 17   Photodynamic therapy for treatment of malignant mesothelioma
2015, 2Q, 31   Thoracoscopic talc pleurodesis

AHA Coding Clinic for table ØB9
2017, 3Q, 15   Bronchoscopy with suctioning for removal of retained secretions
2017, 1Q, 51   Bronchoalveolar lavage
2016, 1Q, 26   Bronchoalveolar lavage, endobronchial biopsy and transbronchial biopsy
2016, 1Q, 27   Fiberoptic bronchoscopy with brushings and bronchoalveolar lavage

AHA Coding Clinic for table ØBB
2016, 1Q, 26   Bronchoalveolar lavage, endobronchial biopsy and transbronchial biopsy
2016, 1Q, 27   Fiberoptic bronchoscopy with brushings and bronchoalveolar lavage
2014, 1Q, 20   Fiducial marker placement

AHA Coding Clinic for table ØBC
2017, 3Q, 14   Bronchoscopy with suctioning and washings for removal of mucus plug

AHA Coding Clinic for table ØBH
2014, 4Q, 3-10   Mechanical ventilation

AHA Coding Clinic for table ØBJ
2015, 2Q, 31   Thoracoscopic talc pleurodesis
2014, 1Q, 20   Fiducial marker placement

AHA Coding Clinic for table ØBN
2015, 3Q, 15   Vascular ring surgery with release of esophagus and trachea

AHA Coding Clinic for table ØBQ
2016, 2Q, 22   Esophageal lengthening Collis gastroplasty with Nissen fundoplication and hiatal hernia
2014, 3Q, 28   Laparoscopic Nissen fundoplication and diaphragmatic hernia repair

AHA Coding Clinic for table ØBU
2015, 1Q, 28   Repair of bronchopleural fistula using omental pedicle graft

Respiratory System

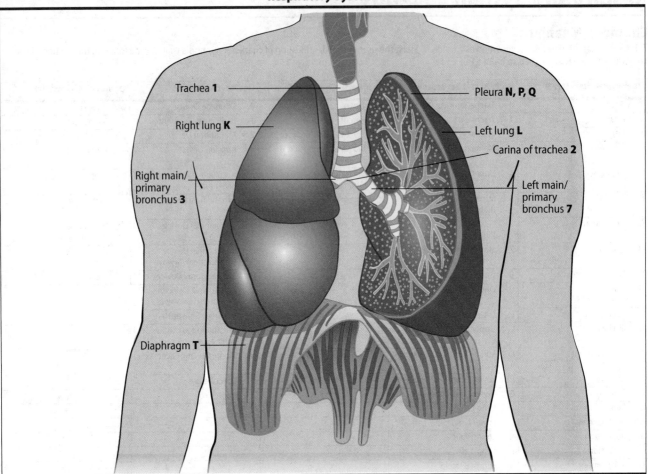

Trachea **1**

Right lung **K**

Right main/
primary
bronchus **3**

Diaphragm **T**

Pleura **N, P, Q**

Left lung **L**

Carina of trachea **2**

Left main/
primary
bronchus **7**

Right Lung Bronchi

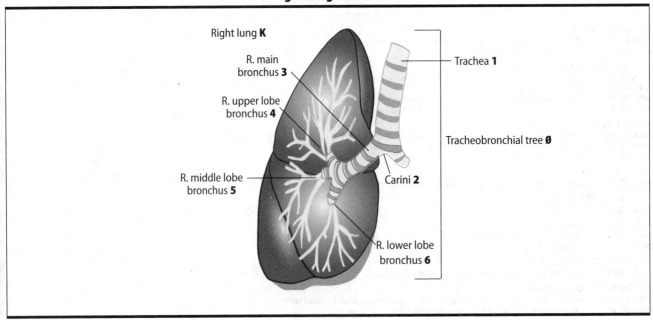

Right lung **K**

R. main
bronchus **3**

R. upper lobe
bronchus **4**

R. middle lobe
bronchus **5**

R. lower lobe
bronchus **6**

Trachea **1**

Tracheobronchial tree **Ø**

Carini **2**

Ø　Medical and Surgical
B　Respiratory System
1　Bypass　　　Definition: Altering the route of passage of the contents of a tubular body part

　　　　　　　　　Explanation: Rerouting contents of a body part to a downstream area of the normal route, to a similar route and body part, or to an abnormal route and dissimilar body part. Includes one or more anastomoses, with or without the use of a device.

Body Part Character 4	Approach Character 5	Device Character 6	Qualifier Character 7
1 Trachea 　Cricoid cartilage	**Ø** Open	**D** Intraluminal Device	**6** Esophagus
1 Trachea 　Cricoid cartilage	**Ø** Open	**F** Tracheostomy Device **Z** No Device	**4** Cutaneous
1 Trachea 　Cricoid cartilage	**3** Percutaneous **4** Percutaneous Endoscopic	**F** Tracheostomy Device **Z** No Device	**4** Cutaneous

DRG Non-OR　ØB113[F,Z]4
Non-OR　　　ØB11ØD6

Ø　Medical and Surgical
B　Respiratory System
2　Change　　　Definition: Taking out or off a device from a body part and putting back an identical or similar device in or on the same body part without cutting or puncturing the skin or a mucous membrane

　　　　　　　　　Explanation: All CHANGE procedures are coded using the approach EXTERNAL

Body Part Character 4	Approach Character 5	Device Character 6	Qualifier Character 7
Ø Tracheobronchial Tree **K** Lung, Right **L** Lung, Left **Q** Pleura **T** Diaphragm	**X** External	**Ø** Drainage Device **Y** Other Device	**Z** No Qualifier
1 Trachea 　Cricoid cartilage	**X** External	**Ø** Drainage Device **E** Intraluminal Device, Endotracheal Airway **F** Tracheostomy Device **Y** Other Device	**Z** No Qualifier

Non-OR　All body part, approach, device, and qualifier values

Ø　Medical and Surgical
B　Respiratory System
5　Destruction　　Definition: Physical eradication of all or a portion of a body part by the direct use of energy, force, or a destructive agent

　　　　　　　　　Explanation: None of the body part is physically taken out

Body Part Character 4	Approach Character 5	Device Character 6	Qualifier Character 7
1 Trachea 　Cricoid cartilage **2** Carina **3** Main Bronchus, Right 　Bronchus intermedius 　Intermediate bronchus **4** Upper Lobe Bronchus, Right **5** Middle Lobe Bronchus, Right **6** Lower Lobe Bronchus, Right **7** Main Bronchus, Left **8** Upper Lobe Bronchus, Left **9** Lingula Bronchus **B** Lower Lobe Bronchus, Left **C** Upper Lung Lobe, Right **D** Middle Lung Lobe, Right **F** Lower Lung Lobe, Right **G** Upper Lung Lobe, Left **H** Lung Lingula **J** Lower Lung Lobe, Left **K** Lung, Right **L** Lung, Left **M** Lungs, Bilateral	**Ø** Open **3** Percutaneous **4** Percutaneous Endoscopic **7** Via Natural or Artificial Opening **8** Via Natural or Artificial Opening Endoscopic	**Z** No Device	**Z** No Qualifier
N Pleura, Right **P** Pleura, Left **T** Diaphragm	**Ø** Open **3** Percutaneous **4** Percutaneous Endoscopic	**Z** No Device	**Z** No Qualifier

Non-OR　ØB5[3,4,5,6,7,8,9,B][4,8]ZZ
Non-OR　ØB5[C,D,F,G,H,J,K,L,M]8ZZ

LC Limited Coverage　**NC** Noncovered　⊞ Combination Member　HAC associated procedure　Combination Only　DRG Non-OR　Non-OR　New/Revised in GREEN

Ø   Medical and Surgical
B   Respiratory System
7   Dilation   Definition: Expanding an orifice or the lumen of a tubular body part

Explanation: The orifice can be a natural orifice or an artificially created orifice. Accomplished by stretching a tubular body part using intraluminal pressure or by cutting part of the orifice or wall of the tubular body part.

Body Part Character 4	Approach Character 5	Device Character 6	Qualifier Character 7

1   Trachea
     Cricoid cartilage
2   Carina
3   Main Bronchus, Right
     Bronchus intermedius
     Intermediate bronchus
4   Upper Lobe Bronchus, Right
5   Middle Lobe Bronchus, Right
6   Lower Lobe Bronchus, Right
7   Main Bronchus, Left
8   Upper Lobe Bronchus, Left
9   Lingula Bronchus
B   Lower Lobe Bronchus, Left
	Ø Open
	3 Percutaneous
	4 Percutaneous Endoscopic
	7 Via Natural or Artificial Opening
	8 Via Natural or Artificial Opening Endoscopic
		D Intraluminal Device
		Z No Device
			Z No Qualifier

Non-OR   ØB7[3,4,5,6,7,8,9,B][Ø,3,4,7,8][D,Z]Z

Ø   Medical and Surgical
B   Respiratory System
9   Drainage   Definition: Taking or letting out fluids and/or gases from a body part

Explanation: The qualifier DIAGNOSTIC is used to identify drainage procedures that are biopsies

Body Part Character 4		Approach Character 5	Device Character 6	Qualifier Character 7

1   Trachea
     Cricoid cartilage
2   Carina
3   Main Bronchus, Right
     Bronchus intermedius
     Intermediate bronchus
4   Upper Lobe Bronchus, Right
5   Middle Lobe Bronchus, Right
6   Lower Lobe Bronchus, Right
7   Main Bronchus, Left
	8 Upper Lobe Bronchus, Left
	9 Lingula Bronchus
	B Lower Lobe Bronchus, Left
	C Upper Lung Lobe, Right
	D Middle Lung Lobe, Right
	F Lower Lung Lobe, Right
	G Upper Lung Lobe, Left
	H Lung Lingula
	J Lower Lung Lobe, Left
	K Lung, Right
	L Lung, Left
	M Lungs, Bilateral
		Ø Open
		3 Percutaneous
		4 Percutaneous Endoscopic
		7 Via Natural or Artificial Opening
		8 Via Natural or Artificial Opening Endoscopic
			Ø Drainage Device	Z No Qualifier

1   Trachea
     Cricoid cartilage
2   Carina
3   Main Bronchus, Right
     Bronchus intermedius
     Intermediate bronchus
4   Upper Lobe Bronchus, Right
5   Middle Lobe Bronchus, Right
6   Lower Lobe Bronchus, Right
7   Main Bronchus, Left
	8 Upper Lobe Bronchus, Left
	9 Lingula Bronchus
	B Lower Lobe Bronchus, Left
	C Upper Lung Lobe, Right
	D Middle Lung Lobe, Right
	F Lower Lung Lobe, Right
	G Upper Lung Lobe, Left
	H Lung Lingula
	J Lower Lung Lobe, Left
	K Lung, Right
	L Lung, Left
	M Lungs, Bilateral
		Ø Open
		3 Percutaneous
		4 Percutaneous Endoscopic
		7 Via Natural or Artificial Opening
		8 Via Natural or Artificial Opening Endoscopic
			Z No Device	X Diagnostic
				Z No Qualifier

N Pleura, Right P Pleura, Left		Ø Open 3 Percutaneous 4 Percutaneous Endoscopic 8 Via Natural or Artificial Opening Endoscopic	Ø Drainage Device	Z No Qualifier
N Pleura, Right P Pleura, Left		Ø Open 3 Percutaneous 4 Percutaneous Endoscopic 8 Via Natural or Artificial Opening Endoscopic	Z No Device	X Diagnostic Z No Qualifier
T Diaphragm		Ø Open 3 Percutaneous 4 Percutaneous Endoscopic	Ø Drainage Device	Z No Qualifier
T Diaphragm		Ø Open 3 Percutaneous 4 Percutaneous Endoscopic	Z No Device	X Diagnostic Z No Qualifier

Non-OR ØB9[1,2,3,4,5,6,7,8,9,B][7,8]ØZ **Non-OR** ØB9[1,2,3,4,5,6,7,8,9,B][3,4]ZX **Non-OR** ØB9[1,2,3,4,5,6,7,8,9,B][7,8]Z[X,Z] **Non-OR** ØB9[C,D,F,G,H,J,K,L,M][3,4,7]ZX **Non-OR** ØB9[N,P][Ø,3,8]ØZ	**Non-OR** ØB9[N,P][Ø,3,8]Z[X,Z] **Non-OR** ØB9[N,P]4ZX **Non-OR** ØB9T[3,4]ØZ **Non-OR** ØB9T[3,4]Z[X,Z]

0   **Medical and Surgical**
B   **Respiratory System**
B   **Excision**   Definition: Cutting out or off, without replacement, a portion of a body part

                         Explanation: The qualifier DIAGNOSTIC is used to identify excision procedures that are biopsies

Body Part Character 4	Approach Character 5	Device Character 6	Qualifier Character 7

1 Trachea
    Cricoid cartilage
2 Carina
3 Main Bronchus, Right
    Bronchus intermedius
    Intermediate bronchus
4 Upper Lobe Bronchus, Right
5 Middle Lobe Bronchus, Right
6 Lower Lobe Bronchus, Right
7 Main Bronchus, Left
8 Upper Lobe Bronchus, Left
9 Lingula Bronchus
B Lower Lobe Bronchus, Left
C Upper Lung Lobe, Right
D Middle Lung Lobe, Right
F Lower Lung Lobe, Right
G Upper Lung Lobe, Left
H Lung Lingula
J Lower Lung Lobe, Left
K Lung, Right
L Lung, Left
M Lungs, Bilateral
	0 Open
	3 Percutaneous
	4 Percutaneous Endoscopic
	7 Via Natural or Artificial Opening
	8 Via Natural or Artificial Opening
	    Endoscopic
		Z No Device	**X** Diagnostic
			Z No Qualifier

N Pleura, Right **P** Pleura, Left	**0** Open **3** Percutaneous **4** Percutaneous Endoscopic **8** Via Natural or Artificial Opening Endoscopic	**Z** No Device	**X** Diagnostic **Z** No Qualifier
T Diaphragm	**0** Open **3** Percutaneous **4** Percutaneous Endoscopic	**Z** No Device	**X** Diagnostic **Z** No Qualifier

    Non-OR   0BB[1,2,3,4,5,6,7,8,9,B][3,4,7,8]ZX   **Non-OR**   0BB[C,D,F,G,H,J,K,L]8ZZ
    Non-OR   0BB[3,4,5,6,7,8,9,B,M][4,8]ZZ   **Non-OR**   0BB[N,P][0,3]ZX
    Non-OR   0BB[C,D,F,G,H,J,K,L,M]3ZX

---

0   **Medical and Surgical**
B   **Respiratory System**
C   **Extirpation**   Definition: Taking or cutting out solid matter from a body part

                         Explanation: The solid matter may be an abnormal byproduct of a biological function or a foreign body; it may be imbedded in a body part or in
                         the lumen of a tubular body part. The solid matter may or may not have been previously broken into pieces.

Body Part Character 4	Approach Character 5	Device Character 6	Qualifier Character 7

1 Trachea
    Cricoid cartilage
2 Carina
3 Main Bronchus, Right
    Bronchus intermedius
    Intermediate bronchus
4 Upper Lobe Bronchus, Right
5 Middle Lobe Bronchus, Right
6 Lower Lobe Bronchus, Right
7 Main Bronchus, Left
8 Upper Lobe Bronchus, Left
9 Lingula Bronchus
B Lower Lobe Bronchus, Left
C Upper Lung Lobe, Right
D Middle Lung Lobe, Right
F Lower Lung Lobe, Right
G Upper Lung Lobe, Left
H Lung Lingula
J Lower Lung Lobe, Left
K Lung, Right
L Lung, Left
M Lungs, Bilateral
	0 Open
	3 Percutaneous
	4 Percutaneous Endoscopic
	7 Via Natural or Artificial Opening
	8 Via Natural or Artificial Opening
	    Endoscopic
		Z No Device	**Z** No Qualifier

N Pleura, Right **P** Pleura, Left **T** Diaphragm	**0** Open **3** Percutaneous **4** Percutaneous Endoscopic	**Z** No Device	**Z** No Qualifier

    Non-OR   0BC[1,2,3,4,5,6,7,8,9,B][7,8]ZZ
    Non-OR   0BC[N,P][0,3,4]ZZ

LC Limited Coverage   **NC** Noncovered   ⊞ Combination Member   HAC associated procedure   Combination Only   DRG Non-OR   Non-OR   New/Revised in GREEN

ICD-10-PCS 2019   **329**

Respiratory System

Ø   Medical and Surgical
B   Respiratory System
D   Extraction   Definition: Pulling or stripping out or off all or a portion of a body part by the use of force
                 Explanation: The qualifier DIAGNOSTIC is used to identify extraction procedures that are biopsies

Body Part Character 4	Approach Character 5	Device Character 6	Qualifier Character 7

1   Trachea
     Cricoid cartilage
2   Carina
3   Main Bronchus, Right
     Bronchus intermedius
     Intermediate bronchus
4   Upper Lobe Bronchus, Right
5   Middle Lobe Bronchus, Right
6   Lower Lobe Bronchus, Right
7   Main Bronchus, Left
8   Upper Lobe Bronchus, Left
9   Lingula Bronchus
B   Lower Lobe Bronchus, Left
C   Upper Lung Lobe, Right
D   Middle Lung Lobe, Right
F   Lower Lung Lobe, Right
G   Upper Lung Lobe, Left
H   Lung Lingula
J   Lower Lung Lobe, Left
K   Lung, Right
L   Lung, Left
M   Lungs, Bilateral
	4 Percutaneous Endoscopic
	8 Via Natural or Artificial Opening
	     Endoscopic
		Z No Device	X Diagnostic

N Pleura, Right P Pleura, Left	Ø Open 3 Percutaneous 4 Percutaneous Endoscopic	Z No Device	X Diagnostic Z No Qualifier

Non-OR   ØBD[1,2,3,4,5,6,7,8,9,B,C,D,F,G,H,J,K,L,M][4,8]ZX

Ø   Medical and Surgical
B   Respiratory System
F   Fragmentation   Definition: Breaking solid matter in a body part into pieces
                 Explanation: Physical force (e.g., manual, ultrasonic) applied directly or indirectly is used to break the solid matter into pieces. The solid matter may be an abnormal byproduct of a biological function or a foreign body. The pieces of solid matter are not taken out.

Body Part Character 4	Approach Character 5	Device Character 6	Qualifier Character 7

1   Trachea   `NC`
     Cricoid cartilage
2   Carina   `NC`
3   Main Bronchus, Right   `NC`
     Bronchus intermedius
     Intermediate bronchus
4   Upper Lobe Bronchus, Right   `NC`
5   Middle Lobe Bronchus, Right   `NC`
6   Lower Lobe Bronchus, Right   `NC`
7   Main Bronchus, Left   `NC`
8   Upper Lobe Bronchus, Left   `NC`
9   Lingula Bronchus   `NC`
B   Lower Lobe Bronchus, Left   `NC`
	Ø Open
	3 Percutaneous
	4 Percutaneous Endoscopic
	7 Via Natural or Artificial Opening
	8 Via Natural or Artificial Opening
	     Endoscopic
	X External
		Z No Device	Z No Qualifier

Non-OR   ØBF[1,2,3,4,5,6,7,8,9,B]XZZ
Non-OR   ØBF[3,4,5,6,7,8,9,B][7,8]ZZ
`NC`   ØBF[1,2,3,4,5,6,7,8,9,B]XZZ

Ø   Medical and Surgical
B   Respiratory System
H   Insertion   Definition: Putting in a nonbiological appliance that monitors, assists, performs, or prevents a physiological function but does not physically take the place of a body part
                 Explanation: None

Body Part Character 4	Approach Character 5	Device Character 6	Qualifier Character 7
Ø Tracheobronchial Tree	Ø Open 3 Percutaneous 4 Percutaneous Endoscopic 7 Via Natural or Artificial Opening 8 Via Natural or Artificial Opening Endoscopic	1 Radioactive Element 2 Monitoring Device 3 Infusion Device D Intraluminal Device Y Other Device	Z No Qualifier
1 Trachea Cricoid cartilage	Ø Open	2 Monitoring Device D Intraluminal Device Y Other Device	Z No Qualifier
1 Trachea Cricoid cartilage	3 Percutaneous	D Intraluminal Device E Intraluminal Device, Endotracheal Airway Y Other Device	Z No Qualifier
1 Trachea Cricoid cartilage	4 Percutaneous Endoscopic	D Intraluminal Device Y Other Device	Z No Qualifier
1 Trachea Cricoid cartilage	7 Via Natural or Artificial Opening 8 Via Natural or Artificial Opening Endoscopic	2 Monitoring Device D Intraluminal Device E Intraluminal Device, Endotracheal Airway Y Other Device	Z No Qualifier

3   Main Bronchus, Right
     Bronchus intermedius
     Intermediate bronchus
4   Upper Lobe Bronchus, Right
5   Middle Lobe Bronchus, Right
6   Lower Lobe Bronchus, Right
7   Main Bronchus, Left
8   Upper Lobe Bronchus, Left
9   Lingula Bronchus
B   Lower Lobe Bronchus, Left
	Ø Open
	3 Percutaneous
	4 Percutaneous Endoscopic
	7 Via Natural or Artificial Opening
	8 Via Natural or Artificial Opening Endoscopic
		G Intraluminal Device, Endobronchial Valve	Z No Qualifier

K Lung, Right L Lung, Left	Ø Open 3 Percutaneous 4 Percutaneous Endoscopic 7 Via Natural or Artificial Opening 8 Via Natural or Artificial Opening Endoscopic	1 Radioactive Element 2 Monitoring Device 3 Infusion Device Y Other Device	Z No Qualifier
Q Pleura	Ø Open 3 Percutaneous 4 Percutaneous Endoscopic 7 Via Natural or Artificial Opening 8 Via Natural or Artificial Opening Endoscopic	Y Other Device	Z No Qualifier
T Diaphragm	Ø Open 3 Percutaneous 4 Percutaneous Endoscopic	2 Monitoring Device M Diaphragmatic Pacemaker Lead Y Other Device	Z No Qualifier
T Diaphragm	7 Via Natural or Artificial Opening 8 Via Natural or Artificial Opening Endoscopic	Y Other Device	Z No Qualifier

Non-OR   ØBHØ3YZ
Non-OR   ØBHØ[7,8][2,3,D,Y]Z
Non-OR   ØBH13[E,Y]Z
Non-OR   ØBH1[7,8][2,D,E,Y]Z
Non-OR   ØBH[3,4,5,6,7,8,9,B]8GZ
Non-OR   ØBH[K,L]3YZ
Non-OR   ØBH[K,L]7[2,3,Y]Z
Non-OR   ØBH[K,L]8[2,3]Z
Non-OR   ØBHQ[3,7]YZ
Non-OR   ØBHT3YZ
Non-OR   ØBHT[7,8]YZ

LC Limited Coverage   NC Noncovered   ⊞ Combination Member   HAC associated procedure   Combination Only   DRG Non-OR   Non-OR   New/Revised in GREEN
ICD-10-PCS 2019   331

ØBH–ØBH

Ø   **Medical and Surgical**
B   **Respiratory System**
J   **Inspection**   Definition: Visually and/or manually exploring a body part

         Explanation: Visual exploration may be performed with or without optical instrumentation. Manual exploration may be performed directly or through intervening body layers.

Body Part Character 4	Approach Character 5	Device Character 6	Qualifier Character 7

Ø Tracheobronchial Tree
1 Trachea
   Cricoid cartilage
K Lung, Right
L Lung, Left
Q Pleura
T Diaphragm
	Ø Open
	3 Percutaneous
	4 Percutaneous Endoscopic
	7 Via Natural or Artificial Opening
	8 Via Natural or Artificial Opening
	   Endoscopic
	X External
		Z No Device	**Z** No Qualifier

Non-OR   ØBJ[Ø,K,L,Q,T][3,7,8,X]ZZ
Non-OR   ØBJ1[3,4,7,8,X]ZZ

Ø   **Medical and Surgical**
B   **Respiratory System**
L   **Occlusion**   Definition: Completely closing an orifice or the lumen of a tubular body part

         Explanation: The orifice can be a natural orifice or an artificially created orifice

Body Part Character 4	Approach Character 5	Device Character 6	Qualifier Character 7

1 Trachea
   Cricoid cartilage
2 Carina
3 Main Bronchus, Right
   Bronchus intermedius
   Intermediate bronchus
4 Upper Lobe Bronchus, Right
5 Middle Lobe Bronchus, Right
6 Lower Lobe Bronchus, Right
7 Main Bronchus, Left
8 Upper Lobe Bronchus, Left
9 Lingula Bronchus
B Lower Lobe Bronchus, Left
	Ø Open
	3 Percutaneous
	4 Percutaneous Endoscopic
		C Extraluminal Device
		D Intraluminal Device
		Z No Device
			Z No Qualifier

1 Trachea
   Cricoid cartilage
2 Carina
3 Main Bronchus, Right
   Bronchus intermedius
   Intermediate bronchus
4 Upper Lobe Bronchus, Right
5 Middle Lobe Bronchus, Right
6 Lower Lobe Bronchus, Right
7 Main Bronchus, Left
8 Upper Lobe Bronchus, Left
9 Lingula Bronchus
B Lower Lobe Bronchus, Left
	7 Via Natural or Artificial Opening
	8 Via Natural or Artificial Opening
	   Endoscopic
		D Intraluminal Device
		Z No Device
			Z No Qualifier

🔲 Limited Coverage   🔲 Noncovered   ⊞ Combination Member   HAC associated procedure   Combination Only   DRG Non-OR   Non-OR   New/Revised in GREEN

332   ICD-10-PCS 2019

Ø Medical and Surgical
B Respiratory System
M Reattachment   Definition: Putting back in or on all or a portion of a separated body part to its normal location or other suitable location
     Explanation: Vascular circulation and nervous pathways may or may not be reestablished

Body Part Character 4	Approach Character 5	Device Character 6	Qualifier Character 7

1 Trachea
    Cricoid cartilage
 2 Carina
 3 Main Bronchus, Right
    Bronchus intermedius
    Intermediate bronchus
 4 Upper Lobe Bronchus, Right
 5 Middle Lobe Bronchus, Right
 6 Lower Lobe Bronchus, Right
 7 Main Bronchus, Left
 8 Upper Lobe Bronchus, Left
 9 Lingula Bronchus
 B Lower Lobe Bronchus, Left
 C Upper Lung Lobe, Right
 D Middle Lung Lobe, Right
 F Lower Lung Lobe, Right
 G Upper Lung Lobe, Left
 H Lung Lingula
 J Lower Lung Lobe, Left
 K Lung, Right
 L Lung, Left
 T Diaphragm
	Ø Open	Z No Device	Z No Qualifier

Ø Medical and Surgical
B Respiratory System
N Release   Definition: Freeing a body part from an abnormal physical constraint by cutting or by the use of force
     Explanation: Some of the restraining tissue may be taken out but none of the body part is taken out

Body Part Character 4	Approach Character 5	Device Character 6	Qualifier Character 7

1 Trachea
    Cricoid cartilage
 2 Carina
 3 Main Bronchus, Right
    Bronchus intermedius
    Intermediate bronchus
 4 Upper Lobe Bronchus, Right
 5 Middle Lobe Bronchus, Right
 6 Lower Lobe Bronchus, Right
 7 Main Bronchus, Left
 8 Upper Lobe Bronchus, Left
 9 Lingula Bronchus
 B Lower Lobe Bronchus, Left
 C Upper Lung Lobe, Right
 D Middle Lung Lobe, Right
 F Lower Lung Lobe, Right
 G Upper Lung Lobe, Left
 H Lung Lingula
 J Lower Lung Lobe, Left
 K Lung, Right
 L Lung, Left
 M Lungs, Bilateral
	Ø Open
	 3 Percutaneous
	 4 Percutaneous Endoscopic
	 7 Via Natural or Artificial Opening
	 8 Via Natural or Artificial Opening Endoscopic
		Z No Device	Z No Qualifier

N Pleura, Right P Pleura, Left T Diaphragm	Ø Open 3 Percutaneous 4 Percutaneous Endoscopic	Z No Device	Z No Qualifier

Ø   Medical and Surgical
B   Respiratory System
P   Removal   Definition: Taking out or off a device from a body part

Explanation: If a device is taken out and a similar device put in without cutting or puncturing the skin or mucous membrane, the procedure is coded to the root operation CHANGE. Otherwise, the procedure for taking out a device is coded to the root operation REMOVAL.

Body Part Character 4	Approach Character 5	Device Character 6	Qualifier Character 7
Ø Tracheobronchial Tree	**Ø** Open **3** Percutaneous **4** Percutaneous Endoscopic **7** Via Natural or Artificial Opening **8** Via Natural or Artificial Opening Endoscopic	**Ø** Drainage Device **1** Radioactive Element **2** Monitoring Device **3** Infusion Device **7** Autologous Tissue Substitute **C** Extraluminal Device **D** Intraluminal Device **J** Synthetic Substitute **K** Nonautologous Tissue Substitute **Y** Other Device	**Z** No Qualifier
Ø Tracheobronchial Tree	**X** External	**Ø** Drainage Device **1** Radioactive Element **2** Monitoring Device **3** Infusion Device **D** Intraluminal Device	**Z** No Qualifier

1 Trachea
   Cricoid cartilage
	Ø Open
	3 Percutaneous
	4 Percutaneous Endoscopic
	7 Via Natural or Artificial Opening
	8 Via Natural or Artificial Opening
	    Endoscopic
		Ø Drainage Device
		2 Monitoring Device
		7 Autologous Tissue Substitute
		C Extraluminal Device
		D Intraluminal Device
		F Tracheostomy Device
		J Synthetic Substitute
		K Nonautologous Tissue Substitute
			Z No Qualifier

1 Trachea Cricoid cartilage	**X** External	**Ø** Drainage Device **2** Monitoring Device **D** Intraluminal Device **F** Tracheostomy Device	**Z** No Qualifier
K Lung, Right **L Lung, Left**	**Ø** Open **3** Percutaneous **4** Percutaneous Endoscopic **7** Via Natural or Artificial Opening **8** Via Natural or Artificial Opening Endoscopic	**Ø** Drainage Device **1** Radioactive Element **2** Monitoring Device **3** Infusion Device **Y** Other Device	**Z** No Qualifier
K Lung, Right **L Lung, Left**	**X** External	**Ø** Drainage Device **1** Radioactive Element **2** Monitoring Device **3** Infusion Device	**Z** No Qualifier
Q Pleura	**Ø** Open **3** Percutaneous **4** Percutaneous Endoscopic **7** Via Natural or Artificial Opening **8** Via Natural or Artificial Opening Endoscopic	**Ø** Drainage Device **1** Radioactive Element **2** Monitoring Device **Y** Other Device	**Z** No Qualifier
Q Pleura	**X** External	**Ø** Drainage Device **1** Radioactive Element **2** Monitoring Device	**Z** No Qualifier
T Diaphragm	**Ø** Open **3** Percutaneous **4** Percutaneous Endoscopic **7** Via Natural or Artificial Opening **8** Via Natural or Artificial Opening Endoscopic	**Ø** Drainage Device **2** Monitoring Device **7** Autologous Tissue Substitute **J** Synthetic Substitute **K** Nonautologous Tissue Substitute **M** Diaphragmatic Pacemaker Lead **Y** Other Device	**Z** No Qualifier
T Diaphragm	**X** External	**Ø** Drainage Device **2** Monitoring Device **M** Diaphragmatic Pacemaker Lead	**Z** No Qualifier

Non-OR	ØBPØ[3,4]YZ	**Non-OR**	ØBPL7[Ø,2,3,Y]Z
Non-OR	ØBPØ[7,8][Ø,2,3,D,Y]Z	**Non-OR**	ØBPL8[Ø,2,3]Z
Non-OR	ØBPØX[Ø,1,2,3,D]Z	**Non-OR**	ØBP[K,L]X[Ø,1,2,3]Z
Non-OR	ØBP1[Ø,3,4]FZ	**Non-OR**	ØBPQ[Ø,3,4,7,8][Ø,1,2,]Z
Non-OR	ØBP1[7,8][Ø,2,D,F]Z	**Non-OR**	ØBPQ[3,7]YZ
Non-OR	ØBP1X[Ø,2,D,F]Z	**Non-OR**	ØBPQX[Ø,1,2]Z
Non-OR	ØBP[K,L]3YZ	**Non-OR**	ØBPT3YZ
Non-OR	ØBPK7[Ø,1,2,3,Y]Z	**Non-OR**	ØBPT[7,8][Ø,2,Y]Z
Non-OR	ØBPK8[Ø,1,2,3]Z	**Non-OR**	ØBPTX[Ø,2,M]Z

LC Limited Coverage   **NC** Noncovered   ⊞ Combination Member   HAC associated procedure   Combination Only   DRG Non-OR   Non-OR   New/Revised in GREEN

334   ICD-10-PCS 2019

Ø   Medical and Surgical
B   Respiratory System
Q   Repair   Definition: Restoring, to the extent possible, a body part to its normal anatomic structure and function

                        Explanation: Used only when the method to accomplish the repair is not one of the other root operations

Body Part Character 4	Approach Character 5	Device Character 6	Qualifier Character 7

1   Trachea
     Cricoid cartilage
2   Carina
3   Main Bronchus, Right
     Bronchus intermedius
     Intermediate bronchus
4   Upper Lobe Bronchus, Right
5   Middle Lobe Bronchus, Right
6   Lower Lobe Bronchus, Right
7   Main Bronchus, Left
8   Upper Lobe Bronchus, Left
9   Lingula Bronchus
B   Lower Lobe Bronchus, Left
C   Upper Lung Lobe, Right
D   Middle Lung Lobe, Right
F   Lower Lung Lobe, Right
G   Upper Lung Lobe, Left
H   Lung Lingula
J   Lower Lung Lobe, Left
K   Lung, Right
L   Lung, Left
M   Lungs, Bilateral
	Ø Open
	3 Percutaneous
	4 Percutaneous Endoscopic
	7 Via Natural or Artificial Opening
	8 Via Natural or Artificial Opening
	     Endoscopic
		Z No Device	**Z** No Qualifier

N Pleura, Right **P** Pleura, Left **T** Diaphragm	**Ø** Open **3** Percutaneous **4** Percutaneous Endoscopic	**Z** No Device	**Z** No Qualifier

Ø   Medical and Surgical
B   Respiratory System
R   Replacement   Definition: Putting in or on biological or synthetic material that physically takes the place and/or function of all or a portion of a body part

Explanation: The body part may have been taken out or replaced, or may be taken out, physically eradicated, or rendered nonfunctional during the REPLACEMENT procedure. A REMOVAL procedure is coded for taking out the device used in a previous replacement procedure.

Body Part Character 4	Approach Character 5	Device Character 6	Qualifier Character 7

1   Trachea
    Cricoid cartilage
2   Carina
3   Main Bronchus, Right
    Bronchus intermedius
    Intermediate bronchus
4   Upper Lobe Bronchus, Right
5   Middle Lobe Bronchus, Right
6   Lower Lobe Bronchus, Right
7   Main Bronchus, Left
8   Upper Lobe Bronchus, Left
9   Lingula Bronchus
B   Lower Lobe Bronchus, Left
T   Diaphragm
	Ø Open
	4 Percutaneous Endoscopic
		7 Autologous Tissue Substitute
		J Synthetic Substitute
		K Nonautologous Tissue Substitute
			Z No Qualifier

Ø   Medical and Surgical
B   Respiratory System
S   Reposition   Definition: Moving to its normal location, or other suitable location, all or a portion of a body part

Explanation: The body part is moved to a new location from an abnormal location, or from a normal location where it is not functioning correctly. The body part may or may not be cut out or off to be moved to the new location.

Body Part Character 4	Approach Character 5	Device Character 6	Qualifier Character 7

1   Trachea
    Cricoid cartilage
2   Carina
3   Main Bronchus, Right
    Bronchus intermedius
    Intermediate bronchus
4   Upper Lobe Bronchus, Right
5   Middle Lobe Bronchus, Right
6   Lower Lobe Bronchus, Right
7   Main Bronchus, Left
8   Upper Lobe Bronchus, Left
9   Lingula Bronchus
B   Lower Lobe Bronchus, Left
C   Upper Lung Lobe, Right
D   Middle Lung Lobe, Right
F   Lower Lung Lobe, Right
G   Upper Lung Lobe, Left
H   Lung Lingula
J   Lower Lung Lobe, Left
K   Lung, Right
L   Lung, Left
T   Diaphragm
	Ø Open	Z No Device	Z No Qualifier

LC Limited Coverage   NC Noncovered   ⊞ Combination Member   HAC associated procedure   Combination Only   DRG Non-OR   Non-OR   New/Revised in GREEN

336   ICD-10-PCS 2019

Ø　Medical and Surgical
B　Respiratory System
T　Resection　　Definition: Cutting out or off, without replacement, all of a body part
　　　　　　　　　　　Explanation: None

Body Part Character 4	Approach Character 5	Device Character 6	Qualifier Character 7
1 Trachea 　Cricoid cartilage **2** Carina **3** Main Bronchus, Right 　Bronchus intermedius 　Intermediate bronchus **4** Upper Lobe Bronchus, Right **5** Middle Lobe Bronchus, Right **6** Lower Lobe Bronchus, Right **7** Main Bronchus, Left **8** Upper Lobe Bronchus, Left **9** Lingula Bronchus **B** Lower Lobe Bronchus, Left **C** Upper Lung Lobe, Right **D** Middle Lung Lobe, Right **F** Lower Lung Lobe, Right **G** Upper Lung Lobe, Left **H** Lung Lingula **J** Lower Lung Lobe, Left **K** Lung, Right **L** Lung, Left **M** Lungs, Bilateral **T** Diaphragm	**Ø** Open **4** Percutaneous Endoscopic	**Z** No Device	**Z** No Qualifier

Ø　Medical and Surgical
B　Respiratory System
U　Supplement　　Definition: Putting in or on biological or synthetic material that physically reinforces and/or augments the function of a portion of a body part
　　　　　　　　　　　Explanation: The biological material is non-living, or is living and from the same individual. The body part may have been previously replaced, and the SUPPLEMENT procedure is performed to physically reinforce and/or augment the function of the replaced body part.

Body Part Character 4	Approach Character 5	Device Character 6	Qualifier Character 7
1 Trachea 　Cricoid cartilage **2** Carina **3** Main Bronchus, Right 　Bronchus intermedius 　Intermediate bronchus **4** Upper Lobe Bronchus, Right **5** Middle Lobe Bronchus, Right **6** Lower Lobe Bronchus, Right **7** Main Bronchus, Left **8** Upper Lobe Bronchus, Left **9** Lingula Bronchus **B** Lower Lobe Bronchus, Left	**Ø** Open **4** Percutaneous Endoscopic **8** Via Natural or Artificial Opening 　Endoscopic	**7** Autologous Tissue Substitute **J** Synthetic Substitute **K** Nonautologous Tissue Substitute	**Z** No Qualifier
T Diaphragm	**Ø** Open **4** Percutaneous Endoscopic	**7** Autologous Tissue Substitute **J** Synthetic Substitute **K** Nonautologous Tissue Substitute	**Z** No Qualifier

Respiratory System *(side tab)*

Ø Medical and Surgical
B Respiratory System
V Restriction   Definition: Partially closing an orifice or the lumen of a tubular body part
　　　　　　　　　Explanation: The orifice can be a natural orifice or an artificially created orifice

Body Part Character 4	Approach Character 5	Device Character 6	Qualifier Character 7
1 Trachea 　Cricoid cartilage **2** Carina **3** Main Bronchus, Right 　Bronchus intermedius 　Intermediate bronchus **4** Upper Lobe Bronchus, Right **5** Middle Lobe Bronchus, Right **6** Lower Lobe Bronchus, Right **7** Main Bronchus, Left **8** Upper Lobe Bronchus, Left **9** Lingula Bronchus **B** Lower Lobe Bronchus, Left	**Ø** Open **3** Percutaneous **4** Percutaneous Endoscopic	**C** Extraluminal Device **D** Intraluminal Device **Z** No Device	**Z** No Qualifier
1 Trachea 　Cricoid cartilage **2** Carina **3** Main Bronchus, Right 　Bronchus intermedius 　Intermediate bronchus **4** Upper Lobe Bronchus, Right **5** Middle Lobe Bronchus, Right **6** Lower Lobe Bronchus, Right **7** Main Bronchus, Left **8** Upper Lobe Bronchus, Left **9** Lingula Bronchus **B** Lower Lobe Bronchus, Left	**7** Via Natural or Artificial Opening **8** Via Natural or Artificial Opening Endoscopic	**D** Intraluminal Device **Z** No Device	**Z** No Qualifier

Ø Medical and Surgical
B Respiratory System
W Revision Definition: Correcting, to the extent possible, a portion of a malfunctioning device or the position of a displaced device
Explanation: Revision can include correcting a malfunctioning or displaced device by taking out or putting in components of the device such as a screw or pin

Body Part Character 4	Approach Character 5	Device Character 6	Qualifier Character 7
Ø Tracheobronchial Tree	Ø Open 3 Percutaneous 4 Percutaneous Endoscopic 7 Via Natural or Artificial Opening 8 Via Natural or Artificial Opening Endoscopic	Ø Drainage Device 2 Monitoring Device 3 Infusion Device 7 Autologous Tissue Substitute C Extraluminal Device D Intraluminal Device J Synthetic Substitute K Nonautologous Tissue Substitute Y Other Device	Z No Qualifier
Ø Tracheobronchial Tree	X External	Ø Drainage Device 2 Monitoring Device 3 Infusion Device 7 Autologous Tissue Substitute C Extraluminal Device D Intraluminal Device J Synthetic Substitute K Nonautologous Tissue Substitute	Z No Qualifier
1 Trachea Cricoid cartilage	Ø Open 3 Percutaneous 4 Percutaneous Endoscopic 7 Via Natural or Artificial Opening 8 Via Natural or Artificial Opening Endoscopic X External	Ø Drainage Device 2 Monitoring Device 7 Autologous Tissue Substitute C Extraluminal Device D Intraluminal Device F Tracheostomy Device J Synthetic Substitute K Nonautologous Tissue Substitute	Z No Qualifier
K Lung, Right L Lung, Left	Ø Open 3 Percutaneous 4 Percutaneous Endoscopic 7 Via Natural or Artificial Opening 8 Via Natural or Artificial Opening Endoscopic	Ø Drainage Device 2 Monitoring Device 3 Infusion Device Y Other Device	Z No Qualifier
K Lung, Right L Lung, Left	X External	Ø Drainage Device 2 Monitoring Device 3 Infusion Device	Z No Qualifier
Q Pleura	Ø Open 3 Percutaneous 4 Percutaneous Endoscopic 7 Via Natural or Artificial Opening 8 Via Natural or Artificial Opening Endoscopic	Ø Drainage Device 2 Monitoring Device Y Other Device	Z No Qualifier
Q Pleura	X External	Ø Drainage Device 2 Monitoring Device	Z No Qualifier
T Diaphragm	Ø Open 3 Percutaneous 4 Percutaneous Endoscopic 7 Via Natural or Artificial Opening 8 Via Natural or Artificial Opening Endoscopic	Ø Drainage Device 2 Monitoring Device 7 Autologous Tissue Substitute J Synthetic Substitute K Nonautologous Tissue Substitute M Diaphragmatic Pacemaker Lead Y Other Device	Z No Qualifier
T Diaphragm	X External	Ø Drainage Device 2 Monitoring Device 7 Autologous Tissue Substitute J Synthetic Substitute K Nonautologous Tissue Substitute M Diaphragmatic Pacemaker Lead	Z No Qualifier

Non-OR ØBWØ[3,4]YZ
Non-OR ØBWØ[7,8][2,3,D,Y]Z
Non-OR ØBWØX[Ø,2,3,7,C,D,J,K]Z
Non-OR ØBW1X[Ø,2,7,C,D,F,J,K]Z
Non-OR ØBW[K,L]3YZ
Non-OR ØBW[K,L]7[Ø,2,3,Y]Z
Non-OR ØBW[K,L]8[Ø,2,3]Z
Non-OR ØBW[K,L]X[Ø,2,3]Z
Non-OR ØBWQ[Ø,3,4,7,8][Ø,2]Z
Non-OR ØBWQ[Ø,3,7]YZ
Non-OR ØBWQX[Ø,2]Z
Non-OR ØBWT[3,7,8]YZ
Non-OR ØBWTX[Ø,2,7,J,K,M]Z

Ø   Medical and Surgical
B   Respiratory System
Y   Transplantation   Definition: Putting in or on all or a portion of a living body part taken from another individual or animal to physically take the place and/or
                           function of all or a portion of a similar body part
                           Explanation: The native body part may or may not be taken out, and the transplanted body part may take over all or a portion of its function

Body Part Character 4		Approach Character 5	Device Character 6	Qualifier Character 7
C Upper Lung Lobe, Right	LC	Ø Open	Z No Device	Ø Allogeneic
D Middle Lung Lobe, Right	LC			1 Syngeneic
F Lower Lung Lobe, Right	LC			2 Zooplastic
G Upper Lung Lobe, Left	LC			
H Lung Lingula	LC			
J Lower Lung Lobe, Left	LC			
K Lung, Right	LC			
L Lung, Left	LC			
M Lungs, Bilateral	LC			

LC   ØBY[C,D,F,G,H,J,K,L,M]ØZ[Ø,1,2]

Mouth and Throat 0C0–0CX

Character Meanings

This Character Meaning table is provided as a guide to assist the user in the identification of character members that may be found in this section of code tables. It **SHOULD NOT** be used to build a PCS code.

Operation–Character 3		Body Part–Character 4		Approach–Character 5		Device–Character 6		Qualifier–Character 7	
0	Alteration	0	Upper Lip	0	Open	0	Drainage Device	0	Single
2	Change	1	Lower Lip	3	Percutaneous	1	Radioactive Element	1	Multiple
5	Destruction	2	Hard Palate	4	Percutaneous Endoscopic	5	External Fixation Device	2	All
7	Dilation	3	Soft Palate	7	Via Natural or Artificial Opening	7	Autologous Tissue Substitute	X	Diagnostic
9	Drainage	4	Buccal Mucosa	8	Via Natural or Artificial Opening Endoscopic	B	Intraluminal Device, Airway	Z	No Qualifier
B	Excision	5	Upper Gingiva	X	External	C	Extraluminal Device		
C	Extirpation	6	Lower Gingiva			D	Intraluminal Device		
D	Extraction	7	Tongue			J	Synthetic Substitute		
F	Fragmentation	8	Parotid Gland, Right			K	Nonautologous Tissue Substitute		
H	Insertion	9	Parotid Gland, Left			Y	Other Device		
J	Inspection	A	Salivary Gland			Z	No Device		
L	Occlusion	B	Parotid Duct, Right						
M	Reattachment	C	Parotid Duct, Left						
N	Release	D	Sublingual Gland, Right						
P	Removal	F	Sublingual Gland, Left						
Q	Repair	G	Submaxillary Gland, Right						
R	Replacement	H	Submaxillary Gland, Left						
S	Reposition	J	Minor Salivary Gland						
T	Resection	M	Pharynx						
U	Supplement	N	Uvula						
V	Restriction	P	Tonsils						
W	Revision	Q	Adenoids						
X	Transfer	R	Epiglottis						
		S	Larynx						
		T	Vocal Cord, Right						
		V	Vocal Cord, Left						
		W	Upper Tooth						
		X	Lower Tooth						
		Y	Mouth and Throat						

AHA Coding Clinic for table 0C9
2017, 2Q, 16   Incision and drainage of floor of mouth

AHA Coding Clinic for table 0CB
2017, 2Q, 16   Excision of floor of mouth
2016, 3Q, 28   Lingual tonsillectomy, tongue base excision and epiglottopexy
2016, 2Q, 19   Biopsy of the base of tongue
2014, 3Q, 21   Superficial parotidectomy

AHA Coding Clinic for table 0CC
2016, 2Q, 20   Sialendoscopy with stone removal

AHA Coding Clinic for table 0CQ
2017, 1Q, 20   Preparatory nasal adhesion repair before definitive cleft palate repair

AHA Coding Clinic for table 0CR
2014, 3Q, 25   Excision of soft palate with placement of surgical obturator
2014, 2Q, 5   Oasis acellular matrix graft
2014, 2Q, 6   Composite grafting (synthetic versus nonautologous tissue substitute)

AHA Coding Clinic for table 0CS
2016, 3Q, 28   Lingual tonsillectomy, tongue base excision and epiglottopexy

AHA Coding Clinic for table 0CT
2016, 2Q, 12   Resection of malignant neoplasm of infratemporal fossa
2014, 3Q, 21   Superficial parotidectomy
2014, 3Q, 23   Le Fort I osteotomy

Salivary Glands

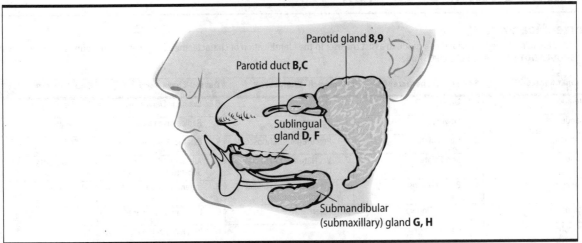

Parotid gland **8,9**

Parotid duct **B,C**

Sublingual gland **D, F**

Submandibular (submaxillary) gland **G, H**

Oral Anatomy

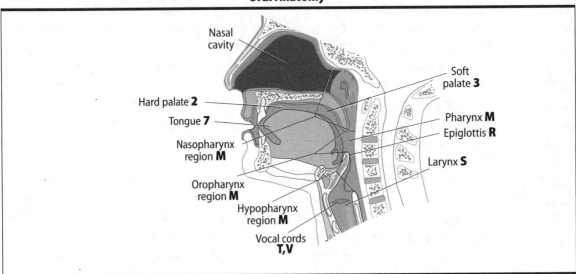

Nasal cavity

Soft palate **3**

Hard palate **2**

Tongue **7**

Pharynx **M**

Epiglottis **R**

Nasopharynx region **M**

Larynx **S**

Oropharynx region **M**

Hypopharynx region **M**

Vocal cords **T,V**

Mouth Frontal View (Upper)

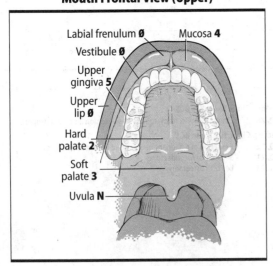

Labial frenulum **Ø**

Mucosa **4**

Vestibule **Ø**

Upper gingiva **5**

Upper lip **Ø**

Hard palate **2**

Soft palate **3**

Uvula **N**

Mouth Frontal View (Lower)

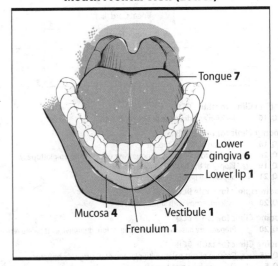

Tongue **7**

Lower gingiva **6**

Lower lip **1**

Mucosa **4**

Vestibule **1**

Frenulum **1**

0   **Medical and Surgical**
C   **Mouth and Throat**
0   **Alteration**   Definition: Modifying the anatomic structure of a body part without affecting the function of the body part

                            Explanation: Principal purpose is to improve appearance

Body Part Character 4	Approach Character 5	Device Character 6	Qualifier Character 7

0 **Upper Lip**
    Frenulum labii superioris
    Labial gland
    Vermilion border
1 **Lower Lip**
    Frenulum labii inferioris
    Labial gland
    Vermilion border
	X External	**7** Autologous Tissue Substitute
		J Synthetic Substitute
		K Nonautologous Tissue Substitute
		Z No Device
			Z No Qualifier

0   **Medical and Surgical**
C   **Mouth and Throat**
2   **Change**   Definition: Taking out or off a device from a body part and putting back an identical or similar device in or on the same body part without cutting or puncturing the skin or a mucous membrane

                            Explanation: All CHANGE procedures are coded using the approach EXTERNAL

Body Part Character 4	Approach Character 5	Device Character 6	Qualifier Character 7

A **Salivary Gland**
S **Larynx**
    Aryepiglottic fold
    Arytenoid cartilage
    Corniculate cartilage
    Cuneiform cartilage
    False vocal cord
    Glottis
    Rima glottidis
    Thyroid cartilage
    Ventricular fold
Y **Mouth and Throat**
	X External	**0** Drainage Device
		Y Other Device
			Z No Qualifier

Non-OR   All body part, approach, device, and qualifier values

LC Limited Coverage   **NC** Noncovered   ⊞ Combination Member   HAC associated procedure   Combination Only   DRG Non-OR   Non-OR   New/Revised in GREEN

ICD-10-PCS 2019   343

0   **Medical and Surgical**
C   **Mouth and Throat**
5   **Destruction**   Definition: Physical eradication of all or a portion of a body part by the direct use of energy, force, or a destructive agent
                      Explanation: None of the body part is physically taken out

Body Part Character 4		Approach Character 5	Device Character 6	Qualifier Character 7
0 Upper Lip Frenulum labii superioris Labial gland Vermilion border **1 Lower Lip** Frenulum labii inferioris Labial gland Vermilion border **2 Hard Palate** **3 Soft Palate** **4 Buccal Mucosa** Buccal gland Molar gland Palatine gland	**5 Upper Gingiva** **6 Lower Gingiva** **7 Tongue** Frenulum linguae **N Uvula** Palatine uvula **P Tonsils** Palatine tonsil **Q Adenoids** Pharyngeal tonsil	**0 Open** **3 Percutaneous** **X External**	**Z No Device**	**Z No Qualifier**
8 Parotid Gland, Right **9 Parotid Gland, Left** **B Parotid Duct, Right** Stensen's duct **C Parotid Duct, Left** *See B Parotid Duct, Right* **D Sublingual Gland, Right**	**F Sublingual Gland, Left** **G Submaxillary Gland, Right** Submandibular gland **H Submaxillary Gland, Left** *See G Submaxillary Gland, Right* **J Minor Salivary Gland** Anterior lingual gland	**0 Open** **3 Percutaneous**	**Z No Device**	**Z No Qualifier**
M Pharynx Base of tongue Hypopharynx Laryngopharynx Lingual tonsil Oropharynx Piriform recess (sinus) Tongue, base of **R Epiglottis** Glossoepiglottic fold	**S Larynx** Aryepiglottic fold Arytenoid cartilage Corniculate cartilage Cuneiform cartilage False vocal cord Glottis Rima glottidis Thyroid cartilage Ventricular fold **T Vocal Cord, Right** Vocal fold **V Vocal Cord, Left** *See T Vocal Cord, Right*	**0 Open** **3 Percutaneous** **4 Percutaneous Endoscopic** **7 Via Natural or Artificial Opening** **8 Via Natural or Artificial Opening Endoscopic**	**Z No Device**	**Z No Qualifier**
W Upper Tooth **X Lower Tooth**		**0 Open** **X External**	**Z No Device**	**0 Single** **1 Multiple** **2 All**

Non-OR   0C5[5,6][0,3,X]ZZ
Non-OR   0C5[W,X][0,X]Z[0,1,2]

0   **Medical and Surgical**
C   **Mouth and Throat**
7   **Dilation**   Definition: Expanding an orifice or the lumen of a tubular body part
                    Explanation: The orifice can be a natural orifice or an artificially created orifice. Accomplished by stretching a tubular body part using intraluminal pressure or by cutting part of the orifice or wall of the tubular body part.

Body Part Character 4	Approach Character 5	Device Character 6	Qualifier Character 7
B Parotid Duct, Right Stensen's duct **C Parotid Duct, Left** *See B Parotid Duct, Right*	**0 Open** **3 Percutaneous** **7 Via Natural or Artificial Opening**	**D Intraluminal Device** **Z No Device**	**Z No Qualifier**
M Pharynx Base of tongue Hypopharynx Laryngopharynx Lingual tonsil Oropharynx Piriform recess (sinus) Tongue, base of	**7 Via Natural or Artificial Opening** **8 Via Natural or Artificial Opening Endoscopic**	**D Intraluminal Device** **Z No Device**	**Z No Qualifier**
S Larynx Aryepiglottic fold Arytenoid cartilage Corniculate cartilage Cuneiform cartilage False vocal cord Glottis Rima glottidis Thyroid cartilage Ventricular fold	**0 Open** **3 Percutaneous** **4 Percutaneous Endoscopic** **7 Via Natural or Artificial Opening** **8 Via Natural or Artificial Opening Endoscopic**	**D Intraluminal Device** **Z No Device**	**Z No Qualifier**

Non-OR   0C7[B,C][0,3,7][D,Z]Z
Non-OR   0C7M[7,8][D,Z]Z

LC Limited Coverage   NC Noncovered   ⊞ Combination Member   HAC associated procedure   Combination Only   DRG Non-OR   Non-OR   New/Revised in **GREEN**

0   **Medical and Surgical**
C   **Mouth and Throat**
9   **Drainage**   Definition: Taking or letting out fluids and/or gases from a body part
                  Explanation: The qualifier DIAGNOSTIC is used to identify drainage procedures that are biopsies

Body Part — Character 4		Approach — Character 5	Device — Character 6	Qualifier — Character 7
0 Upper Lip Frenulum labii superioris Labial gland Vermilion border **1 Lower Lip** Frenulum labii inferioris Labial gland Vermilion border **2 Hard Palate** **3 Soft Palate** **4 Buccal Mucosa** Buccal gland Molar gland Palatine gland	**5 Upper Gingiva** **6 Lower Gingiva** **7 Tongue** Frenulum linguae **N Uvula** Palatine uvula **P Tonsils** Palatine tonsil **Q Adenoids** Pharyngeal tonsil	**0 Open** **3 Percutaneous** **X External**	**0 Drainage Device**	**Z No Qualifier**
0 Upper Lip Frenulum labii superioris Labial gland Vermilion border **1 Lower Lip** Frenulum labii inferioris Labial gland Vermilion border **2 Hard Palate** **3 Soft Palate** **4 Buccal Mucosa** Buccal gland Molar gland Palatine gland	**5 Upper Gingiva** **6 Lower Gingiva** **7 Tongue** Frenulum linguae **N Uvula** Palatine uvula **P Tonsils** Palatine tonsil **Q Adenoids** Pharyngeal tonsil	**0 Open** **3 Percutaneous** **X External**	**Z No Device**	**X Diagnostic** **Z No Qualifier**
8 Parotid Gland, Right **9 Parotid Gland, Left** **B Parotid Duct, Right** Stensen's duct **C Parotid Duct, Left** See B Parotid Duct, Right **D Sublingual Gland, Right**	**F Sublingual Gland, Left** **G Submaxillary Gland, Right** Submandibular gland **H Submaxillary Gland, Left** See G Submaxillary Gland, Right **J Minor Salivary Gland** Anterior lingual gland	**0 Open** **3 Percutaneous**	**0 Drainage Device**	**Z No Qualifier**
8 Parotid Gland, Right **9 Parotid Gland, Left** **B Parotid Duct, Right** Stensen's duct **C Parotid Duct, Left** See B Parotid Duct, Right	**D Sublingual Gland, Right** **F Sublingual Gland, Left** **G Submaxillary Gland, Right** Submandibular gland **H Submaxillary Gland, Left** See G Submaxillary Gland, Right **J Minor Salivary Gland** Anterior lingual gland	**0 Open** **3 Percutaneous**	**Z No Device**	**X Diagnostic** **Z No Qualifier**
M Pharynx Base of tongue Hypopharynx Laryngopharynx Lingual tonsil Oropharynx Piriform recess (sinus) Tongue, base of **R Epiglottis** Glossoepiglottic fold	**S Larynx** Aryepiglottic fold Arytenoid cartilage Corniculate cartilage Cuneiform cartilage False vocal cord Glottis Rima glottidis Thyroid cartilage Ventricular fold **T Vocal Cord, Right** Vocal fold **V Vocal Cord, Left** See T Vocal Cord, Right	**0 Open** **3 Percutaneous** **4 Percutaneous Endoscopic** **7 Via Natural or Artificial Opening** **8 Via Natural or Artificial Opening Endoscopic**	**0 Drainage Device**	**Z No Qualifier**

0C9 Continued on next page

Non-OR	0C9[0,1,2,3,4,7,N,P,Q]30Z
Non-OR	0C9[5,6][0,3,X]0Z
Non-OR	0C9[0,1,4][0,3,X]ZX
Non-OR	0C9[0,1,2,3,4,7,N,P,Q]3ZZ
Non-OR	0C9[5,6][0,3,X]Z[X,Z]
Non-OR	0C97[3,X]ZX
Non-OR	0C9[8,9,B,C,D,F,G,H,J][0,3]0Z
Non-OR	0C9[8,9,B,C,D,F,G,H,J]3ZX
Non-OR	0C9[8,9,B,C,D,F,G,H,J][0,3]ZZ
Non-OR	0C9[M,R,S,T,V]30Z

LC Limited Coverage   NC Noncovered   ⊞ Combination Member   HAC associated procedure   Combination Only   DRG Non-OR   Non-OR   New/Revised in GREEN

ØC9 Continued

Ø **Medical and Surgical**
C **Mouth and Throat**
9 **Drainage** — Definition: Taking or letting out fluids and/or gases from a body part
　　Explanation: The qualifier DIAGNOSTIC is used to identify drainage procedures that are biopsies

Body Part Character 4		Approach Character 5	Device Character 6	Qualifier Character 7
M Pharynx 　Base of tongue 　Hypopharynx 　Laryngopharynx 　Lingual tonsil 　Oropharynx 　Piriform recess (sinus) 　Tongue, base of R Epiglottis 　Glossoepiglottic fold	S Larynx 　Aryepiglottic fold 　Arytenoid cartilage 　Corniculate cartilage 　Cuneiform cartilage 　False vocal cord 　Glottis 　Rima glottidis 　Thyroid cartilage 　Ventricular fold T Vocal Cord, Right 　Vocal fold V Vocal Cord, Left 　See T Vocal Cord, Right	Ø Open 3 Percutaneous 4 Percutaneous Endoscopic 7 Via Natural or Artificial Opening 8 Via Natural or Artificial Opening Endoscopic	Z No Device	X Diagnostic Z No Qualifier
W Upper Tooth X Lower Tooth		Ø Open X External	Ø Drainage Device Z No Device	Ø Single 1 Multiple 2 All

Non-OR　ØC9M[Ø,3,4,7,8]ZX
Non-OR　ØC9[M,R,S,T,V]3ZZ
Non-OR　ØC9[R,S,T,V][3,4,7,8]ZX
Non-OR　ØC9[W,X][Ø,X][Ø,Z][Ø,1,2]

Ø **Medical and Surgical**
C **Mouth and Throat**
B **Excision** — Definition: Cutting out or off, without replacement, a portion of a body part
　　Explanation: The qualifier DIAGNOSTIC is used to identify excision procedures that are biopsies

Body Part Character 4		Approach Character 5	Device Character 6	Qualifier Character 7
Ø Upper Lip 　Frenulum labii superioris 　Labial gland 　Vermilion border 1 Lower Lip 　Frenulum labii inferioris 　Labial gland 　Vermilion border 2 Hard Palate 3 Soft Palate 4 Buccal Mucosa 　Buccal gland 　Molar gland 　Palatine gland	5 Upper Gingiva 6 Lower Gingiva 7 Tongue 　Frenulum linguae N Uvula 　Palatine uvula P Tonsils 　Palatine tonsil Q Adenoids 　Pharyngeal tonsil	Ø Open 3 Percutaneous X External	Z No Device	X Diagnostic Z No Qualifier
8 Parotid Gland, Right 9 Parotid Gland, Left B Parotid Duct, Right 　Stensen's duct C Parotid Duct, Left 　See B Parotid Duct, Right D Sublingual Gland, Right	F Sublingual Gland, Left G Submaxillary Gland, Right 　Submandibular gland H Submaxillary Gland, Left 　See G Submaxillary Gland, Right J Minor Salivary Gland 　Anterior lingual gland	Ø Open 3 Percutaneous	Z No Device	X Diagnostic Z No Qualifier
M Pharynx 　Base of tongue 　Hypopharynx 　Laryngopharynx 　Lingual tonsil 　Oropharynx 　Piriform recess (sinus) 　Tongue, base of R Epiglottis 　Glossoepiglottic fold	S Larynx 　Aryepiglottic fold 　Arytenoid cartilage 　Corniculate cartilage 　Cuneiform cartilage 　False vocal cord 　Glottis 　Rima glottidis 　Thyroid cartilage 　Ventricular fold T Vocal Cord, Right 　Vocal fold V Vocal Cord, Left 　See T Vocal Cord, Right	Ø Open 3 Percutaneous 4 Percutaneous Endoscopic 7 Via Natural or Artificial Opening 8 Via Natural or Artificial Opening Endoscopic	Z No Device	X Diagnostic Z No Qualifier
W Upper Tooth X Lower Tooth		Ø Open X External	Z No Device	Ø Single 1 Multiple 2 All

Non-OR　ØCB[Ø,1,4][Ø,3,X]ZX　　　　Non-OR　ØCBM[Ø,3,4,7,8]ZX
Non-OR　ØCB[5,6][Ø,3,X]Z[X,Z]　　　Non-OR　ØCB[R,S,T,V][3,4,7,8]ZX
Non-OR　ØCB7[3,X]ZX　　　　　　　　Non-OR　ØCB[W,X][Ø,X]Z[Ø,1,2]
Non-OR　ØCB[8,9,B,C,D,F,G,H,J]3ZX

LC Limited Coverage　NC Noncovered　⊞ Combination Member　HAC associated procedure　Combination Only　DRG Non-OR　Non-OR　New/Revised in GREEN

Ø   **Medical and Surgical**
C   **Mouth and Throat**
C   **Extirpation**   Definition: Taking or cutting out solid matter from a body part

Explanation: The solid matter may be an abnormal byproduct of a biological function or a foreign body; it may be imbedded in a body part or in the lumen of a tubular body part. The solid matter may or may not have been previously broken into pieces.

Body Part Character 4		Approach Character 5	Device Character 6	Qualifier Character 7
Ø **Upper Lip** Frenulum labii superioris Labial gland Vermilion border 1 **Lower Lip** Frenulum labii inferioris Labial gland Vermilion border 2 **Hard Palate** 3 **Soft Palate** 4 **Buccal Mucosa** Buccal gland Molar gland Palatine gland	5 **Upper Gingiva** 6 **Lower Gingiva** 7 **Tongue** Frenulum linguae N **Uvula** Palatine uvula P **Tonsils** Palatine tonsil Q **Adenoids** Pharyngeal tonsil	Ø Open 3 Percutaneous X External	Z No Device	Z No Qualifier
8 **Parotid Gland, Right** 9 **Parotid Gland, Left** B **Parotid Duct, Right** Stensen's duct C **Parotid Duct, Left** *See B Parotid Duct, Right* D **Sublingual Gland, Right**	F **Sublingual Gland, Left** G **Submaxillary Gland, Right** Submandibular gland H **Submaxillary Gland, Left** *See G Submaxillary Gland, Right* J **Minor Salivary Gland** Anterior lingual gland	Ø Open 3 Percutaneous	Z No Device	Z No Qualifier

M **Pharynx**
Base of tongue
Hypopharynx
Laryngopharynx
Lingual tonsil
Oropharynx
Piriform recess (sinus)
Tongue, base of
R **Epiglottis**
Glossoepiglottic fold
	S **Larynx**
	Aryepiglottic fold
	Arytenoid cartilage
	Corniculate cartilage
	Cuneiform cartilage
	False vocal cord
	Glottis
	Rima glottidis
	Thyroid cartilage
	Ventricular fold
	T **Vocal Cord, Right**
	Vocal fold
	V **Vocal Cord, Left**
	See T Vocal Cord, Right
		Ø Open
		3 Percutaneous
		4 Percutaneous Endoscopic
		7 Via Natural or Artificial
		   Opening
		8 Via Natural or Artificial
		   Opening Endoscopic
			Z No Device	Z No Qualifier

W **Upper Tooth** X **Lower Tooth**		Ø Open X External	Z No Device	Ø Single 1 Multiple 2 All

Non-OR	ØCC[Ø,1,2,3,4,7,N,P,Q]XZZ
Non-OR	ØCC[5,6][Ø,3,X]ZZ
Non-OR	ØCC[8,9,B,C,D,F,G,H,J][Ø,3]ZZ
Non-OR	ØCC[M,S][7,8]ZZ
Non-OR	ØCC[W,X][Ø,X]Z[Ø,1,2]

Ø   **Medical and Surgical**
C   **Mouth and Throat**
D   **Extraction**   Definition: Pulling or stripping out or off all or a portion of a body part by the use of force

Explanation: The qualifier DIAGNOSTIC is used to identify extraction procedures that are biopsies

Body Part Character 4	Approach Character 5	Device Character 6	Qualifier Character 7
T **Vocal Cord, Right** Vocal fold V **Vocal Cord, Left** *See T Vocal Cord, Right*	Ø Open 3 Percutaneous 4 Percutaneous Endoscopic 7 Via Natural or Artificial Opening 8 Via Natural or Artificial Opening Endoscopic	Z No Device	Z No Qualifier
W **Upper Tooth** X **Lower Tooth**	X External	Z No Device	Ø Single 1 Multiple 2 All

Non-OR	ØCD[W,X]XZ[Ø,1,2]

Mouth and Throat (side tab)

Ø Medical and Surgical
C Mouth and Throat
F Fragmentation   Definition: Breaking solid matter in a body part into pieces

Explanation: Physical force (e.g., manual, ultrasonic) applied directly or indirectly is used to break the solid matter into pieces. The solid matter may be an abnormal byproduct of a biological function or a foreign body. The pieces of solid matter are not taken out.

Body Part Character 4	Approach Character 5	Device Character 6	Qualifier Character 7
B Parotid Duct, Right **NC** Stensen's duct C Parotid Duct, Left **NC** *See B Parotid Duct, Right*	Ø Open 3 Percutaneous 7 Via Natural or Artificial Opening X External	Z No Device	Z No Qualifier

Non-OR   All body part, approach, device, and qualifier values
NC   ØCF[B,C]XZZ

Ø Medical and Surgical
C Mouth and Throat
H Insertion   Definition: Putting in a nonbiological appliance that monitors, assists, performs, or prevents a physiological function but does not physically take the place of a body part

Explanation: None

Body Part Character 4	Approach Character 5	Device Character 6	Qualifier Character 7
7 Tongue Frenulum linguae	Ø Open 3 Percutaneous X External	1 Radioactive Element	Z No Qualifier

A Salivary Gland
 S Larynx
   Aryepiglottic fold
   Arytenoid cartilage
   Corniculate cartilage
   Cuneiform cartilage
   False vocal cord
   Glottis
   Rima glottidis
   Thyroid cartilage
   Ventricular fold
	Ø Open
	 3 Percutaneous
	 7 Via Natural or Artificial Opening
	 8 Via Natural or Artificial Opening Endoscopic
		Y Other Device	Z No Qualifier

Y Mouth and Throat	Ø Open 3 Percutaneous	Y Other Device	Z No Qualifier
Y Mouth and Throat	7 Via Natural or Artificial Opening 8 Via Natural or Artificial Opening Endoscopic	B Intraluminal Device, Airway Y Other Device	Z No Qualifier

Non-OR   ØCH[A,S][3,7,8]YZ
Non-OR   ØCHSØYZ
Non-OR   ØCHY[Ø,3]YZ
Non-OR   ØCHY[7,8][B,Y]Z

Ø Medical and Surgical
C Mouth and Throat
J Inspection   Definition: Visually and/or manually exploring a body part

Explanation: Visual exploration may be performed with or without optical instrumentation. Manual exploration may be performed directly or through intervening body layers.

Body Part Character 4	Approach Character 5	Device Character 6	Qualifier Character 7
A Salivary Gland	Ø Open 3 Percutaneous X External	Z No Device	Z No Qualifier

S Larynx
   Aryepiglottic fold
   Arytenoid cartilage
   Corniculate cartilage
   Cuneiform cartilage
   False vocal cord
   Glottis
   Rima glottidis
   Thyroid cartilage
   Ventricular fold
 Y Mouth and Throat
	Ø Open
	 3 Percutaneous
	 4 Percutaneous Endoscopic
	 7 Via Natural or Artificial Opening
	 8 Via Natural or Artificial Opening Endoscopic
	 X External
		Z No Device	Z No Qualifier

Non-OR   All body part, approach, device, and qualifier values

LC Limited Coverage   **NC** Noncovered   ⊞ Combination Member   HAC associated procedure   Combination Only   DRG Non-OR   Non-OR   New/Revised in GREEN

348   ICD-10-PCS 2019

ØCF–ØCJ (side tab)

Ø   **Medical and Surgical**
C   **Mouth and Throat**
L   **Occlusion**   Definition: Completely closing an orifice or the lumen of a tubular body part
                      Explanation: The orifice can be a natural orifice or an artificially created orifice

Body Part Character 4	Approach Character 5	Device Character 6	Qualifier Character 7

B Parotid Duct, Right
    Stensen's duct
C Parotid Duct, Left
    See B Parotid Duct, Right
	Ø Open
	3 Percutaneous
	4 Percutaneous Endoscopic
		C Extraluminal Device
		D Intraluminal Device
		Z No Device
			Z No Qualifier

B Parotid Duct, Right
    Stensen's duct
C Parotid Duct, Left
    See B Parotid Duct, Right
	7 Via Natural or Artificial Opening
	8 Via Natural or Artificial Opening
	    Endoscopic
		D Intraluminal Device
		Z No Device
			Z No Qualifier

Ø   **Medical and Surgical**
C   **Mouth and Throat**
M   **Reattachment**   Definition: Putting back in or on all or a portion of a separated body part to its normal location or other suitable location
                         Explanation: Vascular circulation and nervous pathways may or may not be reestablished

Body Part Character 4	Approach Character 5	Device Character 6	Qualifier Character 7

Ø Upper Lip
    Frenulum labii superioris
    Labial gland
    Vermilion border
1 Lower Lip
    Frenulum labii inferioris
    Labial gland
    Vermilion border
3 Soft Palate
7 Tongue
    Frenulum linguae
N Uvula
    Palatine uvula
	Ø Open	**Z** No Device	**Z** No Qualifier

W Upper Tooth **X** Lower Tooth	**Ø** Open **X** External	**Z** No Device	**Ø** Single **1** Multiple **2** All

Non-OR   ØCM[W,X][Ø,X]Z[Ø,1,2]

Mouth and Throat

Ø   **Medical and Surgical**
C   **Mouth and Throat**
N   **Release**   Definition: Freeing a body part from an abnormal physical constraint by cutting or by the use of force
                       Explanation: Some of the restraining tissue may be taken out but none of the body part is taken out

Body Part Character 4	Approach Character 5	Device Character 6	Qualifier Character 7

Ø **Upper Lip**
  Frenulum labii superioris
  Labial gland
  Vermilion border
1 **Lower Lip**
  Frenulum labii inferioris
  Labial gland
  Vermilion border
2 **Hard Palate**
3 **Soft Palate**
4 **Buccal Mucosa**
  Buccal gland
  Molar gland
  Palatine gland
5 **Upper Gingiva**
6 **Lower Gingiva**
7 **Tongue**
  Frenulum linguae
N **Uvula**
  Palatine uvula
P **Tonsils**
  Palatine tonsil
Q **Adenoids**
  Pharyngeal tonsil
	Ø Open
	3 Percutaneous
	X External
		Z No Device	Z No Qualifier

8 **Parotid Gland, Right**
9 **Parotid Gland, Left**
B **Parotid Duct, Right**
  Stensen's duct
C **Parotid Duct, Left**
  See B Parotid Duct, Right
D **Sublingual Gland, Right**
F **Sublingual Gland, Left**
G **Submaxillary Gland, Right**
  Submandibular gland
H **Submaxillary Gland, Left**
  See G Submaxillary Gland, Right
J **Minor Salivary Gland**
  Anterior lingual gland
	Ø Open
	3 Percutaneous
		Z No Device	Z No Qualifier

M **Pharynx**
  Base of tongue
  Hypopharynx
  Laryngopharynx
  Lingual tonsil
  Oropharynx
  Piriform recess (sinus)
  Tongue, base of
R **Epiglottis**
  Glossoepiglottic fold
S **Larynx**
  Aryepiglottic fold
  Arytenoid cartilage
  Corniculate cartilage
  Cuneiform cartilage
  False vocal cord
  Glottis
  Rima glottidis
  Thyroid cartilage
  Ventricular fold
T **Vocal Cord, Right**
  Vocal fold
V **Vocal Cord, Left**
  See T Vocal Cord, Right
	Ø Open
	3 Percutaneous
	4 Percutaneous Endoscopic
	7 Via Natural or Artificial Opening
	8 Via Natural or Artificial Opening
	  Endoscopic
		Z No Device	Z No Qualifier

W **Upper Tooth** X **Lower Tooth**	Ø Open X External	Z No Device	Ø Single 1 Multiple 2 All

Non-OR   ØCN[Ø,1,5,6,7][Ø,3,X]ZZ
Non-OR   ØCN[W,X][Ø,X]Z[Ø,1,2]

0   **Medical and Surgical**
C   **Mouth and Throat**
P   **Removal**   Definition: Taking out or off a device from a body part

Explanation: If a device is taken out and a similar device put in without cutting or puncturing the skin or mucous membrane, the procedure is coded to the root operation CHANGE. Otherwise, the procedure for taking out a device is coded to the root operation REMOVAL.

Body Part Character 4	Approach Character 5	Device Character 6	Qualifier Character 7
A Salivary Gland	**0** Open **3** Percutaneous	**0** Drainage Device **C** Extraluminal Device **Y** Other Device	**Z** No Qualifier
A Salivary Gland	**7** Via Natural or Artificial Opening **8** Via Natural or Artificial Opening Endoscopic	**Y** Other Device	**Z** No Qualifier
S Larynx 　Aryepiglottic fold 　Arytenoid cartilage 　Corniculate cartilage 　Cuneiform cartilage 　False vocal cord 　Glottis 　Rima glottidis 　Thyroid cartilage 　Ventricular fold	**0** Open **3** Percutaneous **7** Via Natural or Artificial Opening **8** Via Natural or Artificial Opening Endoscopic	**0** Drainage Device **7** Autologous Tissue Substitute **D** Intraluminal Device **J** Synthetic Substitute **K** Nonautologous Tissue Substitute **Y** Other Device	**Z** No Qualifier
S Larynx 　Aryepiglottic fold 　Arytenoid cartilage 　Corniculate cartilage 　Cuneiform cartilage 　False vocal cord 　Glottis 　Rima glottidis 　Thyroid cartilage 　Ventricular fold	**X** External	**0** Drainage Device **7** Autologous Tissue Substitute **D** Intraluminal Device **J** Synthetic Substitute **K** Nonautologous Tissue Substitute	**Z** No Qualifier
Y Mouth and Throat	**0** Open **3** Percutaneous **7** Via Natural or Artificial Opening **8** Via Natural or Artificial Opening Endoscopic	**0** Drainage Device **1** Radioactive Element **7** Autologous Tissue Substitute **D** Intraluminal Device **J** Synthetic Substitute **K** Nonautologous Tissue Substitute **Y** Other Device	**Z** No Qualifier
Y Mouth and Throat	**X** External	**0** Drainage Device **1** Radioactive Element **7** Autologous Tissue Substitute **D** Intraluminal Device **J** Synthetic Substitute **K** Nonautologous Tissue Substitute	**Z** No Qualifier

Non-OR   0CPA[0,3][0,C,Y]Z
Non-OR   0CPA[7,8]YZ
Non-OR   0CPS3YZ
Non-OR   0CPS[7,8][0,D,Y]Z
Non-OR   0CPSX[0,7,D,J,K]Z
Non-OR   0CPY3YZ
Non-OR   0CPY[7,8][0,D,Y]Z
Non-OR   0CPYX[0,1,7,D,J,K]Z

Mouth and Throat

Ø   Medical and Surgical
C   Mouth and Throat
Q   Repair   Definition: Restoring, to the extent possible, a body part to its normal anatomic structure and function
                    Explanation: Used only when the method to accomplish the repair is not one of the other root operations

Body Part Character 4	Approach Character 5	Device Character 6	Qualifier Character 7

Ø   **Upper Lip**
    Frenulum labii superioris
    Labial gland
    Vermilion border
1   **Lower Lip**
    Frenulum labii inferioris
    Labial gland
    Vermilion border
2   **Hard Palate**
3   **Soft Palate**
4   **Buccal Mucosa**
    Buccal gland
    Molar gland
    Palatine gland
5   **Upper Gingiva**
6   **Lower Gingiva**
7   **Tongue**
    Frenulum linguae
N   **Uvula**
    Palatine uvula
P   **Tonsils**
    Palatine tonsil
Q   **Adenoids**
    Pharyngeal tonsil
	Ø Open
	3 Percutaneous
	X External
		Z No Device	Z No Qualifier

8   **Parotid Gland, Right**
9   **Parotid Gland, Left**
B   **Parotid Duct, Right**
    Stensen's duct
C   **Parotid Duct, Left**
    See B Parotid Duct, Right
D   **Sublingual Gland, Right**
F   **Sublingual Gland, Left**
G   **Submaxillary Gland, Right**
    Submandibular gland
H   **Submaxillary Gland, Left**
    See G Submaxillary Gland, Right
J   **Minor Salivary Gland**
    Anterior lingual gland
	Ø Open
	3 Percutaneous
		Z No Device	Z No Qualifier

M   **Pharynx**
    Base of tongue
    Hypopharynx
    Laryngopharynx
    Lingual tonsil
    Oropharynx
    Piriform recess (sinus)
    Tongue, base of
R   **Epiglottis**
    Glossoepiglottic fold
S   **Larynx**
    Aryepiglottic fold
    Arytenoid cartilage
    Corniculate cartilage
    Cuneiform cartilage
    False vocal cord
    Glottis
    Rima glottidis
    Thyroid cartilage
    Ventricular fold
T   **Vocal Cord, Right**
    Vocal fold
V   **Vocal Cord, Left**
    See T Vocal Cord, Right
	Ø Open
	3 Percutaneous
	4 Percutaneous Endoscopic
	7 Via Natural or Artificial Opening
	8 Via Natural or Artificial Opening
	      Endoscopic
		Z No Device	Z No Qualifier

W **Upper Tooth** X **Lower Tooth**	Ø Open X External	Z No Device	Ø Single 1 Multiple 2 All

Non-OR   ØCQ[Ø,1,4,7]XZZ
Non-OR   ØCQ[5,6][Ø,3,X]ZZ
Non-OR   ØCQ[W,X][Ø,X]Z[Ø,1,2]

Ø Medical and Surgical
C Mouth and Throat
R Replacement Definition: Putting in or on biological or synthetic material that physically takes the place and/or function of all or a portion of a body part

Explanation: The body part may have been taken out or replaced, or may be taken out, physically eradicated, or rendered nonfunctional during the REPLACEMENT procedure. A REMOVAL procedure is coded for taking out the device used in a previous replacement procedure.

Body Part Character 4	Approach Character 5	Device Character 6	Qualifier Character 7
Ø **Upper Lip** Frenulum labii superioris Labial gland Vermilion border **1** **Lower Lip** Frenulum labii inferioris Labial gland Vermilion border **2** **Hard Palate** **3** **Soft Palate** **4** **Buccal Mucosa** Buccal gland Molar gland Palatine gland **5** **Upper Gingiva** **6** **Lower Gingiva** **7** **Tongue** Frenulum linguae **N** **Uvula** Palatine uvula	**Ø** Open **3** Percutaneous **X** External	**7** Autologous Tissue Substitute **J** Synthetic Substitute **K** Nonautologous Tissue Substitute	**Z** No Qualifier
B **Parotid Duct, Right** Stensen's duct **C** **Parotid Duct, Left** *See B Parotid Duct, Right*	**Ø** Open **3** Percutaneous	**7** Autologous Tissue Substitute **J** Synthetic Substitute **K** Nonautologous Tissue Substitute	**Z** No Qualifier
M **Pharynx** Base of tongue Hypopharynx Laryngopharynx Lingual tonsil Oropharynx Piriform recess (sinus) Tongue, base of **R** **Epiglottis** Glossoepiglottic fold **S** **Larynx** Aryepiglottic fold Arytenoid cartilage Corniculate cartilage Cuneiform cartilage False vocal cord Glottis Rima glottidis Thyroid cartilage Ventricular fold **T** **Vocal Cord, Right** Vocal fold **V** **Vocal Cord, Left** *See T Vocal Cord, Right*	**Ø** Open **7** Via Natural or Artificial Opening **8** Via Natural or Artificial Opening Endoscopic	**7** Autologous Tissue Substitute **J** Synthetic Substitute **K** Nonautologous Tissue Substitute	**Z** No Qualifier
W **Upper Tooth** **X** **Lower Tooth**	**Ø** Open **X** External	**7** Autologous Tissue Substitute **J** Synthetic Substitute **K** Nonautologous Tissue Substitute	**Ø** Single **1** Multiple **2** All

Non-OR ØCR[W,X][Ø,X][7,J,K][Ø,1,2]

Mouth and Throat

Ø   Medical and Surgical
C   Mouth and Throat
S   Reposition   Definition: Moving to its normal location, or other suitable location, all or a portion of a body part

Explanation: The body part is moved to a new location from an abnormal location, or from a normal location where it is not functioning correctly. The body part may or may not be cut out or off to be moved to the new location.

Body Part Character 4	Approach Character 5	Device Character 6	Qualifier Character 7
Ø Upper Lip Frenulum labii superioris Labial gland Vermilion border **1 Lower Lip** Frenulum labii inferioris Labial gland Vermilion border **2 Hard Palate** **3 Soft Palate** **7 Tongue** Frenulum linguae **N Uvula** Palatine uvula	**Ø Open** **X External**	**Z No Device**	**Z No Qualifier**
B Parotid Duct, Right Stensen's duct **C Parotid Duct, Left** *See B Parotid Duct, Right*	**Ø Open** **3 Percutaneous**	**Z No Device**	**Z No Qualifier**
R Epiglottis Glossoepiglottic fold **T Vocal Cord, Right** Vocal fold **V Vocal Cord, Left** *See T Vocal Cord, Right*	**Ø Open** **7 Via Natural or Artificial Opening** **8 Via Natural or Artificial Opening Endoscopic**	**Z No Device**	**Z No Qualifier**
W Upper Tooth **X Lower Tooth**	**Ø Open** **X External**	**5 External Fixation Device** **Z No Device**	**Ø Single** **1 Multiple** **2 All**

Non-OR   ØCS[W,X][Ø,X][5,Z][Ø,1,2]

LC Limited Coverage   NC Noncovered   ⊞ Combination Member   HAC associated procedure   Combination Only   DRG Non-OR   Non-OR   New/Revised in GREEN

354 | ICD-10-PCS 2019

Ø   **Medical and Surgical**
C   **Mouth and Throat**
T   **Resection**   Definition: Cutting out or off, without replacement, all of a body part
                   Explanation: None

Body Part Character 4	Approach Character 5	Device Character 6	Qualifier Character 7

Ø **Upper Lip**
   Frenulum labii superioris
   Labial gland
   Vermilion border
1 **Lower Lip**
   Frenulum labii inferioris
   Labial gland
   Vermilion border
2 **Hard Palate**
3 **Soft Palate**
7 **Tongue**
   Frenulum linguae
N **Uvula**
   Palatine uvula
P **Tonsils**
   Palatine tonsil
Q **Adenoids**
   Pharyngeal tonsil
	Ø Open
	X External
		Z No Device	**Z** No Qualifier

8 **Parotid Gland, Right**
9 **Parotid Gland, Left**
B **Parotid Duct, Right**
   Stensen's duct
C **Parotid Duct, Left**
   See B Parotid Duct, Right
D **Sublingual Gland, Right**
F **Sublingual Gland, Left**
G **Submaxillary Gland, Right**
   Submandibular gland
H **Submaxillary Gland, Left**
   See G Submaxillary Gland, Right
J **Minor Salivary Gland**
   Anterior lingual gland
	Ø Open	**Z** No Device	**Z** No Qualifier

M **Pharynx**
   Base of tongue
   Hypopharynx
   Laryngopharynx
   Lingual tonsil
   Oropharynx
   Piriform recess (sinus)
   Tongue, base of
R **Epiglottis**
   Glossoepiglottic fold
S **Larynx**
   Aryepiglottic fold
   Arytenoid cartilage
   Corniculate cartilage
   Cuneiform cartilage
   False vocal cord
   Glottis
   Rima glottidis
   Thyroid cartilage
   Ventricular fold
T **Vocal Cord, Right**
   Vocal fold
V **Vocal Cord, Left**
   See T Vocal Cord, Right
	Ø Open
	4 Percutaneous Endoscopic
	7 Via Natural or Artificial Opening
	8 Via Natural or Artificial Opening
	   Endoscopic
		Z No Device	**Z** No Qualifier

W **Upper Tooth** **X** **Lower Tooth**	**Ø** Open	**Z** No Device	**Ø** Single **1** Multiple **2** All

Non-OR   ØCT[W,X]ØZ[Ø,1,2]

LC Limited Coverage   **NC** Noncovered   ⊞ Combination Member   HAC associated procedure   Combination Only   DRG Non-OR   Non-OR   New/Revised in GREEN

Mouth and Throat *(side margin)*

Ø   **Medical and Surgical**
C   **Mouth and Throat**
U   **Supplement**   Definition: Putting in or on biological or synthetic material that physically reinforces and/or augments the function of a portion of a body part

          Explanation: The biological material is non-living, or is living and from the same individual. The body part may have been previously replaced, and the SUPPLEMENT procedure is performed to physically reinforce and/or augment the function of the replaced body part.

Body Part Character 4	Approach Character 5	Device Character 6	Qualifier Character 7

Ø **Upper Lip**
   Frenulum labii superioris
   Labial gland
   Vermilion border
1 **Lower Lip**
   Frenulum labii inferioris
   Labial gland
   Vermilion border
2 **Hard Palate**
3 **Soft Palate**
4 **Buccal Mucosa**
   Buccal gland
   Molar gland
   Palatine gland
5 **Upper Gingiva**
6 **Lower Gingiva**
7 **Tongue**
   Frenulum linguae
N **Uvula**
   Palatine uvula
	Ø Open
	3 Percutaneous
	X External
		7 Autologous Tissue Substitute
		J Synthetic Substitute
		K Nonautologous Tissue Substitute
			Z No Qualifier

M **Pharynx**
   Base of tongue
   Hypopharynx
   Laryngopharynx
   Lingual tonsil
   Oropharynx
   Piriform recess (sinus)
   Tongue, base of
R **Epiglottis**
   Glossoepiglottic fold
S **Larynx**
   Aryepiglottic fold
   Arytenoid cartilage
   Corniculate cartilage
   Cuneiform cartilage
   False vocal cord
   Glottis
   Rima glottidis
   Thyroid cartilage
   Ventricular fold
T **Vocal Cord, Right**
   Vocal fold
V **Vocal Cord, Left**
   See T Vocal Cord, Right
	Ø Open
	7 Via Natural or Artificial Opening
	8 Via Natural or Artificial Opening Endoscopic
		7 Autologous Tissue Substitute
		J Synthetic Substitute
		K Nonautologous Tissue Substitute
			Z No Qualifier

Non-OR   ØCU2[Ø,3]JZ

Ø   **Medical and Surgical**
C   **Mouth and Throat**
V   **Restriction**   Definition: Partially closing an orifice or the lumen of a tubular body part

          Explanation: The orifice can be a natural orifice or an artificially created orifice

Body Part Character 4	Approach Character 5	Device Character 6	Qualifier Character 7

B **Parotid Duct, Right**
   Stensen's duct
C **Parotid Duct, Left**
   See B Parotid Duct, Right
	Ø Open
	3 Percutaneous
		C Extraluminal Device
		D Intraluminal Device
		Z No Device
			Z No Qualifier

B **Parotid Duct, Right**
   Stensen's duct
C **Parotid Duct, Left**
   See B Parotid Duct, Right
	7 Via Natural or Artificial Opening
	8 Via Natural or Artificial Opening Endoscopic
		D Intraluminal Device
		Z No Device
			Z No Qualifier

LC Limited Coverage   NC Noncovered   ⊞ Combination Member   HAC associated procedure   Combination Only   DRG Non-OR   Non-OR   New/Revised in GREEN

356   ICD-10-PCS 2019

0   **Medical and Surgical**
C   **Mouth and Throat**
W   **Revision**   Definition: Correcting, to the extent possible, a portion of a malfunctioning device or the position of a displaced device
                           Explanation: Revision can include correcting a malfunctioning or displaced device by taking out or putting in components of the device such as a screw or pin

Body Part Character 4	Approach Character 5	Device Character 6	Qualifier Character 7
A Salivary Gland	**0** Open **3** Percutaneous	**0** Drainage Device **C** Extraluminal Device **Y** Other Device	**Z** No Qualifier
A Salivary Gland	**7** Via Natural or Artificial Opening **8** Via Natural or Artificial Opening Endoscopic	**Y** Other Device	**Z** No Qualifier
A Salivary Gland	**X** External	**0** Drainage Device **C** Extraluminal Device	**Z** No Qualifier

S Larynx
   Aryepiglottic fold
   Arytenoid cartilage
   Corniculate cartilage
   Cuneiform cartilage
   False vocal cord
   Glottis
   Rima glottidis
   Thyroid cartilage
   Ventricular fold
	0 Open
	3 Percutaneous
	7 Via Natural or Artificial Opening
	8 Via Natural or Artificial Opening Endoscopic
		0 Drainage Device
		7 Autologous Tissue Substitute
		D Intraluminal Device
		J Synthetic Substitute
		K Nonautologous Tissue Substitute
		Y Other Device
			Z No Qualifier

S Larynx
   Aryepiglottic fold
   Arytenoid cartilage
   Corniculate cartilage
   Cuneiform cartilage
   False vocal cord
   Glottis
   Rima glottidis
   Thyroid cartilage
   Ventricular fold
	X External	**0** Drainage Device
		7 Autologous Tissue Substitute
		D Intraluminal Device
		J Synthetic Substitute
		K Nonautologous Tissue Substitute
			Z No Qualifier

Y Mouth and Throat	**0** Open **3** Percutaneous **7** Via Natural or Artificial Opening **8** Via Natural or Artificial Opening Endoscopic	**0** Drainage Device **1** Radioactive Element **7** Autologous Tissue Substitute **D** Intraluminal Device **J** Synthetic Substitute **K** Nonautologous Tissue Substitute **Y** Other Device	**Z** No Qualifier
Y Mouth and Throat	**X** External	**0** Drainage Device **1** Radioactive Element **7** Autologous Tissue Substitute **D** Intraluminal Device **J** Synthetic Substitute **K** Nonautologous Tissue Substitute	**Z** No Qualifier

Non-OR   0CWA[0,3][0,C,Y]Z
Non-OR   0CWA[7,8]YZ
Non-OR   0CWAX[0,C]Z
Non-OR   0CWS[3,7,8]YZ
Non-OR   0CWSX[0,7,D,J,K]Z
Non-OR   0CWY07Z
Non-OR   0CWY[3,7,8]YZ
Non-OR   0CWYX[0,1,7,D,J,K]Z

Ø   **Medical and Surgical**
C   **Mouth and Throat**
X   **Transfer**   Definition: Moving, without taking out, all or a portion of a body part to another location to take over the function of all or a portion of a body part
                Explanation: The body part transferred remains connected to its vascular and nervous supply

Body Part Character 4	Approach Character 5	Device Character 6	Qualifier Character 7

Ø **Upper Lip**
    Frenulum labii superioris
    Labial gland
    Vermilion border
1 **Lower Lip**
    Frenulum labii inferioris
    Labial gland
    Vermilion border
3 **Soft Palate**
4 **Buccal Mucosa**
    Buccal gland
    Molar gland
    Palatine gland
5 **Upper Gingiva**
6 **Lower Gingiva**
7 **Tongue**
    Frenulum linguae
	Ø Open
	X External
		Z No Device	**Z** No Qualifier

LC Limited Coverage   **NC** Noncovered   ⊞ Combination Member   HAC associated procedure   Combination Only   DRG Non-OR   Non-OR   New/Revised in GREEN

358   ICD-10-PCS 2019

Gastrointestinal System ØD1–ØDY

Character Meanings

This Character Meaning table is provided as a guide to assist the user in the identification of character members that may be found in this section of code tables. It **SHOULD NOT** be used to build a PCS code.

Operation–Character 3	Body Part–Character 4	Approach–Character 5	Device–Character 6	Qualifier–Character 7
1 Bypass	Ø Upper Intestinal Tract	Ø Open	Ø Drainage Device	Ø Allogeneic
2 Change	1 Esophagus, Upper	3 Percutaneous	1 Radioactive Element	1 Syngeneic
5 Destruction	2 Esophagus, Middle	4 Percutaneous Endoscopic	2 Monitoring Device	2 Zooplastic
7 Dilation	3 Esophagus, Lower	7 Via Natural or Artificial Opening	3 Infusion Device	3 Vertical
8 Division	4 Esophagogastric Junction	8 Via Natural or Artificial Opening Endoscopic	7 Autologous Tissue Substitute	4 Cutaneous
9 Drainage	5 Esophagus	F Via Natural or Artificial Opening with Percutaneous Endoscopic Assistance	B Intraluminal Device, Airway	5 Esophagus
B Excision	6 Stomach	X External	C Extraluminal Device	6 Stomach
C Extirpation	7 Stomach, Pylorus		D Intraluminal Device	9 Duodenum
D Extraction	8 Small Intestine		J Synthetic Substitute	A Jejunum
F Fragmentation	9 Duodenum		K Nonautologous Tissue Substitute	B Ileum
H Insertion	A Jejunum		L Artificial Sphincter	H Cecum
J Inspection	B Ileum		M Stimulator Lead	K Ascending Colon
L Occlusion	C Ileocecal Valve		U Feeding Device	L Transverse Colon
M Reattachment	D Lower Intestinal Tract		Y Other Device	M Descending Colon
N Release	E Large Intestine		Z No Device	N Sigmoid Colon
P Removal	F Large Intestine, Right			P Rectum
Q Repair	G Large Intestine, Left			Q Anus
R Replacement	H Cecum			X Diagnostic
S Reposition	J Appendix			Z No Qualifier
T Resection	K Ascending Colon			
U Supplement	L Transverse Colon			
V Restriction	M Descending Colon			
W Revision	N Sigmoid Colon			
X Transfer	P Rectum			
Y Transplantation	Q Anus			
	R Anal Sphincter			
	U Omentum			
	V Mesentery			
	W Peritoneum			

AHA Coding Clinic for table 0D1

2017, 2Q, 17	Billroth II (distal gastrectomy and gastrojejunostomy)
2016, 2Q, 31	Laparoscopic biliopancreatic diversion with duodenal switch
2014, 4Q, 41	Abdominoperineal resection (APR) with flap closure of perineum and colostomy

AHA Coding Clinic for table 0D5

2017, 1Q, 34	Debulking of tumor and peritoneum ablation

AHA Coding Clinic for table 0D7

2017, 3Q, 23	Laparoscopic pyloromyotomy
2014, 4Q, 40	Dilation of gastrojejunostomy anastomosis stricture

AHA Coding Clinic for table 0D8

2017, 3Q, 22	Laparoscopic esophagomyotomy (Heller type) and Toupet fundoplication
2017, 3Q, 23	Laparoscopic pyloromyotomy

AHA Coding Clinic for table 0D9

2015, 2Q, 29	Insertion of nasogastric tube for drainage and feeding

AHA Coding Clinic for table 0DB

2017, 2Q, 17	Billroth II (distal gastrectomy and gastrojejunostomy)
2017, 1Q, 16	Hepatic flexure versus transverse colon
2016, 3Q, 3-7	Stoma creation & takedown procedures
2016, 2Q, 31	Laparoscopic biliopancreatic diversion with duodenal switch
2016, 1Q, 22	Perineal proctectomy
2016, 1Q, 24	Endoscopic brush biopsy of esophagus
2014, 4Q, 40	Abdominoperineal resection (APR) with flap closure of perineum and colostomy
2014, 3Q, 28	Ileostomy takedown and parastomal hernia repair
2014, 3Q, 32	Pyloric-sparing Whipple procedure

AHA Coding Clinic for table 0DD

2017, 4Q, 41-42	Extraction procedures

AHA Coding Clinic for table 0DH

2016, 3Q, 26	Insertion of gastrostomy tube
2013, 4Q, 117	Percutaneous endoscopic placement of gastrostomy tube

AHA Coding Clinic for table 0DJ

2017, 2Q, 15	Low anterior resection with sigmoidoscopy
2016, 2Q, 20	Capsule endoscopy of small intestine
2015, 3Q, 24	Esophagogastroduodenoscopy with epinephrine injection for control of bleeding

AHA Coding Clinic for table 0DL

2013, 4Q, 112	Endoscopic banding of esophageal varices

AHA Coding Clinic for table 0DN

2017, 4Q, 49-50	New and revised body part values - Repositioning of the intestine
2017, 1Q, 35	Lysis of omental and peritoneal adhesions
2015, 3Q, 15	Vascular ring surgery with release of esophagus and trachea
2015, 3Q, 16	Vascular ring surgery and double aortic arch

AHA Coding Clinic for table 0DQ

2018, 2Q, 25	Third and fourth degree obstetric lacerations
2018, 1Q, 11	Repair of internal hernia at Petersen space
2017, 3Q, 17	Posterior sagittal anorectoplasty
2016, 3Q, 3-7	Stoma creation & takedown procedures
2016, 3Q, 26	Insertion of gastrostomy tube
2016, 1Q, 7	Obstetrical perineal laceration repair
2016, 1Q, 8	Obstetrical perineal laceration repair
2014, 4Q, 20	Control of bleeding duodenal ulcer

AHA Coding Clinic for table 0DS

2017, 4Q, 49-50	New and revised body part values - Repositioning of the intestine
2017, 3Q, 9	Ileocolic intussusception reduction via air enema
2017, 3Q, 17	Posterior sagittal anorectoplasty
2016, 3Q, 3-5	Stoma creation & takedown procedures

AHA Coding Clinic for table 0DT

2017, 4Q, 49-50	New and revised body part values - Repositioning of the intestine
2014, 4Q, 40	Abdominoperineal resection (APR) with flap closure of perineum and colostomy
2014, 4Q, 42	Right colectomy with side-to-side functional end-to-end anastomosis
2014, 3Q, 6	Ileocecectomy including cecum, terminal ileum and appendix
2014, 3Q, 6	Right colectomy

AHA Coding Clinic for table 0DV

2017, 3Q, 22	Laparoscopic esophagomyotomy (Heller type) and Toupet fundoplication
2016, 2Q, 22	Esophageal lengthening Collis gastroplasty with Nissen fundoplication and hiatal hernia
2014, 3Q, 28	Laparoscopic Nissen fundoplication and diaphragmatic hernia repair

AHA Coding Clinic for table 0DW

2018, 1Q, 20	Adjustment of gastric band

AHA Coding Clinic for table 0DX

2017, 2Q, 18	Esophagectomy and esophagogastrectomy with cervical esophagogastrostomy
2016, 2Q, 22	Esophageal lengthening Collis gastroplasty with Nissen fundoplication and hiatal hernia
2015, 1Q, 28	Repair of bronchopleural fistula using omental pedicle graft

Upper Intestinal Tract (Ø) and Lower Intestinal Tract (D)

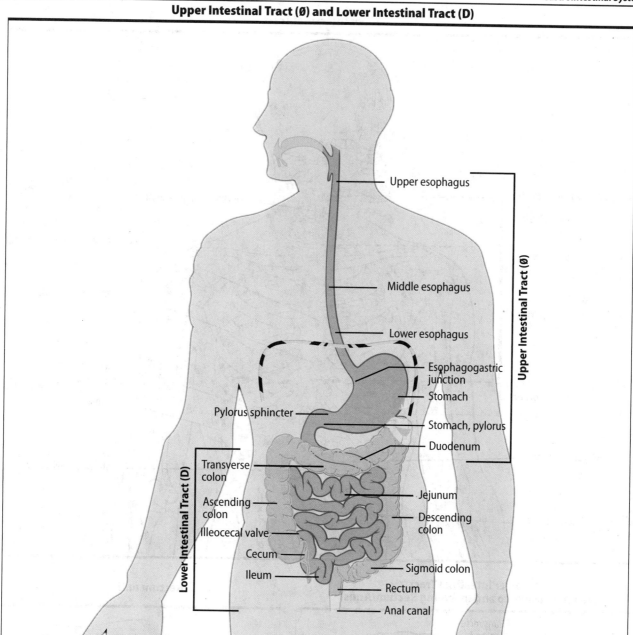

Gastrointestinal System

Upper Intestinal Tract

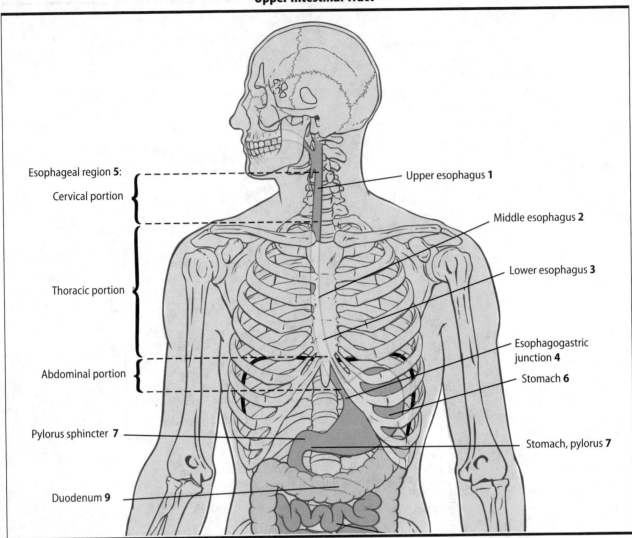

Esophageal region **5**:
Cervical portion
Thoracic portion
Abdominal portion
Pylorus sphincter **7**
Duodenum **9**

Upper esophagus **1**
Middle esophagus **2**
Lower esophagus **3**
Esophagogastric junction **4**
Stomach **6**
Stomach, pylorus **7**

Lower Intestinal Tract
(Jejunum Down to and Including Rectum/Anus)

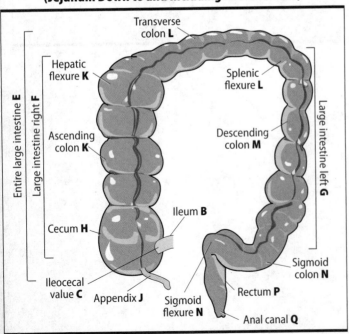

Transverse colon **L**
Hepatic flexure **K**
Splenic flexure **L**
Entire large intestine **E**
Large intestine right **F**
Ascending colon **K**
Descending colon **M**
Large intestine left **G**
Cecum **H**
Ileum **B**
Ileocecal value **C**
Appendix **J**
Sigmoid flexure **N**
Rectum **P**
Anal canal **Q**
Sigmoid colon **N**

Rectum and Anus

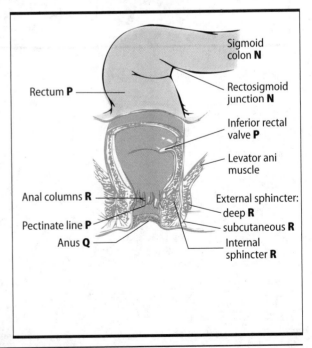

Sigmoid colon **N**
Rectum **P**
Rectosigmoid junction **N**
Inferior rectal valve **P**
Levator ani muscle
Anal columns **R**
Pectinate line **P**
Anus **Q**
External sphincter:
deep **R**
subcutaneous **R**
Internal sphincter **R**

Ø Medical and Surgical
D Gastrointestinal System
1 Bypass   Definition: Altering the route of passage of the contents of a tubular body part

Explanation: Rerouting contents of a body part to a downstream area of the normal route, to a similar route and body part, or to an abnormal route and dissimilar body part. Includes one or more anastomoses, with or without the use of a device.

Body Part Character 4	Approach Character 5	Device Character 6	Qualifier Character 7

1 Esophagus, Upper
  Cervical esophagus
2 Esophagus, Middle
  Thoracic esophagus
3 Esophagus, Lower
  Abdominal esophagus
5 Esophagus
	Ø Open
	4 Percutaneous Endoscopic
	8 Via Natural or Artificial Opening
	  Endoscopic
		7 Autologous Tissue Substitute
		J Synthetic Substitute
		K Nonautologous Tissue Substitute
		Z No Device
			4 Cutaneous
			6 Stomach
			9 Duodenum
			A Jejunum
			B Ileum

1 Esophagus, Upper
  Cervical esophagus
2 Esophagus, Middle
  Thoracic esophagus
3 Esophagus, Lower
  Abdominal esophagus
5 Esophagus
	3 Percutaneous	J Synthetic Substitute	4 Cutaneous

6 Stomach 9 Duodenum	Ø Open 4 Percutaneous Endoscopic 8 Via Natural or Artificial Opening Endoscopic	7 Autologous Tissue Substitute J Synthetic Substitute K Nonautologous Tissue Substitute Z No Device	4 Cutaneous 9 Duodenum A Jejunum B Ileum L Transverse Colon
6 Stomach 9 Duodenum	3 Percutaneous	J Synthetic Substitute	4 Cutaneous

A Jejunum
  Duodenojejunal flexure
	Ø Open
	4 Percutaneous Endoscopic
	8 Via Natural or Artificial Opening
	  Endoscopic
		7 Autologous Tissue Substitute
		J Synthetic Substitute
		K Nonautologous Tissue Substitute
		Z No Device
			4 Cutaneous
			A Jejunum
			B Ileum
			H Cecum
			K Ascending Colon
			L Transverse Colon
			M Descending Colon
			N Sigmoid Colon
			P Rectum
			Q Anus

A Jejunum Duodenojejunal flexure	3 Percutaneous	J Synthetic Substitute	4 Cutaneous
B Ileum	Ø Open 4 Percutaneous Endoscopic 8 Via Natural or Artificial Opening Endoscopic	7 Autologous Tissue Substitute J Synthetic Substitute K Nonautologous Tissue Substitute Z No Device	4 Cutaneous B Ileum H Cecum K Ascending Colon L Transverse Colon M Descending Colon N Sigmoid Colon P Rectum Q Anus
B Ileum	3 Percutaneous	J Synthetic Substitute	4 Cutaneous
H Cecum	Ø Open 4 Percutaneous Endoscopic 8 Via Natural or Artificial Opening Endoscopic	7 Autologous Tissue Substitute J Synthetic Substitute K Nonautologous Tissue Substitute Z No Device	4 Cutaneous H Cecum K Ascending Colon L Transverse Colon M Descending Colon N Sigmoid Colon P Rectum
H Cecum	3 Percutaneous	J Synthetic Substitute	4 Cutaneous
K Ascending Colon	Ø Open 4 Percutaneous Endoscopic 8 Via Natural or Artificial Opening Endoscopic	7 Autologous Tissue Substitute J Synthetic Substitute K Nonautologous Tissue Substitute Z No Device	4 Cutaneous K Ascending Colon L Transverse Colon M Descending Colon N Sigmoid Colon P Rectum

ØD1 Continued on next page

Non-OR   ØD16[Ø,4,8][7,J,K,Z]4
Non-OR   ØD163J4
HAC   ØD16[Ø,4,8][7,J,K,Z][9,A,B,L] when reported with PDx E66.Ø1 and SDx K68.11 or K95.Ø1 or K95.81 or T81.4XXA

LC Limited Coverage   NC Noncovered   ⊞ Combination Member   HAC associated procedure   Combination Only   DRG Non-OR   Non-OR   New/Revised in GREEN

ICD-10-PCS 2019   363

ØD1–ØD1

Gastrointestinal System (side tab)

ØD1 Continued

Ø   **Medical and Surgical**
D   **Gastrointestinal System**
1   **Bypass**   Definition: Altering the route of passage of the contents of a tubular body part

Explanation: Rerouting contents of a body part to a downstream area of the normal route, to a similar route and body part, or to an abnormal route and dissimilar body part. Includes one or more anastomoses, with or without the use of a device.

Body Part Character 4	Approach Character 5	Device Character 6	Qualifier Character 7
K Ascending Colon	3 Percutaneous	J Synthetic Substitute	4 Cutaneous

L Transverse Colon
     Hepatic flexure
     Splenic flexure
	Ø Open
	4 Percutaneous Endoscopic
	8 Via Natural or Artificial Opening
	    Endoscopic
		7 Autologous Tissue Substitute
		J Synthetic Substitute
		K Nonautologous Tissue Substitute
		Z No Device
			4 Cutaneous
			L Transverse Colon
			M Descending Colon
			N Sigmoid Colon
			P Rectum

L Transverse Colon
     Hepatic flexure
     Splenic flexure
	3 Percutaneous	J Synthetic Substitute	4 Cutaneous

M Descending Colon	Ø Open 4 Percutaneous Endoscopic 8 Via Natural or Artificial Opening Endoscopic	7 Autologous Tissue Substitute J Synthetic Substitute K Nonautologous Tissue Substitute Z No Device	4 Cutaneous M Descending Colon N Sigmoid Colon P Rectum
M Descending Colon	3 Percutaneous	J Synthetic Substitute	4 Cutaneous

N Sigmoid Colon
     Rectosigmoid junction
     Sigmoid flexure
	Ø Open
	4 Percutaneous Endoscopic
	8 Via Natural or Artificial Opening
	    Endoscopic
		7 Autologous Tissue Substitute
		J Synthetic Substitute
		K Nonautologous Tissue Substitute
		Z No Device
			4 Cutaneous
			N Sigmoid Colon
			P Rectum

N Sigmoid Colon
     Rectosigmoid junction
     Sigmoid flexure
	3 Percutaneous	J Synthetic Substitute	4 Cutaneous

Ø   **Medical and Surgical**
D   **Gastrointestinal System**
2   **Change**   Definition: Taking out or off a device from a body part and putting back an identical or similar device in or on the same body part without cutting or puncturing the skin or a mucous membrane

Explanation: All CHANGE procedures are coded using the approach EXTERNAL

Body Part Character 4	Approach Character 5	Device Character 6	Qualifier Character 7
Ø Upper Intestinal Tract D Lower Intestinal Tract	X External	Ø Drainage Device U Feeding Device Y Other Device	Z No Qualifier

U Omentum
     Gastrocolic ligament
     Gastrocolic omentum
     Gastrohepatic omentum
     Gastrophrenic ligament
     Gastrosplenic ligament
     Greater Omentum
     Hepatogastric ligament
     Lesser Omentum
V Mesentery
     Mesoappendix
     Mesocolon
W Peritoneum
     Epiploic foramen
	X External	Ø Drainage Device
		Y Other Device
			Z No Qualifier

Non-OR   All body part, approach, device, and qualifier values

LC Limited Coverage   NC Noncovered   ⊞ Combination Member   HAC associated procedure   Combination Only   DRG Non-OR   Non-OR   New/Revised in GREEN
364   ICD-10-PCS 2019

ØD1–ØD2 (side tab)

Ø   **Medical and Surgical**
D   **Gastrointestinal System**
5   **Destruction**   Definition: Physical eradication of all or a portion of a body part by the direct use of energy, force, or a destructive agent
                     Explanation: None of the body part is physically taken out

Body Part Character 4	Approach Character 5	Device Character 6	Qualifier Character 7

1 **Esophagus, Upper**
   Cervical esophagus
2 **Esophagus, Middle**
   Thoracic esophagus
3 **Esophagus, Lower**
   Abdominal esophagus
4 **Esophagogastric Junction**
   Cardia
   Cardioesophageal junction
   Gastroesophageal (GE) junction
5 **Esophagus**
6 **Stomach**
7 **Stomach, Pylorus**
   Pyloric antrum
   Pyloric canal
   Pyloric sphincter
8 **Small Intestine**
9 **Duodenum**
A **Jejunum**
   Duodenojejunal flexure
B **Ileum**
C **Ileocecal Valve**
E **Large Intestine**
F **Large Intestine, Right**
G **Large Intestine, Left**
H **Cecum**
J **Appendix**
   Vermiform appendix
K **Ascending Colon**
L **Transverse Colon**
   Hepatic flexure
   Splenic flexure
M **Descending Colon**
N **Sigmoid Colon**
   Rectosigmoid junction
   Sigmoid flexure
P **Rectum**
   Anorectal junction
	Ø Open
	3 Percutaneous
	4 Percutaneous Endoscopic
	7 Via Natural or Artificial Opening
	8 Via Natural or Artificial Opening
	     Endoscopic
		Z No Device	Z No Qualifier

Q **Anus**
   Anal orifice
	Ø Open
	3 Percutaneous
	4 Percutaneous Endoscopic
	7 Via Natural or Artificial Opening
	8 Via Natural or Artificial Opening
	     Endoscopic
	X External
		Z No Device	Z No Qualifier

R **Anal Sphincter**
   External anal sphincter
   Internal anal sphincter
U **Omentum**
   Gastrocolic ligament
   Gastrocolic omentum
   Gastrohepatic omentum
   Gastrophrenic ligament
   Gastrosplenic ligament
   Greater Omentum
   Hepatogastric ligament
   Lesser Omentum
V **Mesentery**
   Mesoappendix
   Mesocolon
W **Peritoneum**
   Epiploic foramen
	Ø Open
	3 Percutaneous
	4 Percutaneous Endoscopic
		Z No Device	Z No Qualifier

Non-OR   ØD5[1,2,3,4,5,6,7,9,E,F,G,H,K,L,M,N][4,8]ZZ
Non-OR   ØD5P[Ø,3,4,7,8]ZZ
Non-OR   ØD5Q[4,8]ZZ
Non-OR   ØD5R4ZZ

LC Limited Coverage **NC** Noncovered ⊞ Combination Member HAC associated procedure Combination Only DRG Non-OR Non-OR New/Revised in GREEN

ICD-10-PCS 2019   **365**

ØD5–ØD5

Gastrointestinal System

Ø   Medical and Surgical
D   Gastrointestinal System
7   Dilation   Definition: Expanding an orifice or the lumen of a tubular body part

Explanation: The orifice can be a natural orifice or an artificially created orifice. Accomplished by stretching a tubular body part using intraluminal pressure or by cutting part of the orifice or wall of the tubular body part.

Body Part Character 4	Approach Character 5	Device Character 6	Qualifier Character 7

1 **Esophagus, Upper**
  Cervical esophagus
2 **Esophagus, Middle**
  Thoracic esophagus
3 **Esophagus, Lower**
  Abdominal esophagus
4 **Esophagogastric Junction**
  Cardia
  Cardioesophageal junction
  Gastroesophageal (GE) junction
5 **Esophagus**
6 **Stomach**
7 **Stomach, Pylorus**
  Pyloric antrum
  Pyloric canal
  Pyloric sphincter
8 **Small Intestine**
9 **Duodenum**
A **Jejunum**
  Duodenojejunal flexure
B **Ileum**
C **Ileocecal Valve**
E **Large Intestine**
F **Large Intestine, Right**
G **Large Intestine, Left**
H **Cecum**
K **Ascending Colon**
L **Transverse Colon**
  Hepatic flexure
  Splenic flexure
M **Descending Colon**
N **Sigmoid Colon**
  Rectosigmoid junction
  Sigmoid flexure
P **Rectum**
  Anorectal junction
Q **Anus**
  Anal orifice
	Ø Open
	3 Percutaneous
	4 Percutaneous Endoscopic
	7 Via Natural or Artificial Opening
	8 Via Natural or Artificial Opening
	  Endoscopic
		D Intraluminal Device
		Z No Device
			Z No Qualifier

Non-OR   ØD7[1,2,3,4,5,6,8,9,A,B,C,E,F,G,H,K,L,M,N,P,Q][7,8][D,Z]Z
Non-OR   ØD77[4,8]DZ
Non-OR   ØD777[D,Z]Z
Non-OR   ØD7[8,9,A,B,C,E,F,G,H,K,L,M,N][Ø,3,4]DZ

Ø   Medical and Surgical
D   Gastrointestinal System
8   Division   Definition: Cutting into a body part, without draining fluids and/or gases from the body part, in order to separate or transect a body part

Explanation: All or a portion of the body part is separated into two or more portions

Body Part Character 4	Approach Character 5	Device Character 6	Qualifier Character 7

4 **Esophagogastric Junction**
  Cardia
  Cardioesophageal junction
  Gastroesophageal (GE) junction
7 **Stomach, Pylorus**
  Pyloric antrum
  Pyloric canal
  Pyloric sphincter
	Ø Open
	3 Percutaneous
	4 Percutaneous Endoscopic
	7 Via Natural or Artificial Opening
	8 Via Natural or Artificial Opening
	  Endoscopic
		Z No Device	Z No Qualifier

R **Anal Sphincter**
  External anal sphincter
  Internal anal sphincter
	Ø Open
	3 Percutaneous
		Z No Device	Z No Qualifier

LC Limited Coverage   NC Noncovered   ⊞ Combination Member   HAC associated procedure   Combination Only   DRG Non-OR   Non-OR   New/Revised in GREEN

Ø   **Medical and Surgical**
D   **Gastrointestinal System**
9   **Drainage**   Definition: Taking or letting out fluids and/or gases from a body part
                          Explanation: The qualifier DIAGNOSTIC is used to identify drainage procedures that are biopsies

Body Part Character 4		Approach Character 5	Device Character 6	Qualifier Character 7

1 **Esophagus, Upper**
  Cervical esophagus
2 **Esophagus, Middle**
  Thoracic esophagus
3 **Esophagus, Lower**
  Abdominal esophagus
4 **Esophagogastric Junction**
  Cardia
  Cardioesophageal junction
  Gastroesophageal (GE) junction
5 **Esophagus**
6 **Stomach**
7 **Stomach, Pylorus**
  Pyloric antrum
  Pyloric canal
  Pyloric sphincter
8 **Small Intestine**
9 **Duodenum**
	A **Jejunum**
	  Duodenojejunal flexure
	B **Ileum**
	C **Ileocecal Valve**
	E **Large Intestine**
	F **Large Intestine, Right**
	G **Large Intestine, Left**
	H **Cecum**
	J **Appendix**
	  Vermiform appendix
	K **Ascending Colon**
	L **Transverse Colon**
	  Hepatic flexure
	  Splenic flexure
	M **Descending Colon**
	N **Sigmoid Colon**
	  Rectosigmoid junction
	  Sigmoid flexure
	P **Rectum**
	  Anorectal junction
		Ø **Open**
		3 **Percutaneous**
		4 **Percutaneous Endoscopic**
		7 **Via Natural or Artificial Opening**
		8 **Via Natural or Artificial Opening Endoscopic**
			Ø **Drainage Device**	Z **No Qualifier**

1 **Esophagus, Upper**
  Cervical esophagus
2 **Esophagus, Middle**
  Thoracic esophagus
3 **Esophagus, Lower**
  Abdominal esophagus
4 **Esophagogastric Junction**
  Cardia
  Cardioesophageal junction
  Gastroesophageal (GE) junction
5 **Esophagus**
6 **Stomach**
7 **Stomach, Pylorus**
  Pyloric antrum
  Pyloric canal
  Pyloric sphincter
8 **Small Intestine**
9 **Duodenum**
	A **Jejunum**
	  Duodenojejunal flexure
	B **Ileum**
	C **Ileocecal Valve**
	E **Large Intestine**
	F **Large Intestine, Right**
	G **Large Intestine, Left**
	H **Cecum**
	J **Appendix**
	  Vermiform appendix
	K **Ascending Colon**
	L **Transverse Colon**
	  Hepatic flexure
	  Splenic flexure
	M **Descending Colon**
	N **Sigmoid Colon**
	  Rectosigmoid junction
	  Sigmoid flexure
	P **Rectum**
	  Anorectal junction
		Ø **Open**
		3 **Percutaneous**
		4 **Percutaneous Endoscopic**
		7 **Via Natural or Artificial Opening**
		8 **Via Natural or Artificial Opening Endoscopic**
			Z **No Device**	X **Diagnostic**
				Z **No Qualifier**

Q **Anus** Anal orifice		Ø **Open** 3 **Percutaneous** 4 **Percutaneous Endoscopic** 7 **Via Natural or Artificial Opening** 8 **Via Natural or Artificial Opening Endoscopic** X **External**	Ø **Drainage Device**	Z **No Qualifier**
Q **Anus** Anal orifice		Ø **Open** 3 **Percutaneous** 4 **Percutaneous Endoscopic** 7 **Via Natural or Artificial Opening** 8 **Via Natural or Artificial Opening Endoscopic** X **External**	Z **No Device**	X **Diagnostic** Z **No Qualifier**

ØD9 Continued on next page

Non-OR	ØD9[1,2,3,4,5,C,J]3ØZ
Non-OR	ØD9[6,7,8,9,A,B,E,F,G,H,K,L,M,N,P][3,7,8]ØZ
Non-OR	ØD9[1,2,3,4,5,6,7,8,9,A,B,C,E,F,G,H,K,L,M,N,P][3,4,7,8]ZX
Non-OR	ØD9[1,2,3,4,5,6,7,8,9,A,B,C,E,F,G,H,J,K,L,M,N,P]3ZZ
Non-OR	ØD9Q3ØZ
Non-OR	ØD9Q[Ø,4,7,8,X]ZX
Non-OR	ØD9Q3Z[X,Z]

Ø Medical and Surgical
D Gastrointestinal System
9 Drainage   Definition: Taking or letting out fluids and/or gases from a body part

ØD9 Continued

Explanation: The qualifier DIAGNOSTIC is used to identify drainage procedures that are biopsies

Body Part Character 4	Approach Character 5	Device Character 6	Qualifier Character 7
R Anal Sphincter External anal sphincter Internal anal sphincter **U Omentum** Gastrocolic ligament Gastrocolic omentum Gastrohepatic omentum Gastrophrenic ligament Gastrosplenic ligament Greater Omentum Hepatogastric ligament Lesser Omentum **V Mesentery** Mesoappendix Mesocolon **W Peritoneum** Epiploic foramen	**Ø** Open **3** Percutaneous **4** Percutaneous Endoscopic	**Ø** Drainage Device	**Z** No Qualifier
R Anal Sphincter External anal sphincter Internal anal sphincter **U Omentum** Gastrocolic ligament Gastrocolic omentum Gastrohepatic omentum Gastrophrenic ligament Gastrosplenic ligament Greater Omentum Hepatogastric ligament Lesser Omentum **V Mesentery** Mesoappendix Mesocolon **W Peritoneum** Epiploic foramen	**Ø** Open **3** Percutaneous **4** Percutaneous Endoscopic	**Z** No Device	**X** Diagnostic **Z** No Qualifier

Non-OR	ØD9R3ØZ
Non-OR	ØD9[U,V,W][3,4]ØZ
Non-OR	ØD9R[Ø,4]ZX
Non-OR	ØD9[R,U,V,W]3Z[X,Z]
Non-OR	ØD9[U,V,W]4ZZ

Ø   Medical and Surgical
D   Gastrointestinal System
B   Excision   Definition: Cutting out or off, without replacement, a portion of a body part
                 Explanation: The qualifier DIAGNOSTIC is used to identify excision procedures that are biopsies

Body Part Character 4		Approach Character 5	Device Character 6	Qualifier Character 7

1 Esophagus, Upper
  Cervical esophagus
2 Esophagus, Middle
  Thoracic esophagus
3 Esophagus, Lower
  Abdominal esophagus
4 Esophagogastric
  Junction
  Cardia
  Cardioesophageal
    junction
  Gastroesophageal (GE)
    junction
5 Esophagus
7 Stomach, Pylorus
  Pyloric antrum
  Pyloric canal
  Pyloric sphincter
	8 Small Intestine
	9 Duodenum
	A Jejunum
	  Duodenojejunal flexure
	B Ileum
	C Ileocecal Valve
	E Large Intestine
	F Large Intestine, Right
	H Cecum
	J Appendix
	  Vermiform appendix
	K Ascending Colon
	P Rectum
	  Anorectal junction
		Ø Open
		3 Percutaneous
		4 Percutaneous Endoscopic
		7 Via Natural or Artificial
		  Opening
		8 Via Natural or Artificial
		  Opening Endoscopic
			Z No Device	X Diagnostic
				Z No Qualifier

6 Stomach		Ø Open
		3 Percutaneous
		4 Percutaneous Endoscopic
		7 Via Natural or Artificial
		  Opening
		8 Via Natural or Artificial
		  Opening Endoscopic
			Z No Device	3 Vertical
				X Diagnostic
				Z No Qualifier

G Large Intestine, Left
L Transverse Colon
  Hepatic flexure
  Splenic flexure
M Descending Colon
N Sigmoid Colon
  Rectosigmoid junction
  Sigmoid flexure
		Ø Open
		3 Percutaneous
		4 Percutaneous Endoscopic
		7 Via Natural or Artificial
		  Opening
		8 Via Natural or Artificial
		  Opening Endoscopic
			Z No Device	X Diagnostic
				Z No Qualifier

G Large Intestine, Left
L Transverse Colon
  Hepatic flexure
  Splenic flexure
M Descending Colon
N Sigmoid Colon
  Rectosigmoid junction
  Sigmoid flexure
		F Via Natural or Artificial
		  Opening with Percutaneous
		  Endoscopic Assistance
			Z No Device	Z No Qualifier

Q Anus
  Anal orifice
		Ø Open
		3 Percutaneous
		4 Percutaneous Endoscopic
		7 Via Natural or Artificial
		  Opening
		8 Via Natural or Artificial
		  Opening Endoscopic
		X External
			Z No Device	X Diagnostic
				Z No Qualifier

R Anal Sphincter
  External anal sphincter
  Internal anal sphincter
U Omentum
  Gastrocolic ligament
  Gastrocolic omentum
  Gastrohepatic omentum
  Gastrophrenic ligament
  Gastrosplenic ligament
  Greater Omentum
  Hepatogastric ligament
  Lesser Omentum
V Mesentery
  Mesoappendix
  Mesocolon
W Peritoneum
  Epiploic foramen
		Ø Open
		3 Percutaneous
		4 Percutaneous Endoscopic
			Z No Device	X Diagnostic
				Z No Qualifier

Non-OR   ØDB[1,2,3,4,5,7,8,9,A,B,C,E,F,H,K,P][3,4,7,8]ZX
Non-OR   ØDB[1,2,3,5,7,9][4,8]ZZ
Non-OR   ØDB[4,E,F,H,K,P]8ZZ
Non-OR   ØDB6[3,4,7,8]ZX
Non-OR   ØDB6[4,8]ZZ
Non-OR   ØDB[G,L,M,N][3,4,7,8]ZX

Non-OR   ØDB[G,L,M,N]8ZZ
Non-OR   ØDBQ[Ø,3,4,7,8,X]ZX
Non-OR   ØDBQ8ZZ
Non-OR   ØDBR[Ø,3,4]ZX
Non-OR   ØDB[U,V,W][3,4]ZX

LC Limited Coverage   NC Noncovered   ⊞ Combination Member   HAC associated procedure   Combination Only   DRG Non-OR   Non-OR   New/Revised in GREEN

ICD-10-PCS 2019   369

ØDB–ØDB

Gastrointestinal System

Ø　**Medical and Surgical**
D　**Gastrointestinal System**
C　**Extirpation**　　Definition: Taking or cutting out solid matter from a body part

Explanation: The solid matter may be an abnormal byproduct of a biological function or a foreign body; it may be imbedded in a body part or in the lumen of a tubular body part. The solid matter may or may not have been previously broken into pieces.

Body Part Character 4	Approach Character 5	Device Character 6	Qualifier Character 7
1　Esophagus, Upper 　　Cervical esophagus 2　Esophagus, Middle 　　Thoracic esophagus 3　Esophagus, Lower 　　Abdominal esophagus 4　Esophagogastric Junction 　　Cardia 　　Cardioesophageal junction 　　Gastroesophageal (GE) junction 5　Esophagus 6　Stomach 7　Stomach, Pylorus 　　Pyloric antrum 　　Pyloric canal 　　Pyloric sphincter 8　Small Intestine 9　Duodenum A　Jejunum 　　Duodenojejunal flexure B　Ileum C　Ileocecal Valve E　Large Intestine F　Large Intestine, Right G　Large Intestine, Left H　Cecum J　Appendix 　　Vermiform appendix K　Ascending Colon L　Transverse Colon 　　Hepatic flexure 　　Splenic flexure M　Descending Colon N　Sigmoid Colon 　　Rectosigmoid junction 　　Sigmoid flexure P　Rectum 　　Anorectal junction	Ø　Open 3　Percutaneous 4　Percutaneous Endoscopic 7　Via Natural or Artificial Opening 8　Via Natural or Artificial Opening 　　Endoscopic	Z　No Device	Z　No Qualifier
Q　Anus 　　Anal orifice	Ø　Open 3　Percutaneous 4　Percutaneous Endoscopic 7　Via Natural or Artificial Opening 8　Via Natural or Artificial Opening 　　Endoscopic X　External	Z　No Device	Z　No Qualifier
R　Anal Sphincter 　　External anal sphincter 　　Internal anal sphincter U　Omentum 　　Gastrocolic ligament 　　Gastrocolic omentum 　　Gastrohepatic omentum 　　Gastrophrenic ligament 　　Gastrosplenic ligament 　　Greater Omentum 　　Hepatogastric ligament 　　Lesser Omentum V　Mesentery 　　Mesoappendix 　　Mesocolon W　Peritoneum 　　Epiploic foramen	Ø　Open 3　Percutaneous 4　Percutaneous Endoscopic	Z　No Device	Z　No Qualifier

Non-OR　ØDC[1,2,3,4,5,6,7,8,9,A,B,C,E,F,G,H,K,L,M,N,P][7,8]ZZ
Non-OR　ØDCQ[7,8,X]ZZ

Ø　Medical and Surgical
D　Gastrointestinal System
D　Extraction　　　Definition: Pulling or stripping out or off all or a portion of a body part by the use of force
　　　　　　　　　　Explanation: The qualifier DIAGNOSTIC is used to identify extraction procedures that are biopsies

Body Part Character 4	Approach Character 5	Device Character 6	Qualifier Character 7
1　Esophagus, Upper 　　Cervical esophagus **2　Esophagus, Middle** 　　Thoracic esophagus **3　Esophagus, Lower** 　　Abdominal esophagus **4　Esophagogastric Junction** 　　Cardia 　　Cardioesophageal junction 　　Gastroesophageal (GE) junction **5　Esophagus** **6　Stomach** **7　Stomach, Pylorus** 　　Pyloric antrum 　　Pyloric canal 　　Pyloric sphincter **8　Small Intestine** **9　Duodenum** **A　Jejunum** 　　Duodenojejunal flexure **B　Ileum** **C　Ileocecal Valve** **E　Large Intestine** **F　Large Intestine, Right** **G　Large Intestine, Left** **H　Cecum** **J　Appendix** 　　Vermiform appendix **K　Ascending Colon** **L　Transverse Colon** 　　Hepatic flexure 　　Splenic flexure **M　Descending Colon** **N　Sigmoid Colon** 　　Rectosigmoid junction 　　Sigmoid flexure **P　Rectum** 　　Anorectal junction	**3　Percutaneous** **4　Percutaneous Endoscopic** **8　Via Natural or Artificial Opening 　　Endoscopic**	**Z　No Device**	**X　Diagnostic**
Q　Anus 　　Anal orifice	**3　Percutaneous** **4　Percutaneous Endoscopic** **8　Via Natural or Artificial Opening 　　Endoscopic** **X　External**	**Z　No Device**	**X　Diagnostic**

Non-OR　ØDD[1,2,3,4,5,6,7,8,9,A,B,C,E,F,G,H,K,L,M,N,P][3,4,8]ZX
Non-OR　ØDDQ[3,4,8,X]ZX

Ø   Medical and Surgical
D   Gastrointestinal System
F   Fragmentation   Definition: Breaking solid matter in a body part into pieces
Explanation: Physical force (e.g., manual, ultrasonic) applied directly or indirectly is used to break the solid matter into pieces. The solid matter may be an abnormal byproduct of a biological function or a foreign body. The pieces of solid matter are not taken out.

Body Part Character 4	Approach Character 5	Device Character 6	Qualifier Character 7

5 Esophagus   NC
6 Stomach   NC
8 Small Intestine   NC
9 Duodenum   NC
A Jejunum   NC
   Duodenojejunal flexure
B Ileum   NC
E Large Intestine   NC
F Large Intestine, Right   NC
G Large Intestine, Left   NC
H Cecum   NC
J Appendix   NC
   Vermiform appendix
K Ascending Colon   NC
L Transverse Colon   NC
   Hepatic flexure
   Splenic flexure
M Descending Colon   NC
N Sigmoid Colon   NC
   Rectosigmoid junction
   Sigmoid flexure
P Rectum   NC
   Anorectal junction
Q Anus   NC
   Anal orifice
	Ø Open
	3 Percutaneous
	4 Percutaneous Endoscopic
	7 Via Natural or Artificial Opening
	8 Via Natural or Artificial Opening
	   Endoscopic
	X External
		Z No Device	Z No Qualifier

Non-OR   ØDF[5,6,8,9,A,B,E,F,G,H,J,K,L,M,N,P,Q]XZZ
NC   ØDF[5,6,8,9,A,B,E,F,G,H,J,K,L,M,N,P,Q]XZZ

Ø   Medical and Surgical
D   Gastrointestinal System
H   Insertion   Definition: Putting in a nonbiological appliance that monitors, assists, performs, or prevents a physiological function but does not physically take the place of a body part
                Explanation: None

Body Part Character 4	Approach Character 5	Device Character 6	Qualifier Character 7
Ø Upper Intestinal Tract **D** Lower Intestinal Tract	**Ø** Open **3** Percutaneous **4** Percutaneous Endoscopic **7** Via Natural or Artificial Opening **8** Via Natural or Artificial Opening Endoscopic	**Y** Other Device	**Z** No Qualifier
5 Esophagus	**Ø** Open **3** Percutaneous **4** Percutaneous Endoscopic	**1** Radioactive Element **2** Monitoring Device **3** Infusion Device **D** Intraluminal Device **U** Feeding Device **Y** Other Device	**Z** No Qualifier
5 Esophagus	**7** Via Natural or Artificial Opening **8** Via Natural or Artificial Opening Endoscopic	**1** Radioactive Element **2** Monitoring Device **3** Infusion Device **B** Intraluminal Device, Airway **D** Intraluminal Device **U** Feeding Device **Y** Other Device	**Z** No Qualifier
6 Stomach ⊞	**Ø** Open **3** Percutaneous **4** Percutaneous Endoscopic	**2** Monitoring Device **3** Infusion Device **D** Intraluminal Device **M** Stimulator Lead **U** Feeding Device **Y** Other Device	**Z** No Qualifier
6 Stomach	**7** Via Natural or Artificial Opening **8** Via Natural or Artificial Opening Endoscopic	**2** Monitoring Device **3** Infusion Device **D** Intraluminal Device **U** Feeding Device **Y** Other Device	**Z** No Qualifier
8 Small Intestine **9** Duodenum **A** Jejunum Duodenojejunal flexure **B** Ileum	**Ø** Open **3** Percutaneous **4** Percutaneous Endoscopic **7** Via Natural or Artificial Opening **8** Via Natural or Artificial Opening Endoscopic	**2** Monitoring Device **3** Infusion Device **D** Intraluminal Device **U** Feeding Device	**Z** No Qualifier
E Large Intestine	**Ø** Open **3** Percutaneous **4** Percutaneous Endoscopic **7** Via Natural or Artificial Opening **8** Via Natural or Artificial Opening Endoscopic	**D** Intraluminal Device	**Z** No Qualifier
P Rectum Anorectal junction	**Ø** Open **3** Percutaneous **4** Percutaneous Endoscopic **7** Via Natural or Artificial Opening **8** Via Natural or Artificial Opening Endoscopic	**1** Radioactive Element **D** Intraluminal Device	**Z** No Qualifier
Q Anus Anal orifice	**Ø** Open **3** Percutaneous **4** Percutaneous Endoscopic	**D** Intraluminal Device **L** Artificial Sphincter	**Z** No Qualifier
Q Anus Anal orifice	**7** Via Natural or Artificial Opening **8** Via Natural or Artificial Opening Endoscopic	**D** Intraluminal Device	**Z** No Qualifier

R Anal Sphincter
     External anal sphincter
     Internal anal sphincter
	Ø Open
	3 Percutaneous
	4 Percutaneous Endoscopic
		M Stimulator Lead	**Z** No Qualifier

Non-OR   ØDH[Ø,D][Ø,3,4,7,8]YZ
Non-OR   ØDH5[Ø,3,4][D,U]Z
Non-OR   ØDH5[3,4]YZ
Non-OR   ØDH5[7,8][2,3,B,D,U,Y]Z
Non-OR   ØDH6[3,4][U,Y]Z
Non-OR   ØDH6[7,8][2,3,D,U,Y]Z
Non-OR   ØDH[8,9,A,B][Ø,3,4][D,U]Z
Non-OR   ØDH[8,9,A,B][7,8][2,3,D,U]Z
Non-OR   ØDHE[Ø,3,4,7,8]DZ
Non-OR   ØDHP[Ø,3,4,7,8]DZ

See Appendix L for Procedure Combinations
⊞   ØDH6[Ø,3,4]MZ

LC Limited Coverage   **NC** Noncovered   ⊞ Combination Member   HAC associated procedure   Combination Only   DRG Non-OR   Non-OR   New/Revised in GREEN

Gastrointestinal System (sidebar)

Ø   Medical and Surgical
D   Gastrointestinal System
J   Inspection   Definition: Visually and/or manually exploring a body part

          Explanation: Visual exploration may be performed with or without optical instrumentation. Manual exploration may be performed directly or through intervening body layers.

Body Part Character 4	Approach Character 5	Device Character 6	Qualifier Character 7
Ø Upper Intestinal Tract **6** Stomach **D** Lower Intestinal Tract	**Ø** Open **3** Percutaneous **4** Percutaneous Endoscopic **7** Via Natural or Artificial Opening **8** Via Natural or Artificial Opening Endoscopic **X** External	**Z** No Device	**Z** No Qualifier

U Omentum
    Gastrocolic ligament
    Gastrocolic omentum
    Gastrohepatic omentum
    Gastrophrenic ligament
    Gastrosplenic ligament
    Greater Omentum
    Hepatogastric ligament
    Lesser Omentum
V Mesentery
    Mesoappendix
    Mesocolon
W Peritoneum
    Epiploic foramen
	Ø Open
	3 Percutaneous
	4 Percutaneous Endoscopic
	X External
		Z No Device	**Z** No Qualifier

Non-OR	ØDJ[Ø,6,D][3,7,8,X]ZZ
Non-OR	ØDJ[U,V,W][3,X]ZZ

LC Limited Coverage   NC Noncovered   ⊞ Combination Member   HAC associated procedure   Combination Only   DRG Non-OR   Non-OR   New/Revised in GREEN
374   ICD-10-PCS 2019

ØDJ–ØDJ (sidebar)

Ø **Medical and Surgical**
D **Gastrointestinal System**
L **Occlusion**   Definition: Completely closing an orifice or the lumen of a tubular body part
                  Explanation: The orifice can be a natural orifice or an artificially created orifice

Body Part Character 4		Approach Character 5	Device Character 6	Qualifier Character 7
1 **Esophagus, Upper** Cervical esophagus 2 **Esophagus, Middle** Thoracic esophagus 3 **Esophagus, Lower** Abdominal esophagus 4 **Esophagogastric Junction** Cardia Cardioesophageal junction Gastroesophageal (GE) junction 5 **Esophagus** 6 **Stomach** 7 **Stomach, Pylorus** Pyloric antrum Pyloric canal Pyloric sphincter 8 **Small Intestine**	9 **Duodenum** A **Jejunum** Duodenojejunal flexure B **Ileum** C **Ileocecal Valve** E **Large Intestine** F **Large Intestine, Right** G **Large Intestine, Left** H **Cecum** K **Ascending Colon** L **Transverse Colon** Hepatic flexure Splenic flexure M **Descending Colon** N **Sigmoid Colon** Rectosigmoid junction Sigmoid flexure P **Rectum** Anorectal junction	Ø **Open** 3 **Percutaneous** 4 **Percutaneous Endoscopic**	C **Extraluminal Device** D **Intraluminal Device** Z **No Device**	Z **No Qualifier**
1 **Esophagus, Upper** Cervical esophagus 2 **Esophagus, Middle** Thoracic esophagus 3 **Esophagus, Lower** Abdominal esophagus 4 **Esophagogastric Junction** Cardia Cardioesophageal junction Gastroesophageal (GE) junction 5 **Esophagus** 6 **Stomach** 7 **Stomach, Pylorus** Pyloric antrum Pyloric canal Pyloric sphincter 8 **Small Intestine**	9 **Duodenum** A **Jejunum** Duodenojejunal flexure B **Ileum** C **Ileocecal Valve** E **Large Intestine** F **Large Intestine, Right** G **Large Intestine, Left** H **Cecum** K **Ascending Colon** L **Transverse Colon** Hepatic flexure Splenic flexure M **Descending Colon** N **Sigmoid Colon** Rectosigmoid junction Sigmoid flexure P **Rectum** Anorectal junction	7 **Via Natural or Artificial Opening** 8 **Via Natural or Artificial Opening Endoscopic**	D **Intraluminal Device** Z **No Device**	Z **No Qualifier**
Q **Anus** Anal orifice		Ø **Open** 3 **Percutaneous** 4 **Percutaneous Endoscopic** X **External**	C **Extraluminal Device** D **Intraluminal Device** Z **No Device**	Z **No Qualifier**
Q **Anus** Anal orifice		7 **Via Natural or Artificial Opening** 8 **Via Natural or Artificial Opening Endoscopic**	D **Intraluminal Device** Z **No Device**	Z **No Qualifier**

Non-OR   ØDL[1,2,3,4,5][Ø,3,4][C,D,Z]Z
Non-OR   ØDL[1,2,3,4,5][7,8][D,Z]Z

Gastrointestinal System

Ø   **Medical and Surgical**
D   **Gastrointestinal System**
M   **Reattachment**   Definition: Putting back in or on all or a portion of a separated body part to its normal location or other suitable location
                     Explanation: Vascular circulation and nervous pathways may or may not be reestablished

Body Part Character 4	Approach Character 5	Device Character 6	Qualifier Character 7

5 Esophagus
6 Stomach
8 Small Intestine
9 Duodenum
A Jejunum
    Duodenojejunal flexure
B Ileum
E Large Intestine
F Large Intestine, Right
G Large Intestine, Left
H Cecum
K Ascending Colon
L Transverse Colon
    Hepatic flexure
    Splenic flexure
M Descending Colon
N Sigmoid Colon
    Rectosigmoid junction
    Sigmoid flexure
P Rectum
    Anorectal junction
	Ø Open
	4 Percutaneous Endoscopic
		Z No Device	**Z** No Qualifier

Ø   **Medical and Surgical**
D   **Gastrointestinal System**
N   **Release**   Definition: Freeing a body part from an abnormal physical constraint by cutting or by the use of force
                     Explanation: Some of the restraining tissue may be taken out but none of the body part is taken out

Body Part Character 4		Approach Character 5	Device Character 6	Qualifier Character 7

1 Esophagus, Upper
    Cervical esophagus
2 Esophagus, Middle
    Thoracic esophagus
3 Esophagus, Lower
    Abdominal esophagus
4 Esophagogastric
    Junction
    Cardia
    Cardioesophageal
      junction
    Gastroesophageal (GE)
      junction
5 Esophagus
6 Stomach
7 Stomach, Pylorus
    Pyloric antrum
    Pyloric canal
    Pyloric sphincter
8 Small Intestine
9 Duodenum
	A Jejunum
	    Duodenojejunal flexure
	B Ileum
	C Ileocecal Valve
	E Large Intestine
	F Large Intestine, Right
	G Large Intestine, Left
	H Cecum
	J Appendix
	    Vermiform appendix
	K Ascending Colon
	L Transverse Colon
	    Hepatic flexure
	    Splenic flexure
	M Descending Colon
	N Sigmoid Colon
	    Rectosigmoid junction
	    Sigmoid flexure
	P Rectum
	    Anorectal junction
		Ø Open
		3 Percutaneous
		4 Percutaneous Endoscopic
		7 Via Natural or Artificial
		    Opening
		8 Via Natural or Artificial
		    Opening Endoscopic
			Z No Device	**Z** No Qualifier

Q Anus
    Anal orifice
		Ø Open
		3 Percutaneous
		4 Percutaneous Endoscopic
		7 Via Natural or Artificial
		    Opening
		8 Via Natural or Artificial
		    Opening Endoscopic
		X External
			Z No Device	**Z** No Qualifier

R Anal Sphincter
    External anal sphincter
    Internal anal sphincter
U Omentum
    Gastrocolic ligament
    Gastrocolic omentum
    Gastrohepatic omentum
    Gastrophrenic ligament
    Gastrosplenic ligament
    Greater Omentum
    Hepatogastric ligament
    Lesser Omentum
V Mesentery
    Mesoappendix
    Mesocolon
W Peritoneum
    Epiploic foramen
		Ø Open
		3 Percutaneous
		4 Percutaneous Endoscopic
			Z No Device	**Z** No Qualifier

Non-OR   ØDN[8,9,A,B,E,F,G,H,K,L,M,N][7,8]ZZ

LC Limited Coverage   **NC** Noncovered   ⊞ Combination Member   HAC associated procedure   Combination Only   DRG Non-OR   Non-OR   New/Revised in GREEN

376   ICD-10-PCS 2019

Ø   **Medical and Surgical**
D   **Gastrointestinal System**
P   **Removal**   Definition: Taking out or off a device from a body part

Explanation: If a device is taken out and a similar device put in without cutting or puncturing the skin or mucous membrane, the procedure is coded to the root operation CHANGE. Otherwise, the procedure for taking out a device is coded to the root operation REMOVAL.

Body Part Character 4	Approach Character 5	Device Character 6	Qualifier Character 7
Ø Upper Intestinal Tract D Lower Intestinal Tract	Ø Open 3 Percutaneous 4 Percutaneous Endoscopic 7 Via Natural or Artificial Opening 8 Via Natural or Artificial Opening Endoscopic	Ø Drainage Device 2 Monitoring Device 3 Infusion Device 7 Autologous Tissue Substitute C Extraluminal Device D Intraluminal Device J Synthetic Substitute K Nonautologous Tissue Substitute U Feeding Device Y Other Device	Z No Qualifier
Ø Upper Intestinal Tract D Lower Intestinal Tract	X External	Ø Drainage Device 2 Monitoring Device 3 Infusion Device D Intraluminal Device U Feeding Device	Z No Qualifier
5 Esophagus	Ø Open 3 Percutaneous 4 Percutaneous Endoscopic	1 Radioactive Element 2 Monitoring Device 3 Infusion Device U Feeding Device Y Other Device	Z No Qualifier
5 Esophagus	7 Via Natural or Artificial Opening 8 Via Natural or Artificial Opening Endoscopic	1 Radioactive Element D Intraluminal Device Y Other Device	Z No Qualifier
5 Esophagus	X External	1 Radioactive Element 2 Monitoring Device 3 Infusion Device D Intraluminal Device U Feeding Device	Z No Qualifier
6 Stomach	Ø Open 3 Percutaneous 4 Percutaneous Endoscopic	Ø Drainage Device 2 Monitoring Device 3 Infusion Device 7 Autologous Tissue Substitute C Extraluminal Device D Intraluminal Device J Synthetic Substitute K Nonautologous Tissue Substitute M Stimulator Lead U Feeding Device Y Other Device	Z No Qualifier
6 Stomach	7 Via Natural or Artificial Opening 8 Via Natural or Artificial Opening Endoscopic	Ø Drainage Device 2 Monitoring Device 3 Infusion Device 7 Autologous Tissue Substitute C Extraluminal Device D Intraluminal Device J Synthetic Substitute K Nonautologous Tissue Substitute U Feeding Device Y Other Device	Z No Qualifier
6 Stomach	X External	Ø Drainage Device 2 Monitoring Device 3 Infusion Device D Intraluminal Device U Feeding Device	Z No Qualifier

ØDP Continued on next page

Non-OR	ØDP[Ø,D][3,4]YZ
Non-OR	ØDP[Ø,D][7,8][Ø,2,3,D,U,Y]Z
Non-OR	ØDP[Ø,D]X[Ø,2,3,D,U]Z
Non-OR	ØDP5[3,4]YZ
Non-OR	ØDP5[7,8][1,D,Y]Z
Non-OR	ØDP5X[1,2,3,D,U]Z
Non-OR	ØDP6[3,4]YZ
Non-OR	ØDP6[7,8][Ø,2,3,D,U,Y]Z
Non-OR	ØDP6X[Ø,2,3,D,U]Z

LC Limited Coverage   **NC** Noncovered   ⊞ Combination Member   HAC associated procedure   Combination Only   DRG Non-OR   Non-OR   New/Revised in GREEN

ICD-10-PCS 2019   377

ØDP–ØDP

ØDP Continued

Ø   **Medical and Surgical**
D   **Gastrointestinal System**
P   **Removal**   Definition: Taking out or off a device from a body part

> Explanation: If a device is taken out and a similar device put in without cutting or puncturing the skin or mucous membrane, the procedure is coded to the root operation CHANGE. Otherwise, the procedure for taking out a device is coded to the root operation REMOVAL.

Body Part Character 4	Approach Character 5	Device Character 6	Qualifier Character 7
P Rectum Anorectal junction	Ø Open 3 Percutaneous 4 Percutaneous Endoscopic 7 Via Natural or Artificial Opening 8 Via Natural or Artificial Opening Endoscopic X External	1 Radioactive Element	Z No Qualifier
Q Anus Anal orifice	Ø Open 3 Percutaneous 4 Percutaneous Endoscopic 7 Via Natural or Artificial Opening 8 Via Natural or Artificial Opening Endoscopic	L Artificial Sphincter	Z No Qualifier
R Anal Sphincter External anal sphincter Internal anal sphincter	Ø Open 3 Percutaneous 4 Percutaneous Endoscopic	M Stimulator Lead	Z No Qualifier
U Omentum Gastrocolic ligament Gastrocolic omentum Gastrohepatic omentum Gastrophrenic ligament Gastrosplenic ligament Greater Omentum Hepatogastric ligament Lesser Omentum **V Mesentery** Mesoappendix Mesocolon **W Peritoneum** Epiploic foramen	Ø Open 3 Percutaneous 4 Percutaneous Endoscopic	Ø Drainage Device 1 Radioactive Element 7 Autologous Tissue Substitute J Synthetic Substitute K Nonautologous Tissue Substitute	Z No Qualifier

Non-OR   ØDPP[7,8,X]1Z

LC Limited Coverage   NC Noncovered   ⊞ Combination Member   HAC associated procedure   Combination Only   DRG Non-OR   Non-OR   New/Revised in GREEN

378   ICD-10-PCS 2019

Ø   Medical and Surgical
D   Gastrointestinal System
Q   Repair   Definition: Restoring, to the extent possible, a body part to its normal anatomic structure and function

                    Explanation: Used only when the method to accomplish the repair is not one of the other root operations

Body Part Character 4	Approach Character 5	Device Character 6	Qualifier Character 7

1 Esophagus, Upper
    Cervical esophagus
2 Esophagus, Middle
    Thoracic esophagus
3 Esophagus, Lower
    Abdominal esophagus
4 Esophagogastric Junction
    Cardia
    Cardioesophageal junction
    Gastroesophageal (GE) junction
5 Esophagus
6 Stomach
7 Stomach, Pylorus
    Pyloric antrum
    Pyloric canal
    Pyloric sphincter
8 Small Intestine ⊞
9 Duodenum ⊞
A Jejunum ⊞
    Duodenojejunal flexure
B Ileum ⊞
C Ileocecal Valve
E Large Intestine ⊞
F Large Intestine, Right ⊞
G Large Intestine, Left ⊞
H Cecum ⊞
J Appendix
    Vermiform appendix
K Ascending Colon ⊞
L Transverse Colon ⊞
    Hepatic flexure
    Splenic flexure
M Descending Colon ⊞
N Sigmoid Colon ⊞
    Rectosigmoid junction
    Sigmoid flexure
P Rectum
    Anorectal junction
	Ø Open
	3 Percutaneous
	4 Percutaneous Endoscopic
	7 Via Natural or Artificial Opening
	8 Via Natural or Artificial Opening
	    Endoscopic
		Z No Device	Z No Qualifier

Q Anus
    Anal orifice
	Ø Open
	3 Percutaneous
	4 Percutaneous Endoscopic
	7 Via Natural or Artificial Opening
	8 Via Natural or Artificial Opening
	    Endoscopic
	X External
		Z No Device	Z No Qualifier

R Anal Sphincter
    External anal sphincter
    Internal anal sphincter
U Omentum
    Gastrocolic ligament
    Gastrocolic omentum
    Gastrohepatic omentum
    Gastrophrenic ligament
    Gastrosplenic ligament
    Greater Omentum
    Hepatogastric ligament
    Lesser Omentum
V Mesentery
    Mesoappendix
    Mesocolon
W Peritoneum
    Epiploic foramen
	Ø Open
	3 Percutaneous
	4 Percutaneous Endoscopic
		Z No Device	Z No Qualifier

See Appendix L for Procedure Combinations
⊞   ØDQ[8,9,A,B,E,F,G,H,K,L,M,N]ØZZ

LC Limited Coverage   NC Noncovered   ⊞ Combination Member   HAC associated procedure   Combination Only   DRG Non-OR   Non-OR   New/Revised in GREEN

Ø   Medical and Surgical
D   Gastrointestinal System
R   Replacement   Definition: Putting in or on biological or synthetic material that physically takes the place and/or function of all or a portion of a body part

Explanation: The body part may have been taken out or replaced, or may be taken out, physically eradicated, or rendered nonfunctional during the REPLACEMENT procedure. A REMOVAL procedure is coded for taking out the device used in a previous replacement procedure.

Body Part Character 4	Approach Character 5	Device Character 6	Qualifier Character 7
5 Esophagus	Ø Open 4 Percutaneous Endoscopic 7 Via Natural or Artificial Opening 8 Via Natural or Artificial Opening Endoscopic	7 Autologous Tissue Substitute J Synthetic Substitute K Nonautologous Tissue Substitute	Z No Qualifier

R   Anal Sphincter
     External anal sphincter
     Internal anal sphincter
U   Omentum
     Gastrocolic ligament
     Gastrocolic omentum
     Gastrohepatic omentum
     Gastrophrenic ligament
     Gastrosplenic ligament
     Greater Omentum
     Hepatogastric ligament
     Lesser Omentum
V   Mesentery
     Mesoappendix
     Mesocolon
W   Peritoneum
     Epiploic foramen
	Ø Open
	4 Percutaneous Endoscopic
		7 Autologous Tissue Substitute
		J Synthetic Substitute
		K Nonautologous Tissue Substitute
			Z No Qualifier

Ø   Medical and Surgical
D   Gastrointestinal System
S   Reposition   Definition: Moving to its normal location, or other suitable location, all or a portion of a body part

Explanation: The body part is moved to a new location from an abnormal location, or from a normal location where it is not functioning correctly. The body part may or may not be cut out or off to be moved to the new location.

Body Part Character 4	Approach Character 5	Device Character 6	Qualifier Character 7

5   Esophagus
6   Stomach
9   Duodenum
A   Jejunum
     Duodenojejunal flexure
B   Ileum
H   Cecum
K   Ascending Colon
L   Transverse Colon
     Hepatic flexure
     Splenic flexure
M   Descending Colon
N   Sigmoid Colon
     Rectosigmoid junction
     Sigmoid flexure
P   Rectum
     Anorectal junction
Q   Anus
     Anal orifice
	Ø Open
	4 Percutaneous Endoscopic
	7 Via Natural or Artificial Opening
	8 Via Natural or Artificial Opening Endoscopic
	X External
		Z No Device	Z No Qualifier

8 Small Intestine E Large Intestine	Ø Open 4 Percutaneous Endoscopic 7 Via Natural or Artificial Opening 8 Via Natural or Artificial Opening Endoscopic	Z No Device	Z No Qualifier

Non-OR   ØDS[5,6,9,A,B,H,K,L,M,N,P,Q]XZZ

LC Limited Coverage   NC Noncovered   ⊞ Combination Member   HAC associated procedure   Combination Only   DRG Non-OR   Non-OR   New/Revised in GREEN

ICD-10-PCS 2019

Ø   Medical and Surgical
D   Gastrointestinal System
T   Resection   Definition: Cutting out or off, without replacement, all of a body part
                  Explanation: None

Body Part Character 4	Approach Character 5	Device Character 6	Qualifier Character 7
1 Esophagus, Upper Cervical esophagus **2 Esophagus, Middle** Thoracic esophagus **3 Esophagus, Lower** Abdominal esophagus **4 Esophagogastric Junction** Cardia Cardioesophageal junction Gastroesophageal (GE) junction **5 Esophagus** **6 Stomach** **7 Stomach, Pylorus** Pyloric antrum Pyloric canal Pyloric sphincter **8 Small Intestine** **9 Duodenum** ⊞ **A Jejunum** Duodenojejunal flexure **B Ileum** **C Ileocecal Valve** **E Large Intestine** **F Large Intestine, Right** **H Cecum** **J Appendix** Vermiform appendix **K Ascending Colon** **P Rectum** Anorectal junction **Q Anus** Anal orifice	**Ø** Open **4** Percutaneous Endoscopic **7** Via Natural or Artificial Opening **8** Via Natural or Artificial Opening Endoscopic	**Z** No Device	**Z** No Qualifier
G Large Intestine, Left **L Transverse Colon** Hepatic flexure Splenic flexure **M Descending Colon** **N Sigmoid Colon** Rectosigmoid junction Sigmoid flexure	**Ø** Open **4** Percutaneous Endoscopic **7** Via Natural or Artificial Opening **8** Via Natural or Artificial Opening Endoscopic **F** Via Natural or Artificial Opening with Percutaneous Endoscopic Assistance	**Z** No Device	**Z** No Qualifier
R Anal Sphincter External anal sphincter Internal anal sphincter **U Omentum** Gastrocolic ligament Gastrocolic omentum Gastrohepatic omentum Gastrophrenic ligament Gastrosplenic ligament Greater Omentum Hepatogastric ligament Lesser Omentum	**Ø** Open **4** Percutaneous Endoscopic	**Z** No Device	**Z** No Qualifier

See Appendix L for Procedure Combinations
  ⊞   ØDT9ØZZ

Ø Medical and Surgical
D Gastrointestinal System
U Supplement   Definition: Putting in or on biological or synthetic material that physically reinforces and/or augments the function of a portion of a body part
                   Explanation: The biological material is non-living, or is living and from the same individual. The body part may have been previously replaced, and the SUPPLEMENT procedure is performed to physically reinforce and/or augment the function of the replaced body part.

Body Part — Character 4	Approach — Character 5	Device — Character 6	Qualifier — Character 7

1 Esophagus, Upper
   Cervical esophagus
2 Esophagus, Middle
   Thoracic esophagus
3 Esophagus, Lower
   Abdominal esophagus
4 Esophagogastric Junction
   Cardia
   Cardioesophageal junction
   Gastroesophageal (GE) junction
5 Esophagus
6 Stomach
7 Stomach, Pylorus
   Pyloric antrum
   Pyloric canal
   Pyloric sphincter
8 Small Intestine
9 Duodenum
A Jejunum
   Duodenojejunal flexure
B Ileum
C Ileocecal Valve
E Large Intestine
F Large Intestine, Right
G Large Intestine, Left
H Cecum
K Ascending Colon
L Transverse Colon
   Hepatic flexure
   Splenic flexure
M Descending Colon
N Sigmoid Colon
   Rectosigmoid junction
   Sigmoid flexure
P Rectum
   Anorectal junction
	Ø Open
	4 Percutaneous Endoscopic
	7 Via Natural or Artificial Opening
	8 Via Natural or Artificial Opening Endoscopic
		7 Autologous Tissue Substitute
		J Synthetic Substitute
		K Nonautologous Tissue Substitute
			Z No Qualifier

Q Anus Anal orifice	Ø Open 4 Percutaneous Endoscopic 7 Via Natural or Artificial Opening 8 Via Natural or Artificial Opening Endoscopic X External	7 Autologous Tissue Substitute J Synthetic Substitute K Nonautologous Tissue Substitute	Z No Qualifier

R Anal Sphincter
   External anal sphincter
   Internal anal sphincter
U Omentum
   Gastrocolic ligament
   Gastrocolic omentum
   Gastrohepatic omentum
   Gastrophrenic ligament
   Gastrosplenic ligament
   Greater Omentum
   Hepatogastric ligament
   Lesser Omentum
V Mesentery
   Mesoappendix
   Mesocolon
W Peritoneum
   Epiploic foramen
	Ø Open
	4 Percutaneous Endoscopic
		7 Autologous Tissue Substitute
		J Synthetic Substitute
		K Nonautologous Tissue Substitute
			Z No Qualifier

LC Limited Coverage   NC Noncovered   ⊞ Combination Member   HAC associated procedure   Combination Only   DRG Non-OR   Non-OR   New/Revised in GREEN

382   ICD-10-PCS 2019

Ø   **Medical and Surgical**
D   **Gastrointestinal System**
V   **Restriction**   Definition: Partially closing an orifice or the lumen of a tubular body part
                       Explanation: The orifice can be a natural orifice or an artificially created orifice

Body Part Character 4		Approach Character 5	Device Character 6	Qualifier Character 7

1 Esophagus, Upper
   Cervical esophagus
2 Esophagus, Middle
   Thoracic esophagus
3 Esophagus, Lower
   Abdominal esophagus
4 Esophagogastric
   Junction
   Cardia
   Cardioesophageal
     junction
   Gastroesophageal (GE)
     junction
5 Esophagus
6 Stomach
7 Stomach, Pylorus
   Pyloric antrum
   Pyloric canal
   Pyloric sphincter
8 Small Intestine
	9 Duodenum
	A Jejunum
	   Duodenojejunal flexure
	B Ileum
	C Ileocecal Valve
	E Large Intestine
	F Large Intestine, Right
	G Large Intestine, Left
	H Cecum
	K Ascending Colon
	L Transverse Colon
	   Hepatic flexure
	   Splenic flexure
	M Descending Colon
	N Sigmoid Colon
	   Rectosigmoid junction
	   Sigmoid flexure
	P Rectum
	   Anorectal junction
		Ø Open
		3 Percutaneous
		4 Percutaneous Endoscopic
			C Extraluminal Device
			D Intraluminal Device
			Z No Device
				Z No Qualifier

1 Esophagus, Upper
   Cervical esophagus
2 Esophagus, Middle
   Thoracic esophagus
3 Esophagus, Lower
   Abdominal esophagus
4 Esophagogastric
   Junction
   Cardia
   Cardioesophageal
     junction
   Gastroesophageal (GE)
     junction
5 Esophagus
6 Stomach   NC
7 Stomach, Pylorus
   Pyloric antrum
   Pyloric canal
   Pyloric sphincter
8 Small Intestine
	9 Duodenum
	A Jejunum
	   Duodenojejunal flexure
	B Ileum
	C Ileocecal Valve
	E Large Intestine
	F Large Intestine, Right
	G Large Intestine, Left
	H Cecum
	K Ascending Colon
	L Transverse Colon
	   Hepatic flexure
	   Splenic flexure
	M Descending Colon
	N Sigmoid Colon
	   Rectosigmoid junction
	   Sigmoid flexure
	P Rectum
	   Anorectal junction
		7 Via Natural or Artificial
		   Opening
		8 Via Natural or Artificial
		   Opening Endoscopic
			D Intraluminal Device
			Z No Device
				Z No Qualifier

Q Anus Anal orifice		**Ø** Open **3** Percutaneous **4** Percutaneous Endoscopic **X** External	**C** Extraluminal Device **D** Intraluminal Device **Z** No Device	**Z** No Qualifier

Q Anus
   Anal orifice
		7 Via Natural or Artificial
		   Opening
		8 Via Natural or Artificial
		   Opening Endoscopic
			D Intraluminal Device
			Z No Device
				Z No Qualifier

Non-OR   ØDV6[7,8]DZ
HAC   ØDV64CZ when reported with PDx E66.Ø1 and SDx K68.11 or K95.Ø1 or K95.81 or T81.4XXA
NC   ØDV6[7,8]DZ

LC Limited Coverage   **NC** Noncovered   ⊞ Combination Member   HAC associated procedure   Combination Only   DRG Non-OR   Non-OR   New/Revised in GREEN
ICD-10-PCS 2019   383

ØDV–ØDV

Ø   Medical and Surgical
D   Gastrointestinal System
W   Revision   Definition: Correcting, to the extent possible, a portion of a malfunctioning device or the position of a displaced device
Explanation: Revision can include correcting a malfunctioning or displaced device by taking out or putting in components of the device such as a screw or pin

Body Part Character 4	Approach Character 5	Device Character 6	Qualifier Character 7
Ø Upper Intestinal Tract D Lower Intestinal Tract	Ø Open 3 Percutaneous 4 Percutaneous Endoscopic 7 Via Natural or Artificial Opening 8 Via Natural or Artificial Opening Endoscopic	Ø Drainage Device 2 Monitoring Device 3 Infusion Device 7 Autologous Tissue Substitute C Extraluminal Device D Intraluminal Device J Synthetic Substitute K Nonautologous Tissue Substitute U Feeding Device Y Other Device	Z No Qualifier
Ø Upper Intestinal Tract D Lower Intestinal Tract	X External	Ø Drainage Device 2 Monitoring Device 3 Infusion Device 7 Autologous Tissue Substitute C Extraluminal Device D Intraluminal Device J Synthetic Substitute K Nonautologous Tissue Substitute U Feeding Device	Z No Qualifier
5 Esophagus	Ø Open 3 Percutaneous 4 Percutaneous Endoscopic	Y Other Device	Z No Qualifier
5 Esophagus	7 Via Natural or Artificial Opening 8 Via Natural or Artificial Opening Endoscopic	D Intraluminal Device Y Other Device	Z No Qualifier
5 Esophagus	X External	D Intraluminal Device	Z No Qualifier
6 Stomach	Ø Open 3 Percutaneous 4 Percutaneous Endoscopic	Ø Drainage Device 2 Monitoring Device 3 Infusion Device 7 Autologous Tissue Substitute C Extraluminal Device D Intraluminal Device J Synthetic Substitute K Nonautologous Tissue Substitute M Stimulator Lead U Feeding Device Y Other Device	Z No Qualifier
6 Stomach	7 Via Natural or Artificial Opening 8 Via Natural or Artificial Opening Endoscopic	Ø Drainage Device 2 Monitoring Device 3 Infusion Device 7 Autologous Tissue Substitute C Extraluminal Device D Intraluminal Device J Synthetic Substitute K Nonautologous Tissue Substitute U Feeding Device Y Other Device	Z No Qualifier
6 Stomach	X External	Ø Drainage Device 2 Monitoring Device 3 Infusion Device 7 Autologous Tissue Substitute C Extraluminal Device D Intraluminal Device J Synthetic Substitute K Nonautologous Tissue Substitute U Feeding Device	Z No Qualifier

ØDW Continued on next page

Non-OR	ØDW[Ø,D][3,4,7,8]YZ
Non-OR	ØDW[Ø,D]X[Ø,2,3,7,C,D,J,K,U]Z
Non-OR	ØDW5[Ø,3,4]YZ
Non-OR	ØDW5[7,8]YZ
Non-OR	ØDW5XDZ
Non-OR	ØDW6[3,4]YZ
Non-OR	ØDW6[7,8]YZ
Non-OR	ØDW6X[Ø,2,3,7,C,D,J,K,U]Z

Ø   Medical and Surgical
D   Gastrointestinal System
W   Revision   Definition: Correcting, to the extent possible, a portion of a malfunctioning device or the position of a displaced device

ØDW Continued

Explanation: Revision can include correcting a malfunctioning or displaced device by taking out or putting in components of the device such as a screw or pin

Body Part Character 4	Approach Character 5	Device Character 6	Qualifier Character 7
8 Small Intestine E Large Intestine	Ø Open 4 Percutaneous Endoscopic 7 Via Natural or Artificial Opening 8 Via Natural or Artificial Opening Endoscopic	7 Autologous Tissue Substitute J Synthetic Substitute K Nonautologous Tissue Substitute	Z No Qualifier
Q Anus Anal orifice	Ø Open 3 Percutaneous 4 Percutaneous Endoscopic 7 Via Natural or Artificial Opening 8 Via Natural or Artificial Opening Endoscopic	L Artificial Sphincter	Z No Qualifier

R   Anal Sphincter
     External anal sphincter
     Internal anal sphincter
	Ø Open
	3 Percutaneous
	4 Percutaneous Endoscopic
		M Stimulator Lead	Z No Qualifier

U   Omentum
     Gastrocolic ligament
     Gastrocolic omentum
     Gastrohepatic omentum
     Gastrophrenic ligament
     Gastrosplenic ligament
     Greater Omentum
     Hepatogastric ligament
     Lesser Omentum
V   Mesentery
     Mesoappendix
     Mesocolon
W   Peritoneum
     Epiploic foramen
	Ø Open
	3 Percutaneous
	4 Percutaneous Endoscopic
		Ø Drainage Device
		7 Autologous Tissue Substitute
		J Synthetic Substitute
		K Nonautologous Tissue Substitute
			Z No Qualifier

Non-OR   ØDW[U,V,W][Ø,3,4]ØZ

Ø   Medical and Surgical
D   Gastrointestinal System
X   Transfer   Definition: Moving, without taking out, all or a portion of a body part to another location to take over the function of all or a portion of a body part

Explanation: The body part transferred remains connected to its vascular and nervous supply

Body Part Character 4	Approach Character 5	Device Character 6	Qualifier Character 7
6 Stomach 8 Small Intestine E Large Intestine	Ø Open 4 Percutaneous Endoscopic	Z No Device	5 Esophagus

---

Ø   Medical and Surgical
D   Gastrointestinal System
Y   Transplantation   Definition: Putting in or on all or a portion of a living body part taken from another individual or animal to physically take the place and/or function of all or a portion of a similar body part

Explanation: The native body part may or may not be taken out, and the transplanted body part may take over all or a portion of its function

Body Part Character 4	Approach Character 5	Device Character 6	Qualifier Character 7
5 Esophagus 6 Stomach 8 Small Intestine LC E Large Intestine LC	Ø Open	Z No Device	Ø Allogeneic 1 Syngeneic 2 Zooplastic

Non-OR   ØDY5ØZ[Ø,1,2]
LC   ØDY[8,E]ØZ[Ø,1,2]

LC Limited Coverage   **NC** Noncovered   ⊞ Combination Member   HAC associated procedure   Combination Only   DRG Non-OR   Non-OR   New/Revised in GREEN

Hepatobiliary System and Pancreas ØF1–ØFY

Character Meanings

This Character Meaning table is provided as a guide to assist the user in the identification of character members that may be found in this section of code tables. It **SHOULD NOT** be used to build a PCS code.

Operation–Character 3	Body Part–Character 4	Approach–Character 5	Device–Character 6	Qualifier–Character 7
1 Bypass	Ø Liver	Ø Open	Ø Drainage Device	Ø Allogeneic
2 Change	1 Liver, Right Lobe	3 Percutaneous	1 Radioactive Element	1 Syngeneic
5 Destruction	2 Liver, Left Lobe	4 Percutaneous Endoscopic	2 Monitoring Device	2 Zooplastic
7 Dilation	4 Gallbladder	7 Via Natural or Artificial Opening	3 Infusion Device	3 Duodenum
8 Division	5 Hepatic Duct, Right	8 Via Natural or Artificial Opening Endoscopic	7 Autologous Tissue Substitute	4 Stomach
9 Drainage	6 Hepatic Duct, Left	X External	C Extraluminal Device	5 Hepatic Duct, Right
B Excision	7 Hepatic Duct, Common		D Intraluminal Device	6 Hepatic Duct, Left
C Extirpation	8 Cystic Duct		J Synthetic Substitute	7 Hepatic Duct, Caudate
D Extraction	9 Common Bile Duct		K Nonautologous Tissue Substitute	
F Fragmentation	B Hepatobiliary Duct		Y Other Device	8 Cystic Duct
H Insertion	C Ampulla of Vater		Z No Device	9 Common Bile Duct
J Inspection	D Pancreatic Duct			B Small Intestine
L Occlusion	F Pancreatic Duct, Accessory			C Large Intestine
M Reattachment	G Pancreas			F Irreversible Electroporation
N Release				X Diagnostic
P Removal				Z No Qualifier
Q Repair				
R Replacement				
S Reposition				
T Resection				
U Supplement				
V Restriction				
W Revision				
Y Transplantation				

AHA Coding Clinic for table ØF7
2016, 3Q, 27   Endoscopic retrograde cholangiopancreatography with sphincterotomy and insertion of pancreatic stent
2016, 1Q, 25   Endoscopic retrograde cholangiopancreatography with brush biopsy of pancreatic and common bile ducts
2015, 1Q, 32   Percutaneous transhepatic biliary drainage catheter placement
2014, 3Q, 15   Drainage of pancreatic pseudocyst

AHA Coding Clinic for table ØF9
2015, 1Q, 32   Percutaneous transhepatic biliary drainage catheter placement
2014, 3Q, 15   Drainage of pancreatic pseudocyst

AHA Coding Clinic for table ØFB
2016, 3Q, 41   Open cholecystectomy with needle biopsy of liver
2016, 1Q, 23   Endoscopic ultrasound with aspiration biopsy of common hepatic duct
2016, 1Q, 25   Endoscopic retrograde cholangiopancreatography with brush biopsy of pancreatic and common bile ducts
2014, 3Q, 32   Pyloric-sparing Whipple procedure

AHA Coding Clinic for table ØFC
2016, 3Q, 27   Endoscopic retrograde cholangiopancreatography with sphincterotomy and insertion of pancreatic stent

AHA Coding Clinic for table ØFQ
2016, 3Q, 27   Revision of common bile duct anastomosis
2013, 4Q, 109   Separating conjoined twins

AHA Coding Clinic for table ØFT
2012, 4Q, 99   Domino liver transplant

AHA Coding Clinic for table ØFY
2014, 3Q, 13   Orthotopic liver transplant with end to side cavoplasty
2012, 4Q, 99   Domino liver transplant

Liver

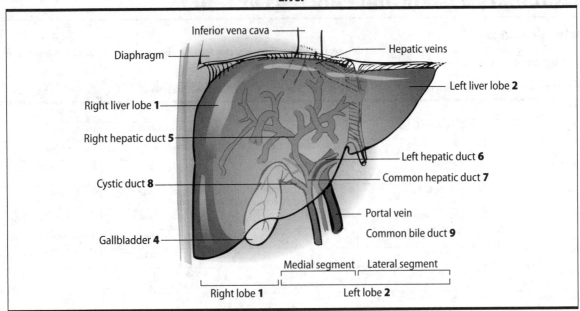

Inferior vena cava
Diaphragm
Hepatic veins
Left liver lobe **2**
Right liver lobe **1**
Right hepatic duct **5**
Left hepatic duct **6**
Common hepatic duct **7**
Cystic duct **8**
Portal vein
Common bile duct **9**
Gallbladder **4**
Medial segment   Lateral segment
Right lobe **1**   Left lobe **2**

Pancreas

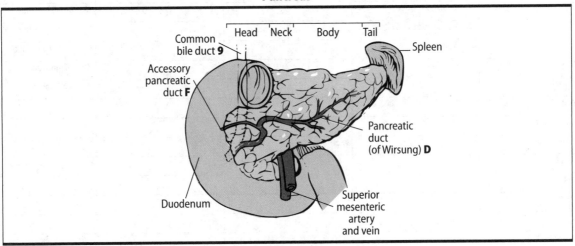

Head   Neck   Body   Tail
Common bile duct **9**
Spleen
Accessory pancreatic duct **F**
Pancreatic duct (of Wirsung) **D**
Duodenum
Superior mesenteric artery and vein

Gallbladder and Ducts

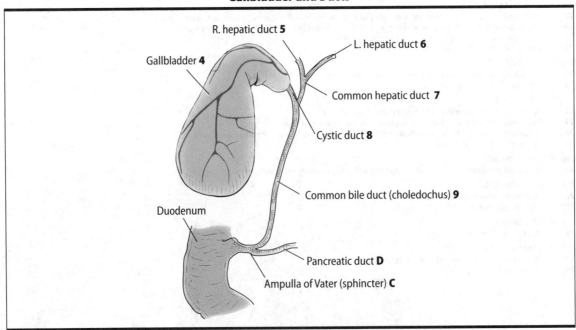

R. hepatic duct **5**
L. hepatic duct **6**
Gallbladder **4**
Common hepatic duct **7**
Cystic duct **8**
Common bile duct (choledochus) **9**
Duodenum
Pancreatic duct **D**
Ampulla of Vater (sphincter) **C**

Ø   **Medical and Surgical**
F   **Hepatobiliary System and Pancreas**
1   **Bypass**   Definition: Altering the route of passage of the contents of a tubular body part

Explanation: Rerouting contents of a body part to a downstream area of the normal route, to a similar route and body part, or to an abnormal route and dissimilar body part. Includes one or more anastomoses, with or without the use of a device.

Body Part Character 4	Approach Character 5	Device Character 6	Qualifier Character 7
4 Gallbladder 5 Hepatic Duct, Right 6 Hepatic Duct, Left 7 Hepatic Duct, Common 8 Cystic Duct 9 Common Bile Duct	Ø Open 4 Percutaneous Endoscopic	D Intraluminal Device Z No Device	3 Duodenum 4 Stomach 5 Hepatic Duct, Right 6 Hepatic Duct, Left 7 Hepatic Duct, Caudate 8 Cystic Duct 9 Common Bile Duct B Small Intestine

D Pancreatic Duct
   Duct of Wirsung
F Pancreatic Duct, Accessory
   Duct of Santorini
G Pancreas
	Ø Open
	4 Percutaneous Endoscopic
		D Intraluminal Device
		Z No Device
			3 Duodenum
			B Small Intestine
			C Large Intestine

Ø   **Medical and Surgical**
F   **Hepatobiliary System and Pancreas**
2   **Change**   Definition: Taking out or off a device from a body part and putting back an identical or similar device in or on the same body part without cutting or puncturing the skin or a mucous membrane

Explanation: All CHANGE procedures are coded using the approach EXTERNAL

Body Part Character 4	Approach Character 5	Device Character 6	Qualifier Character 7

Ø Liver
   Quadrate lobe
4 Gallbladder
B Hepatobiliary Duct
D Pancreatic Duct
   Duct of Wirsung
G Pancreas
	X External	Ø Drainage Device
		Y Other Device
			Z No Qualifier

Non-OR   All body part, approach, device, and qualifier values

Ø   **Medical and Surgical**
F   **Hepatobiliary System and Pancreas**
5   **Destruction**   Definition: Physical eradication of all or a portion of a body part by the direct use of energy, force, or a destructive agent

Explanation: None of the body part is physically taken out

Body Part Character 4	Approach Character 5	Device Character 6	Qualifier Character 7
Ø Liver Quadrate lobe 1 Liver, Right Lobe 2 Liver, Left Lobe	Ø Open 3 Percutaneous 4 Percutaneous Endoscopic	Z No Device	F Irreversible Electroporation Z No Qualifier
4 Gallbladder	Ø Open 3 Percutaneous 4 Percutaneous Endoscopic 8 Via Natural or Artificial Opening Endoscopic	Z No Device	Z No Qualifier

5 Hepatic Duct, Right
6 Hepatic Duct, Left
7 Hepatic Duct, Common
8 Cystic Duct
9 Common Bile Duct
C Ampulla of Vater
   Duodenal ampulla
   Hepatopancreatic ampulla
D Pancreatic Duct
   Duct of Wirsung
F Pancreatic Duct, Accessory
   Duct of Santorini
	Ø Open
	3 Percutaneous
	4 Percutaneous Endoscopic
	7 Via Natural or Artificial Opening
	8 Via Natural or Artificial Opening
	   Endoscopic
		Z No Device	Z No Qualifier

G Pancreas	Ø Open 3 Percutaneous 4 Percutaneous Endoscopic	Z No Device	F Irreversible Electroporation Z No Qualifier
G Pancreas	8 Via Natural or Artificial Opening Endoscopic	Z No Device	Z No Qualifier

Non-OR   ØF5[5,6,7,8,9,C,D,F][4,8]ZZ
Non-OR   ØF5G4ZZ
Non-OR   ØF5G8ZZ

Ø   Medical and Surgical
F   Hepatobiliary System and Pancreas
7   Dilation   Definition: Expanding an orifice or the lumen of a tubular body part

Explanation: The orifice can be a natural orifice or an artificially created orifice. Accomplished by stretching a tubular body part using intraluminal pressure or by cutting part of the orifice or wall of the tubular body part.

Body Part Character 4	Approach Character 5	Device Character 6	Qualifier Character 7

5   Hepatic Duct, Right
6   Hepatic Duct, Left
7   Hepatic Duct, Common
8   Cystic Duct
9   Common Bile Duct
C   Ampulla of Vater
    Duodenal ampulla
    Hepatopancreatic ampulla
D   Pancreatic Duct
    Duct of Wirsung
F   Pancreatic Duct, Accessory
    Duct of Santorini
	Ø Open
	3 Percutaneous
	4 Percutaneous Endoscopic
	7 Via Natural or Artificial Opening
	8 Via Natural or Artificial Opening
	    Endoscopic
		D Intraluminal Device
		Z No Device
			Z No Qualifier

Non-OR	ØF7[5,6,7,8,9][3,4][D,Z]Z		
Non-OR	ØF7[5,6,7,8,9,D][7,8]DZ	**See Appendix L for Procedure Combinations**	
Non-OR	ØF7[5,6,7,8,9,C,D,F]8ZZ	**Combo-only** ØF7[5,6,8,9,D][7,8]DZ	
Non-OR	ØF7[D,F]4[D,Z]Z		
Non-OR	ØF7[C,F]8DZ		

Ø   Medical and Surgical
F   Hepatobiliary System and Pancreas
8   Division   Definition: Cutting into a body part, without draining fluids and/or gases from the body part, in order to separate or transect a body part

Explanation: All or a portion of the body part is separated into two or more portions

Body Part Character 4	Approach Character 5	Device Character 6	Qualifier Character 7
G Pancreas	Ø Open 3 Percutaneous 4 Percutaneous Endoscopic	Z No Device	Z No Qualifier

LC Limited Coverage   **NC** Noncovered   ⊞ Combination Member   HAC associated procedure   Combination Only   DRG Non-OR   Non-OR   New/Revised in GREEN

Ø   **Medical and Surgical**
F   **Hepatobiliary System and Pancreas**
9   **Drainage**   Definition: Taking or letting out fluids and/or gases from a body part
                         Explanation: The qualifier DIAGNOSTIC is used to identify drainage procedures that are biopsies

Body Part Character 4	Approach Character 5	Device Character 6	Qualifier Character 7
Ø **Liver** Quadrate lobe 1 **Liver, Right Lobe** 2 **Liver, Left Lobe**	Ø **Open** 3 **Percutaneous** 4 **Percutaneous Endoscopic**	Ø **Drainage Device**	Z **No Qualifier**
Ø **Liver** Quadrate lobe 1 **Liver, Right Lobe** 2 **Liver, Left Lobe**	Ø **Open** 3 **Percutaneous** 4 **Percutaneous Endoscopic**	Z **No Device**	X **Diagnostic** Z **No Qualifier**
4 **Gallbladder** G **Pancreas**	Ø **Open** 3 **Percutaneous** 4 **Percutaneous Endoscopic** 8 **Via Natural or Artificial Opening Endoscopic**	Ø **Drainage Device**	Z **No Qualifier**
4 **Gallbladder** G **Pancreas**	Ø **Open** 3 **Percutaneous** 4 **Percutaneous Endoscopic** 8 **Via Natural or Artificial Opening Endoscopic**	Z **No Device**	X **Diagnostic** Z **No Qualifier**

5 **Hepatic Duct, Right**
6 **Hepatic Duct, Left**
7 **Hepatic Duct, Common**
8 **Cystic Duct**
9 **Common Bile Duct**
C **Ampulla of Vater**
    Duodenal ampulla
    Hepatopancreatic ampulla
D **Pancreatic Duct**
    Duct of Wirsung
F **Pancreatic Duct, Accessory**
    Duct of Santorini
	Ø **Open**
	3 **Percutaneous**
	4 **Percutaneous Endoscopic**
	7 **Via Natural or Artificial Opening**
	8 **Via Natural or Artificial Opening Endoscopic**
		Ø **Drainage Device**	Z **No Qualifier**

5 **Hepatic Duct, Right**
6 **Hepatic Duct, Left**
7 **Hepatic Duct, Common**
8 **Cystic Duct**
9 **Common Bile Duct**
C **Ampulla of Vater**
    Duodenal ampulla
    Hepatopancreatic ampulla
D **Pancreatic Duct**
    Duct of Wirsung
F **Pancreatic Duct, Accessory**
    Duct of Santorini
	Ø **Open**
	3 **Percutaneous**
	4 **Percutaneous Endoscopic**
	7 **Via Natural or Artificial Opening**
	8 **Via Natural or Artificial Opening Endoscopic**
		Z **No Device**	X **Diagnostic**
			Z **No Qualifier**

Non-OR ØF9[Ø,1,2][3,4]ØZ	**Non-OR** ØF99[3,8]ØZ	
Non-OR ØF9[Ø,1,2][3,4]Z[X,Z]	**Non-OR** ØF9C[3,4,8]ØZ	
Non-OR ØF9[4,G]8ØZ	**Non-OR** ØF9[D,F][3,8]ØZ	
Non-OR ØF9G3ØZ	**Non-OR** ØF9[5,6,8,9,C,D,F]3Z[X,Z]	
Non-OR ØF9[4,G]8Z[X,Z]	**Non-OR** ØF9[5,6,8,9,C,D,F][4,7,8]ZX	
Non-OR ØF9G3Z[XZ]	**Non-OR** ØF9[5,6,8,D,F]8ZZ	
Non-OR ØF9G4ZX	**Non-OR** ØF97[3,4,7,8]Z[X,Z]	
Non-OR ØF9[5,6,8][3,8]ØZ	**Non-OR** ØF99[4,7,8]ZZ	
Non-OR ØF97[3,4,7,8]ØZ	**Non-OR** ØF9C[4,8]ZZ	

LC Limited Coverage   NC Noncovered   ⊞ Combination Member   HAC associated procedure   Combination Only   DRG Non-OR   Non-OR   New/Revised in GREEN

ICD-10-PCS 2019   391

ØF9–ØF9

Hepatobiliary System and Pancreas

0   **Medical and Surgical**
F   **Hepatobiliary System and Pancreas**
B   **Excision**   Definition: Cutting out or off, without replacement, a portion of a body part

Explanation: The qualifier DIAGNOSTIC is used to identify excision procedures that are biopsies

Body Part Character 4	Approach Character 5	Device Character 6	Qualifier Character 7
0 Liver Quadrate lobe **1** Liver, Right Lobe **2** Liver, Left Lobe	**0** Open **3** Percutaneous **4** Percutaneous Endoscopic	**Z** No Device	**X** Diagnostic **Z** No Qualifier
4 Gallbladder **G** Pancreas	**0** Open **3** Percutaneous **4** Percutaneous Endoscopic **8** Via Natural or Artificial Opening Endoscopic	**Z** No Device	**X** Diagnostic **Z** No Qualifier

5   Hepatic Duct, Right
6   Hepatic Duct, Left
7   Hepatic Duct, Common
8   Cystic Duct
9   Common Bile Duct
C   Ampulla of Vater
     Duodenal ampulla
     Hepatopancreatic ampulla
D   Pancreatic Duct
     Duct of Wirsung
F   Pancreatic Duct, Accessory
     Duct of Santorini
	0 Open
	3 Percutaneous
	4 Percutaneous Endoscopic
	7 Via Natural or Artificial Opening
	8 Via Natural or Artificial Opening
	     Endoscopic
		Z No Device	**X** Diagnostic
			Z No Qualifier

Non-OR   0FB[0,1,2]3ZX
Non-OR   0FB[4,G][3,4,8]ZX
Non-OR   0FB[5,6,7,8,9,C,D,F][3,4,7,8]ZX
Non-OR   0FB[5,6,7,8,9,C,D,F][4,8]ZZ

0   **Medical and Surgical**
F   **Hepatobiliary System and Pancreas**
C   **Extirpation**   Definition: Taking or cutting out solid matter from a body part

Explanation: The solid matter may be an abnormal byproduct of a biological function or a foreign body; it may be imbedded in a body part or in the lumen of a tubular body part. The solid matter may or may not have been previously broken into pieces.

Body Part Character 4	Approach Character 5	Device Character 6	Qualifier Character 7
0 Liver Quadrate lobe **1** Liver, Right Lobe **2** Liver, Left Lobe	**0** Open **3** Percutaneous **4** Percutaneous Endoscopic	**Z** No Device	**Z** No Qualifier
4 Gallbladder **G** Pancreas	**0** Open **3** Percutaneous **4** Percutaneous Endoscopic **8** Via Natural or Artificial Opening Endoscopic	**Z** No Device	**Z** No Qualifier

5   Hepatic Duct, Right
6   Hepatic Duct, Left
7   Hepatic Duct, Common
8   Cystic Duct
9   Common Bile Duct
C   Ampulla of Vater
     Duodenal ampulla
     Hepatopancreatic ampulla
D   Pancreatic Duct
     Duct of Wirsung
F   Pancreatic Duct, Accessory
     Duct of Santorini
	0 Open
	3 Percutaneous
	4 Percutaneous Endoscopic
	7 Via Natural or Artificial Opening
	8 Via Natural or Artificial Opening
	     Endoscopic
		Z No Device	**Z** No Qualifier

Non-OR   0FC[5,6,7,8,9][3,4,7,8]ZZ
Non-OR   0FCC[4,8]ZZ
Non-OR   0FC[D,F][3,4,8]ZZ

LC Limited Coverage   **NC** Noncovered   ⊞ Combination Member   HAC associated procedure   Combination Only   DRG Non-OR   Non-OR   New/Revised in GREEN

392   ICD-10-PCS 2019

Ø   **Medical and Surgical**
F   **Hepatobiliary System and Pancreas**
D   **Extraction**   Definition: Pulling or stripping out or off all or a portion of a body part by the use of force
                             Explanation: The qualifier DIAGNOSTIC is used to identify extraction procedures that are biopsies

Body Part Character 4	Approach Character 5	Device Character 6	Qualifier Character 7
Ø Liver Quadrate lobe **1** Liver, Right Lobe **2** Liver, Left Lobe	**3** Percutaneous **4** Percutaneous Endoscopic	**Z** No Device	**X** Diagnostic

4   Gallbladder
5   Hepatic Duct, Right
6   Hepatic Duct, Left
7   Hepatic Duct, Common
8   Cystic Duct
9   Common Bile Duct
C   Ampulla of Vater
     Duodenal ampulla
     Hepatopancreatic ampulla
D   Pancreatic Duct
     Duct of Wirsung
F   Pancreatic Duct, Accessory
     Duct of Santorini
G   Pancreas
	3 Percutaneous
	4 Percutaneous Endoscopic
	8 Via Natural or Artificial Opening
	     Endoscopic
		Z No Device	**X** Diagnostic

Ø   **Medical and Surgical**
F   **Hepatobiliary System and Pancreas**
F   **Fragmentation**   Definition: Breaking solid matter in a body part into pieces
                             Explanation: Physical force (e.g., manual, ultrasonic) applied directly or indirectly is used to break the solid matter into pieces. The solid matter may be an abnormal byproduct of a biological function or a foreign body. The pieces of solid matter are not taken out.

Body Part Character 4	Approach Character 5	Device Character 6	Qualifier Character 7

4   **Gallbladder**   NC
5   **Hepatic Duct, Right**   NC
6   **Hepatic Duct, Left**   NC
7   **Hepatic Duct, Common**
8   **Cystic Duct**
9   **Common Bile Duct**   NC
C   **Ampulla of Vater**   NC
     Duodenal ampulla
     Hepatopancreatic ampulla
D   **Pancreatic Duct**   NC
     Duct of Wirsung
F   **Pancreatic Duct, Accessory**   NC
     Duct of Santorini
	Ø Open
	3 Percutaneous
	4 Percutaneous Endoscopic
	7 Via Natural or Artificial Opening
	8 Via Natural or Artificial Opening
	     Endoscopic
	X External
		Z No Device	**Z** No Qualifier

Non-OR   ØFF[4,5,6,7,8,9,C,D,F][8,X]ZZ
NC   ØFF[4,5,6,8,9,C,D,F]XZZ

Ø   **Medical and Surgical**
F   **Hepatobiliary System and Pancreas**
H   **Insertion**   Definition: Putting in a nonbiological appliance that monitors, assists, performs, or prevents a physiological function but does not physically take the place of a body part
                           Explanation: None

Body Part Character 4	Approach Character 5	Device Character 6	Qualifier Character 7
Ø Liver Quadrate lobe **4** Gallbladder **G** Pancreas	**Ø** Open **3** Percutaneous **4** Percutaneous Endoscopic	**2** Monitoring Device **3** Infusion Device **Y** Other Device	**Z** No Qualifier
1 Liver, Right Lobe **2** Liver, Left Lobe	**Ø** Open **3** Percutaneous **4** Percutaneous Endoscopic	**2** Monitoring Device **3** Infusion Device	**Z** No Qualifier

B   Hepatobiliary Duct
D   Pancreatic Duct
     Duct of Wirsung
	Ø Open
	3 Percutaneous
	4 Percutaneous Endoscopic
	7 Via Natural or Artificial Opening
	8 Via Natural or Artificial Opening
	     Endoscopic
		1 Radioactive Element
		2 Monitoring Device
		3 Infusion Device
		D Intraluminal Device
		Y Other Device
			Z No Qualifier

Non-OR   ØFH[Ø,4,G][Ø,3,4]3Z
Non-OR   ØFH[Ø,4,G][3,4]YZ
Non-OR   ØFH[1,2][Ø,3,4]3Z
Non-OR   ØFH[B,D][Ø,3,4]3Z
Non-OR   ØFH[B,D]4DZ
Non-OR   ØFH[B,D][7,8][2,3]Z
Non-OR   ØFH[B,D]8DZ
Non-OR   ØFH[B,D][3,4,7,8]YZ

See Appendix L for Procedure Combinations
Combo-only   ØFHB8DZ

LC Limited Coverage   NC Noncovered   ⊞ Combination Member   HAC associated procedure   Combination Only   DRG Non-OR   Non-OR   New/Revised in GREEN
ICD-10-PCS 2019   **393**

ØFD–ØFH

Ø   Medical and Surgical
F   Hepatobiliary System and Pancreas
J   Inspection   Definition: Visually and/or manually exploring a body part

Explanation: Visual exploration may be performed with or without optical instrumentation. Manual exploration may be performed directly or through intervening body layers.

Body Part Character 4	Approach Character 5	Device Character 6	Qualifier Character 7
Ø Liver Quadrate lobe	Ø Open 3 Percutaneous 4 Percutaneous Endoscopic X External	Z No Device	Z No Qualifier
4 Gallbladder G Pancreas	Ø Open 3 Percutaneous 4 Percutaneous Endoscopic 8 Via Natural or Artificial Opening Endoscopic X External	Z No Device	Z No Qualifier

B   Hepatobiliary Duct
D   Pancreatic Duct
     Duct of Wirsung
	Ø Open
	3 Percutaneous
	4 Percutaneous Endoscopic
	7 Via Natural or Artificial Opening
	8 Via Natural or Artificial Opening
	     Endoscopic
		Z No Device	Z No Qualifier

Non-OR	ØFJØ[3,X]ZZ
Non-OR	ØFJ[4,G][3,8,X]ZZ
Non-OR	ØFJ[B,D][3,7,8]ZZ

Ø   Medical and Surgical
F   Hepatobiliary System and Pancreas
L   Occlusion   Definition: Completely closing an orifice or the lumen of a tubular body part

Explanation: The orifice can be a natural orifice or an artificially created orifice

Body Part Character 4	Approach Character 5	Device Character 6	Qualifier Character 7

5   Hepatic Duct, Right
6   Hepatic Duct, Left
7   Hepatic Duct, Common
8   Cystic Duct
9   Common Bile Duct
C   Ampulla of Vater
     Duodenal ampulla
     Hepatopancreatic ampulla
D   Pancreatic Duct
     Duct of Wirsung
F   Pancreatic Duct, Accessory
     Duct of Santorini
	Ø Open
	3 Percutaneous
	4 Percutaneous Endoscopic
		C Extraluminal Device
		D Intraluminal Device
		Z No Device
			Z No Qualifier

5   Hepatic Duct, Right
6   Hepatic Duct, Left
7   Hepatic Duct, Common
8   Cystic Duct
9   Common Bile Duct
C   Ampulla of Vater
     Duodenal ampulla
     Hepatopancreatic ampulla
D   Pancreatic Duct
     Duct of Wirsung
F   Pancreatic Duct, Accessory
     Duct of Santorini
	7 Via Natural or Artificial Opening
	8 Via Natural or Artificial Opening
	     Endoscopic
		D Intraluminal Device
		Z No Device
			Z No Qualifier

Non-OR	ØFL[5,6,7,8,9][3,4][C,D,Z]Z
Non-OR	ØFL[5,6,7,8,9][7,8][D,Z]Z

LC Limited Coverage   NC Noncovered   ⊞ Combination Member   HAC associated procedure   Combination Only   DRG Non-OR   Non-OR   New/Revised in GREEN

394   ICD-10-PCS 2019

Ø **Medical and Surgical**
F **Hepatobiliary System and Pancreas**
M **Reattachment** Definition: Putting back in or on all or a portion of a separated body part to its normal location or other suitable location
　　　　　　　　Explanation: Vascular circulation and nervous pathways may or may not be reestablished

Body Part Character 4	Approach Character 5	Device Character 6	Qualifier Character 7
Ø Liver 　Quadrate lobe **1** Liver, Right Lobe **2** Liver, Left Lobe **4** Gallbladder **5** Hepatic Duct, Right **6** Hepatic Duct, Left **7** Hepatic Duct, Common **8** Cystic Duct **9** Common Bile Duct **C** Ampulla of Vater 　Duodenal ampulla 　Hepatopancreatic ampulla **D** Pancreatic Duct 　Duct of Wirsung **F** Pancreatic Duct, Accessory 　Duct of Santorini **G** Pancreas	**Ø** Open **4** Percutaneous Endoscopic	**Z** No Device	**Z** No Qualifier

Non-OR ØFM[4,5,6,7,8,9]4ZZ

Ø **Medical and Surgical**
F **Hepatobiliary System and Pancreas**
N **Release** Definition: Freeing a body part from an abnormal physical constraint by cutting or by the use of force
　　　　　Explanation: Some of the restraining tissue may be taken out but none of the body part is taken out

Body Part Character 4	Approach Character 5	Device Character 6	Qualifier Character 7
Ø Liver 　Quadrate lobe **1** Liver, Right Lobe **2** Liver, Left Lobe	**Ø** Open **3** Percutaneous **4** Percutaneous Endoscopic	**Z** No Device	**Z** No Qualifier
4 Gallbladder **G** Pancreas	**Ø** Open **3** Percutaneous **4** Percutaneous Endoscopic **8** Via Natural or Artificial Opening 　Endoscopic	**Z** No Device	**Z** No Qualifier
5 Hepatic Duct, Right **6** Hepatic Duct, Left **7** Hepatic Duct, Common **8** Cystic Duct **9** Common Bile Duct **C** Ampulla of Vater 　Duodenal ampulla 　Hepatopancreatic ampulla **D** Pancreatic Duct 　Duct of Wirsung **F** Pancreatic Duct, Accessory 　Duct of Santorini	**Ø** Open **3** Percutaneous **4** Percutaneous Endoscopic **7** Via Natural or Artificial Opening **8** Via Natural or Artificial Opening 　Endoscopic	**Z** No Device	**Z** No Qualifier

Ø   Medical and Surgical
F   Hepatobiliary System and Pancreas
P   Removal   Definition: Taking out or off a device from a body part

Explanation: If a device is taken out and a similar device put in without cutting or puncturing the skin or mucous membrane, the procedure is coded to the root operation CHANGE. Otherwise, the procedure for taking out a device is coded to the root operation REMOVAL.

Body Part Character 4	Approach Character 5	Device Character 6	Qualifier Character 7
Ø Liver Quadrate lobe	Ø Open 3 Percutaneous 4 Percutaneous Endoscopic	Ø Drainage Device 2 Monitoring Device 3 Infusion Device Y Other Device	Z No Qualifier
Ø Liver Quadrate lobe	X External	Ø Drainage Device 2 Monitoring Device 3 Infusion Device	Z No Qualifier
4 Gallbladder G Pancreas	Ø Open 3 Percutaneous 4 Percutaneous Endoscopic	Ø Drainage Device 2 Monitoring Device 3 Infusion Device D Intraluminal Device Y Other Device	Z No Qualifier
4 Gallbladder G Pancreas	X External	Ø Drainage Device 2 Monitoring Device 3 Infusion Device D Intraluminal Device	Z No Qualifier

B Hepatobiliary Duct
D Pancreatic Duct
   Duct of Wirsung
	Ø Open
	3 Percutaneous
	4 Percutaneous Endoscopic
	7 Via Natural or Artificial Opening
	8 Via Natural or Artificial Opening
	   Endoscopic
		Ø Drainage Device
		1 Radioactive Element
		2 Monitoring Device
		3 Infusion Device
		7 Autologous Tissue Substitute
		C Extraluminal Device
		D Intraluminal Device
		J Synthetic Substitute
		K Nonautologous Tissue Substitute
		Y Other Device
			Z No Qualifier

B Hepatobiliary Duct D Pancreatic Duct Duct of Wirsung	X External	Ø Drainage Device 1 Radioactive Element 2 Monitoring Device 3 Infusion Device D Intraluminal Device	Z No Qualifier

Non-OR	ØFPØ[3,4]YZ	
Non-OR	ØFPØX[Ø,2,3]Z	
Non-OR	ØFP[4,G][3,4]YZ	
Non-OR	ØFP4X[Ø,2,3,D]Z	
Non-OR	ØFPGX[Ø,2,3]Z	
Non-OR	ØFP[B,D][3,4]YZ	
Non-OR	ØFP[B,D][7,8][Ø,2,3,D,Y]Z	
Non-OR	ØFP[B,D]X[Ø,1,2,3,D]Z	

See Appendix L for Procedure Combinations
Combo-only   ØFP[B,D]XDZ

Ø   Medical and Surgical
F   Hepatobiliary System and Pancreas
Q   Repair   Definition: Restoring, to the extent possible, a body part to its normal anatomic structure and function

Explanation: Used only when the method to accomplish the repair is not one of the other root operations

Body Part Character 4	Approach Character 5	Device Character 6	Qualifier Character 7
Ø Liver Quadrate lobe **1** Liver, Right Lobe **2** Liver, Left Lobe	**Ø** Open **3** Percutaneous **4** Percutaneous Endoscopic	**Z** No Device	**Z** No Qualifier
4 Gallbladder **G** Pancreas	**Ø** Open **3** Percutaneous **4** Percutaneous Endoscopic **8** Via Natural or Artificial Opening Endoscopic	**Z** No Device	**Z** No Qualifier

5 Hepatic Duct, Right
6 Hepatic Duct, Left
7 Hepatic Duct, Common
8 Cystic Duct
9 Common Bile Duct
C Ampulla of Vater
   Duodenal ampulla
   Hepatopancreatic ampulla
D Pancreatic Duct
   Duct of Wirsung
F Pancreatic Duct, Accessory
   Duct of Santorini
	Ø Open
	3 Percutaneous
	4 Percutaneous Endoscopic
	7 Via Natural or Artificial Opening
	8 Via Natural or Artificial Opening
	   Endoscopic
		Z No Device	**Z** No Qualifier

Ø   Medical and Surgical
F   Hepatobiliary System and Pancreas
R   Replacement   Definition: Putting in or on biological or synthetic material that physically takes the place and/or function of all or a portion of a body part

Explanation: The body part may have been taken out or replaced, or may be taken out, physically eradicated, or rendered nonfunctional during the REPLACEMENT procedure. A REMOVAL procedure is coded for taking out the device used in a previous replacement procedure.

Body Part Character 4	Approach Character 5	Device Character 6	Qualifier Character 7

5 Hepatic Duct, Right
6 Hepatic Duct, Left
7 Hepatic Duct, Common
8 Cystic Duct
9 Common Bile Duct
C Ampulla of Vater
   Duodenal ampulla
   Hepatopancreatic ampulla
D Pancreatic Duct
   Duct of Wirsung
F Pancreatic Duct, Accessory
   Duct of Santorini
	Ø Open
	4 Percutaneous Endoscopic
	8 Via Natural or Artificial Opening
	   Endoscopic
		7 Autologous Tissue Substitute
		J Synthetic Substitute
		K Nonautologous Tissue Substitute
			Z No Qualifier

Ø   Medical and Surgical
F   Hepatobiliary System and Pancreas
S   Reposition   Definition: Moving to its normal location, or other suitable location, all or a portion of a body part

Explanation: The body part is moved to a new location from an abnormal location, or from a normal location where it is not functioning correctly. The body part may or may not be cut out or off to be moved to the new location.

Body Part Character 4	Approach Character 5	Device Character 6	Qualifier Character 7

Ø Liver
   Quadrate lobe
4 Gallbladder
5 Hepatic Duct, Right
6 Hepatic Duct, Left
7 Hepatic Duct, Common
8 Cystic Duct
9 Common Bile Duct
C Ampulla of Vater
   Duodenal ampulla
   Hepatopancreatic ampulla
D Pancreatic Duct
   Duct of Wirsung
F Pancreatic Duct, Accessory
   Duct of Santorini
G Pancreas
	Ø Open
	4 Percutaneous Endoscopic
		Z No Device	**Z** No Qualifier

LC Limited Coverage   **NC** Noncovered   ⊞ Combination Member   HAC associated procedure   Combination Only   DRG Non-OR   Non-OR   New/Revised in GREEN

ICD-10-PCS 2019   397

Ø   Medical and Surgical
F   Hepatobiliary System and Pancreas
T   Resection   Definition: Cutting out or off, without replacement, all of a body part

               Explanation: None

Body Part Character 4	Approach Character 5	Device Character 6	Qualifier Character 7
Ø Liver Quadrate lobe **1** Liver, Right Lobe **2** Liver, Left Lobe **4** Gallbladder **G** Pancreas ⊞	**Ø** Open **4** Percutaneous Endoscopic	**Z** No Device	**Z** No Qualifier

5 Hepatic Duct, Right
6 Hepatic Duct, Left
7 Hepatic Duct, Common
8 Cystic Duct
9 Common Bile Duct
C Ampulla of Vater
    Duodenal ampulla
    Hepatopancreatic ampulla
D Pancreatic Duct
    Duct of Wirsung
F Pancreatic Duct, Accessory
    Duct of Santorini
	Ø Open
	4 Percutaneous Endoscopic
	7 Via Natural or Artificial Opening
	8 Via Natural or Artificial Opening
	    Endoscopic
		Z No Device	**Z** No Qualifier

Non-OR   ØFT[D,F][4,8]ZZ

See Appendix L for Procedure Combinations
    ⊞   ØFTGØZZ

Ø   Medical and Surgical
F   Hepatobiliary System and Pancreas
U   Supplement   Definition: Putting in or on biological or synthetic material that physically reinforces and/or augments the function of a portion of a body part

               Explanation: The biological material is non-living, or is living and from the same individual. The body part may have been previously replaced, and the SUPPLEMENT procedure is performed to physically reinforce and/or augment the function of the replaced body part.

Body Part Character 4	Approach Character 5	Device Character 6	Qualifier Character 7

5 Hepatic Duct, Right
6 Hepatic Duct, Left
7 Hepatic Duct, Common
8 Cystic Duct
9 Common Bile Duct
C Ampulla of Vater
    Duodenal ampulla
    Hepatopancreatic ampulla
D Pancreatic Duct
    Duct of Wirsung
F Pancreatic Duct, Accessory
    Duct of Santorini
	Ø Open
	3 Percutaneous
	4 Percutaneous Endoscopic
	8 Via Natural or Artificial Opening
	    Endoscopic
		7 Autologous Tissue Substitute
		J Synthetic Substitute
		K Nonautologous Tissue Substitute
			Z No Qualifier

LG Limited Coverage   NC Noncovered   ⊞ Combination Member   HAC associated procedure   Combination Only   DRG Non-OR   Non-OR   New/Revised in GREEN

Ø　**Medical and Surgical**
F　**Hepatobiliary System and Pancreas**
V　**Restriction**　　　Definition: Partially closing an orifice or the lumen of a tubular body part
　　　　　　　　　　　　Explanation: The orifice can be a natural orifice or an artificially created orifice

Body Part Character 4	Approach Character 5	Device Character 6	Qualifier Character 7
5　Hepatic Duct, Right 6　Hepatic Duct, Left 7　Hepatic Duct, Common 8　Cystic Duct 9　Common Bile Duct C　Ampulla of Vater 　　Duodenal ampulla 　　Hepatopancreatic ampulla D　Pancreatic Duct 　　Duct of Wirsung F　Pancreatic Duct, Accessory 　　Duct of Santorini	Ø　Open 3　Percutaneous 4　Percutaneous Endoscopic	C　Extraluminal Device D　Intraluminal Device Z　No Device	Z　No Qualifier
5　Hepatic Duct, Right 6　Hepatic Duct, Left 7　Hepatic Duct, Common 8　Cystic Duct 9　Common Bile Duct C　Ampulla of Vater 　　Duodenal ampulla 　　Hepatopancreatic ampulla D　Pancreatic Duct 　　Duct of Wirsung F　Pancreatic Duct, Accessory 　　Duct of Santorini	7　Via Natural or Artificial Opening 8　Via Natural or Artificial Opening 　　Endoscopic	D　Intraluminal Device Z　No Device	Z　No Qualifier

Non-OR　ØFV[5,6,7,8,9][3,4][C,D,Z]Z
Non-OR　ØFV[5,6,7,8,9][7,8][D,Z]Z

Ø   **Medical and Surgical**
F   **Hepatobiliary System and Pancreas**
W   **Revision**   Definition: Correcting, to the extent possible, a portion of a malfunctioning device or the position of a displaced device .

                 Explanation: Revision can include correcting a malfunctioning or displaced device by taking out or putting in components of the device such as a screw or pin

Body Part Character 4	Approach Character 5	Device Character 6	Qualifier Character 7
Ø Liver Quadrate lobe	**Ø** Open **3** Percutaneous **4** Percutaneous Endoscopic	**Ø** Drainage Device **2** Monitoring Device **3** Infusion Device **Y** Other Device	**Z** No Qualifier
Ø Liver Quadrate lobe	**X** External	**Ø** Drainage Device **2** Monitoring Device **3** Infusion Device	**Z** No Qualifier
4 Gallbladder **G** Pancreas	**Ø** Open **3** Percutaneous **4** Percutaneous Endoscopic	**Ø** Drainage Device **2** Monitoring Device **3** Infusion Device **D** Intraluminal Device **Y** Other Device	**Z** No Qualifier
4 Gallbladder **G** Pancreas	**X** External	**Ø** Drainage Device **2** Monitoring Device **3** Infusion Device **D** Intraluminal Device	**Z** No Qualifier

B Hepatobiliary Duct
D Pancreatic Duct
   Duct of Wirsung
	Ø Open
	3 Percutaneous
	4 Percutaneous Endoscopic
	7 Via Natural or Artificial Opening
	8 Via Natural or Artificial Opening
	   Endoscopic
		Ø Drainage Device
		2 Monitoring Device
		3 Infusion Device
		7 Autologous Tissue Substitute
		C Extraluminal Device
		D Intraluminal Device
		J Synthetic Substitute
		K Nonautologous Tissue Substitute
		Y Other Device
			Z No Qualifier

B Hepatobiliary Duct **D** Pancreatic Duct Duct of Wirsung	**X** External	**Ø** Drainage Device **2** Monitoring Device **3** Infusion Device **7** Autologous Tissue Substitute **C** Extraluminal Device **D** Intraluminal Device **J** Synthetic Substitute **K** Nonautologous Tissue Substitute	**Z** No Qualifier

Non-OR	ØFWØ[3,4]YZ
Non-OR	ØFWØX[Ø,2,3]Z
Non-OR	ØFW[4,G][3,4]YZ
Non-OR	ØFW[4,G]X[Ø,2,3,D]Z
Non-OR	ØFW[B,D][3,4,7,8]YZ
Non-OR	ØFW[B,D]X[Ø,2,3,7,C,D,J,K]Z

Ø   **Medical and Surgical**
F   **Hepatobiliary System and Pancreas**
Y   **Transplantation**   Definition: Putting in or on all or a portion of a living body part taken from another individual or animal to physically take the place and/or function of all or a portion of a similar body part

                 Explanation: The native body part may or may not be taken out, and the transplanted body part may take over all or a portion of its function

Body Part Character 4	Approach Character 5	Device Character 6	Qualifier Character 7
Ø Liver [LC] Quadrate lobe **G** Pancreas [⊞][LC][NC]	**Ø** Open	**Z** No Device	**Ø** Allogeneic **1** Syngeneic **2** Zooplastic

[LC]	ØFYØØZ[Ø,1,2]
[LC]	ØFYGØZ[Ø,1]
[NC]	ØFYGØZ2

[NC]	ØFYGØZ[Ø,1] If reported alone without one of the following procedures
	    ØTYØØZ[Ø,1,2], ØTY1ØZ[Ø,1,2] and without one of the following
	    diagnoses E1Ø.1Ø-E1Ø.9, E89.1

See Appendix L for Procedure Combinations
   [⊞]   ØFYGØZ[Ø,1,2]

[LC] Limited Coverage   [NC] Noncovered   [⊞] Combination Member   HAC associated procedure   Combination Only   DRG Non-OR   Non-OR   New/Revised in GREEN

Endocrine System ØG2–ØGW

Character Meanings

This Character Meaning table is provided as a guide to assist the user in the identification of character members that may be found in this section of code tables. It **SHOULD NOT** be used to build a PCS code.

Operation–Character 3		Body Part–Character 4		Approach–Character 5		Device–Character 6		Qualifier–Character 7	
2	Change	Ø	Pituitary Gland	Ø	Open	Ø	Drainage Device	X	Diagnostic
5	Destruction	1	Pineal Body	3	Percutaneous	2	Monitoring Device	Z	No Qualifier
8	Division	2	Adrenal Gland, Left	4	Percutaneous Endoscopic	3	Infusion Device		
9	Drainage	3	Adrenal Gland, Right	X	External	Y	Other Device		
B	Excision	4	Adrenal Glands, Bilateral			Z	No Device		
C	Extirpation	5	Adrenal Gland						
H	Insertion	6	Carotid Body, Left						
J	Inspection	7	Carotid Body, Right						
M	Reattachment	8	Carotid Bodies, Bilateral						
N	Release	9	Para-aortic Body						
P	Removal	B	Coccygeal Glomus						
Q	Repair	C	Glomus Jugulare						
S	Reposition	D	Aortic Body						
T	Resection	F	Paraganglion Extremity						
W	Revision	G	Thyroid Gland Lobe, Left						
		H	Thyroid Gland Lobe, Right						
		J	Thyroid Gland Isthmus						
		K	Thyroid Gland						
		L	Superior Parathyroid Gland, Right						
		M	Superior Parathyroid Gland, Left						
		N	Inferior Parathyroid Gland, Right						
		P	Inferior Parathyroid Gland, Left						
		Q	Parathyroid Glands, Multiple						
		R	Parathyroid Gland						
		S	Endocrine Gland						

AHA Coding Clinic for table ØGB

| 2017, 2Q, 20 | Near total thyroidectomy |
| 2014, 3Q, 22 | Transsphenoidal removal of pituitary tumor and fat graft placement |

AHA Coding Clinic for table ØGT

| 2017, 2Q, 20 | Near total thyroidectomy |

Endocrine System

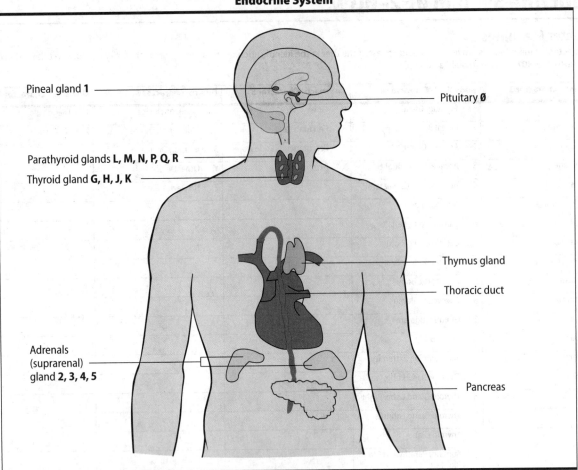

Pineal gland **1**

Pituitary **Ø**

Parathyroid glands **L, M, N, P, Q, R**

Thyroid gland **G, H, J, K**

Thymus gland

Thoracic duct

Adrenals
(suprarenal)
gland **2, 3, 4, 5**

Pancreas

Left Adrenal Gland

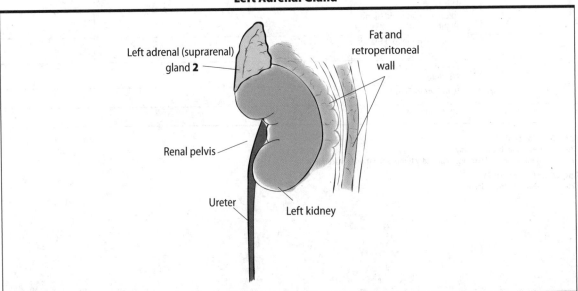

Left adrenal (suprarenal)
gland **2**

Fat and
retroperitoneal
wall

Renal pelvis

Ureter

Left kidney

Thyroid

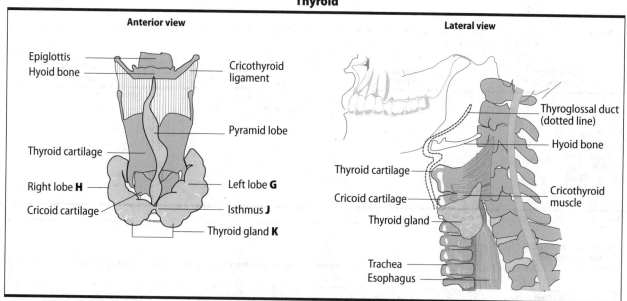

Anterior view

Epiglottis
Hyoid bone
Cricothyroid ligament
Pyramid lobe
Thyroid cartilage
Right lobe **H**
Left lobe **G**
Cricoid cartilage
Isthmus **J**
Thyroid gland **K**

Lateral view

Thyroglossal duct (dotted line)
Hyoid bone
Thyroid cartilage
Cricoid cartilage
Cricothyroid muscle
Thyroid gland
Trachea
Esophagus

Thyroid and Parathyroid Glands

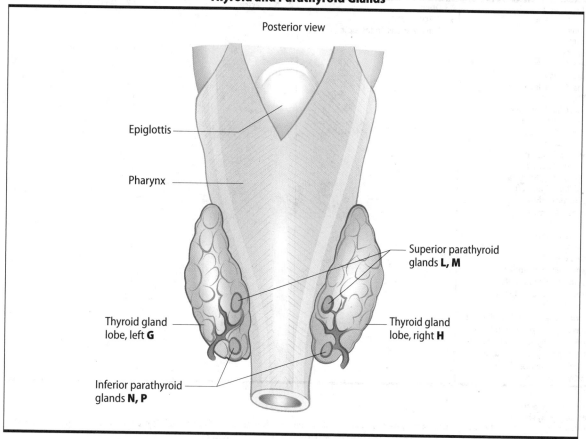

Posterior view

Epiglottis
Pharynx
Superior parathyroid glands **L, M**
Thyroid gland lobe, left **G**
Thyroid gland lobe, right **H**
Inferior parathyroid glands **N, P**

Endocrine System

Ø   **Medical and Surgical**
G   **Endocrine System**
2   **Change**   Definition: Taking out or off a device from a body part and putting back an identical or similar device in or on the same body part without cutting or puncturing the skin or a mucous membrane
                   Explanation: All CHANGE procedures are coded using the approach EXTERNAL

Body Part Character 4	Approach Character 5	Device Character 6	Qualifier Character 7

Ø **Pituitary Gland**
    Adenohypophysis
    Hypophysis
    Neurohypophysis
1 **Pineal Body**
5 **Adrenal Gland**
    Suprarenal gland
K **Thyroid Gland**
R **Parathyroid Gland**
S **Endocrine Gland**
	X External	**Ø** Drainage Device
		Y Other Device
			Z No Qualifier

Non-OR   All body part, approach, device, and qualifier values

Ø   **Medical and Surgical**
G   **Endocrine System**
5   **Destruction**   Definition: Physical eradication of all or a portion of a body part by the direct use of energy, force, or a destructive agent
                   Explanation: None of the body part is physically taken out

Body Part Character 4	Approach Character 5	Device Character 6	Qualifier Character 7

Ø **Pituitary Gland**
    Adenohypophysis
    Hypophysis
    Neurohypophysis
1 **Pineal Body**
2 **Adrenal Gland, Left**
    Suprarenal gland
3 **Adrenal Gland, Right**
    See 2 Adrenal Gland, Left
4 **Adrenal Glands, Bilateral**
    See 2 Adrenal Gland, Left
6 **Carotid Body, Left**
    Carotid glomus
7 **Carotid Body, Right**
    See 6 Carotid Body, Left
8 **Carotid Bodies, Bilateral**
    See 6 Carotid Body, Left
9 **Para-aortic Body**
B **Coccygeal Glomus**
    Coccygeal body
C **Glomus Jugulare**
    Jugular body
D **Aortic Body**
F **Paraganglion Extremity**
G **Thyroid Gland Lobe, Left**
H **Thyroid Gland Lobe, Right**
K **Thyroid Gland**
L **Superior Parathyroid Gland, Right**
M **Superior Parathyroid Gland, Left**
N **Inferior Parathyroid Gland, Right**
P **Inferior Parathyroid Gland, Left**
Q **Parathyroid Glands, Multiple**
R **Parathyroid Gland**
	Ø Open
	3 Percutaneous
	4 Percutaneous Endoscopic
		Z No Device	**Z** No Qualifier

Ø   **Medical and Surgical**
G   **Endocrine System**
8   **Division**   Definition: Cutting into a body part, without draining fluids and/or gases from the body part, in order to separate or transect a body part
                   Explanation: All or a portion of the body part is separated into two or more portions

Body Part Character 4	Approach Character 5	Device Character 6	Qualifier Character 7

Ø **Pituitary Gland**
    Adenohypophysis
    Hypophysis
    Neurohypophysis
J **Thyroid Gland Isthmus**
	Ø Open
	3 Percutaneous
	4 Percutaneous Endoscopic
		Z No Device	**Z** No Qualifier

LC Limited Coverage   NC Noncovered   ⊞ Combination Member   HAC associated procedure   Combination Only   DRG Non-OR   Non-OR   New/Revised in GREEN

404   ICD-10-PCS 2019

Ø   Medical and Surgical
G   Endocrine System
9   Drainage   Definition: Taking or letting out fluids and/or gases from a body part

Explanation: The qualifier DIAGNOSTIC is used to identify drainage procedures that are biopsies

Body Part Character 4	Approach Character 5	Device Character 6	Qualifier Character 7

Ø Pituitary Gland
   Adenohypophysis
   Hypophysis
   Neurohypophysis
1 Pineal Body
2 Adrenal Gland, Left
   Suprarenal gland
3 Adrenal Gland, Right
   See 2 Adrenal Gland, Left
4 Adrenal Glands, Bilateral
   See 2 Adrenal Gland, Left
6 Carotid Body, Left
   Carotid glomus
7 Carotid Body, Right
   See 6 Carotid Body, Left
8 Carotid Bodies, Bilateral
   See 6 Carotid Body, Left
9 Para-aortic Body
B Coccygeal Glomus
   Coccygeal body
C Glomus Jugulare
   Jugular body
D Aortic Body
F Paraganglion Extremity
G Thyroid Gland Lobe, Left
H Thyroid Gland Lobe, Right
K Thyroid Gland
L Superior Parathyroid Gland, Right
M Superior Parathyroid Gland, Left
N Inferior Parathyroid Gland, Right
P Inferior Parathyroid Gland, Left
Q Parathyroid Glands, Multiple
R Parathyroid Gland
	Ø Open
	3 Percutaneous
	4 Percutaneous Endoscopic
		Ø Drainage Device	**Z** No Qualifier

Ø Pituitary Gland
   Adenohypophysis
   Hypophysis
   Neurohypophysis
1 Pineal Body
2 Adrenal Gland, Left
   Suprarenal gland
3 Adrenal Gland, Right
   See 2 Adrenal Gland, Left
4 Adrenal Glands, Bilateral
   See 2 Adrenal Gland, Left
6 Carotid Body, Left
   Carotid glomus
7 Carotid Body, Right
   See 6 Carotid Body, Left
8 Carotid Bodies, Bilateral
   See 6 Carotid Body, Left
9 Para-aortic Body
B Coccygeal Glomus
   Coccygeal body
C Glomus Jugulare
   Jugular body
D Aortic Body
F Paraganglion Extremity
G Thyroid Gland Lobe, Left
H Thyroid Gland Lobe, Right
K Thyroid Gland
L Superior Parathyroid Gland, Right
M Superior Parathyroid Gland, Left
N Inferior Parathyroid Gland, Right
P Inferior Parathyroid Gland, Left
Q Parathyroid Glands, Multiple
R Parathyroid Gland
	Ø Open
	3 Percutaneous
	4 Percutaneous Endoscopic
		Z No Device	**X** Diagnostic
			Z No Qualifier

Non-OR   ØG9[Ø,1,2,3,4,6,7,8,9,B,C,D,F,G,H,K,L,M,N,P,Q,R]3ØZ
Non-OR   ØG9[G,H,K,L,M,N,P,Q,R]4ØZ
Non-OR   ØG9[2,3,4,G,H,K][3,4]ZX
Non-OR   ØG9[Ø,1,2,3,4,6,7,8,9,B,C,D,F,G,H,K,L,M,N,P,Q,R]3ZZ
Non-OR   ØG9[G,H,K,L,M,N,P,Q,R]4ZZ

LC Limited Coverage   NC Noncovered   ⊞ Combination Member   HAC associated procedure   Combination Only   DRG Non-OR   Non-OR   New/Revised in GREEN
ICD-10-PCS 2019   405

ØG9–ØG9

Ø   **Medical and Surgical**
G   **Endocrine System**
B   **Excision**   Definition: Cutting out or off, without replacement, a portion of a body part
                        Explanation: The qualifier DIAGNOSTIC is used to identify excision procedures that are biopsies

Body Part Character 4	Approach Character 5	Device Character 6	Qualifier Character 7

Ø   Pituitary Gland
    Adenohypophysis
    Hypophysis
    Neurohypophysis
1   Pineal Body
2   Adrenal Gland, Left
    Suprarenal gland
3   Adrenal Gland, Right
    See 2 Adrenal Gland, Left
4   Adrenal Glands, Bilateral
    See 2 Adrenal Gland, Left
6   Carotid Body, Left
    Carotid glomus
7   Carotid Body, Right
    See 6 Carotid Body, Left
8   Carotid Bodies, Bilateral
    See 6 Carotid Body, Left
9   Para-aortic Body
B   Coccygeal Glomus
    Coccygeal body
C   Glomus Jugulare
    Jugular body
D   Aortic Body
F   Paraganglion Extremity
G   Thyroid Gland Lobe, Left
H   Thyroid Gland Lobe, Right
J   Thyroid Gland Isthmus
L   Superior Parathyroid Gland, Right
M   Superior Parathyroid Gland, Left
N   Inferior Parathyroid Gland, Right
P   Inferior Parathyroid Gland, Left
Q   Parathyroid Glands, Multiple
R   Parathyroid Gland
	Ø Open
	3 Percutaneous
	4 Percutaneous Endoscopic
		Z No Device	X Diagnostic
			Z No Qualifier

Non-OR   ØGB[2,3,4,G,H,J][3,4]ZX

Ø   **Medical and Surgical**
G   **Endocrine System**
C   **Extirpation**   Definition: Taking or cutting out solid matter from a body part
                        Explanation: The solid matter may be an abnormal byproduct of a biological function or a foreign body; it may be imbedded in a body part or in the lumen of a tubular body part. The solid matter may or may not have been previously broken into pieces.

Body Part Character 4	Approach Character 5	Device Character 6	Qualifier Character 7

Ø   Pituitary Gland
    Adenohypophysis
    Hypophysis
    Neurohypophysis
1   Pineal Body
2   Adrenal Gland, Left
    Suprarenal gland
3   Adrenal Gland, Right
    See 2 Adrenal Gland, Left
4   Adrenal Glands, Bilateral
    See 2 Adrenal Gland, Left
6   Carotid Body, Left
    Carotid glomus
7   Carotid Body, Right
    See 6 Carotid Body, Left
8   Carotid Bodies, Bilateral
    See 6 Carotid Body, Left
9   Para-aortic Body
B   Coccygeal Glomus
    Coccygeal body
C   Glomus Jugulare
    Jugular body
D   Aortic Body
F   Paraganglion Extremity
G   Thyroid Gland Lobe, Left
H   Thyroid Gland Lobe, Right
K   Thyroid Gland
L   Superior Parathyroid Gland, Right
M   Superior Parathyroid Gland, Left
N   Inferior Parathyroid Gland, Right
P   Inferior Parathyroid Gland, Left
Q   Parathyroid Glands, Multiple
R   Parathyroid Gland
	Ø Open
	3 Percutaneous
	4 Percutaneous Endoscopic
		Z No Device	Z No Qualifier

ØGB–ØGC

LC Limited Coverage   NC Noncovered   ⊞ Combination Member   HAC associated procedure   Combination Only   DRG Non-OR   Non-OR   New/Revised in GREEN

406   ICD-10-PCS 2019

Ø   **Medical and Surgical**
G   **Endocrine System**
H   **Insertion**   Definition: Putting in a nonbiological appliance that monitors, assists, performs, or prevents a physiological function but does not physically take the place of a body part
                        Explanation: None

Body Part Character 4	Approach Character 5	Device Character 6	Qualifier Character 7
S Endocrine Gland	Ø Open 3 Percutaneous 4 Percutaneous Endoscopic	2 Monitoring Device 3 Infusion Device Y Other Device	Z No Qualifier

Non-OR   ØGHS[3,4]YZ

Ø   **Medical and Surgical**
G   **Endocrine System**
J   **Inspection**   Definition: Visually and/or manually exploring a body part
                        Explanation: Visual exploration may be performed with or without optical instrumentation. Manual exploration may be performed directly or through intervening body layers.

Body Part Character 4	Approach Character 5	Device Character 6	Qualifier Character 7

Ø   Pituitary Gland
    Adenohypophysis
    Hypophysis
    Neurohypophysis
1   Pineal Body
5   Adrenal Gland
    Suprarenal gland
K   Thyroid Gland
R   Parathyroid Gland
S   Endocrine Gland
	Ø Open
	3 Percutaneous
	4 Percutaneous Endoscopic
		Z No Device	Z No Qualifier

Non-OR   ØGJ[Ø,1,5,K,R,S]3ZZ

Ø   **Medical and Surgical**
G   **Endocrine System**
M   **Reattachment**   Definition: Putting back in or on all or a portion of a separated body part to its normal location or other suitable location
                        Explanation: Vascular circulation and nervous pathways may or may not be reestablished

Body Part Character 4	Approach Character 5	Device Character 6	Qualifier Character 7

2   Adrenal Gland, Left
    Suprarenal gland
3   Adrenal Gland, Right
    See 2 Adrenal Gland, Left
G   Thyroid Gland Lobe, Left
H   Thyroid Gland Lobe, Right
L   Superior Parathyroid Gland, Right
M   Superior Parathyroid Gland, Left
N   Inferior Parathyroid Gland, Right
P   Inferior Parathyroid Gland, Left
Q   Parathyroid Glands, Multiple
R   Parathyroid Gland
	Ø Open
	4 Percutaneous Endoscopic
		Z No Device	Z No Qualifier

Endocrine System *(left margin)*

Ø　Medical and Surgical
G　Endocrine System
N　Release　　Definition: Freeing a body part from an abnormal physical constraint by cutting or by the use of force

Explanation: Some of the restraining tissue may be taken out but none of the body part is taken out

Body Part Character 4	Approach Character 5	Device Character 6	Qualifier Character 7
Ø　Pituitary Gland 　　Adenohypophysis 　　Hypophysis 　　Neurohypophysis **1　Pineal Body** **2　Adrenal Gland, Left** 　　Suprarenal gland **3　Adrenal Gland, Right** 　　*See 2 Adrenal Gland, Left* **4　Adrenal Glands, Bilateral** 　　*See 2 Adrenal Gland, Left* **6　Carotid Body, Left** 　　Carotid glomus **7　Carotid Body, Right** 　　*See 6 Carotid Body, Left* **8　Carotid Bodies, Bilateral** 　　*See 6 Carotid Body, Left* **9　Para-aortic Body** **B　Coccygeal Glomus** 　　Coccygeal body **C　Glomus Jugulare** 　　Jugular body **D　Aortic Body** **F　Paraganglion Extremity** **G　Thyroid Gland Lobe, Left** **H　Thyroid Gland Lobe, Right** **K　Thyroid Gland** **L　Superior Parathyroid Gland, Right** **M　Superior Parathyroid Gland, Left** **N　Inferior Parathyroid Gland, Right** **P　Inferior Parathyroid Gland, Left** **Q　Parathyroid Glands, Multiple** **R　Parathyroid Gland**	**Ø　Open** **3　Percutaneous** **4　Percutaneous Endoscopic**	**Z　No Device**	**Z　No Qualifier**

Non-OR　ØGN[6,7,8,9,B,C,D,F][Ø,3,4]ZZ

Ø　Medical and Surgical
G　Endocrine System
P　Removal　　Definition: Taking out or off a device from a body part

Explanation: If a device is taken out and a similar device put in without cutting or puncturing the skin or mucous membrane, the procedure is coded to the root operation CHANGE. Otherwise, the procedure for taking out a device is coded to the root operation REMOVAL.

Body Part Character 4	Approach Character 5	Device Character 6	Qualifier Character 7
Ø　Pituitary Gland 　　Adenohypophysis 　　Hypophysis 　　Neurohypophysis **1　Pineal Body** **5　Adrenal Gland** 　　Suprarenal gland **K　Thyroid Gland** **R　Parathyroid Gland**	**Ø　Open** **3　Percutaneous** **4　Percutaneous Endoscopic** **X　External**	**Ø　Drainage Device**	**Z　No Qualifier**
S　Endocrine Gland	**Ø　Open** **3　Percutaneous** **4　Percutaneous Endoscopic**	**Ø　Drainage Device** **2　Monitoring Device** **3　Infusion Device** **Y　Other Device**	**Z　No Qualifier**
S　Endocrine Gland	**X　External**	**Ø　Drainage Device** **2　Monitoring Device** **3　Infusion Device**	**Z　No Qualifier**

Non-OR　ØGP[Ø,1,5,K,R]XØZ
Non-OR　ØGPS[3,4]YZ
Non-OR　ØGPSX[Ø,2,3]Z

LC Limited Coverage　NC Noncovered　⊞ Combination Member　HAC associated procedure　Combination Only　DRG Non-OR　Non-OR　New/Revised in GREEN

408　　　　　　　　　　　　　　　　　　　　　　　　　　　　　　　　　　　　ICD-10-PCS 2019

(left margin bottom) ØGN–ØGP

Ø Medical and Surgical
G Endocrine System
Q Repair
           Definition: Restoring, to the extent possible, a body part to its normal anatomic structure and function
           Explanation: Used only when the method to accomplish the repair is not one of the other root operations

Body Part Character 4	Approach Character 5	Device Character 6	Qualifier Character 7

Ø **Pituitary Gland**
   Adenohypophysis
   Hypophysis
   Neurohypophysis
1 **Pineal Body**
2 **Adrenal Gland, Left**
   Suprarenal gland
3 **Adrenal Gland, Right**
   See 2 Adrenal Gland, Left
4 **Adrenal Glands, Bilateral**
   See 2 Adrenal Gland, Left
6 **Carotid Body, Left**
   Carotid glomus
7 **Carotid Body, Right**
   See 6 Carotid Body, Left
8 **Carotid Bodies, Bilateral**
   See 6 Carotid Body, Left
9 **Para-aortic Body**
B **Coccygeal Glomus**
   Coccygeal body
C **Glomus Jugulare**
   Jugular body
D **Aortic Body**
F **Paraganglion Extremity**
G **Thyroid Gland Lobe, Left**
H **Thyroid Gland Lobe, Right**
J **Thyroid Gland Isthmus**
K **Thyroid Gland**
L **Superior Parathyroid Gland, Right**
M **Superior Parathyroid Gland, Left**
N **Inferior Parathyroid Gland, Right**
P **Inferior Parathyroid Gland, Left**
Q **Parathyroid Glands, Multiple**
R **Parathyroid Gland**
	Ø Open
	3 Percutaneous
	4 Percutaneous Endoscopic
		Z No Device	**Z** No Qualifier

Ø Medical and Surgical
G Endocrine System
S Reposition
           Definition: Moving to its normal location, or other suitable location, all or a portion of a body part
           Explanation: The body part is moved to a new location from an abnormal location, or from a normal location where it is not functioning correctly. The body part may or may not be cut out or off to be moved to the new location.

Body Part Character 4	Approach Character 5	Device Character 6	Qualifier Character 7

2 **Adrenal Gland, Left**
   Suprarenal gland
3 **Adrenal Gland, Right**
   See 2 Adrenal Gland, Left
G **Thyroid Gland Lobe, Left**
H **Thyroid Gland Lobe, Right**
L **Superior Parathyroid Gland, Right**
M **Superior Parathyroid Gland, Left**
N **Inferior Parathyroid Gland, Right**
P **Inferior Parathyroid Gland, Left**
Q **Parathyroid Glands, Multiple**
R **Parathyroid Gland**
	Ø Open
	4 Percutaneous Endoscopic
		Z No Device	**Z** No Qualifier

Endocrine System

Ø   Medical and Surgical
G   Endocrine System
T   Resection   Definition: Cutting out or off, without replacement, all of a body part

Explanation: None

Body Part Character 4	Approach Character 5	Device Character 6	Qualifier Character 7

Ø   **Pituitary Gland**
     Adenohypophysis
     Hypophysis
     Neurohypophysis
1   **Pineal Body**
2   **Adrenal Gland, Left**
     Suprarenal gland
3   **Adrenal Gland, Right**
     See 2 Adrenal Gland, Left
4   **Adrenal Glands, Bilateral**
     See 2 Adrenal Gland, Left
6   **Carotid Body, Left**
     Carotid glomus
7   **Carotid Body, Right**
     See 6 Carotid Body, Left
8   **Carotid Bodies, Bilateral**
     See 6 Carotid Body, Left
9   **Para-aortic Body**
B   **Coccygeal Glomus**
     Coccygeal body
C   **Glomus Jugulare**
     Jugular body
D   **Aortic Body**
F   **Paraganglion Extremity**
G   Thyroid Gland Lobe, Left
H   Thyroid Gland Lobe, Right
J   Thyroid Gland Isthmus
K   Thyroid Gland
L   Superior Parathyroid Gland, Right
M   Superior Parathyroid Gland, Left
N   Inferior Parathyroid Gland, Right
P   Inferior Parathyroid Gland, Left
Q   Parathyroid Glands, Multiple
R   Parathyroid Gland
	Ø Open
	4 Percutaneous Endoscopic
		Z No Device	**Z** No Qualifier

Non-OR   ØGT[6,7,8,9,B,C,D,F][Ø,4]ZZ

Ø   Medical and Surgical
G   Endocrine System
W   Revision   Definition: Correcting, to the extent possible, a portion of a malfunctioning device or the position of a displaced device

Explanation: Revision can include correcting a malfunctioning or displaced device by taking out or putting in components of the device such as a screw or pin

Body Part Character 4	Approach Character 5	Device Character 6	Qualifier Character 7

Ø   **Pituitary Gland**
     Adenohypophysis
     Hypophysis
     Neurohypophysis
1   **Pineal Body**
5   **Adrenal Gland**
     Suprarenal gland
K   **Thyroid Gland**
R   **Parathyroid Gland**
	Ø Open
	3 Percutaneous
	4 Percutaneous Endoscopic
	X External
		Ø Drainage Device	**Z** No Qualifier

S **Endocrine Gland**	**Ø** Open **3** Percutaneous **4** Percutaneous Endoscopic	**Ø** Drainage Device **2** Monitoring Device **3** Infusion Device **Y** Other Device	**Z** No Qualifier
S **Endocrine Gland**	**X** External	**Ø** Drainage Device **2** Monitoring Device **3** Infusion Device	**Z** No Qualifier

Non-OR   ØGW[Ø,1,5,K,R]XØZ
Non-OR   ØGWS[3,4]YZ
Non-OR   ØGWSX[Ø,2,3]Z

LC Limited Coverage   NC Noncovered   ⊞ Combination Member   HAC associated procedure   Combination Only   DRG Non-OR   Non-OR   New/Revised in GREEN

410   ICD-10-PCS 2019

Skin and Breast ØHØ–ØHX

Character Meanings*

This Character Meaning table is provided as a guide to assist the user in the identification of character members that may be found in this section of code tables. It **SHOULD NOT** be used to build a PCS code.

Operation–Character 3		Body Part–Character 4		Approach–Character 5		Device–Character 6		Qualifier–Character 7	
Ø	Alteration	Ø	Skin, Scalp	Ø	Open	Ø	Drainage Device	3	Full Thickness
2	Change	1	Skin, Face	3	Percutaneous	1	Radioactive Element	4	Partial Thickness
5	Destruction	2	Skin, Right Ear	7	Via Natural or Artificial Opening	7	Autologous Tissue Substitute	5	Latissimus Dorsi Myocutaneous Flap
8	Division	3	Skin, Left Ear	8	Via Natural or Artificial Opening Endoscopic	J	Synthetic Substitute	6	Transverse Rectus Abdominis Myocutaneous Flap
9	Drainage	4	Skin, Neck	X	External	K	Nonautologous Tissue Substitute	7	Deep Inferior Epigastric Artery Perforator Flap
B	Excision	5	Skin, Chest			N	Tissue Expander	8	Superficial Inferior Epigastric Artery Flap
C	Extirpation	6	Skin, Back			Y	Other Device	9	Gluteal Artery Perforator Flap
D	Extraction	7	Skin, Abdomen			Z	No Device	D	Multiple
H	Insertion	8	Skin, Buttock					X	Diagnostic
J	Inspection	9	Skin, Perineum					Z	No Qualifier
M	Reattachment	A	Skin, Inguinal						
N	Release	B	Skin, Right Upper Arm						
P	Removal	C	Skin, Left Upper Arm						
Q	Repair	D	Skin, Right Lower Arm						
R	Replacement	E	Skin, Left Lower Arm						
S	Reposition	F	Skin, Right Hand						
T	Resection	G	Skin, Left Hand						
U	Supplement	H	Skin, Right Upper Leg						
W	Revision	J	Skin, Left Upper Leg						
X	Transfer	K	Skin, Right Lower Leg						
		L	Skin, Left Lower Leg						
		M	Skin, Right Foot						
		N	Skin, Left Foot						
		P	Skin						
		Q	Finger Nail						
		R	Toe Nail						
		S	Hair						
		T	Breast, Right						
		U	Breast, Left						
		V	Breast, Bilateral						
		W	Nipple, Right						
		X	Nipple, Left						
		Y	Supernumerary Breast						

* Includes skin and breast glands and ducts.

AHA Coding Clinic for table ØHB
2018, 1Q, 14   Excisional debridement of breast tissue and skin
2016, 3Q, 29   Closure of bilateral alveolar clefts
2015, 3Q, 3-8   Excisional and nonexcisional debridement

AHA Coding Clinic for table ØHD
2016, 1Q, 40   Nonexcisional debridement of skin and subcutaneous tissue
2015, 3Q, 3-8   Excisional and nonexcisional debridement

AHA Coding Clinic for table ØHH
2017, 4Q, 67   New qualifier values - Pedicle flap procedures
2014, 2Q, 12   Pedicle latissimus myocutaneous flap with placement of breast tissue expanders
2013, 4Q, 107   Breast tissue expander placement using acellular dermal matrix

AHA Coding Clinic for table ØHP
2016, 2Q, 27   Removal of nonviable transverse rectus abdominis myocutaneous (TRAM) flaps

AHA Coding Clinic for table ØHQ
2018, 2Q, 25   Third and fourth degree obstetric lacerations
2016, 1Q, 7   Obstetrical perineal laceration repair
2014, 4Q, 31   Delayed wound closure following fracture treatment

AHA Coding Clinic for table ØHR
2017, 1Q, 35   Epifix® allograft
2014, 3Q, 14   Application of TheraSkin® and excisional debridement

AHA Coding Clinic for table ØHT
2014, 4Q, 34   Skin-sparing mastectomy

Integumentary Anatomy

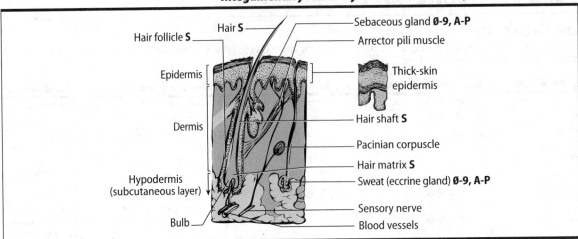

Hair follicle **S**

Hair **S**

Sebaceous gland **Ø-9, A-P**

Arrector pili muscle

Epidermis

Thick-skin epidermis

Dermis

Hair shaft **S**

Pacinian corpuscle

Hair matrix **S**

Hypodermis (subcutaneous layer)

Sweat (eccrine gland) **Ø-9, A-P**

Sensory nerve

Bulb

Blood vessels

Nail Anatomy

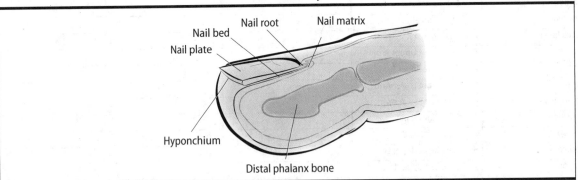

Nail bed

Nail root

Nail matrix

Nail plate

Hyponchium

Distal phalanx bone

Breast

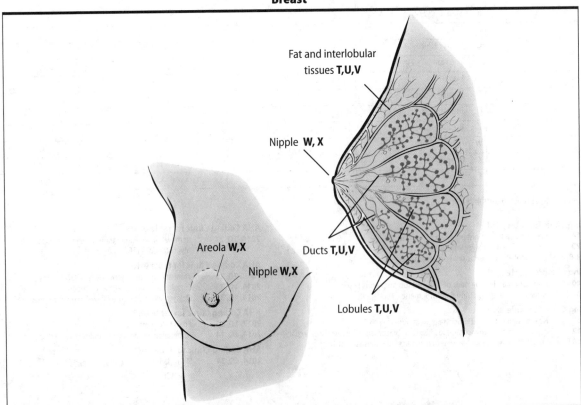

Fat and interlobular tissues **T,U,V**

Nipple **W, X**

Areola **W,X**

Nipple **W,X**

Ducts **T,U,V**

Lobules **T,U,V**

Ø   **Medical and Surgical**
H   **Skin and Breast**
Ø   **Alteration**   Definition: Modifying the anatomic structure of a body part without affecting the function of the body part
                         Explanation: Principal purpose is to improve appearance

Body Part Character 4	Approach Character 5	Device Character 6	Qualifier Character 7

T Breast, Right
    Mammary duct
    Mammary gland
U Breast, Left
    See T Breast, Right
V Breast, Bilateral
    See T Breast, Right
	Ø Open
	3 Percutaneous
	X External
		7 Autologous Tissue
		    Substitute
		J Synthetic Substitute
		K Nonautologous Tissue
		    Substitute
		Z No Device
			Z No Qualifier

Non-OR   ØHØ[T,U,V]3JZ

Ø   **Medical and Surgical**
H   **Skin and Breast**
2   **Change**   Definition: Taking out or off a device from a body part and putting back an identical or similar device in or on the same body part without
                        cutting or puncturing the skin or a mucous membrane
                        Explanation: All CHANGE procedures are coded using the approach EXTERNAL

Body Part Character 4	Approach Character 5	Device Character 6	Qualifier Character 7

P Skin
    Dermis
    Epidermis
    Sebaceous gland
    Sweat gland
T Breast, Right
    Mammary duct
    Mammary gland
U Breast, Left
    See T Breast, Right
	X External	**Ø** Drainage Device
		Y Other Device
			Z No Qualifier

Non-OR   All body part, approach, device, and qualifier values

---

Ø   **Medical and Surgical**
H   **Skin and Breast**
5   **Destruction**   Definition: Physical eradication of all or a portion of a body part by the direct use of energy, force, or a destructive agent
                        Explanation: None of the body part is physically taken out

Body Part Character 4	Approach Character 5	Device Character 6	Qualifier Character 7
Ø Skin, Scalp **C** Skin, Left Upper Arm **1** Skin, Face **D** Skin, Right Lower Arm **2** Skin, Right Ear **E** Skin, Left Lower Arm **3** Skin, Left Ear **F** Skin, Right Hand **4** Skin, Neck **G** Skin, Left Hand **5** Skin, Chest **H** Skin, Right Upper Leg **6** Skin, Back **J** Skin, Left Upper Leg **7** Skin, Abdomen **K** Skin, Right Lower Leg **8** Skin, Buttock **L** Skin, Left Lower Leg **9** Skin, Perineum **M** Skin, Right Foot **A** Skin, Inguinal **N** Skin, Left Foot **B** Skin, Right Upper Arm	**X** External	**Z** No Device	**D** Multiple **Z** No Qualifier

Q Finger Nail   **R** Toe Nail
    Nail bed   *See Q Finger Nail*
    Nail plate
	X External	**Z** No Device	**Z** No Qualifier

T Breast, Right   **W** Nipple, Right
    Mammary duct   Areola
    Mammary gland   **X** Nipple, Left
U Breast, Left   *See W Nipple, Right*
    See T Breast, Right
V Breast, Bilateral
    See T Breast, Right
	Ø Open
	3 Percutaneous
	7 Via Natural or Artificial
	    Opening
	8 Via Natural or Artificial
	    Opening Endoscopic
	X External
		Z No Device	**Z** No Qualifier

DRG Non-OR   ØH5[Ø,1,4,5,6,7,8,9,A,B,C,D,E,F,G,H,J,K,L,M,N]XZ[D,Z]
DRG Non-OR   ØH5[Q,R]XZZ
Non-OR   ØH5[2,3]XZ[D,Z]

Skin and Breast

Ø Medical and Surgical
H Skin and Breast
8 Division Definition: Cutting into a body part, without draining fluids and/or gases from the body part, in order to separate or transect a body part

Explanation: All or a portion of the body part is separated into two or more portions

Body Part — Character 4	Approach — Character 5	Device — Character 6	Qualifier — Character 7
Ø Skin, Scalp C Skin, Left Upper Arm 1 Skin, Face D Skin, Right Lower Arm 2 Skin, Right Ear E Skin, Left Lower Arm 3 Skin, Left Ear F Skin, Right Hand 4 Skin, Neck G Skin, Left Hand 5 Skin, Chest H Skin, Right Upper Leg 6 Skin, Back J Skin, Left Upper Leg 7 Skin, Abdomen K Skin, Right Lower Leg 8 Skin, Buttock L Skin, Left Lower Leg 9 Skin, Perineum M Skin, Right Foot A Skin, Inguinal N Skin, Left Foot B Skin, Right Upper Arm	X External	Z No Device	Z No Qualifier

Non-OR All body part, approach, device, and qualifier values

Ø Medical and Surgical
H Skin and Breast
9 Drainage Definition: Taking or letting out fluids and/or gases from a body part

Explanation: The qualifier DIAGNOSTIC is used to identify drainage procedures that are biopsies

Body Part — Character 4	Approach — Character 5	Device — Character 6	Qualifier — Character 7
Ø Skin, Scalp E Skin, Left Lower Arm 1 Skin, Face F Skin, Right Hand 2 Skin, Right Ear G Skin, Left Hand 3 Skin, Left Ear H Skin, Right Upper Leg 4 Skin, Neck J Skin, Left Upper Leg 5 Skin, Chest K Skin, Right Lower Leg 6 Skin, Back L Skin, Left Lower Leg 7 Skin, Abdomen M Skin, Right Foot 8 Skin, Buttock N Skin, Left Foot 9 Skin, Perineum Q Finger Nail A Skin, Inguinal Nail bed B Skin, Right Upper Arm Nail plate C Skin, Left Upper Arm R Toe Nail D Skin, Right Lower Arm See Q Finger Nail	X External	Ø Drainage Device	Z No Qualifier
Ø Skin, Scalp E Skin, Left Lower Arm 1 Skin, Face F Skin, Right Hand 2 Skin, Right Ear G Skin, Left Hand 3 Skin, Left Ear H Skin, Right Upper Leg 4 Skin, Neck J Skin, Left Upper Leg 5 Skin, Chest K Skin, Right Lower Leg 6 Skin, Back L Skin, Left Lower Leg 7 Skin, Abdomen M Skin, Right Foot 8 Skin, Buttock N Skin, Left Foot 9 Skin, Perineum Q Finger Nail A Skin, Inguinal Nail bed B Skin, Right Upper Arm Nail plate C Skin, Left Upper Arm R Toe Nail D Skin, Right Lower Arm See Q Finger Nail	X External	Z No Device	X Diagnostic Z No Qualifier

T Breast, Right   W Nipple, Right
   Mammary duct   Areola
   Mammary gland   X Nipple, Left
U Breast, Left   See W Nipple, Right
   See T Breast, Right
V Breast, Bilateral
   See T Breast, Right
	Ø Open
	3 Percutaneous
	7 Via Natural or Artificial Opening
	8 Via Natural or Artificial Opening Endoscopic
	X External
		Ø Drainage Device	Z No Qualifier

T Breast, Right   W Nipple, Right
   Mammary duct   Areola
   Mammary gland   X Nipple, Left
U Breast, Left   See W Nipple, Right
   See T Breast, Right
V Breast, Bilateral
   See T Breast, Right
	Ø Open
	3 Percutaneous
	7 Via Natural or Artificial Opening
	8 Via Natural or Artificial Opening Endoscopic
	X External
		Z No Device	X Diagnostic
			Z No Qualifier

Non-OR ØH9[Ø,1,2,3,4,5,6,7,8,A,B,C,D,E,F,G,H,J,K,L,M,N,Q,R]XØZ
Non-OR ØH9[Ø,1,2,3,4,5,6,7,8,A,B,C,D,E,F,G,H,J,K,L,M,N,Q,R]XZ[X,Z]
Non-OR ØH99XZX
Non-OR ØH9[T,U,V,W,X][Ø,3,7,8,X]ØZ
Non-OR ØH9[T,U,V,W,X][3,7,8,X]Z[X,Z]
Non-OR ØH9[T,U,V,W,X]ØZZ

Ø   **Medical and Surgical**
H   **Skin and Breast**
B   **Excision**   Definition: Cutting out or off, without replacement, a portion of a body part
                     Explanation: The qualifier DIAGNOSTIC is used to identify excision procedures that are biopsies

Body Part Character 4	Approach Character 5	Device Character 6	Qualifier Character 7

Ø Skin, Scalp
1 Skin, Face
2 Skin, Right Ear
3 Skin, Left Ear
4 Skin, Neck
5 Skin, Chest
6 Skin, Back
7 Skin, Abdomen
8 Skin, Buttock
9 Skin, Perineum
A Skin, Inguinal
B Skin, Right Upper Arm
C Skin, Left Upper Arm
D Skin, Right Lower Arm
E Skin, Left Lower Arm
F Skin, Right Hand
G Skin, Left Hand
H Skin, Right Upper Leg
J Skin, Left Upper Leg
K Skin, Right Lower Leg
L Skin, Left Lower Leg
M Skin, Right Foot
N Skin, Left Foot
Q Finger Nail
    Nail bed
    Nail plate
R Toe Nail
    See Q Finger Nail
	X External	**Z** No Device	**X** Diagnostic
			Z No Qualifier

T Breast, Right
    Mammary duct
    Mammary gland
U Breast, Left
    See T Breast, Right
V Breast, Bilateral
    See T Breast, Right
W Nipple, Right
    Areola
X Nipple, Left
    See W Nipple, Right
Y Supernumerary Breast
	Ø Open
	3 Percutaneous
	7 Via Natural or Artificial Opening
	8 Via Natural or Artificial Opening
	    Endoscopic
	X External
		Z No Device	**X** Diagnostic
			Z No Qualifier

DRG Non-OR	ØHB9XZZ
Non-OR	ØHB[Ø,1,2,3,4,5,6,7,8,A,B,C,D,E,F,G,H,J,K,L,M,N,Q,R]XZ[X,Z]
Non-OR	ØHB9XZX
Non-OR	ØHB[T,U,V,W,X,Y][3,7,8,X]ZX

Ø   Medical and Surgical
H   Skin and Breast
C   Extirpation   Definition: Taking or cutting out solid matter from a body part

Explanation: The solid matter may be an abnormal byproduct of a biological function or a foreign body; it may be imbedded in a body part or in the lumen of a tubular body part. The solid matter may or may not have been previously broken into pieces.

Body Part Character 4	Approach Character 5	Device Character 6	Qualifier Character 7
Ø Skin, Scalp	X External	Z No Device	Z No Qualifier
1 Skin, Face			
2 Skin, Right Ear			
3 Skin, Left Ear			
4 Skin, Neck			
5 Skin, Chest			
6 Skin, Back			
7 Skin, Abdomen			
8 Skin, Buttock			
9 Skin, Perineum			
A Skin, Inguinal			
B Skin, Right Upper Arm			
C Skin, Left Upper Arm			
D Skin, Right Lower Arm			
E Skin, Left Lower Arm			
F Skin, Right Hand			
G Skin, Left Hand			
H Skin, Right Upper Leg			
J Skin, Left Upper Leg			
K Skin, Right Lower Leg			
L Skin, Left Lower Leg			
M Skin, Right Foot			
N Skin, Left Foot			

Q   Finger Nail
     Nail bed
     Nail plate			

R Toe Nail *See Q Finger Nail*			

T   Breast, Right
     Mammary duct
     Mammary gland
	Ø Open
	3 Percutaneous
	7 Via Natural or Artificial Opening
	8 Via Natural or Artificial Opening
	     Endoscopic
	X External
		Z No Device	Z No Qualifier

U Breast, Left *See T Breast, Right*			
V Breast, Bilateral *See T Breast, Right*			
W Nipple, Right Areola			
X Nipple, Left *See W Nipple, Right*			

Non-OR   All body part, approach, device and qualifier values

Ø   **Medical and Surgical**
H   **Skin and Breast**
D   **Extraction**   Definition: Pulling or stripping out or off all or a portion of a body part by the use of force
                        Explanation: The qualifier DIAGNOSTIC is used to identify extraction procedures that are biopsies

Body Part Character 4	Approach Character 5	Device Character 6	Qualifier Character 7

Ø Skin, Scalp
1 Skin, Face
2 Skin, Right Ear
3 Skin, Left Ear
4 Skin, Neck
5 Skin, Chest
6 Skin, Back
7 Skin, Abdomen
8 Skin, Buttock
9 Skin, Perineum
A Skin, Inguinal
B Skin, Right Upper Arm
C Skin, Left Upper Arm
D Skin, Right Lower Arm
E Skin, Left Lower Arm
F Skin, Right Hand
G Skin, Left Hand
H Skin, Right Upper Leg
J Skin, Left Upper Leg
K Skin, Right Lower Leg
L Skin, Left Lower Leg
M Skin, Right Foot
N Skin, Left Foot
Q Finger Nail
     Nail bed
     Nail plate
R Toe Nail
     See Q Finger Nail
S Hair
	X External	**Z** No Device	**Z** No Qualifier

Non-OR   All body part, approach, device, and qualifier values

Ø   **Medical and Surgical**
H   **Skin and Breast**
H   **Insertion**   Definition: Putting in a nonbiological appliance that monitors, assists, performs, or prevents a physiological function but does not physically
                        take the place of a body part
                        Explanation: None

Body Part Character 4	Approach Character 5	Device Character 6	Qualifier Character 7
P Skin	**X** External	**Y** Other Device	**Z** No Qualifier

T Breast, Right
     Mammary duct
     Mammary gland
U Breast, Left
     See T Breast, Right
	Ø Open
	3 Percutaneous
	7 Via Natural or Artificial Opening
	8 Via Natural or Artificial Opening
	     Endoscopic
		1 Radioactive Element
		N Tissue Expander
		Y Other Device
			Z No Qualifier

T Breast, Right
     Mammary duct
     Mammary gland
U Breast, Left
     See T Breast, Right
	X External	**1** Radioactive Element	**Z** No Qualifier

V Breast, Bilateral
     See T Breast, Right
W Nipple, Right
     Areola
X Nipple, Left
     See W Nipple, Right
	Ø Open
	3 Percutaneous
	7 Via Natural or Artificial Opening
	8 Via Natural or Artificial Opening
	     Endoscopic
		1 Radioactive Element
		N Tissue Expander
			Z No Qualifier

V Breast, Bilateral
     See T Breast, Right
W Nipple, Right
     Areola
X Nipple, Left
     See W Nipple, Right
	X External	**1** Radioactive Element	**Z** No Qualifier

Non-OR   ØHHPXYZ
Non-OR   ØHH[T,U][3,7,8]YZ

Ø Medical and Surgical
H Skin and Breast
J Inspection Definition: Visually and/or manually exploring a body part

Explanation: Visual exploration may be performed with or without optical instrumentation. Manual exploration may be performed directly or through intervening body layers.

Body Part Character 4	Approach Character 5	Device Character 6	Qualifier Character 7
P Skin Dermis Epidermis Sebaceous gland Sweat gland **Q** Finger Nail Nail bed Nail plate **R** Toe Nail *See Q Finger Nail*	**X** External	**Z** No Device	**Z** No Qualifier
T Breast, Right Mammary duct Mammary gland **U** Breast, Left *See T Breast, Right*	**Ø** Open **3** Percutaneous **7** Via Natural or Artificial Opening **8** Via Natural or Artificial Opening Endoscopic **X** External	**Z** No Device	**Z** No Qualifier

Non-OR All body part, approach, device and qualifier values

Ø Medical and Surgical
H Skin and Breast
M Reattachment Definition: Putting back in or on all or a portion of a separated body part to its normal location or other suitable location

Explanation: Vascular circulation and nervous pathways may or may not be reestablished

Body Part Character 4	Approach Character 5	Device Character 6	Qualifier Character 7
Ø Skin, Scalp **1** Skin, Face **2** Skin, Right Ear **3** Skin, Left Ear **4** Skin, Neck **5** Skin, Chest **6** Skin, Back **7** Skin, Abdomen **8** Skin, Buttock **9** Skin, Perineum **A** Skin, Inguinal **B** Skin, Right Upper Arm **C** Skin, Left Upper Arm **D** Skin, Right Lower Arm **E** Skin, Left Lower Arm **F** Skin, Right Hand **G** Skin, Left Hand **H** Skin, Right Upper Leg **J** Skin, Left Upper Leg **K** Skin, Right Lower Leg **L** Skin, Left Lower Leg **M** Skin, Right Foot **N** Skin, Left Foot **T** Breast, Right Mammary duct Mammary gland **U** Breast, Left *See T Breast, Right* **V** Breast, Bilateral *See T Breast, Right* **W** Nipple, Right Areola **X** Nipple, Left *See W Nipple, Right*	**X** External	**Z** No Device	**Z** No Qualifier

Non-OR ØHMØXZZ

Ø   Medical and Surgical
H   Skin and Breast
N   Release   Definition: Freeing a body part from an abnormal physical constraint by cutting or by the use of force
                         Explanation: Some of the restraining tissue may be taken out but none of the body part is taken out

Body Part Character 4	Approach Character 5	Device Character 6	Qualifier Character 7
Ø Skin, Scalp	**X** External	**Z** No Device	**Z** No Qualifier
1 Skin, Face			
2 Skin, Right Ear			
3 Skin, Left Ear			
4 Skin, Neck			
5 Skin, Chest			
6 Skin, Back			
7 Skin, Abdomen			
8 Skin, Buttock			
9 Skin, Perineum			
A Skin, Inguinal			
B Skin, Right Upper Arm			
C Skin, Left Upper Arm			
D Skin, Right Lower Arm			
E Skin, Left Lower Arm			
F Skin, Right Hand			
G Skin, Left Hand			
H Skin, Right Upper Leg			
J Skin, Left Upper Leg			
K Skin, Right Lower Leg			
L Skin, Left Lower Leg			
M Skin, Right Foot			
N Skin, Left Foot			

Q   Finger Nail
     Nail bed
     Nail plate			

R Toe Nail *See Q Finger Nail*			

T   Breast, Right
     Mammary duct
     Mammary gland
	Ø Open
	3 Percutaneous
	7 Via Natural or Artificial Opening
	8 Via Natural or Artificial Opening
	     Endoscopic
	X External
		Z No Device	**Z** No Qualifier

U Breast, Left *See T Breast, Right*			
V Breast, Bilateral *See T Breast, Right*			
W Nipple, Right Areola			
X Nipple, Left *See W Nipple, Right*			

Ø   Medical and Surgical
H   Skin and Breast
P   Removal   Definition: Taking out or off a device from a body part

Explanation: If a device is taken out and a similar device put in without cutting or puncturing the skin or mucous membrane, the procedure is coded to the root operation CHANGE. Otherwise, the procedure for taking out a device is coded to the root operation REMOVAL.

Body Part Character 4	Approach Character 5	Device Character 6	Qualifier Character 7
P Skin Dermis Epidermis Sebaceous gland Sweat gland	**X** External	**Ø** Drainage Device **7** Autologous Tissue Substitute **J** Synthetic Substitute **K** Nonautologous Tissue Substitute **Y** Other Device	**Z** No Qualifier
Q Finger Nail Nail bed Nail plate **R Toe Nail** *See Q Finger Nail*	**X** External	**Ø** Drainage Device **7** Autologous Tissue Substitute **J** Synthetic Substitute **K** Nonautologous Tissue Substitute	**Z** No Qualifier
S Hair	**X** External	**7** Autologous Tissue Substitute **J** Synthetic Substitute **K** Nonautologous Tissue Substitute	**Z** No Qualifier
T Breast, Right Mammary duct Mammary gland **U Breast, Left** *See T Breast, Right*	**Ø** Open **3** Percutaneous **7** Via Natural or Artificial Opening **8** Via Natural or Artificial Opening Endoscopic	**Ø** Drainage Device **1** Radioactive Element **7** Autologous Tissue Substitute **J** Synthetic Substitute **K** Nonautologous Tissue Substitute **N** Tissue Expander **Y** Other Device	**Z** No Qualifier
T Breast, Right Mammary duct Mammary gland **U Breast, Left** *See T Breast, Right*	**X** External	**Ø** Drainage Device **1** Radioactive Element **7** Autologous Tissue Substitute **J** Synthetic Substitute **K** Nonautologous Tissue Substitute	**Z** No Qualifier

Non-OR   ØHPPX[Ø,7,J,K,Y]Z
Non-OR   ØHP[Q,R]X[Ø,7,J,K]Z
Non-OR   ØHPSX[7,J,K]Z
Non-OR   ØHP[T,U]Ø[Ø,1,7,K]Z
Non-OR   ØHP[T,U]3[Ø,1,7,K,Y]Z
Non-OR   ØHP[T,U][7,8][Ø,1,7,J,K,N,Y]Z
Non-OR   ØHP[T,U]X[Ø,1,7,J,K]Z

Ø   Medical and Surgical
H   Skin and Breast
Q   Repair   Definition: Restoring, to the extent possible, a body part to its normal anatomic structure and function
                         Explanation: Used only when the method to accomplish the repair is not one of the other root operations

Body Part Character 4	Approach Character 5	Device Character 6	Qualifier Character 7

Ø Skin, Scalp
1 Skin, Face
2 Skin, Right Ear
3 Skin, Left Ear
4 Skin, Neck
5 Skin, Chest
6 Skin, Back
7 Skin, Abdomen
8 Skin, Buttock
9 Skin, Perineum
A Skin, Inguinal
B Skin, Right Upper Arm
C Skin, Left Upper Arm
D Skin, Right Lower Arm
E Skin, Left Lower Arm
F Skin, Right Hand
G Skin, Left Hand
H Skin, Right Upper Leg
J Skin, Left Upper Leg
K Skin, Right Lower Leg
L Skin, Left Lower Leg
M Skin, Right Foot
N Skin, Left Foot
Q Finger Nail
    Nail bed
    Nail plate
R Toe Nail
    See Q Finger Nail
	X External	**Z** No Device	**Z** No Qualifier

T Breast, Right
    Mammary duct
    Mammary gland
U Breast, Left
    See T Breast, Right
V Breast, Bilateral
    See T Breast, Right
W Nipple, Right
    Areola
X Nipple, Left
    See W Nipple, Right
Y Supernumerary Breast
	Ø Open
	3 Percutaneous
	7 Via Natural or Artificial Opening
	8 Via Natural or Artificial Opening
	    Endoscopic
	X External
		Z No Device	**Z** No Qualifier

DRG Non-OR	ØHQ9XZZ
Non-OR	ØHQ[Ø,1,2,3,4,5,6,7,8,A,B,C,D,E,F,G,H,J,K,L,M,N]XZZ
Non-OR	ØHQ[T,U,V,Y]XZZ

Ø   **Medical and Surgical**
H   **Skin and Breast**
R   **Replacement**   Definition: Putting in or on biological or synthetic material that physically takes the place and/or function of all or a portion of a body part

Explanation: The body part may have been taken out or replaced, or may be taken out, physically eradicated, or rendered nonfunctional during the REPLACEMENT procedure. A REMOVAL procedure is coded for taking out the device used in a previous replacement procedure.

Body Part Character 4		Approach Character 5	Device Character 6	Qualifier Character 7
0 Skin, Scalp **1** Skin, Face **2** Skin, Right Ear **3** Skin, Left Ear **4** Skin, Neck **5** Skin, Chest **6** Skin, Back **7** Skin, Abdomen **8** Skin, Buttock **9** Skin, Perineum **A** Skin, Inguinal **B** Skin, Right Upper Arm	**C** Skin, Left Upper Arm **D** Skin, Right Lower Arm **E** Skin, Left Lower Arm **F** Skin, Right Hand **G** Skin, Left Hand **H** Skin, Right Upper Leg **J** Skin, Left Upper Leg **K** Skin, Right Lower Leg **L** Skin, Left Lower Leg **M** Skin, Right Foot **N** Skin, Left Foot	**X** External	**7** Autologous Tissue Substitute **K** Nonautologous Tissue Substitute	**3** Full Thickness **4** Partial Thickness
0 Skin, Scalp **1** Skin, Face **2** Skin, Right Ear **3** Skin, Left Ear **4** Skin, Neck **5** Skin, Chest **6** Skin, Back **7** Skin, Abdomen **8** Skin, Buttock **9** Skin, Perineum **A** Skin, Inguinal **B** Skin, Right Upper Arm	**C** Skin, Left Upper Arm **D** Skin, Right Lower Arm **E** Skin, Left Lower Arm **F** Skin, Right Hand **G** Skin, Left Hand **H** Skin, Right Upper Leg **J** Skin, Left Upper Leg **K** Skin, Right Lower Leg **L** Skin, Left Lower Leg **M** Skin, Right Foot **N** Skin, Left Foot	**X** External	**J** Synthetic Substitute	**3** Full Thickness **4** Partial Thickness **Z** No Qualifier

Q Finger Nail
   Nail bed
   Nail plate
R Toe Nail
   See Q Finger Nail
S Hair
		X External	**7** Autologous Tissue Substitute
			J Synthetic Substitute
			K Nonautologous Tissue Substitute
				Z No Qualifier

T Breast, Right
   Mammary duct
   Mammary gland
U Breast, Left
   See T Breast, Right
V Breast, Bilateral
   See T Breast, Right
		0 Open	**7** Autologous Tissue Substitute	**5** Latissimus Dorsi Myocutaneous Flap
				6 Transverse Rectus Abdominis Myocutaneous Flap
				7 Deep Inferior Epigastric Artery Perforator Flap
				8 Superficial Inferior Epigastric Artery Flap
				9 Gluteal Artery Perforator Flap
				Z No Qualifier

T Breast, Right
   Mammary duct
   Mammary gland
U Breast, Left
   See T Breast, Right
V Breast, Bilateral
   See T Breast, Right
		0 Open	**J** Synthetic Substitute
			K Nonautologous Tissue Substitute
				Z No Qualifier

T Breast, Right ⊞
   Mammary duct
   Mammary gland
U Breast, Left ⊞
   See T Breast, Right
V Breast, Bilateral ⊞
   See T Breast, Right
		3 Percutaneous
		X External
			7 Autologous Tissue Substitute
			J Synthetic Substitute
			K Nonautologous Tissue Substitute
				Z No Qualifier

W Nipple, Right
   Areola
X Nipple, Left
   See W Nipple, Right
		0 Open
		3 Percutaneous
		X External
			7 Autologous Tissue Substitute
			J Synthetic Substitute
			K Nonautologous Tissue Substitute
				Z No Qualifier

Non-OR   ØHRSX7Z   **See Appendix L for Procedure Combinations**
                                        ⊞   ØHR[T,U,V]37Z

LC Limited Coverage   NC Noncovered   ⊞ Combination Member   HAC associated procedure   Combination Only   DRG Non-OR   Non-OR   New/Revised in GREEN

422   ICD-10-PCS 2019

ØHR–ØHR

Ø   Medical and Surgical
H   Skin and Breast
S   Reposition   Definition: Moving to its normal location, or other suitable location, all or a portion of a body part

Explanation: The body part is moved to a new location from an abnormal location, or from a normal location where it is not functioning correctly. The body part may or may not be cut out or off to be moved to the new location.

Body Part Character 4	Approach Character 5	Device Character 6	Qualifier Character 7

S Hair
 W Nipple, Right
     Areola
 X Nipple, Left
     See W Nipple, Right
	X External	**Z** No Device	**Z** No Qualifier

T Breast, Right
     Mammary duct
     Mammary gland
 U Breast, Left
     See T Breast, Right
 V Breast, Bilateral
     See T Breast, Right
	Ø Open	**Z** No Device	**Z** No Qualifier

Non-OR   ØHSSXZZ

Ø   Medical and Surgical
H   Skin and Breast
T   Resection   Definition: Cutting out or off, without replacement, all of a body part

Explanation: None

Body Part Character 4	Approach Character 5	Device Character 6	Qualifier Character 7

Q Finger Nail
     Nail bed
     Nail plate
 R Toe Nail
     See Q Finger Nail
 W Nipple, Right
     Areola
 X Nipple, Left
     See W Nipple, Right
	X External	**Z** No Device	**Z** No Qualifier

T Breast, Right ⊞
     Mammary duct
     Mammary gland
 U Breast, Left ⊞
     See T Breast, Right
 V Breast, Bilateral ⊞
     See T Breast, Right
 Y Supernumerary Breast
	Ø Open	**Z** No Device	**Z** No Qualifier

Non-OR   ØHT[Q,R]XZZ

See Appendix L for Procedure Combinations
    ⊞   ØHT[T,U,V]ØZZ

Ø   Medical and Surgical
H   Skin and Breast
U   Supplement   Definition: Putting in or on biological or synthetic material that physically reinforces and/or augments the function of a portion of a body part

Explanation: The biological material is non-living, or is living and from the same individual. The body part may have been previously replaced, and the SUPPLEMENT procedure is performed to physically reinforce and/or augment the function of the replaced body part.

Body Part Character 4	Approach Character 5	Device Character 6	Qualifier Character 7

T Breast, Right
     Mammary duct
     Mammary gland
 U Breast, Left
     See T Breast, Right
 V Breast, Bilateral
     See T Breast, Right
 W Nipple, Right
     Areola
 X Nipple, Left
     See W Nipple, Right
	Ø Open
	 3 Percutaneous
	 7 Via Natural or Artificial Opening
	 8 Via Natural or Artificial Opening Endoscopic
	 X External
		7 Autologous Tissue Substitute
		 J Synthetic Substitute
		 K Nonautologous Tissue Substitute
			Z No Qualifier

Non-OR   ØHU[T,U,V]3JZ

LC Limited Coverage   **NC** Noncovered   ⊞ Combination Member   HAC associated procedure   Combination Only   DRG Non-OR   Non-OR   New/Revised in GREEN

ICD-10-PCS 2019   423

ØHS–ØHU

Skin and Breast

Ø Medical and Surgical
H Skin and Breast
W Revision   Definition: Correcting, to the extent possible, a portion of a malfunctioning device or the position of a displaced device

Explanation: Revision can include correcting a malfunctioning or displaced device by taking out or putting in components of the device such as a screw or pin

Body Part Character 4	Approach Character 5	Device Character 6	Qualifier Character 7
P Skin Dermis Epidermis Sebaceous gland Sweat gland	**X** External	**Ø** Drainage Device **7** Autologous Tissue Substitute **J** Synthetic Substitute **K** Nonautologous Tissue Substitute **Y** Other Device	**Z** No Qualifier
Q Finger Nail Nail bed Nail plate **R** Toe Nail *See Q Finger Nail*	**X** External	**Ø** Drainage Device **7** Autologous Tissue Substitute **J** Synthetic Substitute **K** Nonautologous Tissue Substitute	**Z** No Qualifier
S Hair	**X** External	**7** Autologous Tissue Substitute **J** Synthetic Substitute **K** Nonautologous Tissue Substitute	**Z** No Qualifier
T Breast, Right Mammary duct Mammary gland **U** Breast, Left *See T Breast, Right*	**Ø** Open **3** Percutaneous **7** Via Natural or Artificial Opening **8** Via Natural or Artificial Opening Endoscopic	**Ø** Drainage Device **7** Autologous Tissue Substitute **J** Synthetic Substitute **K** Nonautologous Tissue Substitute **N** Tissue Expander **Y** Other Device	**Z** No Qualifier
T Breast, Right Mammary duct Mammary gland **U** Breast, Left *See T Breast, Right*	**X** External	**Ø** Drainage Device **7** Autologous Tissue Substitute **J** Synthetic Substitute **K** Nonautologous Tissue Substitute	**Z** No Qualifier

Non-OR ØHWPX[Ø,7,J,K,Y]Z
Non-OR ØHW[Q,R]X[Ø,7,J,K]Z
Non-OR ØHWSX[7,J,K]Z
Non-OR ØHW[T,U]Ø[Ø,7,K,N]Z
Non-OR ØHW[T,U]3[Ø,7,K,N,Y]Z
Non-OR ØHW[T,U][7,8][Ø,7,J,K,N,Y]Z
Non-OR ØHW[T,U]X[Ø,7,J,K]Z

Ø Medical and Surgical
H Skin and Breast
X Transfer   Definition: Moving, without taking out, all or a portion of a body part to another location to take over the function of all or a portion of a body part

Explanation: The body part transferred remains connected to its vascular and nervous supply

Body Part Character 4	Approach Character 5	Device Character 6	Qualifier Character 7
Ø Skin, Scalp **1** Skin, Face **2** Skin, Right Ear **3** Skin, Left Ear **4** Skin, Neck **5** Skin, Chest **6** Skin, Back **7** Skin, Abdomen **8** Skin, Buttock **9** Skin, Perineum **A** Skin, Inguinal **B** Skin, Right Upper Arm **C** Skin, Left Upper Arm **D** Skin, Right Lower Arm **E** Skin, Left Lower Arm **F** Skin, Right Hand **G** Skin, Left Hand **H** Skin, Right Upper Leg **J** Skin, Left Upper Leg **K** Skin, Right Lower Leg **L** Skin, Left Lower Leg **M** Skin, Right Foot **N** Skin, Left Foot	**X** External	**Z** No Device	**Z** No Qualifier

LC Limited Coverage **NC** Noncovered ⊞ Combination Member HAC associated procedure Combination Only DRG Non-OR Non-OR New/Revised in GREEN

424 ICD-10-PCS 2019

Subcutaneous Tissue and Fascia ØJØ–ØJX

Character Meanings

This Character Meaning table is provided as a guide to assist the user in the identification of character members that may be found in this section of code tables. It **SHOULD NOT** be used to build a PCS code.

Operation–Character 3	Body Part–Character 4	Approach–Character 5	Device–Character 6	Qualifier–Character 7
Ø Alteration	Ø Subcutaneous Tissue and Fascia, Scalp	Ø Open	Ø Drainage Device OR Monitoring Device, Hemodynamic	B Skin and Subcutaneous Tissue
2 Change	1 Subcutaneous Tissue and Fascia, Face	3 Percutaneous	1 Radioactive Element	C Skin, Subcutaneous Tissue and Fascia
5 Destruction	4 Subcutaneous Tissue and Fascia, Right Neck	X External	2 Monitoring Device	X Diagnostic
8 Division	5 Subcutaneous Tissue and Fascia, Left Neck		3 Infusion Device	Z No Qualifier
9 Drainage	6 Subcutaneous Tissue and Fascia, Chest		4 Pacemaker, Single Chamber	
B Excision	7 Subcutaneous Tissue and Fascia, Back		5 Pacemaker, Single Chamber Rate Responsive	
C Extirpation	8 Subcutaneous Tissue and Fascia, Abdomen		6 Pacemaker, Dual Chamber	
D Extraction	9 Subcutaneous Tissue and Fascia, Buttock		7 Autologous Tissue Substitute OR Cardiac Resynchronization Pacemaker Pulse Generator	
H Insertion	B Subcutaneous Tissue and Fascia, Perineum		8 Defibrillator Generator	
J Inspection	C Subcutaneous Tissue and Fascia, Pelvic Region		9 Cardiac Resynchronization Defibrillator Pulse Generator	
N Release	D Subcutaneous Tissue and Fascia, Right Upper Arm		A Contractility Modulation Device	
P Removal	F Subcutaneous Tissue and Fascia, Left Upper Arm		B Stimulator Generator, Single Array	
Q Repair	G Subcutaneous Tissue and Fascia, Right Lower Arm		C Stimulator Generator, Single Array Rechargeable	
R Replacement	H Subcutaneous Tissue and Fascia, Left Lower Arm		D Stimulator Generator, Multiple Array	
U Supplement	J Subcutaneous Tissue and Fascia, Right Hand		E Stimulator Generator, Multiple Array Rechargeable	
W Revision	K Subcutaneous Tissue and Fascia, Left Hand		H Contraceptive Device	
X Transfer	L Subcutaneous Tissue and Fascia, Right Upper Leg		J Synthetic Substitute	
	M Subcutaneous Tissue and Fascia, Left Upper Leg		K Nonautologous Tissue Substitute	
	N Subcutaneous Tissue and Fascia, Right Lower Leg		M Stimulator Generator	
	P Subcutaneous Tissue and Fascia, Left Lower Leg		N Tissue Expander	
	Q Subcutaneous Tissue and Fascia, Right Foot		P Cardiac Rhythm Related Device	
	R Subcutaneous Tissue and Fascia, Left Foot		V Infusion Device, Pump	
	S Subcutaneous Tissue and Fascia, Head and Neck		W Vascular Access Device, Totally Implantable	
	T Subcutaneous Tissue and Fascia, Trunk		X Vascular Access Device, Tunneled	
	V Subcutaneous Tissue and Fascia, Upper Extremity		Y Other Device	
	W Subcutaneous Tissue and Fascia, Lower Extremity		Z No Device	

AHA Coding Clinic for table 0J2

2017, 2Q, 26	Exchange of tunneled catheter

AHA Coding Clinic for table 0J8

2017, 3Q, 11	Bilateral escharotomy of leg, thigh and foot

AHA Coding Clinic for table 0J9

2015, 3Q, 23	Incision and drainage of multiple abscess cavities using vessel loop

AHA Coding Clinic for table 0JB

2018, 1Q, 7	Placement of fat graft following lumbar decompression surgery
2015, 3Q, 3-8	Excisional and nonexcisional debridement
2015, 2Q, 13	Transfer of free flap to reconstruct orbital defect
2015, 1Q, 29	Fistulectomy with placement of seton
2014, 4Q, 38	Abdominoplasty and abdominal wall plication for hernia repair
2014, 3Q, 22	Transsphenoidal removal of pituitary tumor and fat graft placement

AHA Coding Clinic for table 0JC

2017, 3Q, 22	Replacement of native skull bone flap

AHA Coding Clinic for table 0JD

2016, 3Q, 20	VersaJet™ nonexcisional debridement of leg muscle
2016, 3Q, 21	Nonexcisional debridement of infected lumbar wound
2016, 3Q, 21	Nonexcisional pulsed lavage debridement
2016, 3Q, 22	Debridement of bone and tendon using Tenex ultrasound device
2016, 1Q, 40	Nonexcisional debridement of skin and subcutaneous tissue
2015, 3Q, 3-8	Excisional and nonexcisional debridement
2015, 1Q, 23	Non-Excisional debridement with lavage of wound

AHA Coding Clinic for table 0JH

2017, 4Q, 63-64	Added and revised device values - Vascular access reservoir
2017, 2Q, 24	Tunneled catheter versus totally implantable catheter
2017, 2Q, 26	Exchange of tunneled catheter
2016, 4Q, 97-98	Phrenic neurostimulator
2016, 2Q, 14	Insertion of peritoneal totally implantable venous access device
2016, 2Q, 15	Removal and replacement of tunneled internal jugular catheter
2015, 4Q, 14	New Section X codes—New Technology procedures
2015, 4Q, 30-31	Vascular access devices
2015, 2Q, 33	Totally implantable central venous access device (Port-a-Cath)
2014, 3Q, 19	End of life replacement of Baclofen pump
2013, 4Q, 116	Device character for Port-A-Cath placement
2012, 4Q, 104	Placement of subcutaneous implantable cardioverter defibrillator

AHA Coding Clinic for table 0JN

2017, 3Q, 11	Bilateral escharotomy of leg, thigh and foot

AHA Coding Clinic for table 0JP

2016, 2Q, 15	Removal and replacement of tunneled internal jugular catheter
2015, 4Q, 31	Vascular access devices
2014, 3Q, 19	End of life replacement of Baclofen pump
2013, 4Q, 109	Separating conjoined twins
2012, 4Q, 104	Placement of subcutaneous implantable cardioverter defibrillator

AHA Coding Clinic for table 0JQ

2017, 3Q, 19	Anterior repair of cystocele
2014, 4Q, 44	Posterior colporrhaphy/rectocele repair

AHA Coding Clinic for table 0JR

2015, 2Q, 13	Transfer of free flap to reconstruct orbital defect

AHA Coding Clinic for table 0JU

2018, 2Q, 20	Prelaminated free flap graft using Alloderm™
2018, 1Q, 7	Placement of fat graft following lumbar decompression surgery

AHA Coding Clinic for table 0JW

2018, 1Q, 8	Ventricular peritoneal shunt ligation
2015, 4Q, 33	Externalization of peritoneal dialysis catheter
2015, 2Q, 9	Revision of ventriculoperitoneal (VP) shunt
2012, 4Q, 104	Placement of subcutaneous implantable cardioverter defibrillator

AHA Coding Clinic for table 0JX

2018, 1Q, 10	Complex wound closure using pericranial flap
2014, 3Q, 18	Placement of reverse sural fasciocutaneous pedicle flap
2013, 4Q, 109	Separating conjoined twins

Ø Medical and Surgical
J Subcutaneous Tissue and Fascia
Ø Alteration   Definition: Modifying the anatomic structure of a body part without affecting the function of the body part
           Explanation: Principal purpose is to improve appearance

Body Part Character 4		Approach Character 5	Device Character 6	Qualifier Character 7
1 Subcutaneous Tissue and Fascia, Face Masseteric fascia Orbital fascia	**F** Subcutaneous Tissue and Fascia, Left Upper Arm *See D Subcutaneous Tissue and Fascia, Right Upper Arm*	**Ø** Open **3** Percutaneous	**Z** No Device	**Z** No Qualifier
4 Subcutaneous Tissue and Fascia, Right Neck Deep cervical fascia Pretracheal fascia Prevertebral fascia	**G** Subcutaneous Tissue and Fascia, Right Lower Arm Antebrachial fascia Bicipital aponeurosis			
5 Subcutaneous Tissue and Fascia, Left Neck *See 4 Subcutaneous Tissue and Fascia, Right Neck*	**H** Subcutaneous Tissue and Fascia, Left Lower Arm *See G Subcutaneous Tissue and Fascia, Right Lower Arm*			
6 Subcutaneous Tissue and Fascia, Chest Pectoral fascia	**L** Subcutaneous Tissue and Fascia, Right Upper Leg Crural fascia Fascia lata Iliac fascia Iliotibial tract (band)			
7 Subcutaneous Tissue and Fascia, Back				
8 Subcutaneous Tissue and Fascia, Abdomen	**M** Subcutaneous Tissue and Fascia, Left Upper Leg *See L Subcutaneous Tissue and Fascia, Right Upper Leg*			
9 Subcutaneous Tissue and Fascia, Buttock	**N** Subcutaneous Tissue and Fascia, Right Lower Leg			
D Subcutaneous Tissue and Fascia, Right Upper Arm Axillary fascia Deltoid fascia Infraspinatus fascia Subscapular aponeurosis Supraspinatus fascia	**P** Subcutaneous Tissue and Fascia, Left Lower Leg			

Ø Medical and Surgical
J Subcutaneous Tissue and Fascia
2 Change   Definition: Taking out or off a device from a body part and putting back an identical or similar device in or on the same body part without cutting or puncturing the skin or a mucous membrane
           Explanation: All CHANGE procedures are coded using the approach EXTERNAL

Body Part Character 4	Approach Character 5	Device Character 6	Qualifier Character 7
S Subcutaneous Tissue and Fascia, Head and Neck	**X** External	**Ø** Drainage Device	**Z** No Qualifier
T Subcutaneous Tissue and Fascia, Trunk External oblique aponeurosis Transversalis fascia		**Y** Other Device	
V Subcutaneous Tissue and Fascia, Upper Extremity			
W Subcutaneous Tissue and Fascia, Lower Extremity			

     Non-OR   All body part, approach, device, and qualifier values

Ø Medical and Surgical
J Subcutaneous Tissue and Fascia
5 Destruction   Definition: Physical eradication of all or a portion of a body part by the direct use of energy, force, or a destructive agent
                      Explanation: None of the body part is physically taken out

Body Part Character 4		Approach Character 5	Device Character 6	Qualifier Character 7

Ø **Subcutaneous Tissue and Fascia, Scalp**
    Galea aponeurotica
1 **Subcutaneous Tissue and Fascia, Face**
    Masseteric fascia
    Orbital fascia
4 **Subcutaneous Tissue and Fascia, Right Neck**
    Deep cervical fascia
    Pretracheal fascia
    Prevertebral fascia
5 **Subcutaneous Tissue and Fascia, Left Neck**
    See 4 Subcutaneous Tissue and Fascia, Right Neck
6 **Subcutaneous Tissue and Fascia, Chest**
    Pectoral fascia
7 **Subcutaneous Tissue and Fascia, Back**
8 **Subcutaneous Tissue and Fascia, Abdomen**
9 **Subcutaneous Tissue and Fascia, Buttock**
B **Subcutaneous Tissue and Fascia, Perineum**
C **Subcutaneous Tissue and Fascia, Pelvic Region**
D **Subcutaneous Tissue and Fascia, Right Upper Arm**
    Axillary fascia
    Deltoid fascia
    Infraspinatus fascia
    Subscapular aponeurosis
    Supraspinatus fascia
F **Subcutaneous Tissue and Fascia, Left Upper Arm**
    See D Subcutaneous Tissue and Fascia, Right Upper Arm
	G **Subcutaneous Tissue and Fascia, Right Lower Arm**
	    Antebrachial fascia
	    Bicipital aponeurosis
	H **Subcutaneous Tissue and Fascia, Left Lower Arm**
	    See G Subcutaneous Tissue and Fascia, Right Lower Arm
	J **Subcutaneous Tissue and Fascia, Right Hand**
	    Palmar fascia (aponeurosis)
	K **Subcutaneous Tissue and Fascia, Left Hand**
	    See J Subcutaneous Tissue and Fascia, Right Hand
	L **Subcutaneous Tissue and Fascia, Right Upper Leg**
	    Crural fascia
	    Fascia lata
	    Iliac fascia
	    Iliotibial tract (band)
	M **Subcutaneous Tissue and Fascia, Left Upper Leg**
	    See L Subcutaneous Tissue and Fascia, Right Upper Leg
	N **Subcutaneous Tissue and Fascia, Right Lower Leg**
	P **Subcutaneous Tissue and Fascia, Left Lower Leg**
	Q **Subcutaneous Tissue and Fascia, Right Foot**
	    Plantar fascia (aponeurosis)
	R **Subcutaneous Tissue and Fascia, Left Foot**
	    See Q Subcutaneous Tissue and Fascia, Right Foot
		Ø Open
		3 Percutaneous
			Z No Device	**Z** No Qualifier

DRG Non-OR All body part, approach, device, and qualifier values

---

LC Limited Coverage   **NC** Noncovered   ⊞ Combination Member   HAC associated procedure   Combination Only   DRG Non-OR   Non-OR   New/Revised in GREEN

428   ICD-10-PCS 2019

Ø   **Medical and Surgical**
J   **Subcutaneous Tissue and Fascia**
8   **Division**   Definition: Cutting into a body part, without draining fluids and/or gases from the body part, in order to separate or transect a body part
                       Explanation: All or a portion of the body part is separated into two or more portions

Body Part Character 4		Approach Character 5	Device Character 6	Qualifier Character 7
Ø Subcutaneous Tissue and Fascia, Scalp Galea aponeurotica **1** Subcutaneous Tissue and Fascia, Face Masseteric fascia Orbital fascia **4** Subcutaneous Tissue and Fascia, Right Neck Deep cervical fascia Pretracheal fascia Prevertebral fascia **5** Subcutaneous Tissue and Fascia, Left Neck *See 4 Subcutaneous Tissue and Fascia, Right Neck* **6** Subcutaneous Tissue and Fascia, Chest Pectoral fascia **7** Subcutaneous Tissue and Fascia, Back **8** Subcutaneous Tissue and Fascia, Abdomen **9** Subcutaneous Tissue and Fascia, Buttock **B** Subcutaneous Tissue and Fascia, Perineum **C** Subcutaneous Tissue and Fascia, Pelvic Region **D** Subcutaneous Tissue and Fascia, Right Upper Arm Axillary fascia Deltoid fascia Infraspinatus fascia Subscapular aponeurosis Supraspinatus fascia **F** Subcutaneous Tissue and Fascia, Left Upper Arm *See D Subcutaneous Tissue and Fascia, Right Upper Arm* **G** Subcutaneous Tissue and Fascia, Right Lower Arm Antebrachial fascia Bicipital aponeurosis	**H** Subcutaneous Tissue and Fascia, Left Lower Arm *See G Subcutaneous Tissue and Fascia, Right Lower Arm* **J** Subcutaneous Tissue and Fascia, Right Hand Palmar fascia (aponeurosis) **K** Subcutaneous Tissue and Fascia, Left Hand *See J Subcutaneous Tissue and Fascia, Right Hand* **L** Subcutaneous Tissue and Fascia, Right Upper Leg Crural fascia Fascia lata Iliac fascia Iliotibial tract (band) **M** Subcutaneous Tissue and Fascia, Left Upper Leg *See L Subcutaneous Tissue and Fascia, Right Upper Leg* **N** Subcutaneous Tissue and Fascia, Right Lower Leg **P** Subcutaneous Tissue and Fascia, Left Lower Leg **Q** Subcutaneous Tissue and Fascia, Right Foot Plantar fascia (aponeurosis) **R** Subcutaneous Tissue and Fascia, Left Foot *See Q Subcutaneous Tissue and Fascia, Right Foot* **S** Subcutaneous Tissue and Fascia, Head and Neck **T** Subcutaneous Tissue and Fascia, Trunk External oblique aponeurosis Transversalis fascia **V** Subcutaneous Tissue and Fascia, Upper Extremity **W** Subcutaneous Tissue and Fascia, Lower Extremity	**Ø** Open **3** Percutaneous	**Z** No Device	**Z** No Qualifier

Ø   Medical and Surgical
J   Subcutaneous Tissue and Fascia
9   Drainage   Definition: Taking or letting out fluids and/or gases from a body part
                       Explanation: The qualifier DIAGNOSTIC is used to identify drainage procedures that are biopsies

Body Part Character 4		Approach Character 5	Device Character 6	Qualifier Character 7
Ø Subcutaneous Tissue and Fascia, Scalp Galea aponeurotica	**G Subcutaneous Tissue and Fascia, Right Lower Arm** Antebrachial fascia Bicipital aponeurosis	**Ø Open** **3 Percutaneous**	**Ø Drainage Device**	**Z No Qualifier**
1 Subcutaneous Tissue and Fascia, Face Masseteric fascia Orbital fascia	**H Subcutaneous Tissue and Fascia, Left Lower Arm** *See G Subcutaneous Tissue and Fascia, Right Lower Arm*			
4 Subcutaneous Tissue and Fascia, Right Neck Deep cervical fascia Pretracheal fascia Prevertebral fascia	**J Subcutaneous Tissue and Fascia, Right Hand** Palmar fascia (aponeurosis)			
5 Subcutaneous Tissue and Fascia, Left Neck *See 4 Subcutaneous Tissue and Fascia, Right Neck*	**K Subcutaneous Tissue and Fascia, Left Hand** *See J Subcutaneous Tissue and Fascia, Right Hand*			
6 Subcutaneous Tissue and Fascia, Chest Pectoral fascia	**L Subcutaneous Tissue and Fascia, Right Upper Leg** Crural fascia Fascia lata Iliac fascia Iliotibial tract (band)			
7 Subcutaneous Tissue and Fascia, Back				
8 Subcutaneous Tissue and Fascia, Abdomen	**M Subcutaneous Tissue and Fascia, Left Upper Leg** *See L Subcutaneous Tissue and Fascia, Right Upper Leg*			
9 Subcutaneous Tissue and Fascia, Buttock	**N Subcutaneous Tissue and Fascia, Right Lower Leg**			
B Subcutaneous Tissue and Fascia, Perineum	**P Subcutaneous Tissue and Fascia, Left Lower Leg**			
C Subcutaneous Tissue and Fascia, Pelvic Region	**Q Subcutaneous Tissue and Fascia, Right Foot** Plantar fascia (aponeurosis)			
D Subcutaneous Tissue and Fascia, Right Upper Arm Axillary fascia Deltoid fascia Infraspinatus fascia Subscapular aponeurosis Supraspinatus fascia	**R Subcutaneous Tissue and Fascia, Left Foot** *See Q Subcutaneous Tissue and Fascia, Right Foot*			
F Subcutaneous Tissue and Fascia, Left Upper Arm *See D Subcutaneous Tissue and Fascia, Right Upper Arm*				

ØJ9 Continued on next page

Non-OR   ØJ9[Ø,1,4,5,6,7,8,9,B,C,D,F,G,H,J,K,L,M,N,P,Q,R][Ø,3]ØZ

0   **Medical and Surgical**   *0J9 Continued*
J   **Subcutaneous Tissue and Fascia**
9   **Drainage**   Definition: Taking or letting out fluids and/or gases from a body part
                        Explanation: The qualifier DIAGNOSTIC is used to identify drainage procedures that are biopsies

Body Part Character 4		Approach Character 5	Device Character 6	Qualifier Character 7

0 Subcutaneous Tissue and Fascia, Scalp
   Galea aponeurotica
	G Subcutaneous Tissue and Fascia, Right Lower Arm
	   Antebrachial fascia
	   Bicipital aponeurosis
		0 Open
		3 Percutaneous
			Z No Device	**X** Diagnostic
				Z No Qualifier

1 Subcutaneous Tissue and Fascia, Face
   Masseteric fascia
   Orbital fascia
	H Subcutaneous Tissue and Fascia, Left Lower Arm
	   See G Subcutaneous Tissue and Fascia, Right Lower Arm			

4 Subcutaneous Tissue and Fascia, Right Neck
   Deep cervical fascia
   Pretracheal fascia
   Prevertebral fascia
	J Subcutaneous Tissue and Fascia, Right Hand
	   Palmar fascia (aponeurosis)			

5 Subcutaneous Tissue and Fascia, Left Neck
   See 4 Subcutaneous Tissue and Fascia, Right Neck
	K Subcutaenous Tissue and Fascia, Left Hand
	   See J Subcutaneous Tissue and Fascia, Right Hand			

6 Subcutaneous Tissue and Fascia, Chest
   Pectoral fascia
	L Subcutaneous Tissue and Fascia, Right Upper Leg
	   Crural fascia
	   Fascia lata
	   Iliac fascia
	   Iliotibial tract (band)			

7 Subcutaneous Tissue and Fascia, Back	**M** Subcutaneous Tissue and Fascia, Left Upper Leg *See L Subcutaneous Tissue and Fascia, Right Upper Leg*			
8 Subcutaneous Tissue and Fascia, Abdomen	**N** Subcutaneous Tissue and Fascia, Right Lower Leg			
9 Subcutaneous Tissue and Fascia, Buttock	**P** Subcutaneous Tissue and Fascia, Left Lower Leg			
B Subcutaneous Tissue and Fascia, Perineum	**Q** Subcutaneous Tissue and Fascia, Right Foot Plantar fascia (aponeurosis)			
C Subcutaneous Tissue and Fascia, Pelvic Region	**R** Subcutaneous Tissue and Fascia, Left Foot *See Q Subcutaneous Tissue and Fascia, Right Foot*			

D Subcutaneous Tissue and Fascia, Right Upper Arm
   Axillary fascia
   Deltoid fascia
   Infraspinatus fascia
   Subscapular aponeurosis
   Supraspinatus fascia				

F Subcutaneous Tissue and Fascia, Left Upper Arm *See D Subcutaneous Tissue and Fascia, Right Upper Arm*				

Non-OR   0J9[0,1,4,5,6,7,8,9,B,C,D,F,G,H,J,K,L,M,N,P,Q,R][0,3]ZX
Non-OR   0J9[0,1,4,5,6,7,8,9,B,C,D,F,G,H,J,K,L,M,N,P,Q,R]3ZZ

Ø   Medical and Surgical
J   Subcutaneous Tissue and Fascia
B   Excision   Definition: Cutting out or off, without replacement, a portion of a body part
                 Explanation: The qualifier DIAGNOSTIC is used to identify excision procedures that are biopsies

Body Part Character 4		Approach Character 5	Device Character 6	Qualifier Character 7

Ø **Subcutaneous Tissue and Fascia, Scalp**
   Galea aponeurotica
	G **Subcutaneous Tissue and Fascia, Right Lower Arm**
	   Antebrachial fascia
	   Bicipital aponeurosis
		Ø Open
		3 Percutaneous
			Z No Device	**X** Diagnostic
				Z No Qualifier

1 **Subcutaneous Tissue and Fascia, Face**
   Masseteric fascia
   Orbital fascia
	H **Subcutaneous Tissue and Fascia, Left Lower Arm**
	   See G Subcutaneous Tissue and Fascia, Right Lower Arm			

4 **Subcutaneous Tissue and Fascia, Right Neck**
   Deep cervical fascia
   Pretracheal fascia
   Prevertebral fascia
	J **Subcutaneous Tissue and Fascia, Right Hand**
	   Palmar fascia (aponeurosis)			

5 **Subcutaneous Tissue and Fascia, Left Neck**
   See 4 Subcutaneous Tissue and Fascia, Right Neck
	K **Subcutaneous Tissue and Fascia, Left Hand**
	   See J Subcutaneous Tissue and Fascia, Right Hand			

6 **Subcutaneous Tissue and Fascia, Chest**
   Pectoral fascia
	L **Subcutaneous Tissue and Fascia, Right Upper Leg**
	   Crural fascia
	   Fascia lata
	   Iliac fascia
	   Iliotibial tract (band)			

7 **Subcutaneous Tissue and Fascia, Back**	**M** **Subcutaneous Tissue and Fascia, Left Upper Leg** *See L Subcutaneous Tissue and Fascia, Right Upper Leg*			
8 **Subcutaneous Tissue and Fascia, Abdomen**	**N** **Subcutaneous Tissue and Fascia, Right Lower Leg**			
9 **Subcutaneous Tissue and Fascia, Buttock**	**P** **Subcutaneous Tissue and Fascia, Left Lower Leg**			
B **Subcutaneous Tissue and Fascia, Perineum**	**Q** **Subcutaneous Tissue and Fascia, Right Foot** Plantar fascia (aponeurosis)			
C **Subcutaneous Tissue and Fascia, Pelvic Region**	**R** **Subcutaneous Tissue and Fascia, Left Foot** *See Q Subcutaneous Tissue and Fascia, Right Foot*			

D **Subcutaneous Tissue and Fascia, Right Upper Arm**
   Axillary fascia
   Deltoid fascia
   Infraspinatus fascia
   Subscapular aponeurosis
   Supraspinatus fascia				

F **Subcutaneous Tissue and Fascia, Left Upper Arm** *See D Subcutaneous Tissue and Fascia, Right Upper Arm*				

DRG Non-OR   ØJB[Ø,4,5,6,7,8,9,B,C,D,F,G,H,L,M,N,P,Q,R]3ZZ
Non-OR   ØJB[Ø,1,4,5,6,7,8,9,B,C,D,F,G,H,J,K,L,M,N,P,Q,R][Ø,3]ZX

Ø   Medical and Surgical
J   Subcutaneous Tissue and Fascia
C   Extirpation   Definition: Taking or cutting out solid matter from a body part

                Explanation: The solid matter may be an abnormal byproduct of a biological function or a foreign body; it may be imbedded in a body part or in the lumen of a tubular body part. The solid matter may or may not have been previously broken into pieces.

Body Part Character 4		Approach Character 5	Device Character 6	Qualifier Character 7
Ø Subcutaneous Tissue and Fascia, Scalp Galea aponeurotica **1 Subcutaneous Tissue and Fascia, Face** Masseteric fascia Orbital fascia **4 Subcutaneous Tissue and Fascia, Right Neck** Deep cervical fascia Pretracheal fascia Prevertebral fascia **5 Subcutaneous Tissue and Fascia, Left Neck** *See 4 Subcutaneous Tissue and Fascia, Right Neck* **6 Subcutaneous Tissue and Fascia, Chest** Pectoral fascia **7 Subcutaneous Tissue and Fascia, Back** **8 Subcutaneous Tissue and Fascia, Abdomen** **9 Subcutaneous Tissue and Fascia, Buttock** **B Subcutaneous Tissue and Fascia, Perineum** **C Subcutaneous Tissue and Fascia, Pelvic Region** **D Subcutaneous Tissue and Fascia, Right Upper Arm** Axillary fascia Deltoid fascia Infraspinatus fascia Subscapular aponeurosis Supraspinatus fascia **F Subcutaneous Tissue and Fascia, Left Upper Arm** *See D Subcutaneous Tissue and Fascia, Right Upper Arm*	**G Subcutaneous Tissue and Fascia, Right Lower Arm** Antebrachial fascia Bicipital aponeurosis **H Subcutaneous Tissue and Fascia, Left Lower Arm** *See G Subcutaneous Tissue and Fascia, Right Lower Arm* **J Subcutaneous Tissue and Fascia, Right Hand** Palmar fascia (aponeurosis) **K Subcutaneous Tissue and Fascia, Left Hand** *See J Subcutaneous Tissue and Fascia, Right Hand* **L Subcutaneous Tissue and Fascia, Right Upper Leg** Crural fascia Fascia lata Iliac fascia Iliotibial tract (band) **M Subcutaneous Tissue and Fascia, Left Upper Leg** *See L Subcutaneous Tissue and Fascia, Right Upper Leg* **N Subcutaneous Tissue and Fascia, Right Lower Leg** **P Subcutaneous Tissue and Fascia, Left Lower Leg** **Q Subcutaneous Tissue and Fascia, Right Foot** Plantar fascia (aponeurosis) **R Subcutaneous Tissue and Fascia, Left Foot** *See Q Subcutaneous Tissue and Fascia, Right Foot*	**Ø Open** **3 Percutaneous**	**Z No Device**	**Z No Qualifier**

Non-OR   All body part, approach, device, and qualifier values

LC Limited Coverage   **NC** Noncovered   ⊞ Combination Member   HAC associated procedure   Combination Only   DRG Non-OR   Non-OR   New/Revised in GREEN

ICD-10-PCS 2019   433

Subcutaneous Tissue and Fascia *(left margin)*

Ø   Medical and Surgical
J   Subcutaneous Tissue and Fascia
D   Extraction   Definition: Pulling or stripping out or off all or a portion of a body part by the use of force
                  Explanation: The qualifier DIAGNOSTIC is used to identify extraction procedures that are biopsies

Body Part Character 4		Approach Character 5	Device Character 6	Qualifier Character 7

Ø Subcutaneous Tissue and
   Fascia, Scalp
   Galea aponeurotica
1 Subcutaneous Tissue and
   Fascia, Face
   Masseteric fascia
   Orbital fascia
4 Subcutaneous Tissue and
   Fascia, Right Neck
   Deep cervical fascia
   Pretracheal fascia
   Prevertebral fascia
5 Subcutaneous Tissue and
   Fascia, Left Neck
   See 4 Subcutaneous Tissue and
     Fascia, Right Neck
6 Subcutaneous Tissue and
   Fascia, Chest
   Pectoral fascia
7 Subcutaneous Tissue and
   Fascia, Back
8 Subcutaneous Tissue and
   Fascia, Abdomen
9 Subcutaneous Tissue and
   Fascia, Buttock
B Subcutaneous Tissue and
   Fascia, Perineum
C Subcutaneous Tissue and
   Fascia, Pelvic Region
D Subcutaneous Tissue and
   Fascia, Right Upper Arm
   Axillary fascia
   Deltoid fascia
   Infraspinatus fascia
   Subscapular aponeurosis
   Supraspinatus fascia
F Subcutaneous Tissue and
   Fascia, Left Upper Arm
   See D Subcutaneous Tissue and
     Fascia, Right Upper Arm
	G Subcutaneous Tissue and
	   Fascia, Right Lower Arm
	   Antebrachial fascia
	   Bicipital aponeurosis
	H Subcutaneous Tissue and
	   Fascia, Left Lower Arm
	   See G Subcutaneous Tissue and
	     Fascia, Right Lower Arm
	J Subcutaneous Tissue and
	   Fascia, Right Hand
	   Palmar fascia (aponeurosis)
	K Subcutaneous Tissue and
	   Fascia, Left Hand
	   See J Subcutaneous Tissue and
	     Fascia, Right Hand
	L Subcutaneous Tissue and
	   Fascia, Right Upper Leg
	   Crural fascia
	   Fascia lata
	   Iliac fascia
	   Iliotibial tract (band)
	M Subcutaneous Tissue and
	   Fascia, Left Upper Leg
	   See L Subcutaneous Tissue and
	     Fascia, Right Upper Leg
	N Subcutaneous Tissue and
	   Fascia, Right Lower Leg
	P Subcutaneous Tissue and
	   Fascia, Left Lower Leg
	Q Subcutaneous Tissue and
	   Fascia, Right Foot
	   Plantar fascia (aponeurosis)
	R Subcutaneous Tissue and
	   Fascia, Left Foot
	   See Q Subcutaneous Tissue and
	     Fascia, Right Foot
		Ø Open
		3 Percutaneous
			Z No Device	**Z** No Qualifier

Non-OR   ØJD[Ø,1,4,5,B,C,D,F,G,H,J,K,N,P,Q,R]3ZZ

See Appendix L for Procedure Combinations
Combo-only   ØJD[6,7,8,9,L,M]3ZZ

Ø   Medical and Surgical
J   Subcutaneous Tissue and Fascia
H   Insertion   Definition: Putting in a nonbiological appliance that monitors, assists, performs, or prevents a physiological function but does not physically
                take the place of a body part
                Explanation: None

Body Part Character 4		Approach Character 5	Device Character 6	Qualifier Character 7

Ø Subcutaneous Tissue and
   Fascia, Scalp
   Galea aponeurotica
1 Subcutaneous Tissue and
   Fascia, Face
   Masseteric fascia
   Orbital fascia
4 Subcutaneous Tissue and
   Fascia, Right Neck
   Deep cervical fascia
   Pretracheal fascia
   Prevertebral fascia
5 Subcutaneous Tissue and
   Fascia, Left Neck
   See 4 Subcutaneous Tissue and
     Fascia, Right Neck
9 Subcutaneous Tissue and
   Fascia, Buttock
B Subcutaneous Tissue and
   Fascia, Perineum
	C Subcutaneous Tissue and
	   Fascia, Pelvic Region
	J Subcutaneous Tissue and
	   Fascia, Right Hand
	   Palmar fascia (aponeurosis)
	K Subcutaneous Tissue and
	   Fascia, Left Hand
	   See J Subcutaneous Tissue and
	     Fascia, Right Hand
	Q Subcutaneous Tissue and
	   Fascia, Right Foot
	   Plantar fascia (aponeurosis)
	R Subcutaneous Tissue and
	   Fascia, Left Foot
	   See Q Subcutaneous Tissue
	     and Fascia, Right Foot
		Ø Open
		3 Percutaneous
			N Tissue Expander	**Z** No Qualifier

ØJH Continued on next page

LC Limited Coverage   **NC** Noncovered   ⊞ Combination Member   HAC associated procedure   Combination Only   DRG Non-OR   Non-OR   New/Revised in GREEN

Ø   Medical and Surgical
J   Subcutaneous Tissue and Fascia
H   Insertion   Definition: Putting in a nonbiological appliance that monitors, assists, performs, or prevents a physiological function but does not physically
                            take the place of a body part
                            Explanation: None

ØJH Continued

Body Part Character 4	Approach Character 5	Device Character 6	Qualifier Character 7

6 Subcutaneous Tissue and Fascia, Chest ⊞
    Pectoral fascia
8 Subcutaneous Tissue and Fascia, Abdomen ⊞ NC
	Ø Open
	3 Percutaneous
		Ø Monitoring Device, Hemodynamic
		2 Monitoring Device
		4 Pacemaker, Single Chamber
		5 Pacemaker, Single Chamber Rate
		    Responsive
		6 Pacemaker, Dual Chamber
		7 Cardiac Resynchronization
		    Pacemaker Pulse Generator
		8 Defibrillator Generator
		9 Cardiac Resynchronization
		    Defibrillator Pulse Generator
		A Contractility Modulation Device
		B Stimulator Generator, Single Array
		C Stimulator Generator, Single Array
		    Rechargeable
		D Stimulator Generator, Multiple Array
		E Stimulator Generator, Multiple Array
		    Rechargeable
		H Contraceptive Device
		M Stimulator Generator
		N Tissue Expander
		P Cardiac Rhythm Related Device
		V Infusion Device, Pump
		W Vascular Access Device, Totally
		    Implantable
		X Vascular Access Device, Tunneled
			Z No Qualifier

7 Subcutaneous Tissue and Fascia, Back ⊞ NC	**Ø Open**
	3 Percutaneous
		B Stimulator Generator, Single Array
		C Stimulator Generator, Single Array
		    Rechargeable
		D Stimulator Generator, Multiple Array
		E Stimulator Generator, Multiple Array
		    Rechargeable
		M Stimulator Generator
		N Tissue Expander
		V Infusion Device, Pump
			Z No Qualifier

D Subcutaneous Tissue and
    Fascia, Right Upper Arm
    Axillary fascia
    Deltoid fascia
    Infraspinatus fascia
    Subscapular aponeurosis
    Supraspinatus fascia
F Subcutaneous Tissue and
    Fascia, Left Upper Arm
    See D Subcutaneous Tissue
    and Fascia, Right Upper
    Arm
G Subcutaneous Tissue and
    Fascia, Right Lower Arm
    Antebrachial fascia
    Bicipital aponeurosis
H Subcutaneous Tissue and
    Fascia, Left Lower Arm
    See G Subcutaneous Tissue
    and Fascia, Right Lower
    Arm
	L Subcutaneous Tissue and
	    Fascia, Right Upper Leg
	    Crural fascia
	    Fascia lata
	    Iliac fascia
	    Iliotibial tract (band)
	M Subcutaneous Tissue and
	    Fascia, Left Upper Leg
	    See L Subcutaneous Tissue
	    and Fascia, Right Upper
	    Leg
	N Subcutaneous Tissue and
	    Fascia, Right Lower Leg
	P Subcutaneous Tissue and
	    Fascia, Left Lower Leg
		Ø Open
		3 Percutaneous
			H Contraceptive Device
			N Tissue Expander
			V Infusion Device, Pump
			W Vascular Access Device, Totally
			    Implantable
			X Vascular Access Device, Tunneled
				Z No Qualifier

S Subcutaneous Tissue and Fascia, Head and Neck **V Subcutaneous Tissue and Fascia, Upper Extremity** **W Subcutaneous Tissue and Fascia, Lower Extremity**	**Ø Open** **3 Percutaneous**	**1 Radioactive Element** **3 Infusion Device** **Y Other Device**	**Z No Qualifier**

T Subcutaneous Tissue and Fascia, Trunk
    External oblique aponeurosis
    Transversalis fascia
	Ø Open
	3 Percutaneous
		1 Radioactive Element
		3 Infusion Device
		V Infusion Device, Pump
		Y Other Device
			Z No Qualifier

DRG Non-OR	ØJH6[Ø,3][4,5,6,H,W,X]Z	**HAC**	ØJH[6,8][Ø,3][4,5,6,7,8,9,P]Z when reported with SDx K68.11 or
DRG Non-OR	ØJH8[Ø,3][2,4,5,6,H,W,X]Z		T81.4XXA or T82.6XXA or T82.7XXA
DRG Non-OR	ØJH[D,F,G,H,L,M][Ø,3][W,X]Z	**HAC**	ØJH63XZ when reported with SDx J95.811
DRG Non-OR	ØJHNØ[W,X]Z	NC	ØJH8[Ø,3]MZ
DRG Non-OR	ØJHN3[H,W,X]Z	NC	ØJH7[Ø,3]MZ
DRG Non-OR	ØJHP[Ø,3][H,W,X]Z		
Non-OR	ØJH[D,F,G,H,L,M][Ø,3]HZ		**See Appendix L for Procedure Combinations**
Non-OR	ØJHNØHZ	⊞	ØJH[6,8][Ø,3][8,9,A,B,C,D,E]Z
Non-OR	ØJH[S,V,W]Ø3Z	⊞	ØJH7[Ø,3][B,C,D,E]Z
Non-OR	ØJH[S,V,W]3[3,Y]Z		
Non-OR	ØJHTØ3Z		
Non-OR	ØJHT3[3,Y]Z		

LC Limited Coverage   NC Noncovered   ⊞ Combination Member   HAC associated procedure   Combination Only   DRG Non-OR   Non-OR   New/Revised in GREEN

Subcutaneous Tissue and Fascia

Ø Medical and Surgical
J Subcutaneous Tissue and Fascia
J Inspection   Definition: Visually and/or manually exploring a body part
Explanation: Visual exploration may be performed with or without optical instrumentation. Manual exploration may be performed directly or through intervening body layers.

Body Part Character 4	Approach Character 5	Device Character 6	Qualifier Character 7

S Subcutaneous Tissue and Fascia, Head and Neck
T Subcutaneous Tissue and Fascia, Trunk
  External oblique aponeurosis
  Transversalis fascia
V Subcutaneous Tissue and Fascia, Upper Extremity
W Subcutaneous Tissue and Fascia, Lower Extremity
	Ø Open
	3 Percutaneous
	X External
		Z No Device	Z No Qualifier

Non-OR   All body part, approach, device, and qualifier values

Ø Medical and Surgical
J Subcutaneous Tissue and Fascia
N Release   Definition: Freeing a body part from an abnormal physical constraint by cutting or by the use of force
Explanation: Some of the restraining tissue may be taken out but none of the body part is taken out

Body Part Character 4	Approach Character 5	Device Character 6	Qualifier Character 7

Ø Subcutaneous Tissue and Fascia, Scalp
  Galea aponeurotica
1 Subcutaneous Tissue and Fascia, Face
  Masseteric fascia
  Orbital fascia
4 Subcutaneous Tissue and Fascia, Right Neck
  Deep cervical fascia
  Pretracheal fascia
  Prevertebral fascia
5 Subcutaneous Tissue and Fascia, Left Neck
  See 4 Subcutaneous Tissue and Fascia, Right Neck
6 Subcutaneous Tissue and Fascia, Chest
  Pectoral fascia
7 Subcutaneous Tissue and Fascia, Back
8 Subcutaneous Tissue and Fascia, Abdomen
9 Subcutaneous Tissue and Fascia, Buttock
B Subcutaneous Tissue and Fascia, Perineum
C Subcutaneous Tissue and Fascia, Pelvic Region
D Subcutaneous Tissue and Fascia, Right Upper Arm
  Axillary fascia
  Deltoid fascia
  Infraspinatus fascia
  Subscapular aponeurosis
  Supraspinatus fascia
F Subcutaneous Tissue and Fascia, Left Upper Arm
  See D Subcutaneous Tissue and Fascia, Right Upper Arm
 	
G Subcutaneous Tissue and Fascia, Right Lower Arm
  Antebrachial fascia
  Bicipital aponeurosis
H Subcutaneous Tissue and Fascia, Left Lower Arm
  See G Subcutaneous Tissue and Fascia, Right Lower Arm
J Subcutaneous Tissue and Fascia, Right Hand
  Palmar fascia (aponeurosis)
K Subcutaneous Tissue and Fascia, Left Hand
  See J Subcutaneous Tissue and Fascia, Right Hand
L Subcutaneous Tissue and Fascia, Right Upper Leg
  Crural fascia
  Fascia lata
  Iliac fascia
  Iliotibial tract (band)
M Subcutaneous Tissue and Fascia, Left Upper Leg
  See L Subcutaneous Tissue and Fascia, Right Upper Leg
N Subcutaneous Tissue and Fascia, Right Lower Leg
P Subcutaneous Tissue and Fascia, Left Lower Leg
Q Subcutaneous Tissue and Fascia, Right Foot
  Plantar fascia (aponeurosis)
R Subcutaneous Tissue and Fascia, Left Foot
  See Q Subcutaneous Tissue and Fascia, Right Foot
	Ø Open
	3 Percutaneous
	X External
		Z No Device	Z No Qualifier

Non-OR   ØJN[Ø,1,4,5,6,7,8,9,B,C,D,F,G,H,J,K,L,M,N,P,Q,R]XZZ

Ø   Medical and Surgical
J   Subcutaneous Tissue and Fascia
P   Removal   Definition: Taking out or off a device from a body part

                Explanation: If a device is taken out and a similar device put in without cutting or puncturing the skin or mucous membrane, the procedure is coded to the root operation CHANGE. Otherwise, the procedure for taking out a device is coded to the root operation REMOVAL.

Body Part Character 4	Approach Character 5	Device Character 6	Qualifier Character 7
S Subcutaneous Tissue and Fascia, Head and Neck	**Ø** Open **3** Percutaneous	**Ø** Drainage Device **1** Radioactive Element **3** Infusion Device **7** Autologous Tissue Substitute **J** Synthetic Substitute **K** Nonautologous Tissue Substitute **N** Tissue Expander **Y** Other Device	**Z** No Qualifier
S Subcutaneous Tissue and Fascia, Head and Neck	**X** External	**Ø** Drainage Device **1** Radioactive Element **3** Infusion Device	**Z** No Qualifier
T Subcutaneous Tissue and Fascia, Trunk External oblique aponeurosis Transversalis fascia	**Ø** Open **3** Percutaneous	**Ø** Drainage Device **1** Radioactive Element **2** Monitoring Device **3** Infusion Device **7** Autologous Tissue Substitute **H** Contraceptive Device **J** Synthetic Substitute **K** Nonautologous Tissue Substitute **M** Stimulator Generator **N** Tissue Expander **P** Cardiac Rhythm Related Device **V** Infusion Device, Pump **W** Vascular Access Device, Totally Implantable **X** Vascular Access Device, Tunneled **Y** Other Device	**Z** No Qualifier
T Subcutaneous Tissue and Fascia, Trunk External oblique aponeurosis Transversalis fascia	**X** External	**Ø** Drainage Device **1** Radioactive Element **2** Monitoring Device **3** Infusion Device **H** Contraceptive Device **V** Infusion Device, Pump **X** Vascular Access Device, Tunneled	**Z** No Qualifier
V Subcutaneous Tissue and Fascia, Upper Extremity **W** Subcutaneous Tissue and Fascia, Lower Extremity	**Ø** Open **3** Percutaneous	**Ø** Drainage Device **1** Radioactive Element **3** Infusion Device **7** Autologous Tissue Substitute **H** Contraceptive Device **J** Synthetic Substitute **K** Nonautologous Tissue Substitute **N** Tissue Expander **V** Infusion Device, Pump **W** Vascular Access Device, Totally Implantable **X** Vascular Access Device, Tunneled **Y** Other Device	**Z** No Qualifier
V Subcutaneous Tissue and Fascia, Upper Extremity **W** Subcutaneous Tissue and Fascia, Lower Extremity	**X** External	**Ø** Drainage Device **1** Radioactive Element **3** Infusion Device **H** Contraceptive Device **V** Infusion Device, Pump **X** Vascular Access Device, Tunneled	**Z** No Qualifier

Non-OR   ØJPS[Ø,3][Ø,1,3,7,J,K,N,Y]Z
Non-OR   ØJPSX[Ø,1,3]Z
Non-OR   ØJPT[Ø,3][Ø,1,2,3,7,H,J,K,M,N,V,W,X,Y]Z
Non-OR   ØJPTX[Ø,1,2,3,H,V,X]Z
Non-OR   ØJP[V,W][Ø,3][Ø,1,3,7,H,J,K,N,V,W,X,Y]Z
Non-OR   ØJP[V,W]X[Ø,1,3,H,V,X]Z
HAC   ØJPT[Ø,3]PZ when reported with SDx K68.11 or T81.4XXA or
           T82.6XXA or T82.7XXA

Ø Medical and Surgical
J Subcutaneous Tissue and Fascia
Q Repair Definition: Restoring, to the extent possible, a body part to its normal anatomic structure and function
Explanation: Used only when the method to accomplish the repair is not one of the other root operations

Body Part Character 4		Approach Character 5	Device Character 6	Qualifier Character 7
Ø Subcutaneous Tissue and Fascia, Scalp Galea aponeurotica	**G Subcutaneous Tissue and Fascia, Right Lower Arm** Antebrachial fascia Bicipital aponeurosis	**Ø Open** **3 Percutaneous**	**Z No Device**	**Z No Qualifier**
1 Subcutaneous Tissue and Fascia, Face Masseteric fascia Orbital fascia	**H Subcutaneous Tissue and Fascia, Left Lower Arm** *See G Subcutaneous Tissue and Fascia, Right Lower Arm*			
4 Subcutaneous Tissue and Fascia, Right Neck Deep cervical fascia Pretracheal fascia Prevertebral fascia	**J Subcutaneous Tissue and Fascia, Right Hand** Palmar fascia (aponeurosis)			
5 Subcutaneous Tissue and Fascia, Left Neck *See 4 Subcutaneous Tissue and Fascia, Right Neck*	**K Subcutaneous Tissue and Fascia, Left Hand** *See J Subcutaneous Tissue and Fascia, Right Hand*			
6 Subcutaneous Tissue and Fascia, Chest Pectoral fascia	**L Subcutaneous Tissue and Fascia, Right Upper Leg** Crural fascia Fascia lata Iliac fascia Iliotibial tract (band)			
7 Subcutaneous Tissue and Fascia, Back	**M Subcutaneous Tissue and Fascia, Left Upper Leg** *See L Subcutaneous Tissue and Fascia, Right Upper Leg*			
8 Subcutaneous Tissue and Fascia, Abdomen	**N Subcutaneous Tissue and Fascia, Right Lower Leg**			
9 Subcutaneous Tissue and Fascia, Buttock	**P Subcutaneous Tissue and Fascia, Left Lower Leg**			
B Subcutaneous Tissue and Fascia, Perineum	**Q Subcutaneous Tissue and Fascia, Right Foot** Plantar fascia (aponeurosis)			
C Subcutaneous Tissue and Fascia, Pelvic Region	**R Subcutaneous Tissue and Fascia, Left Foot** *See Q Subcutaneous Tissue and Fascia, Right Foot*			
D Subcutaneous Tissue and Fascia, Right Upper Arm Axillary fascia Deltoid fascia Infraspinatus fascia Subscapular aponeurosis Supraspinatus fascia				
F Subcutaneous Tissue and Fascia, Left Upper Arm *See D Subcutaneous Tissue and Fascia, Right Upper Arm*				

Non-OR ØJQ[Ø,1,4,5,6,7,8,9,B,C,D,F,G,H,J,K,L,M,N,P,Q,R]3ZZ

Ø   Medical and Surgical
J   Subcutaneous Tissue and Fascia
R   Replacement   Definition: Putting in or on biological or synthetic material that physically takes the place and/or function of all or a portion of a body part

                Explanation: The body part may have been taken out or replaced, or may be taken out, physically eradicated, or rendered nonfunctional during the REPLACEMENT procedure. A REMOVAL procedure is coded for taking out the device used in a previous replacement procedure.

Body Part Character 4		Approach Character 5	Device Character 6	Qualifier Character 7
Ø Subcutaneous Tissue and Fascia, Scalp Galea aponeurotica	**G** Subcutaneous Tissue and Fascia, Right Lower Arm Antebrachial fascia Bicipital aponeurosis	**Ø** Open **3** Percutaneous	**7** Autologous Tissue Substitute **J** Synthetic Substitute **K** Nonautologous Tissue Substitute	**Z** No Qualifier
1 Subcutaneous Tissue and Fascia, Face Masseteric fascia Orbital fascia	**H** Subcutaneous Tissue and Fascia, Left Lower Arm *See G Subcutaneous Tissue and Fascia, Right Lower Arm*			
4 Subcutaneous Tissue and Fascia, Right Neck Deep cervical fascia Pretracheal fascia Prevertebral fascia	**J** Subcutaneous Tissue and Fascia, Right Hand Palmar fascia (aponeurosis)			
5 Subcutaneous Tissue and Fascia, Left Neck *See 4 Subcutaneous Tissue and Fascia, Right Neck*	**K** Subcutaneous Tissue and Fascia, Left Hand *See J Subcutaneous Tissue and Fascia, Right Hand*			
6 Subcutaneous Tissue and Fascia, Chest Pectoral fascia	**L** Subcutaneous Tissue and Fascia, Right Upper Leg Crural fascia Fascia lata Iliac fascia Iliotibial tract (band)			
7 Subcutaneous Tissue and Fascia, Back	**M** Subcutaneous Tissue and Fascia, Left Upper Leg *See L Subcutaneous Tissue and Fascia, Right Upper Leg*			
8 Subcutaneous Tissue and Fascia, Abdomen	**N** Subcutaneous Tissue and Fascia, Right Lower Leg			
9 Subcutaneous Tissue and Fascia, Buttock	**P** Subcutaneous Tissue and Fascia, Left Lower Leg			
B Subcutaneous Tissue and Fascia, Perineum	**Q** Subcutaneous Tissue and Fascia, Right Foot Plantar fascia (aponeurosis)			
C Subcutaneous Tissue and Fascia, Pelvic Region	**R** Subcutaneous Tissue and Fascia, Left Foot *See Q Subcutaneous Tissue and Fascia, Right Foot*			
D Subcutaneous Tissue and Fascia, Right Upper Arm Axillary fascia Deltoid fascia Infraspinatus fascia Subscapular aponeurosis Supraspinatus fascia				
F Subcutaneous Tissue and Fascia, Left Upper Arm *See D Subcutaneous Tissue and Fascia, Right Upper Arm*				

LC Limited Coverage   **NC** Noncovered   ⊞ Combination Member   HAC associated procedure   Combination Only   DRG Non-OR   Non-OR   New/Revised in GREEN

ICD-10-PCS 2019   439

Ø   Medical and Surgical
J   Subcutaneous Tissue and Fascia
U   Supplement: Definition: Putting in or on biological or synthetic material that physically reinforces and/or augments the function of a portion of a body part
       Explanation: The biological material is non-living, or is living and from the same individual. The body part may have been previously replaced, and the SUPPLEMENT procedure is performed to physically reinforce and/or augment the function of the replaced body part.

Body Part Character 4		Approach Character 5	Device Character 6	Qualifier Character 7

Ø Subcutaneous Tissue and Fascia, Scalp
   Galea aponeurotica
1 Subcutaneous Tissue and Fascia, Face
   Masseteric fascia
   Orbital fascia
4 Subcutaneous Tissue and Fascia, Right Neck
   Deep cervical fascia
   Pretracheal fascia
   Prevertebral fascia
5 Subcutaneous Tissue and Fascia, Left Neck
   See 4 Subcutaneous Tissue and Fascia, Right Neck
6 Subcutaneous Tissue and Fascia, Chest
   Pectoral fascia
7 Subcutaneous Tissue and Fascia, Back
8 Subcutaneous Tissue and Fascia, Abdomen
9 Subcutaneous Tissue and Fascia, Buttock
B Subcutaneous Tissue and Fascia, Perineum
C Subcutaneous Tissue and Fascia, Pelvic Region
D Subcutaneous Tissue and Fascia, Right Upper Arm
   Axillary fascia
   Deltoid fascia
   Infraspinatus fascia
   Subscapular aponeurosis
   Supraspinatus fascia
F Subcutaneous Tissue and Fascia, Left Upper Arm
   See D Subcutaneous Tissue and Fascia, Right Upper Arm
	G Subcutaneous Tissue and Fascia, Right Lower Arm
	   Antebrachial fascia
	   Bicipital aponeurosis
	H Subcutaneous Tissue and Fascia, Left Lower Arm
	   See G Subcutaneous Tissue and Fascia, Right Lower Arm
	J Subcutaneous Tissue and Fascia, Right Hand
	   Palmar fascia (aponeurosis)
	K Subcutaneous Tissue and Fascia, Left Hand
	   See J Subcutaneous Tissue and Fascia, Right Hand
	L Subcutaneous Tissue and Fascia, Right Upper Leg
	   Crural fascia
	   Fascia lata
	   Iliac fascia
	   Iliotibial tract (band)
	M Subcutaneous Tissue and Fascia, Left Upper Leg
	   See L Subcutaneous Tissue and Fascia, Right Upper Leg
	N Subcutaneous Tissue and Fascia, Right Lower Leg
	P Subcutaneous Tissue and Fascia, Left Lower Leg
	Q Subcutaneous Tissue and Fascia, Right Foot
	   Plantar fascia (aponeurosis)
	R Subcutaneous Tissue and Fascia, Left Foot
	   See Q Subcutaneous Tissue and Fascia, Right Foot
		Ø Open
		3 Percutaneous
			7 Autologous Tissue Substitute
			J Synthetic Substitute
			K Nonautologous Tissue Substitute
				Z No Qualifier

Ø   Medical and Surgical
J   Subcutaneous Tissue and Fascia
W   Revision   Definition: Correcting, to the extent possible, a portion of a malfunctioning device or the position of a displaced device
                 Explanation: Revision can include correcting a malfunctioning or displaced device by taking out or putting in components of the device such as a screw or pin

Body Part Character 4	Approach Character 5	Device Character 6	Qualifier Character 7
S Subcutaneous Tissue and Fascia, Head and Neck	**Ø** Open **3** Percutaneous	**Ø** Drainage Device **3** Infusion Device **7** Autologous Tissue Substitute **J** Synthetic Substitute **K** Nonautologous Tissue Substitute **N** Tissue Expander **Y** Other Device	**Z** No Qualifier
S Subcutaneous Tissue and Fascia, Head and Neck	**X** External	**Ø** Drainage Device **3** Infusion Device **7** Autologous Tissue Substitute **J** Synthetic Substitute **K** Nonautologous Tissue Substitute **N** Tissue Expander	**Z** No Qualifier
T Subcutaneous Tissue and Fascia, Trunk External oblique aponeurosis Transversalis fascia	**Ø** Open **3** Percutaneous	**Ø** Drainage Device **2** Monitoring Device **3** Infusion Device **7** Autologous Tissue Substitute **H** Contraceptive Device **J** Synthetic Substitute **K** Nonautologous Tissue Substitute **M** Stimulator Generator **N** Tissue Expander **P** Cardiac Rhythm Related Device **V** Infusion Device, Pump **W** Vascular Access Device, Totally Implantable **X** Vascular Access Device, Tunneled **Y** Other Device	**Z** No Qualifier
T Subcutaneous Tissue and Fascia, Trunk External oblique aponeurosis Transversalis fascia	**X** External	**Ø** Drainage Device **2** Monitoring Device **3** Infusion Device **7** Autologous Tissue Substitute **H** Contraceptive Device **J** Synthetic Substitute **K** Nonautologous Tissue Substitute **M** Stimulator Generator **N** Tissue Expander **P** Cardiac Rhythm Related Device **V** Infusion Device, Pump **W** Vascular Access Device, Totally Implantable **X** Vascular Access Device, Tunneled	**Z** No Qualifier
V Subcutaneous Tissue and Fascia, Upper Extremity **W** Subcutaneous Tissue and Fascia, Lower Extremity	**Ø** Open **3** Percutaneous	**Ø** Drainage Device **3** Infusion Device **7** Autologous Tissue Substitute **H** Contraceptive Device **J** Synthetic Substitute **K** Nonautologous Tissue Substitute **N** Tissue Expander **V** Infusion Device, Pump **W** Vascular Access Device, Totally Implantable **X** Vascular Access Device, Tunneled **Y** Other Device	**Z** No Qualifier
V Subcutaneous Tissue and Fascia, Upper Extremity **W** Subcutaneous Tissue and Fascia, Lower Extremity	**X** External	**Ø** Drainage Device **3** Infusion Device **7** Autologous Tissue Substitute **H** Contraceptive Device **J** Synthetic Substitute **K** Nonautologous Tissue Substitute **N** Tissue Expander **V** Infusion Device, Pump **W** Vascular Access Device, Totally Implantable **X** Vascular Access Device, Tunneled	**Z** No Qualifier

DRG Non-OR	ØJWS[Ø,3][Ø,3,7,J,K,N,Y]Z	**HAC**	ØJWT[Ø,3]PZ when reported with SDx K68.11 or T81.4XXA or T82.6XXA or
DRG Non-OR	ØJWT[Ø,3][Ø,3,7,H,J,K,M,N,V,W,X]Z		T82.7XXA
DRG Non-OR	ØJWTXMZ		
DRG Non-OR	ØJW[V,W][Ø,3][Ø,3,7,H,J,K,N,V,W,X,Y]Z		
Non-OR	ØJWSX[Ø,3,7,J,K,N]Z		
Non-OR	ØJWT3YZ		
Non-OR	ØJWTX[Ø,2,3,7,H,J,K,N,P,V,W,X]Z		
Non-OR	ØJW[V,W]X[Ø,3,7,H,J,K,N,V,W,X]Z		

Subcutaneous Tissue and Fascia *(left margin)*

Ø Medical and Surgical
J Subcutaneous Tissue and Fascia
X Transfer   Definition: Moving, without taking out, all or a portion of a body part to another location to take over the function of all or a portion of a body part
       Explanation: The body part transferred remains connected to its vascular and nervous supply

Body Part Character 4		Approach Character 5	Device Character 6	Qualifier Character 7
Ø Subcutaneous Tissue and Fascia, Scalp Galea aponeurotica **1 Subcutaneous Tissue and Fascia, Face** Masseteric fascia Orbital fascia **4 Subcutaneous Tissue and Fascia, Right Neck** Deep cervical fascia Pretracheal fascia Prevertebral fascia **5 Subcutaneous Tissue and Fascia, Left Neck** *See 4 Subcutaneous Tissue and Fascia, Right Neck* **6 Subcutaneous Tissue and Fascia, Chest** Pectoral fascia **7 Subcutaneous Tissue and Fascia, Back** **8 Subcutaneous Tissue and Fascia, Abdomen** **9 Subcutaneous Tissue and Fascia, Buttock** **B Subcutaneous Tissue and Fascia, Perineum** **C Subcutaneous Tissue and Fascia, Pelvic Region** **D Subcutaneous Tissue and Fascia, Right Upper Arm** Axillary fascia Deltoid fascia Infraspinatus fascia Subscapular aponeurosis Supraspinatus fascia **F Subcutaneous Tissue and Fascia, Left Upper Arm** *See D Subcutaneous Tissue and Fascia, Right Upper Arm*	**G Subcutaneous Tissue and Fascia, Right Lower Arm** Antebrachial fascia Bicipital aponeurosis **H Subcutaneous Tissue and Fascia, Left Lower Arm** *See G Subcutaneous Tissue and Fascia, Right Lower Arm* **J Subcutaneous Tissue and Fascia, Right Hand** Palmar fascia (aponeurosis) **K Subcutaneous Tissue and Fascia, Left Hand** *See J Subcutaneous Tissue and Fascia, Right Hand* **L Subcutaneous Tissue and Fascia, Right Upper Leg** Crural fascia Fascia lata Iliac fascia Iliotibial tract (band) **M Subcutaneous Tissue and Fascia, Left Upper Leg** *See L Subcutaneous Tissue and Fascia, Right Upper Leg* **N Subcutaneous Tissue and Fascia, Right Lower Leg** **P Subcutaneous Tissue and Fascia, Left Lower Leg** **Q Subcutaneous Tissue and Fascia, Right Foot** Plantar fascia (aponeurosis) **R Subcutaneous Tissue and Fascia, Left Foot** *See Q Subcutaneous Tissue and Fascia, Right Foot*	**Ø Open** **3 Percutaneous**	**Z No Device**	**B Skin and Subcutaneous Tissue** **C Skin, Subcutaneous Tissue and Fascia** **Z No Qualifier**

Muscles ØK2–ØKX

Character Meanings

This Character Meaning table is provided as a guide to assist the user in the identification of character members that may be found in this section of code tables. It **SHOULD NOT** be used to build a PCS code.

Operation–Character 3	Body Part–Character 4	Approach–Character 5	Device–Character 6	Qualifier–Character 7
2 Change	Ø Head Muscle	Ø Open	Ø Drainage Device	Ø Skin
5 Destruction	1 Facial Muscle	3 Percutaneous	7 Autologous Tissue Substitute	1 Subcutaneous Tissue
8 Division	2 Neck Muscle, Right	4 Percutaneous Endoscopic	J Synthetic Substitute	2 Skin and Subcutaneous Tissue
9 Drainage	3 Neck Muscle, Left	X External	K Nonautologous Tissue Substitute	5 Latissimus Dorsi Myocutaneous Flap
B Excision	4 Tongue, Palate, Pharynx Muscle		M Stimulator Lead	6 Transverse Rectus Abdominis Myocutaneous Flap
C Extirpation	5 Shoulder Muscle, Right		Y Other Device	7 Deep Inferior Epigastric Artery Perforator Flap
D Extraction	6 Shoulder Muscle, Left		Z No Device	8 Superficial Inferior Epigastric Artery Flap
H Insertion	7 Upper Arm Muscle, Right			9 Gluteal Artery Perforator Flap
J Inspection	8 Upper Arm Muscle, Left			X Diagnostic
M Reattachment	9 Lower Arm and Wrist Muscle, Right			Z No Qualifier
N Release	B Lower Arm and Wrist Muscle, Left			
P Removal	C Hand Muscle, Right			
Q Repair	D Hand Muscle, Left			
R Replacement	F Trunk Muscle, Right			
S Reposition	G Trunk Muscle, Left			
T Resection	H Thorax Muscle, Right			
U Supplement	J Thorax Muscle, Left			
W Revision	K Abdomen Muscle, Right			
X Transfer	L Abdomen Muscle, Left			
	M Perineum Muscle			
	N Hip Muscle, Right			
	P Hip Muscle, Left			
	Q Upper Leg Muscle, Right			
	R Upper Leg Muscle, Left			
	S Lower Leg Muscle, Right			
	T Lower Leg Muscle, Left			
	V Foot Muscle, Right			
	W Foot Muscle, Left			
	X Upper Muscle			
	Y Lower Muscle			

AHA Coding Clinic for table ØKB
2016, 3Q, 20   Excisional debridement of sacrum
2015, 3Q, 3-8   Excisional and nonexcisional debridement

AHA Coding Clinic for table ØKD
2017, 4Q, 41-42   Extraction procedures

AHA Coding Clinic for table ØKN
2017, 2Q, 12   Compartment syndrome and fasciotomy of foot
2017, 2Q, 13   Compartment syndrome and fasciotomy of leg
2015, 2Q, 22   Arthroscopic subacromial decompression
2014, 4Q, 39   Abdominal component release with placement of mesh for hernia repair

AHA Coding Clinic for table ØKQ
2018, 2Q, 25   Third and fourth degree obstetric lacerations
2016, 2Q, 34   Assisted vaginal delivery
2016, 1Q, 7   Obstetrical perineal laceration repair
2014, 4Q, 43   Second degree obstetric perineal laceration
2013, 4Q, 120   Repair of second degree perineum obstetric laceration

AHA Coding Clinic for table ØKS
2017, 1Q, 41   Manual reduction of hernia

AHA Coding Clinic for table ØKT
2016, 2Q, 12   Resection of malignant neoplasm of infratemporal fossa
2015, 1Q, 38   Abdominoperineal resection with flap closure of the perineum and colostomy

AHA Coding Clinic for table ØKX
2018, 2Q, 18   Transverse rectus abdominis myocutaneous (TRAM) delay
2017, 4Q, 67   New qualifier values - Pedicle flap procedures
2016, 3Q, 30   Resection of femur with interposition arthroplasty
2015, 3Q, 33   Cleft lip repair using Millard rotation advancement
2015, 2Q, 26   Pharyngeal flap to soft palate
2014, 4Q, 41   Abdominoperineal resection (APR) with flap closure of perineum and colostomy
2014, 2Q, 10   Transverse abdominomyocutaneous (TRAM) breast reconstruction
2014, 2Q, 12   Pedicle latissimus myocutaneous flap with placement of breast tissue expanders

Muscles

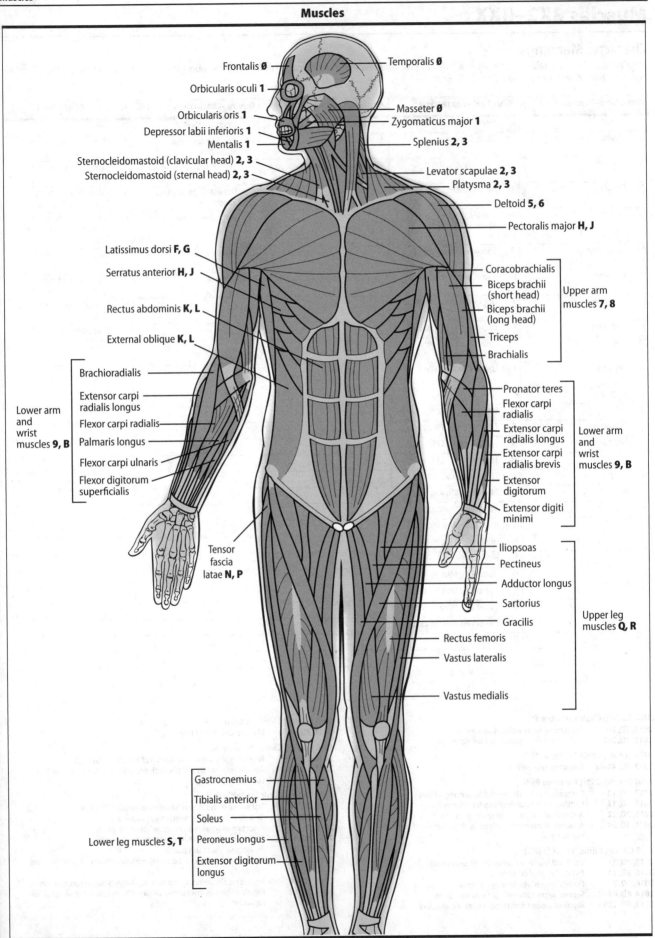

Frontalis **Ø**

Temporalis **Ø**

Orbicularis oculi **1**

Masseter **Ø**

Orbicularis oris **1**

Zygomaticus major **1**

Depressor labii inferioris **1**

Mentalis **1**

Splenius **2, 3**

Sternocleidomastoid (clavicular head) **2, 3**

Sternocleidomastoid (sternal head) **2, 3**

Levator scapulae **2, 3**

Platysma **2, 3**

Deltoid **5, 6**

Pectoralis major **H, J**

Latissimus dorsi **F, G**

Coracobrachialis

Serratus anterior **H, J**

Biceps brachii (short head)

Upper arm muscles **7, 8**

Rectus abdominis **K, L**

Biceps brachii (long head)

External oblique **K, L**

Triceps

Brachialis

Brachioradialis

Pronator teres

Extensor carpi radialis longus

Flexor carpi radialis

Flexor carpi radialis

Extensor carpi radialis longus

Lower arm and wrist muscles **9, B**

Palmaris longus

Extensor carpi radialis brevis

Lower arm and wrist muscles **9, B**

Flexor carpi ulnaris

Extensor digitorum

Flexor digitorum superficialis

Extensor digiti minimi

Iliopsoas

Pectineus

Adductor longus

Tensor fascia latae **N, P**

Sartorius

Gracilis

Upper leg muscles **Q, R**

Rectus femoris

Vastus lateralis

Vastus medialis

Gastrocnemius

Tibialis anterior

Soleus

Lower leg muscles **S, T**

Peroneus longus

Extensor digitorum longus

Ø   Medical and Surgical
K   Muscles
2   Change   Definition: Taking out or off a device from a body part and putting back an identical or similar device in or on the same body part without cutting or puncturing the skin or a mucous membrane

Explanation: All CHANGE procedures are coded using the approach EXTERNAL

Body Part Character 4	Approach Character 5	Device Character 6	Qualifier Character 7
X Upper Muscle Y Lower Muscle	X External	Ø Drainage Device Y Other Device	Z No Qualifier

Non-OR   All body part, approach, device, and qualifier values

Ø   Medical and Surgical
K   Muscles
5   Destruction   Definition: Physical eradication of all or a portion of a body part by the direct use of energy, force, or a destructive agent

Explanation: None of the body part is physically taken out

Body Part Character 4			Approach Character 5	Device Character 6	Qualifier Character 7

Ø Head Muscle
  Auricularis muscle
  Masseter muscle
  Pterygoid muscle
  Splenius capitis muscle
  Temporalis muscle
  Temporoparietalis muscle
1 Facial Muscle
  Buccinator muscle
  Corrugator supercilii muscle
  Depressor anguli oris muscle
  Depressor labii inferioris muscle
  Depressor septi nasi muscle
  Depressor supercilii muscle
  Levator anguli oris muscle
  Levator labii superioris alaeque
    nasi muscle
  Levator labii superioris muscle
  Mentalis muscle
  Nasalis muscle
  Occipitofrontalis muscle
  Orbicularis oris muscle
  Procerus muscle
  Risorius muscle
  Zygomaticus muscle
2 Neck Muscle, Right
  Anterior vertebral muscle
  Arytenoid muscle
  Cricothyroid muscle
  Infrahyoid muscle
  Levator scapulae muscle
  Platysma muscle
  Scalene muscle
  Splenius cervicis muscle
  Sternocleidomastoid muscle
  Suprahyoid muscle
  Thyroarytenoid muscle
3 Neck Muscle, Left
  See 2 Neck Muscle, Right
**4 Tongue, Palate, Pharynx
  Muscle**
  Chondroglossus muscle
  Genioglossus muscle
  Hyoglossus muscle
  Inferior longitudinal muscle
  Levator veli palatini muscle
  Palatoglossal muscle
  Palatopharyngeal muscle
  Pharyngeal constrictor muscle
  Salpingopharyngeus muscle
  Styloglossus muscle
  Stylopharyngeus muscle
  Superior longitudinal muscle
  Tensor veli palatini muscle
5 Shoulder Muscle, Right
  Deltoid muscle
  Infraspinatus muscle
  Subscapularis muscle
  Supraspinatus muscle
  Teres major muscle
  Teres minor muscle
6 Shoulder Muscle, Left
  See 5 Shoulder Muscle, Right
	7 Upper Arm Muscle, Right
	  Biceps brachii muscle
	  Brachialis muscle
	  Coracobrachialis muscle
	  Triceps brachii muscle
	8 Upper Arm Muscle, Left
	  See 7 Upper Arm Muscle, Right
	**9 Lower Arm and Wrist Muscle,
	  Right**
	  Anatomical snuffbox
	  Brachioradialis muscle
	  Extensor carpi radialis muscle
	  Extensor carpi ulnaris muscle
	  Flexor carpi radialis muscle
	  Flexor carpi ulnaris muscle
	  Flexor pollicis longus muscle
	  Palmaris longus muscle
	  Pronator quadratus muscle
	  Pronator teres muscle
	**B Lower Arm and Wrist Muscle,
	  Left**
	  *See 9 Lower Arm and Wrist
	    Muscle, Right*
	C Hand Muscle, Right
	  Hypothenar muscle
	  Palmar interosseous muscle
	  Thenar muscle
	D Hand Muscle, Left
	  See C Hand Muscle, Right
	F Trunk Muscle, Right
	  Coccygeus muscle
	  Erector spinae muscle
	  Interspinalis muscle
	  Intertransversarius muscle
	  Latissimus dorsi muscle
	  Quadratus lumborum muscle
	  Rhomboid major muscle
	  Rhomboid minor muscle
	  Serratus posterior muscle
	  Transversospinalis muscle
	  Trapezius muscle
	G Trunk Muscle, Left
	  See F Trunk Muscle, Right
	H Thorax Muscle, Right
	  Intercostal muscle
	  Levatores costarum muscle
	  Pectoralis major muscle
	  Pectoralis minor muscle
	  Serratus anterior muscle
	  Subclavius muscle
	  Subcostal muscle
	  Transverse thoracis muscle
	J Thorax Muscle, Left
	  See H Thorax Muscle, Right
	K Abdomen Muscle, Right
	  External oblique muscle
	  Internal oblique muscle
	  Pyramidalis muscle
	  Rectus abdominis muscle
	  Transversus abdominis muscle
	L Abdomen Muscle, Left
	  See K Abdomen Muscle, Right
		M Perineum Muscle
		  Bulbospongiosus muscle
		  Cremaster muscle
		  Deep transverse perineal muscle
		  Ischiocavernosus muscle
		  Levator ani muscle
		  Superficial transverse perineal
		    muscle
		N Hip Muscle, Right
		  Gemellus muscle
		  Gluteus maximus muscle
		  Gluteus medius muscle
		  Gluteus minimus muscle
		  Iliacus muscle
		  Obturator muscle
		  Piriformis muscle
		  Psoas muscle
		  Quadratus femoris muscle
		  Tensor fasciae latae muscle
		P Hip Muscle, Left
		  See N Hip Muscle, Right
		Q Upper Leg Muscle, Right
		  Adductor brevis muscle
		  Adductor longus muscle
		  Adductor magnus muscle
		  Biceps femoris muscle
		  Gracilis muscle
		  Pectineus muscle
		  Quadriceps (femoris)
		  Rectus femoris muscle
		  Sartorius muscle
		  Semimembranosus muscle
		  Semitendinosus muscle
		  Vastus intermedius muscle
		  Vastus lateralis muscle
		  Vastus medialis muscle
		R Upper Leg Muscle, Left
		  See Q Upper Leg Muscle, Right
		S Lower Leg Muscle, Right
		  Extensor digitorum longus muscle
		  Extensor hallucis longus muscle
		  Fibularis brevis muscle
		  Fibularis longus muscle
		  Flexor digitorum longus muscle
		  Flexor hallucis longus muscle
		  Gastrocnemius muscle
		  Peroneus brevis muscle
		  Peroneus longus muscle
		  Popliteus muscle
		  Soleus muscle
		  Tibialis anterior muscle
		  Tibialis posterior muscle
		T Lower Leg Muscle, Left
		  See S Lower Leg Muscle, Right
		V Foot Muscle, Right
		  Abductor hallucis muscle
		  Adductor hallucis muscle
		  Extensor digitorum brevis muscle
		  Extensor hallucis brevis muscle
		  Flexor digitorum brevis muscle
		  Flexor hallucis brevis muscle
		  Quadratus plantae muscle
		W Foot Muscle, Left
		  See V Foot Muscle, Right
			Ø Open
			3 Percutaneous
			4 Percutaneous
			     Endoscopic
				Z No Device	**Z** No Qualifier

LC Limited Coverage   **NC** Noncovered   ⊞ Combination Member   HAC associated procedure   Combination Only   DRG Non-OR   Non-OR   New/Revised in GREEN

ICD-10-PCS 2019   445

Ø   Medical and Surgical
K   Muscles
8   Division   Definition: Cutting into a body part, without draining fluids and/or gases from the body part, in order to separate or transect a body part
Explanation: All or a portion of the body part is separated into two or more portions

Body Part Character 4			Approach Character 5	Device Character 6	Qualifier Character 7
Ø Head Muscle Auricularis muscle Masseter muscle Pterygoid muscle Splenius capitis muscle Temporalis muscle Temporoparietalis muscle **1 Facial Muscle** Buccinator muscle Corrugator supercilii muscle Depressor anguli oris muscle Depressor labii inferioris muscle Depressor septi nasi muscle Depressor supercilii muscle Levator anguli oris muscle Levator labii superioris alaeque nasi muscle Levator labii superioris muscle Mentalis muscle Nasalis muscle Occipitofrontalis muscle Orbicularis oris muscle Procerus muscle Risorius muscle Zygomaticus muscle **2 Neck Muscle, Right** Anterior vertebral muscle Arytenoid muscle Cricothyroid muscle Infrahyoid muscle Levator scapulae muscle Platysma muscle Scalene muscle Splenius cervicis muscle Sternocleidomastoid muscle Suprahyoid muscle Thyroarytenoid muscle **3 Neck Muscle, Left** *See 2 Neck Muscle, Right* **4 Tongue, Palate, Pharynx Muscle** Chondroglossus muscle Genioglossus muscle Hyoglossus muscle Inferior longitudinal muscle Levator veli palatini muscle Palatoglossal muscle Palatopharyngeal muscle Pharyngeal constrictor muscle Salpingopharyngeus muscle Styloglossus muscle Stylopharyngeus muscle Superior longitudinal muscle Tensor veli palatini muscle **5 Shoulder Muscle, Right** Deltoid muscle Infraspinatus muscle Subscapularis muscle Supraspinatus muscle Teres major muscle Teres minor muscle **6 Shoulder Muscle, Left** *See 5 Shoulder Muscle, Right*	**7 Upper Arm Muscle, Right** Biceps brachii muscle Brachialis muscle Coracobrachialis muscle Triceps brachii muscle **8 Upper Arm Muscle, Left** *See 7 Upper Arm Muscle, Right* **9 Lower Arm and Wrist Muscle, Right** Anatomical snuffbox Brachioradialis muscle Extensor carpi radialis muscle Extensor carpi ulnaris muscle Flexor carpi radialis muscle Flexor carpi ulnaris muscle Flexor pollicis longus muscle Palmaris longus muscle Pronator quadratus muscle Pronator teres muscle **B Lower Arm and Wrist Muscle, Left** *See 9 Lower Arm and Wrist Muscle, Right* **C Hand Muscle, Right** Hypothenar muscle Palmar interosseous muscle Thenar muscle **D Hand Muscle, Left** *See C Hand Muscle, Right* **F Trunk Muscle, Right** Coccygeus muscle Erector spinae muscle Interspinalis muscle Intertransversarius muscle Latissimus dorsi muscle Quadratus lumborum muscle Rhomboid major muscle Rhomboid minor muscle Serratus posterior muscle Transversospinalis muscle Trapezius muscle **G Trunk Muscle, Left** *See F Trunk Muscle, Right* **H Thorax Muscle, Right** Intercostal muscle Levatores costarum muscle Pectoralis major muscle Pectoralis minor muscle Serratus anterior muscle Subclavius muscle Subcostal muscle Transverse thoracis muscle **J Thorax Muscle, Left** *See H Thorax Muscle, Right* **K Abdomen Muscle, Right** External oblique muscle Internal oblique muscle Pyramidalis muscle Rectus abdominis muscle Transversus abdominis muscle **L Abdomen Muscle, Left** *See K Abdomen Muscle, Right*	**M Perineum Muscle** Bulbospongiosus muscle Cremaster muscle Deep transverse perineal muscle Ischiocavernosus muscle Levator ani muscle Superficial transverse perineal muscle **N Hip Muscle, Right** Gemellus muscle Gluteus maximus muscle Gluteus medius muscle Gluteus minimus muscle Iliacus muscle Obturator muscle Piriformis muscle Psoas muscle Quadratus femoris muscle Tensor fasciae latae muscle **P Hip Muscle, Left** *See N Hip Muscle, Right* **Q Upper Leg Muscle, Right** Adductor brevis muscle Adductor longus muscle Adductor magnus muscle Biceps femoris muscle Gracilis muscle Pectineus muscle Quadriceps (femoris) Rectus femoris muscle Sartorius muscle Semimembranosus muscle Semitendinosus muscle Vastus intermedius muscle Vastus lateralis muscle Vastus medialis muscle **R Upper Leg Muscle, Left** *See Q Upper Leg Muscle, Right* **S Lower Leg Muscle, Right** Extensor digitorum longus muscle Extensor hallucis longus muscle Fibularis brevis muscle Fibularis longus muscle Flexor digitorum longus muscle Flexor hallucis longus muscle Gastrocnemius muscle Peroneus brevis muscle Peroneus longus muscle Popliteus muscle Soleus muscle Tibialis anterior muscle Tibialis posterior muscle **T Lower Leg Muscle, Left** *See S Lower Leg Muscle, Right* **V Foot Muscle, Right** Abductor hallucis muscle Adductor hallucis muscle Extensor digitorum brevis muscle Extensor hallucis brevis muscle Flexor digitorum brevis muscle Flexor hallucis brevis muscle Quadratus plantae muscle **W Foot Muscle, Left** *See V Foot Muscle, Right*	**Ø** Open **3** Percutaneous **4** Percutaneous Endoscopic	**Z** No Device	**Z** No Qualifier

LC Limited Coverage   **NC** Noncovered   ⊞ Combination Member   HAC associated procedure   Combination Only   DRG Non-OR   Non-OR   New/Revised in GREEN
ICD-10-PCS 2019

Ø Medical and Surgical
K Muscles
9 Drainage   Definition: Taking or letting out fluids and/or gases from a body part
Explanation: The qualifier DIAGNOSTIC is used to identify drainage procedures that are biopsies

Body Part – Character 4			Approach – Character 5	Device – Character 6	Qualifier – Character 7
Ø Head Muscle Auricularis muscle Masseter muscle Pterygoid muscle Splenius capitis muscle Temporalis muscle Temporoparietalis muscle **1 Facial Muscle** Buccinator muscle Corrugator supercilii muscle Depressor anguli oris muscle Depressor labii inferioris muscle Depressor septi nasi muscle Depressor supercilii muscle Levator anguli oris muscle Levator labii superioris alaeque nasi muscle Levator labii superioris muscle Mentalis muscle Nasalis muscle Occipitofrontalis muscle Orbicularis oris muscle Procerus muscle Risorius muscle Zygomaticus muscle **2 Neck Muscle, Right** Anterior vertebral muscle Arytenoid muscle Cricothyroid muscle Infrahyoid muscle Levator scapulae muscle Platysma muscle Scalene muscle Splenius cervicis muscle Sternocleidomastoid muscle Suprahyoid muscle Thyroarytenoid muscle **3 Neck Muscle, Left** *See 2 Neck Muscle, Right* **4 Tongue, Palate, Pharynx Muscle** Chondroglossus muscle Genioglossus muscle Hyoglossus muscle Inferior longitudinal muscle Levator veli palatini muscle Palatoglossal muscle Palatopharyngeal muscle Pharyngeal constrictor muscle Salpingopharyngeus muscle Styloglossus muscle Stylopharyngeus muscle Superior longitudinal muscle Tensor veli palatini muscle **5 Shoulder Muscle, Right** Deltoid muscle Infraspinatus muscle Subscapularis muscle Supraspinatus muscle Teres major muscle Teres minor muscle **6 Shoulder Muscle, Left** *See 5 Shoulder Muscle, Right*	**7 Upper Arm Muscle, Right** Biceps brachii muscle Brachialis muscle Coracobrachialis muscle Triceps brachii muscle **8 Upper Arm Muscle, Left** *See 7 Upper Arm Muscle, Right* **9 Lower Arm and Wrist Muscle, Right** Anatomical snuffbox Brachioradialis muscle Extensor carpi radialis muscle Extensor carpi ulnaris muscle Flexor carpi radialis muscle Flexor carpi ulnaris muscle Flexor pollicis longus muscle Palmaris longus muscle Pronator quadratus muscle Pronator teres muscle **B Lower Arm and Wrist Muscle, Left** *See 9 Lower Arm and Wrist Muscle, Right* **C Hand Muscle, Right** Hypothenar muscle Palmar interosseous muscle Thenar muscle **D Hand Muscle, Left** *See C Hand Muscle, Right* **F Trunk Muscle, Right** Coccygeus muscle Erector spinae muscle Interspinalis muscle Intertransversarius muscle Latissimus dorsi muscle Quadratus lumborum muscle Rhomboid major muscle Rhomboid minor muscle Serratus posterior muscle Transversospinalis muscle Trapezius muscle **G Trunk Muscle, Left** *See F Trunk Muscle, Right* **H Thorax Muscle, Right** Intercostal muscle Levatores costarum muscle Pectoralis major muscle Pectoralis minor muscle Serratus anterior muscle Subclavius muscle Subcostal muscle Transverse thoracis muscle **J Thorax Muscle, Left** *See H Thorax Muscle, Right* **K Abdomen Muscle, Right** External oblique muscle Internal oblique muscle Pyramidalis muscle Rectus abdominis muscle Transversus abdominis muscle **L Abdomen Muscle, Left** *See K Abdomen Muscle, Right*	**M Perineum Muscle** Bulbospongiosus muscle Cremaster muscle Deep transverse perineal muscle Ischiocavernosus muscle Levator ani muscle Superficial transverse perineal muscle **N Hip Muscle, Right** Gemellus muscle Gluteus maximus muscle Gluteus medius muscle Gluteus minimus muscle Iliacus muscle Obturator muscle Piriformis muscle Psoas muscle Quadratus femoris muscle Tensor fasciae latae muscle **P Hip Muscle, Left** *See N Hip Muscle, Right* **Q Upper Leg Muscle, Right** Adductor brevis muscle Adductor longus muscle Adductor magnus muscle Biceps femoris muscle Gracilis muscle Pectineus muscle Quadriceps (femoris) Rectus femoris muscle Sartorius muscle Semimembranosus muscle Semitendinosus muscle Vastus intermedius muscle Vastus lateralis muscle Vastus medialis muscle **R Upper Leg Muscle, Left** *See Q Upper Leg Muscle, Right* **S Lower Leg Muscle, Right** Extensor digitorum longus muscle Extensor hallucis longus muscle Fibularis brevis muscle Fibularis longus muscle Flexor digitorum longus muscle Flexor hallucis longus muscle Gastrocnemius muscle Peroneus brevis muscle Peroneus longus muscle Popliteus muscle Soleus muscle Tibialis anterior muscle Tibialis posterior muscle **T Lower Leg Muscle, Left** *See S Lower Leg Muscle, Right* **V Foot Muscle, Right** Abductor hallucis muscle Adductor hallucis muscle Extensor digitorum brevis muscle Extensor hallucis brevis muscle Flexor digitorum brevis muscle Flexor hallucis brevis muscle Quadratus plantae muscle **W Foot Muscle, Left** *See V Foot Muscle, Right*	**Ø Open** **3 Percutaneous** **4 Percutaneous Endoscopic**	**Ø Drainage Device**	**Z No Qualifier**

Non-OR   ØK9[Ø,1,2,3,4,5,6,7,8,9,B,C,D,F,G,H,J,K,L,M,N,P,Q,R,S,T,V,W]3ØZ

ØK9 Continued on next page

0 **Medical and Surgical**
K **Muscles**
9 **Drainage**

0K9 Continued

Definition: Taking or letting out fluids and/or gases from a body part
Explanation: The qualifier DIAGNOSTIC is used to identify drainage procedures that are biopsies

Body Part Character 4		Approach Character 5	Device Character 6	Qualifier Character 7
0 **Head Muscle** Auricularis muscle Masseter muscle Pterygoid muscle Splenius capitis muscle Temporalis muscle Temporoparietalis muscle **1** **Facial Muscle** Buccinator muscle Corrugator supercilii muscle Depressor anguli oris muscle Depressor labii inferioris muscle Depressor septi nasi muscle Depressor supercilii muscle Levator anguli oris muscle Levator labii superioris alaeque nasi muscle Levator labii superioris muscle Mentalis muscle Nasalis muscle Occipitofrontalis muscle Orbicularis oris muscle Procerus muscle Risorius muscle Zygomaticus muscle **2** **Neck Muscle, Right** Anterior vertebral muscle Arytenoid muscle Cricothyroid muscle Infrahyoid muscle Levator scapulae muscle Platysma muscle Scalene muscle Splenius cervicis muscle Sternocleidomastoid muscle Suprahyoid muscle Thyroarytenoid muscle **3** **Neck Muscle, Left** *See 2 Neck Muscle, Right* **4** **Tongue, Palate, Pharynx Muscle** Chondroglossus muscle Genioglossus muscle Hyoglossus muscle Inferior longitudinal muscle Levator veli palatini muscle Palatoglossal muscle Palatopharyngeal muscle Pharyngeal constrictor muscle Salpingopharyngeus muscle Styloglossus muscle Stylopharyngeus muscle Superior longitudinal muscle Tensor veli palatini muscle **5** **Shoulder Muscle, Right** Deltoid muscle Infraspinatus muscle Subscapularis muscle Supraspinatus muscle Teres major muscle Teres minor muscle **6** **Shoulder Muscle, Left** *See 5 Shoulder Muscle, Right*	**7** **Upper Arm Muscle, Right** Biceps brachii muscle Brachialis muscle Coracobrachialis muscle Triceps brachii muscle **8** **Upper Arm Muscle, Left** *See 7 Upper Arm Muscle, Right* **9** **Lower Arm and Wrist Muscle, Right** Anatomical snuffbox Brachioradialis muscle Extensor carpi radialis muscle Extensor carpi ulnaris muscle Flexor carpi radialis muscle Flexor carpi ulnaris muscle Flexor pollicis longus muscle Palmaris longus muscle Pronator quadratus muscle Pronator teres muscle **B** **Lower Arm and Wrist Muscle, Left** *See 9 Lower Arm and Wrist Muscle, Right* **C** **Hand Muscle, Right** Hypothenar muscle Palmar interosseous muscle Thenar muscle **D** **Hand Muscle, Left** *See C Hand Muscle, Right* **F** **Trunk Muscle, Right** Coccygeus muscle Erector spinae muscle Interspinalis muscle Intertransversarius muscle Latissimus dorsi muscle Quadratus lumborum muscle Rhomboid major muscle Rhomboid minor muscle Serratus posterior muscle Transversospinalis muscle Trapezius muscle **G** **Trunk Muscle, Left** *See F Trunk Muscle, Right* **H** **Thorax Muscle, Right** Intercostal muscle Levatores costarum muscle Pectoralis major muscle Pectoralis minor muscle Serratus anterior muscle Subclavius muscle Subcostal muscle Transverse thoracis muscle **J** **Thorax Muscle, Left** *See H Thorax Muscle, Right* **K** **Abdomen Muscle, Right** External oblique muscle Internal oblique muscle Pyramidalis muscle Rectus abdominis muscle Transversus abdominis muscle **L** **Abdomen Muscle, Left** *See K Abdomen Muscle, Right*	**M** **Perineum Muscle** Bulbospongiosus muscle Cremaster muscle Deep transverse perineal muscle Ischiocavernosus muscle Levator ani muscle Superficial transverse perineal muscle **N** **Hip Muscle, Right** Gemellus muscle Gluteus maximus muscle Gluteus medius muscle Gluteus minimus muscle Iliacus muscle Obturator muscle Piriformis muscle Psoas muscle Quadratus femoris muscle Tensor fasciae latae muscle **P** **Hip Muscle, Left** *See N Hip Muscle, Right* **Q** **Upper Leg Muscle, Right** Adductor brevis muscle Adductor longus muscle Adductor magnus muscle Biceps femoris muscle Gracilis muscle Pectineus muscle Quadriceps (femoris) Rectus femoris muscle Sartorius muscle Semimembranosus muscle Semitendinosus muscle Vastus intermedius muscle Vastus lateralis muscle Vastus medialis muscle **R** **Upper Leg Muscle, Left** *See Q Upper Leg Muscle, Right* **S** **Lower Leg Muscle, Right** Extensor digitorum longus muscle Extensor hallucis longus muscle Fibularis brevis muscle Fibularis longus muscle Flexor digitorum longus muscle Flexor hallucis longus muscle Gastrocnemius muscle Peroneus brevis muscle Peroneus longus muscle Popliteus muscle Soleus muscle Tibialis anterior muscle Tibialis posterior muscle **T** **Lower Leg Muscle, Left** *See S Lower Leg Muscle, Right* **V** **Foot Muscle, Right** Abductor hallucis muscle Adductor hallucis muscle Extensor digitorum brevis muscle Extensor hallucis brevis muscle Flexor digitorum brevis muscle Flexor hallucis brevis muscle Quadratus plantae muscle **W** **Foot Muscle, Left** *See V Foot Muscle, Right*	**0** Open **3** Percutaneous **4** Percutaneous Endoscopic	**Z** No Device	**X** Diagnostic **Z** No Qualifier

Non-OR   0K9[0,1,2,3,4,5,6,7,8,9,B,F,G,H,J,K,L,M,N,P,Q,R,S,T,V,W]3ZZ
Non-OR   0K9[C,D][3,4]ZZ

LC Limited Coverage   NC Noncovered   ⊞ Combination Member   HAC associated procedure   Combination Only   DRG Non-OR   Non-OR   New/Revised in GREEN

448

ICD-10-PCS 2019

Ø **Medical and Surgical**
K **Muscles**
B **Excision**   Definition: Cutting out or off, without replacement, a portion of a body part
              Explanation: The qualifier DIAGNOSTIC is used to identify excision procedures that are biopsies

Body Part Character 4			Approach Character 5	Device Character 6	Qualifier Character 7
Ø Head Muscle Auricularis muscle Masseter muscle Pterygoid muscle Splenius capitis muscle Temporalis muscle Temporoparietalis muscle **1 Facial Muscle** Buccinator muscle Corrugator supercilii muscle Depressor anguli oris muscle Depressor labii inferioris muscle Depressor septi nasi muscle Depressor supercilii muscle Levator anguli oris muscle Levator labii superioris alaeque nasi muscle Levator labii superioris muscle Mentalis muscle Nasalis muscle Occipitofrontalis muscle Orbicularis oris muscle Procerus muscle Risorius muscle Zygomaticus muscle **2 Neck Muscle, Right** Anterior vertebral muscle Arytenoid muscle Cricothyroid muscle Infrahyoid muscle Levator scapulae muscle Platysma muscle Scalene muscle Splenius cervicis muscle Sternocleidomastoid muscle Suprahyoid muscle Thyroarytenoid muscle **3 Neck Muscle, Left** *See 2 Neck Muscle, Right* **4 Tongue, Palate, Pharynx Muscle** Chondroglossus muscle Genioglossus muscle Hyoglossus muscle Inferior longitudinal muscle Levator veli palatini muscle Palatoglossal muscle Palatopharyngeal muscle Pharyngeal constrictor muscle Salpingopharyngeus muscle Styloglossus muscle Stylopharyngeus muscle Superior longitudinal muscle Tensor veli palatini muscle **5 Shoulder Muscle, Right** Deltoid muscle Infraspinatus muscle Subscapularis muscle Supraspinatus muscle Teres major muscle Teres minor muscle **6 Shoulder Muscle, Left** *See 5 Shoulder Muscle, Right*	**7 Upper Arm Muscle, Right** Biceps brachii muscle Brachialis muscle Coracobrachialis muscle Triceps brachii muscle **8 Upper Arm Muscle, Left** *See 7 Upper Arm Muscle, Right* **9 Lower Arm and Wrist Muscle, Right** Anatomical snuffbox Brachioradialis muscle Extensor carpi radialis muscle Extensor carpi ulnaris muscle Flexor carpi radialis muscle Flexor carpi ulnaris muscle Flexor pollicis longus muscle Palmaris longus muscle Pronator quadratus muscle Pronator teres muscle **B Lower Arm and Wrist Muscle, Left** *See 9 Lower Arm and Wrist Muscle, Right* **C Hand Muscle, Right** Hypothenar muscle Palmar interosseous muscle Thenar muscle **D Hand Muscle, Left** *See C Hand Muscle, Right* **F Trunk Muscle, Right** Coccygeus muscle Erector spinae muscle Interspinalis muscle Intertransversarius muscle Latissimus dorsi muscle Quadratus lumborum muscle Rhomboid major muscle Rhomboid minor muscle Serratus posterior muscle Transversospinalis muscle Trapezius muscle **G Trunk Muscle, Left** *See F Trunk Muscle, Right* **H Thorax Muscle, Right** Intercostal muscle Levatores costarum muscle Pectoralis major muscle Pectoralis minor muscle Serratus anterior muscle Subclavius muscle Subcostal muscle Transverse thoracis muscle **J Thorax Muscle, Left** *See H Thorax Muscle, Right* **K Abdomen Muscle, Right** External oblique muscle Internal oblique muscle Pyramidalis muscle Rectus abdominis muscle Transversus abdominis muscle **L Abdomen Muscle, Left** *See K Abdomen Muscle, Right*	**M Perineum Muscle** Bulbospongiosus muscle Cremaster muscle Deep transverse perineal muscle Ischiocavernosus muscle Levator ani muscle Superficial transverse perineal muscle **N Hip Muscle, Right** Gemellus muscle Gluteus maximus muscle Gluteus medius muscle Gluteus minimus muscle Iliacus muscle Obturator muscle Piriformis muscle Psoas muscle Quadratus femoris muscle Tensor fasciae latae muscle **P Hip Muscle, Left** *See N Hip Muscle, Right* **Q Upper Leg Muscle, Right** Adductor brevis muscle Adductor longus muscle Adductor magnus muscle Biceps femoris muscle Gracilis muscle Pectineus muscle Quadriceps (femoris) Rectus femoris muscle Sartorius muscle Semimembranosus muscle Semitendinosus muscle Vastus intermedius muscle Vastus lateralis muscle Vastus medialis muscle **R Upper Leg Muscle, Left** *See Q Upper Leg Muscle, Right* **S Lower Leg Muscle, Right** Extensor digitorum longus muscle Extensor hallucis longus muscle Fibularis brevis muscle Fibularis longus muscle Flexor digitorum longus muscle Flexor hallucis longus muscle Gastrocnemius muscle Peroneus brevis muscle Peroneus longus muscle Popliteus muscle Soleus muscle Tibialis anterior muscle Tibialis posterior muscle **T Lower Leg Muscle, Left** *See S Lower Leg Muscle, Right* **V Foot Muscle, Right** Abductor hallucis muscle Adductor hallucis muscle Extensor digitorum brevis muscle Extensor hallucis brevis muscle Flexor digitorum brevis muscle Flexor hallucis brevis muscle Quadratus plantae muscle **W Foot Muscle, Left** *See V Foot Muscle, Right*	**Ø Open** **3 Percutaneous** **4 Percutaneous Endoscopic**	**Z No Device**	**X Diagnostic** **Z No Qualifier**

LC Limited Coverage   NC Noncovered   ⊞ Combination Member   HAC associated procedure   Combination Only   DRG Non-OR   Non-OR   New/Revised in GREEN

ICD-10-PCS 2019   449

ØKB–ØKB

Muscles

Ø   Medical and Surgical
K   Muscles
C   Extirpation   Definition: Taking or cutting out solid matter from a body part

Explanation: The solid matter may be an abnormal byproduct of a biological function or a foreign body; it may be imbedded in a body part or in the lumen of a tubular body part. The solid matter may or may not have been previously broken into pieces.

Body Part Character 4		Approach Character 5	Device Character 6	Qualifier Character 7
Ø Head Muscle Auricularis muscle Masseter muscle Pterygoid muscle Splenius capitis muscle Temporalis muscle Temporoparietalis muscle **1 Facial Muscle** Buccinator muscle Corrugator supercilii muscle Depressor anguli oris muscle Depressor labii inferioris muscle Depressor septi nasi muscle Depressor supercilii muscle Levator anguli oris muscle Levator labii superioris alaeque nasi muscle Levator labii superioris muscle Mentalis muscle Nasalis muscle Occipitofrontalis muscle Orbicularis oris muscle Procerus muscle Risorius muscle Zygomaticus muscle **2 Neck Muscle, Right** Anterior vertebral muscle Arytenoid muscle Cricothyroid muscle Infrahyoid muscle Levator scapulae muscle Platysma muscle Scalene muscle Splenius cervicis muscle Sternocleidomastoid muscle Suprahyoid muscle Thyroarytenoid muscle **3 Neck Muscle, Left** *See 2 Neck Muscle, Right* **4 Tongue, Palate, Pharynx Muscle** Chondroglossus muscle Genioglossus muscle Hyoglossus muscle Inferior longitudinal muscle Levator veli palatini muscle Palatoglossal muscle Palatopharyngeal muscle Pharyngeal constrictor muscle Salpingopharyngeus muscle Styloglossus muscle Stylopharyngeus muscle Superior longitudinal muscle Tensor veli palatini muscle **5 Shoulder Muscle, Right** Deltoid muscle Infraspinatus muscle Subscapularis muscle Supraspinatus muscle Teres major muscle Teres minor muscle **6 Shoulder Muscle, Left** *See 5 Shoulder Muscle, Right*	**7 Upper Arm Muscle, Right** Biceps brachii muscle Brachialis muscle Coracobrachialis muscle Triceps brachii muscle **8 Upper Arm Muscle, Left** *See 7 Upper Arm Muscle, Right* **9 Lower Arm and Wrist Muscle, Right** Anatomical snuffbox Brachioradialis muscle Extensor carpi radialis muscle Extensor carpi ulnaris muscle Flexor carpi radialis muscle Flexor carpi ulnaris muscle Flexor pollicis longus muscle Palmaris longus muscle Pronator quadratus muscle Pronator teres muscle **B Lower Arm and Wrist Muscle, Left** *See 9 Lower Arm and Wrist Muscle, Right* **C Hand Muscle, Right** Hypothenar muscle Palmar interosseous muscle Thenar muscle **D Hand Muscle, Left** *See C Hand Muscle, Right* **F Trunk Muscle, Right** Coccygeus muscle Erector spinae muscle Interspinalis muscle Intertransversarius muscle Latissimus dorsi muscle Quadratus lumborum muscle Rhomboid major muscle Rhomboid minor muscle Serratus posterior muscle Transversospinalis muscle Trapezius muscle **G Trunk Muscle, Left** *See F Trunk Muscle, Right* **H Thorax Muscle, Right** Intercostal muscle Levatores costarum muscle Pectoralis major muscle Pectoralis minor muscle Serratus anterior muscle Subclavius muscle Subcostal muscle Transverse thoracis muscle **J Thorax Muscle, Left** *See H Thorax Muscle, Right* **K Abdomen Muscle, Right** External oblique muscle Internal oblique muscle Pyramidalis muscle Rectus abdominis muscle Transversus abdominis muscle **L Abdomen Muscle, Left** *See K Abdomen Muscle, Right*	**M Perineum Muscle** Bulbospongiosus muscle Cremaster muscle Deep transverse perineal muscle Ischiocavernosus muscle Levator ani muscle Superficial transverse perineal muscle **N Hip Muscle, Right** Gemellus muscle Gluteus maximus muscle Gluteus medius muscle Gluteus minimus muscle Iliacus muscle Obturator muscle Piriformis muscle Psoas muscle Quadratus femoris muscle Tensor fasciae latae muscle **P Hip Muscle, Left** *See N Hip Muscle, Right* **Q Upper Leg Muscle, Right** Adductor brevis muscle Adductor longus muscle Adductor magnus muscle Biceps femoris muscle Gracilis muscle Pectineus muscle Quadriceps (femoris) Rectus femoris muscle Sartorius muscle Semimembranosus muscle Semitendinosus muscle Vastus intermedius muscle Vastus lateralis muscle Vastus medialis muscle **R Upper Leg Muscle, Left** *See Q Upper Leg Muscle, Right* **S Lower Leg Muscle, Right** Extensor digitorum longus muscle Extensor hallucis longus muscle Fibularis brevis muscle Fibularis longus muscle Flexor digitorum longus muscle Flexor hallucis longus muscle Gastrocnemius muscle Peroneus brevis muscle Peroneus longus muscle Popliteus muscle Soleus muscle Tibialis anterior muscle Tibialis posterior muscle **T Lower Leg Muscle, Left** *See S Lower Leg Muscle, Right* **V Foot Muscle, Right** Abductor hallucis muscle Adductor hallucis muscle Extensor digitorum brevis muscle Extensor hallucis brevis muscle Flexor digitorum brevis muscle Flexor hallucis brevis muscle Quadratus plantae muscle **W Foot Muscle, Left** *See V Foot Muscle, Right*	**Ø Open** **3 Percutaneous** **4 Percutaneous Endoscopic**	**Z No Device**	**Z No Qualifier**

LC Limited Coverage   **NC** Noncovered   ⊞ Combination Member   HAC associated procedure   Combination Only   DRG Non-OR   Non-OR   New/Revised in GREEN

450   ICD-10-PCS 2019

Ø   **Medical and Surgical**
K   **Muscles**
D   **Extraction**   Definition: Pulling or stripping out or off all or a portion of a body part by the use of force

                          Explanation: The qualifier DIAGNOSTIC is used to identify extraction procedures that are biopsies

Body Part Character 4			Approach Character 5	Device Character 6	Qualifier Character 7
Ø **Head Muscle** Auricularis muscle Masseter muscle Pterygoid muscle Splenius capitis muscle Temporalis muscle Temporoparietalis muscle **1** **Facial Muscle** Buccinator muscle Corrugator supercilii muscle Depressor anguli oris muscle Depressor labii inferioris muscle Depressor septi nasi muscle Depressor supercilii muscle Levator anguli oris muscle Levator labii superioris alaeque nasi muscle Levator labii superioris muscle Mentalis muscle Nasalis muscle Occipitofrontalis muscle Orbicularis oris muscle Procerus muscle Risorius muscle Zygomaticus muscle **2** **Neck Muscle, Right** Anterior vertebral muscle Arytenoid muscle Cricothyroid muscle Infrahyoid muscle Levator scapulae muscle Platysma muscle Scalene muscle Splenius cervicis muscle Sternocleidomastoid muscle Suprahyoid muscle Thyroarytenoid muscle **3** **Neck Muscle, Left** *See 2 Neck Muscle, Right* **4** **Tongue, Palate, Pharynx Muscle** Chondroglossus muscle Genioglossus muscle Hyoglossus muscle Inferior longitudinal muscle Levator veli palatini muscle Palatoglossal muscle Palatopharyngeal muscle Pharyngeal constrictor muscle Salpingopharyngeus muscle Styloglossus muscle Stylopharyngeus muscle Superior longitudinal muscle Tensor veli palatini muscle **5** **Shoulder Muscle, Right** Deltoid muscle Infraspinatus muscle Subscapularis muscle Supraspinatus muscle Teres major muscle Teres minor muscle **6** **Shoulder Muscle, Left** *See 5 Shoulder Muscle, Right*	**7** **Upper Arm Muscle, Right** Biceps brachii muscle Brachialis muscle Coracobrachialis muscle Triceps brachii muscle **8** **Upper Arm Muscle, Left** *See 7 Upper Arm Muscle, Right* **9** **Lower Arm and Wrist Muscle, Right** Anatomical snuffbox Brachioradialis muscle Extensor carpi radialis muscle Extensor carpi ulnaris muscle Flexor carpi radialis muscle Flexor carpi ulnaris muscle Flexor pollicis longus muscle Palmaris longus muscle Pronator quadratus muscle Pronator teres muscle **B** **Lower Arm and Wrist Muscle, Left** *See 9 Lower Arm and Wrist Muscle, Right* **C** **Hand Muscle, Right** Hypothenar muscle Palmar interosseous muscle Thenar muscle **D** **Hand Muscle, Left** *See C Hand Muscle, Right* **F** **Trunk Muscle, Right** Coccygeus muscle Erector spinae muscle Interspinalis muscle Intertransversarius muscle Latissimus dorsi muscle Quadratus lumborum muscle Rhomboid major muscle Rhomboid minor muscle Serratus posterior muscle Transversospinalis muscle Trapezius muscle **G** **Trunk Muscle, Left** *See F Trunk Muscle, Right* **H** **Thorax Muscle, Right** Intercostal muscle Levatores costarum muscle Pectoralis major muscle Pectoralis minor muscle Serratus anterior muscle Subclavius muscle Subcostal muscle Transverse thoracis muscle **J** **Thorax Muscle, Left** *See H Thorax Muscle, Right* **K** **Abdomen Muscle, Right** External oblique muscle Internal oblique muscle Pyramidalis muscle Rectus abdominis muscle Transversus abdominis muscle **L** **Abdomen Muscle, Left** *See K Abdomen Muscle, Right*	**M** **Perineum Muscle** Bulbospongiosus muscle Cremaster muscle Deep transverse perineal muscle Ischiocavernosus muscle Levator ani muscle Superficial transverse perineal muscle **N** **Hip Muscle, Right** Gemellus muscle Gluteus maximus muscle Gluteus medius muscle Gluteus minimus muscle Iliacus muscle Obturator muscle Piriformis muscle Psoas muscle Quadratus femoris muscle Tensor fasciae latae muscle **P** **Hip Muscle, Left** *See N Hip Muscle, Right* **Q** **Upper Leg Muscle, Right** Adductor brevis muscle Adductor longus muscle Adductor magnus muscle Biceps femoris muscle Gracilis muscle Pectineus muscle Quadriceps (femoris) Rectus femoris muscle Sartorius muscle Semimembranosus muscle Semitendinosus muscle Vastus intermedius muscle Vastus lateralis muscle Vastus medialis muscle **R** **Upper Leg Muscle, Left** *See Q Upper Leg Muscle, Right* **S** **Lower Leg Muscle, Right** Extensor digitorum longus muscle Extensor hallucis longus muscle Fibularis brevis muscle Fibularis longus muscle Flexor digitorum longus muscle Flexor hallucis longus muscle Gastrocnemius muscle Peroneus brevis muscle Peroneus longus muscle Popliteus muscle Soleus muscle Tibialis anterior muscle Tibialis posterior muscle **T** **Lower Leg Muscle, Left** *See S Lower Leg Muscle, Right* **V** **Foot Muscle, Right** Abductor hallucis muscle Adductor hallucis muscle Extensor digitorum brevis muscle Extensor hallucis brevis muscle Flexor digitorum brevis muscle Flexor hallucis brevis muscle Quadratus plantae muscle **W** **Foot Muscle, Left** *See V Foot Muscle, Right*	**Ø** Open	**Z** No Device	**Z** No Qualifier

LC Limited Coverage   NC Noncovered   ⊞ Combination Member   HAC associated procedure   Combination Only   DRG Non-OR   Non-OR   New/Revised in GREEN

ICD-10-PCS 2019

451

ØKD–ØKD

Ø   Medical and Surgical
K   Muscles
H   Insertion   Definition: Putting in a nonbiological appliance that monitors, assists, performs, or prevents a physiological function but does not physically take the place of a body part

Explanation: None

Body Part Character 4	Approach Character 5	Device Character 6	Qualifier Character 7
X Upper Muscle Y Lower Muscle	Ø Open 3 Percutaneous 4 Percutaneous Endoscopic	M Stimulator Lead Y Other Device	Z No Qualifier

Non-OR   ØKH[X,Y][3,4]YZ

Ø   Medical and Surgical
K   Muscles
J   Inspection   Definition: Visually and/or manually exploring a body part

Explanation: Visual exploration may be performed with or without optical instrumentation. Manual exploration may be performed directly or through intervening body layers.

Body Part Character 4	Approach Character 5	Device Character 6	Qualifier Character 7
X Upper Muscle Y Lower Muscle	Ø Open 3 Percutaneous 4 Percutaneous Endoscopic X External	Z No Device	Z No Qualifier

Non-OR   ØKJ[X,Y][3,X]ZZ

Ø   **Medical and Surgical**
K   **Muscles**
M   **Reattachment**   Definition: Putting back in or on all or a portion of a separated body part to its normal location or other suitable location
                      Explanation: Vascular circulation and nervous pathways may or may not be reestablished

Body Part Character 4			Approach Character 5	Device Character 6	Qualifier Character 7

Ø   **Head Muscle**
    Auricularis muscle
    Masseter muscle
    Pterygoid muscle
    Splenius capitis muscle
    Temporalis muscle
    Temporoparietalis muscle
1   **Facial Muscle**
    Buccinator muscle
    Corrugator supercilii
      muscle
    Depressor anguli oris
      muscle
    Depressor labii inferioris
      muscle
    Depressor septi nasi
      muscle
    Depressor supercilii
      muscle
    Levator anguli oris muscle
    Levator labii superioris
      alaeque nasi muscle
    Levator labii superioris
      muscle
    Mentalis muscle
    Nasalis muscle
    Occipitofrontalis muscle
    Orbicularis oris muscle
    Procerus muscle
    Risorius muscle
    Zygomaticus muscle
2   **Neck Muscle, Right**
    Anterior vertebral muscle
    Arytenoid muscle
    Cricothyroid muscle
    Infrahyoid muscle
    Levator scapulae muscle
    Platysma muscle
    Scalene muscle
    Splenius cervicis muscle
    Sternocleidomastoid
      muscle
    Suprahyoid muscle
    Thyroarytenoid muscle
3   **Neck Muscle, Left**
    See 2 Neck Muscle, Right
4   **Tongue, Palate, Pharynx**
    Muscle
    Chondroglossus muscle
    Genioglossus muscle
    Hyoglossus muscle
    Inferior longitudinal
      muscle
    Levator veli palatini
      muscle
    Palatoglossal muscle
    Palatopharyngeal muscle
    Pharyngeal constrictor
      muscle
    Salpingopharyngeus
      muscle
    Styloglossus muscle
    Stylopharyngeus muscle
    Superior longitudinal
      muscle
    Tensor veli palatini muscle
5   **Shoulder Muscle, Right**
    Deltoid muscle
    Infraspinatus muscle
    Subscapularis muscle
    Supraspinatus muscle
    Teres major muscle
    Teres minor muscle
6   **Shoulder Muscle, Left**
    See 5 Shoulder Muscle,
      Right
	7 **Upper Arm Muscle, Right**
	    Biceps brachii muscle
	    Brachialis muscle
	    Coracobrachialis muscle
	    Triceps brachii muscle
	8 **Upper Arm Muscle, Left**
	    See 7 Upper Arm Muscle,
	      Right
	9 **Lower Arm and Wrist**
	    Muscle, Right
	    Anatomical snuffbox
	    Brachioradialis muscle
	    Extensor carpi radialis
	      muscle
	    Extensor carpi ulnaris
	      muscle
	    Flexor carpi radialis muscle
	    Flexor carpi ulnaris muscle
	    Flexor pollicis longus
	      muscle
	    Palmaris longus muscle
	    Pronator quadratus
	      muscle
	    Pronator teres muscle
	B **Lower Arm and Wrist**
	    Muscle, Left
	    See 9 Lower Arm and Wrist
	      Muscle, Right
	C **Hand Muscle, Right**
	    Hypothenar muscle
	    Palmar interosseous
	      muscle
	    Thenar muscle
	D **Hand Muscle, Left**
	    See C Hand Muscle, Right
	F **Trunk Muscle, Right**
	    Coccygeus muscle
	    Erector spinae muscle
	    Interspinalis muscle
	    Intertransversarius muscle
	    Latissimus dorsi muscle
	    Quadratus lumborum
	      muscle
	    Rhomboid major muscle
	    Rhomboid minor muscle
	    Serratus posterior muscle
	    Transversospinalis muscle
	    Trapezius muscle
	G **Trunk Muscle, Left**
	    See F Trunk Muscle, Right
	H **Thorax Muscle, Right**
	    Intercostal muscle
	    Levatores costarum
	      muscle
	    Pectoralis major muscle
	    Pectoralis minor muscle
	    Serratus anterior muscle
	    Subclavius muscle
	    Subcostal muscle
	    Transverse thoracis muscle
	J **Thorax Muscle, Left**
	    See H Thorax Muscle, Right
	K **Abdomen Muscle, Right**
	    External oblique muscle
	    Internal oblique muscle
	    Pyramidalis muscle
	    Rectus abdominis muscle
	    Transversus abdominis
	      muscle
	L **Abdomen Muscle, Left**
	    See K Abdomen Muscle,
	      Right
		M **Perineum Muscle**
		    Bulbospongiosus muscle
		    Cremaster muscle
		    Deep transverse perineal
		      muscle
		    Ischiocavernosus muscle
		    Levator ani muscle
		    Superficial transverse
		      perineal muscle
		N **Hip Muscle, Right**
		    Gemellus muscle
		    Gluteus maximus muscle
		    Gluteus medius muscle
		    Gluteus minimus muscle
		    Iliacus muscle
		    Obturator muscle
		    Piriformis muscle
		    Psoas muscle
		    Quadratus femoris muscle
		    Tensor fasciae latae
		      muscle
		P **Hip Muscle, Left**
		    See N Hip Muscle, Right
		Q **Upper Leg Muscle, Right**
		    Adductor brevis muscle
		    Adductor longus muscle
		    Adductor magnus muscle
		    Biceps femoris muscle
		    Gracilis muscle
		    Pectineus muscle
		    Quadriceps (femoris)
		    Rectus femoris muscle
		    Sartorius muscle
		    Semimembranosus
		      muscle
		    Semitendinosus muscle
		    Vastus intermedius muscle
		    Vastus lateralis muscle
		    Vastus medialis muscle
		R **Upper Leg Muscle, Left**
		    See Q Upper Leg Muscle,
		      Right
		S **Lower Leg Muscle, Right**
		    Extensor digitorum longus
		      muscle
		    Extensor hallucis longus
		      muscle
		    Fibularis brevis muscle
		    Fibularis longus muscle
		    Flexor digitorum longus
		      muscle
		    Flexor hallucis longus
		      muscle
		    Gastrocnemius muscle
		    Peroneus brevis muscle
		    Peroneus longus muscle
		    Popliteus muscle
		    Soleus muscle
		    Tibialis anterior muscle
		    Tibialis posterior muscle
		T **Lower Leg Muscle, Left**
		    See S Lower Leg Muscle,
		      Right
		V **Foot Muscle, Right**
		    Abductor hallucis muscle
		    Adductor hallucis muscle
		    Extensor digitorum brevis
		      muscle
		    Extensor hallucis brevis
		      muscle
		    Flexor digitorum brevis
		      muscle
		    Flexor hallucis brevis
		      muscle
		    Quadratus plantae muscle
		W **Foot Muscle, Left**
		    See V Foot Muscle, Right
			Ø Open
			4 Percutaneous
			    Endoscopic
				Z No Device	**Z** No Qualifier

LC Limited Coverage   **NC** Noncovered   ⊞ Combination Member   HAC associated procedure   Combination Only   DRG Non-OR   Non-OR   New/Revised in GREEN

ICD-10-PCS 2019   453

ØKM–ØKM

Ø Medical and Surgical
K Muscles
N Release

Definition: Freeing a body part from an abnormal physical constraint by cutting or by the use of force
Explanation: Some of the restraining tissue may be taken out but none of the body part is taken out

Body Part Character 4		Approach Character 5	Device Character 6	Qualifier Character 7

Ø Head Muscle
Auricularis muscle
Masseter muscle
Pterygoid muscle
Splenius capitis muscle
Temporalis muscle
Temporoparietalis muscle
1 Facial Muscle
Buccinator muscle
Corrugator supercilii
  muscle
Depressor anguli oris
  muscle
Depressor labii inferioris
  muscle
Depressor septi nasi
  muscle
Depressor supercilii
  muscle
Levator anguli oris muscle
Levator labii superioris
  alaeque nasi muscle
Levator labii superioris
  muscle
Mentalis muscle
Nasalis muscle
Occipitofrontalis muscle
Orbicularis oris muscle
Procerus muscle
Risorius muscle
Zygomaticus muscle
2 Neck Muscle, Right
Anterior vertebral muscle
Arytenoid muscle
Cricothyroid muscle
Infrahyoid muscle
Levator scapulae muscle
Platysma muscle
Scalene muscle
Splenius cervicis muscle
Sternocleidomastoid
  muscle
Suprahyoid muscle
Thyroarytenoid muscle
3 Neck Muscle, Left
See 2 Neck Muscle, Right
**4 Tongue, Palate, Pharynx
Muscle**
Chondroglossus muscle
Genioglossus muscle
Hyoglossus muscle
Inferior longitudinal
  muscle
Levator veli palatini
  muscle
Palatoglossal muscle
Palatopharyngeal muscle
Pharyngeal constrictor
  muscle
Salpingopharyngeus
  muscle
Styloglossus muscle
Stylopharyngeus muscle
Superior longitudinal
  muscle
Tensor veli palatini muscle
5 Shoulder Muscle, Right
Deltoid muscle
Infraspinatus muscle
Subscapularis muscle
Supraspinatus muscle
Teres major muscle
Teres minor muscle
6 Shoulder Muscle, Left
*See 5 Shoulder Muscle,
  Right*
	7 Upper Arm Muscle, Right
	Biceps brachii muscle
	Brachialis muscle
	Coracobrachialis muscle
	Triceps brachii muscle
	8 Upper Arm Muscle, Left
	*See 7 Upper Arm Muscle,
	  Right*
	**9 Lower Arm and Wrist
	Muscle, Right**
	Anatomical snuffbox
	Brachioradialis muscle
	Extensor carpi radialis
	  muscle
	Extensor carpi ulnaris
	  muscle
	Flexor carpi radialis muscle
	Flexor carpi ulnaris muscle
	Flexor pollicis longus
	  muscle
	Palmaris longus muscle
	Pronator quadratus
	  muscle
	Pronator teres muscle
	**B Lower Arm and Wrist
	Muscle, Left**
	*See 9 Lower Arm and Wrist
	  Muscle, Right*
	C Hand Muscle, Right
	Hypothenar muscle
	Palmar interosseous
	  muscle
	Thenar muscle
	D Hand Muscle, Left
	See C Hand Muscle, Right
	F Trunk Muscle, Right
	Coccygeus muscle
	Erector spinae muscle
	Interspinalis muscle
	Intertransversarius muscle
	Latissimus dorsi muscle
	Quadratus lumborum
	  muscle
	Rhomboid major muscle
	Rhomboid minor muscle
	Serratus posterior muscle
	Transversospinalis muscle
	Trapezius muscle
	G Trunk Muscle, Left
	See F Trunk Muscle, Right
	H Thorax Muscle, Right
	Intercostal muscle
	Levatores costarum
	  muscle
	Pectoralis major muscle
	Pectoralis minor muscle
	Serratus anterior muscle
	Subclavius muscle
	Subcostal muscle
	Transverse thoracis muscle
	J Thorax Muscle, Left
	See H Thorax Muscle, Right
	K Abdomen Muscle, Right
	External oblique muscle
	Internal oblique muscle
	Pyramidalis muscle
	Rectus abdominis muscle
	Transversus abdominis
	  muscle
	L Abdomen Muscle, Left
	*See K Abdomen Muscle,
	  Right*
		M Perineum Muscle
		Bulbospongiosus muscle
		Cremaster muscle
		Deep transverse perineal
		  muscle
		Ischiocavernosus muscle
		Levator ani muscle
		Superficial transverse
		  perineal muscle
		N Hip Muscle, Right
		Gemellus muscle
		Gluteus maximus muscle
		Gluteus medius muscle
		Gluteus minimus muscle
		Iliacus muscle
		Obturator muscle
		Piriformis muscle
		Psoas muscle
		Quadratus femoris muscle
		Tensor fasciae latae
		  muscle
		P Hip Muscle, Left
		See N Hip Muscle, Right
		Q Upper Leg Muscle, Right
		Adductor brevis muscle
		Adductor longus muscle
		Adductor magnus muscle
		Biceps femoris muscle
		Gracilis muscle
		Pectineus muscle
		Quadriceps (femoris)
		Rectus femoris muscle
		Sartorius muscle
		Semimembranosus
		  muscle
		Semitendinosus muscle
		Vastus intermedius muscle
		Vastus lateralis muscle
		Vastus medialis muscle
		R Upper Leg Muscle, Left
		*See Q Upper Leg Muscle,
		  Right*
		S Lower Leg Muscle, Right
		Extensor digitorum longus
		  muscle
		Extensor hallucis longus
		  muscle
		Fibularis brevis muscle
		Fibularis longus muscle
		Flexor digitorum longus
		  muscle
		Flexor hallucis longus
		  muscle
		Gastrocnemius muscle
		Peroneus brevis muscle
		Peroneus longus muscle
		Popliteus muscle
		Soleus muscle
		Tibialis anterior muscle
		Tibialis posterior muscle
		T Lower Leg Muscle, Left
		*See S Lower Leg Muscle,
		  Right*
		V Foot Muscle, Right
		Abductor hallucis muscle
		Adductor hallucis muscle
		Extensor digitorum brevis
		  muscle
		Extensor hallucis brevis
		  muscle
		Flexor digitorum brevis
		  muscle
		Flexor hallucis brevis
		  muscle
		Quadratus plantae muscle
		W Foot Muscle, Left
		See V Foot Muscle, Right
			Ø Open
			3 Percutaneous
			**4 Percutaneous
			Endoscopic**
			X External
				Z No Device	**Z No Qualifier**

Non-OR   ØKN[Ø,1,2,3,4,5,6,7,8,9,B,C,D,F,G,H,J,K,L,M,N,P,Q,R,S,T,V,W]XZZ

LC Limited Coverage   NC Noncovered   ⊞ Combination Member   HAC associated procedure   Combination Only   DRG Non-OR   Non-OR   New/Revised in GREEN

454   ICD-10-PCS 2019

ØKN–ØKN

Ø   Medical and Surgical
K   Muscles
P   Removal   Definition: Taking out or off a device from a body part

Explanation: If a device is taken out and a similar device put in without cutting or puncturing the skin or mucous membrane, the procedure is coded to the root operation CHANGE. Otherwise, the procedure for taking out a device is coded to the root operation REMOVAL.

Body Part Character 4	Approach Character 5	Device Character 6	Qualifier Character 7
X Upper Muscle **Y** Lower Muscle	**Ø** Open **3** Percutaneous **4** Percutaneous Endoscopic	**Ø** Drainage Device **7** Autologous Tissue Substitute **J** Synthetic Substitute **K** Nonautologous Tissue Substitute **M** Stimulator Lead **Y** Other Device	**Z** No Qualifier
X Upper Muscle **Y** Lower Muscle	**X** External	**Ø** Drainage Device **M** Stimulator Lead	**Z** No Qualifier

Non-OR   ØKP[X,Y][3,4]YZ
Non-OR   ØKP[X,Y]X[Ø,M]Z

Muscles

Ø　**Medical and Surgical**
K　**Muscles**
Q　**Repair**　Definition: Restoring, to the extent possible, a body part to its normal anatomic structure and function
　　　　Explanation: Used only when the method to accomplish the repair is not one of the other root operations

Body Part Character 4			Approach Character 5	Device Character 6	Qualifier Character 7
Ø **Head Muscle** 　Auricularis muscle 　Masseter muscle 　Pterygoid muscle 　Splenius capitis muscle 　Temporalis muscle 　Temporoparietalis muscle 1 **Facial Muscle** 　Buccinator muscle 　Corrugator supercilii 　　muscle 　Depressor anguli oris 　　muscle 　Depressor labii inferioris 　　muscle 　Depressor septi nasi 　　muscle 　Depressor supercilii 　　muscle 　Levator anguli oris muscle 　Levator labii superioris 　　alaeque nasi muscle 　Levator labii superioris 　　muscle 　Mentalis muscle 　Nasalis muscle 　Occipitofrontalis muscle 　Orbicularis oris muscle 　Procerus muscle 　Risorius muscle 　Zygomaticus muscle 2 **Neck Muscle, Right** 　Anterior vertebral muscle 　Arytenoid muscle 　Cricothyroid muscle 　Infrahyoid muscle 　Levator scapulae muscle 　Platysma muscle 　Scalene muscle 　Splenius cervicis muscle 　Sternocleidomastoid 　　muscle 　Suprahyoid muscle 　Thyroarytenoid muscle 3 **Neck Muscle, Left** 　*See 2 Neck Muscle, Right* 4 **Tongue, Palate, Pharynx** 　**Muscle** 　Chondroglossus muscle 　Genioglossus muscle 　Hyoglossus muscle 　Inferior longitudinal 　　muscle 　Levator veli palatini 　　muscle 　Palatoglossal muscle 　Palatopharyngeal muscle 　Pharyngeal constrictor 　　muscle 　Salpingopharyngeus 　　muscle 　Styloglossus muscle 　Stylopharyngeus muscle 　Superior longitudinal 　　muscle 　Tensor veli palatini muscle 5 **Shoulder Muscle, Right** 　Deltoid muscle 　Infraspinatus muscle 　Subscapularis muscle 　Supraspinatus muscle 　Teres major muscle 　Teres minor muscle 6 **Shoulder Muscle, Left** 　*See 5 Shoulder Muscle,* 　　*Right*	7 **Upper Arm Muscle, Right** 　Biceps brachii muscle 　Brachialis muscle 　Coracobrachialis muscle 　Triceps brachii muscle 8 **Upper Arm Muscle, Left** 　*See 7 Upper Arm Muscle,* 　　*Right* 9 **Lower Arm and Wrist** 　**Muscle, Right** 　Anatomical snuffbox 　Brachioradialis muscle 　Extensor carpi radialis 　　muscle 　Extensor carpi ulnaris 　　muscle 　Flexor carpi radialis muscle 　Flexor carpi ulnaris muscle 　Flexor pollicis longus 　　muscle 　Palmaris longus muscle 　Pronator quadratus 　　muscle 　Pronator teres muscle B **Lower Arm and Wrist** 　**Muscle, Left** 　*See 9 Lower Arm and Wrist* 　　*Muscle, Right* C **Hand Muscle, Right** 　Hypothenar muscle 　Palmar interosseous 　　muscle 　Thenar muscle D **Hand Muscle, Left** 　*See C Hand Muscle, Right* F **Trunk Muscle, Right** 　Coccygeus muscle 　Erector spinae muscle 　Interspinalis muscle 　Intertransversarius muscle 　Latissimus dorsi muscle 　Quadratus lumborum 　　muscle 　Rhomboid major muscle 　Rhomboid minor muscle 　Serratus posterior muscle 　Transversospinalis muscle 　Trapezius muscle G **Trunk Muscle, Left** 　*See F Trunk Muscle, Right* H **Thorax Muscle, Right** 　Intercostal muscle 　Levatores costarum 　　muscle 　Pectoralis major muscle 　Pectoralis minor muscle 　Serratus anterior muscle 　Subclavius muscle 　Subcostal muscle 　Transverse thoracis muscle J **Thorax Muscle, Left** 　*See H Thorax Muscle, Right* K **Abdomen Muscle, Right** 　External oblique muscle 　Internal oblique muscle 　Pyramidalis muscle 　Rectus abdominis muscle 　Transversus abdominis 　　muscle L **Abdomen Muscle, Left** 　*See K Abdomen Muscle,* 　　*Right*	M **Perineum Muscle** 　Bulbospongiosus muscle 　Cremaster muscle 　Deep transverse perineal 　　muscle 　Ischiocavernosus muscle 　Levator ani muscle 　Superficial transverse 　　perineal muscle N **Hip Muscle, Right** 　Gemellus muscle 　Gluteus maximus muscle 　Gluteus medius muscle 　Gluteus minimus muscle 　Iliacus muscle 　Obturator muscle 　Piriformis muscle 　Psoas muscle 　Quadratus femoris muscle 　Tensor fasciae latae 　　muscle P **Hip Muscle, Left** 　*See N Hip Muscle, Right* Q **Upper Leg Muscle, Right** 　Adductor brevis muscle 　Adductor longus muscle 　Adductor magnus muscle 　Biceps femoris muscle 　Gracilis muscle 　Pectineus muscle 　Quadriceps (femoris) 　Rectus femoris muscle 　Sartorius muscle 　Semimembranosus 　　muscle 　Semitendinosus muscle 　Vastus intermedius muscle 　Vastus lateralis muscle 　Vastus medialis muscle R **Upper Leg Muscle, Left** 　*See Q Upper Leg Muscle,* 　　*Right* S **Lower Leg Muscle, Right** 　Extensor digitorum longus 　　muscle 　Extensor hallucis longus 　　muscle 　Fibularis brevis muscle 　Fibularis longus muscle 　Flexor digitorum longus 　　muscle 　Flexor hallucis longus 　　muscle 　Gastrocnemius muscle 　Peroneus brevis muscle 　Peroneus longus muscle 　Popliteus muscle 　Soleus muscle 　Tibialis anterior muscle 　Tibialis posterior muscle T **Lower Leg Muscle, Left** 　*See S Lower Leg Muscle,* 　　*Right* V **Foot Muscle, Right** 　Abductor hallucis muscle 　Adductor hallucis muscle 　Extensor digitorum brevis 　　muscle 　Extensor hallucis brevis 　　muscle 　Flexor digitorum brevis 　　muscle 　Flexor hallucis brevis 　　muscle 　Quadratus plantae muscle W **Foot Muscle, Left** 　*See V Foot Muscle, Right*	Ø Open 3 Percutaneous 4 Percutaneous 　Endoscopic	Z No Device	Z No Qualifier

Ø   Medical and Surgical
K   Muscles
R   Replacement   Definition: Putting in or on biological or synthetic material that physically takes the place and/or function of all or a portion of a body part

Explanation: The body part may have been taken out or replaced, or may be taken out, physically eradicated, or rendered nonfunctional during the REPLACEMENT procedure. A REMOVAL procedure is coded for taking out the device used in a previous replacement procedure.

Body Part Character 4			Approach Character 5	Device Character 6	Qualifier Character 7
Ø Head Muscle Auricularis muscle Masseter muscle Pterygoid muscle Splenius capitis muscle Temporalis muscle Temporoparietalis muscle **1 Facial Muscle** Buccinator muscle Corrugator supercilii muscle Depressor anguli oris muscle Depressor labii inferioris muscle Depressor septi nasi muscle Depressor supercilii muscle Levator anguli oris muscle Levator labii superioris alaeque nasi muscle Levator labii superioris muscle Mentalis muscle Nasalis muscle Occipitofrontalis muscle Orbicularis oris muscle Procerus muscle Risorius muscle Zygomaticus muscle **2 Neck Muscle, Right** Anterior vertebral muscle Arytenoid muscle Cricothyroid muscle Infrahyoid muscle Levator scapulae muscle Platysma muscle Scalene muscle Splenius cervicis muscle Sternocleidomastoid muscle Suprahyoid muscle Thyroarytenoid muscle **3 Neck Muscle, Left** *See 2 Neck Muscle, Right* **4 Tongue, Palate, Pharynx Muscle** Chondroglossus muscle Genioglossus muscle Hyoglossus muscle Inferior longitudinal muscle Levator veli palatini muscle Palatoglossal muscle Palatopharyngeal muscle Pharyngeal constrictor muscle Salpingopharyngeus muscle Styloglossus muscle Stylopharyngeus muscle Superior longitudinal muscle Tensor veli palatini muscle **5 Shoulder Muscle, Right** Deltoid muscle Infraspinatus muscle Subscapularis muscle Supraspinatus muscle Teres major muscle Teres minor muscle **6 Shoulder Muscle, Left** *See 5 Shoulder Muscle, Right*	**7 Upper Arm Muscle, Right** Biceps brachii muscle Brachialis muscle Coracobrachialis muscle Triceps brachii muscle **8 Upper Arm Muscle, Left** *See 7 Upper Arm Muscle, Right* **9 Lower Arm and Wrist Muscle, Right** Anatomical snuffbox Brachioradialis muscle Extensor carpi radialis muscle Extensor carpi ulnaris muscle Flexor carpi radialis muscle Flexor carpi ulnaris muscle Flexor pollicis longus muscle Palmaris longus muscle Pronator quadratus muscle Pronator teres muscle **B Lower Arm and Wrist Muscle, Left** *See 9 Lower Arm and Wrist Muscle, Right* **C Hand Muscle, Right** Hypothenar muscle Palmar interosseous muscle Thenar muscle **D Hand Muscle, Left** *See C Hand Muscle, Right* **F Trunk Muscle, Right** Coccygeus muscle Erector spinae muscle Interspinalis muscle Intertransversarius muscle Latissimus dorsi muscle Quadratus lumborum muscle Rhomboid major muscle Rhomboid minor muscle Serratus posterior muscle Transversospinalis muscle Trapezius muscle **G Trunk Muscle, Left** *See F Trunk Muscle, Right* **H Thorax Muscle, Right** Intercostal muscle Levatores costarum muscle Pectoralis major muscle Pectoralis minor muscle Serratus anterior muscle Subclavius muscle Subcostal muscle Transverse thoracis muscle **J Thorax Muscle, Left** *See H Thorax Muscle, Right* **K Abdomen Muscle, Right** External oblique muscle Internal oblique muscle Pyramidalis muscle Rectus abdominis muscle Transversus abdominis muscle **L Abdomen Muscle, Left** *See K Abdomen Muscle, Right*	**M Perineum Muscle** Bulbospongiosus muscle Cremaster muscle Deep transverse perineal muscle Ischiocavernosus muscle Levator ani muscle Superficial transverse perineal muscle **N Hip Muscle, Right** Gemellus muscle Gluteus maximus muscle Gluteus medius muscle Gluteus minimus muscle Iliacus muscle Obturator muscle Piriformis muscle Psoas muscle Quadratus femoris muscle Tensor fasciae latae muscle **P Hip Muscle, Left** *See N Hip Muscle, Right* **Q Upper Leg Muscle, Right** Adductor brevis muscle Adductor longus muscle Adductor magnus muscle Biceps femoris muscle Gracilis muscle Pectineus muscle Quadriceps (femoris) Rectus femoris muscle Sartorius muscle Semimembranosus muscle Semitendinosus muscle Vastus intermedius muscle Vastus lateralis muscle Vastus medialis muscle **R Upper Leg Muscle, Left** *See Q Upper Leg Muscle, Right* **S Lower Leg Muscle, Right** Extensor digitorum longus muscle Extensor hallucis longus muscle Fibularis brevis muscle Fibularis longus muscle Flexor digitorum longus muscle Flexor hallucis longus muscle Gastrocnemius muscle Peroneus brevis muscle Peroneus longus muscle Popliteus muscle Soleus muscle Tibialis anterior muscle Tibialis posterior muscle **T Lower Leg Muscle, Left** *See S Lower Leg Muscle, Right* **V Foot Muscle, Right** Abductor hallucis muscle Adductor hallucis muscle Extensor digitorum brevis muscle Extensor hallucis brevis muscle Flexor digitorum brevis muscle Flexor hallucis brevis muscle Quadratus plantae muscle **W Foot Muscle, Left** *See V Foot Muscle, Right*	**Ø Open** **4 Percutaneous Endoscopic**	**7 Autologous Tissue Substitute** **J Synthetic Substitute** **K Nonautologous Tissue Substitute**	**Z No Qualifier**

LC Limited Coverage   **NC** Noncovered   ⊞ Combination Member   HAC associated procedure   Combination Only   DRG Non-OR   Non-OR   New/Revised in GREEN

ICD-10-PCS 2019   457

ØKR–ØKR

Muscles

Ø   **Medical and Surgical**
K   **Muscles**
S   **Reposition**   Definition: Moving to its normal location, or other suitable location, all or a portion of a body part
                         Explanation: The body part is moved to a new location from an abnormal location, or from a normal location where it is not functioning
                         correctly. The body part may or may not be cut out or off to be moved to the new location.

Body Part Character 4			Approach Character 5	Device Character 6	Qualifier Character 7

Ø **Head Muscle**
   Auricularis muscle
   Masseter muscle
   Pterygoid muscle
   Splenius capitis muscle
   Temporalis muscle
   Temporoparietalis muscle
1 **Facial Muscle**
   Buccinator muscle
   Corrugator supercilii
     muscle
   Depressor anguli oris
     muscle
   Depressor labii inferioris
     muscle
   Depressor septi nasi
     muscle
   Depressor supercilii
     muscle
   Levator anguli oris muscle
   Levator labii superioris
     alaeque nasi muscle
   Levator labii superioris
     muscle
   Mentalis muscle
   Nasalis muscle
   Occipitofrontalis muscle
   Orbicularis oris muscle
   Procerus muscle
   Risorius muscle
   Zygomaticus muscle
2 **Neck Muscle, Right**
   Anterior vertebral muscle
   Arytenoid muscle
   Cricothyroid muscle
   Infrahyoid muscle
   Levator scapulae muscle
   Platysma muscle
   Scalene muscle
   Splenius cervicis muscle
   Sternocleidomastoid
     muscle
   Suprahyoid muscle
   Thyroarytenoid muscle
3 **Neck Muscle, Left**
   See 2 Neck Muscle, Right
4 **Tongue, Palate, Pharynx**
   Muscle
   Chondroglossus muscle
   Genioglossus muscle
   Hyoglossus muscle
   Inferior longitudinal
     muscle
   Levator veli palatini
     muscle
   Palatoglossal muscle
   Palatopharyngeal muscle
   Pharyngeal constrictor
     muscle
   Salpingopharyngeus
     muscle
   Styloglossus muscle
   Stylopharyngeus muscle
   Superior longitudinal
     muscle
   Tensor veli palatini muscle
5 **Shoulder Muscle, Right**
   Deltoid muscle
   Infraspinatus muscle
   Subscapularis muscle
   Supraspinatus muscle
   Teres major muscle
   Teres minor muscle
6 **Shoulder Muscle, Left**
   See 5 Shoulder Muscle,
   Right
	7 **Upper Arm Muscle, Right**
	   Biceps brachii muscle
	   Brachialis muscle
	   Coracobrachialis muscle
	   Triceps brachii muscle
	8 **Upper Arm Muscle, Left**
	   See 7 Upper Arm Muscle,
	   Right
	9 **Lower Arm and Wrist**
	   Muscle, Right
	   Anatomical snuffbox
	   Brachioradialis muscle
	   Extensor carpi radialis
	     muscle
	   Extensor carpi ulnaris
	     muscle
	   Flexor carpi radialis muscle
	   Flexor carpi ulnaris muscle
	   Flexor pollicis longus
	     muscle
	   Palmaris longus muscle
	   Pronator quadratus
	     muscle
	   Pronator teres muscle
	B **Lower Arm and Wrist**
	   Muscle, Left
	   See 9 Lower Arm and Wrist
	   Muscle, Right
	C **Hand Muscle, Right**
	   Hypothenar muscle
	   Palmar interosseous
	     muscle
	   Thenar muscle
	D **Hand Muscle, Left**
	   See C Hand Muscle, Right
	F **Trunk Muscle, Right**
	   Coccygeus muscle
	   Erector spinae muscle
	   Interspinalis muscle
	   Intertransversarius muscle
	   Latissimus dorsi muscle
	   Quadratus lumborum
	     muscle
	   Rhomboid major muscle
	   Rhomboid minor muscle
	   Serratus posterior muscle
	   Transversospinalis muscle
	   Trapezius muscle
	G **Trunk Muscle, Left**
	   See F Trunk Muscle, Right
	H **Thorax Muscle, Right**
	   Intercostal muscle
	   Levatores costarum
	     muscle
	   Pectoralis major muscle
	   Pectoralis minor muscle
	   Serratus anterior muscle
	   Subclavius muscle
	   Subcostal muscle
	   Transverse thoracis muscle
	J **Thorax Muscle, Left**
	   See H Thorax Muscle, Right
	K **Abdomen Muscle, Right**
	   External oblique muscle
	   Internal oblique muscle
	   Pyramidalis muscle
	   Rectus abdominis muscle
	   Transversus abdominis
	     muscle
	L **Abdomen Muscle, Left**
	   See K Abdomen Muscle,
	   Right
		M **Perineum Muscle**
		   Bulbospongiosus muscle
		   Cremaster muscle
		   Deep transverse perineal
		     muscle
		   Ischiocavernosus muscle
		   Levator ani muscle
		   Superficial transverse
		     perineal muscle
		N **Hip Muscle, Right**
		   Gemellus muscle
		   Gluteus maximus muscle
		   Gluteus medius muscle
		   Gluteus minimus muscle
		   Iliacus muscle
		   Obturator muscle
		   Piriformis muscle
		   Psoas muscle
		   Quadratus femoris muscle
		   Tensor fasciae latae
		     muscle
		P **Hip Muscle, Left**
		   See N Hip Muscle, Right
		Q **Upper Leg Muscle, Right**
		   Adductor brevis muscle
		   Adductor longus muscle
		   Adductor magnus muscle
		   Biceps femoris muscle
		   Gracilis muscle
		   Pectineus muscle
		   Quadriceps (femoris)
		   Rectus femoris muscle
		   Sartorius muscle
		   Semimembranosus
		     muscle
		   Semitendinosus muscle
		   Vastus intermedius muscle
		   Vastus lateralis muscle
		   Vastus medialis muscle
		R **Upper Leg Muscle, Left**
		   See Q Upper Leg Muscle,
		   Right
		S **Lower Leg Muscle, Right**
		   Extensor digitorum longus
		     muscle
		   Extensor hallucis longus
		     muscle
		   Fibularis brevis muscle
		   Fibularis longus muscle
		   Flexor digitorum longus
		     muscle
		   Flexor hallucis longus
		     muscle
		   Gastrocnemius muscle
		   Peroneus brevis muscle
		   Peroneus longus muscle
		   Popliteus muscle
		   Soleus muscle
		   Tibialis anterior muscle
		   Tibialis posterior muscle
		T **Lower Leg Muscle, Left**
		   See S Lower Leg Muscle,
		   Right
		V **Foot Muscle, Right**
		   Abductor hallucis muscle
		   Adductor hallucis muscle
		   Extensor digitorum brevis
		     muscle
		   Extensor hallucis brevis
		     muscle
		   Flexor digitorum brevis
		     muscle
		   Flexor hallucis brevis
		     muscle
		   Quadratus plantae muscle
		W **Foot Muscle, Left**
		   See V Foot Muscle, Right
			Ø **Open**
			4 **Percutaneous**
			   Endoscopic
				Z **No Device**	Z **No Qualifier**

LC Limited Coverage   **NC** Noncovered   ⊞ Combination Member   HAC associated procedure   Combination Only   DRG Non-OR   Non-OR   New/Revised in GREEN

458   ICD-10-PCS 2019

Ø   **Medical and Surgical**
K   **Muscles**
T   **Resection**   Definition: Cutting out or off, without replacement, all of a body part
                    Explanation: None

Body Part Character 4			Approach Character 5	Device Character 6	Qualifier Character 7
Ø Head Muscle	**7 Upper Arm Muscle, Right**	**M Perineum Muscle**	**Ø Open**	**Z No Device**	**Z No Qualifier**
Auricularis muscle	Biceps brachii muscle	Bulbospongiosus muscle	**4 Percutaneous Endoscopic**		
Masseter muscle	Brachialis muscle	Cremaster muscle			
Pterygoid muscle	Coracobrachialis muscle	Deep transverse perineal muscle			
Splenius capitis muscle	Triceps brachii muscle	Ischiocavernosus muscle			
Temporalis muscle	**8 Upper Arm Muscle, Left**	Levator ani muscle			
Temporoparietalis muscle	*See 7 Upper Arm Muscle, Right*	Superficial transverse perineal muscle			
1 Facial Muscle	**9 Lower Arm and Wrist Muscle, Right**	**N Hip Muscle, Right**			
Buccinator muscle	Anatomical snuffbox	Gemellus muscle			
Corrugator supercilii muscle	Brachioradialis muscle	Gluteus maximus muscle			
Depressor anguli oris muscle	Extensor carpi radialis muscle	Gluteus medius muscle			
Depressor labii inferioris muscle	Extensor carpi ulnaris muscle	Gluteus minimus muscle			
Depressor septi nasi muscle	Flexor carpi radialis muscle	Iliacus muscle			
Depressor supercilii muscle	Flexor carpi ulnaris muscle	Obturator muscle			
Levator anguli oris muscle	Flexor pollicis longus muscle	Piriformis muscle			
Levator labii superioris alaeque nasi muscle	Palmaris longus muscle	Psoas muscle			
Levator labii superioris muscle	Pronator quadratus muscle	Quadratus femoris muscle			
Mentalis muscle	Pronator teres muscle	Tensor fasciae latae muscle			
Nasalis muscle	**B Lower Arm and Wrist Muscle, Left**	**P Hip Muscle, Left**			
Occipitofrontalis muscle	*See 9 Lower Arm and Wrist Muscle, Right*	*See N Hip Muscle, Right*			
Orbicularis oris muscle	**C Hand Muscle, Right**	**Q Upper Leg Muscle, Right**			
Procerus muscle	Hypothenar muscle	Adductor brevis muscle			
Risorius muscle	Palmar interosseous muscle	Adductor longus muscle			
Zygomaticus muscle	Thenar muscle	Adductor magnus muscle			
2 Neck Muscle, Right	**D Hand Muscle, Left**	Biceps femoris muscle			
Anterior vertebral muscle	*See C Hand Muscle, Right*	Gracilis muscle			
Arytenoid muscle	**F Trunk Muscle, Right**	Pectineus muscle			
Cricothyroid muscle	Coccygeus muscle	Quadriceps (femoris)			
Infrahyoid muscle	Erector spinae muscle	Rectus femoris muscle			
Levator scapulae muscle	Interspinalis muscle	Sartorius muscle			
Platysma muscle	Intertransversarius muscle	Semimembranosus muscle			
Scalene muscle	Latissimus dorsi muscle	Semitendinosus muscle			
Splenius cervicis muscle	Quadratus lumborum muscle	Vastus intermedius muscle			
Sternocleidomastoid muscle	Rhomboid major muscle	Vastus lateralis muscle			
Suprahyoid muscle	Rhomboid minor muscle	Vastus medialis muscle			
Thyroarytenoid muscle	Serratus posterior muscle	**R Upper Leg Muscle, Left**			
3 Neck Muscle, Left	Transversospinalis muscle	*See Q Upper Leg Muscle, Right*			
See 2 Neck Muscle, Right	Trapezius muscle	**S Lower Leg Muscle, Right**			
4 Tongue, Palate, Pharynx Muscle	**G Trunk Muscle, Left**	Extensor digitorum longus muscle			
Chondroglossus muscle	*See F Trunk Muscle, Right*	Extensor hallucis longus muscle			
Genioglossus muscle	**H Thorax Muscle, Right** ⊞	Fibularis brevis muscle			
Hyoglossus muscle	Intercostal muscle	Fibularis longus muscle			
Inferior longitudinal muscle	Levatores costarum muscle	Flexor digitorum longus muscle			
Levator veli palatini muscle	Pectoralis major muscle	Flexor hallucis longus muscle			
Palatoglossal muscle	Pectoralis minor muscle	Gastrocnemius muscle			
Palatopharyngeal muscle	Serratus anterior muscle	Peroneus brevis muscle			
Pharyngeal constrictor muscle	Subclavius muscle	Peroneus longus muscle			
Salpingopharyngeus muscle	Subcostal muscle	Popliteus muscle			
Styloglossus muscle	Transverse thoracis muscle	Soleus muscle			
Stylopharyngeus muscle	**J Thorax Muscle, Left** ⊞	Tibialis anterior muscle			
Superior longitudinal muscle	*See H Thorax Muscle, Right*	Tibialis posterior muscle			
Tensor veli palatini muscle	**K Abdomen Muscle, Right**	**T Lower Leg Muscle, Left**			
5 Shoulder Muscle, Right	External oblique muscle	*See S Lower Leg Muscle, Right*			
Deltoid muscle	Internal oblique muscle	**V Foot Muscle, Right**			
Infraspinatus muscle	Pyramidalis muscle	Abductor hallucis muscle			
Subscapularis muscle	Rectus abdominis muscle	Adductor hallucis muscle			
Supraspinatus muscle	Transversus abdominis muscle	Extensor digitorum brevis muscle			
Teres major muscle	**L Abdomen Muscle, Left**	Extensor hallucis brevis muscle			
Teres minor muscle	*See K Abdomen Muscle, Right*	Flexor digitorum brevis muscle			
6 Shoulder Muscle, Left		Flexor hallucis brevis muscle			
See 5 Shoulder Muscle, Right		Quadratus plantae muscle			
		W Foot Muscle, Left			
		See V Foot Muscle, Right			

See Appendix L for Procedure Combinations
⊞   ØKT[H,J]ØZZ

Muscles

Ø   **Medical and Surgical**
K   **Muscles**
U   **Supplement**   Definition: Putting in or on biological or synthetic material that physically reinforces and/or augments the function of a portion of a body part
                    Explanation: The biological material is non-living, or is living and from the same individual. The body part may have been previously replaced, and the SUPPLEMENT procedure is performed to physically reinforce and/or augment the function of the replaced body part.

Body Part Character 4			Approach Character 5	Device Character 6	Qualifier Character 7
Ø Head Muscle Auricularis muscle Masseter muscle Pterygoid muscle Splenius capitis muscle Temporalis muscle Temporoparietalis muscle **1 Facial Muscle** Buccinator muscle Corrugator supercilii muscle Depressor anguli oris muscle Depressor labii inferioris muscle Depressor septi nasi muscle Depressor supercilii muscle Levator anguli oris muscle Levator labii superioris alaeque nasi muscle Levator labii superioris muscle Mentalis muscle Nasalis muscle Occipitofrontalis muscle Orbicularis oris muscle Procerus muscle Risorius muscle Zygomaticus muscle **2 Neck Muscle, Right** Anterior vertebral muscle Arytenoid muscle Cricothyroid muscle Infrahyoid muscle Levator scapulae muscle Platysma muscle Scalene muscle Splenius cervicis muscle Sternocleidomastoid muscle Suprahyoid muscle Thyroarytenoid muscle **3 Neck Muscle, Left** *See 2 Neck Muscle, Right* **4 Tongue, Palate, Pharynx Muscle** Chondroglossus muscle Genioglossus muscle Hyoglossus muscle Inferior longitudinal muscle Levator veli palatini muscle Palatoglossus muscle Palatopharyngeal muscle Pharyngeal constrictor muscle Salpingopharyngeus muscle Styloglossus muscle Stylopharyngeus muscle Superior longitudinal muscle Tensor veli palatini muscle **5 Shoulder Muscle, Right** Deltoid muscle Infraspinatus muscle Subscapularis muscle Supraspinatus muscle Teres major muscle Teres minor muscle **6 Shoulder Muscle, Left** *See 5 Shoulder Muscle, Right*	**7 Upper Arm Muscle, Right** Biceps brachii muscle Brachialis muscle Coracobrachialis muscle Triceps brachii muscle **8 Upper Arm Muscle, Left** *See 7 Upper Arm Muscle, Right* **9 Lower Arm and Wrist Muscle, Right** Anatomical snuffbox Brachioradialis muscle Extensor carpi radialis muscle Extensor carpi ulnaris muscle Flexor carpi radialis muscle Flexor carpi ulnaris muscle Flexor pollicis longus muscle Palmaris longus muscle Pronator quadratus muscle Pronator teres muscle **B Lower Arm and Wrist Muscle, Left** *See 9 Lower Arm and Wrist Muscle, Right* **C Hand Muscle, Right** Hypothenar muscle Palmar interosseous muscle Thenar muscle **D Hand Muscle, Left** *See C Hand Muscle, Right* **F Trunk Muscle, Right** Coccygeus muscle Erector spinae muscle Interspinalis muscle Intertransversarius muscle Latissimus dorsi muscle Quadratus lumborum muscle Rhomboid major muscle Rhomboid minor muscle Serratus posterior muscle Transversospinalis muscle Trapezius muscle **G Trunk Muscle, Left** *See F Trunk Muscle, Right* **H Thorax Muscle, Right** Intercostal muscle Levatores costarum muscle Pectoralis major muscle Pectoralis minor muscle Serratus anterior muscle Subclavius muscle Subcostal muscle Transverse thoracis muscle **J Thorax Muscle, Left** *See H Thorax Muscle, Right* **K Abdomen Muscle, Right** External oblique muscle Internal oblique muscle Pyramidalis muscle Rectus abdominis muscle Transversus abdominis muscle **L Abdomen Muscle, Left** *See K Abdomen Muscle, Right*	**M Perineum Muscle** Bulbospongiosus muscle Cremaster muscle Deep transverse perineal muscle Ischiocavernosus muscle Levator ani muscle Superficial transverse perineal muscle **N Hip Muscle, Right** Gemellus muscle Gluteus maximus muscle Gluteus medius muscle Gluteus minimus muscle Iliacus muscle Obturator muscle Piriformis muscle Psoas muscle Quadratus femoris muscle Tensor fasciae latae muscle **P Hip Muscle, Left** *See N Hip Muscle, Right* **Q Upper Leg Muscle, Right** Adductor brevis muscle Adductor longus muscle Adductor magnus muscle Biceps femoris muscle Gracilis muscle Pectineus muscle Quadriceps (femoris) Rectus femoris muscle Sartorius muscle Semimembranosus muscle Semitendinosus muscle Vastus intermedius muscle Vastus lateralis muscle Vastus medialis muscle **R Upper Leg Muscle, Left** *See Q Upper Leg Muscle, Right* **S Lower Leg Muscle, Right** Extensor digitorum longus muscle Extensor hallucis longus muscle Fibularis brevis muscle Fibularis longus muscle Flexor digitorum longus muscle Flexor hallucis longus muscle Gastrocnemius muscle Peroneus brevis muscle Peroneus longus muscle Popliteus muscle Soleus muscle Tibialis anterior muscle Tibialis posterior muscle **T Lower Leg Muscle, Left** *See S Lower Leg Muscle, Right* **V Foot Muscle, Right** Abductor hallucis muscle Adductor hallucis muscle Extensor digitorum brevis muscle Extensor hallucis brevis muscle Flexor digitorum brevis muscle Flexor hallucis brevis muscle Quadratus plantae muscle **W Foot Muscle, Left** *See V Foot Muscle, Right*	**Ø Open** **4 Percutaneous Endoscopic**	**7 Autologous Tissue Substitute** **J Synthetic Substitute** **K Nonautologous Tissue Substitute**	**Z No Qualifier**

Ø   Medical and Surgical
K   Muscles
W   Revision   Definition: Correcting, to the extent possible, a portion of a malfunctioning device or the position of a displaced device

Explanation: Revision can include correcting a malfunctioning or displaced device by taking out or putting in components of the device such as a screw or pin

Body Part Character 4	Approach Character 5	Device Character 6	Qualifier Character 7
X Upper Muscle Y Lower Muscle	Ø Open 3 Percutaneous 4 Percutaneous Endoscopic	Ø Drainage Device 7 Autologous Tissue Substitute J Synthetic Substitute K Nonautologous Tissue Substitute M Stimulator Lead Y Other Device	Z No Qualifier
X Upper Muscle Y Lower Muscle	X External	Ø Drainage Device 7 Autologous Tissue Substitute J Synthetic Substitute K Nonautologous Tissue Substitute M Stimulator Lead	Z No Qualifier

Non-OR   ØKW[X,Y][3,4]YZ
Non-OR   ØKW[X,Y]X[Ø,7,J,K,M]Z

Ø Medical and Surgical
K Muscles
X Transfer

Definition: Moving, without taking out, all or a portion of a body part to another location to take over the function of all or a portion of a body part
Explanation: The body part transferred remains connected to its vascular and nervous supply

Body Part — Character 4			Approach — Character 5	Device — Character 6	Qualifier — Character 7
Ø Head Muscle	**6 Shoulder Muscle, Left** *See 5 Shoulder Muscle, Right*	**P Hip Muscle, Left** *See N Hip Muscle, Right*	**Ø Open**	**Z No Device**	**Ø Skin**
Auricularis muscle		**Q Upper Leg Muscle, Right**	**4 Percutaneous Endoscopic**		**1 Subcutaneous Tissue**
Masseter muscle	**7 Upper Arm Muscle, Right**	Adductor brevis muscle			**2 Skin and Subcutaneous Tissue**
Pterygoid muscle	Biceps brachii muscle	Adductor longus muscle			**Z No Qualifier**
Splenius capitis muscle	Brachialis muscle	Adductor magnus muscle			
Temporalis muscle	Coracobrachialis muscle	Biceps femoris muscle			
Temporoparietalis muscle	Triceps brachii muscle	Gracilis muscle			
1 Facial Muscle	**8 Upper Arm Muscle, Left** *See 7 Upper Arm Muscle, Right*	Pectineus muscle			
Buccinator muscle		Quadriceps (femoris)			
Corrugator supercilii muscle	**9 Lower Arm and Wrist Muscle, Right**	Rectus femoris muscle			
Depressor anguli oris muscle	Anatomical snuffbox	Sartorius muscle			
Depressor labii inferioris muscle	Brachioradialis muscle	Semimembranosus muscle			
Depressor septi nasi muscle	Extensor carpi radialis muscle	Semitendinosus muscle			
Depressor supercilii muscle	Extensor carpi ulnaris muscle	Vastus intermedius muscle			
Levator anguli oris muscle	Flexor carpi radialis muscle	Vastus lateralis muscle			
Levator labii superioris alaeque nasi muscle	Flexor carpi ulnaris muscle	Vastus medialis muscle			
Levator labii superioris muscle	Flexor pollicis longus muscle	**R Upper Leg Muscle, Left** *See Q Upper Leg Muscle, Right*			
Mentalis muscle	Palmaris longus muscle	**S Lower Leg Muscle, Right**			
Nasalis muscle	Pronator quadratus muscle	Extensor digitorum longus muscle			
Occipitofrontalis muscle	Pronator teres muscle	Extensor hallucis longus muscle			
Orbicularis oris muscle	**B Lower Arm and Wrist Muscle, Left** *See 9 Lower Arm and Wrist Muscle, Right*	Fibularis brevis muscle			
Procerus muscle		Fibularis longus muscle			
Risorius muscle	**C Hand Muscle, Right**	Flexor digitorum longus muscle			
Zygomaticus muscle	Hypothenar muscle	Flexor hallucis longus muscle			
2 Neck Muscle, Right	Palmar interosseous muscle	Gastrocnemius muscle			
Anterior vertebral muscle	Thenar muscle	Peroneus brevis muscle			
Arytenoid muscle	**D Hand Muscle, Left** *See C Hand Muscle, Right*	Peroneus longus muscle			
Cricothyroid muscle		Popliteus muscle			
Infrahyoid muscle	**H Thorax Muscle, Right**	Soleus muscle			
Levator scapulae muscle	Intercostal muscle	Tibialis anterior muscle			
Platysma muscle	Levatores costarum muscle	Tibialis posterior muscle			
Scalene muscle	Pectoralis major muscle	**T Lower Leg Muscle, Left** *See S Lower Leg Muscle, Right*			
Splenius cervicis muscle	Pectoralis minor muscle				
Sternocleidomastoid muscle	Serratus anterior muscle	**V Foot Muscle, Right**			
Suprahyoid muscle	Subclavius muscle	Abductor hallucis muscle			
Thyroarytenoid muscle	Subcostal muscle	Adductor hallucis muscle			
3 Neck Muscle, Left *See 2 Neck Muscle, Right*	Transverse thoracis muscle	Extensor digitorum brevis muscle			
4 Tongue, Palate, Pharynx Muscle	**J Thorax Muscle, Left** *See H Thorax Muscle, Right*	Extensor hallucis brevis muscle			
Chondroglossus muscle	**M Perineum Muscle**	Flexor digitorum brevis muscle			
Genioglossus muscle	Bulbospongiosus muscle	Flexor hallucis brevis muscle			
Hyoglossus muscle	Cremaster muscle	Quadratus plantae muscle			
Inferior longitudinal muscle	Deep transverse perineal muscle	**W Foot Muscle, Left** *See V Foot Muscle, Right*			
Levator veli palatini muscle	Ischiocavernosus muscle				
Palatoglossal muscle	Levator ani muscle				
Palatopharyngeal muscle	Superficial transverse perineal muscle				
Pharyngeal constrictor muscle	**N Hip Muscle, Right**				
Salpingopharyngeus muscle	Gemellus muscle				
Styloglossus muscle	Gluteus maximus muscle				
Stylopharyngeus muscle	Gluteus medius muscle				
Superior longitudinal muscle	Gluteus minimus muscle				
Tensor veli palatini muscle	Iliacus muscle				
5 Shoulder Muscle, Right	Obturator muscle				
Deltoid muscle	Piriformis muscle				
Infraspinatus muscle	Psoas muscle				
Subscapularis muscle	Quadratus femoris muscle				
Supraspinatus muscle	Tensor fasciae latae muscle				
Teres major muscle					
Teres minor muscle					

ØKX Continued on next page

LC Limited Coverage   **NC** Noncovered   ⊞ Combination Member   HAC associated procedure   Combination Only   DRG Non-OR   Non-OR   New/Revised in GREEN

462   ICD-10-PCS 2019

Ø **Medical and Surgical**
K **Muscles**
X **Transfer**

ØKX Continued

Definition: Moving, without taking out, all or a portion of a body part to another location to take over the function of all or a portion of a body part
Explanation: The body part transferred remains connected to its vascular and nervous supply

Body Part Character 4	Approach Character 5	Device Character 6	Qualifier Character 7

F **Trunk Muscle, Right**
  Coccygeus muscle
  Erector spinae muscle
  Interspinalis muscle
  Intertransversarius muscle
  Latissimus dorsi muscle
  Quadratus lumborum muscle
  Rhomboid major muscle
  Rhomboid minor muscle
  Serratus posterior muscle
  Transversospinalis muscle
  Trapezius muscle
G **Trunk Muscle, Left**
  See F Trunk Muscle, Right
	Ø Open
	4 Percutaneous Endoscopic
		Z No Device	Ø Skin
			1 Subcutaneous Tissue
			2 Skin and Subcutaneous Tissue
			5 Latissimus Dorsi Myocutaneous
			   Flap
			7 Deep Inferior Epigastric Artery
			   Perforator Flap
			8 Superficial Inferior Epigastric
			   Artery Flap
			9 Gluteal Artery Perforator Flap
			Z No Qualifier

K **Abdomen Muscle, Right**
  External oblique muscle
  Internal oblique muscle
  Pyramidalis muscle
  Rectus abdominis muscle
  Transversus abdominis muscle
L **Abdomen Muscle, Left**
  See K Abdomen Muscle, Right
	Ø Open
	4 Percutaneous Endoscopic
		Z No Device	Ø Skin
			1 Subcutaneous Tissue
			2 Skin and Subcutaneous Tissue
			6 Transverse Rectus Abdominis
			   Myocutaneous Flap
			Z No Qualifier

LC Limited Coverage   **NC** Noncovered   ⊞ Combination Member   HAC associated procedure   Combination Only   DRG Non-OR   Non-OR   New/Revised in GREEN

ICD-10-PCS 2019   **463**

ØKX–ØKX

Tendons ØL2–ØLX

Character Meanings*

This Character Meaning table is provided as a guide to assist the user in the identification of character members that may be found in this section of code tables. It **SHOULD NOT** be used to build a PCS code.

Operation–Character 3	Body Part–Character 4	Approach–Character 5	Device–Character 6	Qualifier–Character 7
2 Change	Ø Head and Neck Tendon	Ø Open	Ø Drainage Device	X Diagnostic
5 Destruction	1 Shoulder Tendon, Right	3 Percutaneous	7 Autologous Tissue Substitute	Z No Qualifier
8 Division	2 Shoulder Tendon, Left	4 Percutaneous Endoscopic	J Synthetic Substitute	
9 Drainage	3 Upper Arm Tendon, Right	X External	K Nonautologous Tissue Substitute	
B Excision	4 Upper Arm Tendon, Left		Y Other Device	
C Extirpation	5 Lower Arm and Wrist Tendon, Right		Z No Device	
D Extraction	6 Lower Arm and Wrist Tendon, Left			
H Insertion	7 Hand Tendon, Right			
J Inspection	8 Hand Tendon, Left			
M Reattachment	9 Trunk Tendon, Right			
N Release	B Trunk Tendon, Left			
P Removal	C Thorax Tendon, Right			
Q Repair	D Thorax Tendon, Left			
R Replacement	F Abdomen Tendon, Right			
S Reposition	G Abdomen Tendon, Left			
T Resection	H Perineum Tendon			
U Supplement	J Hip Tendon, Right			
W Revision	K Hip Tendon, Left			
X Transfer	L Upper Leg Tendon, Right			
	M Upper Leg Tendon, Left			
	N Lower Leg Tendon, Right			
	P Lower Leg Tendon, Left			
	Q Knee Tendon, Right			
	R Knee Tendon, Left			
	S Ankle Tendon, Right			
	T Ankle Tendon, Left			
	V Foot Tendon, Right			
	W Foot Tendon, Left			
	X Upper Tendon			
	Y Lower Tendon			

* Includes synovial membrane.

AHA Coding Clinic for table ØL8
2016, 3Q, 30   Resection of femur with interposition arthroplasty

AHA Coding Clinic for table ØLB
2017, 2Q, 21   Arthroscopic anterior cruciate ligament revision using autograft with anterolateral ligament reconstruction
2015, 3Q, 26   Thumb arthroplasty with resection of trapezium
2014, 3Q, 14   Application of TheraSkin® and excisional debridement
2014, 3Q, 18   Placement of reverse sural fasciocutaneous pedicle flap

AHA Coding Clinic for table ØLD
2017, 4Q, 41   Extraction procedures

AHA Coding Clinic for table ØLQ
2016, 3Q, 32   Rotator cuff repair, tenodesis, decompression, acromioplasty and coracoplasty
2015, 2Q, 11   Repair of patellar and quadriceps tendons with allograft
2013, 3Q, 20   Superior labrum anterior posterior (SLAP) repair and subacromial decompression

AHA Coding Clinic for table ØLS
2016, 3Q, 32   Rotator cuff repair, tenodesis, decompression, acromioplasty and coracoplasty
2015, 3Q, 14   Endoprosthetic replacement of humerus and tendon reattachment

AHA Coding Clinic for table ØLU
2015, 2Q, 11   Repair of patellar and quadriceps tendons with allograft

Foot Tendons

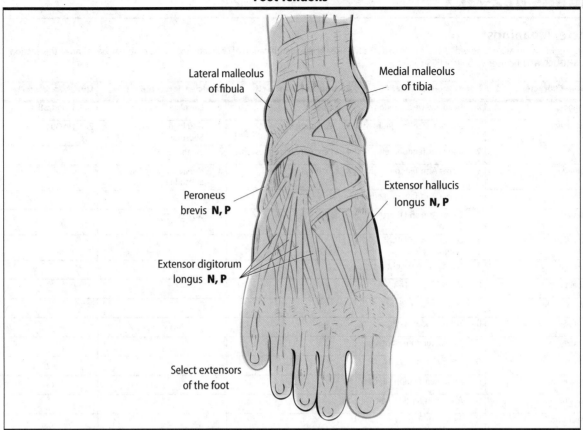

Lateral malleolus of fibula

Medial malleolus of tibia

Peroneus brevis **N, P**

Extensor hallucis longus **N, P**

Extensor digitorum longus **N, P**

Select extensors of the foot

Shoulder Tendons

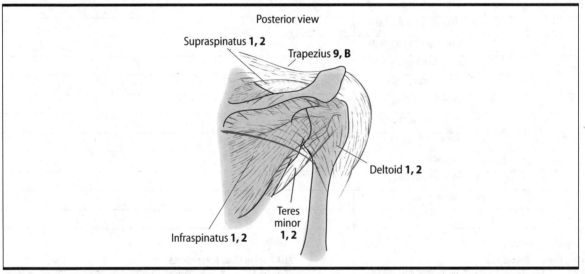

Posterior view

Supraspinatus **1, 2**

Trapezius **9, B**

Deltoid **1, 2**

Infraspinatus **1, 2**

Teres minor **1, 2**

Tendons of Wrist and Hand

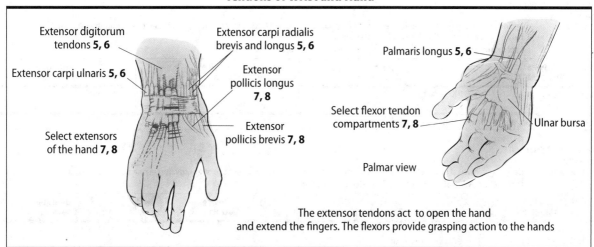

Extensor digitorum tendons **5, 6**

Extensor carpi radialis brevis and longus **5, 6**

Extensor carpi ulnaris **5, 6**

Extensor pollicis longus **7, 8**

Select extensors of the hand **7, 8**

Extensor pollicis brevis **7, 8**

Palmaris longus **5, 6**

Select flexor tendon compartments **7, 8**

Ulnar bursa

Palmar view

The extensor tendons act to open the hand and extend the fingers. The flexors provide grasping action to the hands

Leg Muscles and Tendons

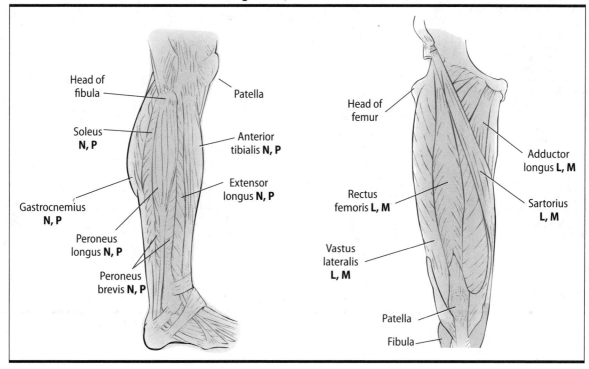

Head of fibula

Patella

Soleus **N, P**

Anterior tibialis **N, P**

Gastrocnemius **N, P**

Extensor longus **N, P**

Peroneus longus **N, P**

Peroneus brevis **N, P**

Head of femur

Adductor longus **L, M**

Rectus femoris **L, M**

Sartorius **L, M**

Vastus lateralis **L, M**

Patella

Fibula

Ø Medical and Surgical
L Tendons
2 Change Definition: Taking out or off a device from a body part and putting back an identical or similar device in or on the same body part without cutting or puncturing the skin or a mucous membrane

Explanation: All CHANGE procedures are coded using the approach EXTERNAL

Body Part Character 4	Approach Character 5	Device Character 6	Qualifier Character 7
X Upper Tendon Y Lower Tendon	X External	Ø Drainage Device Y Other Device	Z No Qualifier

Non-OR All body part, approach, device, and qualifier values

Ø Medical and Surgical
L Tendons
5 Destruction Definition: Physical eradication of all or a portion of a body part by the direct use of energy, force, or a destructive agent

Explanation: None of the body part is physically taken out

Body Part Character 4	Approach Character 5	Device Character 6	Qualifier Character 7

Ø Head and Neck Tendon
1 Shoulder Tendon, Right
2 Shoulder Tendon, Left
3 Upper Arm Tendon, Right
4 Upper Arm Tendon, Left
5 Lower Arm and Wrist Tendon, Right
6 Lower Arm and Wrist Tendon, Left
7 Hand Tendon, Right
8 Hand Tendon, Left
9 Trunk Tendon, Right
B Trunk Tendon, Left
C Thorax Tendon, Right
D Thorax Tendon, Left
F Abdomen Tendon, Right
G Abdomen Tendon, Left
H Perineum Tendon
J Hip Tendon, Right
K Hip Tendon, Left
L Upper Leg Tendon, Right
M Upper Leg Tendon, Left
N Lower Leg Tendon, Right
   Achilles tendon
P Lower Leg Tendon, Left
   See N Lower Leg Tendon, Right
Q Knee Tendon, Right
   Patellar tendon
R Knee Tendon, Left
   See Q Knee Tendon, Right
S Ankle Tendon, Right
T Ankle Tendon, Left
V Foot Tendon, Right
W Foot Tendon, Left
	Ø Open
	3 Percutaneous
	4 Percutaneous Endoscopic
		Z No Device	Z No Qualifier

LC Limited Coverage   NC Noncovered   ⊞ Combination Member   HAC associated procedure   Combination Only   DRG Non-OR   Non-OR   New/Revised in GREEN

468

ICD-10-PCS 2019

0　Medical and Surgical
L　Tendons
8　Division　　Definition: Cutting into a body part, without draining fluids and/or gases from the body part, in order to separate or transect a body part
　　　　　　　　　Explanation: All or a portion of the body part is separated into two or more portions

Body Part Character 4	Approach Character 5	Device Character 6	Qualifier Character 7
0　Head and Neck Tendon	0　Open	Z　No Device	Z　No Qualifier
1　Shoulder Tendon, Right	3　Percutaneous		
2　Shoulder Tendon, Left	4　Percutaneous Endoscopic		
3　Upper Arm Tendon, Right			
4　Upper Arm Tendon, Left			
5　Lower Arm and Wrist Tendon, Right			
6　Lower Arm and Wrist Tendon, Left			
7　Hand Tendon, Right			
8　Hand Tendon, Left			
9　Trunk Tendon, Right			
B　Trunk Tendon, Left			
C　Thorax Tendon, Right			
D　Thorax Tendon, Left			
F　Abdomen Tendon, Right			
G　Abdomen Tendon, Left			
H　Perineum Tendon			
J　Hip Tendon, Right			
K　Hip Tendon, Left			
L　Upper Leg Tendon, Right			
M　Upper Leg Tendon, Left			
N　Lower Leg Tendon, Right 　　Achilles tendon			
P　Lower Leg Tendon, Left 　　See N Lower Leg Tendon, Right			
Q　Knee Tendon, Right 　　Patellar tendon			
R　Knee Tendon, Left 　　See Q Knee Tendon, Right			
S　Ankle Tendon, Right			
T　Ankle Tendon, Left			
V　Foot Tendon, Right			
W　Foot Tendon, Left			

LC Limited Coverage　NC Noncovered　⊞ Combination Member　HAC associated procedure　Combination Only　DRG Non-OR　Non-OR　New/Revised in GREEN
ICD-10-PCS 2019　　　　　　　　　　　　　　　　　　　　　　　　　　　　　　　　　　469

0L8–0L8

Ø Medical and Surgical
L Tendons
9 Drainage   Definition: Taking or letting out fluids and/or gases from a body part
                      Explanation: The qualifier DIAGNOSTIC is used to identify drainage procedures that are biopsies

Body Part Character 4	Approach Character 5	Device Character 6	Qualifier Character 7

Ø Head and Neck Tendon
1 Shoulder Tendon, Right
2 Shoulder Tendon, Left
3 Upper Arm Tendon, Right
4 Upper Arm Tendon, Left
5 Lower Arm and Wrist Tendon, Right
6 Lower Arm and Wrist Tendon, Left
7 Hand Tendon, Right
8 Hand Tendon, Left
9 Trunk Tendon, Right
B Trunk Tendon, Left
C Thorax Tendon, Right
D Thorax Tendon, Left
F Abdomen Tendon, Right
G Abdomen Tendon, Left
H Perineum Tendon
J Hip Tendon, Right
K Hip Tendon, Left
L Upper Leg Tendon, Right
M Upper Leg Tendon, Left
N Lower Leg Tendon, Right
   Achilles tendon
P Lower Leg Tendon, Left
   See N Lower Leg Tendon, Right
Q Knee Tendon, Right
   Patellar tendon
R Knee Tendon, Left
   See Q Knee Tendon, Right
S Ankle Tendon, Right
T Ankle Tendon, Left
V Foot Tendon, Right
W Foot Tendon, Left
	Ø Open
	3 Percutaneous
	4 Percutaneous Endoscopic
		Ø Drainage Device	Z No Qualifier

Ø Head and Neck Tendon
1 Shoulder Tendon, Right
2 Shoulder Tendon, Left
3 Upper Arm Tendon, Right
4 Upper Arm Tendon, Left
5 Lower Arm and Wrist Tendon, Right
6 Lower Arm and Wrist Tendon, Left
7 Hand Tendon, Right
8 Hand Tendon, Left
9 Trunk Tendon, Right
B Trunk Tendon, Left
C Thorax Tendon, Right
D Thorax Tendon, Left
F Abdomen Tendon, Right
G Abdomen Tendon, Left
H Perineum Tendon
J Hip Tendon, Right
K Hip Tendon, Left
L Upper Leg Tendon, Right
M Upper Leg Tendon, Left
N Lower Leg Tendon, Right
   Achilles tendon
P Lower Leg Tendon, Left
   See N Lower Leg Tendon, Right
Q Knee Tendon, Right
   Patellar tendon
R Knee Tendon, Left
   See Q Knee Tendon, Right
S Ankle Tendon, Right
T Ankle Tendon, Left
V Foot Tendon, Right
W Foot Tendon, Left
	Ø Open
	3 Percutaneous
	4 Percutaneous Endoscopic
		Z No Device	X Diagnostic
			Z No Qualifier

Non-OR   ØL9[Ø,1,2,3,4,5,6,7,8,9,B,C,D,F,G,H,J,K,L,M,N,P,Q,R,S,T,V,W]3ØZ   Non-OR   ØL9[7,8]4ZZ
Non-OR   ØL9[Ø,1,2,3,4,5,6,7,8,9,B,C,D,F,G,H,J,K,L,M,N,P,Q,R,S,T,V,W]3ZZ

0   **Medical and Surgical**
L   **Tendons**
B   **Excision**   Definition: Cutting out or off, without replacement, a portion of a body part
                       Explanation: The qualifier DIAGNOSTIC is used to identify excision procedures that are biopsies

Body Part Character 4	Approach Character 5	Device Character 6	Qualifier Character 7

0 Head and Neck Tendon
1 Shoulder Tendon, Right
2 Shoulder Tendon, Left
3 Upper Arm Tendon, Right
4 Upper Arm Tendon, Left
5 Lower Arm and Wrist Tendon, Right
6 Lower Arm and Wrist Tendon, Left
7 Hand Tendon, Right
8 Hand Tendon, Left
9 Trunk Tendon, Right
B Trunk Tendon, Left
C Thorax Tendon, Right
D Thorax Tendon, Left
F Abdomen Tendon, Right
G Abdomen Tendon, Left
H Perineum Tendon
J Hip Tendon, Right
K Hip Tendon, Left
L Upper Leg Tendon, Right
M Upper Leg Tendon, Left
N Lower Leg Tendon, Right
    Achilles tendon
P Lower Leg Tendon, Left
    See N Lower Leg Tendon, Right
Q Knee Tendon, Right
    Patellar tendon
R Knee Tendon, Left
    See Q Knee Tendon, Right
S Ankle Tendon, Right
T Ankle Tendon, Left
V Foot Tendon, Right
W Foot Tendon, Left
	0 Open
	3 Percutaneous
	4 Percutaneous Endoscopic
		Z No Device	**X** Diagnostic
			Z No Qualifier

Ø   **Medical and Surgical**
L   **Tendons**
C   **Extirpation**   Definition: Taking or cutting out solid matter from a body part

Explanation: The solid matter may be an abnormal byproduct of a biological function or a foreign body; it may be imbedded in a body part or in the lumen of a tubular body part. The solid matter may or may not have been previously broken into pieces.

Body Part Character 4	Approach Character 5	Device Character 6	Qualifier Character 7

Ø   Head and Neck Tendon
1   Shoulder Tendon, Right
2   Shoulder Tendon, Left
3   Upper Arm Tendon, Right
4   Upper Arm Tendon, Left
5   Lower Arm and Wrist Tendon, Right
6   Lower Arm and Wrist Tendon, Left
7   Hand Tendon, Right
8   Hand Tendon, Left
9   Trunk Tendon, Right
B   Trunk Tendon, Left
C   Thorax Tendon, Right
D   Thorax Tendon, Left
F   Abdomen Tendon, Right
G   Abdomen Tendon, Left
H   Perineum Tendon
J   Hip Tendon, Right
K   Hip Tendon, Left
L   Upper Leg Tendon, Right
M   Upper Leg Tendon, Left
N   Lower Leg Tendon, Right
    Achilles tendon
P   Lower Leg Tendon, Left
    See N Lower Leg Tendon, Right
Q   Knee Tendon, Right
    Patellar tendon
R   Knee Tendon, Left
    See Q Knee Tendon, Right
S   Ankle Tendon, Right
T   Ankle Tendon, Left
V   Foot Tendon, Right
W   Foot Tendon, Left
	Ø Open
	3 Percutaneous
	4 Percutaneous Endoscopic
		Z No Device	Z No Qualifier

Ø **Medical and Surgical**
L **Tendons**
D **Extraction**　　　　Definition: Pulling or stripping out or off all or a portion of a body part by the use of force
　　　　　　　　　　　　Explanation: The qualifier DIAGNOSTIC is used to identify extraction procedures that are biopsies

Body Part Character 4	Approach Character 5	Device Character 6	Qualifier Character 7
Ø Head and Neck Tendon **1** Shoulder Tendon, Right **2** Shoulder Tendon, Left **3** Upper Arm Tendon, Right **4** Upper Arm Tendon, Left **5** Lower Arm and Wrist Tendon, Right **6** Lower Arm and Wrist Tendon, Left **7** Hand Tendon, Right **8** Hand Tendon, Left **9** Trunk Tendon, Right **B** Trunk Tendon, Left **C** Thorax Tendon, Right **D** Thorax Tendon, Left **F** Abdomen Tendon, Right **G** Abdomen Tendon, Left **H** Perineum Tendon **J** Hip Tendon, Right **K** Hip Tendon, Left **L** Upper Leg Tendon, Right **M** Upper Leg Tendon, Left **N** Lower Leg Tendon, Right 　　Achilles tendon **P** Lower Leg Tendon, Left 　　*See N Lower Leg Tendon, Right* **Q** Knee Tendon, Right 　　Patellar tendon **R** Knee Tendon, Left 　　*See Q Knee Tendon, Right* **S** Ankle Tendon, Right **T** Ankle Tendon, Left **V** Foot Tendon, Right **W** Foot Tendon, Left	**Ø** Open	**Z** No Device	**Z** No Qualifier

Ø **Medical and Surgical**
L **Tendons**
H **Insertion**　　　　Definition: Putting in a nonbiological appliance that monitors, assists, performs, or prevents a physiological function but does not physically
　　　　　　　　　　　take the place of a body part
　　　　　　　　　　　Explanation: None

Body Part Character 4	Approach Character 5	Device Character 6	Qualifier Character 7
X Upper Tendon **Y** Lower Tendon	**Ø** Open **3** Percutaneous **4** Percutaneous Endoscopic	**Y** Other Device	**Z** No Qualifier

　　Non-OR ØLH[X,Y][3,4]YZ

Ø **Medical and Surgical**
L **Tendons**
J **Inspection**　　　　Definition: Visually and/or manually exploring a body part
　　　　　　　　　　　Explanation: Visual exploration may be performed with or without optical instrumentation. Manual exploration may be performed directly or
　　　　　　　　　　　through intervening body layers.

Body Part Character 4	Approach Character 5	Device Character 6	Qualifier Character 7
X Upper Tendon **Y** Lower Tendon	**Ø** Open **3** Percutaneous **4** Percutaneous Endoscopic **X** External	**Z** No Device	**Z** No Qualifier

　　Non-OR ØLJ[X,Y][3,X]ZZ

LC Limited Coverage　**NC** Noncovered　⊞ Combination Member　HAC associated procedure　Combination Only　DRG Non-OR　Non-OR　New/Revised in GREEN
ICD-10-PCS 2019　　473

ØLD–ØLJ

Ø   **Medical and Surgical**
L   **Tendons**
M   **Reattachment**   Definition: Putting back in or on all or a portion of a separated body part to its normal location or other suitable location
                      Explanation: Vascular circulation and nervous pathways may or may not be reestablished

Body Part Character 4	Approach Character 5	Device Character 6	Qualifier Character 7
Ø Head and Neck Tendon	Ø Open	Z No Device	Z No Qualifier
1 Shoulder Tendon, Right	4 Percutaneous Endoscopic		
2 Shoulder Tendon, Left			
3 Upper Arm Tendon, Right			
4 Upper Arm Tendon, Left			
5 Lower Arm and Wrist Tendon, Right			
6 Lower Arm and Wrist Tendon, Left			
7 Hand Tendon, Right			
8 Hand Tendon, Left			
9 Trunk Tendon, Right			
B Trunk Tendon, Left			
C Thorax Tendon, Right			
D Thorax Tendon, Left			
F Abdomen Tendon, Right			
G Abdomen Tendon, Left			
H Perineum Tendon			
J Hip Tendon, Right			
K Hip Tendon, Left			
L Upper Leg Tendon, Right			
M Upper Leg Tendon, Left			
N Lower Leg Tendon, Right Achilles tendon			
P Lower Leg Tendon, Left See N Lower Leg Tendon, Right			
Q Knee Tendon, Right Patellar tendon			
R Knee Tendon, Left See Q Knee Tendon, Right			
S Ankle Tendon, Right			
T Ankle Tendon, Left			
V Foot Tendon, Right			
W Foot Tendon, Left			

Ø   **Medical and Surgical**
L   **Tendons**
N   **Release**   Definition: Freeing a body part from an abnormal physical constraint by cutting or by the use of force
              Explanation: Some of the restraining tissue may be taken out but none of the body part is taken out

Body Part Character 4	Approach Character 5	Device Character 6	Qualifier Character 7
Ø Head and Neck Tendon	Ø Open	Z No Device	Z No Qualifier
1 Shoulder Tendon, Right	3 Percutaneous		
2 Shoulder Tendon, Left	4 Percutaneous Endoscopic		
3 Upper Arm Tendon, Right	X External		
4 Upper Arm Tendon, Left			
5 Lower Arm and Wrist Tendon, Right			
6 Lower Arm and Wrist Tendon, Left			
7 Hand Tendon, Right			
8 Hand Tendon, Left			
9 Trunk Tendon, Right			
B Trunk Tendon, Left			
C Thorax Tendon, Right			
D Thorax Tendon, Left			
F Abdomen Tendon, Right			
G Abdomen Tendon, Left			
H Perineum Tendon			
J Hip Tendon, Right			
K Hip Tendon, Left			
L Upper Leg Tendon, Right			
M Upper Leg Tendon, Left			
N Lower Leg Tendon, Right Achilles tendon			
P Lower Leg Tendon, Left See N Lower Leg Tendon, Right			
Q Knee Tendon, Right Patellar tendon			
R Knee Tendon, Left See Q Knee Tendon, Right			
S Ankle Tendon, Right			
T Ankle Tendon, Left			
V Foot Tendon, Right			
W Foot Tendon, Left			

Non-OR   ØLN[Ø,1,2,3,4,5,6,7,8,9,B,C,D,F,G,H,J,K,L,M,N,P,Q,R,S,T,V,W]XZZ

Ø Medical and Surgical
L Tendons
P Removal

Definition: Taking out or off a device from a body part

Explanation: If a device is taken out and a similar device put in without cutting or puncturing the skin or mucous membrane, the procedure is coded to the root operation CHANGE. Otherwise, the procedure for taking out a device is coded to the root operation REMOVAL.

Body Part Character 4	Approach Character 5	Device Character 6	Qualifier Character 7
X Upper Tendon Y Lower Tendon	Ø Open 3 Percutaneous 4 Percutaneous Endoscopic	Ø Drainage Device 7 Autologous Tissue Substitute J Synthetic Substitute K Nonautologous Tissue Substitute Y Other Device	Z No Qualifier
X Upper Tendon Y Lower Tendon	X External	Ø Drainage Device	Z No Qualifier

Non-OR   ØLP[X,Y]3ØZ
Non-OR   ØLP[X,Y][3,4]YZ
Non-OR   ØLP[X,Y]XØZ

Ø Medical and Surgical
L Tendons
Q Repair

Definition: Restoring, to the extent possible, a body part to its normal anatomic structure and function

Explanation: Used only when the method to accomplish the repair is not one of the other root operations

Body Part Character 4	Approach Character 5	Device Character 6	Qualifier Character 7

Ø Head and Neck Tendon
1 Shoulder Tendon, Right
2 Shoulder Tendon, Left
3 Upper Arm Tendon, Right
4 Upper Arm Tendon, Left
5 Lower Arm and Wrist Tendon, Right
6 Lower Arm and Wrist Tendon, Left
7 Hand Tendon, Right
8 Hand Tendon, Left
9 Trunk Tendon, Right
B Trunk Tendon, Left
C Thorax Tendon, Right
D Thorax Tendon, Left
F Abdomen Tendon, Right
G Abdomen Tendon, Left
H Perineum Tendon
J Hip Tendon, Right
K Hip Tendon, Left
L Upper Leg Tendon, Right
M Upper Leg Tendon, Left
N Lower Leg Tendon, Right
   Achilles tendon
P Lower Leg Tendon, Left
   See N Lower Leg Tendon, Right
Q Knee Tendon, Right
   Patellar tendon
R Knee Tendon, Left
   See Q Knee Tendon, Right
S Ankle Tendon, Right
T Ankle Tendon, Left
V Foot Tendon, Right
W Foot Tendon, Left
	Ø Open
	3 Percutaneous
	4 Percutaneous Endoscopic
		Z No Device	Z No Qualifier

LC Limited Coverage   NC Noncovered   ⊞ Combination Member   HAC associated procedure   Combination Only   DRG Non-OR   Non-OR   New/Revised in GREEN

ICD-10-PCS 2019   475

Ø   **Medical and Surgical**
L   **Tendons**
R   **Replacement**   Definition: Putting in or on biological or synthetic material that physically takes the place and/or function of all or a portion of a body part

Explanation: The body part may have been taken out or replaced, or may be taken out, physically eradicated, or rendered nonfunctional during the REPLACEMENT procedure. A REMOVAL procedure is coded for taking out the device used in a previous replacement procedure.

Body Part Character 4	Approach Character 5	Device Character 6	Qualifier Character 7

Ø   Head and Neck Tendon
1   Shoulder Tendon, Right
2   Shoulder Tendon, Left
3   Upper Arm Tendon, Right
4   Upper Arm Tendon, Left
5   Lower Arm and Wrist Tendon, Right
6   Lower Arm and Wrist Tendon, Left
7   Hand Tendon, Right
8   Hand Tendon, Left
9   Trunk Tendon, Right
B   Trunk Tendon, Left
C   Thorax Tendon, Right
D   Thorax Tendon, Left
F   Abdomen Tendon, Right
G   Abdomen Tendon, Left
H   Perineum Tendon
J   Hip Tendon, Right
K   Hip Tendon, Left
L   Upper Leg Tendon, Right
M   Upper Leg Tendon, Left
N   Lower Leg Tendon, Right
     Achilles tendon
P   Lower Leg Tendon, Left
     See N Lower Leg Tendon, Right
Q   Knee Tendon, Right
     Patellar tendon
R   Knee Tendon, Left
     See Q Knee Tendon, Right
S   Ankle Tendon, Right
T   Ankle Tendon, Left
V   Foot Tendon, Right
W   Foot Tendon, Left
	Ø Open
	4 Percutaneous Endoscopic
		7 Autologous Tissue Substitute
		J Synthetic Substitute
		K Nonautologous Tissue Substitute
			Z No Qualifier

Ø   **Medical and Surgical**
L   **Tendons**
S   **Reposition**   Definition: Moving to its normal location, or other suitable location, all or a portion of a body part

Explanation: The body part is moved to a new location from an abnormal location, or from a normal location where it is not functioning correctly. The body part may or may not be cut out or off to be moved to the new location.

Body Part Character 4	Approach Character 5	Device Character 6	Qualifier Character 7

Ø   Head and Neck Tendon
1   Shoulder Tendon, Right
2   Shoulder Tendon, Left
3   Upper Arm Tendon, Right
4   Upper Arm Tendon, Left
5   Lower Arm and Wrist Tendon, Right
6   Lower Arm and Wrist Tendon, Left
7   Hand Tendon, Right
8   Hand Tendon, Left
9   Trunk Tendon, Right
B   Trunk Tendon, Left
C   Thorax Tendon, Right
D   Thorax Tendon, Left
F   Abdomen Tendon, Right
G   Abdomen Tendon, Left
H   Perineum Tendon
J   Hip Tendon, Right
K   Hip Tendon, Left
L   Upper Leg Tendon, Right
M   Upper Leg Tendon, Left
N   Lower Leg Tendon, Right
     Achilles tendon
P   Lower Leg Tendon, Left
     See N Lower Leg Tendon, Right
Q   Knee Tendon, Right
     Patellar tendon
R   Knee Tendon, Left
     See Q Knee Tendon, Right
S   Ankle Tendon, Right
T   Ankle Tendon, Left
V   Foot Tendon, Right
W   Foot Tendon, Left
	Ø Open
	4 Percutaneous Endoscopic
		Z No Device	Z No Qualifier

ØLR–ØLS

LC Limited Coverage   NC Noncovered   ⊞ Combination Member   HAC associated procedure   Combination Only   DRG Non-OR   Non-OR   New/Revised in GREEN

476   **ICD-10-PCS 2019**

Ø   Medical and Surgical
L   Tendons
T   Resection   Definition: Cutting out or off, without replacement, all of a body part
                       Explanation: None

Body Part Character 4	Approach Character 5	Device Character 6	Qualifier Character 7

Ø   Head and Neck Tendon
1   Shoulder Tendon, Right
2   Shoulder Tendon, Left
3   Upper Arm Tendon, Right
4   Upper Arm Tendon, Left
5   Lower Arm and Wrist Tendon, Right
6   Lower Arm and Wrist Tendon, Left
7   Hand Tendon, Right
8   Hand Tendon, Left
9   Trunk Tendon, Right
B   Trunk Tendon, Left
C   Thorax Tendon, Right
D   Thorax Tendon, Left
F   Abdomen Tendon, Right
G   Abdomen Tendon, Left
H   Perineum Tendon
J   Hip Tendon, Right
K   Hip Tendon, Left
L   Upper Leg Tendon, Right
M   Upper Leg Tendon, Left
N   Lower Leg Tendon, Right
     Achilles tendon
P   Lower Leg Tendon, Left
     See N Lower Leg Tendon, Right
Q   Knee Tendon, Right
     Patellar tendon
R   Knee Tendon, Left
     See Q Knee Tendon, Right
S   Ankle Tendon, Right
T   Ankle Tendon, Left
V   Foot Tendon, Right
W   Foot Tendon, Left
	Ø Open
	4 Percutaneous Endoscopic
		Z No Device	Z No Qualifier

Ø   Medical and Surgical
L   Tendons
U   Supplement   Definition: Putting in or on biological or synthetic material that physically reinforces and/or augments the function of a portion of a body part
                       Explanation: The biological material is non-living, or is living and from the same individual. The body part may have been previously replaced, and the SUPPLEMENT procedure is performed to physically reinforce and/or augment the function of the replaced body part.

Body Part Character 4	Approach Character 5	Device Character 6	Qualifier Character 7

Ø   Head and Neck Tendon
1   Shoulder Tendon, Right
2   Shoulder Tendon, Left
3   Upper Arm Tendon, Right
4   Upper Arm Tendon, Left
5   Lower Arm and Wrist Tendon, Right
6   Lower Arm and Wrist Tendon, Left
7   Hand Tendon, Right
8   Hand Tendon, Left
9   Trunk Tendon, Right
B   Trunk Tendon, Left
C   Thorax Tendon, Right
D   Thorax Tendon, Left
F   Abdomen Tendon, Right
G   Abdomen Tendon, Left
H   Perineum Tendon
J   Hip Tendon, Right
K   Hip Tendon, Left
L   Upper Leg Tendon, Right
M   Upper Leg Tendon, Left
N   Lower Leg Tendon, Right
     Achilles tendon
P   Lower Leg Tendon, Left
     See N Lower Leg Tendon, Right
Q   Knee Tendon, Right
     Patellar tendon
R   Knee Tendon, Left
     See Q Knee Tendon, Right
S   Ankle Tendon, Right
T   Ankle Tendon, Left
V   Foot Tendon, Right
W   Foot Tendon, Left
	Ø Open
	4 Percutaneous Endoscopic
		7 Autologous Tissue Substitute
		J Synthetic Substitute
		K Nonautologous Tissue Substitute
			Z No Qualifier

Ø   Medical and Surgical
L   Tendons
W   Revision   Definition: Correcting, to the extent possible, a portion of a malfunctioning device or the position of a displaced device
                           Explanation: Revision can include correcting a malfunctioning or displaced device by taking out or putting in components of the device such as
                           a screw or pin

Body Part Character 4	Approach Character 5	Device Character 6	Qualifier Character 7
X Upper Tendon Y Lower Tendon	Ø Open 3 Percutaneous 4 Percutaneous Endoscopic	Ø Drainage Device 7 Autologous Tissue Substitute J Synthetic Substitute K Nonautologous Tissue Substitute Y Other Device	Z No Qualifier
X Upper Tendon Y Lower Tendon	X External	Ø Drainage Device 7 Autologous Tissue Substitute J Synthetic Substitute K Nonautologous Tissue Substitute	Z No Qualifier

Non-OR   ØLW[X,Y][3,4]YZ
Non-OR   ØLW[X,Y]X[Ø,7,J,K]Z

Ø   Medical and Surgical
L   Tendons
X   Transfer   Definition: Moving, without taking out, all or a portion of a body part to another location to take over the function of all or a portion of a body part
                          Explanation: The body part transferred remains connected to its vascular and nervous supply

Body Part Character 4	Approach Character 5	Device Character 6	Qualifier Character 7

Ø Head and Neck Tendon
1 Shoulder Tendon, Right
2 Shoulder Tendon, Left
3 Upper Arm Tendon, Right
4 Upper Arm Tendon, Left
5 Lower Arm and Wrist Tendon, Right
6 Lower Arm and Wrist Tendon, Left
7 Hand Tendon, Right
8 Hand Tendon, Left
9 Trunk Tendon, Right
B Trunk Tendon, Left
C Thorax Tendon, Right
D Thorax Tendon, Left
F Abdomen Tendon, Right
G Abdomen Tendon, Left
H Perineum Tendon
J Hip Tendon, Right
K Hip Tendon, Left
L Upper Leg Tendon, Right
M Upper Leg Tendon, Left
N Lower Leg Tendon, Right
   Achilles tendon
P Lower Leg Tendon, Left
   See N Lower Leg Tendon, Right
Q Knee Tendon, Right
   Patellar tendon
R Knee Tendon, Left
   See Q Knee Tendon, Right
S Ankle Tendon, Right
T Ankle Tendon, Left
V Foot Tendon, Right
W Foot Tendon, Left
	Ø Open
	4 Percutaneous Endoscopic
		Z No Device	Z No Qualifier

ØLW–ØLX

LC Limited Coverage   NC Noncovered   ⊞ Combination Member   HAC associated procedure   Combination Only   DRG Non-OR   Non-OR   New/Revised in GREEN
478   ICD-10-PCS 2019

Bursae and Ligaments ØM2–ØMX

Character Meanings*

This Character Meaning table is provided as a guide to assist the user in the identification of character members that may be found in this section of code tables. It **SHOULD NOT** be used to build a PCS code.

Operation–Character 3		Body Part–Character 4		Approach–Character 5		Device–Character 6		Qualifier–Character 7	
2	Change	Ø	Head and Neck Bursa and Ligament	Ø	Open	Ø	Drainage Device	X	Diagnostic
5	Destruction	1	Shoulder Bursa and Ligament, Right	3	Percutaneous	7	Autologous Tissue Substitute	Z	No Qualifier
8	Division	2	Shoulder Bursa and Ligament, Left	4	Percutaneous Endoscopic	J	Synthetic Substitute		
9	Drainage	3	Elbow Bursa and Ligament, Right	X	External	K	Nonautologous Tissue Substitute		
B	Excision	4	Elbow Bursa and Ligament, Left			Y	Other Device		
C	Extirpation	5	Wrist Bursa and Ligament, Right			Z	No Device		
D	Extraction	6	Wrist Bursa and Ligament, Left						
H	Insertion	7	Hand Bursa and Ligament, Right						
J	Inspection	8	Hand Bursa and Ligament, Left						
M	Reattachment	9	Upper Extremity Bursa and Ligament, Right						
N	Release	B	Upper Extremity Bursa and Ligament, Left						
P	Removal	C	Upper Spine Bursa and Ligament						
Q	Repair	D	Lower Spine Bursa and Ligament						
R	Replacement	F	Sternum Bursa and Ligament						
S	Reposition	G	Rib(s) Bursa and Ligament						
T	Resection	H	Abdomen Bursa and Ligament, Right						
U	Supplement	J	Abdomen Bursa and Ligament, Left						
W	Revision	K	Perineum Bursa and Ligament						
X	Transfer	L	Hip Bursa and Ligament, Right						
		M	Hip Bursa and Ligament, Left						
		N	Knee Bursa and Ligament, Right						
		P	Knee Bursa and Ligament, Left						
		Q	Ankle Bursa and Ligament, Right						
		R	Ankle Bursa and Ligament, Left						
		S	Foot Bursa and Ligament, Right						
		T	Foot Bursa and Ligament, Left						
		V	Lower Extremity Bursa and Ligament, Right						
		W	Lower Extremity Bursa and Ligament, Left						
		X	Upper Bursa and Ligament						
		Y	Lower Bursa and Ligament						

* Includes synovial membrane.

AHA Coding Clinic for table ØMM
2013, 3Q, 20   Superior labrum anterior posterior (SLAP) repair and subacromial decompression

AHA Coding Clinic for table ØMQ
2014, 3Q, 9   Interspinous ligamentoplasty

AHA Coding Clinic for table ØMT
2017, 2Q, 21   Arthroscopic anterior cruciate ligament revision using autograft with anterolateral ligament reconstruction

AHA Coding Clinic for table ØMU
2017, 2Q, 21   Arthroscopic anterior cruciate ligament revision using autograft with anterolateral ligament reconstruction

Shoulder Ligaments

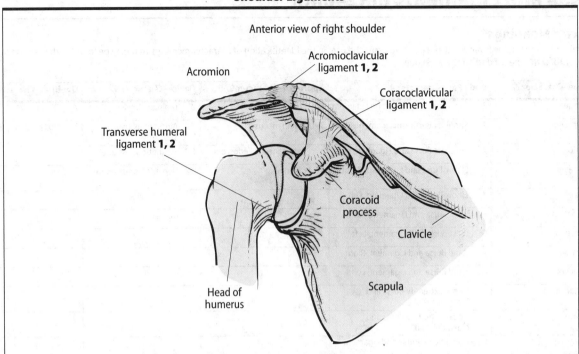

Anterior view of right shoulder

Acromion

Acromioclavicular ligament **1, 2**

Coracoclavicular ligament **1, 2**

Transverse humeral ligament **1, 2**

Coracoid process

Clavicle

Head of humerus

Scapula

Knee Bursae

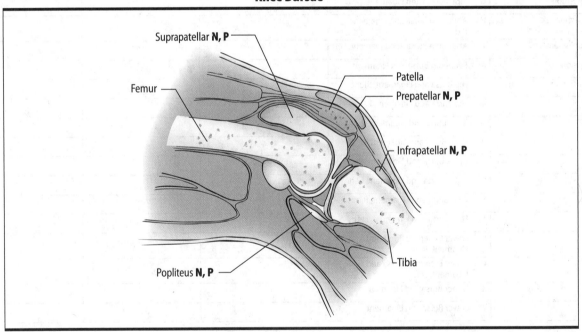

Suprapatellar **N, P**

Patella

Femur

Prepatellar **N, P**

Infrapatellar **N, P**

Popliteus **N, P**

Tibia

Knee Ligaments

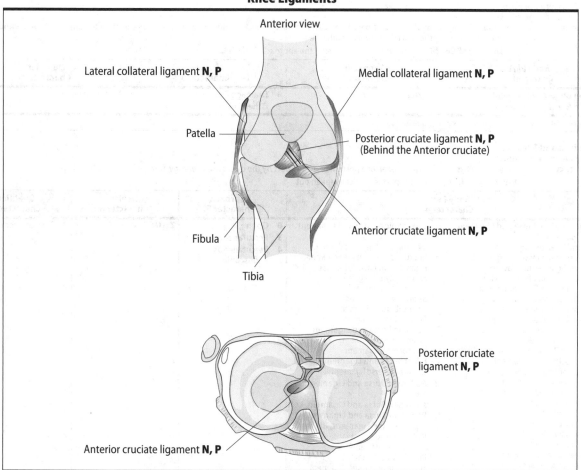

Anterior view

Lateral collateral ligament **N, P**

Medial collateral ligament **N, P**

Patella

Posterior cruciate ligament **N, P**
(Behind the Anterior cruciate)

Anterior cruciate ligament **N, P**

Fibula

Tibia

Posterior cruciate ligament **N, P**

Anterior cruciate ligament **N, P**

Wrist Ligaments

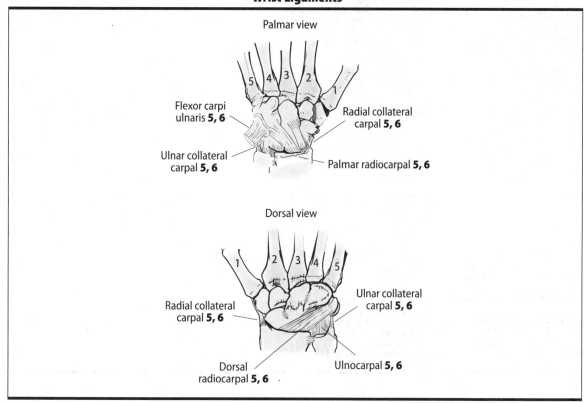

Palmar view

Flexor carpi ulnaris **5, 6**

Radial collateral carpal **5, 6**

Ulnar collateral carpal **5, 6**

Palmar radiocarpal **5, 6**

Dorsal view

Radial collateral carpal **5, 6**

Ulnar collateral carpal **5, 6**

Dorsal radiocarpal **5, 6**

Ulnocarpal **5, 6**

Bursae and Ligaments

Ø   Medical and Surgical
M   Bursae and Ligaments
2   Change   Definition: Taking out or off a device from a body part and putting back an identical or similar device in or on the same body part without cutting or puncturing the skin or a mucous membrane

               Explanation: All CHANGE procedures are coded using the approach EXTERNAL

Body Part Character 4	Approach Character 5	Device Character 6	Qualifier Character 7
X Upper Bursa and Ligament Y Lower Bursa and Ligament	X External	Ø Drainage Device Y Other Device	Z No Qualifier

Non-OR   All body part, approach, device, and qualifier values

Ø   Medical and Surgical
M   Bursae and Ligaments
5   Destruction   Definition: Physical eradication of all or a portion of a body part by the direct use of energy, force, or a destructive agent

               Explanation: None of the body part is physically taken out

Body Part Character 4	Approach Character 5	Device Character 6	Qualifier Character 7

Ø **Head and Neck Bursa and Ligament**
   Alar ligament of axis
   Cervical interspinous ligament
   Cervical intertransverse ligament
   Cervical ligamentum flavum
   Interspinous ligament, cervical
   Intertransverse ligament, cervical
   Lateral temporomandibular ligament
   Ligamentum flavum, cervical
   Sphenomandibular ligament
   Stylomandibular ligament
   Transverse ligament of atlas
1 **Shoulder Bursa and Ligament, Right**
   Acromioclavicular ligament
   Coracoacromial ligament
   Coracoclavicular ligament
   Coracohumeral ligament
   Costoclavicular ligament
   Glenohumeral ligament
   Interclavicular ligament
   Sternoclavicular ligament
   Subacromial bursa
   Transverse humeral ligament
   Transverse scapular ligament
2 **Shoulder Bursa and Ligament, Left**
   See 1 Shoulder Bursa and Ligament, Right
3 **Elbow Bursa and Ligament, Right**
   Annular ligament
   Olecranon bursa
   Radial collateral ligament
   Ulnar collateral ligament
4 **Elbow Bursa and Ligament, Left**
   See 3 Elbow Bursa and Ligament, Right
5 **Wrist Bursa and Ligament, Right**
   Palmar ulnocarpal ligament
   Radial collateral carpal ligament
   Radiocarpal ligament
   Radioulnar ligament
   Ulnar collateral carpal ligament
6 **Wrist Bursa and Ligament, Left**
   See 5 Wrist Bursa and Ligament, Right
7 **Hand Bursa and Ligament, Right**
   Carpometacarpal ligament
   Intercarpal ligament
   Interphalangeal ligament
   Lunotriquetral ligament
   Metacarpal ligament
   Metacarpophalangeal ligament
   Pisohamate ligament
   Pisometacarpal ligament
   Scapholunate ligament
   Scaphotrapezium ligament
8 **Hand Bursa and Ligament, Left**
   See 7 Hand Bursa and Ligament, Right
9 **Upper Extremity Bursa and Ligament, Right**
B **Upper Extremity Bursa and Ligament, Left**
C **Upper Spine Bursa and Ligament**
   Interspinous ligament, thoracic
   Intertransverse ligament, thoracic
   Ligamentum flavum, thoracic
   Supraspinous ligament
	D **Lower Spine Bursa and Ligament**
	   Iliolumbar ligament
	   Interspinous ligament, lumbar
	   Intertransverse ligament, lumbar
	   Ligamentum flavum, lumbar
	   Sacrococcygeal ligament
	   Sacroiliac ligament
	   Sacrospinous ligament
	   Sacrotuberous ligament
	   Supraspinous ligament
	F **Sternum Bursa and Ligament**
	   Costoxiphoid ligament
	   Sternocostal ligament
	G **Rib(s) Bursa and Ligament**
	   Costotransverse ligament
	H **Abdomen Bursa and Ligament, Right**
	J **Abdomen Bursa and Ligament, Left**
	K **Perineum Bursa and Ligament**
	L **Hip Bursa and Ligament, Right**
	   Iliofemoral ligament
	   Ischiofemoral ligament
	   Pubofemoral ligament
	   Transverse acetabular ligament
	   Trochanteric bursa
	M **Hip Bursa and Ligament, Left**
	   See L Hip Bursa and Ligament, Right
	N **Knee Bursa and Ligament, Right**
	   Anterior cruciate ligament (ACL)
	   Lateral collateral ligament (LCL)
	   Ligament of head of fibula
	   Medial collateral ligament (MCL)
	   Patellar ligament
	   Popliteal ligament
	   Posterior cruciate ligament (PCL)
	   Prepatellar bursa
	P **Knee Bursa and Ligament, Left**
	   See N Knee Bursa and Ligament, Right
	Q **Ankle Bursa and Ligament, Right**
	   Calcaneofibular ligament
	   Deltoid ligament
	   Ligament of the lateral malleolus
	   Talofibular ligament
	R **Ankle Bursa and Ligament, Left**
	   See Q Ankle Bursa and Ligament, Right
	S **Foot Bursa and Ligament, Right**
	   Calcaneocuboid ligament
	   Cuneonavicular ligament
	   Intercuneiform ligament
	   Interphalangeal ligament
	   Metatarsal ligament
	   Metatarsophalangeal ligament
	   Subtalar ligament
	   Talocalcaneal ligament
	   Talocalcaneonavicular ligament
	   Tarsometatarsal ligament
	T **Foot Bursa and Ligament, Left**
	   See S Foot Bursa and Ligament, Right
	V **Lower Extremity Bursa and Ligament, Right**
	W **Lower Extremity Bursa and Ligament, Left**
		Ø Open
		3 Percutaneous
		4 Percutaneous Endoscopic
			Z No Device	Z No Qualifier

LC Limited Coverage   NC Noncovered   ⊞ Combination Member   HAC associated procedure   Combination Only   DRG Non-OR   Non-OR   New/Revised in GREEN

482   ICD-10-PCS 2019

Ø   **Medical and Surgical**
M   **Bursae and Ligaments**
8   **Division**   Definition: Cutting into a body part, without draining fluids and/or gases from the body part, in order to separate or transect a body part
                        Explanation: All or a portion of the body part is separated into two or more portions

Body Part Character 4		Approach Character 5	Device Character 6	Qualifier Character 7
Ø **Head and Neck Bursa and Ligament** Alar ligament of axis Cervical interspinous ligament Cervical intertransverse ligament Cervical ligamentum flavum Interspinous ligament, cervical Intertransverse ligament, cervical Lateral temporomandibular ligament Ligamentum flavum, cervical Sphenomandibular ligament Stylomandibular ligament Transverse ligament of atlas **1** **Shoulder Bursa and Ligament, Right** Acromioclavicular ligament Coracoacromial ligament Coracoclavicular ligament Coracohumeral ligament Costoclavicular ligament Glenohumeral ligament Interclavicular ligament Sternoclavicular ligament Subacromial bursa Transverse humeral ligament Transverse scapular ligament **2** **Shoulder Bursa and Ligament, Left** *See 1 Shoulder Bursa and Ligament, Right* **3** **Elbow Bursa and Ligament, Right** Annular ligament Olecranon bursa Radial collateral ligament Ulnar collateral ligament **4** **Elbow Bursa and Ligament, Left** *See 3 Elbow Bursa and Ligament, Right* **5** **Wrist Bursa and Ligament, Right** Palmar ulnocarpal ligament Radial collateral carpal ligament Radiocarpal ligament Radioulnar ligament Ulnar collateral carpal ligament **6** **Wrist Bursa and Ligament, Left** *See 5 Wrist Bursa and Ligament, Right* **7** **Hand Bursa and Ligament, Right** Carpometacarpal ligament Intercarpal ligament Interphalangeal ligament Lunotriquetral ligament Metacarpal ligament Metacarpophalangeal ligament Pisohamate ligament Pisometacarpal ligament Scapholunate ligament Scaphotrapezium ligament **8** **Hand Bursa and Ligament, Left** *See 7 Hand Bursa and Ligament, Right* **9** **Upper Extremity Bursa and Ligament, Right** **B** **Upper Extremity Bursa and Ligament, Left** **C** **Upper Spine Bursa and Ligament** Interspinous ligament, thoracic Intertransverse ligament, thoracic Ligamentum flavum, thoracic Supraspinous ligament	**D** **Lower Spine Bursa and Ligament** Iliolumbar ligament Interspinous ligament, lumbar Intertransverse ligament, lumbar Ligamentum flavum, lumbar Sacrococcygeal ligament Sacroiliac ligament Sacrospinous ligament Sacrotuberous ligament Supraspinous ligament **F** **Sternum Bursa and Ligament** Costoxiphoid ligament Sternocostal ligament **G** **Rib(s) Bursa and Ligament** Costotransverse ligament **H** **Abdomen Bursa and Ligament, Right** **J** **Abdomen Bursa and Ligament, Left** **K** **Perineum Bursa and Ligament** **L** **Hip Bursa and Ligament, Right** Iliofemoral ligament Ischiofemoral ligament Pubofemoral ligament Transverse acetabular ligament Trochanteric bursa **M** **Hip Bursa and Ligament, Left** *See L Hip Bursa and Ligament, Right* **N** **Knee Bursa and Ligament, Right** Anterior cruciate ligament (ACL) Lateral collateral ligament (LCL) Ligament of head of fibula Medial collateral ligament (MCL) Patellar ligament Popliteal ligament Posterior cruciate ligament (PCL) Prepatellar bursa **P** **Knee Bursa and Ligament, Left** *See N Knee Bursa and Ligament, Right* **Q** **Ankle Bursa and Ligament, Right** Calcaneofibular ligament Deltoid ligament Ligament of the lateral malleolus Talofibular ligament **R** **Ankle Bursa and Ligament, Left** *See Q Ankle Bursa and Ligament, Right* **S** **Foot Bursa and Ligament, Right** Calcaneocuboid ligament Cuneonavicular ligament Intercuneiform ligament Interphalangeal ligament Metatarsal ligament Metatarsophalangeal ligament Subtalar ligament Talocalcaneal ligament Talocalcaneonavicular ligament Tarsometatarsal ligament **T** **Foot Bursa and Ligament, Left** *See S Foot Bursa and Ligament, Right* **V** **Lower Extremity Bursa and Ligament, Right** **W** **Lower Extremity Bursa and Ligament, Left**	**Ø** Open **3** Percutaneous **4** Percutaneous Endoscopic	**Z** No Device	**Z** No Qualifier

LC Limited Coverage   NC Noncovered   ⊞ Combination Member   HAC associated procedure   Combination Only   DRG Non-OR   Non-OR   New/Revised in GREEN

ICD-10-PCS 2019   483

Bursae and Ligaments

Ø   **Medical and Surgical**
M   **Bursae and Ligaments**
9   **Drainage**   Definition: Taking or letting out fluids and/or gases from a body part
                    Explanation: The qualifier DIAGNOSTIC is used to identify drainage procedures that are biopsies

Body Part Character 4		Approach Character 5	Device Character 6	Qualifier Character 7

Ø Head and Neck Bursa and Ligament
  Alar ligament of axis
  Cervical interspinous ligament
  Cervical intertransverse ligament
  Cervical ligamentum flavum
  Interspinous ligament, cervical
  Intertransverse ligament, cervical
  Lateral temporomandibular
    ligament
  Ligamentum flavum, cervical
  Sphenomandibular ligament
  Stylomandibular ligament
  Transverse ligament of atlas
1 Shoulder Bursa and Ligament, Right
  Acromioclavicular ligament
  Coracoacromial ligament
  Coracoclavicular ligament
  Coracohumeral ligament
  Costoclavicular ligament
  Glenohumeral ligament
  Interclavicular ligament
  Sternoclavicular ligament
  Subacromial bursa
  Transverse humeral ligament
  Transverse scapular ligament
2 Shoulder Bursa and Ligament, Left
  See 1 Shoulder Bursa and Ligament, Right
3 Elbow Bursa and Ligament, Right
  Annular ligament
  Olecranon bursa
  Radial collateral ligament
  Ulnar collateral ligament
4 Elbow Bursa and Ligament, Left
  See 3 Elbow Bursa and Ligament, Right
5 Wrist Bursa and Ligament, Right
  Palmar ulnocarpal ligament
  Radial collateral carpal ligament
  Radiocarpal ligament
  Radioulnar ligament
  Ulnar collateral carpal ligament
6 Wrist Bursa and Ligament, Left
  See 5 Wrist Bursa and Ligament, Right
7 Hand Bursa and Ligament, Right
  Carpometacarpal ligament
  Intercarpal ligament
  Interphalangeal ligament
  Lunotriquetral ligament
  Metacarpal ligament
  Metacarpophalangeal ligament
  Pisohamate ligament
  Pisometacarpal ligament
  Scapholunate ligament
  Scaphotrapezium ligament
8 Hand Bursa and Ligament, Left
  See 7 Hand Bursa and Ligament, Right
9 Upper Extremity Bursa and Ligament, Right
B Upper Extremity Bursa and Ligament, Left
C Upper Spine Bursa and Ligament
  Interspinous ligament, thoracic
  Intertransverse ligament, thoracic
  Ligamentum flavum, thoracic
  Supraspinous ligament
	D Lower Spine Bursa and Ligament
	  Iliolumbar ligament
	  Interspinous ligament, lumbar
	  Intertransverse ligament, lumbar
	  Ligamentum flavum, lumbar
	  Sacrococcygeal ligament
	  Sacroiliac ligament
	  Sacrospinous ligament
	  Sacrotuberous ligament
	  Supraspinous ligament
	F Sternum Bursa and Ligament
	  Costoxiphoid ligament
	  Sternocostal ligament
	G Rib(s) Bursa and Ligament
	  Costotransverse ligament
	H Abdomen Bursa and Ligament, Right
	J Abdomen Bursa and Ligament, Left
	K Perineum Bursa and Ligament
	L Hip Bursa and Ligament, Right
	  Iliofemoral ligament
	  Ischiofemoral ligament
	  Pubofemoral ligament
	  Transverse acetabular ligament
	  Trochanteric bursa
	M Hip Bursa and Ligament, Left
	  See L Hip Bursa and Ligament, Right
	N Knee Bursa and Ligament, Right
	  Anterior cruciate ligament (ACL)
	  Lateral collateral ligament (LCL)
	  Ligament of head of fibula
	  Medial collateral ligament (MCL)
	  Patellar ligament
	  Popliteal ligament
	  Posterior cruciate ligament (PCL)
	  Prepatellar bursa
	P Knee Bursa and Ligament, Left
	  See N Knee Bursa and Ligament, Right
	Q Ankle Bursa and Ligament, Right
	  Calcaneofibular ligament
	  Deltoid ligament
	  Ligament of the lateral malleolus
	  Talofibular ligament
	R Ankle Bursa and Ligament, Left
	  See Q Ankle Bursa and Ligament, Right
	S Foot Bursa and Ligament, Right
	  Calcaneocuboid ligament
	  Cuneonavicular ligament
	  Intercuneiform ligament
	  Interphalangeal ligament
	  Metatarsal ligament
	  Metatarsophalangeal ligament
	  Subtalar ligament
	  Talocalcaneal ligament
	  Talocalcaneonavicular ligament
	  Tarsometatarsal ligament
	T Foot Bursa and Ligament, Left
	  See S Foot Bursa and Ligament, Right
	V Lower Extremity Bursa and Ligament, Right
	W Lower Extremity Bursa and Ligament, Left
		Ø Open
		3 Percutaneous
		4 Percutaneous Endoscopic
			Ø Drainage Device	**Z No Qualifier**

ØM9 Continued on next page

Non-OR	ØM9[Ø,1,2,3,4,5,6,7,8,9,B,C,D,F,G,H,J,K,L,M,N,P,Q,R,S,T,V,W]30Z
Non-OR	ØM9[1,2,3,4,7,8,9,B,C,D,F,G,H,J,K,L,M,V,W]40Z

Ø   **Medical and Surgical**   ***ØM9 Continued***
M   **Bursae and Ligaments**
9   **Drainage**   Definition: Taking or letting out fluids and/or gases from a body part
                        Explanation: The qualifier DIAGNOSTIC is used to identify drainage procedures that are biopsies

Body Part Character 4		Approach Character 5	Device Character 6	Qualifier Character 7

Ø   **Head and Neck Bursa and Ligament**
    Alar ligament of axis
    Cervical interspinous ligament
    Cervical intertransverse ligament
    Cervical ligamentum flavum
    Interspinous ligament, cervical
    Intertransverse ligament, cervical
    Lateral temporomandibular
      ligament
    Ligamentum flavum, cervical
    Sphenomandibular ligament
    Stylomandibular ligament
    Transverse ligament of atlas
1   **Shoulder Bursa and Ligament, Right**
    Acromioclavicular ligament
    Coracoacromial ligament
    Coracoclavicular ligament
    Coracohumeral ligament
    Costoclavicular ligament
    Glenohumeral ligament
    Interclavicular ligament
    Sternoclavicular ligament
    Subacromial bursa
    Transverse humeral ligament
    Transverse scapular ligament
2   **Shoulder Bursa and Ligament, Left**
    See 1 Shoulder Bursa and
      Ligament, Right
3   **Elbow Bursa and Ligament, Right**
    Annular ligament
    Olecranon bursa
    Radial collateral ligament
    Ulnar collateral ligament
4   **Elbow Bursa and Ligament, Left**
    See 3 Elbow Bursa and Ligament,
      Right
5   **Wrist Bursa and Ligament, Right**
    Palmar ulnocarpal ligament
    Radial collateral carpal ligament
    Radiocarpal ligament
    Radioulnar ligament
    Ulnar collateral carpal ligament
6   **Wrist Bursa and Ligament, Left**
    See 5 Wrist Bursa and Ligament,
      Right
7   **Hand Bursa and Ligament, Right**
    Carpometacarpal ligament
    Intercarpal ligament
    Interphalangeal ligament
    Lunotriquetral ligament
    Metacarpal ligament
    Metacarpophalangeal ligament
    Pisohamate ligament
    Pisometacarpal ligament
    Scapholunate ligament
    Scaphotrapezium ligament
8   **Hand Bursa and Ligament, Left**
    See 7 Hand Bursa and Ligament,
      Right
9   **Upper Extremity Bursa and Ligament, Right**
B   **Upper Extremity Bursa and Ligament, Left**
C   **Upper Spine Bursa and Ligament**
    Interspinous ligament, thoracic
    Intertransverse ligament, thoracic
    Ligamentum flavum, thoracic
    Supraspinous ligament
	D **Lower Spine Bursa and Ligament**
	    Iliolumbar ligament
	    Interspinous ligament, lumbar
	    Intertransverse ligament, lumbar
	    Ligamentum flavum, lumbar
	    Sacrococcygeal ligament
	    Sacroiliac ligament
	    Sacrospinous ligament
	    Sacrotuberous ligament
	    Supraspinous ligament
	F **Sternum Bursa and Ligament**
	    Costoxiphoid ligament
	    Sternocostal ligament
	G **Rib(s) Bursa and Ligament**
	    Costotransverse ligament
	H **Abdomen Bursa and Ligament, Right**
	J **Abdomen Bursa and Ligament, Left**
	K **Perineum Bursa and Ligament**
	L **Hip Bursa and Ligament, Right**
	    Iliofemoral ligament
	    Ischiofemoral ligament
	    Pubofemoral ligament
	    Transverse acetabular ligament
	    Trochanteric bursa
	M **Hip Bursa and Ligament, Left**
	    See L Hip Bursa and Ligament,
	      Right
	N **Knee Bursa and Ligament, Right**
	    Anterior cruciate ligament (ACL)
	    Lateral collateral ligament (LCL)
	    Ligament of head of fibula
	    Medial collateral ligament (MCL)
	    Patellar ligament
	    Popliteal ligament
	    Posterior cruciate ligament (PCL)
	    Prepatellar bursa
	P **Knee Bursa and Ligament, Left**
	    See N Knee Bursa and Ligament,
	      Right
	Q **Ankle Bursa and Ligament, Right**
	    Calcaneofibular ligament
	    Deltoid ligament
	    Ligament of the lateral malleolus
	    Talofibular ligament
	R **Ankle Bursa and Ligament, Left**
	    See Q Ankle Bursa and Ligament,
	      Right
	S **Foot Bursa and Ligament, Right**
	    Calcaneocuboid ligament
	    Cuneonavicular ligament
	    Intercuneiform ligament
	    Interphalangeal ligament
	    Metatarsal ligament
	    Metatarsophalangeal ligament
	    Subtalar ligament
	    Talocalcaneal ligament
	    Talocalcaneonavicular ligament
	    Tarsometatarsal ligament
	T **Foot Bursa and Ligament, Left**
	    See S Foot Bursa and Ligament,
	      Right
	V **Lower Extremity Bursa and Ligament, Right**
	W **Lower Extremity Bursa and Ligament, Left**
		Ø Open
		3 Percutaneous
		4 Percutaneous Endoscopic
			Z No Device	**X** Diagnostic
				Z No Qualifier

Non-OR   ØM9[Ø,1,2,3,4,5,6,7,8,C,D,F,G,L,M,N,P,Q,R,S,T][Ø,3,4]ZX
Non-OR   ØM9[Ø,1,2,3,4,5,6,7,8,9,B,C,D,F,G,H,J,K,L,M,N,P,Q,R,S,T,V,W]3ZZ
Non-OR   ØM9[Ø,5,6,7,8,9,B,C,D,F,G,H,J,K,N,P,Q,R,S,T,V,W]4ZZ

Bursae and Ligaments *(side tab)*

Ø   **Medical and Surgical**
M   **Bursae and Ligaments**
B   **Excision**   Definition: Cutting out or off, without replacement, a portion of a body part
                   Explanation: The qualifier DIAGNOSTIC is used to identify excision procedures that are biopsies

Body Part Character 4		Approach Character 5	Device Character 6	Qualifier Character 7

Ø Head and Neck Bursa and Ligament
Alar ligament of axis
Cervical interspinous ligament
Cervical intertransverse ligament
Cervical ligamentum flavum
Interspinous ligament, cervical
Intertransverse ligament, cervical
Lateral temporomandibular
  ligament
Ligamentum flavum, cervical
Sphenomandibular ligament
Stylomandibular ligament
Transverse ligament of atlas
1 Shoulder Bursa and Ligament, Right
Acromioclavicular ligament
Coracoacromial ligament
Coracoclavicular ligament
Coracohumeral ligament
Costoclavicular ligament
Glenohumeral ligament
Interclavicular ligament
Sternoclavicular ligament
Subacromial bursa
Transverse humeral ligament
Transverse scapular ligament
2 Shoulder Bursa and Ligament, Left
*See 1 Shoulder Bursa and
  Ligament, Right*
3 Elbow Bursa and Ligament, Right
Annular ligament
Olecranon bursa
Radial collateral ligament
Ulnar collateral ligament
4 Elbow Bursa and Ligament, Left
*See 3 Elbow Bursa and Ligament,
  Right*
5 Wrist Bursa and Ligament, Right
Palmar ulnocarpal ligament
Radial collateral carpal ligament
Radiocarpal ligament
Radioulnar ligament
Ulnar collateral carpal ligament
6 Wrist Bursa and Ligament, Left
*See 5 Wrist Bursa and Ligament,
  Right*
7 Hand Bursa and Ligament, Right
Carpometacarpal ligament
Intercarpal ligament
Interphalangeal ligament
Lunotriquetral ligament
Metacarpal ligament
Metacarpophalangeal ligament
Pisohamate ligament
Pisometacarpal ligament
Scapholunate ligament
Scaphotrapezium ligament
8 Hand Bursa and Ligament, Left
*See 7 Hand Bursa and Ligament,
  Right*
9 Upper Extremity Bursa and Ligament, Right
B Upper Extremity Bursa and Ligament, Left
C Upper Spine Bursa and Ligament
Interspinous ligament, thoracic
Intertransverse ligament, thoracic
Ligamentum flavum, thoracic
Supraspinous ligament
	D Lower Spine Bursa and Ligament
	Iliolumbar ligament
	Interspinous ligament, lumbar
	Intertransverse ligament, lumbar
	Ligamentum flavum, lumbar
	Sacrococcygeal ligament
	Sacroiliac ligament
	Sacrospinous ligament
	Sacrotuberous ligament
	Supraspinous ligament
	F Sternum Bursa and Ligament
	Costoxiphoid ligament
	Sternocostal ligament
	G Rib(s) Bursa and Ligament
	Costotransverse ligament
	H Abdomen Bursa and Ligament, Right
	J Abdomen Bursa and Ligament, Left
	K Perineum Bursa and Ligament
	L Hip Bursa and Ligament, Right
	Iliofemoral ligament
	Ischiofemoral ligament
	Pubofemoral ligament
	Transverse acetabular ligament
	Trochanteric bursa
	M Hip Bursa and Ligament, Left
	*See L Hip Bursa and Ligament,
	  Right*
	N Knee Bursa and Ligament, Right
	Anterior cruciate ligament (ACL)
	Lateral collateral ligament (LCL)
	Ligament of head of fibula
	Medial collateral ligament (MCL)
	Patellar ligament
	Popliteal ligament
	Posterior cruciate ligament (PCL)
	Prepatellar bursa
	P Knee Bursa and Ligament, Left
	*See N Knee Bursa and Ligament,
	  Right*
	Q Ankle Bursa and Ligament, Right
	Calcaneofibular ligament
	Deltoid ligament
	Ligament of the lateral malleolus
	Talofibular ligament
	R Ankle Bursa and Ligament, Left
	*See Q Ankle Bursa and Ligament,
	  Right*
	S Foot Bursa and Ligament, Right
	Calcaneocuboid ligament
	Cuneonavicular ligament
	Intercuneiform ligament
	Interphalangeal ligament
	Metatarsal ligament
	Metatarsophalangeal ligament
	Subtalar ligament
	Talocalcaneal ligament
	Talocalcaneonavicular ligament
	Tarsometatarsal ligament
	T Foot Bursa and Ligament, Left
	*See S Foot Bursa and Ligament,
	  Right*
	V Lower Extremity Bursa and Ligament, Right
	W Lower Extremity Bursa and Ligament, Left
		Ø Open
		3 Percutaneous
		4 Percutaneous Endoscopic
			Z No Device	**X Diagnostic**
				Z No Qualifier

Non-OR   ØMB[Ø,1,2,3,4,5,6,7,8,B,C,D,F,G,L,M,N,P,Q,R,S,T][Ø,3,4]ZX
Non-OR   ØMB94ZX

Ø   **Medical and Surgical**
M   **Bursae and Ligaments**
C   **Extirpation**   Definition: Taking or cutting out solid matter from a body part

Explanation: The solid matter may be an abnormal byproduct of a biological function or a foreign body; it may be imbedded in a body part or in the lumen of a tubular body part. The solid matter may or may not have been previously broken into pieces.

Body Part Character 4		Approach Character 5	Device Character 6	Qualifier Character 7

Ø   **Head and Neck Bursa and Ligament**
    Alar ligament of axis
    Cervical interspinous ligament
    Cervical intertransverse ligament
    Cervical ligamentum flavum
    Interspinous ligament, cervical
    Intertransverse ligament, cervical
    Lateral temporomandibular
       ligament
    Ligamentum flavum, cervical
    Sphenomandibular ligament
    Stylomandibular ligament
    Transverse ligament of atlas
1   **Shoulder Bursa and Ligament, Right**
    Acromioclavicular ligament
    Coracoacromial ligament
    Coracoclavicular ligament
    Coracohumeral ligament
    Costoclavicular ligament
    Glenohumeral ligament
    Interclavicular ligament
    Sternoclavicular ligament
    Subacromial bursa
    Transverse humeral ligament
    Transverse scapular ligament
2   **Shoulder Bursa and Ligament, Left**
    See 1 Shoulder Bursa and Ligament, Right
3   **Elbow Bursa and Ligament, Right**
    Annular ligament
    Olecranon bursa
    Radial collateral ligament
    Ulnar collateral ligament
4   **Elbow Bursa and Ligament, Left**
    See 3 Elbow Bursa and Ligament, Right
5   **Wrist Bursa and Ligament, Right**
    Palmar ulnocarpal ligament
    Radial collateral carpal ligament
    Radiocarpal ligament
    Radioulnar ligament
    Ulnar collateral carpal ligament
6   **Wrist Bursa and Ligament, Left**
    See 5 Wrist Bursa and Ligament, Right
7   **Hand Bursa and Ligament, Right**
    Carpometacarpal ligament
    Intercarpal ligament
    Interphalangeal ligament
    Lunotriquetral ligament
    Metacarpal ligament
    Metacarpophalangeal ligament
    Pisohamate ligament
    Pisometacarpal ligament
    Scapholunate ligament
    Scaphotrapezium ligament
8   **Hand Bursa and Ligament, Left**
    See 7 Hand Bursa and Ligament, Right
9   **Upper Extremity Bursa and Ligament, Right**
B   **Upper Extremity Bursa and Ligament, Left**
C   **Upper Spine Bursa and Ligament**
    Interspinous ligament, thoracic
    Intertransverse ligament, thoracic
    Ligamentum flavum, thoracic
    Supraspinous ligament
	D **Lower Spine Bursa and Ligament**
	    Iliolumbar ligament
	    Interspinous ligament, lumbar
	    Intertransverse ligament, lumbar
	    Ligamentum flavum, lumbar
	    Sacrococcygeal ligament
	    Sacroiliac ligament
	    Sacrospinous ligament
	    Sacrotuberous ligament
	    Supraspinous ligament
	F **Sternum Bursa and Ligament**
	    Costoxiphoid ligament
	    Sternocostal ligament
	G **Rib(s) Bursa and Ligament**
	    Costotransverse ligament
	H **Abdomen Bursa and Ligament, Right**
	J **Abdomen Bursa and Ligament, Left**
	K **Perineum Bursa and Ligament**
	L **Hip Bursa and Ligament, Right**
	    Iliofemoral ligament
	    Ischiofemoral ligament
	    Pubofemoral ligament
	    Transverse acetabular ligament
	    Trochanteric bursa
	M **Hip Bursa and Ligament, Left**
	    See L Hip Bursa and Ligament, Right
	N **Knee Bursa and Ligament, Right**
	    Anterior cruciate ligament (ACL)
	    Lateral collateral ligament (LCL)
	    Ligament of head of fibula
	    Medial collateral ligament (MCL)
	    Patellar ligament
	    Popliteal ligament
	    Posterior cruciate ligament (PCL)
	    Prepatellar bursa
	P **Knee Bursa and Ligament, Left**
	    See N Knee Bursa and Ligament, Right
	Q **Ankle Bursa and Ligament, Right**
	    Calcaneofibular ligament
	    Deltoid ligament
	    Ligament of the lateral malleolus
	    Talofibular ligament
	R **Ankle Bursa and Ligament, Left**
	    See Q Ankle Bursa and Ligament, Right
	S **Foot Bursa and Ligament, Right**
	    Calcaneocuboid ligament
	    Cuneonavicular ligament
	    Intercuneiform ligament
	    Interphalangeal ligament
	    Metatarsal ligament
	    Metatarsophalangeal ligament
	    Subtalar ligament
	    Talocalcaneal ligament
	    Talocalcaneonavicular ligament
	    Tarsometatarsal ligament
	T **Foot Bursa and Ligament, Left**
	    See S Foot Bursa and Ligament, Right
	V **Lower Extremity Bursa and Ligament, Right**
	W **Lower Extremity Bursa and Ligament, Left**
		Ø Open
		3 Percutaneous
		4 Percutaneous Endoscopic
			Z No Device	**Z** No Qualifier

Ø Medical and Surgical
M Bursae and Ligaments
D Extraction   Definition: Pulling or stripping out or off all or a portion of a body part by the use of force
                Explanation: The qualifier DIAGNOSTIC is used to identify extraction procedures that are biopsies

Body Part Character 4		Approach Character 5	Device Character 6	Qualifier Character 7

Ø Head and Neck Bursa and Ligament
Alar ligament of axis
Cervical interspinous ligament
Cervical intertransverse ligament
Cervical ligamentum flavum
Interspinous ligament, cervical
Intertransverse ligament, cervical
Lateral temporomandibular
   ligament
Ligamentum flavum, cervical
Sphenomandibular ligament
Stylomandibular ligament
Transverse ligament of atlas
	D Lower Spine Bursa and Ligament
	Iliolumbar ligament
	Interspinous ligament, lumbar
	Intertransverse ligament, lumbar
	Ligamentum flavum, lumbar
	Sacrococcygeal ligament
	Sacroiliac ligament
	Sacrospinous ligament
	Sacrotuberous ligament
	Supraspinous ligament
	F Sternum Bursa and Ligament
	Costoxiphoid ligament
	Sternocostal ligament
		Ø Open
		3 Percutaneous
		**4 Percutaneous
		   Endoscopic**
			Z No Device	**Z No Qualifier**

1 Shoulder Bursa and Ligament, Right Acromioclavicular ligament Coracoacromial ligament Coracoclavicular ligament Coracohumeral ligament Costoclavicular ligament Glenohumeral ligament Interclavicular ligament Sternoclavicular ligament Subacromial bursa Transverse humeral ligament Transverse scapular ligament	**G Rib(s) Bursa and Ligament** Costotransverse ligament **H Abdomen Bursa and Ligament, Right** **J Abdomen Bursa and Ligament, Left** **K Perineum Bursa and Ligament** **L Hip Bursa and Ligament, Right** Iliofemoral ligament Ischiofemoral ligament Pubofemoral ligament Transverse acetabular ligament Trochanteric bursa			

2 Shoulder Bursa and Ligament, Left
*See 1 Shoulder Bursa and
   Ligament, Right*
	M Hip Bursa and Ligament, Left
	*See L Hip Bursa and Ligament,
	   Right*			

3 Elbow Bursa and Ligament, Right Annular ligament Olecranon bursa Radial collateral ligament Ulnar collateral ligament	**N Knee Bursa and Ligament, Right** Anterior cruciate ligament (ACL) Lateral collateral ligament (LCL) Ligament of head of fibula Medial collateral ligament (MCL) Patellar ligament Popliteal ligament Posterior cruciate ligament (PCL) Prepatellar bursa			

4 Elbow Bursa and Ligament, Left
*See 3 Elbow Bursa and Ligament,
   Right*
	P Knee Bursa and Ligament, Left
	*See N Knee Bursa and Ligament,
	   Right*			

5 Wrist Bursa and Ligament, Right Palmar ulnocarpal ligament Radial collateral carpal ligament Radiocarpal ligament Radioulnar ligament Ulnar collateral carpal ligament	**Q Ankle Bursa and Ligament, Right** Calcaneofibular ligament Deltoid ligament Ligament of the lateral malleolus Talofibular ligament			

6 Wrist Bursa and Ligament, Left
*See 5 Wrist Bursa and Ligament,
   Right*
	R Ankle Bursa and Ligament, Left
	*See Q Ankle Bursa and Ligament,
	   Right*			

7 Hand Bursa and Ligament, Right Carpometacarpal ligament Intercarpal ligament Interphalangeal ligament Lunotriquetral ligament Metacarpal ligament Metacarpophalangeal ligament Pisohamate ligament Pisometacarpal ligament Scapholunate ligament Scaphotrapezium ligament	**S Foot Bursa and Ligament, Right** Calcaneocuboid ligament Cuneonavicular ligament Intercuneiform ligament Interphalangeal ligament Metatarsal ligament Metatarsophalangeal ligament Subtalar ligament Talocalcaneal ligament Talocalcaneonavicular ligament Tarsometatarsal ligament			

8 Hand Bursa and Ligament, Left
*See 7 Hand Bursa and Ligament,
   Right*
	T Foot Bursa and Ligament, Left
	*See S Foot Bursa and Ligament,
	   Right*			

9 Upper Extremity Bursa and Ligament, Right **B Upper Extremity Bursa and Ligament, Left** **C Upper Spine Bursa and Ligament** Interspinous ligament, thoracic Intertransverse ligament, thoracic Ligamentum flavum, thoracic Supraspinous ligament	**V Lower Extremity Bursa and Ligament, Right** **W Lower Extremity Bursa and Ligament, Left**			

Ø   **Medical and Surgical**
M   **Bursae and Ligaments**
H   **Insertion**   Definition: Putting in a nonbiological appliance that monitors, assists, performs, or prevents a physiological function but does not physically take the place of a body part

         Explanation: None

Body Part Character 4	Approach Character 5	Device Character 6	Qualifier Character 7
X Upper Bursa and Ligament Y Lower Bursa and Ligament	Ø Open 3 Percutaneous 4 Percutaneous Endoscopic	Y Other Device	Z No Qualifier

Non-OR   ØMH[X,Y][3,4]YZ

Ø   **Medical and Surgical**
M   **Bursae and Ligaments**
J   **Inspection**   Definition: Visually and/or manually exploring a body part

         Explanation: Visual exploration may be performed with or without optical instrumentation. Manual exploration may be performed directly or through intervening body layers.

Body Part Character 4	Approach Character 5	Device Character 6	Qualifier Character 7
X Upper Bursa and Ligament Y Lower Bursa and Ligament	Ø Open 3 Percutaneous 4 Percutaneous Endoscopic X External	Z No Device	Z No Qualifier

Non-OR   ØMJ[X,Y][3,X]ZZ

LC Limited Coverage   NC Noncovered   ⊞ Combination Member   HAC associated procedure   Combination Only   DRG Non-OR   Non-OR   New/Revised in GREEN

ICD-10-PCS 2019   **489**

Ø Medical and Surgical
M Bursae and Ligaments
M Reattachment Definition: Putting back in or on all or a portion of a separated body part to its normal location or other suitable location
Explanation: Vascular circulation and nervous pathways may or may not be reestablished

Body Part Character 4		Approach Character 5	Device Character 6	Qualifier Character 7
Ø Head and Neck Bursa and Ligament Alar ligament of axis Cervical interspinous ligament Cervical intertransverse ligament Cervical ligamentum flavum Interspinous ligament, cervical Intertransverse ligament, cervical Lateral temporomandibular ligament Ligamentum flavum, cervical Sphenomandibular ligament Stylomandibular ligament Transverse ligament of atlas	**D Lower Spine Bursa and Ligament** Iliolumbar ligament Interspinous ligament, lumbar Intertransverse ligament, lumbar Ligamentum flavum, lumbar Sacrococcygeal ligament Sacroiliac ligament Sacrospinous ligament Sacrotuberous ligament Supraspinous ligament	**Ø Open** **4 Percutaneous Endoscopic**	**Z No Device**	**Z No Qualifier**
1 Shoulder Bursa and Ligament, Right Acromioclavicular ligament Coracoacromial ligament Coracoclavicular ligament Coracohumeral ligament Costoclavicular ligament Glenohumeral ligament Interclavicular ligament Sternoclavicular ligament Subacromial bursa Transverse humeral ligament Transverse scapular ligament	**F Sternum Bursa and Ligament** Costoxiphoid ligament Sternocostal ligament **G Rib(s) Bursa and Ligament** Costotransverse ligament **H Abdomen Bursa and Ligament, Right** **J Abdomen Bursa and Ligament, Left** **K Perineum Bursa and Ligament**			
2 Shoulder Bursa and Ligament, Left See 1 Shoulder Bursa and Ligament, Right	**L Hip Bursa and Ligament, Right** Iliofemoral ligament Ischiofemoral ligament Pubofemoral ligament Transverse acetabular ligament Trochanteric bursa			
3 Elbow Bursa and Ligament, Right Annular ligament Olecranon bursa Radial collateral ligament Ulnar collateral ligament	**M Hip Bursa and Ligament, Left** See L Hip Bursa and Ligament, Right			
4 Elbow Bursa and Ligament, Left See 3 Elbow Bursa and Ligament, Right	**N Knee Bursa and Ligament, Right** Anterior cruciate ligament (ACL) Lateral collateral ligament (LCL) Ligament of head of fibula Medial collateral ligament (MCL) Patellar ligament Popliteal ligament Posterior cruciate ligament (PCL) Prepatellar bursa			
5 Wrist Bursa and Ligament, Right Palmar ulnocarpal ligament Radial collateral carpal ligament Radiocarpal ligament Radioulnar ligament Ulnar collateral carpal ligament	**P Knee Bursa and Ligament, Left** See N Knee Bursa and Ligament, Right			
6 Wrist Bursa and Ligament, Left See 5 Wrist Bursa and Ligament, Right	**Q Ankle Bursa and Ligament, Right** Calcaneofibular ligament Deltoid ligament Ligament of the lateral malleolus Talofibular ligament			
7 Hand Bursa and Ligament, Right Carpometacarpal ligament Intercarpal ligament Interphalangeal ligament Lunotriquetral ligament Metacarpal ligament Metacarpophalangeal ligament Pisohamate ligament Pisometacarpal ligament Scapholunate ligament Scaphotrapezium ligament	**R Ankle Bursa and Ligament, Left** See Q Ankle Bursa and Ligament, Right **S Foot Bursa and Ligament, Right** Calcaneocuboid ligament Cuneonavicular ligament Intercuneiform ligament Interphalangeal ligament Metatarsal ligament Metatarsophalangeal ligament Subtalar ligament Talocalcaneal ligament Talocalcaneonavicular ligament Tarsometatarsal ligament			
8 Hand Bursa and Ligament, Left See 7 Hand Bursa and Ligament, Right	**T Foot Bursa and Ligament, Left** See S Foot Bursa and Ligament, Right			
9 Upper Extremity Bursa and Ligament, Right **B Upper Extremity Bursa and Ligament, Left**	**V Lower Extremity Bursa and Ligament, Right** **W Lower Extremity Bursa and Ligament, Left**			
C Upper Spine Bursa and Ligament Interspinous ligament, thoracic Intertransverse ligament, thoracic Ligamentum flavum, thoracic Supraspinous ligament				

LC Limited Coverage   NC Noncovered   ⊞ Combination Member   HAC associated procedure   Combination Only   DRG Non-OR   Non-OR   New/Revised in GREEN

Bursae and Ligaments

Ø   **Medical and Surgical**
M   **Bursae and Ligaments**
N   **Release**   Definition: Freeing a body part from an abnormal physical constraint by cutting or by the use of force
                   Explanation: Some of the restraining tissue may be taken out but none of the body part is taken out

Body Part Character 4		Approach Character 5	Device Character 6	Qualifier Character 7
Ø Head and Neck Bursa and Ligament Alar ligament of axis Cervical interspinous ligament Cervical intertransverse ligament Cervical ligamentum flavum Interspinous ligament, cervical Intertransverse ligament, cervical Lateral temporomandibular ligament Ligamentum flavum, cervical Sphenomandibular ligament Stylomandibular ligament Transverse ligament of atlas **1 Shoulder Bursa and Ligament, Right** Acromioclavicular ligament Coracoacromial ligament Coracoclavicular ligament Coracohumeral ligament Costoclavicular ligament Glenohumeral ligament Interclavicular ligament Sternoclavicular ligament Subacromial bursa Transverse humeral ligament Transverse scapular ligament **2 Shoulder Bursa and Ligament, Left** *See 1 Shoulder Bursa and Ligament, Right* **3 Elbow Bursa and Ligament, Right** Annular ligament Olecranon bursa Radial collateral ligament Ulnar collateral ligament **4 Elbow Bursa and Ligament, Left** *See 3 Elbow Bursa and Ligament, Right* **5 Wrist Bursa and Ligament, Right** Palmar ulnocarpal ligament Radial collateral carpal ligament Radiocarpal ligament Radioulnar ligament Ulnar collateral carpal ligament **6 Wrist Bursa and Ligament, Left** *See 5 Wrist Bursa and Ligament, Right* **7 Hand Bursa and Ligament, Right** Carpometacarpal ligament Intercarpal ligament Interphalangeal ligament Lunotriquetral ligament Metacarpal ligament Metacarpophalangeal ligament Pisohamate ligament Pisometacarpal ligament Scapholunate ligament Scaphotrapezium ligament **8 Hand Bursa and Ligament, Left** *See 7 Hand Bursa and Ligament, Right* **9 Upper Extremity Bursa and Ligament, Right** **B Upper Extremity Bursa and Ligament, Left** **C Upper Spine Bursa and Ligament** Interspinous ligament, thoracic Intertransverse ligament, thoracic Ligamentum flavum, thoracic Supraspinous ligament.	**D Lower Spine Bursa and Ligament** Iliolumbar ligament Interspinous ligament, lumbar Intertransverse ligament, lumbar Ligamentum flavum, lumbar Sacrococcygeal ligament Sacroiliac ligament Sacrospinous ligament Sacrotuberous ligament Supraspinous ligament **F Sternum Bursa and Ligament** Costoxiphoid ligament Sternocostal ligament **G Rib(s) Bursa and Ligament** Costotransverse ligament **H Abdomen Bursa and Ligament, Right** **J Abdomen Bursa and Ligament, Left** **K Perineum Bursa and Ligament** **L Hip Bursa and Ligament, Right** Iliofemoral ligament Ischiofemoral ligament Pubofemoral ligament Transverse acetabular ligament Trochanteric bursa **M Hip Bursa and Ligament, Left** *See L Hip Bursa and Ligament, Right* **N Knee Bursa and Ligament, Right** Anterior cruciate ligament (ACL) Lateral collateral ligament (LCL) Ligament of head of fibula Medial collateral ligament (MCL) Patellar ligament Popliteal ligament Posterior cruciate ligament (PCL) Prepatellar bursa **P Knee Bursa and Ligament, Left** *See N Knee Bursa and Ligament, Right* **Q Ankle Bursa and Ligament, Right** Calcaneofibular ligament Deltoid ligament Ligament of the lateral malleolus Talofibular ligament **R Ankle Bursa and Ligament, Left** *See Q Ankle Bursa and Ligament, Right* **S Foot Bursa and Ligament, Right** Calcaneocuboid ligament Cuneonavicular ligament Intercuneiform ligament Interphalangeal ligament Metatarsal ligament Metatarsophalangeal ligament Subtalar ligament Talocalcaneal ligament Talocalcaneonavicular ligament Tarsometatarsal ligament **T Foot Bursa and Ligament, Left** *See S Foot Bursa and Ligament, Right* **V Lower Extremity Bursa and Ligament, Right** **W Lower Extremity Bursa and Ligament, Left**	**Ø Open** **3 Percutaneous** **4 Percutaneous Endoscopic** **X External**	**Z No Device**	**Z No Qualifier**

Non-OR   ØMN[Ø,1,2,3,4,5,6,7,8,9,B,C,D,F,G,H,J,K,L,M,N,P,Q,R,S,T,V,W]XZZ

Ø Medical and Surgical
M Bursae and Ligaments
P Removal   Definition: Taking out or off a device from a body part

Explanation: If a device is taken out and a similar device put in without cutting or puncturing the skin or mucous membrane, the procedure is coded to the root operation CHANGE. Otherwise, the procedure for taking out a device is coded to the root operation REMOVAL.

Body Part Character 4	Approach Character 5	Device Character 6	Qualifier Character 7
X Upper Bursa and Ligament Y Lower Bursa and Ligament	Ø Open 3 Percutaneous 4 Percutaneous Endoscopic	Ø Drainage Device 7 Autologous Tissue Substitute J Synthetic Substitute K Nonautologous Tissue Substitute Y Other Device	Z No Qualifier
X Upper Bursa and Ligament Y Lower Bursa and Ligament	X External	Ø Drainage Device	Z No Qualifier

Non-OR   ØMP[X,Y]3ØZ
Non-OR   ØMP[X,Y][3,4]YZ
Non-OR   ØMP[X,Y]XØZ

Ø   Medical and Surgical
M   Bursae and Ligaments
Q   Repair   Definition: Restoring, to the extent possible, a body part to its normal anatomic structure and function
                 Explanation: Used only when the method to accomplish the repair is not one of the other root operations

Body Part Character 4		Approach Character 5	Device Character 6	Qualifier Character 7
Ø Head and Neck Bursa and Ligament Alar ligament of axis Cervical interspinous ligament Cervical intertransverse ligament Cervical ligamentum flavum Interspinous ligament, cervical Intertransverse ligament, cervical Lateral temporomandibular ligament Ligamentum flavum, cervical Sphenomandibular ligament Stylomandibular ligament Transverse ligament of atlas **1 Shoulder Bursa and Ligament, Right** Acromioclavicular ligament Coracoacromial ligament Coracoclavicular ligament Coracohumeral ligament Costoclavicular ligament Glenohumeral ligament Interclavicular ligament Sternoclavicular ligament Subacromial bursa Transverse humeral ligament Transverse scapular ligament **2 Shoulder Bursa and Ligament, Left** *See 1 Shoulder Bursa and Ligament, Right* **3 Elbow Bursa and Ligament, Right** Annular ligament Olecranon bursa Radial collateral ligament Ulnar collateral ligament **4 Elbow Bursa and Ligament, Left** *See 3 Elbow Bursa and Ligament, Right* **5 Wrist Bursa and Ligament, Right** Palmar ulnocarpal ligament Radial collateral carpal ligament Radiocarpal ligament Radioulnar ligament Ulnar collateral carpal ligament **6 Wrist Bursa and Ligament, Left** *See 5 Wrist Bursa and Ligament, Right* **7 Hand Bursa and Ligament, Right** Carpometacarpal ligament Intercarpal ligament Interphalangeal ligament Lunotriquetral ligament Metacarpal ligament Metacarpophalangeal ligament Pisohamate ligament Pisometacarpal ligament Scapholunate ligament Scaphotrapezium ligament **8 Hand Bursa and Ligament, Left** *See 7 Hand Bursa and Ligament, Right* **9 Upper Extremity Bursa and Ligament, Right** **B Upper Extremity Bursa and Ligament, Left** **C Upper Spine Bursa and Ligament** Interspinous ligament, thoracic Intertransverse ligament, thoracic Ligamentum flavum, thoracic Supraspinous ligament	**D Lower Spine Bursa and Ligament** Iliolumbar ligament Interspinous ligament, lumbar Intertransverse ligament, lumbar Ligamentum flavum, lumbar Sacrococcygeal ligament Sacroiliac ligament Sacrospinous ligament Sacrotuberous ligament Supraspinous ligament **F Sternum Bursa and Ligament** Costoxiphoid ligament Sternocostal ligament **G Rib(s) Bursa and Ligament** Costotransverse ligament **H Abdomen Bursa and Ligament, Right** **J Abdomen Bursa and Ligament, Left** **K Perineum Bursa and Ligament** **L Hip Bursa and Ligament, Right** Iliofemoral ligament Ischiofemoral ligament Pubofemoral ligament Transverse acetabular ligament Trochanteric bursa **M Hip Bursa and Ligament, Left** *See L Hip Bursa and Ligament, Right* **N Knee Bursa and Ligament, Right** Anterior cruciate ligament (ACL) Lateral collateral ligament (LCL) Ligament of head of fibula Medial collateral ligament (MCL) Patellar ligament Popliteal ligament Posterior cruciate ligament (PCL) Prepatellar bursa **P Knee Bursa and Ligament, Left** *See N Knee Bursa and Ligament, Right* **Q Ankle Bursa and Ligament, Right** Calcaneofibular ligament Deltoid ligament Ligament of the lateral malleolus Talofibular ligament **R Ankle Bursa and Ligament, Left** *See Q Ankle Bursa and Ligament, Right* **S Foot Bursa and Ligament, Right** Calcaneocuboid ligament Cuneonavicular ligament Intercuneiform ligament Interphalangeal ligament Metatarsal ligament Metatarsophalangeal ligament Subtalar ligament Talocalcaneal ligament Talocalcaneonavicular ligament Tarsometatarsal ligament **T Foot Bursa and Ligament, Left** *See S Foot Bursa and Ligament, Right* **V Lower Extremity Bursa and Ligament, Right** **W Lower Extremity Bursa and Ligament, Left**	**Ø Open** **3 Percutaneous** **4 Percutaneous Endoscopic**	**Z No Device**	**Z No Qualifier**

Ⓛ Limited Coverage   Ⓝ Noncovered   ⊞ Combination Member   HAC associated procedure   Combination Only   DRG Non-OR   Non-OR   New/Revised in GREEN

ICD-10-PCS 2019   493

Bursae and Ligaments

Ø Medical and Surgical
M Bursae and Ligaments
R Replacement   Definition: Putting in or on biological or synthetic material that physically takes the place and/or function of all or a portion of a body part

Explanation: The body part may have been taken out or replaced, or may be taken out, physically eradicated, or rendered nonfunctional during the REPLACEMENT procedure. A REMOVAL procedure is coded for taking out the device used in a previous replacement procedure.

Body Part Character 4		Approach Character 5	Device Character 6	Qualifier Character 7
Ø Head and Neck Bursa and Ligament Alar ligament of axis Cervical interspinous ligament Cervical intertransverse ligament Cervical ligamentum flavum Interspinous ligament, cervical Intertransverse ligament, cervical Lateral temporomandibular ligament Ligamentum flavum, cervical Sphenomandibular ligament Stylomandibular ligament Transverse ligament of atlas **1 Shoulder Bursa and Ligament, Right** Acromioclavicular ligament Coracoacromial ligament Coracoclavicular ligament Coracohumeral ligament Costoclavicular ligament Glenohumeral ligament Interclavicular ligament Sternoclavicular ligament Subacromial bursa Transverse humeral ligament Transverse scapular ligament **2 Shoulder Bursa and Ligament, Left** *See 1 Shoulder Bursa and Ligament, Right* **3 Elbow Bursa and Ligament, Right** Annular ligament Olecranon bursa Radial collateral ligament Ulnar collateral ligament **4 Elbow Bursa and Ligament, Left** *See 3 Elbow Bursa and Ligament, Right* **5 Wrist Bursa and Ligament, Right** Palmar ulnocarpal ligament Radial collateral carpal ligament Radiocarpal ligament Radioulnar ligament Ulnar collateral carpal ligament **6 Wrist Bursa and Ligament, Left** *See 5 Wrist Bursa and Ligament, Right* **7 Hand Bursa and Ligament, Right** Carpometacarpal ligament Intercarpal ligament Interphalangeal ligament Lunotriquetral ligament Metacarpal ligament Metacarpophalangeal ligament Pisohamate ligament Pisometacarpal ligament Scapholunate ligament Scaphotrapezium ligament **8 Hand Bursa and Ligament, Left** *See 7 Hand Bursa and Ligament, Right* **9 Upper Extremity Bursa and Ligament, Right** **B Upper Extremity Bursa and Ligament, Left** **C Upper Spine Bursa and Ligament** Interspinous ligament, thoracic Intertransverse ligament, thoracic Ligamentum flavum, thoracic Supraspinous ligament	**D Lower Spine Bursa and Ligament** Iliolumbar ligament Interspinous ligament, lumbar Intertransverse ligament, lumbar Ligamentum flavum, lumbar Sacrococcygeal ligament Sacroiliac ligament Sacrospinous ligament Sacrotuberous ligament Supraspinous ligament **F Sternum Bursa and Ligament** Costoxiphoid ligament Sternocostal ligament **G Rib(s) Bursa and Ligament** Costotransverse ligament **H Abdomen Bursa and Ligament, Right** **J Abdomen Bursa and Ligament, Left** **K Perineum Bursa and Ligament** **L Hip Bursa and Ligament, Right** Iliofemoral ligament Ischiofemoral ligament Pubofemoral ligament Transverse acetabular ligament Trochanteric bursa **M Hip Bursa and Ligament, Left** *See L Hip Bursa and Ligament, Right* **N Knee Bursa and Ligament, Right** Anterior cruciate ligament (ACL) Lateral collateral ligament (LCL) Ligament of head of fibula Medial collateral ligament (MCL) Patellar ligament Popliteal ligament Posterior cruciate ligament (PCL) Prepatellar bursa **P Knee Bursa and Ligament, Left** *See N Knee Bursa and Ligament, Right* **Q Ankle Bursa and Ligament, Right** Calcaneofibular ligament Deltoid ligament Ligament of the lateral malleolus Talofibular ligament **R Ankle Bursa and Ligament, Left** *See Q Ankle Bursa and Ligament, Right* **S Foot Bursa and Ligament, Right** Calcaneocuboid ligament Cuneonavicular ligament Intercuneiform ligament Interphalangeal ligament Metatarsal ligament Metatarsophalangeal ligament Subtalar ligament Talocalcaneal ligament Talocalcaneonavicular ligament Tarsometatarsal ligament **T Foot Bursa and Ligament, Left** *See S Foot Bursa and Ligament, Right* **V Lower Extremity Bursa and Ligament, Right** **W Lower Extremity Bursa and Ligament, Left**	**Ø Open** **4 Percutaneous Endoscopic**	**7 Autologous Tissue Substitute** **J Synthetic Substitute** **K Nonautologous Tissue Substitute**	**Z No Qualifier**

LC Limited Coverage   NC Noncovered   ⊞ Combination Member   HAC associated procedure   Combination Only   DRG Non-OR   Non-OR   New/Revised in GREEN

494   ICD-10-PCS 2019

Ø   Medical and Surgical
M   Bursae and Ligaments
S   Reposition   Definition: Moving to its normal location, or other suitable location, all or a portion of a body part

Explanation: The body part is moved to a new location from an abnormal location, or from a normal location where it is not functioning correctly. The body part may or may not be cut out or off to be moved to the new location.

Body Part Character 4		Approach Character 5	Device Character 6	Qualifier Character 7
Ø Head and Neck Bursa and Ligament Alar ligament of axis Cervical interspinous ligament Cervical intertransverse ligament Cervical ligamentum flavum Interspinous ligament, cervical Intertransverse ligament, cervical Lateral temporomandibular ligament Ligamentum flavum, cervical Sphenomandibular ligament Stylomandibular ligament Transverse ligament of atlas **1 Shoulder Bursa and Ligament, Right** Acromioclavicular ligament Coracoacromial ligament Coracoclavicular ligament Coracohumeral ligament Costoclavicular ligament Glenohumeral ligament Interclavicular ligament Sternoclavicular ligament Subacromial bursa Transverse humeral ligament Transverse scapular ligament **2 Shoulder Bursa and Ligament, Left** *See 1 Shoulder Bursa and Ligament, Right* **3 Elbow Bursa and Ligament, Right** Annular ligament Olecranon bursa Radial collateral ligament Ulnar collateral ligament **4 Elbow Bursa and Ligament, Left** *See 3 Elbow Bursa and Ligament, Right* **5 Wrist Bursa and Ligament, Right** Palmar ulnocarpal ligament Radial collateral carpal ligament Radiocarpal ligament Radioulnar ligament Ulnar collateral carpal ligament **6 Wrist Bursa and Ligament, Left** *See 5 Wrist Bursa and Ligament, Right* **7 Hand Bursa and Ligament, Right** Carpometacarpal ligament Intercarpal ligament Interphalangeal ligament Lunotriquetral ligament Metacarpal ligament Metacarpophalangeal ligament Pisohamate ligament Pisometacarpal ligament Scapholunate ligament Scaphotrapezium ligament **8 Hand Bursa and Ligament, Left** *See 7 Hand Bursa and Ligament, Right* **9 Upper Extremity Bursa and Ligament, Right** **B Upper Extremity Bursa and Ligament, Left** **C Upper Spine Bursa and Ligament** Interspinous ligament, thoracic Intertransverse ligament, thoracic Ligamentum flavum, thoracic Supraspinous ligament	**D Lower Spine Bursa and Ligament** Iliolumbar ligament Interspinous ligament, lumbar Intertransverse ligament, lumbar Ligamentum flavum, lumbar Sacrococcygeal ligament Sacroiliac ligament Sacrospinous ligament Sacrotuberous ligament Supraspinous ligament **F Sternum Bursa and Ligament** Costoxiphoid ligament Sternocostal ligament **G Rib(s) Bursa and Ligament** Costotransverse ligament **H Abdomen Bursa and Ligament, Right** **J Abdomen Bursa and Ligament, Left** **K Perineum Bursa and Ligament** **L Hip Bursa and Ligament, Right** Iliofemoral ligament Ischiofemoral ligament Pubofemoral ligament Transverse acetabular ligament Trochanteric bursa **M Hip Bursa and Ligament, Left** *See L Hip Bursa and Ligament, Right* **N Knee Bursa and Ligament, Right** Anterior cruciate ligament (ACL) Lateral collateral ligament (LCL) Ligament of head of fibula Medial collateral ligament (MCL) Patellar ligament Popliteal ligament Posterior cruciate ligament (PCL) Prepatellar bursa **P Knee Bursa and Ligament, Left** *See N Knee Bursa and Ligament, Right* **Q Ankle Bursa and Ligament, Right** Calcaneofibular ligament Deltoid ligament Ligament of the lateral malleolus Talofibular ligament **R Ankle Bursa and Ligament, Left** *See Q Ankle Bursa and Ligament, Right* **S Foot Bursa and Ligament, Right** Calcaneocuboid ligament Cuneonavicular ligament Intercuneiform ligament Interphalangeal ligament Metatarsal ligament Metatarsophalangeal ligament Subtalar ligament Talocalcaneal ligament Talocalcaneonavicular ligament Tarsometatarsal ligament **T Foot Bursa and Ligament, Left** *See S Foot Bursa and Ligament, Right* **V Lower Extremity Bursa and Ligament, Right** **W Lower Extremity Bursa and Ligament, Left**	**Ø Open** **4 Percutaneous Endoscopic**	**Z No Device**	**Z No Qualifier**

LC Limited Coverage   **NC** Noncovered   ⊞ Combination Member   HAC associated procedure   Combination Only   DRG Non-OR   Non-OR   New/Revised in GREEN

ICD-10-PCS 2019   495

Ø Medical and Surgical
M Bursae and Ligaments
T Resection Definition: Cutting out or off, without replacement, all of a body part
Explanation: None

Body Part Character 4		Approach Character 5	Device Character 6	Qualifier Character 7
Ø Head and Neck Bursa and Ligament Alar ligament of axis Cervical interspinous ligament Cervical intertransverse ligament Cervical ligamentum flavum Interspinous ligament, cervical Intertransverse ligament, cervical Lateral temporomandibular ligament Ligamentum flavum, cervical Sphenomandibular ligament Stylomandibular ligament Transverse ligament of atlas	**D** Lower Spine Bursa and Ligament Iliolumbar ligament Interspinous ligament, lumbar Intertransverse ligament, lumbar Ligamentum flavum, lumbar Sacrococcygeal ligament Sacroiliac ligament Sacrospinous ligament Sacrotuberous ligament Supraspinous ligament	**Ø** Open **4** Percutaneous Endoscopic	**Z** No Device	**Z** No Qualifier
1 Shoulder Bursa and Ligament, Right Acromioclavicular ligament Coracoacromial ligament Coracoclavicular ligament Coracohumeral ligament Costoclavicular ligament Glenohumeral ligament Interclavicular ligament Sternoclavicular ligament Subacromial bursa Transverse humeral ligament Transverse scapular ligament	**F** Sternum Bursa and Ligament Costoxiphoid ligament Sternocostal ligament **G** Rib(s) Bursa and Ligament Costotransverse ligament **H** Abdomen Bursa and Ligament, Right **J** Abdomen Bursa and Ligament, Left **K** Perineum Bursa and Ligament			
2 Shoulder Bursa and Ligament, Left *See 1 Shoulder Bursa and Ligament, Right*	**L** Hip Bursa and Ligament, Right Iliofemoral ligament Ischiofemoral ligament Pubofemoral ligament Transverse acetabular ligament Trochanteric bursa			
3 Elbow Bursa and Ligament, Right Annular ligament Olecranon bursa Radial collateral ligament Ulnar collateral ligament	**M** Hip Bursa and Ligament, Left *See L Hip Bursa and Ligament, Right*			
4 Elbow Bursa and Ligament, Left *See 3 Elbow Bursa and Ligament, Right*	**N** Knee Bursa and Ligament, Right Anterior cruciate ligament (ACL) Lateral collateral ligament (LCL) Ligament of head of fibula Medial collateral ligament (MCL) Patellar ligament Popliteal ligament Posterior cruciate ligament (PCL) Prepatellar bursa			
5 Wrist Bursa and Ligament, Right Palmar ulnocarpal ligament Radial collateral carpal ligament Radiocarpal ligament Radioulnar ligament Ulnar collateral carpal ligament	**P** Knee Bursa and Ligament, Left *See N Knee Bursa and Ligament, Right*			
6 Wrist Bursa and Ligament, Left *See 5 Wrist Bursa and Ligament, Right*	**Q** Ankle Bursa and Ligament, Right Calcaneofibular ligament Deltoid ligament Ligament of the lateral malleolus Talofibular ligament			
7 Hand Bursa and Ligament, Right Carpometacarpal ligament Intercarpal ligament Interphalangeal ligament Lunotriquetral ligament Metacarpal ligament Metacarpophalangeal ligament Pisohamate ligament Pisometacarpal ligament Scapholunate ligament Scaphotrapezium ligament	**R** Ankle Bursa and Ligament, Left *See Q Ankle Bursa and Ligament, Right*			
8 Hand Bursa and Ligament, Left *See 7 Hand Bursa and Ligament, Right*	**S** Foot Bursa and Ligament, Right Calcaneocuboid ligament Cuneonavicular ligament Intercuneiform ligament Interphalangeal ligament Metatarsal ligament Metatarsophalangeal ligament Subtalar ligament Talocalcaneal ligament Talocalcaneonavicular ligament Tarsometatarsal ligament			
9 Upper Extremity Bursa and Ligament, Right	**T** Foot Bursa and Ligament, Left *See S Foot Bursa and Ligament, Right*			
B Upper Extremity Bursa and Ligament, Left	**V** Lower Extremity Bursa and Ligament, Right			
C Upper Spine Bursa and Ligament Interspinous ligament, thoracic Intertransverse ligament, thoracic Ligamentum flavum, thoracic Supraspinous ligament	**W** Lower Extremity Bursa and Ligament, Left			

Ø   Medical and Surgical
M   Bursae and Ligaments
U   Supplement   Definition: Putting in or on biological or synthetic material that physically reinforces and/or augments the function of a portion of a body part
                     Explanation: The biological material is non-living, or is living and from the same individual. The body part may have been previously replaced, and the SUPPLEMENT procedure is performed to physically reinforce and/or augment the function of the replaced body part.

Body Part Character 4		Approach Character 5	Device Character 6	Qualifier Character 7
Ø Head and Neck Bursa and Ligament Alar ligament of axis Cervical interspinous ligament Cervical intertransverse ligament Cervical ligamentum flavum Interspinous ligament, cervical Intertransverse ligament, cervical Lateral temporomandibular ligament Ligamentum flavum, cervical Sphenomandibular ligament Stylomandibular ligament Transverse ligament of atlas **1 Shoulder Bursa and Ligament, Right** Acromioclavicular ligament Coracoacromial ligament Coracoclavicular ligament Coracohumeral ligament Costoclavicular ligament Glenohumeral ligament Interclavicular ligament Sternoclavicular ligament Subacromial bursa Transverse humeral ligament Transverse scapular ligament **2 Shoulder Bursa and Ligament, Left** *See 1 Shoulder Bursa and Ligament, Right* **3 Elbow Bursa and Ligament, Right** Annular ligament Olecranon bursa Radial collateral ligament Ulnar collateral ligament **4 Elbow Bursa and Ligament, Left** *See 3 Elbow Bursa and Ligament, Right* **5 Wrist Bursa and Ligament, Right** Palmar ulnocarpal ligament Radial collateral carpal ligament Radiocarpal ligament Radioulnar ligament Ulnar collateral carpal ligament **6 Wrist Bursa and Ligament, Left** *See 5 Wrist Bursa and Ligament, Right* **7 Hand Bursa and Ligament, Right** Carpometacarpal ligament Intercarpal ligament Interphalangeal ligament Lunotriquetral ligament Metacarpal ligament Metacarpophalangeal ligament Pisohamate ligament Pisometacarpal ligament Scapholunate ligament Scaphotrapezium ligament **8 Hand Bursa and Ligament, Left** *See 7 Hand Bursa and Ligament, Right* **9 Upper Extremity Bursa and Ligament, Right** **B Upper Extremity Bursa and Ligament, Left** **C Upper Spine Bursa and Ligament** Interspinous ligament, thoracic Intertransverse ligament, thoracic Ligamentum flavum, thoracic Supraspinous ligament	**D Lower Spine Bursa and Ligament** Iliolumbar ligament Interspinous ligament, lumbar Intertransverse ligament, lumbar Ligamentum flavum, lumbar Sacrococcygeal ligament Sacroiliac ligament Sacrospinous ligament Sacrotuberous ligament Supraspinous ligament **F Sternum Bursa and Ligament** Costoxiphoid ligament Sternocostal ligament **G Rib(s) Bursa and Ligament** Costotransverse ligament **H Abdomen Bursa and Ligament, Right** **J Abdomen Bursa and Ligament, Left** **K Perineum Bursa and Ligament** **L Hip Bursa and Ligament, Right** Iliofemoral ligament Ischiofemoral ligament Pubofemoral ligament Transverse acetabular ligament Trochanteric bursa **M Hip Bursa and Ligament, Left** *See L Hip Bursa and Ligament, Right* **N Knee Bursa and Ligament, Right** Anterior cruciate ligament (ACL) Lateral collateral ligament (LCL) Ligament of head of fibula Medial collateral ligament (MCL) Patellar ligament Popliteal ligament Posterior cruciate ligament (PCL) Prepatellar bursa **P Knee Bursa and Ligament, Left** *See N Knee Bursa and Ligament, Right* **Q Ankle Bursa and Ligament, Right** Calcaneofibular ligament Deltoid ligament Ligament of the lateral malleolus Talofibular ligament **R Ankle Bursa and Ligament, Left** *See Q Ankle Bursa and Ligament, Right* **S Foot Bursa and Ligament, Right** Calcaneocuboid ligament Cuneonavicular ligament Intercuneiform ligament Interphalangeal ligament Metatarsal ligament Metatarsophalangeal ligament Subtalar ligament Talocalcaneal ligament Talocalcaneonavicular ligament Tarsometatarsal ligament **T Foot Bursa and Ligament, Left** *See S Foot Bursa and Ligament, Right* **V Lower Extremity Bursa and Ligament, Right** **W Lower Extremity Bursa and Ligament, Left**	**Ø Open** **4 Percutaneous Endoscopic**	**7 Autologous Tissue Substitute** **J Synthetic Substitute** **K Nonautologous Tissue Substitute**	**Z No Qualifier**

Ø   Medical and Surgical
M   Bursae and Ligaments
W   Revision   Definition: Correcting, to the extent possible, a portion of a malfunctioning device or the position of a displaced device

                       Explanation: Revision can include correcting a malfunctioning or displaced device by taking out or putting in components of the device such as a screw or pin

Body Part Character 4	Approach Character 5	Device Character 6	Qualifier Character 7
X Upper Bursa and Ligament Y Lower Bursa and Ligament	Ø Open 3 Percutaneous 4 Percutaneous Endoscopic	Ø Drainage Device 7 Autologous Tissue Substitute J Synthetic Substitute K Nonautologous Tissue Substitute Y Other Device	Z No Qualifier
X Upper Bursa and Ligament Y Lower Bursa and Ligament	X External	Ø Drainage Device 7 Autologous Tissue Substitute J Synthetic Substitute K Nonautologous Tissue Substitute	Z No Qualifier

Non-OR   ØMW[X,Y][3,4]YZ
Non-OR   ØMW[X,Y]X[Ø,7,J,K]Z

Ø   Medical and Surgical
M   Bursae and Ligaments
X   Transfer   Definition: Moving, without taking out, all or a portion of a body part to another location to take over the function of all or a portion of a body part
            Explanation: The body part transferred remains connected to its vascular and nervous supply

Body Part Character 4		Approach Character 5	Device Character 6	Qualifier Character 7
Ø Head and Neck Bursa and Ligament Alar ligament of axis Cervical interspinous ligament Cervical intertransverse ligament Cervical ligamentum flavum Interspinous ligament, cervical Intertransverse ligament, cervical Lateral temporomandibular ligament Ligamentum flavum, cervical Sphenomandibular ligament Stylomandibular ligament Transverse ligament of atlas **1 Shoulder Bursa and Ligament, Right** Acromioclavicular ligament Coracoacromial ligament Coracoclavicular ligament Coracohumeral ligament Costoclavicular ligament Glenohumeral ligament Interclavicular ligament Sternoclavicular ligament Subacromial bursa Transverse humeral ligament Transverse scapular ligament **2 Shoulder Bursa and Ligament, Left** *See 1 Shoulder Bursa and Ligament, Right* **3 Elbow Bursa and Ligament, Right** Annular ligament Olecranon bursa Radial collateral ligament Ulnar collateral ligament **4 Elbow Bursa and Ligament, Left** *See 3 Elbow Bursa and Ligament, Right* **5 Wrist Bursa and Ligament, Right** Palmar ulnocarpal ligament Radial collateral carpal ligament Radiocarpal ligament Radioulnar ligament Ulnar collateral carpal ligament **6 Wrist Bursa and Ligament, Left** *See 5 Wrist Bursa and Ligament, Right* **7 Hand Bursa and Ligament, Right** Carpometacarpal ligament Intercarpal ligament Interphalangeal ligament Lunotriquetral ligament Metacarpal ligament Metacarpophalangeal ligament Pisohamate ligament Pisometacarpal ligament Scapholunate ligament Scaphotrapezium ligament **8 Hand Bursa and Ligament, Left** *See 7 Hand Bursa and Ligament, Right* **9 Upper Extremity Bursa and Ligament, Right** **B Upper Extremity Bursa and Ligament, Left** **C Upper Spine Bursa and Ligament** Interspinous ligament, thoracic Intertransverse ligament, thoracic Ligamentum flavum, thoracic Supraspinous ligament	**D Lower Spine Bursa and Ligament** Iliolumbar ligament Interspinous ligament, lumbar Intertransverse ligament, lumbar Ligamentum flavum, lumbar Sacrococcygeal ligament Sacroiliac ligament Sacrospinous ligament Sacrotuberous ligament Supraspinous ligament **F Sternum Bursa and Ligament** Costoxiphoid ligament Sternocostal ligament **G Rib(s) Bursa and Ligament** Costotransverse ligament **H Abdomen Bursa and Ligament, Right** **J Abdomen Bursa and Ligament, Left** **K Perineum Bursa and Ligament** **L Hip Bursa and Ligament, Right** Iliofemoral ligament Ischiofemoral ligament Pubofemoral ligament Transverse acetabular ligament Trochanteric bursa **M Hip Bursa and Ligament, Left** *See L Hip Bursa and Ligament, Right* **N Knee Bursa and Ligament, Right** Anterior cruciate ligament (ACL) Lateral collateral ligament (LCL) Ligament of head of fibula Medial collateral ligament (MCL) Patellar ligament Popliteal ligament Posterior cruciate ligament (PCL) Prepatellar bursa **P Knee Bursa and Ligament, Left** *See N Knee Bursa and Ligament, Right* **Q Ankle Bursa and Ligament, Right** Calcaneofibular ligament Deltoid ligament Ligament of the lateral malleolus Talofibular ligament **R Ankle Bursa and Ligament, Left** *See Q Ankle Bursa and Ligament, Right* **S Foot Bursa and Ligament, Right** Calcaneocuboid ligament Cuneonavicular ligament Intercuneiform ligament Interphalangeal ligament Metatarsal ligament Metatarsophalangeal ligament Subtalar ligament Talocalcaneal ligament Talocalcaneonavicular ligament Tarsometatarsal ligament **T Foot Bursa and Ligament, Left** *See S Foot Bursa and Ligament, Right* **V Lower Extremity Bursa and Ligament, Right** **W Lower Extremity Bursa and Ligament, Left**	**Ø Open** **4 Percutaneous Endoscopic**	**Z No Device**	**Z No Qualifier**

LC Limited Coverage   NC Noncovered   ⊞ Combination Member   HAC associated procedure   Combination Only   DRG Non-OR   Non-OR   New/Revised in GREEN

Head and Facial Bones ØN2–ØNW

Character Meanings

This Character Meaning table is provided as a guide to assist the user in the identification of character members that may be found in this section of code tables. It **SHOULD NOT** be used to build a PCS code.

Operation–Character 3	Body Part–Character 4	Approach–Character 5	Device–Character 6	Qualifier–Character 7
2 Change	Ø Skull	Ø Open	Ø Drainage Device	X Diagnostic
5 Destruction	1 Frontal Bone	3 Percutaneous	4 Internal Fixation Device	Z No Qualifier
8 Division	3 Parietal Bone, Right	4 Percutaneous Endoscopic	5 External Fixation Device	
9 Drainage	4 Parietal Bone, Left	X External	7 Autologous Tissue Substitute	
B Excision	5 Temporal Bone, Right		J Synthetic Substitute	
C Extirpation	6 Temporal Bone, Left		K Nonautologous Tissue Substitute	
D Extraction	7 Occipital Bone		M Bone Growth Stimulator	
H Insertion	B Nasal Bone		N Neurostimulator Generator	
J Inspection	C Sphenoid Bone		S Hearing Device	
N Release	F Ethmoid Bone, Right		Y Other Device	
P Removal	G Ethmoid Bone, Left		Z No Device	
Q Repair	H Lacrimal Bone, Right			
R Replacement	J Lacrimal Bone, Left			
S Reposition	K Palatine Bone, Right			
T Resection	L Palatine Bone, Left			
U Supplement	M Zygomatic Bone, Right			
W Revision	N Zygomatic Bone, Left			
	P Orbit, Right			
	Q Orbit, Left			
	R Maxilla			
	T Mandible, Right			
	V Mandible, Left			
	W Facial Bone			
	X Hyoid Bone			

AHA Coding Clinic for table ØNB
2017, 1Q, 20   Preparatory nasal adhesion repair before definitive cleft palate repair
2015, 3Q, 3-8   Excisional and nonexcisional debridement
2015, 2Q, 12   Orbital exenteration

AHA Coding Clinic for table ØND
2017, 4Q, 41   Extraction procedures

AHA Coding Clinic for table ØNH
2015, 3Q, 13   Nonexcisional debridement of cranial wound with removal and replacement of hardware

AHA Coding Clinic for table ØNP
2015, 3Q, 13   Nonexcisional debridement of cranial wound with removal and replacement of hardware

AHA Coding Clinic for table ØNQ
2016, 3Q, 29   Closure of bilateral alveolar clefts

AHA Coding Clinic for table ØNR
2017, 3Q, 17   Resection of schwannoma and placement of DuraGen and Lorenz cranial plating system
2017, 3Q, 22   Replacement of native skull bone flap
2017, 1Q, 23   Reconstruction of mandible using titanium and bone
2014, 3Q, 7   Hemi-cranioplasty for repair of cranial defect

AHA Coding Clinic for table ØNS
2017, 3Q, 22   Replacement of native skull bone flap
2017, 1Q, 20   Preparatory nasal adhesion repair before definitive cleft palate repair
2016, 2Q, 30   Clipping (occlusion) of cerebral artery, decompressive craniectomy and storage of bone flap in abdominal wall
2015, 3Q, 17   Craniosynostosis with cranial vault reconstruction
2015, 3Q, 27   Moyamoya disease and hemispheric pial synagiosis with craniotomy
2014, 3Q, 23   Le Fort I osteotomy
2013, 3Q, 24   Distraction osteogenesis
2013, 3Q, 25   Fracture of frontal bone with repair and coagulation for hemostasis

AHA Coding Clinic for table ØNU
2016, 3Q, 29   Closure of bilateral alveolar clefts
2013, 3Q, 24   Distraction osteogenesis

Head and Facial Bones

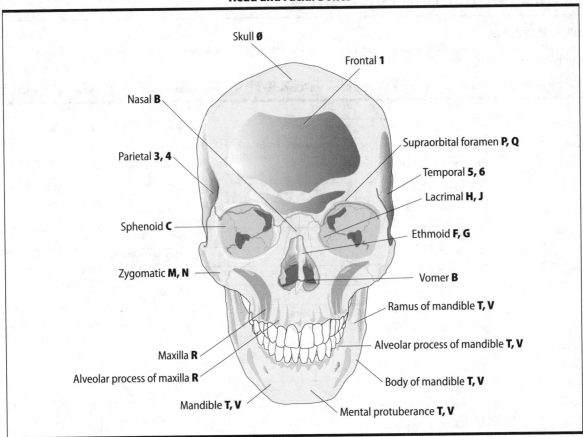

Skull **Ø**

Frontal **1**

Nasal **B**

Supraorbital foramen **P, Q**

Parietal **3, 4**

Temporal **5, 6**

Lacrimal **H, J**

Sphenoid **C**

Ethmoid **F, G**

Zygomatic **M, N**

Vomer **B**

Ramus of mandible **T, V**

Alveolar process of mandible **T, V**

Maxilla **R**

Alveolar process of maxilla **R**

Body of mandible **T, V**

Mandible **T, V**

Mental protuberance **T, V**

Skull Bones

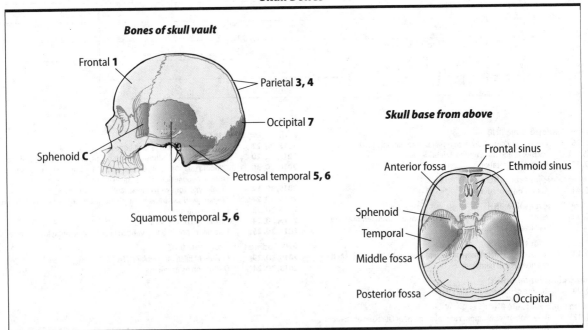

Bones of skull vault

Frontal **1**

Parietal **3, 4**

Occipital **7**

Sphenoid **C**

Petrosal temporal **5, 6**

Squamous temporal **5, 6**

Skull base from above

Frontal sinus

Anterior fossa

Ethmoid sinus

Sphenoid

Temporal

Middle fossa

Posterior fossa

Occipital

Head and Facial Bones

0   **Medical and Surgical**
N   **Head and Facial Bones**
2   **Change**   Definition: Taking out or off a device from a body part and putting back an identical or similar device in or on the same body part without cutting or puncturing the skin or a mucous membrane
                   Explanation: All CHANGE procedures are coded using the approach EXTERNAL

Body Part Character 4	Approach Character 5	Device Character 6	Qualifier Character 7
0 Skull **B** Nasal Bone Vomer of nasal septum **W** Facial Bone	**X** External	**0** Drainage Device **Y** Other Device	**Z** No Qualifier

     Non-OR   All body part, approach, device, and qualifier values

0   **Medical and Surgical**
N   **Head and Facial Bones**
5   **Destruction**   Definition: Physical eradication of all or a portion of a body part by the direct use of energy, force, or a destructive agent
                         Explanation: None of the body part is physically taken out

Body Part Character 4	Approach Character 5	Device Character 6	Qualifier Character 7

0   Skull
1   Frontal Bone
      Zygomatic process of frontal bone
3   Parietal Bone, Right
4   Parietal Bone, Left
5   Temporal Bone, Right
      Mastoid process
      Petrous part of temporal bone
      Tympanic part of temporal bone
      Zygomatic process of temporal bone
6   Temporal Bone, Left
      See 5 Temporal Bone, Right
7   Occipital Bone
      Foramen magnum
B   Nasal Bone
      Vomer of nasal septum
C   Sphenoid Bone
      Greater wing
      Lesser wing
      Optic foramen
      Pterygoid process
      Sella turcica
F   Ethmoid Bone, Right
      Cribriform plate
G   Ethmoid Bone, Left
      See F Ethmoid Bone, Right
H   Lacrimal Bone, Right
J   Lacrimal Bone, Left
K   Palatine Bone, Right
L   Palatine Bone, Left
M   Zygomatic Bone, Right
N   Zygomatic Bone, Left
P   Orbit, Right
      Bony orbit
      Orbital portion of ethmoid bone
      Orbital portion of frontal bone
      Orbital portion of lacrimal bone
      Orbital portion of maxilla
      Orbital portion of palatine bone
      Orbital portion of sphenoid bone
      Orbital portion of zygomatic bone
Q   Orbit, Left
      See P Orbit, Right
R   Maxilla
      Alveolar process of maxilla
T   Mandible, Right
      Alveolar process of mandible
      Condyloid process
      Mandibular notch
      Mental foramen
V   Mandible, Left
      See T Mandible, Right
X   Hyoid Bone
	0 Open
	3 Percutaneous
	4 Percutaneous Endoscopic
		Z No Device	**Z** No Qualifier

Head and Facial Bones

Ø   **Medical and Surgical**
N   **Head and Facial Bones**
8   **Division**   Definition: Cutting into a body part, without draining fluids and/or gases from the body part, in order to separate or transect a body part
                             Explanation: All or a portion of the body part is separated into two or more portions

Body Part Character 4	Approach Character 5	Device Character 6	Qualifier Character 7
Ø Skull	Ø Open	Z No Device	Z No Qualifier
1 Frontal Bone Zygomatic process of frontal bone	3 Percutaneous 4 Percutaneous Endoscopic		
3 Parietal Bone, Right			
4 Parietal Bone, Left			

5   Temporal Bone, Right
     Mastoid process
     Petrous part of temporal bone
     Tympanic part of temporal bone
     Zygomatic process of temporal bone			

6 Temporal Bone, Left *See 5 Temporal Bone, Right*			
7 Occipital Bone Foramen magnum			
B Nasal Bone Vomer of nasal septum			

C   Sphenoid Bone
     Greater wing
     Lesser wing
     Optic foramen
     Pterygoid process
     Sella turcica			

F Ethmoid Bone, Right Cribriform plate			
G Ethmoid Bone, Left *See F Ethmoid Bone, Right*			
H Lacrimal Bone, Right			
J Lacrimal Bone, Left			
K Palatine Bone, Right			
L Palatine Bone, Left			
M Zygomatic Bone, Right			
N Zygomatic Bone, Left			

P   Orbit, Right
     Bony orbit
     Orbital portion of ethmoid bone
     Orbital portion of frontal bone
     Orbital portion of lacrimal bone
     Orbital portion of maxilla
     Orbital portion of palatine bone
     Orbital portion of sphenoid bone
     Orbital portion of zygomatic bone			

Q Orbit, Left *See P Orbit, Right*			
R Maxilla Alveolar process of maxilla			

T   Mandible, Right
     Alveolar process of mandible
     Condyloid process
     Mandibular notch
     Mental foramen			

V Mandible, Left *See T Mandible, Right*			
X Hyoid Bone			

Non-OR   ØN8B[Ø,3,4]ZZ

LC Limited Coverage   NC Noncovered   ⊞ Combination Member   HAC associated procedure   Combination Only   DRG Non-OR   Non-OR   New/Revised in GREEN

504   ICD-10-PCS 2019

0	**Medical and Surgical**
N	**Head and Facial Bones**
9	**Drainage**	Definition: Taking or letting out fluids and/or gases from a body part
	Explanation: The qualifier DIAGNOSTIC is used to identify drainage procedures that are biopsies

Body Part Character 4	Approach Character 5	Device Character 6	Qualifier Character 7
0 Skull	0 Open	0 Drainage Device	Z No Qualifier
1 Frontal Bone	3 Percutaneous		
Zygomatic process of frontal bone	4 Percutaneous Endoscopic		
3 Parietal Bone, Right			
4 Parietal Bone, Left			
5 Temporal Bone, Right			
Mastoid process			
Petrous part of temporal bone			
Tympanic part of temporal bone			
Zygomatic process of temporal bone			
6 Temporal Bone, Left			
See 5 Temporal Bone, Right			
7 Occipital Bone			
Foramen magnum			
B Nasal Bone			
Vomer of nasal septum			
C Sphenoid Bone			
Greater wing			
Lesser wing			
Optic foramen			
Pterygoid process			
Sella turcica			
F Ethmoid Bone, Right			
Cribriform plate			
G Ethmoid Bone, Left			
See F Ethmoid Bone, Right			
H Lacrimal Bone, Right			
J Lacrimal Bone, Left			
K Palatine Bone, Right			
L Palatine Bone, Left			
M Zygomatic Bone, Right			
N Zygomatic Bone, Left			
P Orbit, Right			
Bony orbit			
Orbital portion of ethmoid bone			
Orbital portion of frontal bone			
Orbital portion of lacrimal bone			
Orbital portion of maxilla			
Orbital portion of palatine bone			
Orbital portion of sphenoid bone			
Orbital portion of zygomatic bone			
Q Orbit, Left			
See P Orbit, Right			
R Maxilla			
Alveolar process of maxilla			
T Mandible, Right			
Alveolar process of mandible			
Condyloid process			
Mandibular notch			
Mental foramen			
V Mandible, Left			
See T Mandible, Right			
X Hyoid Bone			

0N9 Continued on next page

Non-OR	0N9[0,1,3,4,5,6,7,C,F,G,H,J,K,L,M,N,P,Q,X]30Z
Non-OR	0N9[B,R,T,V][0,3,4]0Z

ØN9 Continued

Ø   **Medical and Surgical**
N   **Head and Facial Bones**
9   **Drainage**   Definition: Taking or letting out fluids and/or gases from a body part
                          Explanation: The qualifier DIAGNOSTIC is used to identify drainage procedures that are biopsies

Body Part Character 4	Approach Character 5	Device Character 6	Qualifier Character 7
Ø Skull	Ø Open	Z No Device	X Diagnostic
1 Frontal Bone	3 Percutaneous		Z No Qualifier
Zygomatic process of frontal bone	4 Percutaneous Endoscopic		
3 Parietal Bone, Right			
4 Parietal Bone, Left			
5 Temporal Bone, Right			
Mastoid process			
Petrous part of temporal bone			
Tympanic part of temporal bone			
Zygomatic process of temporal bone			
6 Temporal Bone, Left			
See 5 Temporal Bone, Right			
7 Occipital Bone			
Foramen magnum			
B Nasal Bone			
Vomer of nasal septum			
C Sphenoid Bone			
Greater wing			
Lesser wing			
Optic foramen			
Pterygoid process			
Sella turcica			
F Ethmoid Bone, Right			
Cribriform plate			
G Ethmoid Bone, Left			
See F Ethmoid Bone, Right			
H Lacrimal Bone, Right			
J Lacrimal Bone, Left			
K Palatine Bone, Right			
L Palatine Bone, Left			
M Zygomatic Bone, Right			
N Zygomatic Bone, Left			
P Orbit, Right			
Bony orbit			
Orbital portion of ethmoid bone			
Orbital portion of frontal bone			
Orbital portion of lacrimal bone			
Orbital portion of maxilla			
Orbital portion of palatine bone			
Orbital portion of sphenoid bone			
Orbital portion of zygomatic bone			
Q Orbit, Left			
See P Orbit, Right			
R Maxilla			
Alveolar process of maxilla			
T Mandible, Right			
Alveolar process of mandible			
Condyloid process			
Mandibular notch			
Mental foramen			
V Mandible, Left			
See T Mandible, Right			
X Hyoid Bone			

Non-OR	ØN9[Ø,1,3,4,5,6,7,C,F,G,H,J,K,L,M,N,P,Q,X]3ZZ
Non-OR	ØN9B[Ø,3,4]Z[X,Z]
Non-OR	ØN9[R,T,V][Ø,3,4]ZZ

LC Limited Coverage   NC Noncovered   ⊞ Combination Member   HAC associated procedure   Combination Only   DRG Non-OR   Non-OR   New/Revised in GREEN

506   ICD-10-PCS 2019

Ø   **Medical and Surgical**
N   **Head and Facial Bones**
B   **Excision**   Definition: Cutting out or off, without replacement, a portion of a body part
                   Explanation: The qualifier DIAGNOSTIC is used to identify excision procedures that are biopsies

Body Part Character 4	Approach Character 5	Device Character 6	Qualifier Character 7
Ø Skull	**Ø** Open	**Z** No Device	**X** Diagnostic
1 Frontal Bone	**3** Percutaneous		**Z** No Qualifier
Zygomatic process of frontal bone	**4** Percutaneous Endoscopic		
3 Parietal Bone, Right			
4 Parietal Bone, Left			
5 Temporal Bone, Right			
Mastoid process			
Petrous part of temporal bone			
Tympanic part of temporal bone			
Zygomatic process of temporal bone			
6 Temporal Bone, Left			
See 5 Temporal Bone, Right			
7 Occipital Bone			
Foramen magnum			
B Nasal Bone			
Vomer of nasal septum			
C Sphenoid Bone			
Greater wing			
Lesser wing			
Optic foramen			
Pterygoid process			
Sella turcica			
F Ethmoid Bone, Right			
Cribriform plate			
G Ethmoid Bone, Left			
See F Ethmoid Bone, Right			
H Lacrimal Bone, Right			
J Lacrimal Bone, Left			
K Palatine Bone, Right			
L Palatine Bone, Left			
M Zygomatic Bone, Right			
N Zygomatic Bone, Left			
P Orbit, Right			
Bony orbit			
Orbital portion of ethmoid bone			
Orbital portion of frontal bone			
Orbital portion of lacrimal bone			
Orbital portion of maxilla			
Orbital portion of palatine bone			
Orbital portion of sphenoid bone			
Orbital portion of zygomatic bone			
Q Orbit, Left			
See P Orbit, Right			
R Maxilla			
Alveolar process of maxilla			
T Mandible, Right			
Alveolar process of mandible			
Condyloid process			
Mandibular notch			
Mental foramen			
V Mandible, Left			
See T Mandible, Right			
X Hyoid Bone			

Non-OR   ØNB[B,R,T,V][Ø,3,4]ZX

Ø   **Medical and Surgical**
N   **Head and Facial Bones**
C   **Extirpation**   Definition: Taking or cutting out solid matter from a body part

                              Explanation: The solid matter may be an abnormal byproduct of a biological function or a foreign body; it may be imbedded in a body part or in the lumen of a tubular body part. The solid matter may or may not have been previously broken into pieces.

Body Part Character 4	Approach Character 5	Device Character 6	Qualifier Character 7

1   **Frontal Bone**
     Zygomatic process of frontal bone
3   **Parietal Bone, Right**
4   **Parietal Bone, Left**
5   **Temporal Bone, Right**
     Mastoid process
     Petrous part of temporal bone
     Tympanic part of temporal bone
     Zygomatic process of temporal bone
6   **Temporal Bone, Left**
     See 5 Temporal Bone, Right
7   **Occipital Bone**
     Foramen magnum
B   **Nasal Bone**
     Vomer of nasal septum
C   **Sphenoid Bone**
     Greater wing
     Lesser wing
     Optic foramen
     Pterygoid process
     Sella turcica
F   **Ethmoid Bone, Right**
     Cribriform plate
G   **Ethmoid Bone, Left**
     See F Ethmoid Bone, Right
H   **Lacrimal Bone, Right**
J   **Lacrimal Bone, Left**
K   **Palatine Bone, Right**
L   **Palatine Bone, Left**
M   **Zygomatic Bone, Right**
N   **Zygomatic Bone, Left**
P   **Orbit, Right**
     Bony orbit
     Orbital portion of ethmoid bone
     Orbital portion of frontal bone
     Orbital portion of lacrimal bone
     Orbital portion of maxilla
     Orbital portion of palatine bone
     Orbital portion of sphenoid bone
     Orbital portion of zygomatic bone
Q   **Orbit, Left**
     See P Orbit, Right
R   **Maxilla**
     Alveolar process of maxilla
T   **Mandible, Right**
     Alveolar process of mandible
     Condyloid process
     Mandibular notch
     Mental foramen
V   **Mandible, Left**
     See T Mandible, Right
X   **Hyoid Bone**
	Ø Open
	3 Percutaneous
	4 Percutaneous Endoscopic
		Z No Device	**Z** No Qualifier

Non-OR   ØNC[B,R,T,V][Ø,3,4]ZZ

LC Limited Coverage   NC Noncovered   ⊞ Combination Member   HAC associated procedure   Combination Only   DRG Non-OR   Non-OR   New/Revised in GREEN

508   ICD-10-PCS 2019

Ø   **Medical and Surgical**
N   **Head and Facial Bones**
D   **Extraction**   Definition: Pulling or stripping out or off all or a portion of a body part by the use of force
                                   Explanation: The qualifier DIAGNOSTIC is used to identify extraction procedures that are biopsies

Body Part Character 4	Approach Character 5	Device Character 6	Qualifier Character 7
Ø Skull	**Ø** Open	**Z** No Device	**Z** No Qualifier
1 Frontal Bone Zygomatic process of frontal bone			
3 Parietal Bone, Right			
4 Parietal Bone, Left			

5   Temporal Bone, Right
    Mastoid process
    Petrous part of temporal bone
    Tympanic part of temporal bone
    Zygomatic process of temporal bone			

6 Temporal Bone, Left *See 5 Temporal Bone, Right*			
7 Occipital Bone Foramen magnum			
B Nasal Bone Vomer of nasal septum			

C   Sphenoid Bone
    Greater wing
    Lesser wing
    Optic foramen
    Pterygoid process
    Sella turcica			

F Ethmoid Bone, Right Cribriform plate			
G Ethmoid Bone, Left *See F Ethmoid Bone, Right*			
H Lacrimal Bone, Right			
J Lacrimal Bone, Left			
K Palatine Bone, Right			
L Palatine Bone, Left			
M Zygomatic Bone, Right			
N Zygomatic Bone, Left			

P   Orbit, Right
    Bony orbit
    Orbital portion of ethmoid bone
    Orbital portion of frontal bone
    Orbital portion of lacrimal bone
    Orbital portion of maxilla
    Orbital portion of palatine bone
    Orbital portion of sphenoid bone
    Orbital portion of zygomatic bone			

Q Orbit, Left *See P Orbit, Right*			
R Maxilla Alveolar process of maxilla			

T   Mandible, Right
    Alveolar process of mandible
    Condyloid process
    Mandibular notch
    Mental foramen			

V Mandible, Left *See T Mandible, Right*			
X Hyoid Bone			

Head and Facial Bones

Ø   **Medical and Surgical**
N   **Head and Facial Bones**
H   **Insertion**   Definition: Putting in a nonbiological appliance that monitors, assists, performs, or prevents a physiological function but does not physically take the place of a body part
                  Explanation: None

Body Part Character 4	Approach Character 5	Device Character 6	Qualifier Character 7
Ø Skull ⊞	**Ø** Open	**4** Internal Fixation Device **5** External Fixation Device **M** Bone Growth Stimulator **N** Neurostimulator Generator	**Z** No Qualifier
Ø Skull	**3** Percutaneous **4** Percutaneous Endoscopic	**4** Internal Fixation Device **5** External Fixation Device **M** Bone Growth Stimulator	**Z** No Qualifier
1 Frontal Bone Zygomatic process of frontal bone **3 Parietal Bone, Right** **4 Parietal Bone, Left** **7 Occipital Bone** Foramen magnum **C Sphenoid Bone** Greater wing Lesser wing Optic foramen Pterygoid process Sella turcica **F Ethmoid Bone, Right** Cribriform plate **G Ethmoid Bone, Left** *See F Ethmoid Bone, Right* **H Lacrimal Bone, Right** **J Lacrimal Bone, Left** **K Palatine Bone, Right** **L Palatine Bone, Left** **M Zygomatic Bone, Right** **N Zygomatic Bone, Left** **P Orbit, Right** Bony orbit Orbital portion of ethmoid bone Orbital portion of frontal bone Orbital portion of lacrimal bone Orbital portion of maxilla Orbital portion of palatine bone Orbital portion of sphenoid bone Orbital portion of zygomatic bone **Q Orbit, Left** *See P Orbit, Right* **X Hyoid Bone**	**Ø** Open **3** Percutaneous **4** Percutaneous Endoscopic	**4** Internal Fixation Device	**Z** No Qualifier
5 Temporal Bone, Right Mastoid process Petrous part of temporal bone Tympanic part of temporal bone Zygomatic process of temporal bone **6 Temporal Bone, Left** *See 5 Temporal Bone, Right*	**Ø** Open **3** Percutaneous **4** Percutaneous Endoscopic	**4** Internal Fixation Device **S** Hearing Device	**Z** No Qualifier
B Nasal Bone Vomer of nasal septum	**Ø** Open **3** Percutaneous **4** Percutaneous Endoscopic	**4** Internal Fixation Device **M** Bone Growth Stimulator	**Z** No Qualifier
R Maxilla Alveolar process of maxilla **T Mandible, Right** Alveolar process of mandible Condyloid process Mandibular notch Mental foramen **V Mandible, Left** *See T Mandible, Right*	**Ø** Open **3** Percutaneous **4** Percutaneous Endoscopic	**4** Internal Fixation Device **5** External Fixation Device	**Z** No Qualifier
W Facial Bone	**Ø** Open **3** Percutaneous **4** Percutaneous Endoscopic	**M** Bone Growth Stimulator	**Z** No Qualifier

Non-OR   ØNHØØ5Z
Non-OR   ØNHØ[3,4]5Z
Non-OR   ØNHB[Ø,3,4][4,M]Z

See Appendix L for Procedure Combinations
⊞   ØNHØØNZ

🔲 Limited Coverage   🔲 Noncovered   ⊞ Combination Member   HAC associated procedure   Combination Only   DRG Non-OR   Non-OR   New/Revised in GREEN

510   ICD-10-PCS 2019

Ø   **Medical and Surgical**
N   **Head and Facial Bones**
J   **Inspection**   Definition: Visually and/or manually exploring a body part

           Explanation: Visual exploration may be performed with or without optical instrumentation. Manual exploration may be performed directly or through intervening body layers.

Body Part Character 4	Approach Character 5	Device Character 6	Qualifier Character 7
Ø Skull B Nasal Bone Vomer of nasal septum W Facial Bone	Ø Open 3 Percutaneous 4 Percutaneous Endoscopic X External	Z No Device	Z No Qualifier

Non-OR   ØNJ[Ø,B,W][3,X]ZZ

Ø   **Medical and Surgical**
N   **Head and Facial Bones**
N   **Release**   Definition: Freeing a body part from an abnormal physical constraint by cutting or by the use of force

           Explanation: Some of the restraining tissue may be taken out but none of the body part is taken out

Body Part Character 4	Approach Character 5	Device Character 6	Qualifier Character 7

1   Frontal Bone
     Zygomatic process of frontal bone
3   Parietal Bone, Right
4   Parietal Bone, Left
5   Temporal Bone, Right
     Mastoid process
     Petrous part of temporal bone
     Tympanic part of temporal bone
     Zygomatic process of temporal bone
6   Temporal Bone, Left
     See 5 Temporal Bone, Right
7   Occipital Bone
     Foramen magnum
B   Nasal Bone
     Vomer of nasal septum
C   Sphenoid Bone
     Greater wing
     Lesser wing
     Optic foramen
     Pterygoid process
     Sella turcica
F   Ethmoid Bone, Right
     Cribriform plate
G   Ethmoid Bone, Left
     See F Ethmoid Bone, Right
H   Lacrimal Bone, Right
J   Lacrimal Bone, Left
K   Palatine Bone, Right
L   Palatine Bone, Left
M   Zygomatic Bone, Right
N   Zygomatic Bone, Left
P   Orbit, Right
     Bony orbit
     Orbital portion of ethmoid bone
     Orbital portion of frontal bone
     Orbital portion of lacrimal bone
     Orbital portion of maxilla
     Orbital portion of palatine bone
     Orbital portion of sphenoid bone
     Orbital portion of zygomatic bone
Q   Orbit, Left
     See P Orbit, Right
R   Maxilla
     Alveolar process of maxilla
T   Mandible, Right
     Alveolar process of mandible
     Condyloid process
     Mandibular notch
     Mental foramen
V   Mandible, Left
     See T Mandible, Right
X   Hyoid Bone
	Ø Open
	3 Percutaneous
	4 Percutaneous Endoscopic
		Z No Device	Z No Qualifier

Non-OR   ØNNB[Ø,3,4]ZZ

Ø   Medical and Surgical
N   Head and Facial Bones
P   Removal   Definition: Taking out or off a device from a body part

Explanation: If a device is taken out and a similar device put in without cutting or puncturing the skin or mucous membrane, the procedure is coded to the root operation CHANGE. Otherwise, the procedure for taking out a device is coded to the root operation REMOVAL.

Body Part Character 4	Approach Character 5	Device Character 6	Qualifier Character 7
Ø Skull	Ø Open	Ø Drainage Device 4 Internal Fixation Device 5 External Fixation Device 7 Autologous Tissue Substitute J Synthetic Substitute K Nonautologous Tissue Substitute M Bone Growth Stimulator N Neurostimulator Generator S Hearing Device	Z No Qualifier
Ø Skull	3 Percutaneous 4 Percutaneous Endoscopic	Ø Drainage Device 4 Internal Fixation Device 5 External Fixation Device 7 Autologous Tissue Substitute J Synthetic Substitute K Nonautologous Tissue Substitute M Bone Growth Stimulator S Hearing Device	Z No Qualifier
Ø Skull	X External	Ø Drainage Device 4 Internal Fixation Device 5 External Fixation Device M Bone Growth Stimulator S Hearing Device	Z No Qualifier
B Nasal Bone Vomer of nasal septum W Facial Bone	Ø Open 3 Percutaneous 4 Percutaneous Endoscopic	Ø Drainage Device 4 Internal Fixation Device 7 Autologous Tissue Substitute J Synthetic Substitute K Nonautologous Tissue Substitute M Bone Growth Stimulator	Z No Qualifier
B Nasal Bone Vomer of nasal septum W Facial Bone	X External	Ø Drainage Device 4 Internal Fixation Device M Bone Growth Stimulator	Z No Qualifier

Non-OR   ØNPØ[3,4]5Z
Non-OR   ØNPØX[Ø,5]Z
Non-OR   ØNPB[Ø,3,4][Ø,4,7,J,K,M]Z
Non-OR   ØNPBX[Ø,4,M]Z
Non-OR   ØNPWX[Ø,M]Z

Ø   Medical and Surgical
N   Head and Facial Bones
Q   Repair   Definition: Restoring, to the extent possible, a body part to its normal anatomic structure and function

                     Explanation: Used only when the method to accomplish the repair is not one of the other root operations

Body Part Character 4	Approach Character 5	Device Character 6	Qualifier Character 7

Ø   Skull
1   Frontal Bone
     Zygomatic process of frontal bone
3   Parietal Bone, Right
4   Parietal Bone, Left
5   Temporal Bone, Right
     Mastoid process
     Petrous part of temporal bone
     Tympanic part of temporal bone
     Zygomatic process of temporal bone
6   Temporal Bone, Left
     See 5 Temporal Bone, Right
7   Occipital Bone
     Foramen magnum
B   Nasal Bone
     Vomer of nasal septum
C   Sphenoid Bone
     Greater wing
     Lesser wing
     Optic foramen
     Pterygoid process
     Sella turcica
F   Ethmoid Bone, Right
     Cribriform plate
G   Ethmoid Bone, Left
     See F Ethmoid Bone, Right
H   Lacrimal Bone, Right
J   Lacrimal Bone, Left
K   Palatine Bone, Right
L   Palatine Bone, Left
M   Zygomatic Bone, Right
N   Zygomatic Bone, Left
P   Orbit, Right
     Bony orbit
     Orbital portion of ethmoid bone
     Orbital portion of frontal bone
     Orbital portion of lacrimal bone
     Orbital portion of maxilla
     Orbital portion of palatine bone
     Orbital portion of sphenoid bone
     Orbital portion of zygomatic bone
Q   Orbit, Left
     See P Orbit, Right
R   Maxilla
     Alveolar process of maxilla
T   Mandible, Right
     Alveolar process of mandible
     Condyloid process
     Mandibular notch
     Mental foramen
V   Mandible, Left
     See T Mandible, Right
X   Hyoid Bone
	Ø Open
	3 Percutaneous
	4 Percutaneous Endoscopic
	X External
		Z No Device	**Z No Qualifier**

Non-OR   ØNQ[Ø,1,3,4,5,6,7,B,C,F,G,H,J,K,L,M,N,P,Q,R,T,V,X]XZZ

Head and Facial Bones

Ø Medical and Surgical
N Head and Facial Bones
R Replacement   Definition: Putting in or on biological or synthetic material that physically takes the place and/or function of all or a portion of a body part

Explanation: The body part may have been taken out or replaced, or may be taken out, physically eradicated, or rendered nonfunctional during the REPLACEMENT procedure. A REMOVAL procedure is coded for taking out the device used in a previous replacement procedure.

Body Part Character 4	Approach Character 5	Device Character 6	Qualifier Character 7

Ø Skull
1 Frontal Bone
   Zygomatic process of frontal bone
3 Parietal Bone, Right
4 Parietal Bone, Left
5 Temporal Bone, Right
   Mastoid process
   Petrous part of temporal bone
   Tympanic part of temporal bone
   Zygomatic process of temporal bone
6 Temporal Bone, Left
   See 5 Temporal Bone, Right
7 Occipital Bone
   Foramen magnum
B Nasal Bone
   Vomer of nasal septum
C Sphenoid Bone
   Greater wing
   Lesser wing
   Optic foramen
   Pterygoid process
   Sella turcica
F Ethmoid Bone, Right
   Cribriform plate
G Ethmoid Bone, Left
   See F Ethmoid Bone, Right
H Lacrimal Bone, Right
J Lacrimal Bone, Left
K Palatine Bone, Right
L Palatine Bone, Left
M Zygomatic Bone, Right
N Zygomatic Bone, Left
P Orbit, Right
   Bony orbit
   Orbital portion of ethmoid bone
   Orbital portion of frontal bone
   Orbital portion of lacrimal bone
   Orbital portion of maxilla
   Orbital portion of palatine bone
   Orbital portion of sphenoid bone
   Orbital portion of zygomatic bone
Q Orbit, Left
   See P Orbit, Right
R Maxilla
   Alveolar process of maxilla
T Mandible, Right
   Alveolar process of mandible
   Condyloid process
   Mandibular notch
   Mental foramen
V Mandible, Left
   See T Mandible, Right
X Hyoid Bone
	Ø Open
	3 Percutaneous
	4 Percutaneous Endoscopic
		7 Autologous Tissue Substitute
		J Synthetic Substitute
		K Nonautologous Tissue Substitute
			Z No Qualifier

LC Limited Coverage   NC Noncovered   ⊞ Combination Member   HAC associated procedure   Combination Only   DRG Non-OR   Non-OR   New/Revised in GREEN

514   ICD-10-PCS 2019

Ø   **Medical and Surgical**
N   **Head and Facial Bones**
S   **Reposition**   Definition: Moving to its normal location, or other suitable location, all or a portion of a body part

                        Explanation: The body part is moved to a new location from an abnormal location, or from a normal location where it is not functioning correctly. The body part may or may not be cut out or off to be moved to the new location.

Body Part Character 4	Approach Character 5	Device Character 6	Qualifier Character 7

Ø Skull
R Maxilla
   Alveolar process of maxilla
T Mandible, Right
   Alveolar process of mandible
   Condyloid process
   Mandibular notch
   Mental foramen
V Mandible, Left
   See T Mandible, Right
	Ø Open
	3 Percutaneous
	4 Percutaneous Endoscopic
		4 Internal Fixation Device
		5 External Fixation Device
		Z No Device
			Z No Qualifier

Ø Skull
R Maxilla
   Alveolar process of maxilla
T Mandible, Right
   Alveolar process of mandible
   Condyloid process
   Mandibular notch
   Mental foramen
V Mandible, Left
   See T Mandible, Right
	X External	**Z No Device**	**Z No Qualifier**

1 Frontal Bone
   Zygomatic process of frontal bone
3 Parietal Bone, Right
4 Parietal Bone, Left
5 Temporal Bone, Right
   Mastoid process
   Petrous part of temporal bone
   Tympanic part of temporal bone
   Zygomatic process of temporal bone
6 Temporal Bone, Left
   See 5 Temporal Bone, Right
7 Occipital Bone
   Foramen magnum
B Nasal Bone
   Vomer of nasal septum
C Sphenoid Bone
   Greater wing
   Lesser wing
   Optic foramen
   Pterygoid process
   Sella turcica
F Ethmoid Bone, Right
   Cribriform plate
G Ethmoid Bone, Left
   See F Ethmoid Bone, Right
H Lacrimal Bone, Right
J Lacrimal Bone, Left
K Palatine Bone, Right
L Palatine Bone, Left
M Zygomatic Bone, Right
N Zygomatic Bone, Left
P Orbit, Right
   Bony orbit
   Orbital portion of ethmoid bone
   Orbital portion of frontal bone
   Orbital portion of lacrimal bone
   Orbital portion of maxilla
   Orbital portion of palatine bone
   Orbital portion of sphenoid bone
   Orbital portion of zygomatic bone
Q Orbit, Left
   See P Orbit, Right
X Hyoid Bone
	Ø Open
	3 Percutaneous
	4 Percutaneous Endoscopic
		4 Internal Fixation Device
		Z No Device
			Z No Qualifier

ØNS Continued on next page

Non-OR   ØNS[R,T,V][3,4][4,5,Z]Z
Non-OR   ØNS[Ø,R,T,V]XZZ
Non-OR   ØNS[B,C,F,G,H,J,K,L,M,N,P,Q,X][3,4][4,Z]Z

LC Limited Coverage   NC Noncovered   ⊞ Combination Member   HAC associated procedure   Combination Only   DRG Non-OR   Non-OR   New/Revised in GREEN

Head and Facial Bones

ØNS Continued

Ø	**Medical and Surgical**
N	**Head and Facial Bones**
S	**Reposition** Definition: Moving to its normal location, or other suitable location, all or a portion of a body part

Explanation: The body part is moved to a new location from an abnormal location, or from a normal location where it is not functioning correctly. The body part may or may not be cut out or off to be moved to the new location.

Body Part Character 4	Approach Character 5	Device Character 6	Qualifier Character 7

1 Frontal Bone
  Zygomatic process of frontal bone
3 Parietal Bone, Right
4 Parietal Bone, Left
5 Temporal Bone, Right
  Mastoid process
  Petrous part of temporal bone
  Tympanic part of temporal bone
  Zygomatic process of temporal bone
6 Temporal Bone, Left
  See 5 Temporal Bone, Right
7 Occipital Bone
  Foramen magnum
B Nasal Bone
  Vomer of nasal septum
C Sphenoid Bone
  Greater wing
  Lesser wing
  Optic foramen
  Pterygoid process
  Sella turcica
F Ethmoid Bone, Right
  Cribriform plate
G Ethmoid Bone, Left
  See F Ethmoid Bone, Right
H Lacrimal Bone, Right
J Lacrimal Bone, Left
K Palatine Bone, Right
L Palatine Bone, Left
M Zygomatic Bone, Right
N Zygomatic Bone, Left
P Orbit, Right
  Bony orbit
  Orbital portion of ethmoid bone
  Orbital portion of frontal bone
  Orbital portion of lacrimal bone
  Orbital portion of maxilla
  Orbital portion of palatine bone
  Orbital portion of sphenoid bone
  Orbital portion of zygomatic bone
Q Orbit, Left
  See P Orbit, Right
X Hyoid Bone
	X External	**Z No Device**	**Z No Qualifier**

Non-OR   ØNS[1,3,4,5,6,7,B,C,F,G,H,J,K,L,M,N,P,Q,X]XZZ

Ø Medical and Surgical
N Head and Facial Bones
T Resection   Definition: Cutting out or off, without replacement, all of a body part
                 Explanation: None

Body Part Character 4	Approach Character 5	Device Character 6	Qualifier Character 7
1 Frontal Bone Zygomatic process of frontal bone **3 Parietal Bone, Right** **4 Parietal Bone, Left** **5 Temporal Bone, Right** Mastoid process Petrous part of temporal bone Tympanic part of temporal bone Zygomatic process of temporal bone **6 Temporal Bone, Left** *See 5 Temporal Bone, Right* **7 Occipital Bone** Foramen magnum **B Nasal Bone** Vomer of nasal septum **C Sphenoid Bone** Greater wing Lesser wing Optic foramen Pterygoid process Sella turcica **F Ethmoid Bone, Right** Cribriform plate **G Ethmoid Bone, Left** *See F Ethmoid Bone, Right* **H Lacrimal Bone, Right** **J Lacrimal Bone, Left** **K Palatine Bone, Right** **L Palatine Bone, Left** **M Zygomatic Bone, Right** **N Zygomatic Bone, Left** **P Orbit, Right** Bony orbit Orbital portion of ethmoid bone Orbital portion of frontal bone Orbital portion of lacrimal bone Orbital portion of maxilla Orbital portion of palatine bone Orbital portion of sphenoid bone Orbital portion of zygomatic bone **Q Orbit, Left** *See P Orbit, Right* **R Maxilla** Alveolar process of maxilla **T Mandible, Right** Alveolar process of mandible Condyloid process Mandibular notch Mental foramen **V Mandible, Left** *See T Mandible, Right* **X Hyoid Bone**	**Ø Open**	**Z No Device**	**Z No Qualifier**

LC Limited Coverage   **NC** Noncovered   ⊞ Combination Member   HAC associated procedure   Combination Only   DRG Non-OR   Non-OR   New/Revised in GREEN

ICD-10-PCS 2019   **517**

Ø Medical and Surgical
N Head and Facial Bones
U Supplement Definition: Putting in or on biological or synthetic material that physically reinforces and/or augments the function of a portion of a body part
  Explanation: The biological material is non-living, or is living and from the same individual. The body part may have been previously replaced, and the SUPPLEMENT procedure is performed to physically reinforce and/or augment the function of the replaced body part.

Body Part Character 4	Approach Character 5	Device Character 6	Qualifier Character 7
Ø Skull	Ø Open	7 Autologous Tissue Substitute	Z No Qualifier
1 Frontal Bone Zygomatic process of frontal bone	3 Percutaneous 4 Percutaneous Endoscopic	J Synthetic Substitute K Nonautologous Tissue Substitute	
3 Parietal Bone, Right			
4 Parietal Bone, Left			

5 Temporal Bone, Right
  Mastoid process
  Petrous part of temporal bone
  Tympanic part of temporal bone
  Zygomatic process of temporal bone			

6 Temporal Bone, Left *See 5 Temporal Bone, Right*			
7 Occipital Bone Foramen magnum			
B Nasal Bone Vomer of nasal septum			

C Sphenoid Bone
  Greater wing
  Lesser wing
  Optic foramen
  Pterygoid process
  Sella turcica			

F Ethmoid Bone, Right Cribriform plate			
G Ethmoid Bone, Left *See F Ethmoid Bone, Right*			
H Lacrimal Bone, Right			
J Lacrimal Bone, Left			
K Palatine Bone, Right			
L Palatine Bone, Left			
M Zygomatic Bone, Right			
N Zygomatic Bone, Left			

P Orbit, Right
  Bony orbit
  Orbital portion of ethmoid bone
  Orbital portion of frontal bone
  Orbital portion of lacrimal bone
  Orbital portion of maxilla
  Orbital portion of palatine bone
  Orbital portion of sphenoid bone
  Orbital portion of zygomatic bone			

Q Orbit, Left *See P Orbit, Right*			
R Maxilla Alveolar process of maxilla			

T Mandible, Right
  Alveolar process of mandible
  Condyloid process
  Mandibular notch
  Mental foramen			

V Mandible, Left *See T Mandible, Right*			
X Hyoid Bone			

Ø Medical and Surgical
N Head and Facial Bones
W Revision   Definition: Correcting, to the extent possible, a portion of a malfunctioning device or the position of a displaced device

                             Explanation: Revision can include correcting a malfunctioning or displaced device by taking out or putting in components of the device such as a screw or pin

Body Part Character 4	Approach Character 5	Device Character 6	Qualifier Character 7
Ø Skull	**Ø Open**	**Ø Drainage Device** **4 Internal Fixation Device** **5 External Fixation Device** **7 Autologous Tissue Substitute** **J Synthetic Substitute** **K Nonautologous Tissue Substitute** **M Bone Growth Stimulator** **N Neurostimulator Generator** **S Hearing Device**	**Z No Qualifier**
Ø Skull	**3 Percutaneous** **4 Percutaneous Endoscopic** **X External**	**Ø Drainage Device** **4 Internal Fixation Device** **5 External Fixation Device** **7 Autologous Tissue Substitute** **J Synthetic Substitute** **K Nonautologous Tissue Substitute** **M Bone Growth Stimulator** **S Hearing Device**	**Z No Qualifier**
B Nasal Bone Vomer of nasal septum **W Facial Bone**	**Ø Open** **3 Percutaneous** **4 Percutaneous Endoscopic** **X External**	**Ø Drainage Device** **4 Internal Fixation Device** **7 Autologous Tissue Substitute** **J Synthetic Substitute** **K Nonautologous Tissue Substitute** **M Bone Growth Stimulator**	**Z No Qualifier**

Non-OR   ØNWØX[Ø,4,5,7,J,K,M,S]Z
Non-OR   ØNWB[Ø,3,4,X][Ø,4,7,J,K,M]Z
Non-OR   ØNWWX[Ø,4,7,J,K,M]Z

Upper Bones ØP2–ØPW

Character Meanings

This Character Meaning table is provided as a guide to assist the user in the identification of character members that may be found in this section of code tables. It **SHOULD NOT** be used to build a PCS code.

Operation–Character 3	Body Part–Character 4	Approach–Character 5	Device–Character 6	Qualifier–Character 7
2 Change	Ø Sternum	Ø Open	Ø Drainage Device OR Internal Fixation Device, Rigid Plate	X Diagnostic
5 Destruction	1 Ribs, 1 to 2	3 Percutaneous	4 Internal Fixation Device	Z No Qualifier
8 Division	2 Ribs, 3 or more	4 Percutaneous Endoscopic	5 External Fixation Device	
9 Drainage	3 Cervical Vertebra	X External	6 Internal Fixation Device, Intramedullary	
B Excision	4 Thoracic Vertebra		7 Autologous Tissue Substitute	
C Extirpation	5 Scapula, Right		8 External Fixation Device, Limb Lengthening	
D Extraction	6 Scapula, Left		B External Fixation Device, Monoplanar	
H Insertion	7 Glenoid Cavity, Right		C External Fixation Device, Ring	
J Inspection	8 Glenoid Cavity, Left		D External Fixation Device, Hybrid	
N Release	9 Clavicle, Right		J Synthetic Substitute	
P Removal	B Clavicle, Left		K Nonautologous Tissue Substitute	
Q Repair	C Humeral Head, Right		M Bone Growth Stimulator	
R Replacement	D Humeral Head, Left		Y Other Device	
S Reposition	F Humeral Shaft, Right		Z No Device	
T Resection	G Humeral Shaft, Left			
U Supplement	H Radius, Right			
W Revision	J Radius, Left			
	K Ulna, Right			
	L Ulna, Left			
	M Carpal, Right			
	N Carpal, Left			
	P Metacarpal, Right			
	Q Metacarpal, Left			
	R Thumb Phalanx, Right			
	S Thumb Phalanx, Left			
	T Finger Phalanx, Right			
	V Finger Phalanx, Left			
	Y Upper Bone			

AHA Coding Clinic for table ØPB
2015, 3Q, 3-8	Excisional and nonexcisional debridement
2015, 2Q, 34	Decompressive laminectomy
2013, 4Q, 109	Separating conjoined twins
2013, 4Q, 116	Spinal decompression
2013, 3Q, 20	Superior labrum anterior posterior (SLAP) repair and subacromialdecompression
2012, 4Q, 101	Rib resection with reconstruction of anterior chest wall
2012, 2Q, 19	Multiple decompressive cervical laminectomies

AHA Coding Clinic for table ØPD
2017, 4Q, 41	Extraction procedures

AHA Coding Clinic for table ØPH
2017, 2Q, 20	Exchange of intramedullary antibiotic impregnated spacer
2016, 4Q, 117	Placement of magnetic growth rods
2014, 4Q, 28	Removal and replacement of displaced growing rods

AHA Coding Clinic for table ØPP
2017, 2Q, 20	Exchange of intramedullary antibiotic impregnated spacer
2016, 4Q, 117	Placement of magnetic growth rods
2014, 4Q, 28	Removal and replacement of displaced growing rods

AHA Coding Clinic for table ØPS
2017, 4Q, 53	New and revised body part values - Ribs
2016, 1Q, 21	Elongation derotation flexion casting
2015, 4Q, 33	Ravitch operation
2015, 2Q, 35	Application of tongs to reduce and stabilize cervical fracture
2014, 4Q, 26	Placement of vertical expandable prosthetic titanium rib (VEPTR)
2014, 4Q, 32	Open reduction internal fixation of fracture with debridement
2014, 3Q, 33	Radial fracture treatment with open reduction internal fixation, and release of carpal ligament

AHA Coding Clinic for table ØPT
2015, 3Q, 26	Thumb arthroplasty with resection of trapezium

AHA Coding Clinic for table ØPU
2015, 2Q, 20	Cervical laminoplasty
2013, 4Q, 109	Separating conjoined twins

AHA Coding Clinic for table ØPW
2014, 4Q, 26	Adjustment of VEPTR lengthening mechanism
2014, 4Q, 27	Bilateral lengthening of growing rods

Upper Bones

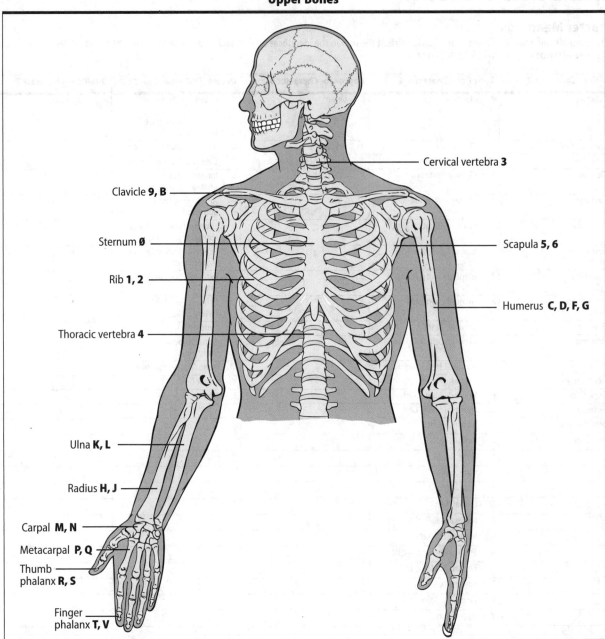

Cervical vertebra **3**

Clavicle **9, B**

Sternum **Ø**

Rib **1, 2**

Thoracic vertebra **4**

Scapula **5, 6**

Humerus **C, D, F, G**

Ulna **K, L**

Radius **H, J**

Carpal **M, N**

Metacarpal **P, Q**

Thumb phalanx **R, S**

Finger phalanx **T, V**

Humerus and Scapula

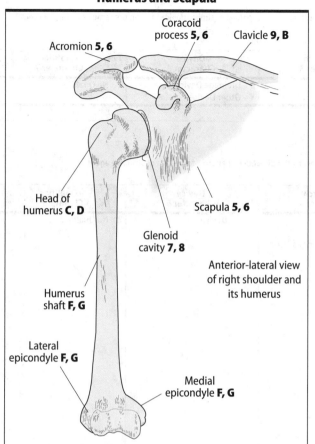

Coracoid
process **5, 6**

Acromion **5, 6**

Clavicle **9, B**

Head of
humerus **C, D**

Scapula **5, 6**

Glenoid
cavity **7, 8**

Anterior-lateral view
of right shoulder and
its humerus

Humerus
shaft **F, G**

Lateral
epicondyle **F, G**

Medial
epicondyle **F, G**

Radius and Ulna

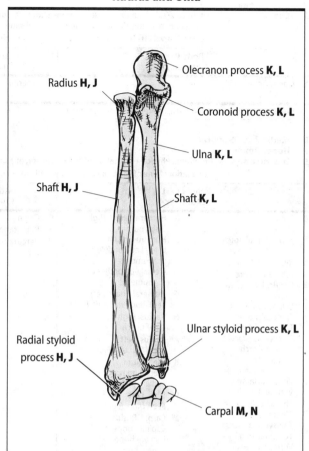

Olecranon process **K, L**

Radius **H, J**

Coronoid process **K, L**

Ulna **K, L**

Shaft **H, J**

Shaft **K, L**

Radial styloid
process **H, J**

Ulnar styloid process **K, L**

Carpal **M, N**

Hand

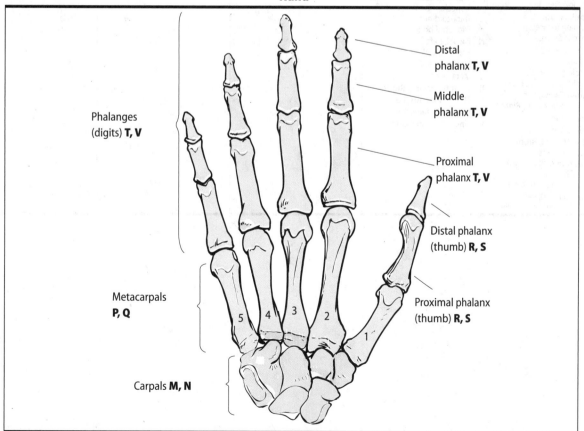

Phalanges
(digits) **T, V**

Distal
phalanx **T, V**

Middle
phalanx **T, V**

Proximal
phalanx **T, V**

Distal phalanx
(thumb) **R, S**

Metacarpals
P, Q

5 4 3 2

1

Proximal phalanx
(thumb) **R, S**

Carpals **M, N**

Ø Medical and Surgical
P Upper Bones
2 Change   Definition: Taking out or off a device from a body part and putting back an identical or similar device in or on the same body part without cutting or puncturing the skin or a mucous membrane

Explanation: ALL CHANGE procedures are coded using the approach EXTERNAL

Body Part Character 4	Approach Character 5	Device Character 6	Qualifier Character 7
Y Upper Bone	X External	Ø Drainage Device Y Other Device	Z No Qualifier

Non-OR   All body part, approach, device, and qualifier values

---

Ø Medical and Surgical
P Upper Bones
5 Destruction   Definition: Physical eradication of all or a portion of a body part by the direct use of energy, force, or a destructive agent

Explanation: None of the body part is physically taken out

Body Part Character 4		Approach Character 5	Device Character 6	Qualifier Character 7

Ø   **Sternum**
    Manubrium
    Suprasternal notch
    Xiphoid process
1   **Ribs, 1 to 2**
2   **Ribs, 3 or More**
3   **Cervical Vertebra**
    Dens
    Odontoid process
    Spinous process
    Transverse foramen
    Transverse process
    Vertebral arch
    Vertebral body
    Vertebral foramen
    Vertebral lamina
    Vertebral pedicle
4   **Thoracic Vertebra**
    Spinous process
    Transverse process
    Vertebral arch
    Vertebral body
    Vertebral foramen
    Vertebral lamina
    Vertebral pedicle
5   **Scapula, Right**
    Acromion (process)
    Coracoid process
6   **Scapula, Left**
    See 5 Scapula, Right
7   **Glenoid Cavity, Right**
    Glenoid fossa (of scapula)
8   **Glenoid Cavity, Left**
    See 7 Glenoid Cavity, Right
9   **Clavicle, Right**
B   **Clavicle, Left**
C   **Humeral Head, Right**
    Greater tuberosity
    Lesser tuberosity
    Neck of humerus
      (anatomical)(surgical)
D   **Humeral Head, Left**
    See C Humeral Head, Right
	F **Humeral Shaft, Right**
	    Distal humerus
	    Humerus, distal
	    Lateral epicondyle of
	      humerus
	    Medial epicondyle of
	      humerus
	G **Humeral Shaft, Left**
	    See F Humeral Shaft, Right
	H **Radius, Right**
	    Ulnar notch
	J **Radius, Left**
	    See H Radius, Right
	K **Ulna, Right**
	    Olecranon process
	    Radial notch
	L **Ulna, Left**
	    See K Ulna, Right
	M **Carpal, Right**
	    Capitate bone
	    Hamate bone
	    Lunate bone
	    Pisiform bone
	    Scaphoid bone
	    Trapezium bone
	    Trapezoid bone
	    Triquetral bone
	N **Carpal, Left**
	    See M Carpal, Right
	P **Metacarpal, Right**
	Q **Metacarpal, Left**
	R **Thumb Phalanx, Right**
	S **Thumb Phalanx, Left**
	T **Finger Phalanx, Right**
	V **Finger Phalanx, Left**
		Ø Open
		3 Percutaneous
		4 Percutaneous Endoscopic
			Z No Device	Z No Qualifier

LC Limited Coverage   **NC** Noncovered   ⊞ Combination Member   HAC associated procedure   Combination Only   DRG Non-OR   Non-OR   New/Revised in GREEN

524   ICD-10-PCS 2019

ØP2–ØP5

0   **Medical and Surgical**
P   **Upper Bones**
8   **Division**

Definition: Cutting into a body part, without draining fluids and/or gases from the body part, in order to separate or transect a body part

Explanation: All or a portion of the body part is separated into two or more portions

Body Part Character 4		Approach Character 5	Device Character 6	Qualifier Character 7

0 Sternum
   Manubrium
   Suprasternal notch
   Xiphoid process
1 Ribs, 1 to 2
2 Ribs, 3 or More
3 Cervical Vertebra
   Dens
   Odontoid process
   Spinous process
   Transverse foramen
   Transverse process
   Vertebral arch
   Vertebral body
   Vertebral foramen
   Vertebral lamina
   Vertebral pedicle
4 Thoracic Vertebra
   Spinous process
   Transverse process
   Vertebral arch
   Vertebral body
   Vertebral foramen
   Vertebral lamina
   Vertebral pedicle
5 Scapula, Right
   Acromion (process)
   Coracoid process
6 Scapula, Left
   See 5 Scapula, Right
7 Glenoid Cavity, Right
   Glenoid fossa (of scapula)
8 Glenoid Cavity, Left
   See 7 Glenoid Cavity, Right
9 Clavicle, Right
B Clavicle, Left
C Humeral Head, Right
   Greater tuberosity
   Lesser tuberosity
   Neck of humerus
     (anatomical)(surgical)
D Humeral Head, Left
   See C Humeral Head, Right
	F Humeral Shaft, Right
	   Distal humerus
	   Humerus, distal
	   Lateral epicondyle of
	     humerus
	   Medial epicondyle of
	     humerus
	G Humeral Shaft, Left
	   See F Humeral Shaft, Right
	H Radius, Right
	   Ulnar notch
	J Radius, Left
	   See H Radius, Right
	K Ulna, Right
	   Olecranon process
	   Radial notch
	L Ulna, Left
	   See K Ulna, Right
	M Carpal, Right
	   Capitate bone
	   Hamate bone
	   Lunate bone
	   Pisiform bone
	   Scaphoid bone
	   Trapezium bone
	   Trapezoid bone
	   Triquetral bone
	N Carpal, Left
	   See M Carpal, Right
	P Metacarpal, Right
	Q Metacarpal, Left
	R Thumb Phalanx, Right
	S Thumb Phalanx, Left
	T Finger Phalanx, Right
	V Finger Phalanx, Left
		0 Open
		3 Percutaneous
		4 Percutaneous Endoscopic
			Z No Device	**Z** No Qualifier

LC Limited Coverage   **NC** Noncovered   ⊞ Combination Member   HAC associated procedure   Combination Only   DRG Non-OR   Non-OR   New/Revised in GREEN

ICD-10-PCS 2019   **525**

0P8–0P8

Upper Bones

Ø Medical and Surgical
P Upper Bones
9 Drainage　　　Definition: Taking or letting out fluids and/or gases from a body part
　　　　　　　　Explanation: The qualifier DIAGNOSTIC is used to identify drainage procedures that are biopsies

Body Part Character 4		Approach Character 5	Device Character 6	Qualifier Character 7
Ø Sternum 　Manubrium 　Suprasternal notch 　Xiphoid process 1 Ribs, 1 to 2 2 Ribs, 3 or More 3 Cervical Vertebra 　Dens 　Odontoid process 　Spinous process 　Transverse foramen 　Transverse process 　Vertebral arch 　Vertebral body 　Vertebral foramen 　Vertebral lamina 　Vertebral pedicle 4 Thoracic Vertebra 　Spinous process 　Transverse process 　Vertebral arch 　Vertebral body 　Vertebral foramen 　Vertebral lamina 　Vertebral pedicle 5 Scapula, Right 　Acromion (process) 　Coracoid process 6 Scapula, Left 　See 5 Scapula, Right 7 Glenoid Cavity, Right 　Glenoid fossa (of scapula) 8 Glenoid Cavity, Left 　See 7 Glenoid Cavity, Right 9 Clavicle, Right B Clavicle, Left C Humeral Head, Right 　Greater tuberosity 　Lesser tuberosity 　Neck of humerus 　　(anatomical)(surgical)	D Humeral Head, Left 　See C Humeral Head, Right F Humeral Shaft, Right 　Distal humerus 　Humerus, distal 　Lateral epicondyle of 　　humerus 　Medial epicondyle of 　　humerus G Humeral Shaft, Left 　See F Humeral Shaft, Right H Radius, Right 　Ulnar notch J Radius, Left 　See H Radius, Right K Ulna, Right 　Olecranon process 　Radial notch L Ulna, Left 　See K Ulna, Right M Carpal, Right 　Capitate bone 　Hamate bone 　Lunate bone 　Pisiform bone 　Scaphoid bone 　Trapezium bone 　Trapezoid bone 　Triquetral bone N Carpal, Left 　See M Carpal, Right P Metacarpal, Right Q Metacarpal, Left R Thumb Phalanx, Right S Thumb Phalanx, Left T Finger Phalanx, Right V Finger Phalanx, Left	Ø Open 3 Percutaneous 4 Percutaneous Endoscopic	Ø Drainage Device	Z No Qualifier

ØP9 Continued on next page

Non-OR ØP9[Ø,1,2,3,4,5,6,7,8,9,B,C,D,F,G,H,J,K,L,M,N,P,Q,R,S,T,V]3ØZ

0   Medical and Surgical   *0P9 Continued*
P   Upper Bones
9   Drainage   Definition: Taking or letting out fluids and/or gases from a body part

Explanation: The qualifier DIAGNOSTIC is used to identify drainage procedures that are biopsies

Body Part Character 4		Approach Character 5	Device Character 6	Qualifier Character 7

0 Sternum
   Manubrium
   Suprasternal notch
   Xiphoid process
1 Ribs, 1 to 2
2 Ribs, 3 or More
3 Cervical Vertebra
   Dens
   Odontoid process
   Spinous process
   Transverse foramen
   Transverse process
   Vertebral arch
   Vertebral body
   Vertebral foramen
   Vertebral lamina
   Vertebral pedicle
4 Thoracic Vertebra
   Spinous process
   Transverse process
   Vertebral arch
   Vertebral body
   Vertebral foramen
   Vertebral lamina
   Vertebral pedicle
5 Scapula, Right
   Acromion (process)
   Coracoid process
6 Scapula, Left
   See 5 Scapula, Right
7 Glenoid Cavity, Right
   Glenoid fossa (of scapula)
8 Glenoid Cavity, Left
   See 7 Glenoid Cavity, Right
9 Clavicle, Right
B Clavicle, Left
C Humeral Head, Right
   Greater tuberosity
   Lesser tuberosity
   Neck of humerus
      (anatomical)(surgical)
	D Humeral Head, Left
	   See C Humeral Head, Right
	F Humeral Shaft, Right
	   Distal humerus
	   Humerus, distal
	   Lateral epicondyle of
	      humerus
	   Medial epicondyle of
	      humerus
	G Humeral Shaft, Left
	   See F Humeral Shaft, Right
	H Radius, Right
	   Ulnar notch
	J Radius, Left
	   See H Radius, Right
	K Ulna, Right
	   Olecranon process
	   Radial notch
	L Ulna, Left
	   See K Ulna, Right
	M Carpal, Right
	   Capitate bone
	   Hamate bone
	   Lunate bone
	   Pisiform bone
	   Scaphoid bone
	   Trapezium bone
	   Trapezoid bone
	   Triquetral bone
	N Carpal, Left
	   See M Carpal, Right
	P Metacarpal, Right
	Q Metacarpal, Left
	R Thumb Phalanx, Right
	S Thumb Phalanx, Left
	T Finger Phalanx, Right
	V Finger Phalanx, Left
		0 Open
		3 Percutaneous
		4 Percutaneous Endoscopic
			Z No Device	**X Diagnostic**
				Z No Qualifier

Non-OR   0P9[0,1,2,3,4,5,6,7,8,9,B,C,D,F,G,H,J,K,L,M,N,P,Q,R,S,T,V]3ZZ

Ø   Medical and Surgical
P   Upper Bones
B   Excision

Definition: Cutting out or off, without replacement, a portion of a body part

Explanation: The qualifier DIAGNOSTIC is used to identify excision procedures that are biopsies

Body Part Character 4		Approach Character 5	Device Character 6	Qualifier Character 7

Ø Sternum
Manubrium
Suprasternal notch
Xiphoid process
1 Ribs, 1 to 2
2 Ribs, 3 or More
3 Cervical Vertebra
Dens
Odontoid process
Spinous process
Transverse foramen
Transverse process
Vertebral arch
Vertebral body
Vertebral foramen
Vertebral lamina
Vertebral pedicle
4 Thoracic Vertebra
Spinous process
Transverse process
Vertebral arch
Vertebral body
Vertebral foramen
Vertebral lamina
Vertebral pedicle
5 Scapula, Right
Acromion (process)
Coracoid process
6 Scapula, Left
See 5 Scapula, Right
7 Glenoid Cavity, Right
Glenoid fossa (of scapula)
8 Glenoid Cavity, Left
See 7 Glenoid Cavity, Right
9 Clavicle, Right
B Clavicle, Left
C Humeral Head, Right
Greater tuberosity
Lesser tuberosity
Neck of humerus
  (anatomical)(surgical)
D Humeral Head, Left
See C Humeral Head, Right
	F Humeral Shaft, Right
	Distal humerus
	Humerus, distal
	Lateral epicondyle of
	  humerus
	Medial epicondyle of
	  humerus
	G Humeral Shaft, Left
	See F Humeral Shaft, Right
	H Radius, Right
	Ulnar notch
	J Radius, Left
	See H Radius, Right
	K Ulna, Right
	Olecranon process
	Radial notch
	L Ulna, Left
	See K Ulna, Right
	M Carpal, Right
	Capitate bone
	Hamate bone
	Lunate bone
	Pisiform bone
	Scaphoid bone
	Trapezium bone
	Trapezoid bone
	Triquetral bone
	N Carpal, Left
	See M Carpal, Right
	P Metacarpal, Right
	Q Metacarpal, Left
	R Thumb Phalanx, Right
	S Thumb Phalanx, Left
	T Finger Phalanx, Right
	V Finger Phalanx, Left
		Ø Open
		3 Percutaneous
		4 Percutaneous Endoscopic
			Z No Device	**X Diagnostic**
				Z No Qualifier

LC Limited Coverage   NC Noncovered   ⊞ Combination Member   HAC associated procedure   Combination Only   DRG Non-OR   Non-OR   New/Revised in GREEN

528   ICD-10-PCS 2019

ØPB–ØPB

0   **Medical and Surgical**
P   **Upper Bones**
C   **Extirpation**   Definition: Taking or cutting out solid matter from a body part

Explanation: The solid matter may be an abnormal byproduct of a biological function or a foreign body; it may be imbedded in a body part or in the lumen of a tubular body part. The solid matter may or may not have been previously broken into pieces.

Body Part Character 4		Approach Character 5	Device Character 6	Qualifier Character 7

0 **Sternum**
     Manubrium
     Suprasternal notch
     Xiphoid process
1 **Ribs, 1 to 2**
2 **Ribs, 3 or More**
3 **Cervical Vertebra**
     Dens
     Odontoid process
     Spinous process
     Transverse foramen
     Transverse process
     Vertebral arch
     Vertebral body
     Vertebral foramen
     Vertebral lamina
     Vertebral pedicle
4 **Thoracic Vertebra**
     Spinous process
     Transverse process
     Vertebral arch
     Vertebral body
     Vertebral foramen
     Vertebral lamina
     Vertebral pedicle
5 **Scapula, Right**
     Acromion (process)
     Coracoid process
6 **Scapula, Left**
     See 5 Scapula, Right
7 **Glenoid Cavity, Right**
     Glenoid fossa (of scapula)
8 **Glenoid Cavity, Left**
     See 7 Glenoid Cavity, Right
9 **Clavicle, Right**
B **Clavicle, Left**
C **Humeral Head, Right**
     Greater tuberosity
     Lesser tuberosity
     Neck of humerus
         (anatomical)(surgical)
D **Humeral Head, Left**
     See C Humeral Head, Right
	F **Humeral Shaft, Right**
	     Distal humerus
	     Humerus, distal
	     Lateral epicondyle of
	         humerus
	     Medial epicondyle of
	         humerus
	G **Humeral Shaft, Left**
	     See F Humeral Shaft, Right
	H **Radius, Right**
	     Ulnar notch
	J **Radius, Left**
	     See H Radius, Right
	K **Ulna, Right**
	     Olecranon process
	     Radial notch
	L **Ulna, Left**
	     See K Ulna, Right
	M **Carpal, Right**
	     Capitate bone
	     Hamate bone
	     Lunate bone
	     Pisiform bone
	     Scaphoid bone
	     Trapezium bone
	     Trapezoid bone
	     Triquetral bone
	N **Carpal, Left**
	     See M Carpal, Right
	P **Metacarpal, Right**
	Q **Metacarpal, Left**
	R **Thumb Phalanx, Right**
	S **Thumb Phalanx, Left**
	T **Finger Phalanx, Right**
	V **Finger Phalanx, Left**
		0 Open
		3 Percutaneous
		4 Percutaneous Endoscopic
			Z No Device	**Z** No Qualifier

LC Limited Coverage   **NC** Noncovered   ⊞ Combination Member   HAC associated procedure   Combination Only   DRG Non-OR   Non-OR   New/Revised in GREEN

ICD-10-PCS 2019   **529**

0PC–0PC

Upper Bones

Ø   Medical and Surgical
P   Upper Bones
D   Extraction   Definition: Pulling or stripping out or off all or a portion of a body part by the use of force
                 Explanation: The qualifier DIAGNOSTIC is used to identify extraction procedures that are biopsies

Body Part Character 4		Approach Character 5	Device Character 6	Qualifier Character 7

Ø   **Sternum**
     Manubrium
     Suprasternal notch
     Xiphoid process
 1   Ribs, 1 to 2
 2   Ribs, 3 or More
 3   Cervical Vertebra
     Dens
     Odontoid process
     Spinous process
     Transverse foramen
     Transverse process
     Vertebral arch
     Vertebral body
     Vertebral foramen
     Vertebral lamina
     Vertebral pedicle
 4   Thoracic Vertebra
     Spinous process
     Transverse process
     Vertebral arch
     Vertebral body
     Vertebral foramen
     Vertebral lamina
     Vertebral pedicle
 5   Scapula, Right
     Acromion (process)
     Coracoid process
 6   Scapula, Left
     See 5 Scapula, Right
 7   Glenoid Cavity, Right
     Glenoid fossa (of scapula)
 8   Glenoid Cavity, Left
     See 7 Glenoid Cavity, Right
 9   Clavicle, Right
 B   Clavicle, Left
 C   Humeral Head, Right
     Greater tuberosity
     Lesser tuberosity
     Neck of humerus
       (anatomical)(surgical)
 D   Humeral Head, Left
     See C Humeral Head, Right
	F Humeral Shaft, Right
	     Distal humerus
	     Humerus, distal
	     Lateral epicondyle of
	       humerus
	     Medial epicondyle of
	       humerus
	 G Humeral Shaft, Left
	     See F Humeral Shaft, Right
	 H Radius, Right
	     Ulnar notch
	 J Radius, Left
	     See H Radius, Right
	 K Ulna, Right
	     Olecranon process
	     Radial notch
	 L Ulna, Left
	     See K Ulna, Right
	 M Carpal, Right
	     Capitate bone
	     Hamate bone
	     Lunate bone
	     Pisiform bone
	     Scaphoid bone
	     Trapezium bone
	     Trapezoid bone
	     Triquetral bone
	 N Carpal, Left
	     See M Carpal, Right
	 P Metacarpal, Right
	 Q Metacarpal, Left
	 R Thumb Phalanx, Right
	 S Thumb Phalanx, Left
	 T Finger Phalanx, Right
	 V Finger Phalanx, Left
		Ø Open	Z No Device	Z No Qualifier

LC Limited Coverage   **NC** Noncovered   ⊞ Combination Member   HAC associated procedure   Combination Only   DRG Non-OR   Non-OR   New/Revised in GREEN

530   ICD-10-PCS 2019

Ø   **Medical and Surgical**
P   **Upper Bones**
H   **Insertion**   Definition: Putting in a nonbiological appliance that monitors, assists, performs, or prevents a physiological function but does not physically take the place of a body part

                   Explanation: None

Body Part Character 4		Approach Character 5	Device Character 6	Qualifier Character 7
Ø Sternum Manubrium Suprasternal notch Xiphoid process		**Ø Open** **3 Percutaneous** **4 Percutaneous Endoscopic**	**Ø Internal Fixation Device, Rigid Plate** **4 Internal Fixation Device**	**Z No Qualifier**
1 Ribs, 1 to 2 **2 Ribs, 3 or More** **3 Cervical Vertebra** Dens Odontoid process Spinous process Transverse foramen Transverse process Vertebral arch Vertebral body Vertebral foramen Vertebral lamina Vertebral pedicle **4 Thoracic Vertebra** Spinous process Transverse process Vertebral arch Vertebral body Vertebral foramen Vertebral lamina Vertebral pedicle	**5 Scapula, Right** Acromion (process) Coracoid process **6 Scapula, Left** *See 5 Scapula, Right* **7 Glenoid Cavity, Right** Glenoid fossa (of scapula) **8 Glenoid Cavity, Left** *See 7 Glenoid Cavity, Right* **9 Clavicle, Right** **B Clavicle, Left**	**Ø Open** **3 Percutaneous** **4 Percutaneous Endoscopic**	**4 Internal Fixation Device**	**Z No Qualifier**
C Humeral Head, Right Greater tuberosity Lesser tuberosity Neck of humerus (anatomical)(surgical) **D Humeral Head, Left** *See C Humeral Head, Right* **F Humeral Shaft, Right** Distal humerus Humerus, distal Lateral epicondyle of humerus Medial epicondyle of humerus	**G Humeral Shaft, Left** *See F Humeral Shaft, Right* **H Radius, Right** Ulnar notch **J Radius, Left** *See H Radius, Right* **K Ulna, Right** Olecranon process Radial notch **L Ulna, Left** *See K Ulna, Right*	**Ø Open** **3 Percutaneous** **4 Percutaneous Endoscopic**	**4 Internal Fixation Device** **5 External Fixation Device** **6 Internal Fixation Device, Intramedullary** **8 External Fixation Device, Limb Lengthening** **B External Fixation Device, Monoplanar** **C External Fixation Device, Ring** **D External Fixation Device, Hybrid**	**Z No Qualifier**
M Carpal, Right Capitate bone Hamate bone Lunate bone Pisiform bone Scaphoid bone Trapezium bone Trapezoid bone Triquetral bone **N Carpal, Left** *See M Carpal, Right*	**P Metacarpal, Right** **Q Metacarpal, Left** **R Thumb Phalanx, Right** **S Thumb Phalanx, Left** **T Finger Phalanx, Right** **V Finger Phalanx, Left**	**Ø Open** **3 Percutaneous** **4 Percutaneous Endoscopic**	**4 Internal Fixation Device** **5 External Fixation Device**	**Z No Qualifier**
Y Upper Bone		**Ø Open** **3 Percutaneous** **4 Percutaneous Endoscopic**	**M Bone Growth Stimulator**	**Z No Qualifier**

Non-OR   ØPH[C,D,F,G,H,J,K,L][Ø,3,4]8Z

LC Limited Coverage   NC Noncovered   ⊞ Combination Member   HAC associated procedure   Combination Only   DRG Non-OR   Non-OR   New/Revised in GREEN

Ø   Medical and Surgical
P   Upper Bones
J   Inspection   Definition: Visually and/or manually exploring a body part

Explanation: Visual exploration may be performed with or without optical instrumentation. Manual exploration may be performed directly or through intervening body layers.

Body Part Character 4	Approach Character 5	Device Character 6	Qualifier Character 7
Y Upper Bone	**Ø** Open **3** Percutaneous **4** Percutaneous Endoscopic **X** External	**Z** No Device	**Z** No Qualifier

Non-OR   ØPJY[3,X]ZZ

Ø   Medical and Surgical
P   Upper Bones
N   Release   Definition: Freeing a body part from an abnormal physical constraint by cutting or by the use of force

Explanation: Some of the restraining tissue may be taken out but none of the body part is taken out

Body Part Character 4	Approach Character 5	Device Character 6	Qualifier Character 7

Ø   Sternum
    Manubrium
    Suprasternal notch
    Xiphoid process
1   Ribs, 1 to 2
2   Ribs, 3 or More
3   Cervical Vertebra
    Dens
    Odontoid process
    Spinous process
    Transverse foramen
    Transverse process
    Vertebral arch
    Vertebral body
    Vertebral foramen
    Vertebral lamina
    Vertebral pedicle
4   Thoracic Vertebra
    Spinous process
    Transverse process
    Vertebral arch
    Vertebral body
    Vertebral foramen
    Vertebral lamina
    Vertebral pedicle
5   Scapula, Right
    Acromion (process)
    Coracoid process
6   Scapula, Left
    See 5 Scapula, Right
7   Glenoid Cavity, Right
    Glenoid fossa (of scapula)
8   Glenoid Cavity, Left
    See 7 Glenoid Cavity, Right
9   Clavicle, Right
B   Clavicle, Left
C   Humeral Head, Right
    Greater tuberosity
    Lesser tuberosity
    Neck of humerus
      (anatomical) (surgical)
D   Humeral Head, Left
    See C Humeral Head, Right
	F Humeral Shaft, Right
	    Distal humerus
	    Humerus, distal
	    Lateral epicondyle of
	      humerus
	    Medial epicondyle of
	      humerus
	G Humeral Shaft, Left
	    See F Humeral Shaft, Right
	H Radius, Right
	    Ulnar notch
	J Radius, Left
	    See H Radius, Right
	K Ulna, Right
	    Olecranon process
	    Radial notch
	L Ulna, Left
	    See K Ulna, Right
	M Carpal, Right
	    Capitate bone
	    Hamate bone
	    Lunate bone
	    Pisiform bone
	    Scaphoid bone
	    Trapezium bone
	    Trapezoid bone
	    Triquetral bone
	N Carpal, Left
	    See M Carpal, Right
	P Metacarpal, Right
	Q Metacarpal, Left
	R Thumb Phalanx, Right
	S Thumb Phalanx, Left
	T Finger Phalanx, Right
	V Finger Phalanx, Left
		Ø Open
		3 Percutaneous
		4 Percutaneous Endoscopic
			Z No Device	**Z** No Qualifier

Ø **Medical and Surgical**
P **Upper Bones**
P **Removal**   Definition: Taking out or off a device from a body part

Explanation: If a device is taken out and a similar device put in without cutting or puncturing the skin or mucous membrane, the procedure is coded to the root operation CHANGE. Otherwise, the procedure for taking out a device is coded to the root operation REMOVAL.

Body Part Character 4		Approach Character 5	Device Character 6	Qualifier Character 7
Ø Sternum Manubrium Suprasternal notch Xiphoid process **1 Ribs, 1 to 2** **2 Ribs, 3 or More** **3 Cervical Vertebra** Dens Odontoid process Spinous process Transverse foramen Transverse process Vertebral arch Vertebral body Vertebral foramen Vertebral lamina Vertebral pedicle	**4 Thoracic Vertebra** Spinous process Transverse process Vertebral arch Vertebral body Vertebral foramen Vertebral lamina Vertebral pedicle **5 Scapula, Right** Acromion (process) Coracoid process **6 Scapula, Left** *See 5 Scapula, Right* **7 Glenoid Cavity, Right** Glenoid fossa (of scapula) **8 Glenoid Cavity, Left** *See 7 Glenoid Cavity, Right* **9 Clavicle, Right** **B Clavicle, Left**	**Ø Open** **3 Percutaneous** **4 Percutaneous Endoscopic**	**4 Internal Fixation Device** **7 Autologous Tissue Substitute** **J Synthetic Substitute** **K Nonautologous Tissue Substitute**	**Z No Qualifier**
Ø Sternum Manubrium Suprasternal notch Xiphoid process **1 Ribs, 1 to 2** **2 Ribs, 3 or More** **3 Cervical Vertebra** Dens Odontoid process Spinous process Transverse foramen Transverse process Vertebral arch Vertebral body Vertebral foramen Vertebral lamina Vertebral pedicle	**4 Thoracic Vertebra** Spinous process Transverse process Vertebral arch Vertebral body Vertebral foramen Vertebral lamina Vertebral pedicle **5 Scapula, Right** Acromion (process) Coracoid process **6 Scapula, Left** *See 5 Scapula, Right* **7 Glenoid Cavity, Right** Glenoid fossa (of scapula) **8 Glenoid Cavity, Left** *See 7 Glenoid Cavity, Right* **9 Clavicle, Right** **B Clavicle, Left**	**X External**	**4 Internal Fixation Device**	**Z No Qualifier**
C Humeral Head, Right Greater tuberosity Lesser tuberosity Neck of humerus (anatomical) (surgical) **D Humeral Head, Left** *See C Humeral Head, Right* **F Humeral Shaft, Right** Distal humerus Humerus, distal Lateral epicondyle of humerus Medial epicondyle of humerus **G Humeral Shaft, Left** *See F Humeral Shaft, Right* **H Radius, Right** Ulnar notch **J Radius, Left** *See H Radius, Right* **K Ulna, Right** Olecranon process Radial notch	**L Ulna, Left** *See K Ulna, Right* **M Carpal, Right** Capitate bone Hamate bone Lunate bone Pisiform bone Scaphoid bone Trapezium bone Trapezoid bone Triquetral bone **N Carpal, Left** *See M Carpal, Right* **P Metacarpal, Right** **Q Metacarpal, Left** **R Thumb Phalanx, Right** **S Thumb Phalanx, Left** **T Finger Phalanx, Right** **V Finger Phalanx, Left**	**Ø Open** **3 Percutaneous** **4 Percutaneous Endoscopic**	**4 Internal Fixation Device** **5 External Fixation Device** **7 Autologous Tissue Substitute** **J Synthetic Substitute** **K Nonautologous Tissue Substitute**	**Z No Qualifier**

ØPP Continued on next page

Non-OR   ØPP[Ø,1,2,3,4,5,6,7,8,9,B]X4Z

LC Limited Coverage   **NC** Noncovered   ⊞ Combination Member   HAC associated procedure   Combination Only   DRG Non-OR   Non-OR   New/Revised in GREEN

ICD-10-PCS 2019   533

ØPP–ØPP

Ø   Medical and Surgical
P   Upper Bones
P   Removal

Definition: Taking out or off a device from a body part

Explanation: If a device is taken out and a similar device put in without cutting or puncturing the skin or mucous membrane, the procedure is coded to the root operation CHANGE. Otherwise, the procedure for taking out a device is coded to the root operation REMOVAL.

Body Part Character 4		Approach Character 5	Device Character 6	Qualifier Character 7
C Humeral Head, Right 　　Greater tuberosity 　　Lesser tuberosity 　　Neck of humerus 　　　(anatomical) (surgical) **D Humeral Head, Left** 　　*See C Humeral Head, Right* **F Humeral Shaft, Right** 　　Distal humerus 　　Humerus, distal 　　Lateral epicondyle of 　　　humerus 　　Medial epicondyle of 　　　humerus **G Humeral Shaft, Left** 　　*See F Humeral Shaft, Right* **H Radius, Right** 　　Ulnar notch **J Radius, Left** 　　*See H Radius, Right* **K Ulna, Right** 　　Olecranon process 　　Radial notch	**L Ulna, Left** 　　*See K Ulna, Right* **M Carpal, Right** 　　Capitate bone 　　Hamate bone 　　Lunate bone 　　Pisiform bone 　　Scaphoid bone 　　Trapezium bone 　　Trapezoid bone 　　Triquetral bone **N Carpal, Left** 　　*See M Carpal, Right* **P Metacarpal, Right** **Q Metacarpal, Left** **R Thumb Phalanx, Right** **S Thumb Phalanx, Left** **T Finger Phalanx, Right** **V Finger Phalanx, Left**	**X External**	**4 Internal Fixation Device** **5 External Fixation Device**	**Z No Qualifier**
Y Upper Bone		**Ø Open** **3 Percutaneous** **4 Percutaneous Endoscopic** **X External**	**Ø Drainage Device** **M Bone Growth Stimulator**	**Z No Qualifier**

Non-OR　ØPP[C,D,F,G,H,J,K,L,M,N,P,Q,R,S,T,V]X[4,5]Z
Non-OR　ØPPY3ØZ
Non-OR　ØPPYX[Ø,M]Z

Ø   Medical and Surgical
P   Upper Bones
Q   Repair   Definition: Restoring, to the extent possible, a body part to its normal anatomic structure and function
                Explanation: Used only when the method to accomplish the repair is not one of the other root operations

Body Part		Approach	Device	Qualifier
Character 4		**Character 5**	**Character 6**	**Character 7**

Ø Sternum
 Manubrium
 Suprasternal notch
 Xiphoid process
 1 Ribs, 1 to 2
 2 Ribs, 3 or More
 3 Cervical Vertebra
 Dens
 Odontoid process
 Spinous process
 Transverse foramen
 Transverse process
 Vertebral arch
 Vertebral body
 Vertebral foramen
 Vertebral lamina
 Vertebral pedicle
 4 Thoracic Vertebra
 Spinous process
 Transverse process
 Vertebral arch
 Vertebral body
 Vertebral foramen
 Vertebral lamina
 Vertebral pedicle
 5 Scapula, Right
 Acromion (process)
 Coracoid process
 6 Scapula, Left
 See 5 Scapula, Right
 7 Glenoid Cavity, Right
 Glenoid fossa (of scapula)
 8 Glenoid Cavity, Left
 See 7 Glenoid Cavity, Right
 9 Clavicle, Right
 B Clavicle, Left
 C Humeral Head, Right
 Greater tuberosity
 Lesser tuberosity
 Neck of humerus
   (anatomical)(surgical)
 D Humeral Head, Left
 See C Humeral Head, Right
	F Humeral Shaft, Right
	 Distal humerus
	 Humerus, distal
	 Lateral epicondyle of
	   humerus
	 Medial epicondyle of
	   humerus
	 G Humeral Shaft, Left
	 See F Humeral Shaft, Right
	 H Radius, Right
	 Ulnar notch
	 J Radius, Left
	 See H Radius, Right
	 K Ulna, Right
	 Olecranon process
	 Radial notch
	 L Ulna, Left
	 See K Ulna, Right
	 M Carpal, Right
	 Capitate bone
	 Hamate bone
	 Lunate bone
	 Pisiform bone
	 Scaphoid bone
	 Trapezium bone
	 Trapezoid bone
	 Triquetral bone
	 N Carpal, Left
	 See M Carpal, Right
	 P Metacarpal, Right
	 Q Metacarpal, Left
	 R Thumb Phalanx, Right
	 S Thumb Phalanx, Left
	 T Finger Phalanx, Right
	 V Finger Phalanx, Left
		Ø Open
		 3 Percutaneous
		 4 Percutaneous Endoscopic
		 X External
			Z No Device	**Z No Qualifier**

Non-OR   ØPQ[Ø,1,2,3,4,5,6,7,8,9,B,C,D,F,G,H,J,K,L,M,N,P,Q,R,S,T,V]XZZ

LC Limited Coverage   NC Noncovered   ⊞ Combination Member   HAC associated procedure   Combination Only   DRG Non-OR   Non-OR   New/Revised in GREEN

ICD-10-PCS 2019   535

ØPQ–ØPQ

Ø   Medical and Surgical
P   Upper Bones
R   Replacement   Definition: Putting in or on biological or synthetic material that physically takes the place and/or function of all or a portion of a body part

Explanation: The body part may have been taken out or replaced, or may be taken out, physically eradicated, or rendered nonfunctional during the REPLACEMENT procedure. A REMOVAL procedure is coded for taking out the device used in a previous replacement procedure.

Body Part Character 4		Approach Character 5	Device Character 6	Qualifier Character 7

Ø   Sternum
    Manubrium
    Suprasternal notch
    Xiphoid process
1   Ribs, 1 to 2
2   Ribs, 3 or More
3   Cervical Vertebra
    Dens
    Odontoid process
    Spinous process
    Transverse foramen
    Transverse process
    Vertebral arch
    Vertebral body
    Vertebral foramen
    Vertebral lamina
    Vertebral pedicle
4   Thoracic Vertebra
    Spinous process
    Transverse process
    Vertebral arch
    Vertebral body
    Vertebral foramen
    Vertebral lamina
    Vertebral pedicle
5   Scapula, Right
    Acromion (process)
    Coracoid process
6   Scapula, Left
    See 5 Scapula, Right
7   Glenoid Cavity, Right
    Glenoid fossa (of scapula)
8   Glenoid Cavity, Left
    See 7 Glenoid Cavity, Right
9   Clavicle, Right
B   Clavicle, Left
C   Humeral Head, Right
    Greater tuberosity
    Lesser tuberosity
    Neck of humerus
      (anatomical)(surgical)
D   Humeral Head, Left
    See C Humeral Head, Right
	F Humeral Shaft, Right
	    Distal humerus
	    Humerus, distal
	    Lateral epicondyle of
	      humerus
	    Medial epicondyle of
	      humerus
	G Humeral Shaft, Left
	    See F Humeral Shaft, Right
	H Radius, Right
	    Ulnar notch
	J Radius, Left
	    See H Radius, Right
	K Ulna, Right
	    Olecranon process
	    Radial notch
	L Ulna, Left
	    See K Ulna, Right
	M Carpal, Right
	    Capitate bone
	    Hamate bone
	    Lunate bone
	    Pisiform bone
	    Scaphoid bone
	    Trapezium bone
	    Trapezoid bone
	    Triquetral bone
	N Carpal, Left
	    See M Carpal, Right
	P Metacarpal, Right
	Q Metacarpal, Left
	R Thumb Phalanx, Right
	S Thumb Phalanx, Left
	T Finger Phalanx, Right
	V Finger Phalanx, Left
		Ø Open
		3 Percutaneous
		4 Percutaneous Endoscopic
			**7 Autologous Tissue
			    Substitute**
			J Synthetic Substitute
			**K Nonautologous Tissue
			    Substitute**
				Z No Qualifier

LC Limited Coverage   NC Noncovered   ⊞ Combination Member   HAC associated procedure   Combination Only   DRG Non-OR   Non-OR   New/Revised in GREEN

536   ICD-10-PCS 2019

ØPR–ØPR

Ø **Medical and Surgical**
P **Upper Bones**
S **Reposition**   Definition: Moving to its normal location, or other suitable location, all or a portion of a body part

Explanation: The body part is moved to a new location from an abnormal location, or from a normal location where it is not functioning correctly. The body part may or may not be cut out or off to be moved to the new location.

Body Part — Character 4		Approach — Character 5	Device — Character 6	Qualifier — Character 7
Ø **Sternum** Manubrium Suprasternal notch Xiphoid process		Ø Open 3 Percutaneous 4 Percutaneous Endoscopic	Ø Internal Fixation Device, Rigid Plate 4 Internal Fixation Device Z No Device	Z No Qualifier
Ø **Sternum** Manubrium Suprasternal notch Xiphoid process		X External	Z No Device	Z No Qualifier
1 **Ribs, 1 to 2** 2 **Ribs, 3 or More** 3 **Cervical Vertebra** ⊞ Dens Odontoid process Spinous process Transverse foramen Transverse process Vertebral arch Vertebral body Vertebral foramen Vertebral lamina Vertebral pedicle 4 **Thoracic Vertebra** ⊞ Spinous process Transverse process Vertebral arch Vertebral body Vertebral foramen Vertebral lamina Vertebral pedicle	5 **Scapula, Right** Acromion (process) Coracoid process 6 **Scapula, Left** *See 5 Scapula, Right* 7 **Glenoid Cavity, Right** Glenoid fossa (of scapula) 8 **Glenoid Cavity, Left** *See 7 Glenoid Cavity, Right* 9 **Clavicle, Right** B **Clavicle, Left**	Ø Open 3 Percutaneous 4 Percutaneous Endoscopic	4 Internal Fixation Device Z No Device	Z No Qualifier
1 **Ribs, 1 to 2** 2 **Ribs, 3 or More** 3 **Cervical Vertebra** Dens Odontoid process Spinous process Transverse foramen Transverse process Vertebral arch Vertebral body Vertebral foramen Vertebral lamina Vertebral pedicle 4 **Thoracic Vertebra** Spinous process Transverse process Vertebral arch Vertebral body Vertebral foramen Vertebral lamina Vertebral pedicle	5 **Scapula, Right** Acromion (process) Coracoid process 6 **Scapula, Left** *See 5 Scapula, Right* 7 **Glenoid Cavity, Right** Glenoid fossa (of scapula) 8 **Glenoid Cavity, Left** *See 7 Glenoid Cavity, Right* 9 **Clavicle, Right** B **Clavicle, Left**	X External	Z No Device	Z No Qualifier
C **Humeral Head, Right** Greater tuberosity Lesser tuberosity Neck of humerus (anatomical)(surgical) D **Humeral Head, Left** *See C Humeral Head, Right* F **Humeral Shaft, Right** Distal humerus Humerus, distal Lateral epicondyle of humerus Medial epicondyle of humerus	G **Humeral Shaft, Left** *See F Humeral Shaft, Right* H **Radius, Right** Ulnar notch J **Radius, Left** *See H Radius, Right* K **Ulna, Right** Olecranon process Radial notch L **Ulna, Left** *See K Ulna, Right*	Ø Open 3 Percutaneous 4 Percutaneous Endoscopic	4 Internal Fixation Device 5 External Fixation Device 6 Internal Fixation Device, Intramedullary B External Fixation Device, Monoplanar C External Fixation Device, Ring D External Fixation Device, Hybrid Z No Device	Z No Qualifier

ØPS Continued on next page

Non-OR ØPSØ[3,4]ZZ	
Non-OR ØPSØXZZ	**See Appendix L for Procedure Combinations**
Non-OR ØPS[1,2,5,6,7,8,9,B][3,4]ZZ	⊞ ØPS[3,4]3ZZ
Non-OR ØPS[1,2,3,4,5,6,7,8,9,B]XZZ	
Non-OR ØPS[C,D,F,G,H,J,K,L][3,4]ZZ	

LC Limited Coverage   **NC** Noncovered   ⊞ Combination Member   HAC associated procedure   Combination Only   DRG Non-OR   Non-OR   New/Revised in GREEN

Upper Bones

ØPS Continued

Ø **Medical and Surgical**
P **Upper Bones**
S **Reposition**   Definition: Moving to its normal location, or other suitable location, all or a portion of a body part

Explanation: The body part is moved to a new location from an abnormal location, or from a normal location where it is not functioning correctly. The body part may or may not be cut out or off to be moved to the new location.

Body Part Character 4		Approach Character 5	Device Character 6	Qualifier Character 7

C Humeral Head, Right
 Greater tuberosity
 Lesser tuberosity
 Neck of humerus
   (anatomical)(surgical)
 D Humeral Head, Left
 See C Humeral Head, Right
 F Humeral Shaft, Right
 Distal humerus
 Humerus, distal
 Lateral epicondyle of
   humerus
 Medial epicondyle of
   humerus
	G Humeral Shaft, Left
	 See F Humeral Shaft, Right
	 H Radius, Right
	 Ulnar notch
	 J Radius, Left
	 See H Radius, Right
	 K Ulna, Right
	 Olecranon process
	 Radial notch
	 L Ulna, Left
	 See K Ulna, Right
		X External	**Z No Device**	**Z No Qualifier**

M Carpal, Right Capitate bone Hamate bone Lunate bone Pisiform bone Scaphoid bone Trapezium bone Trapezoid bone Triquetral bone	**N Carpal, Left** *See M Carpal, Right* **P Metacarpal, Right** **Q Metacarpal, Left** **R Thumb Phalanx, Right** **S Thumb Phalanx, Left** **T Finger Phalanx, Right** **V Finger Phalanx, Left**	**Ø Open** **3 Percutaneous** **4 Percutaneous Endoscopic**	**4 Internal Fixation Device** **5 External Fixation Device** **Z No Device**	**Z No Qualifier**
M Carpal, Right Capitate bone Hamate bone Lunate bone Pisiform bone Scaphoid bone Trapezium bone Trapezoid bone Triquetral bone	**N Carpal, Left** *See M Carpal, Right* **P Metacarpal, Right** **Q Metacarpal, Left** **R Thumb Phalanx, Right** **S Thumb Phalanx, Left** **T Finger Phalanx, Right** **V Finger Phalanx, Left**	**X External**	**Z No Device**	**Z No Qualifier**

Non-OR   ØPS[C,D,F,G,H,J,K,L]XZZ
Non-OR   ØPS[M,N,P,Q,R,S,T,V][3,4]ZZ
Non-OR   ØPS[M,N,P,Q,R,S,T,V]XZZ

Ø **Medical and Surgical**
P **Upper Bones**
T **Resection**   Definition: Cutting out or off, without replacement, all of a body part

Explanation: None

Body Part Character 4		Approach Character 5	Device Character 6	Qualifier Character 7
Ø Sternum Manubrium Suprasternal notch Xiphoid process **1 Ribs, 1 to 2** **2 Ribs, 3 or More** **5 Scapula, Right** Acromion (process) Coracoid process **6 Scapula, Left** *See 5 Scapula, Right* **7 Glenoid Cavity, Right** Glenoid fossa (of scapula) **8 Glenoid Cavity, Left** *See 7 Glenoid Cavity, Right* **9 Clavicle, Right** **B Clavicle, Left** **C Humeral Head, Right** Greater tuberosity Lesser tuberosity Neck of humerus (anatomical) (surgical) **D Humeral Head, Left** *See C Humeral Head, Right* **F Humeral Shaft, Right** Distal humerus Humerus, distal Lateral epicondyle of humerus Medial epicondyle of humerus	**G Humeral Shaft, Left** *See F Humeral Shaft, Right* **H Radius, Right** Ulnar notch **J Radius, Left** *See H Radius, Right* **K Ulna, Right** Olecranon process Radial notch **L Ulna, Left** *See K Ulna, Right* **M Carpal, Right** Capitate bone Hamate bone Lunate bone Pisiform bone Scaphoid bone Trapezium bone Trapezoid bone Triquetral bone **N Carpal, Left** *See M Carpal, Right* **P Metacarpal, Right** **Q Metacarpal, Left** **R Thumb Phalanx, Right** **S Thumb Phalanx, Left** **T Finger Phalanx, Right** **V Finger Phalanx, Left**	**Ø Open**	**Z No Device**	**Z No Qualifier**

LC Limited Coverage   **NC** Noncovered   ⊞ Combination Member   HAC associated procedure   Combination Only   DRG Non-OR   Non-OR   New/Revised in GREEN

538   ICD-10-PCS 2019

ØPS–ØPT

Ø   Medical and Surgical
P   Upper Bones
U   Supplement   Definition: Putting in or on biological or synthetic material that physically reinforces and/or augments the function of a portion of a body part
                              Explanation: The biological material is non-living, or is living and from the same individual. The body part may have been previously replaced, and the SUPPLEMENT procedure is performed to physically reinforce and/or augment the function of the replaced body part.

Body Part Character 4		Approach Character 5	Device Character 6	Qualifier Character 7

Ø Sternum
   Manubrium
   Suprasternal notch
   Xiphoid process
1 Ribs, 1 to 2
2 Ribs, 3 or More
3 Cervical Vertebra ⊞
   Dens
   Odontoid process
   Spinous process
   Transverse foramen
   Transverse process
   Vertebral arch
   Vertebral body
   Vertebral foramen
   Vertebral lamina
   Vertebral pedicle
4 Thoracic Vertebra ⊞
   Spinous process
   Transverse process
   Vertebral arch
   Vertebral body
   Vertebral foramen
   Vertebral lamina
   Vertebral pedicle
5 Scapula, Right
   Acromion (process)
   Coracoid process
6 Scapula, Left
   See 5 Scapula, Right
7 Glenoid Cavity, Right
   Glenoid fossa (of scapula)
8 Glenoid Cavity, Left
   See 7 Glenoid Cavity, Right
9 Clavicle, Right
B Clavicle, Left
C Humeral Head, Right
   Greater tuberosity
   Lesser tuberosity
   Neck of humerus
     (anatomical) (surgical)
	D Humeral Head, Left
	   See C Humeral Head, Right
	F Humeral Shaft, Right
	   Distal humerus
	   Humerus, distal
	   Lateral epicondyle of
	     humerus
	   Medial epicondyle of
	     humerus
	G Humeral Shaft, Left
	   See F Humeral Shaft, Right
	H Radius, Right
	   Ulnar notch
	J Radius, Left
	   See H Radius, Right
	K Ulna, Right
	   Olecranon process
	   Radial notch
	L Ulna, Left
	   See K Ulna, Right
	M Carpal, Right
	   Capitate bone
	   Hamate bone
	   Lunate bone
	   Pisiform bone
	   Scaphoid bone
	   Trapezium bone
	   Trapezoid bone
	   Triquetral bone
	N Carpal, Left
	   See M Carpal, Right
	P Metacarpal, Right
	Q Metacarpal, Left
	R Thumb Phalanx, Right
	S Thumb Phalanx, Left
	T Finger Phalanx, Right
	V Finger Phalanx, Left
		Ø Open
		3 Percutaneous
		4 Percutaneous Endoscopic
			7 Autologous Tissue
			   Substitute
			J Synthetic Substitute
			K Nonautologous Tissue
			   Substitute
				Z No Qualifier

See Appendix L for Procedure Combinations
   ⊞   ØPU[3,4]3JZ

Upper Bones

Ø Medical and Surgical
P Upper Bones
W Revision Definition: Correcting, to the extent possible, a portion of a malfunctioning device or the position of a displaced device

Explanation: Revision can include correcting a malfunctioning or displaced device by taking out or putting in components of the device such as a screw or pin

Body Part Character 4		Approach Character 5	Device Character 6	Qualifier Character 7
Ø Sternum Manubrium Suprasternal notch Xiphoid process **1 Ribs, 1 to 2** **2 Ribs, 3 or More** **3 Cervical Vertebra** Dens Odontoid process Spinous process Transverse foramen Transverse process Vertebral arch Vertebral body Vertebral foramen Vertebral lamina Vertebral pedicle **4 Thoracic Vertebra** Spinous process Transverse process Vertebral arch Vertebral body Vertebral foramen Vertebral lamina Vertebral pedicle	**5 Scapula, Right** Acromion (process) Coracoid process **6 Scapula, Left** *See 5 Scapula, Right* **7 Glenoid Cavity, Right** Glenoid fossa (of scapula) **8 Glenoid Cavity, Left** *See 7 Glenoid Cavity, Right* **9 Clavicle, Right** **B Clavicle, Left**	**Ø Open** **3 Percutaneous** **4 Percutaneous Endoscopic** **X External**	**4 Internal Fixation Device** **7 Autologous Tissue Substitute** **J Synthetic Substitute** **K Nonautologous Tissue Substitute**	**Z No Qualifier**
C Humeral Head, Right Greater tuberosity Lesser tuberosity Neck of humerus (anatomical)(surgical) **D Humeral Head, Left** *See C Humeral Head, Right* **F Humeral Shaft, Right** Distal humerus Humerus, distal Lateral epicondyle of humerus Medial epicondyle of humerus **G Humeral Shaft, Left** *See F Humeral Shaft, Right* **H Radius, Right** Ulnar notch **J Radius, Left** *See H Radius, Right* **K Ulna, Right** Olecranon process Radial notch	**L Ulna, Left** *See K Ulna, Right* **M Carpal, Right** Capitate bone Hamate bone Lunate bone Pisiform bone Scaphoid bone Trapezium bone Trapezoid bone Triquetral bone **N Carpal, Left** *See M Carpal, Right* **P Metacarpal, Right** **Q Metacarpal, Left** **R Thumb Phalanx, Right** **S Thumb Phalanx, Left** **T Finger Phalanx, Right** **V Finger Phalanx, Left**	**Ø Open** **3 Percutaneous** **4 Percutaneous Endoscopic** **X External**	**4 Internal Fixation Device** **5 External Fixation Device** **7 Autologous Tissue Substitute** **J Synthetic Substitute** **K Nonautologous Tissue Substitute**	**Z No Qualifier**
Y Upper Bone		**Ø Open** **3 Percutaneous** **4 Percutaneous Endoscopic** **X External**	**Ø Drainage Device** **M Bone Growth Stimulator**	**Z No Qualifier**

Non-OR ØPW[Ø,1,2,3,4,5,6,7,8,9,B]X[4,7,J,K]Z
Non-OR ØPW[C,D,F,G,H,J,K,L,M,N,P,Q,R,S,T,V]X[4,5,7,J,K]Z
Non-OR ØPWYX[Ø,M]Z

Lower Bones ØQ2–ØQW

Character Meanings

This Character Meaning table is provided as a guide to assist the user in the identification of character members that may be found in this section of code tables. It **SHOULD NOT** be used to build a PCS code.

Operation–Character 3		Body Part–Character 4		Approach–Character 5		Device–Character 6		Qualifier–Character 7	
2	Change	Ø	Lumbar Vertebra	Ø	Open	Ø	Drainage Device	2	Sesamoid Bone(s) 1st Toe
5	Destruction	1	Sacrum	3	Percutaneous	4	Internal Fixation Device	X	Diagnostic
8	Division	2	Pelvic Bone, Right	4	Percutaneous Endoscopic	5	External Fixation Device	Z	No Qualifier
9	Drainage	3	Pelvic Bone, Left	X	External	6	Internal Fixation Device, Intramedullary		
B	Excision	4	Acetabulum, Right			7	Autologous Tissue Substitute		
C	Extirpation	5	Acetabulum, Left			8	External Fixation Device, Limb Lengthening		
D	Extraction	6	Upper Femur, Right			B	External Fixation Device, Monoplanar		
H	Insertion	7	Upper Femur, Left			C	External Fixation Device, Ring		
J	Inspection	8	Femoral Shaft, Right			D	External Fixation Device, Hybrid		
N	Release	9	Femoral Shaft, Left			J	Synthetic Substitute		
P	Removal	B	Lower Femur, Right			K	Nonautologous Tissue Substitute		
Q	Repair	C	Lower Femur, Left			M	Bone Growth Stimulator		
R	Replacement	D	Patella, Right			Y	Other Device		
S	Reposition	F	Patella, Left			Z	No Device		
T	Resection	G	Tibia, Right						
U	Supplement	H	Tibia, Left						
W	Revision	J	Fibula, Right						
		K	Fibula, Left						
		L	Tarsal, Right						
		M	Tarsal, Left						
		N	Metatarsal, Right						
		P	Metatarsal, Left						
		Q	Toe Phalanx, Right						
		R	Toe Phalanx, Left						
		S	Coccyx						
		Y	Lower Bone						

AHA Coding Clinic for table ØQ8

| 2018, 1Q, 25 | Periacetabular ostectomy for repair of congenital hip dysplasia |
| 2016, 2Q, 31 | Periacetabular ostectomy for repair of congenital hip dysplasia |

AHA Coding Clinic for table ØQB

2017, 1Q, 23	Reconstruction of mandible using titanium and bone
2016, 3Q, 30	Resection of femur with interposition arthroplasty
2015, 3Q, 3-8	Excisional and nonexcisional debridement
2015, 3Q, 26	Femoral head resection
2015, 2Q, 34	Decompressive laminectomy
2014, 4Q, 25	Femoroacetabular impingement and labral tear with repair
2014, 2Q, 6	Posterior lumbar fusion with discectomy
2013, 4Q, 116	Spinal decompression
2013, 2Q, 39	Ankle fusion, osteotomy, and removal of hardware
2012, 2Q, 19	Multiple decompressive cervical laminectomies

AHA Coding Clinic for table ØQD

| 2017, 4Q, 41 | Extraction procedures |

AHA Coding Clinic for table ØQH

| 2017, 1Q, 21 | Staged scoliosis surgery with iliac fixation and spinal fusion |
| 2016, 3Q, 34 | Tibial/fibula epiphysiodesis |

AHA Coding Clinic for table ØQP

| 2017, 4Q, 74-75 | Magnetic growth rods |
| 2015, 2Q, 6 | Planned implant break |

AHA Coding Clinic for table ØQQ

| 2018, 1Q, 15 | Pubic symphysis fusion |
| 2014, 3Q, 24 | Repair of lipomyelomeningocele and tethered cord |

AHA Coding Clinic for table ØQR

| 2017, 1Q, 22 | Total knee replacement and patellar component |
| 2016, 3Q, 30 | Resection of femur with interposition arthroplasty |

AHA Coding Clinic for table ØQS

2018, 1Q, 13	Bilateral cuboid osteotomy for repair of congenital talipes equinovarus
2018, 1Q, 25	Periacetabular osteotomy for repair of congenital hip dysplasia
2016, 3Q, 34	Tibial/fibula epiphysiodesis
2014, 4Q, 29	Rotational osteosynthesis
2014, 4Q, 31	Reposition of femur for correction of valgus and recurvatum deformities

AHA Coding Clinic for table ØQT

2017, 1Q, 22	Chopart amputation of foot
2016, 3Q, 30	Resection of femur with interposition arthroplasty
2015, 3Q, 26	Femoral head resection
2014, 4Q, 29	Rotational osteosynthesis

AHA Coding Clinic for table ØQU

2015, 3Q, 18	Total hip replacement with acetabular reconstruction
2014, 4Q, 31	Reposition of femur for correction of valgus and recurvatum deformities
2014, 2Q, 12	Percutaneous vertebroplasty using cement
2013, 2Q, 35	Use of bone void filler in grafting

AHA Coding Clinic for table ØQW

| 2017, 4Q, 74-75 | Magnetic growth rods |

Lower Bones

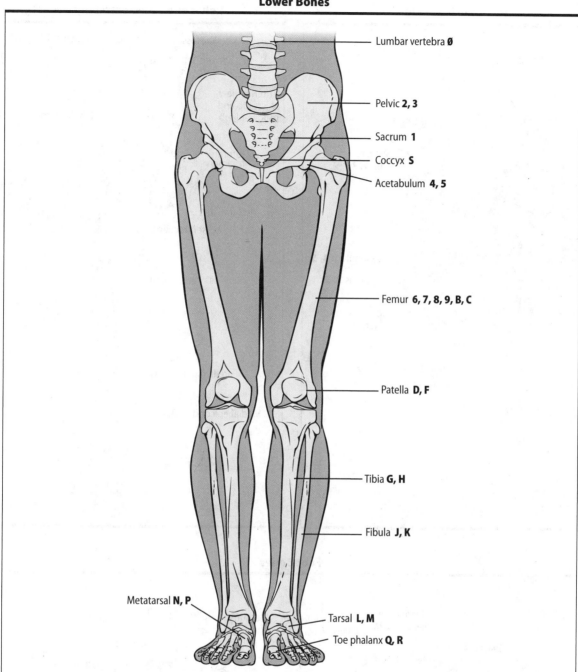

Lumbar vertebra **Ø**

Pelvic **2, 3**

Sacrum **1**

Coccyx **S**

Acetabulum **4, 5**

Femur **6, 7, 8, 9, B, C**

Patella **D, F**

Tibia **G, H**

Fibula **J, K**

Metatarsal **N, P**

Tarsal **L, M**

Toe phalanx **Q, R**

Hip Bone Anatomy

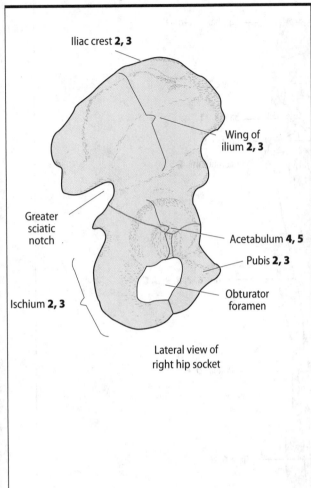

Iliac crest **2, 3**

Wing of ilium **2, 3**

Greater sciatic notch

Acetabulum **4, 5**

Pubis **2, 3**

Obturator foramen

Ischium **2, 3**

Lateral view of right hip socket

Pelvic and Lower Extremity Bones

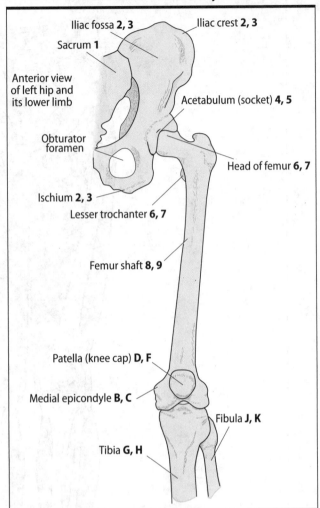

Iliac fossa **2, 3**

Iliac crest **2, 3**

Sacrum **1**

Anterior view of left hip and its lower limb

Obturator foramen

Acetabulum (socket) **4, 5**

Head of femur **6, 7**

Ischium **2, 3**

Lesser trochanter **6, 7**

Femur shaft **8, 9**

Patella (knee cap) **D, F**

Medial epicondyle **B, C**

Fibula **J, K**

Tibia **G, H**

Foot Bones

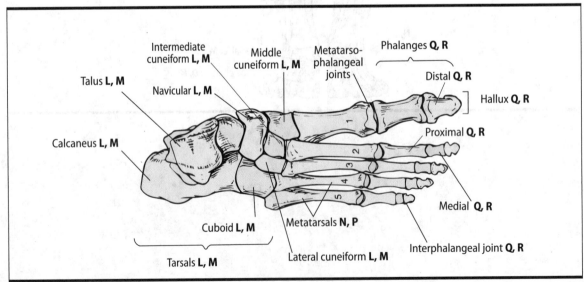

Intermediate cuneiform **L, M**

Middle cuneiform **L, M**

Metatarso-phalangeal joints

Phalanges **Q, R**

Talus **L, M**

Navicular **L, M**

Distal **Q, R**

Hallux **Q, R**

Calcaneus **L, M**

Proximal **Q, R**

Medial **Q, R**

Cuboid **L, M**

Metatarsals **N, P**

Interphalangeal joint **Q, R**

Tarsals **L, M**

Lateral cuneiform **L, M**

0   **Medical and Surgical**
Q   **Lower Bones**
2   **Change**   Definition: Taking out or off a device from a body part and putting back an identical or similar device in or on the same body part without cutting or puncturing the skin or a mucous membrane

           Explanation: All CHANGE procedures are coded using the approach EXTERNAL

Body Part Character 4	Approach Character 5	Device Character 6	Qualifier Character 7
Y Lower Bone	**X** External	**0** Drainage Device **Y** Other Device	**Z** No Qualifier

    Non-OR   All body part, approach, device, and qualifier values

0   **Medical and Surgical**
Q   **Lower Bones**
5   **Destruction**   Definition: Physical eradication of all or a portion of a body part by the direct use of energy, force, or a destructive agent

           Explanation: None of the body part is physically taken out

Body Part Character 4		Approach Character 5	Device Character 6	Qualifier Character 7

0   Lumbar Vertebra
    Spinous process
    Transverse process
    Vertebral arch
    Vertebral body
    Vertebral foramen
    Vertebral lamina
    Vertebral pedicle
1   Sacrum
2   Pelvic Bone, Right
    Iliac crest
    Ilium
    Ischium
    Pubis
3   Pelvic Bone, Left
    See 2 Pelvic Bone, Right
4   Acetabulum, Right
5   Acetabulum, Left
6   Upper Femur, Right
    Femoral head
    Greater trochanter
    Lesser trochanter
    Neck of femur
7   Upper Femur, Left
    See 6 Upper Femur, Right
8   Femoral Shaft, Right
    Body of femur
9   Femoral Shaft, Left
    See 8 Femoral Shaft, Right
B   Lower Femur, Right
    Lateral condyle of femur
    Lateral epicondyle of femur
    Medial condyle of femur
    Medial epicondyle of femur
C   Lower Femur, Left
    See B Lower Femur, Right
	D Patella, Right
	F Patella, Left
	G Tibia, Right
	    Lateral condyle of tibia
	    Medial condyle of tibia
	    Medial malleolus
	H Tibia, Left
	    See G Tibia, Right
	J Fibula, Right
	    Body of fibula
	    Head of fibula
	    Lateral malleolus
	K Fibula, Left
	    See J Fibula, Right
	L Tarsal, Right
	    Calcaneus
	    Cuboid bone
	    Intermediate cuneiform
	       bone
	    Lateral cuneiform bone
	    Medial cuneiform bone
	    Navicular bone
	    Talus bone
	M Tarsal, Left
	    See L Tarsal, Right
	N Metatarsal, Right
	P Metatarsal, Left
	Q Toe Phalanx, Right
	R Toe Phalanx, Left
	S Coccyx
		0 Open
		3 Percutaneous
		4 Percutaneous Endoscopic
			Z No Device	**Z** No Qualifier

0   Medical and Surgical
Q   Lower Bones
8   Division   Definition: Cutting into a body part, without draining fluids and/or gases from the body part, in order to separate or transect a body part
                 Explanation: All or a portion of the body part is separated into two or more portions

Body Part Character 4	Approach Character 5	Device Character 6	Qualifier Character 7

0 Lumbar Vertebra
  Spinous process
  Transverse process
  Vertebral arch
  Vertebral body
  Vertebral foramen
  Vertebral lamina
  Vertebral pedicle
1 Sacrum
2 Pelvic Bone, Right
  Iliac crest
  Ilium
  Ischium
  Pubis
3 Pelvic Bone, Left
  See 2 Pelvic Bone, Right
4 Acetabulum, Right
5 Acetabulum, Left
6 Upper Femur, Right
  Femoral head
  Greater trochanter
  Lesser trochanter
  Neck of femur
7 Upper Femur, Left
  See 6 Upper Femur, Right
8 Femoral Shaft, Right
  Body of femur
9 Femoral Shaft, Left
  See 8 Femoral Shaft, Right
B Lower Femur, Right
  Lateral condyle of femur
  Lateral epicondyle of femur
  Medial condyle of femur
  Medial epicondyle of femur
C Lower Femur, Left
  See B Lower Femur, Right
D Patella, Right
F Patella, Left
G Tibia, Right
  Lateral condyle of tibia
  Medial condyle of tibia
  Medial malleolus
H Tibia, Left
  See G Tibia, Right
J Fibula, Right
  Body of fibula
  Head of fibula
  Lateral malleolus
K Fibula, Left
  See J Fibula, Right
L Tarsal, Right
  Calcaneus
  Cuboid bone
  Intermediate cuneiform bone
  Lateral cuneiform bone
  Medial cuneiform bone
  Navicular bone
  Talus bone
M Tarsal, Left
  See L Tarsal, Right
N Metatarsal, Right
P Metatarsal, Left
Q Toe Phalanx, Right
R Toe Phalanx, Left
S Coccyx
	0 Open
	3 Percutaneous
	4 Percutaneous Endoscopic
		Z No Device	**Z No Qualifier**

LC Limited Coverage   **NC** Noncovered   ⊞ Combination Member   HAC associated procedure   Combination Only   DRG Non-OR   Non-OR   New/Revised in GREEN

546   ICD-10-PCS 2019

0   **Medical and Surgical**
Q   **Lower Bones**
9   **Drainage**   Definition: Taking or letting out fluids and/or gases from a body part

Explanation: The qualifier DIAGNOSTIC is used to identify drainage procedures that are biopsies

Body Part Character 4		Approach Character 5	Device Character 6	Qualifier Character 7
0 Lumbar Vertebra Spinous process Transverse process Vertebral arch Vertebral body Vertebral foramen Vertebral lamina Vertebral pedicle **1 Sacrum** **2 Pelvic Bone, Right** Iliac crest Ilium Ischium Pubis **3 Pelvic Bone, Left** *See 2 Pelvic Bone, Right* **4 Acetabulum, Right** **5 Acetabulum, Left** **6 Upper Femur, Right** Femoral head Greater trochanter Lesser trochanter Neck of femur **7 Upper Femur, Left** *See 6 Upper Femur, Right* **8 Femoral Shaft, Right** Body of femur **9 Femoral Shaft, Left** *See 8 Femoral Shaft, Right* **B Lower Femur, Right** Lateral condyle of femur Lateral epicondyle of femur Medial condyle of femur Medial epicondyle of femur	**C Lower Femur, Left** *See B Lower Femur, Right* **D Patella, Right** **F Patella, Left** **G Tibia, Right** Lateral condyle of tibia Medial condyle of tibia Medial malleolus **H Tibia, Left** *See G Tibia, Right* **J Fibula, Right** Body of fibula Head of fibula Lateral malleolus **K Fibula, Left** *See J Fibula, Right* **L Tarsal, Right** Calcaneus Cuboid bone Intermediate cuneiform bone Lateral cuneiform bone Medial cuneiform bone Navicular bone Talus bone **M Tarsal, Left** *See L Tarsal, Right* **N Metatarsal, Right** **P Metatarsal, Left** **Q Toe Phalanx, Right** **R Toe Phalanx, Left** **S Coccyx**	**0 Open** **3 Percutaneous** **4 Percutaneous Endoscopic**	**0 Drainage Device**	**Z No Qualifier**
0 Lumbar Vertebra Spinous process Transverse process Vertebral arch Vertebral body Vertebral foramen Vertebral lamina Vertebral pedicle **1 Sacrum** **2 Pelvic Bone, Right** Iliac crest Ilium Ischium Pubis **3 Pelvic Bone, Left** *See 2 Pelvic Bone, Right* **4 Acetabulum, Right** **5 Acetabulum, Left** **6 Upper Femur, Right** Femoral head Greater trochanter Lesser trochanter Neck of femur **7 Upper Femur, Left** *See 6 Upper Femur, Right* **8 Femoral Shaft, Right** Body of femur **9 Femoral Shaft, Left** *See 8 Femoral Shaft, Right* **B Lower Femur, Right** Lateral condyle of femur Lateral epicondyle of femur Medial condyle of femur Medial epicondyle of femur	**C Lower Femur, Left** *See B Lower Femur, Right* **D Patella, Right** **F Patella, Left** **G Tibia, Right** Lateral condyle of tibia Medial condyle of tibia Medial malleolus **H Tibia, Left** *See G Tibia, Right* **J Fibula, Right** Body of fibula Head of fibula Lateral malleolus **K Fibula, Left** *See J Fibula, Right* **L Tarsal, Right** Calcaneus Cuboid bone Intermediate cuneiform bone Lateral cuneiform bone Medial cuneiform bone Navicular bone Talus bone **M Tarsal, Left** *See L Tarsal, Right* **N Metatarsal, Right** **P Metatarsal, Left** **Q Toe Phalanx, Right** **R Toe Phalanx, Left** **S Coccyx**	**0 Open** **3 Percutaneous** **4 Percutaneous Endoscopic**	**Z No Device**	**X Diagnostic** **Z No Qualifier**

Non-OR   0Q9[0,1,2,3,4,5,6,7,8,9,B,C,D,F,G,H,J,K,L,M,P,Q,R,S]30Z
Non-OR   0Q9[0,1,2,3,4,5,6,7,8,9,B,C,D,F,G,H,J,K,L,M,P,Q,R,S]3ZZ

Lower Bones

0Q9–0Q9

Lower Bones

Ø **Medical and Surgical**
Q **Lower Bones**
B **Excision**　　　Definition: Cutting out or off, without replacement, a portion of a body part
　　　　　　　　　　　Explanation: The qualifier DIAGNOSTIC is used to identify excision procedures that are biopsies

Body Part Character 4	Approach Character 5	Device Character 6	Qualifier Character 7
Ø **Lumbar Vertebra** 　Spinous process 　Transverse process 　Vertebral arch 　Vertebral body 　Vertebral foramen 　Vertebral lamina 　Vertebral pedicle **1** **Sacrum** **2** **Pelvic Bone, Right** 　Iliac crest 　Ilium 　Ischium 　Pubis **3** **Pelvic Bone, Left** 　*See 2 Pelvic Bone, Right* **4** **Acetabulum, Right** **5** **Acetabulum, Left** **6** **Upper Femur, Right** 　Femoral head 　Greater trochanter 　Lesser trochanter 　Neck of femur **7** **Upper Femur, Left** 　*See 6 Upper Femur, Right* **8** **Femoral Shaft, Right** 　Body of femur **9** **Femoral Shaft, Left** 　*See 8 Femoral Shaft, Right* **B** **Lower Femur, Right** 　Lateral condyle of femur 　Lateral epicondyle of femur 　Medial condyle of femur 　Medial epicondyle of femur **C** **Lower Femur, Left** 　*See B Lower Femur, Right* **D** **Patella, Right** **F** **Patella, Left** **G** **Tibia, Right** 　Lateral condyle of tibia 　Medial condyle of tibia 　Medial malleolus **H** **Tibia, Left** 　*See G Tibia, Right* **J** **Fibula, Right** 　Body of fibula 　Head of fibula 　Lateral malleolus **K** **Fibula, Left** 　*See J Fibula, Right* **L** **Tarsal, Right** 　Calcaneus 　Cuboid bone 　Intermediate cuneiform bone 　Lateral cuneiform bone 　Medial cuneiform bone 　Navicular bone 　Talus bone **M** **Tarsal, Left** 　*See L Tarsal, Right* **N** **Metatarsal, Right** **P** **Metatarsal, Left** **Q** **Toe Phalanx, Right** **R** **Toe Phalanx, Left** **S** **Coccyx**	**Ø** Open **3** Percutaneous **4** Percutaneous Endoscopic	**Z** No Device	**X** Diagnostic **Z** No Qualifier

Lower Bones

0   Medical and Surgical
Q   Lower Bones
C   Extirpation   Definition: Taking or cutting out solid matter from a body part

Explanation: The solid matter may be an abnormal byproduct of a biological function or a foreign body; it may be imbedded in a body part or in the lumen of a tubular body part. The solid matter may or may not have been previously broken into pieces.

Body Part Character 4		Approach Character 5	Device Character 6	Qualifier Character 7

0   **Lumbar Vertebra**
    Spinous process
    Transverse process
    Vertebral arch
    Vertebral body
    Vertebral foramen
    Vertebral lamina
    Vertebral pedicle
1   **Sacrum**
2   **Pelvic Bone, Right**
    Iliac crest
    Ilium
    Ischium
    Pubis
3   **Pelvic Bone, Left**
    See 2 Pelvic Bone, Right
4   **Acetabulum, Right**
5   **Acetabulum, Left**
6   **Upper Femur, Right**
    Femoral head
    Greater trochanter
    Lesser trochanter
    Neck of femur
7   **Upper Femur, Left**
    See 6 Upper Femur, Right
8   **Femoral Shaft, Right**
    Body of femur
9   **Femoral Shaft, Left**
    See 8 Femoral Shaft, Right
B   **Lower Femur, Right**
    Lateral condyle of femur
    Lateral epicondyle of femur
    Medial condyle of femur
    Medial epicondyle of femur
	C **Lower Femur, Left**
	    See B Lower Femur, Right
	D **Patella, Right**
	F **Patella, Left**
	G **Tibia, Right**
	    Lateral condyle of tibia
	    Medial condyle of tibia
	    Medial malleolus
	H **Tibia, Left**
	    See G Tibia, Right
	J **Fibula, Right**
	    Body of fibula
	    Head of fibula
	    Lateral malleolus
	K **Fibula, Left**
	    See J Fibula, Right
	L **Tarsal, Right**
	    Calcaneus
	    Cuboid bone
	    Intermediate cuneiform bone
	    Lateral cuneiform bone
	    Medial cuneiform bone
	    Navicular bone
	    Talus bone
	M **Tarsal, Left**
	    See L Tarsal, Right
	N **Metatarsal, Right**
	P **Metatarsal, Left**
	Q **Toe Phalanx, Right**
	R **Toe Phalanx, Left**
	S **Coccyx**
		0 **Open**
		3 **Percutaneous**
		4 **Percutaneous Endoscopic**
			Z **No Device**	**Z** **No Qualifier**

0   Medical and Surgical
Q   Lower Bones
D   Extraction   Definition: Pulling or stripping out or off all or a portion of a body part by the use of force

Explanation: The qualifier DIAGNOSTIC is used to identify extraction procedures that are biopsies

Body Part Character 4		Approach Character 5	Device Character 6	Qualifier Character 7

0   **Lumbar Vertebra**
    Spinous process
    Transverse process
    Vertebral arch
    Vertebral body
    Vertebral foramen
    Vertebral lamina
    Vertebral pedicle
1   **Sacrum**
2   **Pelvic Bone, Right**
    Iliac crest
    Ilium
    Ischium
    Pubis
3   **Pelvic Bone, Left**
    See 2 Pelvic Bone, Right
4   **Acetabulum, Right**
5   **Acetabulum, Left**
6   **Upper Femur, Right**
    Femoral head
    Greater trochanter
    Lesser trochanter
    Neck of femur
7   **Upper Femur, Left**
    See 6 Upper Femur, Right
8   **Femoral Shaft, Right**
    Body of femur
9   **Femoral Shaft, Left**
    See 8 Femoral Shaft, Right
B   **Lower Femur, Right**
    Lateral condyle of femur
    Lateral epicondyle of femur
    Medial condyle of femur
    Medial epicondyle of femur
	C **Lower Femur, Left**
	    See B Lower Femur, Right
	D **Patella, Right**
	F **Patella, Left**
	G **Tibia, Right**
	    Lateral condyle of tibia
	    Medial condyle of tibia
	    Medial malleolus
	H **Tibia, Left**
	    See G Tibia, Right
	J **Fibula, Right**
	    Body of fibula
	    Head of fibula
	    Lateral malleolus
	K **Fibula, Left**
	    See J Fibula, Right
	L **Tarsal, Right**
	    Calcaneus
	    Cuboid bone
	    Intermediate cuneiform bone
	    Lateral cuneiform bone
	    Medial cuneiform bone
	    Navicular bone
	    Talus bone
	M **Tarsal, Left**
	    See L Tarsal, Right
	N **Metatarsal, Right**
	P **Metatarsal, Left**
	Q **Toe Phalanx, Right**
	R **Toe Phalanx, Left**
	S **Coccyx**
		0 **Open**	**Z** **No Device**	**Z** **No Qualifier**

LC Limited Coverage   NC Noncovered   ⊞ Combination Member   HAC associated procedure   Combination Only   DRG Non-OR   Non-OR   New/Revised in GREEN

ICD-10-PCS 2019   549

0QC–0QD

Lower Bones

Ø   **Medical and Surgical**
Q   **Lower Bones**
H   **Insertion**   Definition: Putting in a nonbiological appliance that monitors, assists, performs, or prevents a physiological function but does not physically take the place of a body part

Explanation: None

Body Part Character 4		Approach Character 5	Device Character 6	Qualifier Character 7

Ø **Lumbar Vertebra**
   Spinous process
   Transverse process
   Vertebral arch
   Vertebral body
   Vertebral foramen
   Vertebral lamina
   Vertebral pedicle
1 **Sacrum**
2 **Pelvic Bone, Right**
   Iliac crest
   Ilium
   Ischium
   Pubis
3 **Pelvic Bone, Left**
   See 2 Pelvic Bone, Right
4 **Acetabulum, Right**
5 **Acetabulum, Left**
	D **Patella, Right**
	F **Patella, Left**
	L **Tarsal, Right**
	   Calcaneus
	   Cuboid bone
	   Intermediate cuneiform bone
	   Lateral cuneiform bone
	   Medial cuneiform bone
	   Navicular bone
	   Talus bone
	M **Tarsal, Left**
	   See L Tarsal, Right
	N **Metatarsal, Right**
	P **Metatarsal, Left**
	Q **Toe Phalanx, Right**
	R **Toe Phalanx, Left**
	S **Coccyx**
		Ø Open
		3 Percutaneous
		4 Percutaneous Endoscopic
			4 Internal Fixation Device
			5 External Fixation Device
				Z No Qualifier

6 **Upper Femur, Right**
   Femoral head
   Greater trochanter
   Lesser trochanter
   Neck of femur
7 **Upper Femur, Left**
   See 6 Upper Femur, Right
8 **Femoral Shaft, Right**
   Body of femur
9 **Femoral Shaft, Left**
   See 8 Femoral Shaft, Right
B **Lower Femur, Right**
   Lateral condyle of femur
   Lateral epicondyle of femur
   Medial condyle of femur
   Medial epicondyle of femur
	C **Lower Femur, Left**
	   See B Lower Femur, Right
	G **Tibia, Right**
	   Lateral condyle of tibia
	   Medial condyle of tibia
	   Medial malleolus
	H **Tibia, Left**
	   See G Tibia, Right
	J **Fibula, Right**
	   Body of fibula
	   Head of fibula
	   Lateral malleolus
	K **Fibula, Left**
	   See J Fibula, Right
		Ø Open
		3 Percutaneous
		4 Percutaneous Endoscopic
			4 Internal Fixation Device
			5 External Fixation Device
			6 Internal Fixation Device, Intramedullary
			8 External Fixation Device, Limb Lengthening
			B External Fixation Device, Monoplanar
			C External Fixation Device, Ring
			D External Fixation Device, Hybrid
				Z No Qualifier

Y **Lower Bone**		**Ø** Open **3** Percutaneous **4** Percutaneous Endoscopic	**M** Bone Growth Stimulator	**Z** No Qualifier

Non-OR   ØQH[6,7,8,9,B,C,G,H,J,K][Ø,3,4]8Z

Ø   **Medical and Surgical**
Q   **Lower Bones**
J   **Inspection**   Definition: Visually and/or manually exploring a body part

Explanation: Visual exploration may be performed with or without optical instrumentation. Manual exploration may be performed directly or through intervening body layers.

Body Part Character 4	Approach Character 5	Device Character 6	Qualifier Character 7
Y **Lower Bone**	**Ø** Open **3** Percutaneous **4** Percutaneous Endoscopic **X** External	**Z** No Device	**Z** No Qualifier

Non-OR   ØQJY[3,X]ZZ

🅛🅒 Limited Coverage   🅝🅒 Noncovered   ⊞ Combination Member   HAC associated procedure   Combination Only   DRG Non-OR   Non-OR   New/Revised in GREEN

550   ICD-10-PCS 2019

Ø   **Medical and Surgical**
Q   **Lower Bones**
N   **Release**   Definition: Freeing a body part from an abnormal physical constraint by cutting or by the use of force

Explanation: Some of the restraining tissue may be taken out but none of the body part is taken out

Body Part Character 4		Approach Character 5	Device Character 6	Qualifier Character 7
Ø Lumbar Vertebra Spinous process Transverse process Vertebral arch Vertebral body Vertebral foramen Vertebral lamina Vertebral pedicle **1 Sacrum** **2 Pelvic Bone, Right** Iliac crest Ilium Ischium Pubis **3 Pelvic Bone, Left** *See 2 Pelvic Bone, Right* **4 Acetabulum, Right** **5 Acetabulum, Left** **6 Upper Femur, Right** Femoral head Greater trochanter Lesser trochanter Neck of femur **7 Upper Femur, Left** *See 6 Upper Femur, Right* **8 Femoral Shaft, Right** Body of femur **9 Femoral Shaft, Left** *See 8 Femoral Shaft, Right* **B Lower Femur, Right** Lateral condyle of femur Lateral epicondyle of femur Medial condyle of femur Medial epicondyle of femur	**C Lower Femur, Left** *See B Lower Femur, Right* **D Patella, Right** **F Patella, Left** **G Tibia, Right** Lateral condyle of tibia Medial condyle of tibia Medial malleolus **H Tibia, Left** *See G Tibia, Right* **J Fibula, Right** Body of fibula Head of fibula Lateral malleolus **K Fibula, Left** *See J Fibula, Right* **L Tarsal, Right** Calcaneus Cuboid bone Intermediate cuneiform bone Lateral cuneiform bone Medial cuneiform bone Navicular bone Talus bone **M Tarsal, Left** *See L Tarsal, Right* **N Metatarsal, Right** **P Metatarsal, Left** **Q Toe Phalanx, Right** **R Toe Phalanx, Left** **S Coccyx**	**Ø Open** **3 Percutaneous** **4 Percutaneous Endoscopic**	**Z No Device**	**Z No Qualifier**

Ø   **Medical and Surgical**
Q   **Lower Bones**
P   **Removal**   Definition: Taking out or off a device from a body part

Explanation: If a device is taken out and a similar device put in without cutting or puncturing the skin or mucous membrane, the procedure is coded to the root operation CHANGE. Otherwise, the procedure for taking out a device is coded to the root operation REMOVAL.

Body Part Character 4	Approach Character 5	Device Character 6	Qualifier Character 7
Ø Lumbar Vertebra Spinous process Transverse process Vertebral arch Vertebral body Vertebral foramen Vertebral lamina Vertebral pedicle **1 Sacrum** **4 Acetabulum, Right** **5 Acetabulum, Left** **S Coccyx**	**Ø Open** **3 Percutaneous** **4 Percutaneous Endoscopic**	**4 Internal Fixation Device** **7 Autologous Tissue Substitute** **J Synthetic Substitute** **K Nonautologous Tissue Substitute**	**Z No Qualifier**
Ø Lumbar Vertebra Spinous process Transverse process Vertebral arch Vertebral body Vertebral foramen Vertebral lamina Vertebral pedicle **1 Sacrum** **4 Acetabulum, Right** **5 Acetabulum, Left** **S Coccyx**	**X External**	**4 Internal Fixation Device**	**Z No Qualifier**

ØQP Continued on next page

Non-OR   ØQP[Ø,1,4,5,S]X4Z

LC Limited Coverage   **NC** Noncovered   ⊞ Combination Member   HAC associated procedure   Combination Only   DRG Non-OR   Non-OR   New/Revised in GREEN

ICD-10-PCS 2019   551

ØQN–ØQP

Lower Bones (side tab)

Ø **Medical and Surgical**
Q **Lower Bones**
P **Removal**   Definition: Taking out or off a device from a body part

Explanation: If a device is taken out and a similar device put in without cutting or puncturing the skin or mucous membrane, the procedure is coded to the root operation CHANGE. Otherwise, the procedure for taking out a device is coded to the root operation REMOVAL.

Body Part Character 4		Approach Character 5	Device Character 6	Qualifier Character 7
2 Pelvic Bone, Right Iliac crest Ilium Ischium Pubis **3 Pelvic Bone, Left** *See 2 Pelvic Bone, Right* **6 Upper Femur, Right** Femoral head Greater trochanter Lesser trochanter Neck of femur **7 Upper Femur, Left** *See 6 Upper Femur, Right* **8 Femoral Shaft, Right** Body of femur **9 Femoral Shaft, Left** *See 8 Femoral Shaft, Right* **B Lower Femur, Right** Lateral condyle of femur Lateral epicondyle of femur Medial condyle of femur Medial epicondyle of femur **C Lower Femur, Left** *See B Lower Femur, Right* **D Patella, Right** **F Patella, Left**	**G Tibia, Right** Lateral condyle of tibia Medial condyle of tibia Medial malleolus **H Tibia, Left** *See G Tibia, Right* **J Fibula, Right** Body of fibula Head of fibula Lateral malleolus **K Fibula, Left** *See J Fibula, Right* **L Tarsal, Right** Calcaneus Cuboid bone Intermediate cuneiform bone Lateral cuneiform bone Medial cuneiform bone Navicular bone Talus bone **M Tarsal, Left** *See L Tarsal, Right* **N Metatarsal, Right** **P Metatarsal, Left** **Q Toe Phalanx, Right** **R Toe Phalanx, Left**	**Ø Open** **3 Percutaneous** **4 Percutaneous Endoscopic**	**4 Internal Fixation Device** **5 External Fixation Device** **7 Autologous Tissue Substitute** **J Synthetic Substitute** **K Nonautologous Tissue Substitute**	**Z No Qualifier**
2 Pelvic Bone, Right Iliac crest Ilium Ischium Pubis **3 Pelvic Bone, Left** *See 2 Pelvic Bone, Right* **6 Upper Femur, Right** Femoral head Greater trochanter Lesser trochanter Neck of femur **7 Upper Femur, Left** *See 6 Upper Femur, Right* **8 Femoral Shaft, Right** Body of femur **9 Femoral Shaft, Left** *See 8 Femoral Shaft, Right* **B Lower Femur, Right** Lateral condyle of femur Lateral epicondyle of femur Medial condyle of femur Medial epicondyle of femur **C Lower Femur, Left** *See B Lower Femur, Right* **D Patella, Right** **F Patella, Left**	**G Tibia, Right** Lateral condyle of tibia Medial condyle of tibia Medial malleolus **H Tibia, Left** *See G Tibia, Right* **J Fibula, Right** Body of fibula Head of fibula Lateral malleolus **K Fibula, Left** *See J Fibula, Right* **L Tarsal, Right** Calcaneus Cuboid bone Intermediate cuneiform bone Lateral cuneiform bone Medial cuneiform bone Navicular bone Talus bone **M Tarsal, Left** *See L Tarsal, Right* **N Metatarsal, Right** **P Metatarsal, Left** **Q Toe Phalanx, Right** **R Toe Phalanx, Left**	**X External**	**4 Internal Fixation Device** **5 External Fixation Device**	**Z No Qualifier**
Y Lower Bone		**Ø Open** **3 Percutaneous** **4 Percutaneous Endoscopic** **X External**	**Ø Drainage Device** **M Bone Growth Stimulator**	**Z No Qualifier**

Non-OR   ØQP[2,3,6,7,8,9,B,C,D,F,G,H,J,K,L,M,N,P,Q,R]X[4,5]Z
Non-OR   ØQPY3ØZ
Non-OR   ØQPYX[Ø,M]Z

0　**Medical and Surgical**
Q　**Lower Bones**
Q　**Repair**　　　Definition: Restoring, to the extent possible, a body part to its normal anatomic structure and function
　　　　　　　　　Explanation: Used only when the method to accomplish the repair is not one of the other root operations

Body Part Character 4	Approach Character 5	Device Character 6	Qualifier Character 7
0 **Lumbar Vertebra** 　Spinous process 　Transverse process 　Vertebral arch 　Vertebral body 　Vertebral foramen 　Vertebral lamina 　Vertebral pedicle	**0** Open **3** Percutaneous **4** Percutaneous Endoscopic **X** External	**Z** No Device	**Z** No Qualifier
1 **Sacrum**			
2 **Pelvic Bone, Right** 　Iliac crest 　Ilium 　Ischium 　Pubis			
3 **Pelvic Bone, Left** 　*See 2 Pelvic Bone, Right*			
4 **Acetabulum, Right**			
5 **Acetabulum, Left**			
6 **Upper Femur, Right** 　Femoral head 　Greater trochanter 　Lesser trochanter 　Neck of femur			
7 **Upper Femur, Left** 　*See 6 Upper Femur, Right*			
8 **Femoral Shaft, Right** 　Body of femur			
9 **Femoral Shaft, Left** 　*See 8 Femoral Shaft, Right*			
B **Lower Femur, Right** 　Lateral condyle of femur 　Lateral epicondyle of femur 　Medial condyle of femur 　Medial epicondyle of femur			
C **Lower Femur, Left** 　*See B Lower Femur, Right*			
D **Patella, Right**			
F **Patella, Left**			
G **Tibia, Right** 　Lateral condyle of tibia 　Medial condyle of tibia 　Medial malleolus			
H **Tibia, Left** 　*See G Tibia, Right*			
J **Fibula, Right** 　Body of fibula 　Head of fibula 　Lateral malleolus			
K **Fibula, Left** 　*See J Fibula, Right*			
L **Tarsal, Right** 　Calcaneus 　Cuboid bone 　Intermediate cuneiform bone 　Lateral cuneiform bone 　Medial cuneiform bone 　Navicular bone 　Talus bone			
M **Tarsal, Left** 　*See L Tarsal, Right*			
N **Metatarsal, Right**			
P **Metatarsal, Left**			
Q **Toe Phalanx, Right**			
R **Toe Phalanx, Left**			
S **Coccyx**			

Non-OR　0QQ[0,1,2,3,4,5,6,7,8,9,B,C,D,F,G,H,J,K,L,M,N,P,Q,R,S]XZZ

LC Limited Coverage　**NC** Noncovered　⊞ Combination Member　HAC associated procedure　Combination Only　DRG Non-OR　Non-OR　New/Revised in GREEN

Lower Bones

Ø   **Medical and Surgical**
Q   **Lower Bones**
R   **Replacement**   **Definition:** Putting in or on biological or synthetic material that physically takes the place and/or function of all or a portion of a body part

                            Explanation: The body part may have been taken out or replaced, or may be taken out, physically eradicated, or rendered nonfunctional during the REPLACEMENT procedure. A REMOVAL procedure is coded for taking out the device used in a previous replacement procedure.

Body Part Character 4	Approach Character 5	Device Character 6	Qualifier Character 7

Ø **Lumbar Vertebra**
   Spinous process
   Transverse process
   Vertebral arch
   Vertebral body
   Vertebral foramen
   Vertebral lamina
   Vertebral pedicle
1 **Sacrum**
2 **Pelvic Bone, Right**
   Iliac crest
   Ilium
   Ischium
   Pubis
3 **Pelvic Bone, Left**
   See 2 Pelvic Bone, Right
4 **Acetabulum, Right**
5 **Acetabulum, Left**
6 **Upper Femur, Right**
   Femoral head
   Greater trochanter
   Lesser trochanter
   Neck of femur
7 **Upper Femur, Left**
   See 6 Upper Femur, Right
8 **Femoral Shaft, Right**
   Body of femur
9 **Femoral Shaft, Left**
   See 8 Femoral Shaft, Right
B **Lower Femur, Right**
   Lateral condyle of femur
   Lateral epicondyle of femur
   Medial condyle of femur
   Medial epicondyle of femur
C **Lower Femur, Left**
   See B Lower Femur, Right
D **Patella, Right**
F **Patella, Left**
G **Tibia, Right**
   Lateral condyle of tibia
   Medial condyle of tibia
   Medial malleolus
H **Tibia, Left**
   See G Tibia, Right
J **Fibula, Right**
   Body of fibula
   Head of fibula
   Lateral malleolus
K **Fibula, Left**
   See J Fibula, Right
L **Tarsal, Right**
   Calcaneus
   Cuboid bone
   Intermediate cuneiform bone
   Lateral cuneiform bone
   Medial cuneiform bone
   Navicular bone
   Talus bone
M **Tarsal, Left**
   See L Tarsal, Right
N **Metatarsal, Right**
P **Metatarsal, Left**
Q **Toe Phalanx, Right**
R **Toe Phalanx, Left**
S **Coccyx**
	Ø Open
	3 Percutaneous
	4 Percutaneous Endoscopic
		7 Autologous Tissue Substitute
		J Synthetic Substitute
		K Nonautologous Tissue Substitute
			Z No Qualifier

LC Limited Coverage   **NC** Noncovered   ⊞ Combination Member   HAC associated procedure   Combination Only   DRG Non-OR   Non-OR   New/Revised in GREEN

554   ICD-10-PCS 2019

Lower Bones

0   **Medical and Surgical**
Q   **Lower Bones**
S   **Reposition**   Definition: Moving to its normal location, or other suitable location, all or a portion of a body part

                            Explanation: The body part is moved to a new location from an abnormal location, or from a normal location where it is not functioning correctly. The body part may or may not be cut out or off to be moved to the new location.

Body Part Character 4	Approach Character 5	Device Character 6	Qualifier Character 7

0 **Lumbar Vertebra** ⊞
   Spinous process
   Transverse process
   Vertebral arch
   Vertebral body
   Vertebral foramen
   Vertebral lamina
   Vertebral pedicle
1 **Sacrum** ⊞
4 **Acetabulum, Right**
5 **Acetabulum, Left**
S **Coccyx** ⊞
	0 Open
	3 Percutaneous
	4 Percutaneous Endoscopic
		4 Internal Fixation Device
		Z No Device
			Z No Qualifier

0 **Lumbar Vertebra**
   Spinous process
   Transverse process
   Vertebral arch
   Vertebral body
   Vertebral foramen
   Vertebral lamina
   Vertebral pedicle
1 **Sacrum**
4 **Acetabulum, Right**
5 **Acetabulum, Left**
S **Coccyx**
	X External	**Z** No Device	**Z** No Qualifier

2 **Pelvic Bone, Right**
   Iliac crest
   Ilium
   Ischium
   Pubis
3 **Pelvic Bone, Left**
   See 2 Pelvic Bone, Right
D **Patella, Right**
F **Patella, Left**
L **Tarsal, Right**
   Calcaneus
   Cuboid bone
   Intermediate cuneiform bone
   Lateral cuneiform bone
   Medial cuneiform bone
   Navicular bone
   Talus bone
M **Tarsal, Left**
   See L Tarsal, Right
Q **Toe Phalanx, Right**
R **Toe Phalanx, Left**
	0 Open
	3 Percutaneous
	4 Percutaneous Endoscopic
		4 Internal Fixation Device
		5 External Fixation Device
		Z No Device
			Z No Qualifier

2 **Pelvic Bone, Right**
   Iliac crest
   Ilium
   Ischium
   Pubis
3 **Pelvic Bone, Left**
   See 2 Pelvic Bone, Right
D **Patella, Right**
F **Patella, Left**
L **Tarsal, Right**
   Calcaneus
   Cuboid bone
   Intermediate cuneiform bone
   Lateral cuneiform bone
   Medial cuneiform bone
   Navicular bone
   Talus bone
M **Tarsal, Left**
   See L Tarsal, Right
Q **Toe Phalanx, Right**
R **Toe Phalanx, Left**
	X External	**Z** No Device	**Z** No Qualifier

0QS Continued on next page

Non-OR	0QS[4,5][3,4]ZZ
Non-OR	0QS[0,1,4,5,S]XZZ
Non-OR	0QS[2,3,D,F,L,M,Q,R][3,4]ZZ
Non-OR	0QS[2,3,D,F,L,M,Q,R]XZZ

See Appendix L for Procedure Combinations
⊞   0QS[0,1,S]3ZZ

Lower Bones

ØQS Continued

Ø **Medical and Surgical**
Q **Lower Bones**
S **Reposition**   Definition: Moving to its normal location, or other suitable location, all or a portion of a body part

Explanation: The body part is moved to a new location from an abnormal location, or from a normal location where it is not functioning correctly. The body part may or may not be cut out or off to be moved to the new location.

Body Part Character 4	Approach Character 5	Device Character 6	Qualifier Character 7
6 Upper Femur, Right Femoral head Greater trochanter Lesser trochanter Neck of femur **7 Upper Femur, Left** *See 6 Upper Femur, Right* **8 Femoral Shaft, Right** Body of femur **9 Femoral Shaft, Left** *See 8 Femoral Shaft, Right* **B Lower Femur, Right** Lateral condyle of femur Lateral epicondyle of femur Medial condyle of femur Medial epicondyle of femur **C Lower Femur, Left** *See B Lower Femur, Right* **G Tibia, Right** Lateral condyle of tibia Medial condyle of tibia Medial malleolus **H Tibia, Left** *See G Tibia, Right* **J Fibula, Right** Body of fibula Head of fibula Lateral malleolus **K Fibula, Left** *See J Fibula, Right*	**Ø Open** **3 Percutaneous** **4 Percutaneous Endoscopic**	**4 Internal Fixation Device** **5 External Fixation Device** **6 Internal Fixation Device, Intramedullary** **B External Fixation Device, Monoplanar** **C External Fixation Device, Ring** **D External Fixation Device, Hybrid** **Z No Device**	**Z No Qualifier**
6 Upper Femur, Right Femoral head Greater trochanter Lesser trochanter Neck of femur **7 Upper Femur, Left** *See 6 Upper Femur, Right* **8 Femoral Shaft, Right** Body of femur **9 Femoral Shaft, Left** *See 8 Femoral Shaft, Right* **B Lower Femur, Right** Lateral condyle of femur Lateral epicondyle of femur Medial condyle of femur Medial epicondyle of femur **C Lower Femur, Left** *See B Lower Femur, Right* **G Tibia, Right** Lateral condyle of tibia Medial condyle of tibia Medial malleolus **H Tibia, Left** *See G Tibia, Right* **J Fibula, Right** Body of fibula Head of fibula Lateral malleolus **K Fibula, Left** *See J Fibula, Right*	**X External**	**Z No Device**	**Z No Qualifier**
N Metatarsal, Right **P Metatarsal, Left**	**Ø Open** **3 Percutaneous** **4 Percutaneous Endoscopic**	**4 Internal Fixation Device** **5 External Fixation Device** **Z No Device**	**2 Sesamoid Bone(s) 1st Toe** **Z No Qualifier**
N Metatarsal, Right **P Metatarsal, Left**	**X External**	**Z No Device**	**2 Sesamoid Bone(s) 1st Toe** **Z No Qualifier**

Non OR   ØQS[6,7,8,9,B,C,G,H,J,K][3,4]ZZ
Non-OR   ØQS[6,7,8,9,B,C,G,H,J,K]XZZ
Non-OR   ØQS[N,P][3,4]Z[2,Z]
Non-OR   ØQS[N,P]XZ[2,Z]

LC Limited Coverage   NC Noncovered   ⊞ Combination Member   HAC associated procedure   Combination Only   DRG Non-OR   Non-OR   New/Revised in GREEN

0   **Medical and Surgical**
Q   **Lower Bones**
T   **Resection**   Definition: Cutting out or off, without replacement, all of a body part
                         Explanation: None

Body Part Character 4	Approach Character 5	Device Character 6	Qualifier Character 7

2 Pelvic Bone, Right
  Iliac crest
  Ilium
  Ischium
  Pubis
3 Pelvic Bone, Left
  See 2 Pelvic Bone, Right
4 Acetabulum, Right
5 Acetabulum, Left
6 Upper Femur, Right
  Femoral head
  Greater trochanter
  Lesser trochanter
  Neck of femur
7 Upper Femur, Left
  See 6 Upper Femur, Right
8 Femoral Shaft, Right
  Body of femur
9 Femoral Shaft, Left
  See 8 Femoral Shaft, Right
B Lower Femur, Right
  Lateral condyle of femur
  Lateral epicondyle of femur
  Medial condyle of femur
  Medial epicondyle of femur
C Lower Femur, Left
  See B Lower Femur, Right
D Patella, Right
 	
F Patella, Left
G Tibia, Right
  Lateral condyle of tibia
  Medial condyle of tibia
  Medial malleolus
H Tibia, Left
  See G Tibia, Right
J Fibula, Right
  Body of fibula
  Head of fibula
  Lateral malleolus
K Fibula, Left
  See J Fibula, Right
L Tarsal, Right
  Calcaneus
  Cuboid bone
  Intermediate cuneiform bone
  Lateral cuneiform bone
  Medial cuneiform bone
  Navicular bone
  Talus bone
M Tarsal, Left
  See L Tarsal, Right
N Metatarsal, Right
P Metatarsal, Left
Q Toe Phalanx, Right
R Toe Phalanx, Left
S Coccyx
	0 Open	Z No Device	Z No Qualifier

0   **Medical and Surgical**
Q   **Lower Bones**
U   **Supplement**   Definition: Putting in or on biological or synthetic material that physically reinforces and/or augments the function of a portion of a body part
           Explanation: The biological material is non-living, or is living and from the same individual. The body part may have been previously replaced, and the SUPPLEMENT procedure is performed to physically reinforce and/or augment the function of the replaced body part.

Body Part Character 4	Approach Character 5	Device Character 6	Qualifier Character 7

0 Lumbar Vertebra ⊞
  Spinous process
  Transverse process
  Vertebral arch
  Vertebral body
  Vertebral foramen
  Vertebral lamina
  Vertebral pedicle
1 Sacrum ⊞
2 Pelvic Bone, Right
  Iliac crest
  Ilium
  Ischium
  Pubis
3 Pelvic Bone, Left
  See 2 Pelvic Bone, Right
4 Acetabulum, Right
5 Acetabulum, Left
6 Upper Femur, Right
  Femoral head
  Greater trochanter
  Lesser trochanter
  Neck of femur
7 Upper Femur, Left
  See 6 Upper Femur, Right
8 Femoral Shaft, Right
  Body of femur
9 Femoral Shaft, Left
  See 8 Femoral Shaft, Right
B Lower Femur, Right
  Lateral condyle of femur
  Lateral epicondyle of femur
  Medial condyle of femur
  Medial epicondyle of femur
C Lower Femur, Left
  See B Lower Femur, Right
D Patella, Right
F Patella, Left
G Tibia, Right
  Lateral condyle of tibia
  Medial condyle of tibia
  Medial malleolus
H Tibia, Left
  See G Tibia, Right
J Fibula, Right
  Body of fibula
  Head of fibula
  Lateral malleolus
K Fibula, Left
  See J Fibula, Right
L Tarsal, Right
  Calcaneus
  Cuboid bone
  Intermediate cuneiform bone
  Lateral cuneiform bone
  Medial cuneiform bone
  Navicular bone
  Talus bone
M Tarsal, Left
  See L Tarsal, Right
N Metatarsal, Right
P Metatarsal, Left
Q Toe Phalanx, Right
R Toe Phalanx, Left
S Coccyx ⊞
	0 Open
	3 Percutaneous
	4 Percutaneous Endoscopic
		7 Autologous Tissue Substitute
		J Synthetic Substitute
		K Nonautologous Tissue Substitute
			Z No Qualifier

See Appendix L for Procedure Combinations
⊞   0QU[0,1,S]3JZ

LC Limited Coverage   NC Noncovered   ⊞ Combination Member   HAC associated procedure   Combination Only   DRG Non-OR   Non-OR   New/Revised in GREEN

ICD-10-PCS 2019   557

0QT–0QU

Lower Bones

Ø　**Medical and Surgical**
Q　**Lower Bones**
W　**Revision**　　Definition: Correcting, to the extent possible, a portion of a malfunctioning device or the position of a displaced device

Explanation: Revision can include correcting a malfunctioning or displaced device by taking out or putting in components of the device such as a screw or pin

Body Part Character 4	Approach Character 5	Device Character 6	Qualifier Character 7
Ø **Lumbar Vertebra** Spinous process Transverse process Vertebral arch Vertebral body Vertebral foramen Vertebral lamina Vertebral pedicle **1** **Sacrum** **4** **Acetabulum, Right** **5** **Acetabulum, Left** **S** **Coccyx**	**Ø** Open **3** Percutaneous **4** Percutaneous Endoscopic **X** External	**4** Internal Fixation Device **7** Autologous Tissue Substitute **J** Synthetic Substitute **K** Nonautologous Tissue Substitute	**Z** No Qualifier
2 **Pelvic Bone, Right** Iliac crest Ilium Ischium Pubis **3** **Pelvic Bone, Left** See 2 Pelvic Bone, Right **6** **Upper Femur, Right** Femoral head Greater trochanter Lesser trochanter Neck of femur **7** **Upper Femur, Left** See 6 Upper Femur, Right **8** **Femoral Shaft, Right** Body of femur **9** **Femoral Shaft, Left** See 8 Femoral Shaft, Right **B** **Lower Femur, Right** Lateral condyle of femur Lateral epicondyle of femur Medial condyle of femur Medial epicondyle of femur **C** **Lower Femur, Left** See B Lower Femur, Right **D** **Patella, Right** **F** **Patella, Left** **G** **Tibia, Right** Lateral condyle of tibia Medial condyle of tibia Medial malleolus **H** **Tibia, Left** See G Tibia, Right **J** **Fibula, Right** Body of fibula Head of fibula Lateral malleolus **K** **Fibula, Left** See J Fibula, Right **L** **Tarsal, Right** Calcaneus Cuboid bone Intermediate cuneiform bone Lateral cuneiform bone Medial cuneiform bone Navicular bone Talus bone **M** **Tarsal, Left** See L Tarsal, Right **N** **Metatarsal, Right** **P** **Metatarsal, Left** **Q** **Toe Phalanx, Right** **R** **Toe Phalanx, Left**	**Ø** Open **3** Percutaneous **4** Percutaneous Endoscopic **X** External	**4** Internal Fixation Device **5** External Fixation Device **7** Autologous Tissue Substitute **J** Synthetic Substitute **K** Nonautologous Tissue Substitute	**Z** No Qualifier
Y **Lower Bone**	**Ø** Open **3** Percutaneous **4** Percutaneous Endoscopic **X** External	**Ø** Drainage Device **M** Bone Growth Stimulator	**Z** No Qualifier

Non-OR　ØQW[Ø,1,4,5,S]X[4,7,J,K]Z
Non-OR　ØQW[2,3,6,7,8,9,B,C,D,F,G,H,J,K,L,M,N,P,Q,R]X[4,5,7,J,K]Z
Non-OR　ØQWYX[Ø,M]Z

LC Limited Coverage　**NC** Noncovered　⊞ Combination Member　HAC associated procedure　Combination Only　DRG Non-OR　Non-OR　New/Revised in GREEN

558　　　　　　　　　　　　　　　　　　　　　　　　　　　　　　　　　　　　　ICD-10-PCS 2019

Upper Joints ØR2–ØRW

Character Meanings*

This Character Meaning table is provided as a guide to assist the user in the identification of character members that may be found in this section of code tables. It **SHOULD NOT** be used to build a PCS code.

Operation–Character 3	Body Part–Character 4	Approach–Character 5	Device–Character 6	Qualifier–Character 7
2 Change	Ø Occipital-cervical Joint	Ø Open	Ø Drainage Device OR Synthetic Substitute, Reverse Ball and Socket	Ø Anterior Approach, Anterior Column
5 Destruction	1 Cervical Vertebral Joint	3 Percutaneous	3 Infusion Device	1 Posterior Approach, Posterior Column
9 Drainage	2 Cervical Vertebral Joint, 2 or more	4 Percutaneous Endoscopic	4 Internal Fixation Device	6 Humeral Surface
B Excision	3 Cervical Vertebral Disc	X External	5 External Fixation Device	7 Glenoid Surface
C Extirpation	4 Cervicothoracic Vertebral Joint		7 Autologous Tissue Substitute	J Posterior Approach, Anterior Column
G Fusion	5 Cervicothoracic Vertebral Disc		8 Spacer	X Diagnostic
H Insertion	6 Thoracic Vertebral Joint		A Interbody Fusion Device	Z No Qualifier
J Inspection	7 Thoracic Vertebral Joint, 2 to 7		B Spinal Stabilization Device, Interspinous Process	
N Release	8 Thoracic Vertebral Joint, 8 or more		C Spinal Stabilization Device, Pedicle-Based	
P Removal	9 Thoracic Vertebral Disc		D Spinal Stabilization Device, Facet Replacement	
Q Repair	A Thoracolumbar Vertebral Joint		J Synthetic Substitute	
R Replacement	B Thoracolumbar Vertebral Disc		K Nonautologous Tissue Substitute	
S Reposition	C Temporomandibular Joint, Right		Y Other Device	
T Resection	D Temporomandibular Joint, Left		Z No Device	
U Supplement	E Sternoclavicular Joint, Right			
W Revision	F Sternoclavicular Joint, Left			
	G Acromioclavicular Joint, Right			
	H Acromioclavicular Joint, Left			
	J Shoulder Joint, Right			
	K Shoulder Joint, Left			
	L Elbow Joint, Right			
	M Elbow Joint, Left			
	N Wrist Joint, Right			
	P Wrist Joint, Left			
	Q Carpal Joint, Right			
	R Carpal Joint, Left			
	S Carpometacarpal Joint, Right			
	T Carpometacarpal Joint, Left			
	U Metacarpophalangeal Joint, Right			
	V Metacarpophalangeal Joint, Left			
	W Finger Phalangeal Joint, Right			
	X Finger Phalangeal Joint, Left			
	Y Upper Joint			

* Includes synovial membrane.

AHA Coding Clinic for table ØRG

2018, 1Q, 22	Spinal fusion procedures without bone graft
2017, 4Q, 62	Added and revised device values - Nerve substitutes
2017, 4Q, 76	Radiolucent porous interbody fusion device
2017, 2Q, 23	Decompression of spinal cord and placement of instrumentation
2014, 3Q, 30	Spinal fusion and fixation instrumentation
2014, 2Q, 7	Anterior cervical thoracic fusion with total discectomy
2013, 1Q, 21-23	Spinal fusion of thoracic and lumbar vertebrae
2013, 1Q, 29	Cervical and thoracic spinal fusion

AHA Coding Clinic for table ØRH

2017, 2Q, 23	Decompression of spinal cord and placement of instrumentation
2016, 3Q, 32	Rotator cuff repair, tenodesis, decompression, acromioplasty and coracoplasty

AHA Coding Clinic for table ØRN

2016, 3Q, 32	Rotator cuff repair, tenodesis, decompression, acromioplasty and coracoplasty
2015, 2Q, 22	Arthroscopic subacromial decompression
2015, 2Q, 23	Arthroscopic release of shoulder joint

AHA Coding Clinic for table ØRP

2017, 4Q, 107	Total ankle replacement versus revision

AHA Coding Clinic for table ØRQ

2016, 1Q, 30	Thermal capsulorrhaphy of shoulder

AHA Coding Clinic for table ØRR

2017, 4Q, 107	Total ankle replacement versus revision
2015, 3Q, 14	Endoprosthetic replacement of humerus and tendon reattachment
2015, 1Q, 27	Reverse total shoulder arthroplasty

AHA Coding Clinic for table ØRS

2015, 2Q, 35	Application of tongs to reduce and stabilize cervical fracture
2014, 4Q, 32	Open reduction internal fixation of fracture with debridement
2014, 3Q, 33	Radial fracture treatment with open reduction internal fixation, and release of carpal ligament
2013, 2Q, 39	Application of cervical tongs for reduction of cervical fracture

AHA Coding Clinic for table ØRT

2014, 2Q, 7	Anterior cervical thoracic fusion with total discectomy

AHA Coding Clinic for table ØRU

2015, 3Q, 26	Thumb arthroplasty with resection of trapezium

AHA Coding Clinic for table ØRW

2017, 4Q, 107	Total ankle replacement versus revision

Upper Joints

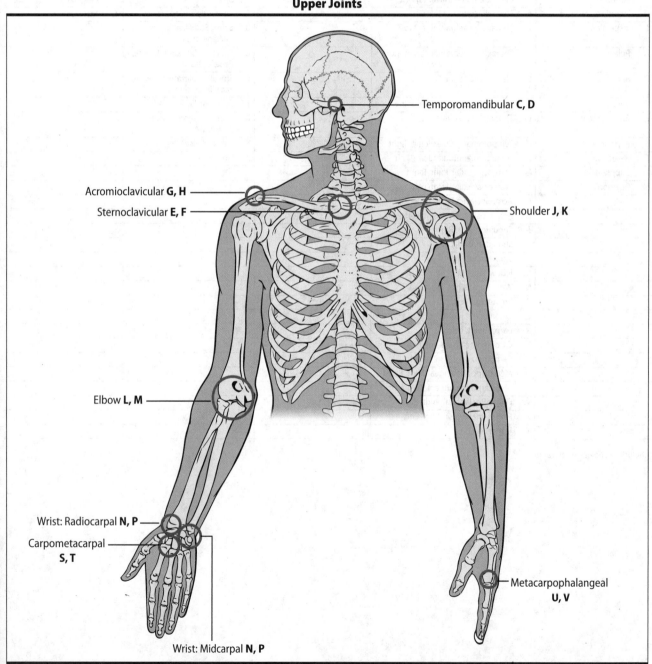

Temporomandibular **C, D**

Acromioclavicular **G, H**

Sternoclavicular **E, F**

Shoulder **J, K**

Elbow **L, M**

Wrist: Radiocarpal **N, P**

Carpometacarpal **S, T**

Metacarpophalangeal **U, V**

Wrist: Midcarpal **N, P**

Hand Joints

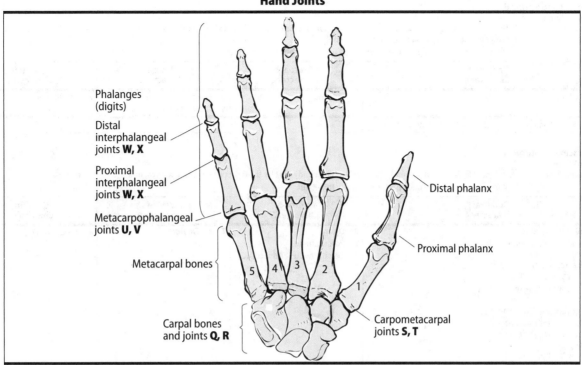

Phalanges (digits)

Distal interphalangeal joints **W, X**

Proximal interphalangeal joints **W, X**

Metacarpophalangeal joints **U, V**

Metacarpal bones

Carpal bones and joints **Q, R**

Distal phalanx

Proximal phalanx

Carpometacarpal joints **S, T**

Shoulder Joints

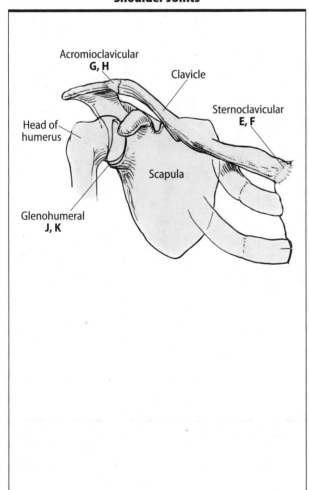

Acromioclavicular **G, H**

Clavicle

Sternoclavicular **E, F**

Head of humerus

Glenohumeral **J, K**

Scapula

Upper Vertebral Joints

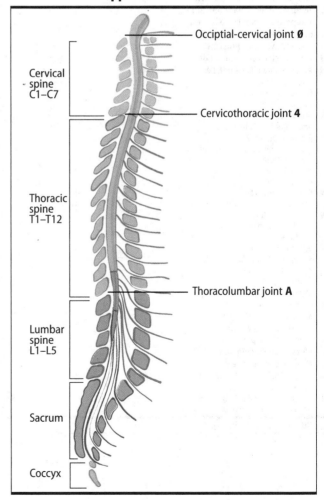

Occiptial-cervical joint **Ø**

Cervical spine C1–C7

Cervicothoracic joint **4**

Thoracic spine T1–T12

Thoracolumbar joint **A**

Lumbar spine L1–L5

Sacrum

Coccyx

0 **Medical and Surgical**
R **Upper Joints**
2 **Change**

Definition: Taking out or off a device from a body part and putting back an identical or similar device in or on the same body part without cutting or puncturing the skin or a mucous membrane

Explanation: All CHANGE procedures are coded using the approach EXTERNAL

Body Part Character 4	Approach Character 5	Device Character 6	Qualifier Character 7
Y Upper Joint	X External	0 Drainage Device Y Other Device	Z No Qualifier

Non-OR All body part, approach, device, and qualifier values

0 **Medical and Surgical**
R **Upper Joints**
5 **Destruction**

Definition: Physical eradication of all or a portion of a body part by the direct use of energy, force, or a destructive agent

Explanation: None of the body part is physically taken out

Body Part Character 4	Approach Character 5	Device Character 6	Qualifier Character 7

0 Occipital-cervical Joint
1 Cervical Vertebral Joint
  Atlantoaxial joint
  Cervical facet joint
3 Cervical Vertebral Disc
4 Cervicothoracic Vertebral Joint
  Cervicothoracic facet joint
5 Cervicothoracic Vertebral Disc
6 Thoracic Vertebral Joint
  Costotransverse joint
  Costovertebral joint
  Thoracic facet joint
9 Thoracic Vertebral Disc
A Thoracolumbar Vertebral Joint
  Thoracolumbar facet joint
B Thoracolumbar Vertebral Disc
C Temporomandibular Joint, Right
D Temporomandibular Joint, Left
E Sternoclavicular Joint, Right
F Sternoclavicular Joint, Left
G Acromioclavicular Joint, Right
H Acromioclavicular Joint, Left
J Shoulder Joint, Right
  Glenohumeral joint
  Glenoid ligament (labrum)
K Shoulder Joint, Left
  See J Shoulder Joint, Right
L Elbow Joint, Right
  Distal humerus, involving joint
  Humeroradial joint
  Humeroulnar joint
  Proximal radioulnar joint
M Elbow Joint, Left
  See L Elbow Joint, Right
N Wrist Joint, Right
  Distal radioulnar joint
  Radiocarpal joint
P Wrist Joint, Left
  See N Wrist Joint, Right
Q Carpal Joint, Right
  Intercarpal joint
  Midcarpal joint
R Carpal Joint, Left
  See Q Carpal Joint, Right
S Carpometacarpal Joint, Right
T Carpometacarpal Joint, Left
U Metacarpophalangeal Joint, Right
V Metacarpophalangeal Joint, Left
W Finger Phalangeal Joint, Right
  Interphalangeal (IP) joint
X Finger Phalangeal Joint, Left
  See W Finger Phalangeal Joint, Right
	0 Open
	3 Percutaneous
	4 Percutaneous Endoscopic
		Z No Device	Z No Qualifier

Non-OR 0R5[3,5,9,B][3,4]ZZ

LC Limited Coverage   NC Noncovered   ⊞ Combination Member   HAC associated procedure   Combination Only   DRG Non-OR   Non-OR   New/Revised in GREEN

562   ICD-10-PCS 2019

0   **Medical and Surgical**
R   **Upper Joints**
9   **Drainage**   Definition: Taking or letting out fluids and/or gases from a body part
                     Explanation: The qualifier DIAGNOSTIC is used to identify drainage procedures that are biopsies

Body Part Character 4		Approach Character 5	Device Character 6	Qualifier Character 7

0 Occipital-cervical Joint
1 Cervical Vertebral Joint
   Atlantoaxial joint
   Cervical facet joint
3 Cervical Vertebral Disc
4 Cervicothoracic Vertebral
   Joint
   Cervicothoracic facet joint
5 Cervicothoracic Vertebral
   Disc
6 Thoracic Vertebral Joint
   Costotransverse joint
   Costovertebral joint
   Thoracic facet joint
9 Thoracic Vertebral Disc
A Thoracolumbar Vertebral
   Joint
   Thoracolumbar facet joint
B Thoracolumbar Vertebral
   Disc
C Temporomandibular Joint,
   Right
D Temporomandibular Joint,
   Left
E Sternoclavicular Joint, Right
F Sternoclavicular Joint, Left
G Acromioclavicular Joint,
   Right
H Acromioclavicular Joint, Left
J Shoulder Joint, Right
   Glenohumeral joint
   Glenoid ligament (labrum)
K Shoulder Joint, Left
   See J Shoulder Joint, Right
	L Elbow Joint, Right
	   Distal humerus, involving
	     joint
	   Humeroradial joint
	   Humeroulnar joint
	   Proximal radioulnar joint
	M Elbow Joint, Left
	   See L Elbow Joint, Right
	N Wrist Joint, Right
	   Distal radioulnar joint
	   Radiocarpal joint
	P Wrist Joint, Left
	   See N Wrist Joint, Right
	Q Carpal Joint, Right
	   Intercarpal joint
	   Midcarpal joint
	R Carpal Joint, Left
	   See Q Carpal Joint, Right
	S Carpometacarpal Joint,
	   Right
	T Carpometacarpal Joint, Left
	U Metacarpophalangeal Joint,
	   Right
	V Metacarpophalangeal Joint,
	   Left
	W Finger Phalangeal Joint,
	   Right
	   Interphalangeal (IP) joint
	X Finger Phalangeal Joint, Left
	   *See W Finger Phalangeal Joint,
	    Right*
		0 Open
		3 Percutaneous
		4 Percutaneous Endoscopic
			0 Drainage Device	**Z** No Qualifier

0 Occipital-cervical Joint
1 Cervical Vertebral Joint
   Atlantoaxial joint
   Cervical facet joint
3 Cervical Vertebral Disc
4 Cervicothoracic Vertebral
   Joint
   Cervicothoracic facet joint
5 Cervicothoracic Vertebral
   Disc
6 Thoracic Vertebral Joint
   Costotransverse joint
   Costovertebral joint
   Thoracic facet joint
9 Thoracic Vertebral Disc
A Thoracolumbar Vertebral
   Joint
   Thoracolumbar facet joint
B Thoracolumbar Vertebral
   Disc
C Temporomandibular Joint,
   Right
D Temporomandibular Joint,
   Left
E Sternoclavicular Joint, Right
F Sternoclavicular Joint, Left
G Acromioclavicular Joint,
   Right
H Acromioclavicular Joint, Left
J Shoulder Joint, Right
   Glenohumeral joint
   Glenoid ligament (labrum)
K Shoulder Joint, Left
   See J Shoulder Joint, Right
	L Elbow Joint, Right
	   Distal humerus, involving
	     joint
	   Humeroradial joint
	   Humeroulnar joint
	   Proximal radioulnar joint
	M Elbow Joint, Left
	   See L Elbow Joint, Right
	N Wrist Joint, Right
	   Distal radioulnar joint
	   Radiocarpal joint
	P Wrist Joint, Left
	   See N Wrist Joint, Right
	Q Carpal Joint, Right
	   Intercarpal joint
	   Midcarpal joint
	R Carpal Joint, Left
	   See Q Carpal Joint, Right
	S Carpometacarpal Joint,
	   Right
	T Carpometacarpal Joint, Left
	U Metacarpophalangeal Joint,
	   Right
	V Metacarpophalangeal Joint,
	   Left
	W Finger Phalangeal Joint,
	   Right
	   Interphalangeal (IP) joint
	X Finger Phalangeal Joint, Left
	   *See W Finger Phalangeal Joint,
	    Right*
		0 Open
		3 Percutaneous
		4 Percutaneous Endoscopic
			Z No Device	**X** Diagnostic
				Z No Qualifier

Non-OR	0R9[0,1,3,4,5,6,9,A,B,E,F,G,H,J,K,L,M,N,P,Q,R,S,T,U,V,W,X][3,4]0Z
Non-OR	0R9[C,D]30Z
Non-OR	0R9[0,1,3,4,5,6,9,A,B,E,F,G,H,J,K,L,M,N,P,Q,R,S,T,U,V,W,X][0,3,4]ZX
Non-OR	0R9[0,1,3,4,5,6,9,A,B,E,F,G,H,J,K,L,M,N,P,Q,R,S,T,U,V,W,X][3,4]ZZ
Non-OR	0R9[C,D]3ZZ

LC Limited Coverage   **NC** Noncovered   ⊞ Combination Member   HAC associated procedure   Combination Only   DRG Non-OR   Non-OR   New/Revised in GREEN
ICD-10-PCS 2019   563

0R9–0R9

Ø   Medical and Surgical
R   Upper Joints
B   Excision   Definition: Cutting out or off, without replacement, a portion of a body part
                 Explanation: The qualifier DIAGNOSTIC is used to identify excision procedures that are biopsies

Body Part Character 4	Approach Character 5	Device Character 6	Qualifier Character 7
Ø **Occipital-cervical Joint**	**Ø** Open	**Z** No Device	**X** Diagnostic
1 **Cervical Vertebral Joint**	**3** Percutaneous		**Z** No Qualifier
Atlantoaxial joint	**4** Percutaneous Endoscopic		
Cervical facet joint			
3 **Cervical Vertebral Disc**			
4 **Cervicothoracic Vertebral Joint**			
Cervicothoracic facet joint			
5 **Cervicothoracic Vertebral Disc**			
6 **Thoracic Vertebral Joint**			
Costotransverse joint			
Costovertebral joint			
Thoracic facet joint			
9 **Thoracic Vertebral Disc**			
A **Thoracolumbar Vertebral Joint**			
Thoracolumbar facet joint			
B **Thoracolumbar Vertebral Disc**			
C **Temporomandibular Joint, Right**			
D **Temporomandibular Joint, Left**			
E **Sternoclavicular Joint, Right**			
F **Sternoclavicular Joint, Left**			
G **Acromioclavicular Joint, Right**			
H **Acromioclavicular Joint, Left**			
J **Shoulder Joint, Right**			
Glenohumeral joint			
Glenoid ligament (labrum)			
K **Shoulder Joint, Left**			
See J Shoulder Joint, Right			
L **Elbow Joint, Right**			
Distal humerus, involving joint			
Humeroradial joint			
Humeroulnar joint			
Proximal radioulnar joint			
M **Elbow Joint, Left**			
See L Elbow Joint, Right			
N **Wrist Joint, Right**			
Distal radioulnar joint			
Radiocarpal joint			
P **Wrist Joint, Left**			
See N Wrist Joint, Right			
Q **Carpal Joint, Right**			
Intercarpal joint			
Midcarpal joint			
R **Carpal Joint, Left**			
See Q Carpal Joint, Right			
S **Carpometacarpal Joint, Right**			
T **Carpometacarpal Joint, Left**			
U **Metacarpophalangeal Joint, Right**			
V **Metacarpophalangeal Joint, Left**			
W **Finger Phalangeal Joint, Right**			
Interphalangeal (IP) joint			
X **Finger Phalangeal Joint, Left**			
See W Finger Phalangeal Joint, Right			

Non-OR   ØRB[Ø,1,3,4,5,6,9,A,B,E,F,G,H,J,K,L,M,N,P,Q,R,S,T,U,V,W,X][Ø,3,4]ZX

🔲 Limited Coverage   🔲 Noncovered   ⊞ Combination Member   HAC associated procedure   Combination Only   DRG Non-OR   Non-OR   New/Revised in GREEN

564   ICD-10-PCS 2019

ØRB–ØRB

Ø Medical and Surgical
R Upper Joints
C Extirpation   Definition: Taking or cutting out solid matter from a body part

Explanation: The solid matter may be an abnormal byproduct of a biological function or a foreign body; it may be imbedded in a body part or in the lumen of a tubular body part. The solid matter may or may not have been previously broken into pieces.

Body Part Character 4	Approach Character 5	Device Character 6	Qualifier Character 7
Ø Occipital-cervical Joint	Ø Open	Z No Device	Z No Qualifier
1 Cervical Vertebral Joint	3 Percutaneous		
Atlantoaxial joint	4 Percutaneous Endoscopic		
Cervical facet joint			
3 Cervical Vertebral Disc			
4 Cervicothoracic Vertebral Joint			
Cervicothoracic facet joint			
5 Cervicothoracic Vertebral Disc			
6 Thoracic Vertebral Joint			
Costotransverse joint			
Costovertebral joint			
Thoracic facet joint			
9 Thoracic Vertebral Disc			
A Thoracolumbar Vertebral Joint			
Thoracolumbar facet joint			
B Thoracolumbar Vertebral Disc			
C Temporomandibular Joint, Right			
D Temporomandibular Joint, Left			
E Sternoclavicular Joint, Right			
F Sternoclavicular Joint, Left			
G Acromioclavicular Joint, Right			
H Acromioclavicular Joint, Left			
J Shoulder Joint, Right			
Glenohumeral joint			
Glenoid ligament (labrum)			
K Shoulder Joint, Left			
See J Shoulder Joint, Right			
L Elbow Joint, Right			
Distal humerus, involving joint			
Humeroradial joint			
Humeroulnar joint			
Proximal radioulnar joint			
M Elbow Joint, Left			
See L Elbow Joint, Right			
N Wrist Joint, Right			
Distal radioulnar joint			
Radiocarpal joint			
P Wrist Joint, Left			
See N Wrist Joint, Right			
Q Carpal Joint, Right			
Intercarpal joint			
Midcarpal joint			
R Carpal Joint, Left			
See Q Carpal Joint, Right			
S Carpometacarpal Joint, Right			
T Carpometacarpal Joint, Left			
U Metacarpophalangeal Joint, Right			
V Metacarpophalangeal Joint, Left			
W Finger Phalangeal Joint, Right			
Interphalangeal (IP) joint			
X Finger Phalangeal Joint, Left			
See W Finger Phalangeal Joint, Right			

LC Limited Coverage   NC Noncovered   ⊞ Combination Member   HAC associated procedure   Combination Only   DRG Non-OR   Non-OR   New/Revised in GREEN
ICD-10-PCS 2019   565

ØRC–ØRC

Ø   Medical and Surgical
R   Upper Joints
G   Fusion   Definition: Joining together portions of an articular body part rendering the articular body part immobile
                    Explanation: The body part is joined together by fixation device, bone graft, or other means

Body Part Character 4	Approach Character 5	Device Character 6	Qualifier Character 7

Ø   Occipital-cervical Joint
1   Cervical Vertebral Joint
     Atlantoaxial joint
     Cervical facet joint
2   Cervical Vertebral Joints, 2 or more
     Cervical facet joint
4   Cervicothoracic Vertebral Joint
     Cervicothoracic facet joint
6   Thoracic Vertebral Joint
     Costotransverse joint
     Costovertebral joint
     Thoracic facet joint
7   Thoracic Vertebral Joints, 2 to 7   ⊞
8   Thoracic Vertebral Joints, 8 or more
A   Thoracolumbar Vertebral Joint
     Thoracolumbar facet joint
	Ø Open
	3 Percutaneous
	4 Percutaneous Endoscopic
		7 Autologous Tissue
		     Substitute
		J Synthetic Substitute
		K Nonautologous Tissue
		     Substitute
			Ø Anterior Approach, Anterior
			     Column
			1 Posterior Approach,
			     Posterior Column
			J Posterior Approach,
			     Anterior Column

Ø   Occipital-cervical Joint
1   Cervical Vertebral Joint
     Atlantoaxial joint
     Cervical facet joint
2   Cervical Vertebral Joints, 2 or more
     Cervical facet joint
4   Cervicothoracic Vertebral Joint
     Cervicothoracic facet joint
6   Thoracic Vertebral Joint
     Costotransverse joint
     Costovertebral joint
     Thoracic facet joint
7   Thoracic Vertebral Joints, 2 to 7   ⊞
8   Thoracic Vertebral Joints, 8 or more
A   Thoracolumbar Vertebral Joint
     Thoracolumbar facet joint
	Ø Open
	3 Percutaneous
	4 Percutaneous Endoscopic
		A Interbody Fusion Device	Ø Anterior Approach, Anterior
			     Column
			J Posterior Approach,
			     Anterior Column

C   Temporomandibular Joint, Right
D   Temporomandibular Joint, Left
E   Sternoclavicular Joint, Right
F   Sternoclavicular Joint, Left
G   Acromioclavicular Joint, Right
H   Acromioclavicular Joint, Left
J   Shoulder Joint, Right
     Glenohumeral joint
     Glenoid ligament (labrum)
K   Shoulder Joint, Left
     See J Shoulder Joint, Right
	Ø Open
	3 Percutaneous
	4 Percutaneous Endoscopic
		4 Internal Fixation Device
		7 Autologous Tissue
		     Substitute
		J Synthetic Substitute
		K Nonautologous Tissue
		     Substitute
			Z No Qualifier

L   Elbow Joint, Right
     Distal humerus, involving
       joint
     Humeroradial joint
     Humeroulnar joint
     Proximal radioulnar joint
M   Elbow Joint, Left
     See L Elbow Joint, Right
N   Wrist Joint, Right
     Distal radioulnar joint
     Radiocarpal joint
P   Wrist Joint, Left
     See N Wrist Joint, Right
Q   Carpal Joint, Right
     Intercarpal joint
     Midcarpal joint
 	
R   Carpal Joint, Left
     See Q Carpal Joint, Right
S   Carpometacarpal Joint,
     Right
T   Carpometacarpal Joint,
     Left
U   Metacarpophalangeal
     Joint, Right
V   Metacarpophalangeal
     Joint, Left
W   Finger Phalangeal Joint,
     Right
     Interphalangeal (IP) joint
X   Finger Phalangeal Joint,
     Left
     *See W Finger Phalangeal
     Joint, Right*
	Ø Open
	3 Percutaneous
	4 Percutaneous Endoscopic
		4 Internal Fixation Device
		5 External Fixation Device
		7 Autologous Tissue
		     Substitute
		J Synthetic Substitute
		K Nonautologous Tissue
		     Substitute
			Z No Qualifier

HAC	ØRG[Ø,1,2,4,6,7,8,A][Ø,3,4][7,J,K][Ø,1,J] when reported with SDx K68.11 or T81.4XXA or T84.60-T84.619, T84.63-T84.7 with 7th character A	**See Appendix L for Procedure Combinations**
HAC	ØRG[Ø,1,2,4,6,7,8,A][Ø,3,4]A[Ø,J] when reported with SDx K68.11 or T81.4XXA or T84.60-T84.619, T84.63-T84.7 with 7th character A	⊞ ØRG7[Ø,3,4][7,J,K][Ø,1,J] ⊞ ØRG7[Ø,3,4]A[Ø,J]
HAC	ØRG[E,F,G,H,J,K][Ø,3,4][4,7,J,K]Z when reported with SDx K68.11 or T81.4XXA or T84.60-T84.619, T84.63-T84.7 with 7th character A	
HAC	ØRG[L,M][Ø,3,4][4,5,7,J,K]Z when reported with SDx K68.11 or T81.4XXA or T84.60-T84.619, T84.63-T84.7 with 7th character A	

🅛🅒 Limited Coverage   🅝🅒 Noncovered   ⊞ Combination Member   HAC associated procedure   Combination Only   DRG Non-OR   Non-OR   New/Revised in GREEN

566   ICD-10-PCS 2019

Ø   **Medical and Surgical**
R   **Upper Joints**
H   **Insertion**   Definition: Putting in a nonbiological appliance that monitors, assists, performs, or prevents a physiological function but does not physically take the place of a body part

                 Explanation: None

Body Part Character 4	Approach Character 5	Device Character 6	Qualifier Character 7

Ø Occipital-cervical Joint
1 Cervical Vertebral Joint
   Atlantoaxial joint
   Cervical facet joint
4 Cervicothoracic Vertebral Joint
   Cervicothoracic facet joint
6 Thoracic Vertebral Joint
   Costotransverse joint
   Costovertebral joint
   Thoracic facet joint
A Thoracolumbar Vertebral Joint
   Thoracolumbar facet joint
	Ø Open
	3 Percutaneous
	4 Percutaneous Endoscopic
		3 Infusion Device
		4 Internal Fixation Device
		8 Spacer
		B Spinal Stabilization Device, Interspinous Process
		C Spinal Stabilization Device, Pedicle-Based
		D Spinal Stabilization Device, Facet Replacement
			Z No Qualifier

3 Cervical Vertebral Disc **5** Cervicothoracic Vertebral Disc **9** Thoracic Vertebral Disc **B** Thoracolumbar Vertebral Disc	**Ø** Open **3** Percutaneous **4** Percutaneous Endoscopic	**3** Infusion Device	**Z** No Qualifier

C Temporomandibular Joint, Right
D Temporomandibular Joint, Left
E Sternoclavicular Joint, Right
F Sternoclavicular Joint, Left
G Acromioclavicular Joint, Right
H Acromioclavicular Joint, Left
J Shoulder Joint, Right
   Glenohumeral joint
   Glenoid ligament (labrum)
K Shoulder Joint, Left
   See J Shoulder Joint, Right
	Ø Open
	3 Percutaneous
	4 Percutaneous Endoscopic
		3 Infusion Device
		4 Internal Fixation Device
		8 Spacer
			Z No Qualifier

L Elbow Joint, Right
   Distal humerus, involving joint
   Humeroradial joint
   Humeroulnar joint
   Proximal radioulnar joint
M Elbow Joint, Left
   See L Elbow Joint, Right
N Wrist Joint, Right
   Distal radioulnar joint
   Radiocarpal joint
P Wrist Joint, Left
   See N Wrist Joint, Right
Q Carpal Joint, Right
   Intercarpal joint
   Midcarpal joint
R Carpal Joint, Left
   See Q Carpal Joint, Right
S Carpometacarpal Joint, Right
T Carpometacarpal Joint, Left
U Metacarpophalangeal Joint, Right
V Metacarpophalangeal Joint, Left
W Finger Phalangeal Joint, Right
   Interphalangeal (IP) joint
X Finger Phalangeal Joint, Left
   See W Finger Phalangeal Joint, Right
	Ø Open
	3 Percutaneous
	4 Percutaneous Endoscopic
		3 Infusion Device
		4 Internal Fixation Device
		5 External Fixation Device
		8 Spacer
			Z No Qualifier

Non-OR	ØRH[Ø,1,4,6,A][Ø,3,4][3,8]Z
Non-OR	ØRH[3,5,9,B][Ø,3,4]3Z
Non-OR	ØRH[C,D][Ø,4]8Z
Non-OR	ØRH[C,D]3[3,8]Z
Non-OR	ØRH[E,F,G,H,J,K][Ø,3,4][3,8]Z
Non-OR	ØRH[L,M,N,P,Q,R,S,T,U,V,W,X][Ø,3,4][3,8]Z

LC Limited Coverage   **NC** Noncovered   ⊞ Combination Member   HAC associated procedure   Combination Only   DRG Non-OR   Non-OR   New/Revised in GREEN

ICD-10-PCS 2019   **567**

ØRH–ØRH

Upper Joints

Ø　Medical and Surgical
R　Upper Joints
J　Inspection　　Definition: Visually and/or manually exploring a body part
　　　　　　　　　　Explanation: Visual exploration may be performed with or without optical instrumentation. Manual exploration may be performed directly or
　　　　　　　　　　through intervening body layers.

Body Part Character 4	Approach Character 5	Device Character 6	Qualifier Character 7
Ø **Occipital-cervical Joint**	**Ø** Open	**Z** No Device	**Z** No Qualifier
1 **Cervical Vertebral Joint**	**3** Percutaneous		
Atlantoaxial joint	**4** Percutaneous Endoscopic		
Cervical facet joint	**X** External		
3 **Cervical Vertebral Disc**			
4 **Cervicothoracic Vertebral Joint**			
Cervicothoracic facet joint			
5 **Cervicothoracic Vertebral Disc**			
6 **Thoracic Vertebral Joint**			
Costotransverse joint			
Costovertebral joint			
Thoracic facet joint			
9 **Thoracic Vertebral Disc**			
A **Thoracolumbar Vertebral Joint**			
Thoracolumbar facet joint			
B **Thoracolumbar Vertebral Disc**			
C **Temporomandibular Joint, Right**			
D **Temporomandibular Joint, Left**			
E **Sternoclavicular Joint, Right**			
F **Sternoclavicular Joint, Left**			
G **Acromioclavicular Joint, Right**			
H **Acromioclavicular Joint, Left**			
J **Shoulder Joint, Right**			
Glenohumeral joint			
Glenoid ligament (labrum)			
K **Shoulder Joint, Left**			
See J Shoulder Joint, Right			
L **Elbow Joint, Right**			
Distal humerus, involving joint			
Humeroradial joint			
Humeroulnar joint			
Proximal radioulnar joint			
M **Elbow Joint, Left**			
See L Elbow Joint, Right			
N **Wrist Joint, Right**			
Distal radioulnar joint			
Radiocarpal joint			
P **Wrist Joint, Left**			
See N Wrist Joint, Right			
Q **Carpal Joint, Right**			
Intercarpal joint			
Midcarpal joint			
R **Carpal Joint, Left**			
See Q Carpal Joint, Right			
S **Carpometacarpal Joint, Right**			
T **Carpometacarpal Joint, Left**			
U **Metacarpophalangeal Joint, Right**			
V **Metacarpophalangeal Joint, Left**			
W **Finger Phalangeal Joint, Right**			
Interphalangeal (IP) joint			
X **Finger Phalangeal Joint, Left**			
See W Finger Phalangeal Joint, Right			

Non-OR　ØRJ[Ø,1,3,4,5,6,9,A,B,C,D,E,F,G,H,J,K,L,M,N,P,Q,R,S,T,U,V,W,X][3,X]ZZ

Ø   Medical and Surgical
R   Upper Joints
N   Release   Definition: Freeing a body part from an abnormal physical constraint by cutting or by the use of force
                     Explanation: Some of the restraining tissue may be taken out but none of the body part is taken out

Body Part Character 4	Approach Character 5	Device Character 6	Qualifier Character 7
Ø **Occipital-cervical Joint**	**Ø** Open	**Z** No Device	**Z** No Qualifier
1 **Cervical Vertebral Joint**	**3** Percutaneous		
Atlantoaxial joint	**4** Percutaneous Endoscopic		
Cervical facet joint	**X** External		
3 **Cervical Vertebral Disc**			
4 **Cervicothoracic Vertebral Joint**			
Cervicothoracic facet joint			
5 **Cervicothoracic Vertebral Disc**			
6 **Thoracic Vertebral Joint**			
Costotransverse joint			
Costovertebral joint			
Thoracic facet joint			
9 **Thoracic Vertebral Disc**			
A **Thoracolumbar Vertebral Joint**			
Thoracolumbar facet joint			
B **Thoracolumbar Vertebral Disc**			
C **Temporomandibular Joint, Right**			
D **Temporomandibular Joint, Left**			
E **Sternoclavicular Joint, Right**			
F **Sternoclavicular Joint, Left**			
G **Acromioclavicular Joint, Right**			
H **Acromioclavicular Joint, Left**			
J **Shoulder Joint, Right**			
Glenohumeral joint			
Glenoid ligament (labrum)			
K **Shoulder Joint, Left**			
See J Shoulder Joint, Right			
L **Elbow Joint, Right**			
Distal humerus, involving joint			
Humeroradial joint			
Humeroulnar joint			
Proximal radioulnar joint			
M **Elbow Joint, Left**			
See L Elbow Joint, Right			
N **Wrist Joint, Right**			
Distal radioulnar joint			
Radiocarpal joint			
P **Wrist Joint, Left**			
See N Wrist Joint, Right			
Q **Carpal Joint, Right**			
Intercarpal joint			
Midcarpal joint			
R **Carpal Joint, Left**			
See Q Carpal Joint, Right			
S **Carpometacarpal Joint, Right**			
T **Carpometacarpal Joint, Left**			
U **Metacarpophalangeal Joint, Right**			
V **Metacarpophalangeal Joint, Left**			
W **Finger Phalangeal Joint, Right**			
Interphalangeal (IP) joint			
X **Finger Phalangeal Joint, Left**			
See W Finger Phalangeal Joint, Right			

Non-OR   ØRN[Ø,1,3,4,5,6,9,A,B,C,D,E,F,G,H,J,K,L,M,N,P,Q,R,S,T,U,V,W,X]XZZ

LC Limited Coverage   NC Noncovered   ⊞ Combination Member   HAC associated procedure   Combination Only   DRG Non-OR   Non-OR   New/Revised in GREEN

ICD-10-PCS 2019   569

Ø   Medical and Surgical
R   Upper Joints
P   Removal   Definition: Taking out or off a device from a body part

Explanation: If a device is taken out and a similar device put in without cutting or puncturing the skin or mucous membrane, the procedure is coded to the root operation CHANGE. Otherwise, the procedure for taking out the device is coded to the root operation REMOVAL.

Body Part Character 4	Approach Character 5	Device Character 6	Qualifier Character 7

Ø   Occipital-cervical Joint
1   Cervical Vertebral Joint
    Atlantoaxial joint
    Cervical facet joint
4   Cervicothoracic Vertebral Joint
    Cervicothoracic facet joint
6   Thoracic Vertebral Joint
    Costotransverse joint
    Costovertebral joint
    Thoracic facet joint
A   Thoracolumbar Vertebral Joint
    Thoracolumbar facet joint
	Ø Open
	3 Percutaneous
	4 Percutaneous Endoscopic
		Ø Drainage Device
		3 Infusion Device
		4 Internal Fixation Device
		7 Autologous Tissue
		    Substitute
		8 Spacer
		A Interbody Fusion Device
		J Synthetic Substitute
		K Nonautologous Tissue
		    Substitute
			Z No Qualifier

Ø   Occipital-cervical Joint
1   Cervical Vertebral Joint
    Atlantoaxial joint
    Cervical facet joint
4   Cervicothoracic Vertebral Joint
    Cervicothoracic facet joint
6   Thoracic Vertebral Joint
    Costotransverse joint
    Costovertebral joint
    Thoracic facet joint
A   Thoracolumbar Vertebral Joint
    Thoracolumbar facet joint
	X External	Ø Drainage Device
		3 Infusion Device
		4 Internal Fixation Device
			Z No Qualifier

3   Cervical Vertebral Disc
5   Cervicothoracic Vertebral Disc
9   Thoracic Vertebral Disc
B   Thoracolumbar Vertebral Disc
	Ø Open
	3 Percutaneous
	4 Percutaneous Endoscopic
		Ø Drainage Device
		3 Infusion Device
		7 Autologous Tissue
		    Substitute
		J Synthetic Substitute
		K Nonautologous Tissue
		    Substitute
			Z No Qualifier

3 Cervical Vertebral Disc 5 Cervicothoracic Vertebral Disc 9 Thoracic Vertebral Disc B Thoracolumbar Vertebral Disc	X External	Ø Drainage Device 3 Infusion Device	Z No Qualifier

C   Temporomandibular Joint, Right
D   Temporomandibular Joint, Left
E   Sternoclavicular Joint, Right
F   Sternoclavicular Joint, Left
G   Acromioclavicular Joint, Right
H   Acromioclavicular Joint, Left
J   Shoulder Joint, Right
    Glenohumeral joint
    Glenoid ligament (labrum)
K   Shoulder Joint, Left
    See J Shoulder Joint, Right
	Ø Open
	3 Percutaneous
	4 Percutaneous Endoscopic
		Ø Drainage Device
		3 Infusion Device
		4 Internal Fixation Device
		7 Autologous Tissue
		    Substitute
		8 Spacer
		J Synthetic Substitute
		K Nonautologous Tissue
		    Substitute
			Z No Qualifier

C   Temporomandibular Joint, Right
D   Temporomandibular Joint, Left
E   Sternoclavicular Joint, Right
F   Sternoclavicular Joint, Left
G   Acromioclavicular Joint, Right
H   Acromioclavicular Joint, Left
J   Shoulder Joint, Right
    Glenohumeral joint
    Glenoid ligament (labrum)
K   Shoulder Joint, Left
    See J Shoulder Joint, Right
	X External	Ø Drainage Device
		3 Infusion Device
		4 Internal Fixation Device
			Z No Qualifier

ØRP Continued on next page

Non-OR	ØRP[Ø,1,4,6,A]3[Ø,3,8]Z
Non-OR	ØRP[Ø,1,4,6,A][Ø,4]8Z
Non-OR	ØRP[Ø,1,4,6,A]X[Ø,3,4]Z
Non-OR	ØRP[3,5,9,B]3[Ø,3]Z
Non-OR	ØRP[3,5,9,B]X[Ø,3]Z
Non-OR	ØRP[C,D,E,F,G,H,J,K]3[Ø,3,8]Z
Non-OR	ØRP[C,D,E,F,G,H,J,K][Ø,4]8Z
Non-OR	ØRP[C,D]X[Ø,3]Z
Non-OR	ØRP[E,F,G,H,J,K]X[Ø,3,4]Z

Ø   Medical and Surgical   *ØRP Continued*
R   Upper Joints
P   Removal   Definition: Taking out or off a device from a body part

Explanation: If a device is taken out and a similar device put in without cutting or puncturing the skin or mucous membrane, the procedure is coded to the root operation CHANGE. Otherwise, the procedure for taking out the device is coded to the root operation REMOVAL.

Body Part Character 4	Approach Character 5	Device Character 6	Qualifier Character 7

L Elbow Joint, Right
   Distal humerus, involving joint
   Humeroradial joint
   Humeroulnar joint
   Proximal radioulnar joint
M Elbow Joint, Left
   See L Elbow Joint, Right
N Wrist Joint, Right
   Distal radioulnar joint
   Radiocarpal joint
P Wrist Joint, Left
   See N Wrist Joint, Right
Q Carpal Joint, Right
   Intercarpal joint
   Midcarpal joint
R Carpal Joint, Left
   See Q Carpal Joint, Right
S Carpometacarpal Joint, Right
T Carpometacarpal Joint, Left
U Metacarpophalangeal Joint, Right
V Metacarpophalangeal Joint, Left
W Finger Phalangeal Joint, Right
   Interphalangeal (IP) joint
X Finger Phalangeal Joint, Left
   See W Finger Phalangeal Joint, Right
	Ø Open
	3 Percutaneous
	4 Percutaneous Endoscopic
		Ø Drainage Device
		3 Infusion Device
		4 Internal Fixation Device
		5 External Fixation Device
		7 Autologous Tissue
		   Substitute
		8 Spacer
		J Synthetic Substitute
		K Nonautologous Tissue
		   Substitute
			Z No Qualifier

L Elbow Joint, Right
   Distal humerus, involving joint
   Humeroradial joint
   Humeroulnar joint
   Proximal radioulnar joint
M Elbow Joint, Left
   See L Elbow Joint, Right
N Wrist Joint, Right
   Distal radioulnar joint
   Radiocarpal joint
P Wrist Joint, Left
   See N Wrist Joint, Right
Q Carpal Joint, Right
   Intercarpal joint
   Midcarpal joint
R Carpal Joint, Left
   See Q Carpal Joint, Right
S Carpometacarpal Joint, Right
T Carpometacarpal Joint, Left
U Metacarpophalangeal Joint, Right
V Metacarpophalangeal Joint, Left
W Finger Phalangeal Joint, Right
   Interphalangeal (IP) joint
X Finger Phalangeal Joint, Left
   See W Finger Phalangeal Joint, Right
	X External	**Ø** Drainage Device
		3 Infusion Device
		4 Internal Fixation Device
		5 External Fixation Device
			Z No Qualifier

Non-OR   ØRP[L,M,N,P,Q,R,S,T,U,V,W,X]3[Ø,3,8]Z
Non-OR   ØRP[L,M,N,P,Q,R,S,T,U,V,W,X][Ø,4]8Z
Non-OR   ØRP[L,M,N,P,Q,R,S,T,U,V,W,X]X[Ø,3,4,5]Z

⬛ Limited Coverage   ⬛ Noncovered   ⊞ Combination Member   HAC associated procedure   Combination Only   DRG Non-OR   Non-OR   New/Revised in GREEN

ICD-10-PCS 2019   571

Upper Joints

Ø   **Medical and Surgical**
R   **Upper Joints**
Q   **Repair**   Definition: Restoring, to the extent possible, a body part to its normal anatomic structure and function
               Explanation: Used only when the method to accomplish the repair is not one of the other root operations

Body Part Character 4	Approach Character 5	Device Character 6	Qualifier Character 7

Ø Occipital-cervical Joint
1 Cervical Vertebral Joint
   Atlantoaxial joint
   Cervical facet joint
3 Cervical Vertebral Disc
4 Cervicothoracic Vertebral Joint
   Cervicothoracic facet joint
5 Cervicothoracic Vertebral Disc
6 Thoracic Vertebral Joint
   Costotransverse joint
   Costovertebral joint
   Thoracic facet joint
9 Thoracic Vertebral Disc
A Thoracolumbar Vertebral Joint
   Thoracolumbar facet joint
B Thoracolumbar Vertebral Disc
C Temporomandibular Joint, Right
D Temporomandibular Joint, Left
E Sternoclavicular Joint, Right
F Sternoclavicular Joint, Left
G Acromioclavicular Joint, Right
H Acromioclavicular Joint, Left
J Shoulder Joint, Right
   Glenohumeral joint
   Glenoid ligament (labrum)
K Shoulder Joint, Left
   See J Shoulder Joint, Right
L Elbow Joint, Right
   Distal humerus, involving joint
   Humeroradial joint
   Humeroulnar joint
   Proximal radioulnar joint
M Elbow Joint, Left
   See L Elbow Joint, Right
N Wrist Joint, Right
   Distal radioulnar joint
   Radiocarpal joint
P Wrist Joint, Left
   See N Wrist Joint, Right
Q Carpal Joint, Right
   Intercarpal joint
   Midcarpal joint
R Carpal Joint, Left
   See Q Carpal Joint, Right
S Carpometacarpal Joint, Right
T Carpometacarpal Joint, Left
U Metacarpophalangeal Joint, Right
V Metacarpophalangeal Joint, Left
W Finger Phalangeal Joint, Right
   Interphalangeal (IP) joint
X Finger Phalangeal Joint, Left
   See W Finger Phalangeal Joint, Right
	Ø Open
	3 Percutaneous
	4 Percutaneous Endoscopic
	X External
		Z No Device	Z No Qualifier

Non-OR   ØRQ[Ø,1,3,4,5,6,9,A,B,C,D,E,F,G,H,J,K,L,M,N,P,Q,R,S,T,U,V,W,X]XZZ
HAC   ØRQ[E,F,G,H,J,K,L,M][Ø,3,4,X]ZZ when reported with SDx K68.11 or T81.4XXA or T84.6Ø-T84.619, T84.63-T84.7 with 7th character A

Ø   **Medical and Surgical**
R   **Upper Joints**
R   **Replacement**   Definition: Putting in or on biological or synthetic material that physically takes the place and/or function of all or a portion of a body part
                                  Explanation: The body part may have been taken out or replaced, or may be taken out, physically eradicated, or rendered nonfunctional during
                                  the REPLACEMENT procedure. A REMOVAL procedure is coded for taking out the device used in a previous replacement procedure.

Body Part Character 4	Approach Character 5	Device Character 6	Qualifier Character 7

Ø Occipital-cervical Joint
1 Cervical Vertebral Joint
   Atlantoaxial joint
   Cervical facet joint
3 Cervical Vertebral Disc
4 Cervicothoracic Vertebral Joint
   Cervicothoracic facet joint
5 Cervicothoracic Vertebral Disc
6 Thoracic Vertebral Joint
   Costotransverse joint
   Costovertebral joint
   Thoracic facet joint
9 Thoracic Vertebral Disc
A Thoracolumbar Vertebral Joint
   Thoracolumbar facet joint
B Thoracolumbar Vertebral Disc
C Temporomandibular Joint, Right
D Temporomandibular Joint, Left
E Sternoclavicular Joint, Right
F Sternoclavicular Joint, Left
G Acromioclavicular Joint, Right
H Acromioclavicular Joint, Left
L Elbow Joint, Right
   Distal humerus, involving joint
   Humeroradial joint
   Humeroulnar joint
   Proximal radioulnar joint
M Elbow Joint, Left
   See L Elbow Joint, Right
N Wrist Joint, Right
   Distal radioulnar joint
   Radiocarpal joint
P Wrist Joint, Left
   See N Wrist Joint, Right
Q Carpal Joint, Right
   Intercarpal joint
   Midcarpal joint
R Carpal Joint, Left
   See Q Carpal Joint, Right
S Carpometacarpal Joint, Right
T Carpometacarpal Joint, Left
U Metacarpophalangeal Joint, Right
V Metacarpophalangeal Joint, Left
W Finger Phalangeal Joint, Right
   Interphalangeal (IP) joint
X Finger Phalangeal Joint, Left
   See W Finger Phalangeal Joint, Right
	Ø Open	**7 Autologous Tissue Substitute**
		J Synthetic Substitute
		K Nonautologous Tissue Substitute
			Z No Qualifier

J Shoulder Joint, Right
   Glenohumeral joint
   Glenoid ligament (labrum)
K Shoulder Joint, Left
   See J Shoulder Joint, Right
	Ø Open	**Ø Synthetic Substitute, Reverse Ball and Socket**
		7 Autologous Tissue Substitute
		K Nonautologous Tissue Substitute
			Z No Qualifier

J Shoulder Joint, Right
   Glenohumeral joint
   Glenoid ligament (labrum)
K Shoulder Joint, Left
   See J Shoulder Joint, Right
	Ø Open	**J Synthetic Substitute**	**6 Humeral Surface**
			7 Glenoid Surface
			Z No Qualifier

LC Limited Coverage   NC Noncovered   ⊞ Combination Member   HAC associated procedure   Combination Only   DRG Non-OR   Non-OR   New/Revised in GREEN

ICD-10-PCS 2019   573

Upper Joints

Ø	Medical and Surgical
R	Upper Joints
S	Reposition

Definition: Moving to its normal location, or other suitable location, all or a portion of a body part

Explanation: The body part is moved to a new location from an abnormal location, or from a normal location where it is not functioning correctly. The body part may or may not be cut out or off to be moved to the new location.

Body Part Character 4	Approach Character 5	Device Character 6	Qualifier Character 7

Ø Occipital-cervical Joint
1 Cervical Vertebral Joint
   Atlantoaxial joint
   Cervical facet joint
4 Cervicothoracic Vertebral Joint
   Cervicothoracic facet joint
6 Thoracic Vertebral Joint
   Costotransverse joint
   Costovertebral joint
   Thoracic facet joint
A Thoracolumbar Vertebral Joint
   Thoracolumbar facet joint
C Temporomandibular Joint, Right
D Temporomandibular Joint, Left
E Sternoclavicular Joint, Right
F Sternoclavicular Joint, Left
G Acromioclavicular Joint, Right
H Acromioclavicular Joint, Left
J Shoulder Joint, Right
   Glenohumeral joint
   Glenoid ligament (labrum)
K Shoulder Joint, Left
   See J Shoulder Joint, Right
	Ø Open
	3 Percutaneous
	4 Percutaneous Endoscopic
	X External
		4 Internal Fixation Device
		Z No Device
			Z No Qualifier

L Elbow Joint, Right
   Distal humerus, involving joint
   Humeroradial joint
   Humeroulnar joint
   Proximal radioulnar joint
M Elbow Joint, Left
   See L Elbow Joint, Right
N Wrist Joint, Right
   Distal radioulnar joint
   Radiocarpal joint
P Wrist Joint, Left
   See N Wrist Joint, Right
Q Carpal Joint, Right
   Intercarpal joint
   Midcarpal joint
R Carpal Joint, Left
   See Q Carpal Joint, Right
S Carpometacarpal Joint, Right
T Carpometacarpal Joint, Left
U Metacarpophalangeal Joint, Right
V Metacarpophalangeal Joint, Left
W Finger Phalangeal Joint, Right
   Interphalangeal (IP) joint
X Finger Phalangeal Joint, Left
   See W Finger Phalangeal Joint, Right
	Ø Open
	3 Percutaneous
	4 Percutaneous Endoscopic
	X External
		4 Internal Fixation Device
		5 External Fixation Device
		Z No Device
			Z No Qualifier

Non-OR	ØRS[Ø,1,4,6,A,C,D,E,F,G,H,J,K][3,4,X][4,Z]Z
Non-OR	ØRS[L,M,N,P,Q,R,S,T,U,V,W,X][3,4,X][4,5,Z]Z

LC Limited Coverage   **NC** Noncovered   ⊞ Combination Member   HAC associated procedure   Combination Only   DRG Non-OR   Non-OR   New/Revised in GREEN

574   ICD-10-PCS 2019

Ø   Medical and Surgical
R   Upper Joints
T   Resection   Definition: Cutting out or off, without replacement, all of a body part
                        Explanation: None

Body Part Character 4		Approach Character 5	Device Character 6	Qualifier Character 7
3 Cervical Vertebral Disc	**M** Elbow Joint, Left	**Ø** Open	**Z** No Device	**Z** No Qualifier
4 Cervicothoracic Vertebral Joint	*See L Elbow Joint, Right*			
Cervicothoracic facet joint	**N** Wrist Joint, Right			
5 Cervicothoracic Vertebral Disc	Distal radioulnar joint			
9 Thoracic Vertebral Disc	Radiocarpal joint			
B Thoracolumbar Vertebral Disc	**P** Wrist Joint, Left			
C Temporomandibular Joint, Right	*See N Wrist Joint, Right*			
D Temporomandibular Joint, Left	**Q** Carpal Joint, Right			
E Sternoclavicular Joint, Right	Intercarpal joint			
F Sternoclavicular Joint, Left	Midcarpal joint			
G Acromioclavicular Joint, Right	**R** Carpal Joint, Left			
H Acromioclavicular Joint, Left	*See Q Carpal Joint, Right*			
J Shoulder Joint, Right	**S** Carpometacarpal Joint, Right			
Glenohumeral joint	**T** Carpometacarpal Joint, Left			
Glenoid ligament (labrum)	**U** Metacarpophalangeal Joint, Right			
K Shoulder Joint, Left	**V** Metacarpophalangeal Joint, Left			
See J Shoulder Joint, Right	**W** Finger Phalangeal Joint, Right			
L Elbow Joint, Right	Interphalangeal (IP) joint			
Distal humerus, involving joint	**X** Finger Phalangeal Joint, Left			
Humeroradial joint	*See W Finger Phalangeal Joint, Right*			
Humeroulnar joint				
Proximal radioulnar joint				

Ø   Medical and Surgical
R   Upper Joints
U   Supplement   Definition: Putting in or on biological or synthetic material that physically reinforces and/or augments the function of a portion of a body part
                        Explanation: The biological material is non-living, or is living and from the same individual. The body part may have been previously replaced, and the SUPPLEMENT procedure is performed to physically reinforce and/or augment the function of the replaced body part.

Body Part Character 4		Approach Character 5	Device Character 6	Qualifier Character 7
Ø Occipital-cervical Joint	**L** Elbow Joint, Right	**Ø** Open	**7** Autologous Tissue Substitute	**Z** No Qualifier
1 Cervical Vertebral Joint	Distal humerus, involving joint	**3** Percutaneous	**J** Synthetic Substitute	
Atlantoaxial joint	Humeroradial joint	**4** Percutaneous Endoscopic	**K** Nonautologous Tissue Substitute	
Cervical facet joint	Humeroulnar joint			
3 Cervical Vertebral Disc	Proximal radioulnar joint			
4 Cervicothoracic Vertebral Joint	**M** Elbow Joint, Left			
Cervicothoracic facet joint	*See L Elbow Joint, Right*			
5 Cervicothoracic Vertebral Disc	**N** Wrist Joint, Right			
6 Thoracic Vertebral Joint	Distal radioulnar joint			
Costotransverse joint	Radiocarpal joint			
Costovertebral joint	**P** Wrist Joint, Left			
Thoracic facet joint	*See N Wrist Joint, Right*			
9 Thoracic Vertebral Disc	**Q** Carpal Joint, Right			
A Thoracolumbar Vertebral Joint	Intercarpal joint			
Thoracolumbar facet joint	Midcarpal joint			
B Thoracolumbar Vertebral Disc	**R** Carpal Joint, Left			
C Temporomandibular Joint, Right	*See Q Carpal Joint, Right*			
D Temporomandibular Joint, Left	**S** Carpometacarpal Joint, Right			
E Sternoclavicular Joint, Right	**T** Carpometacarpal Joint, Left			
F Sternoclavicular Joint, Left	**U** Metacarpophalangeal Joint, Right			
G Acromioclavicular Joint, Right	**V** Metacarpophalangeal Joint, Left			
H Acromioclavicular Joint, Left	**W** Finger Phalangeal Joint, Right			
J Shoulder Joint, Right	Interphalangeal (IP) joint			
Glenohumeral joint	**X** Finger Phalangeal Joint, Left			
Glenoid ligament (labrum)	*See W Finger Phalangeal Joint, Right*			
K Shoulder Joint, Left				
See J Shoulder Joint, Right				

HAC   ØRU[E,F,G,H,J,K,L,M][Ø,3,4][7,J,K]Z when reported with SDx K68.11 or T81.4XXA or T84.6Ø-T84.619, T84.63-T84.7 with 7th character A

Ø   Medical and Surgical
R   Upper Joints
W   Revision   Definition: Correcting, to the extent possible, a portion of a malfunctioning device or the position of a displaced device

Explanation: Revision can include correcting a malfunctioning or displaced device by taking out or putting in components of the device such as a screw or pin

Body Part Character 4	Approach Character 5	Device Character 6	Qualifier Character 7

Ø Occipital-cervical Joint
1 Cervical Vertebral Joint
   Atlantoaxial joint
   Cervical facet joint
4 Cervicothoracic Vertebral Joint
   Cervicothoracic facet joint
6 Thoracic Vertebral Joint
   Costotransverse joint
   Costovertebral joint
   Thoracic facet joint
A Thoracolumbar Vertebral Joint
   Thoracolumbar facet joint
	Ø Open
	3 Percutaneous
	4 Percutaneous Endoscopic
	X External
		Ø Drainage Device
		3 Infusion Device
		4 Internal Fixation Device
		7 Autologous Tissue
		Substitute
		8 Spacer
		A Interbody Fusion Device
		J Synthetic Substitute
		K Nonautologous Tissue
		Substitute
			Z No Qualifier

3 Cervical Vertebral Disc **5 Cervicothoracic Vertebral Disc** **9 Thoracic Vertebral Disc** **B Thoracolumbar Vertebral Disc**	**Ø Open** **3 Percutaneous** **4 Percutaneous Endoscopic** **X External**	**Ø Drainage Device** **3 Infusion Device** **7 Autologous Tissue** **Substitute** **J Synthetic Substitute** **K Nonautologous Tissue** **Substitute**	**Z No Qualifier**

C Temporomandibular Joint, Right
D Temporomandibular Joint, Left
E Sternoclavicular Joint, Right
F Sternoclavicular Joint, Left
G Acromioclavicular Joint, Right
H Acromioclavicular Joint, Left
J Shoulder Joint, Right
   Glenohumeral joint
   Glenoid ligament (labrum)
K Shoulder Joint, Left
   See J Shoulder Joint, Right
	Ø Open
	3 Percutaneous
	4 Percutaneous Endoscopic
	X External
		Ø Drainage Device
		3 Infusion Device
		4 Internal Fixation Device
		7 Autologous Tissue
		Substitute
		8 Spacer
		J Synthetic Substitute
		K Nonautologous Tissue
		Substitute
			Z No Qualifier

L Elbow Joint, Right
   Distal humerus, involving joint
   Humeroradial joint
   Humeroulnar joint
   Proximal radioulnar joint
M Elbow Joint, Left
   See L Elbow Joint, Right
N Wrist Joint, Right
   Distal radioulnar joint
   Radiocarpal joint
P Wrist Joint, Left
   See N Wrist Joint, Right
Q Carpal Joint, Right
   Intercarpal joint
   Midcarpal joint
R Carpal Joint, Left
   See Q Carpal Joint, Right
S Carpometacarpal Joint, Right
T Carpometacarpal Joint, Left
U Metacarpophalangeal Joint, Right
V Metacarpophalangeal Joint, Left
W Finger Phalangeal Joint, Right
   Interphalangeal (IP) joint
X Finger Phalangeal Joint, Left
   See W Finger Phalangeal Joint, Right
	Ø Open
	3 Percutaneous
	4 Percutaneous Endoscopic
	X External
		Ø Drainage Device
		3 Infusion Device
		4 Internal Fixation Device
		5 External Fixation Device
		7 Autologous Tissue
		Substitute
		8 Spacer
		J Synthetic Substitute
		K Nonautologous Tissue
		Substitute
			Z No Qualifier

Non-OR	ØRW[Ø,1,4,6,A]X[Ø,3,4,7,8,A,J,K]Z
Non-OR	ØRW[3,5,9,B]X[Ø,3,7,J,K]Z
Non-OR	ØRW[C,D,E,F,G,H,J,K]X[Ø,3,4,7,8,J,K]Z
Non-OR	ØRW[L,M,N,P,Q,R,S,T,U,V,W,X]X[Ø,3,4,5,7,8,J,K]Z

LC Limited Coverage   **NC** Noncovered   ⊞ Combination Member   HAC associated procedure   Combination Only   DRG Non-OR   Non-OR   New/Revised in GREEN

576   ICD-10-PCS 2019

ØRW–ØRW

Lower Joints ØS2–ØSW

Character Meanings*

This Character Meaning table is provided as a guide to assist the user in the identification of character members that may be found in this section of code tables. It **SHOULD NOT** be used to build a PCS code.

Operation–Character 3	Body Part–Character 4	Approach–Character 5	Device–Character 6	Qualifier–Character 7
2 Change	Ø Lumbar Vertebral Joint	Ø Open	Ø Drainage Device OR Synthetic Substitute, Polyethylene	Ø Anterior Approach, Anterior Column
5 Destruction	1 Lumbar Vertebral Joint, 2 or more	3 Percutaneous	1 Synthetic Substitute, Metal	1 Posterior Approach, Posterior Column
9 Drainage	2 Lumbar Vertebral Disc	4 Percutaneous Endoscopic	2 Synthetic Substitute, Metal on Polyethylene	9 Cemented
B Excision	3 Lumbosacral Joint	X External	3 Infusion Device OR Synthetic Substitute, Ceramic	A Uncemented
C Extirpation	4 Lumbosacral Disc		4 Internal Fixation Device OR Synthetic Substitute, Ceramic on Polyethylene	C Patellar Surface
G Fusion	5 Sacrococcygeal Joint		5 External Fixation Device	J Posterior Approach, Anterior Column
H Insertion	6 Coccygeal Joint		6 Synthetic Substitute, Oxidized Zirconium on Polyethylene	X Diagnostic
J Inspection	7 Sacroiliac Joint, Right		7 Autologous Tissue Substitute	Z No Qualifier
N Release	8 Sacroiliac Joint, Left		8 Spacer	
P Removal	9 Hip Joint, Right		9 Liner	
	A Hip Joint, Acetabular Surface, Right		A Interbody Fusion Device	
Q Repair	B Hip Joint, Left		B Resurfacing Device OR Spinal Stabilization Device, Interspinous Process	
R Replacement	C Knee Joint, Right		C Spinal Stabilization Device, Pedicle-Based	
S Reposition	D Knee Joint, Left		D Spinal Stabilization Device, Facet Replacement	
T Resection	E Hip Joint, Acetabular Surface, Left		E Articulating Spacer	
U Supplement	F Ankle Joint, Right		J Synthetic Substitute	
W Revision	G Ankle Joint, Left		K Nonautologous Tissue Substitute	
	H Tarsal Joint, Right		L Synthetic Substitute, Unicondylar Medial	
	J Tarsal Joint, Left		M Synthetic Substitute, Unicondylar Lateral	
	K Tarsometatarsal Joint, Right		N Synthetic Substitute, Patellofemoral	
	L Tarsometatarsal Joint, Left		Y Other Device	
	M Metatarsal-Phalangeal Joint, Right		Z No Device	
	N Metatarsal-Phalangeal Joint, Left			
	P Toe Phalangeal Joint, Right			
	Q Toe Phalangeal Joint, Left			
	R Hip Joint, Femoral Surface, Right			
	S Hip Joint, Femoral Surface, Left			
	T Knee Joint, Femoral Surface, Right			
	U Knee Joint, Femoral Surface, Left			
	V Knee Joint, Tibial Surface, Right			
	W Knee Joint, Tibial Surface, Left			
	Y Lower Joint			

* Includes synovial membrane.

Lower Joints

AHA Coding Clinic for table ØS9

2018, 2Q, 17	Arthroscopic drainage of knee and nonexcisional debridement
2017, 1Q, 50	Dry aspiration of ankle joint

AHA Coding Clinic for table ØSB

2017, 4Q, 76	Radiolucent porous interbody fusion device
2016, 2Q, 16	Decompressive laminectomy/foraminotomy and lumbar discectomy
2016, 1Q, 20	Metatarsophalangeal joint resection arthroplasty
2015, 1Q, 34	Arthroscopic meniscectomy with debridement and abrasion chondroplasty
2014, 2Q, 6	Posterior lumbar fusion with discectomy

AHA Coding Clinic for table ØSG

2018, 1Q, 22	Spinal fusion procedures without bone graft
2017, 4Q, 76	Radiolucent porous interbody fusion device
2017, 2Q, 23	Decompression of spinal cord and placement of instrumentation
2014, 3Q, 30	Spinal fusion and fixation instrumentation
2014, 3Q, 36	Lumbar interbody fusion of two vertebral levels
2014, 2Q, 6	Posterior lumbar fusion with discectomy
2013, 3Q, 25	360-degree spinal fusion
2013, 2Q, 39	Ankle fusion, osteotomy, and removal of hardware
2013, 1Q, 21-23	Spinal fusion of thoracic and lumbar vertebrae

AHA Coding Clinic for table ØSH

2017, 2Q, 23	Decompression of spinal cord and placement of instrumentation

AHA Coding Clinic for table ØSJ

2017, 1Q, 50	Dry aspiration of ankle joint

AHA Coding Clinic for table ØSP

2018, 2Q, 16	Exchange of tibial polyethylene component with stabilizing insert (tibial tray)
2017, 4Q, 107	Total ankle replacement versus revision
2016, 4Q, 110-112	Removal and revision of hip and knee devices
2015, 2Q, 18	Total knee revision
2015, 2Q, 19	Revision of femoral head and acetabular liner
2013, 2Q, 39	Ankle fusion, osteotomy, and removal of hardware

AHA Coding Clinic for table ØSQ

2014, 4Q, 25	Femoroacetabular impingement and labral tear with repair

AHA Coding Clinic for table ØSR

2018, 2Q, 16	Exchange of tibial polyethylene component with stabilizing insert (tibial tray)
2017, 4Q, 38-39	Oxidized zirconium on polyethylene bearing surface
2017, 4Q, 107	Total ankle replacement versus revision
2017, 1Q, 22	Total knee replacement and patellar component
2016, 4Q, 110-111	Partial (unicondylar) knee replacement
2016, 4Q, 111-112	Removal and revision of hip and knee devices
2016, 3Q, 35	Use of cemented versus uncemented qualifier for joint replacement
2015, 3Q, 18	Total hip replacement with acetabular reconstruction
2015, 2Q, 18	Total knee revision
2015, 2Q, 19	Revision of femoral head and acetabular liner

AHA Coding Clinic for table ØSS

2016, 2Q, 31	Periacetabular ostectomy for repair of congenital hip dysplasia

AHA Coding Clinic for table ØST

2016, 1Q, 20	Metatarsophalangeal joint resection arthroplasty
2014, 4Q, 29	Rotational osteosynthesis

AHA Coding Clinic for table ØSU

2018, 2Q, 16	Exchange of tibial polyethylene component with stabilizing insert (tibial tray)
2016, 4Q, 111	Removal and revision of hip and knee devices
2015, 2Q, 19	Revision of femoral head and acetabular liner

AHA Coding Clinic for table ØSW

2017, 4Q, 107	Total ankle replacement versus revision
2016, 4Q, 110-112	Removal and revision of hip and knee devices
2015, 2Q, 18	Total knee revision
2015, 2Q, 19	Revision of femoral head and acetabular liner

Lower Joints

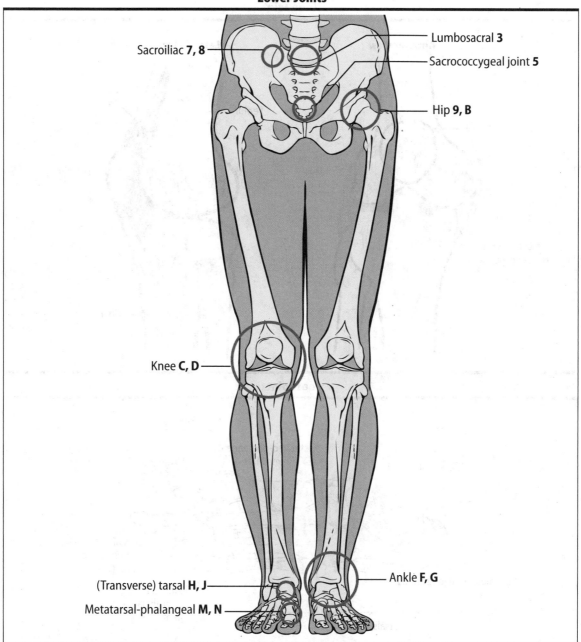

Sacroiliac **7, 8**

Lumbosacral **3**

Sacrococcygeal joint **5**

Hip **9, B**

Knee **C, D**

(Transverse) tarsal **H, J**

Metatarsal-phalangeal **M, N**

Ankle **F, G**

Hip Joint

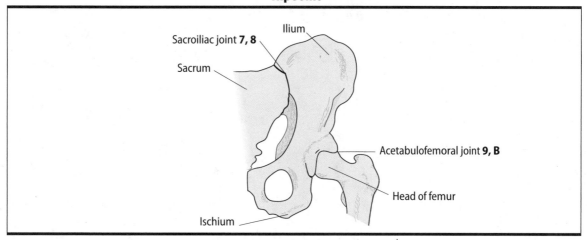

Sacroiliac joint **7, 8**

Ilium

Sacrum

Acetabulofemoral joint **9, B**

Head of femur

Ischium

Knee Joint

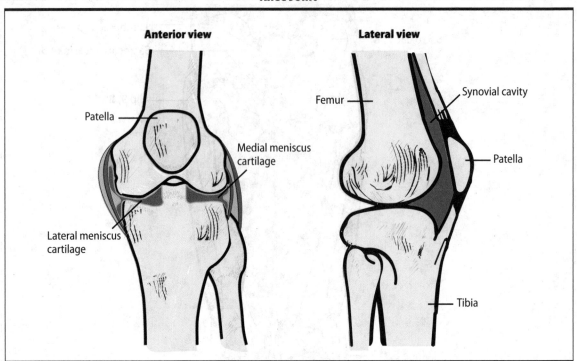

Anterior view

Patella

Medial meniscus cartilage

Lateral meniscus cartilage

Lateral view

Femur

Synovial cavity

Patella

Tibia

Foot Joints

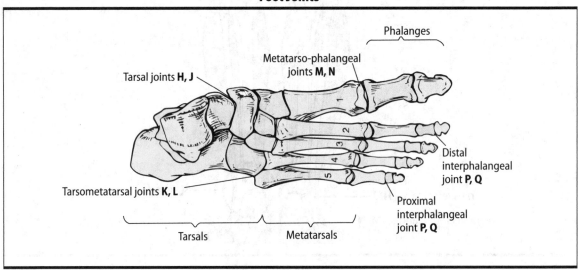

Phalanges

Metatarso-phalangeal joints **M, N**

Tarsal joints **H, J**

Tarsometatarsal joints **K, L**

Distal interphalangeal joint **P, Q**

Proximal interphalangeal joint **P, Q**

Tarsals

Metatarsals

Ø   **Medical and Surgical**
S   **Lower Joints**
2   **Change**   Definition: Taking out or off a device from a body part and putting back an identical or similar device in or on the same body part without cutting or puncturing the skin or a mucous membrane
                            Explanation: All CHANGE procedures are coded using the approach EXTERNAL

Body Part Character 4	Approach Character 5	Device Character 6	Qualifier Character 7
Y Lower Joint	X External	Ø Drainage Device Y Other Device	Z No Qualifier

Non-OR	All body part, approach, device, and qualifier values

Ø   **Medical and Surgical**
S   **Lower Joints**
5   **Destruction**   Definition: Physical eradication of all or a portion of a body part by the direct use of energy, force, or a destructive agent
                              Explanation: None of the body part is physically taken out

Body Part Character 4	Approach Character 5	Device Character 6	Qualifier Character 7

Ø   Lumbar Vertebral Joint
     Lumbar facet joint
2   Lumbar Vertebral Disc
3   Lumbosacral Joint
     Lumbosacral facet joint
4   Lumbosacral Disc
5   Sacrococcygeal Joint
     Sacrococcygeal symphysis
6   Coccygeal Joint
7   Sacroiliac Joint, Right
8   Sacroiliac Joint, Left
9   Hip Joint, Right
     Acetabulofemoral joint
B   Hip Joint, Left
     See 9 Hip Joint, Right
C   Knee Joint, Right
     Femoropatellar joint
     Femorotibial joint
     Lateral meniscus
     Medial meniscus
     Patellofemoral joint
     Tibiofemoral joint
D   Knee Joint, Left
     See C Knee Joint, Right
F   Ankle Joint, Right
     Inferior tibiofibular joint
     Talocrural joint
G   Ankle Joint, Left
     See F Ankle Joint, Right
H   Tarsal Joint, Right
     Calcaneocuboid joint
     Cuboideonavicular joint
     Cuneonavicular joint
     Intercuneiform joint
     Subtalar (talocalcaneal) joint
     Talocalcaneal (subtalar) joint
     Talocalcaneonavicular joint
J   Tarsal Joint, Left
     See H Tarsal Joint, Right
K   Tarsometatarsal Joint, Right
L   Tarsometatarsal Joint, Left
M   Metatarsal-Phalangeal Joint, Right
     Metatarsophalangeal (MTP) joint
N   Metatarsal-Phalangeal Joint, Left
     See M Metatarsal-Phalangeal Joint, Right
P   Toe Phalangeal Joint, Right
     Interphalangeal (IP) joint
Q   Toe Phalangeal Joint, Left
     See P Toe Phalangeal Joint, Right
	Ø Open
	3 Percutaneous
	4 Percutaneous Endoscopic
		Z No Device	Z No Qualifier

Ø   Medical and Surgical
S   Lower Joints
9   Drainage   Definition: Taking or letting out fluids and/or gases from a body part

Explanation: The qualifier DIAGNOSTIC is used to identify drainage procedures that are biopsies

Body Part Character 4		Approach Character 5	Device Character 6	Qualifier Character 7
Ø Lumbar Vertebral Joint	**H** Tarsal Joint, Right	**Ø** Open	**Ø** Drainage Device	**Z** No Qualifier
Lumbar facet joint	Calcaneocuboid joint	**3** Percutaneous		
2 Lumbar Vertebral Disc	Cuboideonavicular joint	**4** Percutaneous Endoscopic		
3 Lumbosacral Joint	Cuneonavicular joint			
Lumbosacral facet joint	Intercuneiform joint			
4 Lumbosacral Disc	Subtalar (talocalcaneal) joint			
5 Sacrococcygeal Joint	Talocalcaneal (subtalar) joint			
Sacrococcygeal symphysis	Talocalcaneonavicular joint			
6 Coccygeal Joint	**J** Tarsal Joint, Left			
7 Sacroiliac Joint, Right	*See H Tarsal Joint, Right*			
8 Sacroiliac Joint, Left	**K** Tarsometatarsal Joint, Right			
9 Hip Joint, Right	**L** Tarsometatarsal Joint, Left			
Acetabulofemoral joint	**M** Metatarsal-Phalangeal Joint, Right			
B Hip Joint, Left	Metatarsophalangeal (MTP) joint			
See 9 Hip Joint, Right	**N** Metatarsal-Phalangeal Joint, Left			
C Knee Joint, Right	*See M Metatarsal-Phalangeal Joint, Right*			
Femoropatellar joint	**P** Toe Phalangeal Joint, Right			
Femorotibial joint	Interphalangeal (IP) joint			
Lateral meniscus	**Q** Toe Phalangeal Joint, Left			
Medial meniscus	*See P Toe Phalangeal Joint, Right*			
Patellofemoral joint				
Tibiofemoral joint				
D Knee Joint, Left				
See C Knee Joint, Right				
F Ankle Joint, Right				
Inferior tibiofibular joint				
Talocrural joint				
G Ankle Joint, Left				
See F Ankle Joint, Right				
Ø Lumbar Vertebral Joint	**H** Tarsal Joint, Right	**Ø** Open	**Z** No Device	**X** Diagnostic
Lumbar facet joint	Calcaneocuboid joint	**3** Percutaneous		**Z** No Qualifier
2 Lumbar Vertebral Disc	Cuboideonavicular joint	**4** Percutaneous Endoscopic		
3 Lumbosacral Joint	Cuneonavicular joint			
Lumbosacral facet joint	Intercuneiform joint			
4 Lumbosacral Disc	Subtalar (talocalcaneal) joint			
5 Sacrococcygeal Joint	Talocalcaneal (subtalar) joint			
Sacrococcygeal symphysis	Talocalcaneonavicular joint			
6 Coccygeal Joint	**J** Tarsal Joint, Left			
7 Sacroiliac Joint, Right	*See H Tarsal Joint, Right*			
8 Sacroiliac Joint, Left	**K** Tarsometatarsal Joint, Right			
9 Hip Joint, Right	**L** Tarsometatarsal Joint, Left			
Acetabulofemoral joint	**M** Metatarsal-Phalangeal Joint, Right			
B Hip Joint, Left	Metatarsophalangeal (MTP) joint			
See 9 Hip Joint, Right	**N** Metatarsal-Phalangeal Joint, Left			
C Knee Joint, Right	*See M Metatarsal-Phalangeal Joint, Right*			
Femoropatellar joint	**P** Toe Phalangeal Joint, Right			
Femorotibial joint	Interphalangeal (IP) joint			
Lateral meniscus	**Q** Toe Phalangeal Joint, Left			
Medial meniscus	*See P Toe Phalangeal Joint, Right*			
Patellofemoral joint				
Tibiofemoral joint				
D Knee Joint, Left				
See C Knee Joint, Right				
F Ankle Joint, Right				
Inferior tibiofibular joint				
Talocrural joint				
G Ankle Joint, Left				
See F Ankle Joint, Right				

Non-OR   ØS9[Ø,2,3,4,5,6,7,8,9,B,C,D,F,G,H,J,K,L,M,N,P,Q][3,4]ØZ
Non-OR   ØS9[Ø,2,3,4,5,6,7,8,9,B,C,D,F,G,H,J,K,L,M,N,P,Q][Ø,3,4]ZX
Non-OR   ØS9[Ø,2,3,4,5,6,7,8,9,B,C,D,F,G,H,J,K,L,M,N,P,Q][3,4]ZZ

Ø   Medical and Surgical
S   Lower Joints
B   Excision   Definition: Cutting out or off, without replacement, a portion of a body part

               Explanation: The qualifier DIAGNOSTIC is used to identify excision procedures that are biopsies

Body Part Character 4		Approach Character 5	Device Character 6	Qualifier Character 7
Ø Lumbar Vertebral Joint Lumbar facet joint	**H Tarsal Joint, Right** Calcaneocuboid joint	**Ø Open**	**Z No Device**	**X Diagnostic**
2 Lumbar Vertebral Disc	Cuboideonavicular joint	**3 Percutaneous**		**Z No Qualifier**
3 Lumbosacral Joint Lumbosacral facet joint	Cuneonavicular joint Intercuneiform joint	**4 Percutaneous Endoscopic**		
4 Lumbosacral Disc	Subtalar (talocalcaneal) joint Talocalcaneal (subtalar) joint			
5 Sacrococcygeal Joint Sacrococcygeal symphysis	Talocalcaneonavicular joint			
6 Coccygeal Joint	**J Tarsal Joint, Left** *See H Tarsal Joint, Right*			
7 Sacroiliac Joint, Right	**K Tarsometatarsal Joint, Right**			
8 Sacroiliac Joint, Left	**L Tarsometatarsal Joint, Left**			
9 Hip Joint, Right Acetabulofemoral joint	**M Metatarsal-Phalangeal Joint, Right**			
B Hip Joint, Left *See 9 Hip Joint, Right*	Metatarsophalangeal (MTP) joint			
C Knee Joint, Right Femoropatellar joint	**N Metatarsal-Phalangeal Joint, Left**			
Femorotibial joint Lateral meniscus	*See M Metatarsal-Phalangeal Joint, Right*			
Medial meniscus Patellofemoral joint	**P Toe Phalangeal Joint, Right** Interphalangeal (IP) joint			
Tibiofemoral joint	**Q Toe Phalangeal Joint, Left**			
D Knee Joint, Left *See C Knee Joint, Right*	*See P Toe Phalangeal Joint, Right*			
F Ankle Joint, Right Inferior tibiofibular joint Talocrural joint				
G Ankle Joint, Left *See F Ankle Joint, Right*				

Non-OR   ØSB[Ø,2,3,4,5,6,7,8,9,B,C,D,F,G,H,J,K,L,M,N,P,Q][Ø,3,4]ZX

Ø   Medical and Surgical
S   Lower Joints
C   Extirpation   Definition: Taking or cutting out solid matter from a body part

               Explanation: The solid matter may be an abnormal byproduct of a biological function or a foreign body; it may be imbedded in a body part or in the lumen of a tubular body part. The solid matter may or may not have been previously broken into pieces.

Body Part Character 4		Approach Character 5	Device Character 6	Qualifier Character 7
Ø Lumbar Vertebral Joint Lumbar facet joint	**H Tarsal Joint, Right** Calcaneocuboid joint	**Ø Open**	**Z No Device**	**Z No Qualifier**
2 Lumbar Vertebral Disc	Cuboideonavicular joint	**3 Percutaneous**		
3 Lumbosacral Joint Lumbosacral facet joint	Cuneonavicular joint Intercuneiform joint	**4 Percutaneous Endoscopic**		
4 Lumbosacral Disc	Subtalar (talocalcaneal) joint Talocalcaneal (subtalar) joint			
5 Sacrococcygeal Joint Sacrococcygeal symphysis	Talocalcaneonavicular joint			
6 Coccygeal Joint	**J Tarsal Joint, Left** *See H Tarsal Joint, Right*			
7 Sacroiliac Joint, Right	**K Tarsometatarsal Joint, Right**			
8 Sacroiliac Joint, Left	**L Tarsometatarsal Joint, Left**			
9 Hip Joint, Right Acetabulofemoral joint	**M Metatarsal-Phalangeal Joint, Right**			
B Hip Joint, Left *See 9 Hip Joint, Right*	Metatarsophalangeal (MTP) joint			
C Knee Joint, Right Femoropatellar joint	**N Metatarsal-Phalangeal Joint, Left**			
Femorotibial joint Lateral meniscus	*See M Metatarsal-Phalangeal Joint, Right*			
Medial meniscus Patellofemoral joint	**P Toe Phalangeal Joint, Right** Interphalangeal (IP) joint			
Tibiofemoral joint	**Q Toe Phalangeal Joint, Left**			
D Knee Joint, Left *See C Knee Joint, Right*	*See P Toe Phalangeal Joint, Right*			
F Ankle Joint, Right Inferior tibiofibular joint Talocrural joint				
G Ankle Joint, Left *See F Ankle Joint, Right*				

LC Limited Coverage   **NC** Noncovered   ⊞ Combination Member   HAC associated procedure   Combination Only   DRG Non-OR   Non-OR   New/Revised in GREEN

ICD-10-PCS 2019   583

ØSB–ØSC

Ø   **Medical and Surgical**
S   **Lower Joints**
G   **Fusion**   Definition: Joining together portions of an articular body part rendering the articular body part immobile

                        Explanation: The body part is joined together by fixation device, bone graft, or other means

Body Part Character 4	Approach Character 5	Device Character 6	Qualifier Character 7

Ø Lumbar Vertebral Joint
   Lumbar facet joint
1 Lumbar Vertebral Joints, 2 or more ⊞
3 Lumbosacral Joint
   Lumbosacral facet joint
	Ø Open
	3 Percutaneous
	4 Percutaneous Endoscopic
		7 Autologous Tissue
		   Substitute
		J Synthetic Substitute
		K Nonautologous Tissue
		   Substitute
			Ø Anterior Approach, Anterior
			   Column
			1 Posterior Approach,
			   Posterior Column
			J Posterior Approach,
			   Anterior Column

Ø Lumbar Vertebral Joint
   Lumbar facet joint
1 Lumbar Vertebral Joints, 2 or more ⊞
3 Lumbosacral Joint
   Lumbosacral facet joint
	Ø Open
	3 Percutaneous
	4 Percutaneous Endoscopic
		A Interbody Fusion Device	**Ø** Anterior Approach, Anterior
			   Column
			J Posterior Approach,
			   Anterior Column

5 Sacrococcygeal Joint
   Sacrococcygeal symphysis
6 Coccygeal Joint
7 Sacroiliac Joint, Right
8 Sacroiliac Joint, Left
	Ø Open
	3 Percutaneous
	4 Percutaneous Endoscopic
		4 Internal Fixation Device
		7 Autologous Tissue
		   Substitute
		J Synthetic Substitute
		K Nonautologous Tissue
		   Substitute
			Z No Qualifier

9 Hip Joint, Right
   Acetabulofemoral joint
B Hip Joint, Left
   See 9 Hip Joint, Right
C Knee Joint, Right
   Femoropatellar joint
   Femorotibial joint
   Lateral meniscus
   Medial meniscus
   Patellofemoral joint
   Tibiofemoral joint
D Knee Joint, Left
   See C Knee Joint, Right
F Ankle Joint, Right
   Inferior tibiofibular joint
   Talocrural joint
G Ankle Joint, Left
   See F Ankle Joint, Right
H Tarsal Joint, Right
   Calcaneocuboid joint
   Cuboideonavicular joint
   Cuneonavicular joint
   Intercuneiform joint
   Subtalar (talocalcaneal) joint
   Talocalcaneal (subtalar) joint
   Talocalcaneonavicular joint
J Tarsal Joint, Left
   See H Tarsal Joint, Right
K Tarsometatarsal Joint, Right
L Tarsometatarsal Joint, Left
M Metatarsal-Phalangeal Joint, Right
   Metatarsophalangeal (MTP) joint
N Metatarsal-Phalangeal Joint, Left
   See M Metatarsal-Phalangeal Joint, Right
P Toe Phalangeal Joint, Right
   Interphalangeal (IP) joint
Q Toe Phalangeal Joint, Left
   See P Toe Phalangeal Joint, Right
	Ø Open
	3 Percutaneous
	4 Percutaneous Endoscopic
		4 Internal Fixation Device
		5 External Fixation Device
		7 Autologous Tissue
		   Substitute
		J Synthetic Substitute
		K Nonautologous Tissue
		   Substitute
			Z No Qualifier

HAC	ØSG[Ø,1,3][Ø,3,4][7,J,K][Ø,1,J] when reported with SDx K68.11 or T81.4XXA or T84.6Ø- T84.619, T84.63-T84.7 with 7th character A
HAC	ØSG[Ø,1,3][Ø,3,4]A[Ø,J] when reported with SDx K68.11 or T81.4XXA or T84.6Ø-T84.619, T84.63-T84.7 with 7th character A
HAC	ØSG[7,8][Ø,3,4][4,7,J,K]Z when reported with SDx K68.11 or T81.4XXA or T84.6Ø-T84.619, T84.63-T84.7 with 7th character A

See Appendix L for Procedure Combinations
  ⊞   ØSG1[Ø,3,4][7,J,K][Ø,1,J]
  ⊞   ØSG1[Ø,3,4]A[Ø,J]

▣ Limited Coverage   NC Noncovered   ⊞ Combination Member   HAC associated procedure   Combination Only   DRG Non-OR   Non-OR   New/Revised in GREEN

584   ICD-10-PCS 2019

ØSG–ØSG

Lower Joints

Ø Medical and Surgical
S Lower Joints
H Insertion   Definition: Putting in a nonbiological appliance that monitors, assists, performs, or prevents a physiological function but does not physically take the place of a body part
                  Explanation: None

Body Part Character 4	Approach Character 5	Device Character 6	Qualifier Character 7
Ø Lumbar Vertebral Joint Lumbar facet joint **3 Lumbosacral Joint** Lumbosacral facet joint	**Ø** Open **3** Percutaneous **4** Percutaneous Endoscopic	**3** Infusion Device **4** Internal Fixation Device **8** Spacer **B** Spinal Stabilization Device, Interspinous Process **C** Spinal Stabilization Device, Pedicle-Based **D** Spinal Stabilization Device, Facet Replacement	**Z** No Qualifier
2 Lumbar Vertebral Disc **4 Lumbosacral Disc**	**Ø** Open **3** Percutaneous **4** Percutaneous Endoscopic	**3** Infusion Device **8** Spacer	**Z** No Qualifier
5 Sacrococcygeal Joint Sacrococcygeal symphysis **6 Coccygeal Joint** **7 Sacroiliac Joint, Right** **8 Sacroiliac Joint, Left**	**Ø** Open **3** Percutaneous **4** Percutaneous Endoscopic	**3** Infusion Device **4** Internal Fixation Device **8** Spacer	**Z** No Qualifier
9 Hip Joint, Right Acetabulofemoral joint **B Hip Joint, Left** *See 9 Hip Joint, Right* **C Knee Joint, Right** Femoropatellar joint Femorotibial joint Lateral meniscus Medial meniscus Patellofemoral joint Tibiofemoral joint **D Knee Joint, Left** *See C Knee Joint, Right* **F Ankle Joint, Right** Inferior tibiofibular joint Talocrural joint **G Ankle Joint, Left** *See F Ankle Joint, Right* **H Tarsal Joint, Right** Calcaneocuboid joint Cuboideonavicular joint Cuneonavicular joint Intercuneiform joint Subtalar (talocalcaneal) joint Talocalcaneal (subtalar) joint Talocalcaneonavicular joint **J Tarsal Joint, Left** *See H Tarsal Joint, Right* **K Tarsometatarsal Joint, Right** **L Tarsometatarsal Joint, Left** **M Metatarsal-Phalangeal Joint, Right** Metatarsophalangeal (MTP) joint **N Metatarsal-Phalangeal Joint, Left** *See M Metatarsal-Phalangeal Joint, Right* **P Toe Phalangeal Joint, Right** Interphalangeal (IP) joint **Q Toe Phalangeal Joint, Left** *See P Toe Phalangeal Joint, Right*	**Ø** Open **3** Percutaneous **4** Percutaneous Endoscopic	**3** Infusion Device **4** Internal Fixation Device **5** External Fixation Device **8** Spacer	**Z** No Qualifier

Non-OR	ØSH[Ø,3][Ø,3,4][3,8]Z
Non-OR	ØSH[2,4][Ø,3,4][3,8]Z
Non-OR	ØSH[5,6,7,8][Ø,3,4][3,8]Z
Non-OR	ØSH[9,B,C,D,F,G,H,J,K,L,M,N,P,Q][Ø,3,4][3,8]Z

Ø **Medical and Surgical**
S **Lower Joints**
J **Inspection** Definition: Visually and/or manually exploring a body part

Explanation: Visual exploration may be performed with or without optical instrumentation. Manual exploration may be performed directly or through intervening body layers.

Body Part Character 4		Approach Character 5	Device Character 6	Qualifier Character 7
Ø Lumbar Vertebral Joint Lumbar facet joint **2 Lumbar Vertebral Disc** **3 Lumbosacral Joint** Lumbosacral facet joint **4 Lumbosacral Disc** **5 Sacrococcygeal Joint** Sacrococcygeal symphysis **6 Coccygeal Joint** **7 Sacroiliac Joint, Right** **8 Sacroiliac Joint, Left** **9 Hip Joint, Right** Acetabulofemoral joint **B Hip Joint, Left** *See 9 Hip Joint, Right* **C Knee Joint, Right** Femoropatellar joint Femorotibial joint Lateral meniscus Medial meniscus Patellofemoral joint Tibiofemoral joint **D Knee Joint, Left** *See C Knee Joint, Right* **F Ankle Joint, Right** Inferior tibiofibular joint Talocrural joint **G Ankle Joint, Left** *See F Ankle Joint, Right*	**H Tarsal Joint, Right** Calcaneocuboid joint Cuboideonavicular joint Cuneonavicular joint Intercuneiform joint Subtalar (talocalcaneal) joint Talocalcaneal (subtalar) joint Talocalcaneonavicular joint **J Tarsal Joint, Left** *See H Tarsal Joint, Right* **K Tarsometatarsal Joint, Right** **L Tarsometatarsal Joint, Left** **M Metatarsal-Phalangeal Joint, Right** Metatarsophalangeal (MTP) joint **N Metatarsal-Phalangeal Joint, Left** *See M Metatarsal-Phalangeal Joint, Right* **P Toe Phalangeal Joint, Right** Interphalangeal (IP) joint **Q Toe Phalangeal Joint, Left** *See P Toe Phalangeal Joint, Right*	**Ø Open** **3 Percutaneous** **4 Percutaneous Endoscopic** **X External**	**Z No Device**	**Z No Qualifier**

Non-OR ØSJ[Ø,2,3,4,5,6,7,8,9,B,C,D,F,G,H,J,K,L,M,N,P,Q][3,X]ZZ

Ø **Medical and Surgical**
S **Lower Joints**
N **Release** Definition: Freeing a body part from an abnormal physical constraint by cutting or by the use of force

Explanation: Some of the restraining tissue may be taken out but none of the body part is taken out

Body Part Character 4		Approach Character 5	Device Character 6	Qualifier Character 7
Ø Lumbar Vertebral Joint Lumbar facet joint **2 Lumbar Vertebral Disc** **3 Lumbosacral Joint** Lumbosacral facet joint **4 Lumbosacral Disc** **5 Sacrococcygeal Joint** Sacrococcygeal symphysis **6 Coccygeal Joint** **7 Sacroiliac Joint, Right** **8 Sacroiliac Joint, Left** **9 Hip Joint, Right** Acetabulofemoral joint **B Hip Joint, Left** *See 9 Hip Joint, Right* **C Knee Joint, Right** Femoropatellar joint Femorotibial joint Lateral meniscus Medial meniscus Patellofemoral joint Tibiofemoral joint **D Knee Joint, Left** *See C Knee Joint, Right* **F Ankle Joint, Right** Inferior tibiofibular joint Talocrural joint **G Ankle Joint, Left** *See F Ankle Joint, Right*	**H Tarsal Joint, Right** Calcaneocuboid joint Cuboideonavicular joint Cuneonavicular joint Intercuneiform joint Subtalar (talocalcaneal) joint Talocalcaneal (subtalar) joint Talocalcaneonavicular joint **J Tarsal Joint, Left** *See H Tarsal Joint, Right* **K Tarsometatarsal Joint, Right** **L Tarsometatarsal Joint, Left** **M Metatarsal-Phalangeal Joint, Right** Metatarsophalangeal (MTP) joint **N Metatarsal-Phalangeal Joint, Left** *See M Metatarsal-Phalangeal Joint, Right* **P Toe Phalangeal Joint, Right** Interphalangeal (IP) joint **Q Toe Phalangeal Joint, Left** *See P Toe Phalangeal Joint, Right*	**Ø Open** **3 Percutaneous** **4 Percutaneous Endoscopic** **X External**	**Z No Device**	**Z No Qualifier**

Non-OR ØSN[Ø,2,3,4,5,6,7,8,9,B,C,D,F,G,H,J,K,L,M,N,P,Q]XZZ

LC Limited Coverage NC Noncovered ⊞ Combination Member HAC associated procedure Combination Only DRG Non-OR Non-OR New/Revised in GREEN

Ø   **Medical and Surgical**
S   **Lower Joints**
P   **Removal**   Definition: Taking out or off a device from a body part

Explanation: If a device is taken out and a similar device put in without cutting or puncturing the skin or mucous membrane, the procedure is coded to the root operation CHANGE. Otherwise, the procedure for taking out the device is coded to the root operation REMOVAL.

Body Part Character 4	Approach Character 5	Device Character 6	Qualifier Character 7

Ø   Lumbar Vertebral Joint
     Lumbar facet joint
3   Lumbosacral Joint
     Lumbosacral facet joint
	Ø Open
	3 Percutaneous
	4 Percutaneous Endoscopic
		Ø Drainage Device
		3 Infusion Device
		4 Internal Fixation Device
		7 Autologous Tissue Substitute
		8 Spacer
		A Interbody Fusion Device
		J Synthetic Substitute
		K Nonautologous Tissue Substitute
			Z No Qualifier

Ø   Lumbar Vertebral Joint
     Lumbar facet joint
3   Lumbosacral Joint
     Lumbosacral facet joint
	X External	Ø Drainage Device
		3 Infusion Device
		4 Internal Fixation Device
			Z No Qualifier

2 Lumbar Vertebral Disc 4 Lumbosacral Disc	Ø Open 3 Percutaneous 4 Percutaneous Endoscopic	Ø Drainage Device 3 Infusion Device 7 Autologous Tissue Substitute J Synthetic Substitute K Nonautologous Tissue Substitute	Z No Qualifier
2 Lumbar Vertebral Disc 4 Lumbosacral Disc	X External	Ø Drainage Device 3 Infusion Device	Z No Qualifier
5 Sacrococcygeal Joint Sacrococcygeal symphysis 6 Coccygeal Joint 7 Sacroiliac Joint, Right 8 Sacroiliac Joint, Left	Ø Open 3 Percutaneous 4 Percutaneous Endoscopic	Ø Drainage Device 3 Infusion Device 4 Internal Fixation Device 7 Autologous Tissue Substitute 8 Spacer J Synthetic Substitute K Nonautologous Tissue Substitute	Z No Qualifier
5 Sacrococcygeal Joint Sacrococcygeal symphysis 6 Coccygeal Joint 7 Sacroiliac Joint, Right 8 Sacroiliac Joint, Left	X External	Ø Drainage Device 3 Infusion Device 4 Internal Fixation Device	Z No Qualifier

9   Hip Joint, Right   ⊞
     Acetabulofemoral joint
B   Hip Joint, Left   ⊞
     See 9 Hip Joint, Right
	Ø Open	Ø Drainage Device
		3 Infusion Device
		4 Internal Fixation Device
		5 External Fixation Device
		7 Autologous Tissue Substitute
		8 Spacer
		9 Liner
		B Resurfacing Device
		E Articulating Spacer
		J Synthetic Substitute
		K Nonautologous Tissue Substitute
			Z No Qualifier

9   Hip Joint, Right   ⊞
     Acetabulofemoral joint
B   Hip Joint, Left   ⊞
     See 9 Hip Joint, Right
	3 Percutaneous
	4 Percutaneous Endoscopic
		Ø Drainage Device
		3 Infusion Device
		4 Internal Fixation Device
		5 External Fixation Device
		7 Autologous Tissue Substitute
		8 Spacer
		J Synthetic Substitute
		K Nonautologous Tissue Substitute
			Z No Qualifier

9   Hip Joint, Right
     Acetabulofemoral joint
B   Hip Joint, Left
     See 9 Hip Joint, Right
	X External	Ø Drainage Device
		3 Infusion Device
		4 Internal Fixation Device
		5 External Fixation Device
			Z No Qualifier

ØSP Continued on next page

Non-OR ØSP[Ø,3][Ø,3,4]8Z	**See Appendix L for Procedure Combinations**	
Non-OR ØSP[Ø,3]3[Ø,3]Z	**Combo-only** ØSP[9,B]Ø8Z	
Non-OR ØSP[Ø,3]X[Ø,3,4]Z	**Combo-only** ØSP[9,B]48Z	
Non-OR ØSP[2,4]3[Ø,3]Z	⊞ ØSP[9,B]Ø[9,B,J]Z	
Non-OR ØSP[2,4]X[Ø,3]Z	⊞ ØSP[9,B]4JZ	
Non-OR ØSP[5,6,7,8][Ø,3,4]8Z		
Non-OR ØSP[5,6,7,8]3[Ø,3]Z		
Non-OR ØSP[5,6,7,8]X[Ø,3,4]Z		
Non-OR ØSP[9,B]3[Ø,3,8]Z		
Non-OR ØSP[9,B]X[Ø,3,4,5]Z		

🔒 Limited Coverage   🚫 Noncovered   ⊞ Combination Member   HAC associated procedure   Combination Only   DRG Non-OR   Non-OR   New/Revised in GREEN

ØSP Continued

Ø	Medical and Surgical
S	Lower Joints
P	Removal	Definition: Taking out or off a device from a body part

Explanation: If a device is taken out and a similar device put in without cutting or puncturing the skin or mucous membrane, the procedure is coded to the root operation CHANGE. Otherwise, the procedure for taking out the device is coded to the root operation REMOVAL.

Body Part Character 4	Approach Character 5	Device Character 6	Qualifier Character 7

A Hip Joint, Acetabular Surface, Right ⊞
E Hip Joint, Acetabular Surface, Left ⊞
R Hip Joint, Femoral Surface, Right ⊞
S Hip Joint, Femoral Surface, Left ⊞
T Knee Joint, Femoral Surface, Right ⊞
  Femoropatellar joint
  Patellofemoral joint
U Knee Joint, Femoral Surface, Left ⊞
  See T Knee Joint, Femoral Surface, Right
V Knee Joint, Tibial Surface, Right ⊞
  Femorotibial joint
  Tibiofemoral joint
W Knee Joint, Tibial Surface, Left ⊞
  See V Knee Joint, Tibial Surface, Right
	Ø Open
	3 Percutaneous
	4 Percutaneous Endoscopic
		J Synthetic Substitute	**Z** No Qualifier

C Knee Joint, Right ⊞
  Femoropatellar joint
  Femorotibial joint
  Lateral meniscus
  Medial meniscus
  Patellofemoral joint
  Tibiofemoral joint
D Knee Joint, Left ⊞
  See C Knee Joint, Right
	Ø Open	**Ø** Drainage Device
		3 Infusion Device
		4 Internal Fixation Device
		5 External Fixation Device
		7 Autologous Tissue Substitute
		8 Spacer
		9 Liner
		E Articulating Spacer
		K Nonautologous Tissue Substitute
		L Synthetic Substitute, Unicondylar Medial
		M Synthetic Substitute, Unicondylar Lateral
		N Synthetic Substitute, Patellofemoral
			Z No Qualifier

C Knee Joint, Right ⊞
  Femoropatellar joint
  Femorotibial joint
  Lateral meniscus
  Medial meniscus
  Patellofemoral joint
  Tibiofemoral joint
D Knee Joint, Left ⊞
  See C Knee Joint, Right
	Ø Open	**J** Synthetic Substitute	**C** Patellar Surface
			Z No Qualifier

C Knee Joint, Right ⊞
  Femoropatellar joint
  Femorotibial joint
  Lateral meniscus
  Medial meniscus
  Patellofemoral joint
  Tibiofemoral joint
D Knee Joint, Left
  See C Knee Joint, Right
	3 Percutaneous
	4 Percutaneous Endoscopic
		Ø Drainage Device
		3 Infusion Device
		4 Internal Fixation Device
		5 External Fixation Device
		7 Autologous Tissue Substitute
		8 Spacer
		K Nonautologous Tissue Substitute
		L Synthetic Substitute, Unicondylar Medial
		M Synthetic Substitute, Unicondylar Lateral
		N Synthetic Substitute, Patellofemoral
			Z No Qualifier

C Knee Joint, Right ⊞
  Femoropatellar joint
  Femorotibial joint
  Lateral meniscus
  Medial meniscus
  Patellofemoral joint
  Tibiofemoral joint
D Knee Joint, Left ⊞
  See C Knee Joint, Right
	3 Percutaneous
	4 Percutaneous Endoscopic
		J Synthetic Substitute	**C** Patellar Surface
			Z No Qualifier

ØSP Continued on next page

Non-OR	ØSP[C,D]3[Ø,3]Z

See Appendix L for Procedure Combinations

Combo-only	ØSP[C,D]Ø8Z	⊞	ØSP[C,D]Ø9Z
Combo-only	ØSP[C,D][3,4]8Z		ØSP[C,D]ØJ[C,Z]
⊞	ØSP[A,E,R,S,T,U,V,W][Ø,4]JZ	⊞	ØSP[C,D]4J[C,Z]

LC Limited Coverage   NC Noncovered   ⊞ Combination Member   HAC associated procedure   Combination Only   DRG Non-OR   Non-OR   New/Revised in GREEN

0 Medical and Surgical
S Lower Joints
P Removal

Definition: Taking out or off a device from a body part

Explanation: If a device is taken out and a similar device put in without cutting or puncturing the skin or mucous membrane, the procedure is coded to the root operation CHANGE. Otherwise, the procedure for taking out the device is coded to the root operation REMOVAL.

Body Part Character 4	Approach Character 5	Device Character 6	Qualifier Character 7
C Knee Joint, Right Femoropatellar joint Femorotibial joint Lateral meniscus Medial meniscus Patellofemoral joint Tibiofemoral joint **D Knee Joint, Left** *See C Knee Joint, Right*	**X External**	**0 Drainage Device** **3 Infusion Device** **4 Internal Fixation Device** **5 External Fixation Device**	**Z No Qualifier**
F Ankle Joint, Right Inferior tibiofibular joint Talocrural joint **G Ankle Joint, Left** *See F Ankle Joint, Right* **H Tarsal Joint, Right** Calcaneocuboid joint Cuboideonavicular joint Cuneonavicular joint Intercuneiform joint Subtalar (talocalcaneal) joint Talocalcaneal (subtalar) joint Talocalcaneonavicular joint **J Tarsal Joint, Left** *See H Tarsal Joint, Right* **K Tarsometatarsal Joint, Right** **L Tarsometatarsal Joint, Left** **M Metatarsal-Phalangeal Joint, Right** Metatarsophalangeal (MTP) joint **N Metatarsal-Phalangeal Joint, Left** *See M Metatarsal-Phalangeal Joint, Right* **P Toe Phalangeal Joint, Right** Interphalangeal (IP) joint **Q Toe Phalangeal Joint, Left** *See P Toe Phalangeal Joint, Right*	**0 Open** **3 Percutaneous** **4 Percutaneous Endoscopic**	**0 Drainage Device** **3 Infusion Device** **4 Internal Fixation Device** **5 External Fixation Device** **7 Autologous Tissue Substitute** **8 Spacer** **J Synthetic Substitute** **K Nonautologous Tissue Substitute**	**Z No Qualifier**
F Ankle Joint, Right Inferior tibiofibular joint Talocrural joint **G Ankle Joint, Left** *See F Ankle Joint, Right* **H Tarsal Joint, Right** Calcaneocuboid joint Cuboideonavicular joint Cuneonavicular joint Intercuneiform joint Subtalar (talocalcaneal) joint Talocalcaneal (subtalar) joint Talocalcaneonavicular joint **J Tarsal Joint, Left** *See H Tarsal Joint, Right* **K Tarsometatarsal Joint, Right** **L Tarsometatarsal Joint, Left** **M Metatarsal-Phalangeal Joint, Right** Metatarsophalangeal (MTP) joint **N Metatarsal-Phalangeal Joint, Left** *See M Metatarsal-Phalangeal Joint, Right* **P Toe Phalangeal Joint, Right** Interphalangeal (IP) joint **Q Toe Phalangeal Joint, Left** *See P Toe Phalangeal Joint, Right*	**X External**	**0 Drainage Device** **3 Infusion Device** **4 Internal Fixation Device** **5 External Fixation Device**	**Z No Qualifier**

Non-OR   0SP[C,D]X[0,3,4,5]Z
Non-OR   0SP[F,G,H,J,K,L,M,N,P,Q]3[0,3,8]Z
Non-OR   0SP[F,G,H,J,K,L,M,N,P,Q][0,4]8Z
Non-OR   0SP[F,G,H,J,K,L,M,N,P,Q]X[0,3,4,5]Z

Lower Joints

0   **Medical and Surgical**
S   **Lower Joints**
Q   **Repair**   Definition: Restoring, to the extent possible, a body part to its normal anatomic structure and function
                     Explanation: Used only when the method to accomplish the repair is not one of the other root operations

Body Part Character 4	Approach Character 5	Device Character 6	Qualifier Character 7

0 **Lumbar Vertebral Joint**
   Lumbar facet joint
2 **Lumbar Vertebral Disc**
3 **Lumbosacral Joint**
   Lumbosacral facet joint
4 **Lumbosacral Disc**
5 **Sacrococcygeal Joint**
   Sacrococcygeal symphysis
6 **Coccygeal Joint**
7 **Sacroiliac Joint, Right**
8 **Sacroiliac Joint, Left**
9 **Hip Joint, Right**
   Acetabulofemoral joint
B **Hip Joint, Left**
   See 9 Hip Joint, Right
C **Knee Joint, Right**
   Femoropatellar joint
   Femorotibial joint
   Lateral meniscus
   Medial meniscus
   Patellofemoral joint
   Tibiofemoral joint
D **Knee Joint, Left**
   See C Knee Joint, Right
F **Ankle Joint, Right**
   Inferior tibiofibular joint
   Talocrural joint
G **Ankle Joint, Left**
   See F Ankle Joint, Right
H **Tarsal Joint, Right**
   Calcaneocuboid joint
   Cuboideonavicular joint
   Cuneonavicular joint
   Intercuneiform joint
   Subtalar (talocalcaneal) joint
   Talocalcaneal (subtalar) joint
   Talocalcaneonavicular joint
J **Tarsal Joint, Left**
   See H Tarsal Joint, Right
K **Tarsometatarsal Joint, Right**
L **Tarsometatarsal Joint, Left**
M **Metatarsal-Phalangeal Joint, Right**
   Metatarsophalangeal (MTP) joint
N **Metatarsal-Phalangeal Joint, Left**
   See M Metatarsal-Phalangeal Joint, Right
P **Toe Phalangeal Joint, Right**
   Interphalangeal (IP) joint
Q **Toe Phalangeal Joint, Left**
   See P Toe Phalangeal Joint, Right
	0 Open
	3 Percutaneous
	4 Percutaneous Endoscopic
	X External
		Z No Device	**Z** No Qualifier

Non-OR   0SQ[0,2,3,4,5,6,7,8,9,B,C,D,F,G,H,J,K,L,M,N,P,Q]XZZ

Lower Joints

Ø   Medical and Surgical
S   Lower Joints
R   Replacement   Definition: Putting in or on biological or synthetic material that physically takes the place and/or function of all or a portion of a body part

Explanation: The body part may have been taken out or replaced, or may be taken out, physically eradicated, or rendered nonfunctional during the REPLACEMENT procedure. A REMOVAL procedure is coded for taking out the device used in a previous replacement procedure.

Body Part Character 4	Approach Character 5	Device Character 6	Qualifier Character 7

Ø Lumbar Vertebral Joint
    Lumbar facet joint
2 Lumbar Vertebral Disc NC
3 Lumbosacral Joint
    Lumbosacral facet joint
4 Lumbosacral Disc NC
5 Sacrococcygeal Joint
    Sacrococcygeal symphysis
6 Coccygeal Joint
7 Sacroiliac Joint, Right
8 Sacroiliac Joint, Left
H Tarsal Joint, Right
    Calcaneocuboid joint
    Cuboideonavicular joint
    Cuneonavicular joint
    Intercuneiform joint
    Subtalar (talocalcaneal) joint
    Talocalcaneal (subtalar) joint
    Talocalcaneonavicular joint
J Tarsal Joint, Left
    See H Tarsal Joint, Right
K Tarsometatarsal Joint, Right
L Tarsometatarsal Joint, Left
M Metatarsal-Phalangeal Joint, Right
    Metatarsophalangeal (MTP) joint
N Metatarsal-Phalangeal Joint, Left
    See M Metatarsal-Phalangeal Joint, Right
P Toe Phalangeal Joint, Right
    Interphalangeal (IP) joint
Q Toe Phalangeal Joint, Left
    See P Toe Phalangeal Joint, Right
	Ø Open	**7** Autologous Tissue Substitute
		J Synthetic Substitute
		K Nonautologous Tissue Substitute
			Z No Qualifier

9 Hip Joint, Right ⊞
    Acetabulofemoral joint
B Hip Joint, Left ⊞
    See 9 Hip Joint, Right
	Ø Open	**1** Synthetic Substitute, Metal
		2 Synthetic Substitute, Metal on Polyethylene
		3 Synthetic Substitute, Ceramic
		4 Synthetic Substitute, Ceramic on Polyethylene
		6 Synthetic Substitute, Oxidized Zirconium on Polyethylene
		J Synthetic Substitute
			9 Cemented
			A Uncemented
			Z No Qualifier

9 Hip Joint, Right
    Acetabulofemoral joint
B Hip Joint, Left
    See 9 Hip Joint, Right
	Ø Open	**7** Autologous Tissue Substitute
		E Articulating Spacer
		K Nonautologous Tissue Substitute
			Z No Qualifier

A Hip Joint, Acetabular Surface, ⊞
    Right
E Hip Joint, Acetabular Surface, ⊞
    Left
	Ø Open	**Ø** Synthetic Substitute, Polyethylene
		1 Synthetic Substitute, Metal
		3 Synthetic Substitute, Ceramic
		J Synthetic Substitute
			9 Cemented
			A Uncemented
			Z No Qualifier

A Hip Joint, Acetabular Surface, Right **E** Hip Joint, Acetabular Surface, Left	**Ø** Open	**7** Autologous Tissue Substitute **K** Nonautologous Tissue Substitute	**Z** No Qualifier

ØSR Continued on next page

HAC ØSR[9,B]Ø[1,2,3,4,6,J][9,A,Z] when reported with SDx of I26.02-I26.09,
        I26.92-I26.99, or I82.401-I82.4Z9
	See Appendix L for Procedure Combinations
	  ⊞ ØSR[9,B]Ø[1,2,3,4,6,J][9,A,Z]
	  ⊞ ØSR[A,E]Ø[Ø,1,3,J][9,A,Z]

HAC ØSR[9,B]Ø[7,K]Z when reported with SDx of I26.02-I26.09, I26.92-I26.99, or I82.401-I82.4Z9	
HAC ØSR[A,E]Ø[Ø,1,3,J][9,A,Z] when reported with SDx of I26.02-I26.09, I26.92-I26.99, or I82.401-I82.4Z9	
HAC ØSR[A,E]Ø[7,K]Z when reported with SDx of I26.02-I26.09, I26.92-I26.99, or I82.401-I82.4Z9	
NC ØSR[2,4]ØJZ when beneficiary age is over 60	

LC Limited Coverage NC Noncovered ⊞ Combination Member HAC associated procedure Combination Only DRG Non-OR Non-OR New/Revised in GREEN

ICD-10-PCS 2019   591

ØSR Continued

Ø	Medical and Surgical
S	Lower Joints
R	Replacement

Definition: Putting in or on biological or synthetic material that physically takes the place and/or function of all or a portion of a body part

Explanation: The body part may have been taken out or replaced, or may be taken out, physically eradicated, or rendered nonfunctional during the REPLACEMENT procedure. A REMOVAL procedure is coded for taking out the device used in a previous replacement procedure.

Body Part Character 4		Approach Character 5	Device Character 6	Qualifier Character 7

C Knee Joint, Right
  Femoropatellar joint
  Femorotibial joint
  Lateral meniscus
  Medial meniscus
  Patellofemoral joint
  Tibiofemoral joint
D Knee Joint, Left
  See C Knee Joint, Right
		Ø Open	6 Synthetic Substitute, Oxidized
			  Zirconium on Polyethylene
			J Synthetic Substitute
			L Synthetic Substitute, Unicondylar
			  Medial
			M Synthetic Substitute, Unicondylar
			  Lateral
			N Synthetic Substitute,
			  Patellofemoral
				9 Cemented
				A Uncemented
				Z No Qualifier

C Knee Joint, Right
  Femoropatellar joint
  Femorotibial joint
  Lateral meniscus
  Medial meniscus
  Patellofemoral joint
  Tibiofemoral joint
D Knee Joint, Left
  See C Knee Joint, Right
	⊞
	
	⊞
		Ø Open	7 Autologous Tissue Substitute
			E Articulating Spacer
			K Nonautologous Tissue Substitute
				Z No Qualifier

F Ankle Joint, Right
  Inferior tibiofibular joint
  Talocrural joint
G Ankle Joint, Left
  See F Ankle Joint, Right
T Knee Joint, Femoral Surface, Right
  Femoropatellar joint
  Patellofemoral joint
U Knee Joint, Femoral Surface, Left
  See T Knee Joint, Femoral Surface, Right
V Knee Joint, Tibial Surface, Right
  Femorotibial joint
  Tibiofemoral joint
W Knee Joint, Tibial Surface, Left
  See V Knee Joint, Tibial Surface, Right
		Ø Open	7 Autologous Tissue Substitute
			K Nonautologous Tissue Substitute
				Z No Qualifier

F Ankle Joint, Right
  Inferior tibiofibular joint
  Talocrural joint
G Ankle Joint, Left
  See F Ankle Joint, Right
T Knee Joint, Femoral Surface, Right
  Femoropatellar joint
  Patellofemoral joint
U Knee Joint, Femoral Surface, Left
  See T Knee Joint, Femoral Surface, Right
V Knee Joint, Tibial Surface, Right
  Femorotibial joint
  Tibiofemoral joint
W Knee Joint, Tibial Surface, Left
  See V Knee Joint, Tibial Surface, Right
	
	⊞
	
	⊞
	
	⊞
	
	⊞
		Ø Open	J Synthetic Substitute	9 Cemented
				A Uncemented
				Z No Qualifier

R Hip Joint, Femoral Surface, Right S Hip Joint, Femoral Surface, Left	⊞ ⊞	Ø Open	1 Synthetic Substitute, Metal 3 Synthetic Substitute, Ceramic J Synthetic Substitute	9 Cemented A Uncemented Z No Qualifier
R Hip Joint, Femoral Surface, Right S Hip Joint, Femoral Surface, Left		Ø Open	7 Autologous Tissue Substitute K Nonautologous Tissue Substitute	Z No Qualifier

HAC	ØSR[C,D]Ø[6,J][9,A,Z] when reported with SDx of I26.02-I26.09, I26.92-I26.99 or I82.401-I82.4Z9
HAC	ØSR[C,D]Ø[7,K]Z when reported with SDx of I26.02-I26.09, I26.92-I26.99 or I82.401-I82.4Z9
HAC	ØSR[T,U,V,W]Ø[7,K]Z when reported with SDx of I26.02-I26.09, I26.92-I26.99 or I82.401-I82.4Z9
HAC	ØSR[T,U,V,W]ØJ[9,A,Z] when reported with SDx of I26.02-I26.09, I26.92-I26.99 or I82.401-I82.4Z9
HAC	ØSR[R,S]Ø[1,3,J][9,A,Z] when reported with SDx of I26.02-I26.09, I26.92-I26.99, or I82.401-I82.4Z9
HAC	ØSR[R,S]Ø[7,K]Z when reported with SDx of I26.02-I26.09, I26.92-I26.99, or I82.401-I82.4Z9

See Appendix L for Procedure Combinations
⊞	ØSR[C,D]Ø[6,J][9,A,Z]
⊞	ØSR[T,U,V,W]ØJ[9,A,Z]
⊞	ØSR[R,S]Ø[1,3,J][9,A,Z]

LC Limited Coverage   NC Noncovered   ⊞ Combination Member   HAC associated procedure   Combination Only   DRG Non-OR   Non-OR   New/Revised in GREEN

592   ICD-10-PCS 2019

ØSR–ØSR

Ø　Medical and Surgical
S　Lower Joints
S　Reposition　Definition: Moving to its normal location, or other suitable location, all or a portion of a body part
　　　　　　　　　Explanation: The body part is moved to a new location from an abnormal location, or from a normal location where it is not functioning correctly. The body part may or may not be cut out or off to be moved to the new location.

Body Part Character 4		Approach Character 5	Device Character 6	Qualifier Character 7
Ø **Lumbar Vertebral Joint** Lumbar facet joint **3** **Lumbosacral Joint** Lumbosacral facet joint **5** **Sacrococcygeal Joint** Sacrococcygeal symphysis **6** **Coccygeal Joint** **7** **Sacroiliac Joint, Right** **8** **Sacroiliac Joint, Left**		**Ø** Open **3** Percutaneous **4** Percutaneous Endoscopic **X** External	**4** Internal Fixation Device **Z** No Device	**Z** No Qualifier
9 **Hip Joint, Right** Acetabulofemoral joint **B** **Hip Joint, Left** *See 9 Hip Joint, Right* **C** **Knee Joint, Right** Femoropatellar joint Femorotibial joint Lateral meniscus Medial meniscus Patellofemoral joint Tibiofemoral joint **D** **Knee Joint, Left** *See C Knee Joint, Right* **F** **Ankle Joint, Right** Inferior tibiofibular joint Talocrural joint **G** **Ankle Joint, Left** *See F Ankle Joint, Right* **H** **Tarsal Joint, Right** Calcaneocuboid joint Cuboideonavicular joint Cuneonavicular joint Intercuneiform joint Subtalar (talocalcaneal) joint Talocalcaneal (subtalar) joint Talocalcaneonavicular joint	**J** **Tarsal Joint, Left** *See H Tarsal Joint, Right* **K** **Tarsometatarsal Joint, Right** **L** **Tarsometatarsal Joint, Left** **M** **Metatarsal-Phalangeal Joint, Right** Metatarsophalangeal (MTP) joint **N** **Metatarsal-Phalangeal Joint, Left** *See M Metatarsal-Phalangeal Joint, Right* **P** **Toe Phalangeal Joint, Right** Interphalangeal (IP) joint **Q** **Toe Phalangeal Joint, Left** *See P Toe Phalangeal Joint, Right*	**Ø** Open **3** Percutaneous **4** Percutaneous Endoscopic **X** External	**4** Internal Fixation Device **5** External Fixation Device **Z** No Device	**Z** No Qualifier

Non-OR　ØSS[Ø,3,5,6,7,8][3,4,X][4,Z]Z
Non-OR　ØSS[9,B,C,D,F,G,H,J,K,L,M,N,P,Q][3,4,X][4,5,Z]Z

Ø　Medical and Surgical
S　Lower Joints
T　Resection　Definition: Cutting out or off, without replacement, all of a body part
　　　　　　　Explanation: None

Body Part Character 4		Approach Character 5	Device Character 6	Qualifier Character 7
2 **Lumbar Vertebral Disc** **4** **Lumbosacral Disc** **5** **Sacrococcygeal Joint** Sacrococcygeal symphysis **6** **Coccygeal Joint** **7** **Sacroiliac Joint, Right** **8** **Sacroiliac Joint, Left** **9** **Hip Joint, Right** Acetabulofemoral joint **B** **Hip Joint, Left** *See 9 Hip Joint, Right* **C** **Knee Joint, Right** Femoropatellar joint Femorotibial joint Lateral meniscus Medial meniscus Patellofemoral joint Tibiofemoral joint **D** **Knee Joint, Left** *See C Knee Joint, Right* **F** **Ankle Joint, Right** Inferior tibiofibular joint Talocrural joint **G** **Ankle Joint, Left** *See F Ankle Joint, Right*	**H** **Tarsal Joint, Right** Calcaneocuboid joint Cuboideonavicular joint Cuneonavicular joint Intercuneiform joint Subtalar (talocalcaneal) joint Talocalcaneal (subtalar) joint Talocalcaneonavicular joint **J** **Tarsal Joint, Left** *See H Tarsal Joint, Right* **K** **Tarsometatarsal Joint, Right** **L** **Tarsometatarsal Joint, Left** **M** **Metatarsal-Phalangeal Joint, Right** Metatarsophalangeal (MTP) joint **N** **Metatarsal-Phalangeal Joint, Left** *See M Metatarsal-Phalangeal Joint, Right* **P** **Toe Phalangeal Joint, Right** Interphalangeal (IP) joint **Q** **Toe Phalangeal Joint, Left** *See P Toe Phalangeal Joint, Right*	**Ø** Open	**Z** No Device	**Z** No Qualifier

Lower Joints

Ø   Medical and Surgical
S   Lower Joints
U   Supplement   Definition: Putting in or on biological or synthetic material that physically reinforces and/or augments the function of a portion of a body part

Explanation: The biological material is non-living, or is living and from the same individual. The body part may have been previously replaced, and the SUPPLEMENT procedure is performed to physically reinforce and/or augment the function of the replaced body part.

Body Part — Character 4		Approach — Character 5	Device — Character 6	Qualifier — Character 7
Ø Lumbar Vertebral Joint Lumbar facet joint **2** Lumbar Vertebral Disc **3** Lumbosacral Joint Lumbosacral facet joint **4** Lumbosacral Disc **5** Sacrococcygeal Joint Sacrococcygeal symphysis **6** Coccygeal Joint **7** Sacroiliac Joint, Right **8** Sacroiliac Joint, Left **F** Ankle Joint, Right Inferior tibiofibular joint Talocrural joint **G** Ankle Joint, Left *See F Ankle Joint, Right* **H** Tarsal Joint, Right Calcaneocuboid joint Cuboideonavicular joint Cuneonavicular joint Intercuneiform joint Subtalar (talocalcaneal) joint Talocalcaneal (subtalar) joint Talocalcaneonavicular joint	**J** Tarsal Joint, Left *See H Tarsal Joint, Right* **K** Tarsometatarsal Joint, Right **L** Tarsometatarsal Joint, Left **M** Metatarsal-Phalangeal Joint, Right Metatarsophalangeal (MTP) joint **N** Metatarsal-Phalangeal Joint, Left *See M Metatarsal-Phalangeal Joint, Right* **P** Toe Phalangeal Joint, Right Interphalangeal (IP) joint **Q** Toe Phalangeal Joint, Left *See P Toe Phalangeal Joint, Right*	**Ø** Open **3** Percutaneous **4** Percutaneous Endoscopic	**7** Autologous Tissue Substitute **J** Synthetic Substitute **K** Nonautologous Tissue Substitute	**Z** No Qualifier
9 Hip Joint, Right ⊞ Acetabulofemoral joint **B** Hip Joint, Left ⊞ *See 9 Hip Joint, Right*		**Ø** Open	**7** Autologous Tissue Substitute **9** Liner **B** Resurfacing Device **J** Synthetic Substitute **K** Nonautologous Tissue Substitute	**Z** No Qualifier
9 Hip Joint, Right Acetabulofemoral joint **B** Hip Joint, Left *See 9 Hip Joint, Right*		**3** Percutaneous **4** Percutaneous Endoscopic	**7** Autologous Tissue Substitute **J** Synthetic Substitute **K** Nonautologous Tissue Substitute	**Z** No Qualifier
A Hip Joint, Acetabular Surface, Right ⊞ **E** Hip Joint, Acetabular Surface, Left ⊞ **R** Hip Joint, Femoral Surface, Right ⊞ **S** Hip Joint, Femoral Surface, Left ⊞		**Ø** Open	**9** Liner **B** Resurfacing Device	**Z** No Qualifier
C Knee Joint, Right Femoropatellar joint Femorotibial joint Lateral meniscus Medial meniscus Patellofemoral joint Tibiofemoral joint **D** Knee Joint, Left *See C Knee Joint, Right*		**Ø** Open	**7** Autologous Tissue Substitute **J** Synthetic Substitute **K** Nonautologous Tissue Substitute	**Z** No Qualifier
C Knee Joint, Right Femoropatellar joint Femorotibial joint Lateral meniscus Medial meniscus Patellofemoral joint Tibiofemoral joint **D** Knee Joint, Left *See C Knee Joint, Right*		**Ø** Open	**9** Liner	**C** Patellar Surface **Z** No Qualifier

ØSU Continued on next page

HAC	ØSU[9,B]ØBZ when reported with SDx of I26.Ø2-I26.Ø9, I26.92-I26.99, or I82.4Ø1-I82.4Z9
HAC	ØSU[A,E,R,S]ØBZ when reported with SDx of I26.Ø2-I26.Ø9, I26.92-I26.99, or I82.4Ø1-I82.4Z9

See Appendix L for Procedure Combinations
⊞   ØSU[9,B]Ø9Z
⊞   ØSU[A,E,R,S]Ø9Z

LC Limited Coverage   NC Noncovered   ⊞ Combination Member   HAC associated procedure   Combination Only   DRG Non-OR   Non-OR   New/Revised in GREEN

594   ICD-10-PCS 2019

Ø **Medical and Surgical**   *ØSU Continued*
S **Lower Joints**
U **Supplement**   Definition: Putting in or on biological or synthetic material that physically reinforces and/or augments the function of a portion of a body part

Explanation: The biological material is non-living, or is living and from the same individual. The body part may have been previously replaced, and the SUPPLEMENT procedure is performed to physically reinforce and/or augment the function of the replaced body part.

Body Part Character 4	Approach Character 5	Device Character 6	Qualifier Character 7
C Knee Joint, Right Femoropatellar joint Femorotibial joint Lateral meniscus Medial meniscus Patellofemoral joint Tibiofemoral joint **D Knee Joint, Left** *See C Knee Joint, Right*	**3** Percutaneous **4** Percutaneous Endoscopic	**7** Autologous Tissue Substitute **J** Synthetic Substitute **K** Nonautologous Tissue Substitute	**Z** No Qualifier
T Knee Joint, Femoral Surface, Right Femoropatellar joint Patellofemoral joint **U Knee Joint, Femoral Surface, Left** *See T Knee Joint, Femoral Surface, Right* **V Knee Joint, Tibial Surface, Right** ⊞ Femorotibial joint Tibiofemoral joint **W Knee Joint, Tibial Surface, Left** ⊞ *See V Knee Joint, Tibial Surface, Right*	**Ø** Open	**9** Liner	**Z** No Qualifier

See Appendix L for Procedure Combinations
⊞   ØSU[V,W]Ø9Z

LC Limited Coverage   NC Noncovered   ⊞ Combination Member   HAC associated procedure   Combination Only   DRG Non-OR   Non-OR   New/Revised in GREEN

ICD-10-PCS 2019   **595**

ØSU–ØSU

Lower Joints

Ø **Medical and Surgical**
S **Lower Joints**
W **Revision**   Definition: Correcting, to the extent possible, a portion of a malfunctioning device or the position of a displaced device

     Explanation: Revision can include correcting a malfunctioning or displaced device by taking out or putting in components of the device such as a screw or pin

Body Part Character 4	Approach Character 5	Device Character 6	Qualifier Character 7

Ø Lumbar Vertebral Joint
  Lumbar facet joint
3 Lumbosacral Joint
  Lumbosacral facet joint
	Ø Open
	3 Percutaneous
	4 Percutaneous Endoscopic
	X External
		Ø Drainage Device
		3 Infusion Device
		4 Internal Fixation Device
		7 Autologous Tissue Substitute
		8 Spacer
		A Interbody Fusion Device
		J Synthetic Substitute
		K Nonautologous Tissue Substitute
			Z No Qualifier

2 Lumbar Vertebral Disc 4 Lumbosacral Disc	Ø Open 3 Percutaneous 4 Percutaneous Endoscopic X External	Ø Drainage Device 3 Infusion Device 7 Autologous Tissue Substitute J Synthetic Substitute K Nonautologous Tissue Substitute	Z No Qualifier
5 Sacrococcygeal Joint Sacrococcygeal symphysis 6 Coccygeal Joint 7 Sacroiliac Joint, Right 8 Sacroiliac Joint, Left	Ø Open 3 Percutaneous 4 Percutaneous Endoscopic X External	Ø Drainage Device 3 Infusion Device 4 Internal Fixation Device 7 Autologous Tissue Substitute 8 Spacer J Synthetic Substitute K Nonautologous Tissue Substitute	Z No Qualifier

9 Hip Joint, Right
  Acetabulofemoral joint
B Hip Joint, Left
  See 9 Hip Joint, Right
	Ø Open	Ø Drainage Device
		3 Infusion Device
		4 Internal Fixation Device
		5 External Fixation Device
		7 Autologous Tissue Substitute
		8 Spacer
		9 Liner
		B Resurfacing Device
		J Synthetic Substitute
		K Nonautologous Tissue Substitute
			Z No Qualifier

9 Hip Joint, Right
  Acetabulofemoral joint
B Hip Joint, Left
  See 9 Hip Joint, Right
	3 Percutaneous
	4 Percutaneous Endoscopic
	X External
		Ø Drainage Device
		3 Infusion Device
		4 Internal Fixation Device
		5 External Fixation Device
		7 Autologous Tissue Substitute
		8 Spacer
		J Synthetic Substitute
		K Nonautologous Tissue Substitute
			Z No Qualifier

A Hip Joint, Acetabular Surface, Right
E Hip Joint, Acetabular Surface, Left
R Hip Joint, Femoral Surface, Right
S Hip Joint, Femoral Surface, Left
T Knee Joint, Femoral Surface, Right
  Femoropatellar joint
  Patellofemoral joint
U Knee Joint, Femoral Surface, Left
  See T Knee Joint, Femoral Surface, Right
V Knee Joint, Tibial Surface, Right
  Femorotibial joint
  Tibiofemoral joint
W Knee Joint, Tibial Surface, Left
  See V Knee Joint, Tibial Surface, Right
	Ø Open
	3 Percutaneous
	4 Percutaneous Endoscopic
	X External
		J Synthetic Substitute	Z No Qualifier

C Knee Joint, Right
  Femoropatellar joint
  Femorotibial joint
  Lateral meniscus
  Medial meniscus
  Patellofemoral joint
  Tibiofemoral joint
D Knee Joint, Left
  See C Knee Joint, Right
	Ø Open	Ø Drainage Device
		3 Infusion Device
		4 Internal Fixation Device
		5 External Fixation Device
		7 Autologous Tissue Substitute
		8 Spacer
		9 Liner
		K Nonautologous Tissue Substitute
			Z No Qualifier

ØSW Continued on next page

Non-OR	ØSW[Ø,3]X[Ø,3,4,7,8,A,J,K]Z
Non-OR	ØSW[2,4]X[Ø,3,7,J,K]Z
Non-OR	ØSW[5,6,7,8]X[Ø,3,4,7,8,J,K]Z
Non-OR	ØSW[9,B]X[Ø,3,4,5,7,8,J,K]Z
Non-OR	ØSW[A,E,R,S,T,U,V,W]XJZ

LC Limited Coverage   NC Noncovered   ⊞ Combination Member   HAC associated procedure   Combination Only   DRG Non-OR   Non-OR   New/Revised in GREEN

596   ICD-10-PCS 2019

Ø   Medical and Surgical
S   Lower Joints
W   Revision

ØSW Continued

Definition: Correcting, to the extent possible, a portion of a malfunctioning device or the position of a displaced device

Explanation: Revision can include correcting a malfunctioning or displaced device by taking out or putting in components of the device such as a screw or pin

Body Part Character 4	Approach Character 5	Device Character 6	Qualifier Character 7
C Knee Joint, Right Femoropatellar joint Femorotibial joint Lateral meniscus Medial meniscus Patellofemoral joint Tibiofemoral joint **D Knee Joint, Left** *See C Knee Joint, Right*	**Ø** Open	**J** Synthetic Substitute	**C** Patellar Surface **Z** No Qualifier
C Knee Joint, Right Femoropatellar joint Femorotibial joint Lateral meniscus Medial meniscus Patellofemoral joint Tibiofemoral joint **D Knee Joint, Left** *See C Knee Joint, Right*	**3** Percutaneous **4** Percutaneous Endoscopic **X** External	**Ø** Drainage Device **3** Infusion Device **4** Internal Fixation Device **5** External Fixation Device **7** Autologous Tissue Substitute **8** Spacer **K** Nonautologous Tissue Substitute	**Z** No Qualifier
C Knee Joint, Right Femoropatellar joint Femorotibial joint Lateral meniscus Medial meniscus Patellofemoral joint Tibiofemoral joint **D Knee Joint, Left** *See C Knee Joint, Right*	**3** Percutaneous **4** Percutaneous Endoscopic **X** External	**J** Synthetic Substitute	**C** Patellar Surface **Z** No Qualifier
F Ankle Joint, Right Inferior tibiofibular joint Talocrural joint **G Ankle Joint, Left** *See F Ankle Joint, Right* **H Tarsal Joint, Right** Calcaneocuboid joint Cuboideonavicular joint Cuneonavicular joint Intercuneiform joint Subtalar (talocalcaneal) joint Talocalcaneal (subtalar) joint Talocalcaneonavicular joint **J Tarsal Joint, Left** *See H Tarsal Joint, Right* **K Tarsometatarsal Joint, Right** **L Tarsometatarsal Joint, Left** **M Metatarsal-Phalangeal Joint, Right** Metatarsophalangeal (MTP) joint **N Metatarsal-Phalangeal Joint, Left** *See M Metatarsal-Phalangeal Joint, Right* **P Toe Phalangeal Joint, Right** Interphalangeal (IP) joint **Q Toe Phalangeal Joint, Left** *See P Toe Phalangeal Joint, Right*	**Ø** Open **3** Percutaneous **4** Percutaneous Endoscopic **X** External	**Ø** Drainage Device **3** Infusion Device **4** Internal Fixation Device **5** External Fixation Device **7** Autologous Tissue Substitute **8** Spacer **J** Synthetic Substitute **K** Nonautologous Tissue Substitute	**Z** No Qualifier

Non-OR   ØSW[C,D]X[Ø,3,4,5,7,8,K]Z
Non-OR   ØSW[C,D]XJ[C,Z]
Non-OR   ØSW[F,G,H,J,K,L,M,N,P,Q]X[Ø,3,4,5,7,8,J,K]Z

Urinary System ØT1–ØTY

Character Meanings

This Character Meaning table is provided as a guide to assist the user in the identification of character members that may be found in this section of code tables. It **SHOULD NOT** be used to build a PCS code.

Operation–Character 3	Body Part–Character 4	Approach–Character 5	Device–Character 6	Qualifier–Character 7
1 Bypass	Ø Kidney, Right	Ø Open	Ø Drainage Device	Ø Allogeneic
2 Change	1 Kidney, Left	3 Percutaneous	2 Monitoring Device	1 Syngeneic
5 Destruction	2 Kidneys, Bilateral	4 Percutaneous Endoscopic	3 Infusion Device	2 Zooplastic
7 Dilation	3 Kidney Pelvis, Right	7 Via Natural or Artificial Opening	7 Autologous Tissue Substitute	3 Kidney Pelvis, Right
8 Division	4 Kidney Pelvis, Left	8 Via Natural or Artificial Opening Endoscopic	C Extraluminal Device	4 Kidney Pelvis, Left
9 Drainage	5 Kidney	X External	D Intraluminal Device	6 Ureter, Right
B Excision	6 Ureter, Right		J Synthetic Substitute	7 Ureter, Left
C Extirpation	7 Ureter, Left		K Nonautologous Tissue Substitute	8 Colon
D Extraction	8 Ureters, Bilateral		L Artificial Sphincter	9 Colocutaneous
F Fragmentation	9 Ureter		M Stimulator Lead	A Ileum
H Insertion	B Bladder		Y Other Device	B Bladder
J Inspection	C Bladder Neck		Z No Device	C Ileocutaneous
L Occlusion	D Urethra			D Cutaneous
M Reattachment				X Diagnostic
N Release				Z No Qualifier
P Removal				
Q Repair				
R Replacement				
S Reposition				
T Resection				
U Supplement				
V Restriction				
W Revision				
Y Transplantation				

AHA Coding Clinic for table ØT1
2017, 3Q, 20   Creation of Indiana pouch
2017, 3Q, 21   Augmentation cystoplasty with Indiana pouch and continent urinary diversion
2017, 1Q, 37   Perineal urethrostomy
2015, 3Q, 34   Redo urinary diversion surgery via left ureteral reimplantation

AHA Coding Clinic for table ØT7
2017, 4Q, 111   Exchange of ureteral stent
2016, 2Q, 27   Exchange of ureteral stents
2015, 2Q, 8   Urinary calculi fragmentation and evacuation
2013, 4Q, 123   Urolift® procedure

AHA Coding Clinic for table ØT9
2017, 3Q, 19   Ureteral stent placement for urinary leakage
2017, 3Q, 20   Creation of Indiana pouch
2017, 3Q, 21   Augmentation cystoplasty with Indiana pouch and continent urinary diversion

AHA Coding Clinic for table ØTB
2016, 1Q, 19   Biopsy of neobladder malignancy
2015, 3Q, 34   Excision of Mitrofanoff polyp
2014, 2Q, 8   Ileoscopy with excision of polyp of Ileal loop urinary diversion

AHA Coding Clinic for table ØTC
2016, 3Q, 23   Ureteral stone migrating into bladder
2015, 2Q, 7   Urinary calculi fragmentation and evacuation
2015, 2Q, 8   Urinary calculi fragmentation and evacuation
2013, 4Q, 122   Laser lithotripsy with removal of fragments

AHA Coding Clinic for table ØTF
2015, 2Q, 7   Urinary calculi fragmentation and evacuation
2013, 4Q, 122   Extracorporeal shock wave lithotripsy
2013, 4Q, 122   Laser lithotripsy with removal of fragments

AHA Coding Clinic for table ØTP
2017, 4Q, 111   Exchange of ureteral stent
2016, 2Q, 27   Exchange of ureteral stents

AHA Coding Clinic for table ØTQ
2018, 2Q, 27   Dismembered pyeloplasty
2017, 1Q, 37   Perineal urethrostomy

AHA Coding Clinic for table ØTR
2017, 3Q, 20   Creation of Indiana pouch

AHA Coding Clinic for table ØTS
2018, 2Q, 27   Dismembered pyeloplasty
2017, 1Q, 36   Dismembered pyeloplasty
2016, 1Q, 15   Pubovaginal sling placement

AHA Coding Clinic for table ØTT
2014, 3Q, 16   Hand-assisted laparoscopy nephroureterectomy

AHA Coding Clinic for table ØTU
2017, 3Q, 21   Augmentation cystoplasty with Indiana pouch and continent urinary diversion

AHA Coding Clinic for table ØTV
2015, 2Q, 11   Cystourethroscopic Deflux® injection

Urinary System

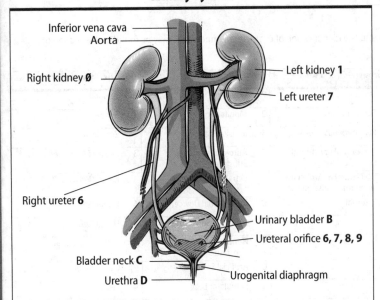

- Inferior vena cava
- Aorta
- Right kidney **Ø**
- Left kidney **1**
- Left ureter **7**
- Right ureter **6**
- Urinary bladder **B**
- Ureteral orifice **6, 7, 8, 9**
- Bladder neck **C**
- Urogenital diaphragm
- Urethra **D**

Kidney

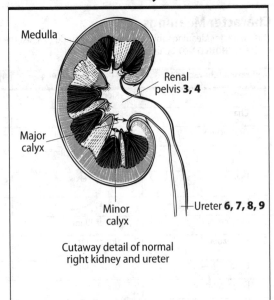

- Medulla
- Renal pelvis **3, 4**
- Major calyx
- Minor calyx
- Ureter **6, 7, 8, 9**

Cutaway detail of normal right kidney and ureter

Bladder

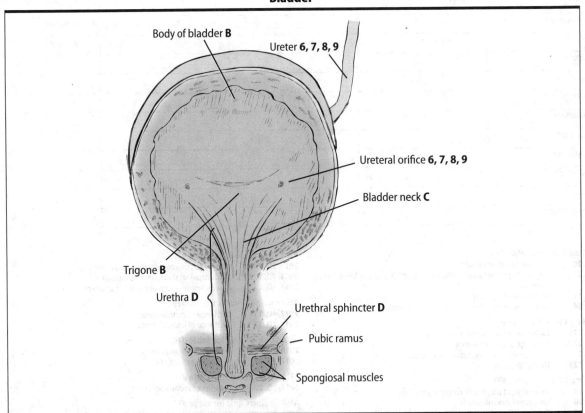

- Body of bladder **B**
- Ureter **6, 7, 8, 9**
- Ureteral orifice **6, 7, 8, 9**
- Bladder neck **C**
- Trigone **B**
- Urethra **D**
- Urethral sphincter **D**
- Pubic ramus
- Spongiosal muscles

Urinary System *(side tab)*

0   **Medical and Surgical**
T   **Urinary System**
1   **Bypass**   Definition: Altering the route of passage of the contents of a tubular body part

                     Explanation: Rerouting contents of a body part to a downstream area of the normal route, to a similar route and body part, or to an abnormal route and dissimilar body part. Includes one or more anastomoses, with or without the use of a device.

Body Part Character 4	Approach Character 5	Device Character 6	Qualifier Character 7

3 Kidney Pelvis, Right
   Ureteropelvic junction (UPJ)
4 Kidney Pelvis, Left
   See 3 Kidney Pelvis, Right
	0 Open
	4 Percutaneous Endoscopic
		7 Autologous Tissue Substitute
		J Synthetic Substitute
		K Nonautologous Tissue Substitute
		Z No Device
			3 Kidney Pelvis, Right
			4 Kidney Pelvis, Left
			6 Ureter, Right
			7 Ureter, Left
			8 Colon
			9 Colocutaneous
			A Ileum
			B Bladder
			C Ileocutaneous
			D Cutaneous

3 Kidney Pelvis, Right
   Ureteropelvic junction (UPJ)
4 Kidney Pelvis, Left
   See 3 Kidney Pelvis, Right
	3 Percutaneous	J Synthetic Substitute	D Cutaneous

6 Ureter, Right
   Ureteral orifice
   Ureterovesical orifice
7 Ureter, Left
   See 6 Ureter, Right
8 Ureters, Bilateral
   See 6 Ureter, Right
	0 Open
	4 Percutaneous Endoscopic
		7 Autologous Tissue Substitute
		J Synthetic Substitute
		K Nonautologous Tissue Substitute
		Z No Device
			6 Ureter, Right
			7 Ureter, Left
			8 Colon
			9 Colocutaneous
			A Ileum
			B Bladder
			C Ileocutaneous
			D Cutaneous

6 Ureter, Right
   Ureteral orifice
   Ureterovesical orifice
7 Ureter, Left
   See 6 Ureter, Right
8 Ureters, Bilateral
   See 6 Ureter, Right
	3 Percutaneous	J Synthetic Substitute	D Cutaneous

B Bladder Trigone of bladder	0 Open 4 Percutaneous Endoscopic	7 Autologous Tissue Substitute J Synthetic Substitute K Nonautologous Tissue Substitute Z No Device	9 Colocutaneous C Ileocutaneous D Cutaneous
B Bladder Trigone of bladder	3 Percutaneous	J Synthetic Substitute	D Cutaneous

0   **Medical and Surgical**
T   **Urinary System**
2   **Change**   Definition: Taking out or off a device from a body part and putting back an identical or similar device in or on the same body part without cutting or puncturing the skin or a mucous membrane

                     Explanation: All CHANGE procedures are coded using the approach EXTERNAL

Body Part Character 4	Approach Character 5	Device Character 6	Qualifier Character 7

5 Kidney
   Renal calyx
   Renal capsule
   Renal cortex
   Renal segment
9 Ureter
   Ureteral orifice
   Ureterovesical orifice
B Bladder
   Trigone of bladder
D Urethra
   Bulbourethral (Cowper's) gland
   Cowper's (bulbourethral) gland
   External urethral sphincter
   Internal urethral sphincter
   Membranous urethra
   Penile urethra
   Prostatic urethra
	X External	0 Drainage Device
		Y Other Device
			Z No Qualifier

Non-OR   All body part, approach, device, and qualifier values

Urinary System

Ø Medical and Surgical
T Urinary System
5 Destruction — Definition: Physical eradication of all or a portion of a body part by the direct use of energy, force, or a destructive agent
Explanation: None of the body part is physically taken out

Body Part Character 4	Approach Character 5	Device Character 6	Qualifier Character 7
Ø **Kidney, Right** Renal calyx Renal capsule Renal cortex Renal segment 1 **Kidney, Left** *See Ø Kidney, Right* 3 **Kidney Pelvis, Right** Ureteropelvic junction (UPJ) 4 **Kidney Pelvis, Left** *See 3 Kidney Pelvis, Right* 6 **Ureter, Right** Ureteral orifice Ureterovesical orifice 7 **Ureter, Left** *See 6 Ureter, Right* B **Bladder** Trigone of bladder C **Bladder Neck**	Ø Open 3 Percutaneous 4 Percutaneous Endoscopic 7 Via Natural or Artificial Opening 8 Via Natural or Artificial Opening Endoscopic	Z No Device	Z No Qualifier
D **Urethra** Bulbourethral (Cowper's) gland Cowper's (bulbourethral) gland External urethral sphincter Internal urethral sphincter Membranous urethra Penile urethra Prostatic urethra	Ø Open 3 Percutaneous 4 Percutaneous Endoscopic 7 Via Natural or Artificial Opening 8 Via Natural or Artificial Opening Endoscopic X External	Z No Device	Z No Qualifier

Non-OR   ØT5D[Ø,3,4,7,8,X]ZZ

Ø Medical and Surgical
T Urinary System
7 Dilation — Definition: Expanding an orifice or the lumen of a tubular body part
Explanation: The orifice can be a natural orifice or an artificially created orifice. Accomplished by stretching a tubular body part using intraluminal pressure or by cutting part of the orifice or wall of the tubular body part.

Body Part Character 4	Approach Character 5	Device Character 6	Qualifier Character 7
3 **Kidney Pelvis, Right** Ureteropelvic junction (UPJ) 4 **Kidney Pelvis, Left** *See 3 Kidney Pelvis, Right* 6 **Ureter, Right** Ureteral orifice Ureterovesical orifice 7 **Ureter, Left** *See 6 Ureter, Right* 8 **Ureters, Bilateral** *See 6 Ureter, Right* B **Bladder** Trigone of bladder C **Bladder Neck** D **Urethra** Bulbourethral (Cowper's) gland Cowper's (bulbourethral) gland External urethral sphincter Internal urethral sphincter Membranous urethra Penile urethra Prostatic urethra	Ø Open 3 Percutaneous 4 Percutaneous Endoscopic 7 Via Natural or Artificial Opening 8 Via Natural or Artificial Opening Endoscopic	D Intraluminal Device Z No Device	Z No Qualifier

Non-OR   ØT7[6,7][Ø,3,4,7,8]DZ
Non-OR   ØT7[6,7][7,8]ZZ
Non-OR   ØT7[8,D][Ø,3,4]DZ

Non-OR   ØT7[8,B,D][7,8][D,Z]Z
Non-OR   ØT7C[Ø,3,4,7,8][D,Z]Z

Ø Medical and Surgical
T Urinary System
8 Division — Definition: Cutting into a body part, without draining fluids and/or gases from the body part, in order to separate or transect a body part
Explanation: All or a portion of the body part is separated into two or more portions

Body Part Character 4	Approach Character 5	Device Character 6	Qualifier Character 7
2 **Kidneys, Bilateral** Renal calyx Renal capsule Renal cortex Renal segment C **Bladder Neck**	Ø Open 3 Percutaneous 4 Percutaneous Endoscopic	Z No Device	Z No Qualifier

LC Limited Coverage   NC Noncovered   ⊞ Combination Member   HAC associated procedure   Combination Only   DRG Non-OR   Non-OR   New/Revised in GREEN

602   ICD-10-PCS 2019

Ø Medical and Surgical
T Urinary System
9 Drainage

Definition: Taking or letting out fluids and/or gases from a body part

Explanation: The qualifier DIAGNOSTIC is used to identify drainage procedures that are biopsies

Body Part Character 4	Approach Character 5	Device Character 6	Qualifier Character 7
Ø Kidney, Right Renal calyx Renal capsule Renal cortex Renal segment **1 Kidney, Left** *See Ø Kidney, Right* **3 Kidney Pelvis, Right** Ureteropelvic junction (UPJ) **4 Kidney Pelvis, Left** *See 3 Kidney Pelvis, Right* **6 Ureter, Right** Ureteral orifice Ureterovesical orifice **7 Ureter, Left** *See 6 Ureter, Right* **8 Ureters, Bilateral** *See 6 Ureter, Right* **B Bladder** Trigone of bladder **C Bladder Neck**	**Ø** Open **3** Percutaneous **4** Percutaneous Endoscopic **7** Via Natural or Artificial Opening **8** Via Natural or Artificial Opening Endoscopic	**Ø** Drainage Device	**Z** No Qualifier
Ø Kidney, Right Renal calyx Renal capsule Renal cortex Renal segment **1 Kidney, Left** *See Ø Kidney, Right* **3 Kidney Pelvis, Right** Ureteropelvic junction (UPJ) **4 Kidney Pelvis, Left** *See 3 Kidney Pelvis, Right* **6 Ureter, Right** Ureteral orifice Ureterovesical orifice **7 Ureter, Left** *See 6 Ureter, Right* **8 Ureters, Bilateral** *See 6 Ureter, Right* **B Bladder** Trigone of bladder **C Bladder Neck**	**Ø** Open **3** Percutaneous **4** Percutaneous Endoscopic **7** Via Natural or Artificial Opening **8** Via Natural or Artificial Opening Endoscopic	**Z** No Device	**X** Diagnostic **Z** No Qualifier
D Urethra Bulbourethral (Cowper's) gland Cowper's (bulbourethral) gland External urethral sphincter Internal urethral sphincter Membranous urethra Penile urethra Prostatic urethra	**Ø** Open **3** Percutaneous **4** Percutaneous Endoscopic **7** Via Natural or Artificial Opening **8** Via Natural or Artificial Opening Endoscopic **X** External	**Ø** Drainage Device	**Z** No Qualifier
D Urethra Bulbourethral (Cowper's) gland Cowper's (bulbourethral) gland External urethral sphincter Internal urethral sphincter Membranous urethra Penile urethra Prostatic urethra	**Ø** Open **3** Percutaneous **4** Percutaneous Endoscopic **7** Via Natural or Artificial Opening **8** Via Natural or Artificial Opening Endoscopic **X** External	**Z** No Device	**X** Diagnostic **Z** No Qualifier

Non-OR	ØT9[Ø,1,3,4]3ØZ
Non-OR	ØT9[6,7,8][Ø,3,4,7,8]ØZ
Non-OR	ØT9[B,C][3,4,7,8]ØZ
Non-OR	ØT9[Ø,1,3,4,6,7,8][3,4,7,8]ZX
Non-OR	ØT9[Ø,1,3,4][3,4]ZZ
Non-OR	ØT9[6,7,8]3ZZ
Non-OR	ØT9[B,C][3,4,7,8]ZZ
Non-OR	ØT9D3ØZ
Non-OR	ØT9D[Ø,3,4,7,8,X]ZX
Non-OR	ØT9D3ZZ

Urinary System *(side tab)*

Ø Medical and Surgical
T Urinary System
B Excision Definition: Cutting out or off, without replacement, a portion of a body part
Explanation: The qualifier DIAGNOSTIC is used to identify excision procedures that are biopsies

Body Part Character 4	Approach Character 5	Device Character 6	Qualifier Character 7
Ø Kidney, Right Renal calyx Renal capsule Renal cortex Renal segment **1 Kidney, Left** *See Ø Kidney, Right* **3 Kidney Pelvis, Right** Ureteropelvic junction (UPJ) **4 Kidney Pelvis, Left** *See 3 Kidney Pelvis, Right* **6 Ureter, Right** Ureteral orifice Ureterovesical orifice **7 Ureter, Left** *See 6 Ureter, Right* **B Bladder** Trigone of bladder **C Bladder Neck**	**Ø** Open **3** Percutaneous **4** Percutaneous Endoscopic **7** Via Natural or Artificial Opening **8** Via Natural or Artificial Opening Endoscopic	**Z** No Device	**X** Diagnostic **Z** No Qualifier
D Urethra Bulbourethral (Cowper's) gland Cowper's (bulbourethral) gland External urethral sphincter Internal urethral sphincter Membranous urethra Penile urethra Prostatic urethra	**Ø** Open **3** Percutaneous **4** Percutaneous Endoscopic **7** Via Natural or Artificial Opening **8** Via Natural or Artificial Opening Endoscopic **X** External	**Z** No Device	**X** Diagnostic **Z** No Qualifier

Non-OR   ØTB[Ø,1,3,4,6,7][3,4,7,8]ZX
Non-OR   ØTBD[Ø,3,4,7,8,X]ZX

Ø Medical and Surgical
T Urinary System
C Extirpation Definition: Taking or cutting out solid matter from a body part
Explanation: The solid matter may be an abnormal byproduct of a biological function or a foreign body; it may be imbedded in a body part or in the lumen of a tubular body part. The solid matter may or may not have been previously broken into pieces.

Body Part Character 4	Approach Character 5	Device Character 6	Qualifier Character 7
Ø Kidney, Right Renal calyx Renal capsule Renal cortex Renal segment **1 Kidney, Left** *See Ø Kidney, Right* **3 Kidney Pelvis, Right** Ureteropelvic junction (UPJ) **4 Kidney Pelvis, Left** *See 3 Kidney Pelvis, Right* **6 Ureter, Right** Ureteral orifice Ureterovesical orifice **7 Ureter, Left** *See 6 Ureter, Right* **B Bladder** Trigone of bladder **C Bladder Neck**	**Ø** Open **3** Percutaneous **4** Percutaneous Endoscopic **7** Via Natural or Artificial Opening **8** Via Natural or Artificial Opening Endoscopic	**Z** No Device	**Z** No Qualifier
D Urethra Bulbourethral (Cowper's) gland Cowper's (bulbourethral) gland External urethral sphincter Internal urethral sphincter Membranous urethra Penile urethra Prostatic urethra	**Ø** Open **3** Percutaneous **4** Percutaneous Endoscopic **7** Via Natural or Artificial Opening **8** Via Natural or Artificial Opening Endoscopic **X** External	**Z** No Device	**Z** No Qualifier

Non-OR   ØTC[B,C][7,8]ZZ
Non-OR   ØTCD[7,8,X]ZZ

LC Limited Coverage   **NC** Noncovered   ⊞ Combination Member   HAC associated procedure   Combination Only   DRG Non-OR   Non-OR   New/Revised in GREEN
604   ICD-10-PCS 2019

ØTB–ØTC *(side tab)*

Ø   **Medical and Surgical**
T   **Urinary System**
D   **Extraction**   Definition: Pulling or stripping out or off all or a portion of a body part by the use of force
                       Explanation: The qualifier DIAGNOSTIC is used to identify extraction procedures that are biopsies

Body Part Character 4	Approach Character 5	Device Character 6	Qualifier Character 7

Ø **Kidney, Right**
    Renal calyx
    Renal capsule
    Renal cortex
    Renal segment
1 **Kidney, Left**
    See Ø *Kidney, Right*
	Ø Open
	3 Percutaneous
	4 Percutaneous Endoscopic
		Z No Device	Z No Qualifier

Ø   **Medical and Surgical**
T   **Urinary System**
F   **Fragmentation**   Definition: Breaking solid matter in a body part into pieces
                       Explanation: Physical force (e.g., manual, ultrasonic) applied directly or indirectly is used to break the solid matter into pieces. The solid matter may be an abnormal byproduct of a biological function or a foreign body. The pieces of solid matter are not taken out.

Body Part Character 4	Approach Character 5	Device Character 6	Qualifier Character 7

3 **Kidney Pelvis, Right**
    Ureteropelvic junction (UPJ)
4 **Kidney Pelvis, Left**
    See 3 *Kidney Pelvis, Right*
6 **Ureter, Right**
    Ureteral orifice
    Ureterovesical orifice
7 **Ureter, Left**
    See 6 *Ureter, Right*
B **Bladder**
    Trigone of bladder
C **Bladder Neck**
D **Urethra**   **NC**
    Bulbourethral (Cowper's) gland
    Cowper's (bulbourethral) gland
    External urethral sphincter
    Internal urethral sphincter
    Membranous urethra
    Penile urethra
    Prostatic urethra
	Ø Open
	3 Percutaneous
	4 Percutaneous Endoscopic
	7 Via Natural or Artificial Opening
	8 Via Natural or Artificial Opening
	    Endoscopic
	X External
		Z No Device	Z No Qualifier

DRG Non-OR	ØTF[3,4,6,7,B,C]XZZ
Non-OR	ØTF[3,4][Ø,7,8]ZZ
Non-OR	ØTF[6,7,B,C][Ø,3,4,7,8]ZZ
Non-OR	ØTFD[Ø,3,4,7,8,X]ZZ
NC	ØTFDXZZ

Urinary System

Ø   Medical and Surgical
T   Urinary System
H   Insertion   Definition: Putting in a nonbiological appliance that monitors, assists, performs, or prevents a physiological function but does not physically take the place of a body part
                         Explanation: None

Body Part Character 4	Approach Character 5	Device Character 6	Qualifier Character 7
5 Kidney Renal calyx Renal capsule Renal cortex Renal segment	Ø Open 3 Percutaneous 4 Percutaneous Endoscopic 7 Via Natural or Artificial Opening 8 Via Natural or Artificial Opening Endoscopic	2 Monitoring Device 3 Infusion Device Y Other Device	Z No Qualifier
9 Ureter Ureteral orifice Ureterovesical orifice	Ø Open 3 Percutaneous 4 Percutaneous Endoscopic 7 Via Natural or Artificial Opening 8 Via Natural or Artificial Opening Endoscopic	2 Monitoring Device 3 Infusion Device M Stimulator Lead Y Other Device	Z No Qualifier
B Bladder NC Trigone of bladder	Ø Open 3 Percutaneous 4 Percutaneous Endoscopic 7 Via Natural or Artificial Opening 8 Via Natural or Artificial Opening Endoscopic	2 Monitoring Device 3 Infusion Device L Artificial Sphincter M Stimulator Lead Y Other Device	Z No Qualifier
C Bladder Neck	Ø Open 3 Percutaneous 4 Percutaneous Endoscopic 7 Via Natural or Artificial Opening 8 Via Natural or Artificial Opening Endoscopic	L Artificial Sphincter	Z No Qualifier
D Urethra Bulbourethral (Cowper's) gland Cowper's (bulbourethral) gland External urethral sphincter Internal urethral sphincter Membranous urethra Penile urethra Prostatic urethra	Ø Open 3 Percutaneous 4 Percutaneous Endoscopic 7 Via Natural or Artificial Opening 8 Via Natural or Artificial Opening Endoscopic	2 Monitoring Device 3 Infusion Device L Artificial Sphincter Y Other Device	Z No Qualifier
D Urethra Bulbourethral (Cowper's) gland Cowper's (bulbourethral) gland External urethral sphincter Internal urethral sphincter Membranous urethra Penile urethra Prostatic urethra	X External	2 Monitoring Device 3 Infusion Device L Artificial Sphincter	Z No Qualifier

Non-OR	ØTH5Ø3Z	**Non-OR**	ØTHB[3,4][3,Y]Z
Non-OR	ØTH5[3,4][3,Y]Z	**Non-OR**	ØTHB7[2,3,Y]Z
Non-OR	ØTH57[2,3,Y]Z	**Non-OR**	ØTHB8[2,3]Z
Non-OR	ØTH58[2,3]Z	**Non-OR**	ØTHDØ3Z
Non-OR	ØTH9Ø3Z	**Non-OR**	ØTHD[3,4][3,Y]Z
Non-OR	ØTH9[3,4][3,Y]Z	**Non-OR**	ØTHD[7,8][2,3,Y]Z
Non-OR	ØTH97[2,3,Y]Z	**Non-OR**	ØTHDX3Z
Non-OR	ØTH98[2,3]Z	**NC**	ØTHB[Ø,3,4,7,8]MZ
Non-OR	ØTHBØ3Z		

LC Limited Coverage   **NC** Noncovered   ⊞ Combination Member   HAC associated procedure   Combination Only   DRG Non-OR   Non-OR   New/Revised in GREEN

606   ICD-10-PCS 2019

Ø   Medical and Surgical
T   Urinary System
J   Inspection   Definition: Visually and/or manually exploring a body part

Explanation: Visual exploration may be performed with or without optical instrumentation. Manual exploration may be performed directly or through intervening body layers.

Body Part Character 4	Approach Character 5	Device Character 6	Qualifier Character 7
5 Kidney Renal calyx Renal capsule Renal cortex Renal segment **9 Ureter** Ureteral orifice Ureterovesical orifice **B Bladder** Trigone of bladder **D Urethra** Bulbourethral (Cowper's) gland Cowper's (bulbourethral) gland External urethral sphincter Internal urethral sphincter Membranous urethra Penile urethra Prostatic urethra	**Ø** Open **3** Percutaneous **4** Percutaneous Endoscopic **7** Via Natural or Artificial Opening **8** Via Natural or Artificial Opening Endoscopic **X** External	**Z** No Device	**Z** No Qualifier

Non-OR   ØTJ[5,9,D][3,4,7,8,X]ZZ
Non-OR   ØTJB[3,7,8,X]ZZ

Ø   Medical and Surgical
T   Urinary System
L   Occlusion   Definition: Completely closing an orifice or the lumen of a tubular body part

Explanation: The orifice can be a natural orifice or an artificially created orifice

Body Part Character 4	Approach Character 5	Device Character 6	Qualifier Character 7
3 Kidney Pelvis, Right Ureteropelvic junction (UPJ) **4 Kidney Pelvis, Left** *See 3 Kidney Pelvis, Right* **6 Ureter, Right** Ureteral orifice Ureterovesical orifice **7 Ureter, Left** *See 6 Ureter, Right* **B Bladder** Trigone of bladder **C Bladder Neck**	**Ø** Open **3** Percutaneous **4** Percutaneous Endoscopic	**C** Extraluminal Device **D** Intraluminal Device **Z** No Device	**Z** No Qualifier
3 Kidney Pelvis, Right Ureteropelvic junction (UPJ) **4 Kidney Pelvis, Left** *See 3 Kidney Pelvis, Right* **6 Ureter, Right** Ureteral orifice Ureterovesical orifice **7 Ureter, Left** *See 6 Ureter, Right* **B Bladder** Trigone of bladder **C Bladder Neck**	**7** Via Natural or Artificial Opening **8** Via Natural or Artificial Opening Endoscopic	**D** Intraluminal Device **Z** No Device	**Z** No Qualifier
D Urethra Bulbourethral (Cowper's) gland Cowper's (bulbourethral) gland External urethral sphincter Internal urethral sphincter Membranous urethra Penile urethra Prostatic urethra	**Ø** Open **3** Percutaneous **4** Percutaneous Endoscopic **X** External	**C** Extraluminal Device **D** Intraluminal Device **Z** No Device	**Z** No Qualifier
D Urethra Bulbourethral (Cowper's) gland Cowper's (bulbourethral) gland External urethral sphincter Internal urethral sphincter Membranous urethra Penile urethra Prostatic urethra	**7** Via Natural or Artificial Opening **8** Via Natural or Artificial Opening Endoscopic	**D** Intraluminal Device **Z** No Device	**Z** No Qualifier

LC Limited Coverage   NC Noncovered   ⊞ Combination Member   HAC associated procedure   Combination Only   DRG Non-OR   Non-OR   New/Revised in GREEN

Ø   Medical and Surgical
T   Urinary System
M   Reattachment   Definition: Putting back in or on all or a portion of a separated body part to its normal location or other suitable location
Explanation: Vascular circulation and nervous pathways may or may not be reestablished

Body Part Character 4	Approach Character 5	Device Character 6	Qualifier Character 7

Ø Kidney, Right
     Renal calyx
     Renal capsule
     Renal cortex
     Renal segment
1 Kidney, Left
     See Ø Kidney, Right
2 Kidneys, Bilateral
     See Ø Kidney, Right
3 Kidney Pelvis, Right
     Ureteropelvic junction (UPJ)
4 Kidney Pelvis, Left
     See 3 Kidney Pelvis, Right
6 Ureter, Right
     Ureteral orifice
     Ureterovesical orifice
7 Ureter, Left
     See 6 Ureter, Right
8 Ureters, Bilateral
     See 6 Ureter, Right
B Bladder
     Trigone of bladder
C Bladder Neck
D Urethra
     Bulbourethral (Cowper's) gland
     Cowper's (bulbourethral) gland
     External urethral sphincter
     Internal urethral sphincter
     Membranous urethra
     Penile urethra
     Prostatic urethra
	Ø Open
	4 Percutaneous Endoscopic
		Z No Device	**Z No Qualifier**

Ø   Medical and Surgical
T   Urinary System
N   Release   Definition: Freeing a body part from an abnormal physical constraint by cutting or by the use of force
Explanation: Some of the restraining tissue may be taken out but none of the body part is taken out

Body Part Character 4	Approach Character 5	Device Character 6	Qualifier Character 7

Ø Kidney, Right
     Renal calyx
     Renal capsule
     Renal cortex
     Renal segment
1 Kidney, Left
     See Ø Kidney, Right
3 Kidney Pelvis, Right
     Ureteropelvic junction (UPJ)
4 Kidney Pelvis, Left
     See 3 Kidney Pelvis, Right
6 Ureter, Right
     Ureteral orifice
     Ureterovesical orifice
7 Ureter, Left
     See 6 Ureter, Right
B Bladder
     Trigone of bladder
C Bladder Neck
	Ø Open
	3 Percutaneous
	4 Percutaneous Endoscopic
	7 Via Natural or Artificial Opening
	8 Via Natural or Artificial Opening Endoscopic
		Z No Device	**Z No Qualifier**

D Urethra
     Bulbourethral (Cowper's) gland
     Cowper's (bulbourethral) gland
     External urethral sphincter
     Internal urethral sphincter
     Membranous urethra
     Penile urethra
     Prostatic urethra
	Ø Open
	3 Percutaneous
	4 Percutaneous Endoscopic
	7 Via Natural or Artificial Opening
	8 Via Natural or Artificial Opening Endoscopic
	X External
		Z No Device	**Z No Qualifier**

LC Limited Coverage   NC Noncovered   ⊞ Combination Member   HAC associated procedure   Combination Only   DRG Non-OR   Non-OR   New/Revised in GREEN

608   ICD-10-PCS 2019

Ø Medical and Surgical
T Urinary System
P Removal   Definition: Taking out or off a device from a body part

Explanation: If a device is taken out and a similar device put in without cutting or puncturing the skin or mucous membrane, the procedure is coded to the root operation CHANGE. Otherwise, the procedure for taking out the device is coded to the root operation REMOVAL.

Body Part Character 4	Approach Character 5	Device Character 6	Qualifier Character 7
5 Kidney Renal calyx Renal capsule Renal cortex Renal segment	Ø Open 3 Percutaneous 4 Percutaneous Endoscopic 7 Via Natural or Artificial Opening 8 Via Natural or Artificial Opening Endoscopic	Ø Drainage Device 2 Monitoring Device 3 Infusion Device 7 Autologous Tissue Substitute C Extraluminal Device D Intraluminal Device J Synthetic Substitute K Nonautologous Tissue Substitute Y Other Device	Z No Qualifier
5 Kidney Renal calyx Renal capsule Renal cortex Renal segment	X External	Ø Drainage Device 2 Monitoring Device 3 Infusion Device D Intraluminal Device	Z No Qualifier
9 Ureter Ureteral orifice Ureterovesical orifice	Ø Open 3 Percutaneous 4 Percutaneous Endoscopic 7 Via Natural or Artificial Opening 8 Via Natural or Artificial Opening Endoscopic	Ø Drainage Device 2 Monitoring Device 3 Infusion Device 7 Autologous Tissue Substitute C Extraluminal Device D Intraluminal Device J Synthetic Substitute K Nonautologous Tissue Substitute M Stimulator Lead Y Other Device	Z No Qualifier
9 Ureter Ureteral orifice Ureterovesical orifice	X External	Ø Drainage Device 2 Monitoring Device 3 Infusion Device D Intraluminal Device M Stimulator Lead	Z No Qualifier
B Bladder NC Trigone of bladder	Ø Open 3 Percutaneous 4 Percutaneous Endoscopic 7 Via Natural or Artificial Opening 8 Via Natural or Artificial Opening Endoscopic	Ø Drainage Device 2 Monitoring Device 3 Infusion Device 7 Autologous Tissue Substitute C Extraluminal Device D Intraluminal Device J Synthetic Substitute K Nonautologous Tissue Substitute L Artificial Sphincter M Stimulator Lead Y Other Device	Z No Qualifier
B Bladder Trigone of bladder	X External	Ø Drainage Device 2 Monitoring Device 3 Infusion Device D Intraluminal Device L Artificial Sphincter M Stimulator Lead	Z No Qualifier
D Urethra Bulbourethral (Cowper's) gland Cowper's (bulbourethral) gland External urethral sphincter Internal urethral sphincter Membranous urethra Penile urethra Prostatic urethra	Ø Open 3 Percutaneous 4 Percutaneous Endoscopic 7 Via Natural or Artificial Opening 8 Via Natural or Artificial Opening Endoscopic	Ø Drainage Device 2 Monitoring Device 3 Infusion Device 7 Autologous Tissue Substitute C Extraluminal Device D Intraluminal Device J Synthetic Substitute K Nonautologous Tissue Substitute L Artificial Sphincter Y Other Device	Z No Qualifier
D Urethra Bulbourethral (Cowper's) gland Cowper's (bulbourethral) gland External urethral sphincter Internal urethral sphincter Membranous urethra Penile urethra Prostatic urethra	X External	Ø Drainage Device 2 Monitoring Device 3 Infusion Device D Intraluminal Device L Artificial Sphincter	Z No Qualifier

Non-OR ØTP5[3,4,7]YZ	**Non-OR** ØTP9[7,8][Ø,2,3,D]Z	**Non-OR** ØTPB[7,8][Ø,2,3,D]Z	**Non-OR** ØTPD[7,8][Ø,2,3,D,Y]Z
Non-OR ØTP5[7,8][Ø,2,3,D]Z	**Non-OR** ØTP9X[Ø,2,3,D]Z	**Non-OR** ØTPBX[Ø,2,3,D,L]Z	**Non-OR** ØTPDX[Ø,2,3,D]Z
Non-OR ØTP5X[Ø,2,3,D]Z	**Non-OR** ØTPB[3,4,7]YZ	**Non-OR** ØTPD[3,4]YZ	**NC** ØTPB[Ø,3,4,7,8]MZ
Non-OR ØTP9[3,4,7]YZ			

LC Limited Coverage   **NC** Noncovered   ⊞ Combination Member   HAC associated procedure   Combination Only   DRG Non-OR   Non-OR   New/Revised in GREEN

ICD-10-PCS 2019   609

ØTP–ØTP

Urinary System

Ø **Medical and Surgical**
T **Urinary System**
Q **Repair**   Definition: Restoring, to the extent possible, a body part to its normal anatomic structure and function
                    Explanation: Used only when the method to accomplish the repair is not one of the other root operations

Body Part Character 4	Approach Character 5	Device Character 6	Qualifier Character 7
Ø **Kidney, Right** Renal calyx Renal capsule Renal cortex Renal segment **1** **Kidney, Left** See Ø Kidney, Right **3** **Kidney Pelvis, Right** Ureteropelvic junction (UPJ) **4** **Kidney Pelvis, Left** See 3 Kidney Pelvis, Right **6** **Ureter, Right** Ureteral orifice Ureterovesical orifice **7** **Ureter, Left** See 6 Ureter, Right **B** **Bladder** ⊞ Trigone of bladder **C** **Bladder Neck**	**Ø** Open **3** Percutaneous **4** Percutaneous Endoscopic **7** Via Natural or Artificial Opening **8** Via Natural or Artificial Opening Endoscopic	**Z** No Device	**Z** No Qualifier
D **Urethra** Bulbourethral (Cowper's) gland Cowper's (bulbourethral) gland External urethral sphincter Internal urethral sphincter Membranous urethra Penile urethra Prostatic urethra	**Ø** Open **3** Percutaneous **4** Percutaneous Endoscopic **7** Via Natural or Artificial Opening **8** Via Natural or Artificial Opening Endoscopic **X** External	**Z** No Device	**Z** No Qualifier

See Appendix L for Procedure Combinations
⊞   ØTQB[Ø,3,4]ZZ

Ø **Medical and Surgical**
T **Urinary System**
R **Replacement**   Definition: Putting in or on biological or synthetic material that physically takes the place and/or function of all or a portion of a body part
                    Explanation: The body part may have been taken out or replaced, or may be taken out, physically eradicated, or rendered nonfunctional during
                    the REPLACEMENT procedure. A REMOVAL procedure is coded for taking out the device used in a previous replacement procedure.

Body Part Character 4	Approach Character 5	Device Character 6	Qualifier Character 7
3 **Kidney Pelvis, Right** Ureteropelvic junction (UPJ) **4** **Kidney Pelvis, Left** See 3 Kidney Pelvis, Right **6** **Ureter, Right** Ureteral orifice Ureterovesical orifice **7** **Ureter, Left** See 6 Ureter, Right **B** **Bladder** Trigone of bladder **C** **Bladder Neck**	**Ø** Open **4** Percutaneous Endoscopic **7** Via Natural or Artificial Opening **8** Via Natural or Artificial Opening Endoscopic	**7** Autologous Tissue Substitute **J** Synthetic Substitute **K** Nonautologous Tissue Substitute	**Z** No Qualifier
D **Urethra** Bulbourethral (Cowper's) gland Cowper's (bulbourethral) gland External urethral sphincter Internal urethral sphincter Membranous urethra Penile urethra Prostatic urethra	**Ø** Open **4** Percutaneous Endoscopic **7** Via Natural or Artificial Opening **8** Via Natural or Artificial Opening Endoscopic **X** External	**7** Autologous Tissue Substitute **J** Synthetic Substitute **K** Nonautologous Tissue Substitute	**Z** No Qualifier

Ø　Medical and Surgical
T　Urinary System
S　Reposition　　Definition: Moving to its normal location, or other suitable location, all or a portion of a body part

Explanation: The body part is moved to a new location from an abnormal location, or from a normal location where it is not functioning correctly. The body part may or may not be cut out or off to be moved to the new location.

Body Part Character 4	Approach Character 5	Device Character 6	Qualifier Character 7
Ø　Kidney, Right 　Renal calyx 　Renal capsule 　Renal cortex 　Renal segment **1　Kidney, Left** 　*See Ø Kidney, Right* **2　Kidneys, Bilateral** 　*See Ø Kidney, Right* **3　Kidney Pelvis, Right** 　Ureteropelvic junction (UPJ) **4　Kidney Pelvis, Left** 　*See 3 Kidney Pelvis, Right* **6　Ureter, Right** 　Ureteral orifice 　Ureterovesical orifice **7　Ureter, Left** 　*See 6 Ureter, Right* **8　Ureters, Bilateral** 　*See 6 Ureter, Right* **B　Bladder** 　Trigone of bladder **C　Bladder Neck** **D　Urethra** 　Bulbourethral (Cowper's) gland 　Cowper's (bulbourethral) gland 　External urethral sphincter 　Internal urethral sphincter 　Membranous urethra 　Penile urethra 　Prostatic urethra	**Ø　Open** **4　Percutaneous Endoscopic**	**Z　No Device**	**Z　No Qualifier**

Ø　Medical and Surgical
T　Urinary System
T　Resection　　Definition: Cutting out or off, without replacement, all of a body part

Explanation: None

Body Part Character 4	Approach Character 5	Device Character 6	Qualifier Character 7
Ø　Kidney, Right 　Renal calyx 　Renal capsule 　Renal cortex 　Renal segment **1　Kidney, Left** 　*See Ø Kidney, Right* **2　Kidneys, Bilateral** 　*See Ø Kidney, Right*	**Ø　Open** **4　Percutaneous Endoscopic**	**Z　No Device**	**Z　No Qualifier**
3　Kidney Pelvis, Right 　Ureteropelvic junction (UPJ) **4　Kidney Pelvis, Left** 　*See 3 Kidney Pelvis, Right* **6　Ureter, Right** 　Ureteral orifice 　Ureterovesical orifice **7　Ureter, Left** 　*See 6 Ureter, Right* **B　Bladder**　⊞ 　Trigone of bladder **C　Bladder Neck** **D　Urethra** 　Bulbourethral (Cowper's) gland 　Cowper's (bulbourethral) gland 　External urethral sphincter 　Internal urethral sphincter 　Membranous urethra 　Penile urethra 　Prostatic urethra	**Ø　Open** **4　Percutaneous Endoscopic** **7　Via Natural or Artificial Opening** **8　Via Natural or Artificial Opening Endoscopic**	**Z　No Device**	**Z　No Qualifier**

Non-OR　ØTTD[4,7,8]ZZ

See Appendix L for Procedure Combinations
Combo-only　ØTTDØZZ
⊞　　　　　ØTTBØZZ

🔳 Limited Coverage　🔳 Noncovered　⊞ Combination Member　HAC associated procedure　Combination Only　DRG Non-OR　Non-OR　New/Revised in GREEN
ICD-10-PCS 2019　　　　　　　　　　　　　　　　　　　　　　　　　　　　611

ØTS–ØTT

Urinary System

Ø   Medical and Surgical
T   Urinary System
U   Supplement   Definition: Putting in or on biological or synthetic material that physically reinforces and/or augments the function of a portion of a body part
Explanation: The biological material is non-living, or is living and from the same individual. The body part may have been previously replaced, and the SUPPLEMENT procedure is performed to physically reinforce and/or augment the function of the replaced body part.

Body Part Character 4	Approach Character 5	Device Character 6	Qualifier Character 7

3   **Kidney Pelvis, Right**
     Ureteropelvic junction (UPJ)
 4   **Kidney Pelvis, Left**
     See 3 Kidney Pelvis, Right
 6   **Ureter, Right**
     Ureteral orifice
     Ureterovesical orifice
 7   **Ureter, Left**
     See 6 Ureter, Right
 B   **Bladder**
     Trigone of bladder
 C   **Bladder Neck**
	Ø **Open**
	 4 **Percutaneous Endoscopic**
	 7 **Via Natural or Artificial Opening**
	 8 **Via Natural or Artificial Opening Endoscopic**
		7 **Autologous Tissue Substitute**
		 J **Synthetic Substitute**
		 K **Nonautologous Tissue Substitute**
			Z **No Qualifier**

D   **Urethra**
     Bulbourethral (Cowper's) gland
     Cowper's (bulbourethral) gland
     External urethral sphincter
     Internal urethral sphincter
     Membranous urethra
     Penile urethra
     Prostatic urethra
	Ø **Open**
	 4 **Percutaneous Endoscopic**
	 7 **Via Natural or Artificial Opening**
	 8 **Via Natural or Artificial Opening Endoscopic**
	 X **External**
		7 **Autologous Tissue Substitute**
		 J **Synthetic Substitute**
		 K **Nonautologous Tissue Substitute**
			Z **No Qualifier**

Ø   Medical and Surgical
T   Urinary System
V   Restriction   Definition: Partially closing an orifice or the lumen of a tubular body part
Explanation: The orifice can be a natural orifice or an artificially created orifice

Body Part Character 4	Approach Character 5	Device Character 6	Qualifier Character 7

3   **Kidney Pelvis, Right**
     Ureteropelvic junction (UPJ)
 4   **Kidney Pelvis, Left**
     See 3 Kidney Pelvis, Right
 6   **Ureter, Right**
     Ureteral orifice
     Ureterovesical orifice
 7   **Ureter, Left**
     See 6 Ureter, Right
 B   **Bladder**
     Trigone of bladder
 C   **Bladder Neck**
	Ø **Open**
	 3 **Percutaneous**
	 4 **Percutaneous Endoscopic**
		C **Extraluminal Device**
		 D **Intraluminal Device**
		 Z **No Device**
			Z **No Qualifier**

3   **Kidney Pelvis, Right**
     Ureteropelvic junction (UPJ)
 4   **Kidney Pelvis, Left**
     See 3 Kidney Pelvis, Right
 6   **Ureter, Right**
     Ureteral orifice
     Ureterovesical orifice
 7   **Ureter, Left**
     See 6 Ureter, Right
 B   **Bladder**
     Trigone of bladder
 C   **Bladder Neck**
	7 **Via Natural or Artificial Opening**
	 8 **Via Natural or Artificial Opening Endoscopic**
		D **Intraluminal Device**
		 Z **No Device**
			Z **No Qualifier**

D   **Urethra**
     Bulbourethral (Cowper's) gland
     Cowper's (bulbourethral) gland
     External urethral sphincter
     Internal urethral sphincter
     Membranous urethra
     Penile urethra
     Prostatic urethra
	Ø **Open**
	 3 **Percutaneous**
	 4 **Percutaneous Endoscopic**
		C **Extraluminal Device**
		 D **Intraluminal Device**
		 Z **No Device**
			Z **No Qualifier**

D   **Urethra**
     Bulbourethral (Cowper's) gland
     Cowper's (bulbourethral) gland
     External urethral sphincter
     Internal urethral sphincter
     Membranous urethra
     Penile urethra
     Prostatic urethra
	7 **Via Natural or Artificial Opening**
	 8 **Via Natural or Artificial Opening Endoscopic**
		D **Intraluminal Device**
		 Z **No Device**
			Z **No Qualifier**

D   **Urethra**
     Bulbourethral (Cowper's) gland
     Cowper's (bulbourethral) gland
     External urethral sphincter
     Internal urethral sphincter
     Membranous urethra
     Penile urethra
     Prostatic urethra
	X **External**	**Z** **No Device**	**Z** **No Qualifier**

LC Limited Coverage   NC Noncovered   ⊞ Combination Member   HAC associated procedure   Combination Only   DRG Non-OR   Non-OR   New/Revised in GREEN

612   ICD-10-PCS 2019

Ø Medical and Surgical
T Urinary System
W Revision Definition: Correcting, to the extent possible, a portion of a malfunctioning device or the position of a displaced device

Explanation: Revision can include correcting a malfunctioning or displaced device by taking out or putting in components of the device such as a screw or pin

Body Part Character 4	Approach Character 5	Device Character 6	Qualifier Character 7
5 Kidney Renal calyx Renal capsule Renal cortex Renal segment	**Ø** Open **3** Percutaneous **4** Percutaneous Endoscopic **7** Via Natural or Artificial Opening **8** Via Natural or Artificial Opening Endoscopic	**Ø** Drainage Device **2** Monitoring Device **3** Infusion Device **7** Autologous Tissue Substitute **C** Extraluminal Device **D** Intraluminal Device **J** Synthetic Substitute **K** Nonautologous Tissue Substitute **Y** Other Device	**Z** No Qualifier
5 Kidney Renal calyx Renal capsule Renal cortex Renal segment	**X** External	**Ø** Drainage Device **2** Monitoring Device **3** Infusion Device **7** Autologous Tissue Substitute **C** Extraluminal Device **D** Intraluminal Device **J** Synthetic Substitute **K** Nonautologous Tissue Substitute	**Z** No Qualifier
9 Ureter Ureteral orifice Ureterovesical orifice	**Ø** Open **3** Percutaneous **4** Percutaneous Endoscopic **7** Via Natural or Artificial Opening **8** Via Natural or Artificial Opening Endoscopic	**Ø** Drainage Device **2** Monitoring Device **3** Infusion Device **7** Autologous Tissue Substitute **C** Extraluminal Device **D** Intraluminal Device **J** Synthetic Substitute **K** Nonautologous Tissue Substitute **M** Stimulator Lead **Y** Other Device	**Z** No Qualifier
9 Ureter Ureteral orifice Ureterovesical orifice	**X** External	**Ø** Drainage Device **2** Monitoring Device **3** Infusion Device **7** Autologous Tissue Substitute **C** Extraluminal Device **D** Intraluminal Device **J** Synthetic Substitute **K** Nonautologous Tissue Substitute **M** Stimulator Lead	**Z** No Qualifier
B Bladder Trigone of bladder	**Ø** Open **3** Percutaneous **4** Percutaneous Endoscopic **7** Via Natural or Artificial Opening **8** Via Natural or Artificial Opening Endoscopic	**Ø** Drainage Device **2** Monitoring Device **3** Infusion Device **7** Autologous Tissue Substitute **C** Extraluminal Device **D** Intraluminal Device **J** Synthetic Substitute **K** Nonautologous Tissue Substitute **L** Artificial Sphincter **M** Stimulator Lead **Y** Other Device	**Z** No Qualifier
B Bladder Trigone of bladder	**X** External	**Ø** Drainage Device **2** Monitoring Device **3** Infusion Device **7** Autologous Tissue Substitute **C** Extraluminal Device **D** Intraluminal Device **J** Synthetic Substitute **K** Nonautologous Tissue Substitute **L** Artificial Sphincter **M** Stimulator Lead	**Z** No Qualifier

ØTW Continued on next page

Non-OR	ØTW5[3,4,7]YZ	Non-OR	ØTW9X[Ø,2,3,7,C,D,J,K,M]Z
Non-OR	ØTW5X[Ø,2,3,7,C,D,J,K]Z	Non-OR	ØTWB[3,4,7]YZ
Non-OR	ØTW9[3,4,7]YZ	Non-OR	ØTWBX[Ø,2,3,7,C,D,J,K,L,M]Z

LC Limited Coverage NC Noncovered ⊞ Combination Member HAC associated procedure Combination Only DRG Non-OR Non-OR New/Revised in GREEN

Urinary System

Ø Medical and Surgical
T Urinary System
W Revision   Definition: Correcting, to the extent possible, a portion of a malfunctioning device or the position of a displaced device

Explanation: Revision can include correcting a malfunctioning or displaced device by taking out or putting in components of the device such as a screw or pin

Body Part Character 4	Approach Character 5	Device Character 6	Qualifier Character 7
D Urethra Bulbourethral (Cowper's) gland Cowper's (bulbourethral) gland External urethral sphincter Internal urethral sphincter Membranous urethra Penile urethra Prostatic urethra	Ø Open 3 Percutaneous 4 Percutaneous Endoscopic 7 Via Natural or Artificial Opening 8 Via Natural or Artificial Opening Endoscopic	Ø Drainage Device 2 Monitoring Device 3 Infusion Device 7 Autologous Tissue Substitute C Extraluminal Device D Intraluminal Device J Synthetic Substitute K Nonautologous Tissue Substitute L Artificial Sphincter Y Other Device	Z No Qualifier
D Urethra Bulbourethral (Cowper's) gland Cowper's (bulbourethral) gland External urethral sphincter Internal urethral sphincter Membranous urethra Penile urethra Prostatic urethra	X External	Ø Drainage Device 2 Monitoring Device 3 Infusion Device 7 Autologous Tissue Substitute C Extraluminal Device D Intraluminal Device J Synthetic Substitute K Nonautologous Tissue Substitute L Artificial Sphincter	Z No Qualifier

Non-OR ØTWD[3,4,7,8]YZ
Non-OR ØTWDX[Ø,2,3,7,C,D,J,K,L]Z

Ø Medical and Surgical
T Urinary System
Y Transplantation Definition: Putting in or on all or a portion of a living body part taken from another individual or animal to physically take the place and/or function of all or a portion of a similar body part

Explanation: The native body part may or may not be taken out, and the transplanted body part may take over all or a portion of its function

Body Part Character 4	Approach Character 5	Device Character 6	Qualifier Character 7
Ø Kidney, Right ⊞ LC Renal calyx Renal capsule Renal cortex Renal segment 1 Kidney, Left ⊞ LC *See Ø Kidney, Right*	Ø Open	Z No Device	Ø Allogeneic 1 Syngeneic 2 Zooplastic

LC ØTY[Ø,1]ØZ[Ø,1,2]

See Appendix L for Procedure Combinations
⊞ ØTY[Ø,1]ØZ[Ø,1,2]

Female Reproductive System ØU1–ØUY

Character Meanings

This Character Meaning table is provided as a guide to assist the user in the identification of character members that may be found in this section of code tables. It **SHOULD NOT** be used to build a PCS code.

Operation–Character 3		Body Part–Character 4		Approach–Character 5		Device–Character 6		Qualifier–Character 7	
1	Bypass	Ø	Ovary, Right	Ø	Open	Ø	Drainage Device	Ø	Allogeneic
2	Change	1	Ovary, Left	3	Percutaneous	1	Radioactive Element	1	Syngeneic
5	Destruction	2	Ovaries, Bilateral	4	Percutaneous Endoscopic	3	Infusion Device	2	Zooplastic
7	Dilation	3	Ovary	7	Via Natural or Artificial Opening	7	Autologous Tissue Substitute	5	Fallopian Tube, Right
8	Division	4	Uterine Supporting Structure	8	Via Natural or Artificial Opening Endoscopic	C	Extraluminal Device	6	Fallopian Tube, Left
9	Drainage	5	Fallopian Tube, Right	F	Via Natural or Artificial Opening With Percutaneous Endoscopic Assistance	D	Intraluminal Device	9	Uterus
B	Excision	6	Fallopian Tube, Left	X	External	G	Intraluminal Device, Pessary	L	Supracervical
C	Extirpation	7	Fallopian Tubes, Bilateral			H	Contraceptive Device	X	Diagnostic
D	Extraction	8	Fallopian Tube			J	Synthetic Substitute	Z	No Qualifier
F	Fragmentation	9	Uterus			K	Nonautologous Tissue Substitute		
H	Insertion	B	Endometrium			Y	Other Device		
J	Inspection	C	Cervix			Z	No Device		
L	Occlusion	D	Uterus and Cervix						
M	Reattachment	F	Cul-de-sac						
N	Release	G	Vagina						
P	Removal	H	Vagina and Cul-de-sac						
Q	Repair	J	Clitoris						
S	Reposition	K	Hymen						
T	Resection	L	Vestibular Gland						
U	Supplement	M	Vulva						
V	Restriction	N	Ova						
W	Revision								
Y	Transplantation								

AHA Coding Clinic for table ØU5
2015, 3Q, 31   Tubal ligation for sterilization

AHA Coding Clinic for table ØU9
2016, 4Q, 58   Longitudinal vaginal septum

AHA Coding Clinic for table ØUB
2018, 1Q, 23   Tubal ligation procedure
2015, 3Q, 31   Laparoscopic partial salpingectomy for ectopic pregnancy
2015, 3Q, 31   Tubal ligation for sterilization
2014, 4Q, 16   Excision of multiple uterine fibroids
2014, 3Q, 12   Excision of skin tag from labia majora

AHA Coding Clinic for table ØUC
2015, 3Q, 30   Removal of cervical cerclage
2013, 2Q, 38   Evacuation of clot post-partum

AHA Coding Clinic for table ØUH
2018, 1Q, 25   Intrauterine brachytherapy & placement of tandems & ovoids
2013, 2Q, 34   Placement of intrauterine device via open approach

AHA Coding Clinic for table ØUJ
2015, 1Q, 33   Robotic-assisted laparoscopic hysterectomy converted to open procedure

AHA Coding Clinic for table ØUL
2018, 1Q, 23   Tubal ligation procedure
2015, 3Q, 31   Tubal ligation for sterilization

AHA Coding Clinic for table ØUQ
2014, 4Q, 18   Obstetrical periurethral laceration
2013, 4Q, 120   Repair of clitoral obstetric laceration

AHA Coding Clinic for table ØUS
2016, 1Q, 9   Anteversion of retroverted pregnant uterus

AHA Coding Clinic for table ØUT
2017, 4Q, 68   New qualifier values - Supracervical hysterectomy
2015, 1Q, 33   Robotic-assisted laparoscopic hysterectomy converted to open procedure
2013, 3Q, 28   Total hysterectomy
2013, 1Q, 24   Excision versus Resection of remaining ovarian remnant following previous excision

AHA Coding Clinic for table ØUV
2015, 3Q, 30   Insertion of cervical cerclage

Female Reproductive System

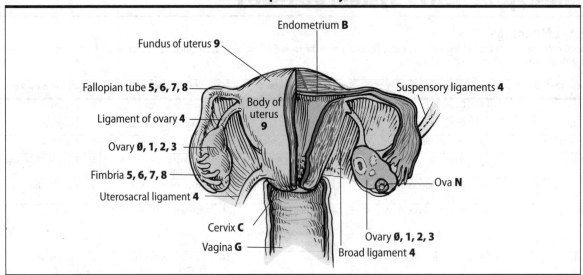

Female Internal/External Structures

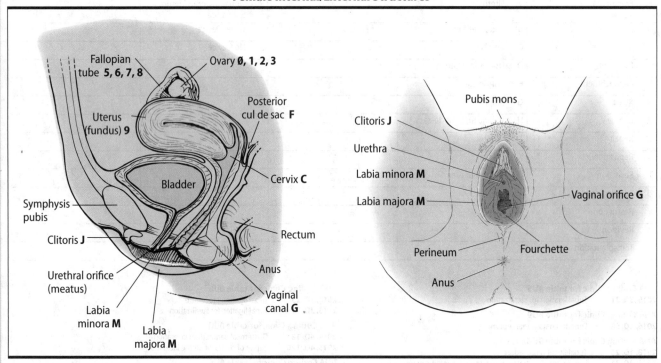

Female Reproductive System

Ø   **Medical and Surgical**
U   **Female Reproductive System**
1   **Bypass**   Definition: Altering the route of passage of the contents of a tubular body part

                     Explanation: Rerouting contents of a body part to a downstream area of the normal route, to a similar route and body part, or to an abnormal route and dissimilar body part. Includes one or more anastomoses, with or without the use of a device.

Body Part Character 4	Approach Character 5	Device Character 6	Qualifier Character 7

5 Fallopian Tube, Right ♀
   Oviduct
   Salpinx
   Uterine tube
6 Fallopian Tube, Left ♀
   See 5 Fallopian Tube, Right
	Ø Open
	4 Percutaneous Endoscopic
		7 Autologous Tissue Substitute
		J Synthetic Substitute
		K Nonautologous Tissue Substitute
		Z No Device
			5 Fallopian Tube, Right
			6 Fallopian Tube, Left
			9 Uterus

    ♀   All body part, approach, device, and qualifier values

Ø   **Medical and Surgical**
U   **Female Reproductive System**
2   **Change**   Definition: Taking out or off a device from a body part and putting back an identical or similar device in or on the same body part without cutting or puncturing the skin or a mucous membrane

                     Explanation: All CHANGE procedures are coded using the approach EXTERNAL

Body Part Character 4	Approach Character 5	Device Character 6	Qualifier Character 7

3 Ovary ♀
8 Fallopian Tube ♀
M Vulva ♀
   Labia majora
   Labia minora
	X External	Ø Drainage Device
		Y Other Device
			Z No Qualifier

D Uterus and Cervix ♀	X External	Ø Drainage Device H Contraceptive Device Y Other Device	Z No Qualifier
H Vagina and Cul-de-sac ♀	X External	Ø Drainage Device G Intraluminal Device, Pessary Y Other Device	Z No Qualifier

   Non-OR   All body part, approach, device, and qualifier values   ♀   All body part, approach, device, and qualifier values

Female Reproductive System

Ø　Medical and Surgical
U　Female Reproductive System
5　Destruction　　Definition: Physical eradication of all or a portion of a body part by the direct use of energy, force, or a destructive agent
　　　　　　　　　　　Explanation: None of the body part is physically taken out

Body Part Character 4	Approach Character 5	Device Character 6	Qualifier Character 7
Ø Ovary, Right ♀ 1 Ovary, Left ♀ 2 Ovaries, Bilateral ♀ 4 Uterine Supporting Structure ♀ 　Broad ligament 　Infundibulopelvic ligament 　Ovarian ligament 　Round ligament of uterus	Ø Open 3 Percutaneous 4 Percutaneous Endoscopic 8 Via Natural or Artificial Opening 　Endoscopic	Z No Device	Z No Qualifier
5 Fallopian Tube, Right ♀ 　Oviduct 　Salpinx 　Uterine tube 6 Fallopian Tube, Left ♀ 　*See 5 Fallopian Tube, Right* 7 Fallopian Tubes, Bilateral NC ♀ 9 Uterus ♀ 　Fundus uteri 　Myometrium 　Perimetrium 　Uterine cornu B Endometrium ♀ C Cervix ♀ F Cul-de-sac ♀	Ø Open 3 Percutaneous 4 Percutaneous Endoscopic 7 Via Natural or Artificial Opening 8 Via Natural or Artificial Opening 　Endoscopic	Z No Device	Z No Qualifier
G Vagina ♀ K Hymen ♀	Ø Open 3 Percutaneous 4 Percutaneous Endoscopic 7 Via Natural or Artificial Opening 8 Via Natural or Artificial Opening 　Endoscopic X External	Z No Device	Z No Qualifier
J Clitoris ♀ L Vestibular Gland ♀ 　Bartholin's (greater vestibular) gland 　Greater vestibular (Bartholin's) gland 　Paraurethral (Skene's) gland 　Skene's (paraurethral) gland M Vulva ♀ 　Labia majora 　Labia minora	Ø Open X External	Z No Device	Z No Qualifier

NC　ØU57[Ø,3,4,7,8]ZZ with principal or secondary diagnosis of Z3Ø.2　　　♀　All body part, approach, device, and qualifier values

0   **Medical and Surgical**
U   **Female Reproductive System**
7   **Dilation**   Definition: Expanding an orifice or the lumen of a tubular body part

Explanation: The orifice can be a natural orifice or an artificially created orifice. Accomplished by stretching a tubular body part using intraluminal pressure or by cutting part of the orifice or wall of the tubular body part.

Body Part Character 4	Approach Character 5	Device Character 6	Qualifier Character 7

5 Fallopian Tube, Right ♀
   Oviduct
   Salpinx
   Uterine tube
6 Fallopian Tube, Left ♀
   See 5 Fallopian Tube, Right
7 Fallopian Tubes, Bilateral ♀
9 Uterus ♀
   Fundus uteri
   Myometrium
   Perimetrium
   Uterine cornu
C Cervix ♀
G Vagina ♀
	0 Open
	3 Percutaneous
	4 Percutaneous Endoscopic
	7 Via Natural or Artificial Opening
	8 Via Natural or Artificial Opening
	   Endoscopic
		D Intraluminal Device
		Z No Device
			Z No Qualifier

K Hymen ♀	**0** Open **3** Percutaneous **4** Percutaneous Endoscopic **7** Via Natural or Artificial Opening **8** Via Natural or Artificial Opening Endoscopic **X** External	**D** Intraluminal Device **Z** No Device	**Z** No Qualifier

Non-OR   0U7C[0,3,4,7,8][D,Z]Z
Non-OR   0U7G[7,8][D,Z]Z

♀   All body part, approach, device, and qualifier values

---

0   **Medical and Surgical**
U   **Female Reproductive System**
8   **Division**   Definition: Cutting into a body part, without draining fluids and/or gases from the body part, in order to separate or transect a body part

Explanation: All or a portion of the body part is separated into two or more portions

Body Part Character 4	Approach Character 5	Device Character 6	Qualifier Character 7

0 Ovary, Right ♀
1 Ovary, Left ♀
2 Ovaries, Bilateral ♀
4 Uterine Supporting Structure ♀
   Broad ligament
   Infundibulopelvic ligament
   Ovarian ligament
   Round ligament of uterus
	0 Open
	3 Percutaneous
	4 Percutaneous Endoscopic
		Z No Device	**Z** No Qualifier

K Hymen ♀	**7** Via Natural or Artificial Opening **8** Via Natural or Artificial Opening Endoscopic **X** External	**Z** No Device	**Z** No Qualifier

Non-OR   0U8K[7,8,X]ZZ

♀   All body part, approach, device, and qualifier values

LC Limited Coverage   NC Noncovered   ⊞ Combination Member   HAC associated procedure   Combination Only   DRG Non-OR   Non-OR   New/Revised in GREEN

Female Reproductive System

Ø   Medical and Surgical
U   Female Reproductive System
9   Drainage   Definition: Taking or letting out fluids and/or gases from a body part
                    Explanation: The qualifier DIAGNOSTIC is used to identify drainage procedures that are biopsies

Body Part Character 4	Approach Character 5	Device Character 6	Qualifier Character 7
Ø Ovary, Right ♀ 1 Ovary, Left ♀ 2 Ovaries, Bilateral ♀	Ø Open 3 Percutaneous 4 Percutaneous Endoscopic 8 Via Natural or Artificial Opening Endoscopic	Ø Drainage Device	Z No Qualifier
Ø Ovary, Right ♀ 1 Ovary, Left ♀ 2 Ovaries, Bilateral ♀	Ø Open 3 Percutaneous 4 Percutaneous Endoscopic 8 Via Natural or Artificial Opening Endoscopic	Z No Device	X Diagnostic Z No Qualifier
Ø Ovary, Right ♀ 1 Ovary, Left ♀ 2 Ovaries, Bilateral ♀	X External	Z No Device	Z No Qualifier

4   Uterine Supporting Structure ♀
      Broad ligament
      Infundibulopelvic ligament
      Ovarian ligament
      Round ligament of uterus
	Ø Open
	3 Percutaneous
	4 Percutaneous Endoscopic
	8 Via Natural or Artificial Opening Endoscopic
		Ø Drainage Device	Z No Qualifier

4   Uterine Supporting Structure ♀
      Broad ligament
      Infundibulopelvic ligament
      Ovarian ligament
      Round ligament of uterus
	Ø Open
	3 Percutaneous
	4 Percutaneous Endoscopic
	8 Via Natural or Artificial Opening Endoscopic
		Z No Device	X Diagnostic
			Z No Qualifier

5   Fallopian Tube, Right ♀
      Oviduct
      Salpinx
      Uterine tube
6   Fallopian Tube, Left ♀
      See 5 Fallopian Tube, Right
7   Fallopian Tubes, Bilateral ♀
9   Uterus ♀
      Fundus uteri
      Myometrium
      Perimetrium
      Uterine cornu
C   Cervix ♀
F   Cul-de-sac ♀
	Ø Open
	3 Percutaneous
	4 Percutaneous Endoscopic
	7 Via Natural or Artificial Opening
	8 Via Natural or Artificial Opening Endoscopic
		Ø Drainage Device	Z No Qualifier

5   Fallopian Tube, Right ♀
      Oviduct
      Salpinx
      Uterine tube
6   Fallopian Tube, Left ♀
      See 5 Fallopian Tube, Right
7   Fallopian Tubes, Bilateral ♀
9   Uterus ♀
      Fundus uteri
      Myometrium
      Perimetrium
      Uterine cornu
C   Cervix ♀
F   Cul-de-sac ♀
	Ø Open
	3 Percutaneous
	4 Percutaneous Endoscopic
	7 Via Natural or Artificial Opening
	8 Via Natural or Artificial Opening Endoscopic
		Z No Device	X Diagnostic
			Z No Qualifier

ØU9 Continued on next page

Non-OR ØU9[Ø,1,2][3,8]ØZ	**Non-OR** ØU9[5,6,7,9,C]3ØZ
Non-OR ØU9[Ø,1,2][3,8]ZZ	**Non-OR** ØU9F[3,4]ØZ
Non-OR ØU9[Ø,1,2]8ZX	**Non-OR** ØU9[5,6,7][3,4,7,8]ZZ
Non-OR ØU94[3,8]ØZ	**Non-OR** ØU9[9,C]3ZZ
Non-OR ØU94[3,8]ZZ	**Non-OR** ØU9F[3,4]ZZ
Non-OR ØU948ZX	♀ All body part, approach, device, and qualifier values

LC Limited Coverage   NC Noncovered   ⊞ Combination Member   HAC associated procedure   Combination Only   DRG Non-OR   Non-OR   New/Revised in GREEN

620   ICD-10-PCS 2019

Ø   **Medical and Surgical**
U   **Female Reproductive System**
9   **Drainage**   Definition: Taking or letting out fluids and/or gases from a body part

ØU9 Continued

                Explanation: The qualifier DIAGNOSTIC is used to identify drainage procedures that are biopsies

Body Part Character 4	Approach Character 5	Device Character 6	Qualifier Character 7
G Vagina ♀ **K** Hymen ♀	**Ø** Open **3** Percutaneous **4** Percutaneous Endoscopic **7** Via Natural or Artificial Opening **8** Via Natural or Artificial Opening Endoscopic **X** External	**Ø** Drainage Device	**Z** No Qualifier
G Vagina ♀ **K** Hymen ♀	**Ø** Open **3** Percutaneous **4** Percutaneous Endoscopic **7** Via Natural or Artificial Opening **8** Via Natural or Artificial Opening Endoscopic **X** External	**Z** No Device	**X** Diagnostic **Z** No Qualifier

J Clitoris ♀
L Vestibular Gland ♀
  Bartholin's (greater vestibular) gland
  Greater vestibular (Bartholin's) gland
  Paraurethral (Skene's) gland
  Skene's (paraurethral) gland
M Vulva ♀
  Labia majora
  Labia minora
	Ø Open
	X External
		Ø Drainage Device	**Z** No Qualifier

J Clitoris ♀
L Vestibular Gland ♀
  Bartholin's (greater vestibular) gland
  Greater vestibular (Bartholin's) gland
  Paraurethral (Skene's) gland
  Skene's (paraurethral) gland
M Vulva ♀
  Labia majora
  Labia minora
	Ø Open
	X External
		Z No Device	**X** Diagnostic
			Z No Qualifier

Non-OR ØU9G3ØZ
Non-OR ØU9K[Ø,3,4,7,8,X]ØZ
Non-OR ØU9G3ZZ
Non-OR ØU9K[Ø,3,4,7,8,X]ZZ

Non-OR ØU9L[Ø,X]ØZ
Non-OR ØU9L[Ø,X]ZZ
♀   All body part, approach, device, and qualifier values

Female Reproductive System

Ø   **Medical and Surgical**
U   **Female Reproductive System**
B   **Excision**   Definition: Cutting out or off, without replacement, a portion of a body part
                Explanation: The qualifier DIAGNOSTIC is used to identify excision procedures that are biopsies

Body Part Character 4	Approach Character 5	Device Character 6	Qualifier Character 7

Ø Ovary, Right ♀
1 Ovary, Left ♀
2 Ovaries, Bilateral ♀
4 Uterine Supporting Structure ♀
   Broad ligament
   Infundibulopelvic ligament
   Ovarian ligament
   Round ligament of uterus
5 Fallopian Tube, Right ♀
   Oviduct
   Salpinx
   Uterine tube
6 Fallopian Tube, Left ♀
   See 5 Fallopian Tube, Right
7 Fallopian Tubes, Bilateral ♀
9 Uterus ♀
   Fundus uteri
   Myometrium
   Perimetrium
   Uterine cornu
C Cervix ♀
F Cul-de-sac ♀
	Ø Open
	3 Percutaneous
	4 Percutaneous Endoscopic
	7 Via Natural or Artificial Opening
	8 Via Natural or Artificial Opening
	   Endoscopic
		Z No Device	X Diagnostic
			Z No Qualifier

G Vagina ♀ K Hymen ♀	Ø Open 3 Percutaneous 4 Percutaneous Endoscopic 7 Via Natural or Artificial Opening 8 Via Natural or Artificial Opening Endoscopic X External	Z No Device	X Diagnostic Z No Qualifier

J Clitoris ♀
L Vestibular Gland ♀
   Bartholin's (greater vestibular) gland
   Greater vestibular (Bartholin's) gland
   Paraurethral (Skene's) gland
   Skene's (paraurethral) gland
M Vulva ♀
   Labia majora
   Labia minora
	Ø Open
	X External
		Z No Device	X Diagnostic
			Z No Qualifier

♀   All body part, approach, device, and qualifier values

Ø   Medical and Surgical
U   Female Reproductive System
C   Extirpation   Definition: Taking or cutting out solid matter from a body part

Explanation: The solid matter may be an abnormal byproduct of a biological function or a foreign body; it may be imbedded in a body part or in the lumen of a tubular body part. The solid matter may or may not have been previously broken into pieces.

Body Part Character 4		Approach Character 5	Device Character 6	Qualifier Character 7

Ø Ovary, Right ♀
1 Ovary, Left ♀
2 Ovaries, Bilateral ♀
4 Uterine Supporting Structure ♀
   Broad ligament
   Infundibulopelvic ligament
   Ovarian ligament
   Round ligament of uterus
		Ø Open
		3 Percutaneous
		4 Percutaneous Endoscopic
		8 Via Natural or Artificial Opening
		   Endoscopic
			Z No Device	Z No Qualifier

5 Fallopian Tube, Right ♀
   Oviduct
   Salpinx
   Uterine tube
6 Fallopian Tube, Left ♀
   See 5 Fallopian Tube, Right
7 Fallopian Tubes, Bilateral ♀
9 Uterus ♀
   Fundus uteri
   Myometrium
   Perimetrium
   Uterine cornu
B Endometrium ♀
C Cervix ♀
F Cul-de-sac ♀
		Ø Open
		3 Percutaneous
		4 Percutaneous Endoscopic
		7 Via Natural or Artificial Opening
		8 Via Natural or Artificial Opening
		   Endoscopic
			Z No Device	Z No Qualifier

G Vagina ♀ K Hymen ♀		Ø Open 3 Percutaneous 4 Percutaneous Endoscopic 7 Via Natural or Artificial Opening 8 Via Natural or Artificial Opening Endoscopic X External	Z No Device	Z No Qualifier

J Clitoris ♀
L Vestibular Gland ♀
   Bartholin's (greater vestibular) gland
   Greater vestibular (Bartholin's) gland
   Paraurethral (Skene's) gland
   Skene's (paraurethral) gland
M Vulva ♀
   Labia majora
   Labia minora
		Ø Open
		X External
			Z No Device	Z No Qualifier

Non-OR   ØUC9[7,8]ZZ
Non-OR   ØUCG[7,8,X]ZZ
Non-OR   ØUCK[Ø,3,4,7,8,X]ZZ

Non-OR   ØUCMXZZ
♀   All body part, approach, device, and qualifier values

Ø   Medical and Surgical
U   Female Reproductive System
D   Extraction   Definition: Pulling or stripping out or off all or a portion of a body part by the use of force

Explanation: The qualifier DIAGNOSTIC is used to identify extraction procedures that are biopsies

Body Part Character 4		Approach Character 5	Device Character 6	Qualifier Character 7
B Endometrium ♀		7 Via Natural or Artificial Opening 8 Via Natural or Artificial Opening Endoscopic	Z No Device	X Diagnostic Z No Qualifier
N Ova ♀		Ø Open 3 Percutaneous 4 Percutaneous Endoscopic	Z No Device	Z No Qualifier

♀   All body part, approach, device, and qualifier values

🔲 Limited Coverage   🔲 Noncovered   ⊞ Combination Member   HAC associated procedure   Combination Only   DRG Non-OR   Non-OR   New/Revised in GREEN
ICD-10-PCS 2019   623

ØUC–ØUD

Female Reproductive System

Ø   **Medical and Surgical**
U   **Female Reproductive System**
F   **Fragmentation**   Definition: Breaking solid matter in a body part into pieces

Explanation: Physical force (e.g., manual, ultrasonic) applied directly or indirectly is used to break the solid matter into pieces. The solid matter may be an abnormal byproduct of a biological function or a foreign body. The pieces of solid matter are not taken out.

Body Part Character 4	Approach Character 5	Device Character 6	Qualifier Character 7

5 **Fallopian Tube, Right** NC ♀
   Oviduct
   Salpinx
   Uterine tube
6 **Fallopian Tube, Left** NC ♀
   See 5 Fallopian Tube, Right
7 **Fallopian Tubes, Bilateral** NC ♀
9 **Uterus** NC ♀
   Fundus uteri
   Myometrium
   Perimetrium
   Uterine cornu
	Ø Open
	3 Percutaneous
	4 Percutaneous Endoscopic
	7 Via Natural or Artificial Opening
	8 Via Natural or Artificial Opening
	   Endoscopic
	X External
		Z No Device	Z No Qualifier

Non-OR   ØUF[5,6,7,9]XZZ
NC   ØUF[5,6,7,9]XZZ
♀   All body part, approach, device, and qualifier values

Ø   **Medical and Surgical**
U   **Female Reproductive System**
H   **Insertion**   Definition: Putting in a nonbiological appliance that monitors, assists, performs, or prevents a physiological function but does not physically take the place of a body part

Explanation: None

Body Part Character 4	Approach Character 5	Device Character 6	Qualifier Character 7
3 Ovary ♀	Ø Open 3 Percutaneous 4 Percutaneous Endoscopic	3 Infusion Device Y Other Device	Z No Qualifier
3 Ovary ♀	7 Via Natural or Artificial Opening 8 Via Natural or Artificial Opening Endoscopic	Y Other Device	Z No Qualifier
8 Fallopian Tube ♀ D Uterus and Cervix ♀ H Vagina and Cul-de-sac ♀	Ø Open 3 Percutaneous 4 Percutaneous Endoscopic 7 Via Natural or Artificial Opening 8 Via Natural or Artificial Opening Endoscopic	3 Infusion Device Y Other Device	Z No Qualifier

9 Uterus ♀
   Fundus uteri
   Myometrium
   Perimetrium
   Uterine cornu
	Ø Open
	7 Via Natural or Artificial Opening
	8 Via Natural or Artificial Opening
	   Endoscopic
		H Contraceptive Device	Z No Qualifier

C Cervix ♀	Ø Open 3 Percutaneous 4 Percutaneous Endoscopic	1 Radioactive Element	Z No Qualifier
C Cervix ♀	7 Via Natural or Artificial Opening 8 Via Natural or Artificial Opening Endoscopic	1 Radioactive Element H Contraceptive Device	Z No Qualifier
F Cul-de-sac ♀	7 Via Natural or Artificial Opening 8 Via Natural or Artificial Opening Endoscopic	G Intraluminal Device, Pessary	Z No Qualifier
G Vagina ♀	Ø Open 3 Percutaneous 4 Percutaneous Endoscopic X External	1 Radioactive Element	Z No Qualifier
G Vagina ♀	7 Via Natural or Artificial Opening 8 Via Natural or Artificial Opening Endoscopic	1 Radioactive Element G Intraluminal Device, Pessary	Z No Qualifier

Non-OR   ØUH3[Ø,3,4][3,Y]Z
Non-OR   ØUH3[7,8]YZ
Non-OR   ØUH[8,D][Ø,3,4,7,8][3,Y]Z
Non-OR   ØUHH[3,4]YZ
Non-OR   ØUHH[7,8][3,Y]Z

Non-OR   ØUH9[Ø,7,8]HZ
Non-OR   ØUHC[7,8]HZ
Non-OR   ØUHF[7,8]GZ
Non-OR   ØUHG[7,8]GZ
♀   All body part, approach, device, and qualifier values

LG Limited Coverage   NC Noncovered   ⊞ Combination Member   HAC associated procedure   Combination Only   DRG Non-OR   Non-OR   New/Revised in GREEN

624   ICD-10-PCS 2019

Ø Medical and Surgical
U Female Reproductive System
J Inspection   Definition: Visually and/or manually exploring a body part

              Explanation: Visual exploration may be performed with or without optical instrumentation. Manual exploration may be performed directly or through intervening body layers.

Body Part Character 4	Approach Character 5	Device Character 6	Qualifier Character 7
3 Ovary ♀	Ø Open 3 Percutaneous 4 Percutaneous Endoscopic 8 Via Natural or Artificial Opening Endoscopic X External	Z No Device	Z No Qualifier
8 Fallopian Tube ♀ D Uterus and Cervix ♀ H Vagina and Cul-de-sac ♀	Ø Open 3 Percutaneous 4 Percutaneous Endoscopic 7 Via Natural or Artificial Opening 8 Via Natural or Artificial Opening Endoscopic X External	Z No Device	Z No Qualifier

M Vulva ♀
   Labia majora
   Labia minora
	Ø Open
	X External
		Z No Device	Z No Qualifier

Non-OR ØUJ3[3,8,X]ZZ		**Non-OR** ØUJMXZZ	
Non-OR ØUJ[8,D,H][3,7,8,X]ZZ		♀ All body part, approach, device, and qualifier values	

Ø Medical and Surgical
U Female Reproductive System
L Occlusion   Definition: Completely closing an orifice or the lumen of a tubular body part

              Explanation: The orifice can be a natural orifice or an artificially created orifice

Body Part Character 4	Approach Character 5	Device Character 6	Qualifier Character 7

5 Fallopian Tube, Right ♀
   Oviduct
   Salpinx
   Uterine tube
6 Fallopian Tube, Left ♀
   See 5 Fallopian Tube, Right
7 Fallopian Tubes, Bilateral NC ♀
	Ø Open
	3 Percutaneous
	4 Percutaneous Endoscopic
		C Extraluminal Device
		D Intraluminal Device
		Z No Device
			Z No Qualifier

5 Fallopian Tube, Right ♀
   Oviduct
   Salpinx
   Uterine tube
6 Fallopian Tube, Left ♀
   See 5 Fallopian Tube, Right
7 Fallopian Tubes, Bilateral NC ♀
	7 Via Natural or Artificial Opening
	8 Via Natural or Artificial Opening Endoscopic
		D Intraluminal Device
		Z No Device
			Z No Qualifier

F Cul-de-sac ♀ G Vagina ♀	7 Via Natural or Artificial Opening 8 Via Natural or Artificial Opening Endoscopic	D Intraluminal Device Z No Device	Z No Qualifier

NC ØUL7[Ø,3,4][C,D,Z]Z with principal or secondary diagnosis of Z3Ø.2	♀	All body part, approach, device, and qualifier values
NC ØUL7[7,8][D,Z]Z with principal or secondary diagnosis of Z3Ø.2		

Female Reproductive System

Ø   **Medical and Surgical**
U   **Female Reproductive System**
M   **Reattachment**   Definition: Putting back in or on all or a portion of a separated body part to its normal location or other suitable location
           Explanation: Vascular circulation and nervous pathways may or may not be reestablished

Body Part Character 4	Approach Character 5	Device Character 6	Qualifier Character 7

Ø   **Ovary, Right** ♀
1   **Ovary, Left** ♀
2   **Ovaries, Bilateral** ♀
4   **Uterine Supporting Structure** ♀
     Broad ligament
     Infundibulopelvic ligament
     Ovarian ligament
     Round ligament of uterus
5   **Fallopian Tube, Right** ♀
     Oviduct
     Salpinx
     Uterine tube
6   **Fallopian Tube, Left** ♀
     See 5 Fallopian Tube, Right
7   **Fallopian Tubes, Bilateral** ♀
9   **Uterus** ♀
     Fundus uteri
     Myometrium
     Perimetrium
     Uterine cornu
C   **Cervix** ♀
F   **Cul-de-sac** ♀
G   **Vagina** ♀
	Ø Open
	4 Percutaneous Endoscopic
		Z No Device	**Z** No Qualifier

J   **Clitoris** ♀
M   **Vulva** ♀
     Labia majora
     Labia minora
	X External	**Z** No Device	**Z** No Qualifier

K **Hymen** ♀	**Ø** Open **4** Percutaneous Endoscopic **X** External	**Z** No Device	**Z** No Qualifier

♀   All body part, approach, device, and qualifier values

Ø   **Medical and Surgical**
U   **Female Reproductive System**
N   **Release**   Definition: Freeing a body part from an abnormal physical constraint by cutting or by the use of force
                 Explanation: Some of the restraining tissue may be taken out but none of the body part is taken out

Body Part Character 4	Approach Character 5	Device Character 6	Qualifier Character 7

Ø **Ovary, Right** ♀
1 **Ovary, Left** ♀
2 **Ovaries, Bilateral** ♀
4 **Uterine Supporting Structure** ♀
      Broad ligament
      Infundibulopelvic ligament
      Ovarian ligament
      Round ligament of uterus
	Ø Open
	3 Percutaneous
	4 Percutaneous Endoscopic
	8 Via Natural or Artificial Opening
	     Endoscopic
		Z No Device	**Z** No Qualifier

5 **Fallopian Tube, Right** ♀
      Oviduct
      Salpinx
      Uterine tube
6 **Fallopian Tube, Left** ♀
      See 5 Fallopian Tube, Right
7 **Fallopian Tubes, Bilateral** ♀
9 **Uterus** ♀
      Fundus uteri
      Myometrium
      Perimetrium
      Uterine cornu
C **Cervix** ♀
F **Cul-de-sac** ♀
	Ø Open
	3 Percutaneous
	4 Percutaneous Endoscopic
	7 Via Natural or Artificial Opening
	8 Via Natural or Artificial Opening
	     Endoscopic
		Z No Device	**Z** No Qualifier

G **Vagina** ♀ **K** **Hymen** ♀	**Ø** Open **3** Percutaneous **4** Percutaneous Endoscopic **7** Via Natural or Artificial Opening **8** Via Natural or Artificial Opening Endoscopic **X** External	**Z** No Device	**Z** No Qualifier

J **Clitoris** ♀
L **Vestibular Gland** ♀
      Bartholin's (greater vestibular) gland
      Greater vestibular (Bartholin's) gland
      Paraurethral (Skene's) gland
      Skene's (paraurethral) gland
M **Vulva** ♀
      Labia majora
      Labia minora
	Ø Open
	X External
		Z No Device	**Z** No Qualifier

♀   All body part, approach, device, and qualifier values

LC Limited Coverage   NC Noncovered   ⊞ Combination Member   HAC associated procedure   Combination Only   DRG Non-OR   Non-OR   New/Revised in GREEN

Ø Medical and Surgical
U Female Reproductive System
P Removal Definition: Taking out or off a device from a body part

Explanation: If a device is taken out and a similar device put in without cutting or puncturing the skin or mucous membrane, the procedure is coded to the root operation CHANGE. Otherwise, the procedure for taking out the device is coded to the root operation REMOVAL.

Body Part Character 4	Approach Character 5	Device Character 6	Qualifier Character 7
3 Ovary ♀	Ø Open 3 Percutaneous 4 Percutaneous Endoscopic	Ø Drainage Device 3 Infusion Device Y Other Device	Z No Qualifier
3 Ovary ♀	7 Via Natural or Artificial Opening 8 Via Natural or Artificial Opening Endoscopic	Y Other Device	Z No Qualifier
3 Ovary ♀	X External	Ø Drainage Device 3 Infusion Device	Z No Qualifier
8 Fallopian Tube ♀	Ø Open 3 Percutaneous 4 Percutaneous Endoscopic 7 Via Natural or Artificial Opening 8 Via Natural or Artificial Opening Endoscopic	Ø Drainage Device 3 Infusion Device 7 Autologous Tissue Substitute C Extraluminal Device D Intraluminal Device J Synthetic Substitute K Nonautologous Tissue Substitute Y Other Device	Z No Qualifier
8 Fallopian Tube ♀	X External	Ø Drainage Device 3 Infusion Device D Intraluminal Device	Z No Qualifier
D Uterus and Cervix ♀	Ø Open 3 Percutaneous 4 Percutaneous Endoscopic 7 Via Natural or Artificial Opening 8 Via Natural or Artificial Opening Endoscopic	Ø Drainage Device 1 Radioactive Element 3 Infusion Device 7 Autologous Tissue Substitute C Extraluminal Device D Intraluminal Device H Contraceptive Device J Synthetic Substitute K Nonautologous Tissue Substitute Y Other Device	Z No Qualifier
D Uterus and Cervix ♀	X External	Ø Drainage Device 3 Infusion Device D Intraluminal Device H Contraceptive Device	Z No Qualifier
H Vagina and Cul-de-sac ♀	Ø Open 3 Percutaneous 4 Percutaneous Endoscopic 7 Via Natural or Artificial Opening 8 Via Natural or Artificial Opening Endoscopic	Ø Drainage Device 1 Radioactive Element 3 Infusion Device 7 Autologous Tissue Substitute D Intraluminal Device J Synthetic Substitute K Nonautologous Tissue Substitute Y Other Device	Z No Qualifier
H Vagina and Cul-de-sac ♀	X External	Ø Drainage Device 1 Radioactive Element 3 Infusion Device D Intraluminal Device	Z No Qualifier
M Vulva ♀ Labia majora Labia minora	Ø Open	Ø Drainage Device 7 Autologous Tissue Substitute J Synthetic Substitute K Nonautologous Tissue Substitute	Z No Qualifier
M Vulva ♀ Labia majora Labia minora	X External	Ø Drainage Device	Z No Qualifier

Non-OR ØUP3[3,4]YZ
Non-OR ØUP3[7,8]YZ
Non-OR ØUP3X[Ø,3]Z
Non-OR ØUP8[3,4]YZ
Non-OR ØUP8[7,8][Ø,3,D,Y]Z
Non-OR ØUP8X[Ø,3,D]Z
Non-OR ØUPD[3,4][C,Y]Z
Non-OR ØUPD[7,8][Ø,3,C,D,H,Y]Z
Non-OR ØUPDX[Ø,3,D,H]Z
Non-OR ØUPH[3,4]YZ
Non-OR ØUPH[7,8][Ø,3,D,Y]Z
Non-OR ØUPHX[Ø,1,3,D]Z
Non-OR ØUPMXØZ
♀ All body part, approach, device, and qualifier values

Ø Medical and Surgical
U Female Reproductive System
Q Repair   Definition: Restoring, to the extent possible, a body part to its normal anatomic structure and function

Explanation: Used only when the method to accomplish the repair is not one of the other root operations

Body Part Character 4	Approach Character 5	Device Character 6	Qualifier Character 7

Ø Ovary, Right ♀
1 Ovary, Left ♀
2 Ovaries, Bilateral ♀
4 Uterine Supporting Structure ♀
  Broad ligament
  Infundibulopelvic ligament
  Ovarian ligament
  Round ligament of uterus
	Ø Open
	3 Percutaneous
	4 Percutaneous Endoscopic
	8 Via Natural or Artificial Opening Endoscopic
		Z No Device	**Z** No Qualifier

5 Fallopian Tube, Right ♀
  Oviduct
  Salpinx
  Uterine tube
6 Fallopian Tube, Left ♀
  See 5 Fallopian Tube, Right
7 Fallopian Tubes, Bilateral ♀
9 Uterus ♀
  Fundus uteri
  Myometrium
  Perimetrium
  Uterine cornu
C Cervix ♀
F Cul-de-sac ♀
	Ø Open
	3 Percutaneous
	4 Percutaneous Endoscopic
	7 Via Natural or Artificial Opening
	8 Via Natural or Artificial Opening Endoscopic
		Z No Device	**Z** No Qualifier

G Vagina ♀ **K** Hymen ♀	**Ø** Open **3** Percutaneous **4** Percutaneous Endoscopic **7** Via Natural or Artificial Opening **8** Via Natural or Artificial Opening Endoscopic **X** External	**Z** No Device	**Z** No Qualifier

J Clitoris ♀
L Vestibular Gland ♀
  Bartholin's (greater vestibular) gland
  Greater vestibular (Bartholin's) gland
  Paraurethral (Skene's) gland
  Skene's (paraurethral) gland
M Vulva ♀
  Labia majora
  Labia minora
	Ø Open
	X External
		Z No Device	**Z** No Qualifier

Non-OR ØUQG[7,X]ZZ
Non-OR ØUQKXZZ
Non-OR ØUQMXZZ
♀ All body part, approach, device, and qualifier values

Ø Medical and Surgical
U Female Reproductive System
S Reposition   Definition: Moving to its normal location, or other suitable location, all or a portion of a body part

Explanation: The body part is moved to a new location from an abnormal location, or from a normal location where it is not functioning correctly. The body part may or may not be cut out or off to be moved to the new location.

Body Part Character 4	Approach Character 5	Device Character 6	Qualifier Character 7

Ø Ovary, Right ♀
1 Ovary, Left ♀
2 Ovaries, Bilateral ♀
4 Uterine Supporting Structure ♀
  Broad ligament
  Infundibulopelvic ligament
  Ovarian ligament
  Round ligament of uterus
5 Fallopian Tube, Right ♀
  Oviduct
  Salpinx
  Uterine tube
6 Fallopian Tube, Left ♀
  See 5 Fallopian Tube, Right
7 Fallopian Tubes, Bilateral ♀
C Cervix ♀
F Cul-de-sac ♀
	Ø Open
	4 Percutaneous Endoscopic
	8 Via Natural or Artificial Opening Endoscopic
		Z No Device	**Z** No Qualifier

9 Uterus ♀
  Fundus uteri
  Myometrium
  Perimetrium
  Uterine cornu
G Vagina ♀
	Ø Open
	4 Percutaneous Endoscopic
	7 Via Natural or Artificial Opening
	8 Via Natural or Artificial Opening Endoscopic
	X External
		Z No Device	**Z** No Qualifier

Non-OR ØUS9XZZ
♀ All body part, approach, device, and qualifier values

LC Limited Coverage   NC Noncovered   ⊞ Combination Member   HAC associated procedure   Combination Only   DRG Non-OR   Non-OR   New/Revised in GREEN

Ø   Medical and Surgical
U   Female Reproductive System
T   Resection   Definition: Cutting out or off, without replacement, all of a body part
                         Explanation: None

Body Part Character 4	Approach Character 5	Device Character 6	Qualifier Character 7
Ø Ovary, Right ♀ **1** Ovary, Left ♀ **2** Ovaries, Bilateral ⊞♀ **5** Fallopian Tube, Right ♀ Oviduct Salpinx Uterine tube **6** Fallopian Tube, Left ♀ *See 5 Fallopian Tube, Right* **7** Fallopian Tubes, Bilateral ⊞♀	**Ø** Open **4** Percutaneous Endoscopic **7** Via Natural or Artificial Opening **8** Via Natural or Artificial Opening Endoscopic **F** Via Natural or Artificial Opening With Percutaneous Endoscopic Assistance	**Z** No Device	**Z** No Qualifier
4 Uterine Supporting Structure ⊞♀ Broad ligament Infundibulopelvic ligament Ovarian ligament Round ligament of uterus **C** Cervix ⊞♀ **F** Cul-de-sac ♀ **G** Vagina ⊞♀	**Ø** Open **4** Percutaneous Endoscopic **7** Via Natural or Artificial Opening **8** Via Natural or Artificial Opening Endoscopic	**Z** No Device	**Z** No Qualifier
9 Uterus ⊞♀ Fundus uteri Myometrium Perimetrium Uterine cornu	**Ø** Open **4** Percutaneous Endoscopic **7** Via Natural or Artificial Opening **8** Via Natural or Artificial Opening Endoscopic **F** Via Natural or Artificial Opening With Percutaneous Endoscopic Assistance	**Z** No Device	**L** Supracervical **Z** No Qualifier
J Clitoris ♀ **L** Vestibular Gland ♀ Bartholin's (greater vestibular) gland Greater vestibular (Bartholin's) gland Paraurethral (Skene's) gland Skene's (paraurethral) gland **M** Vulva ⊞♀ Labia majora Labia minora	**Ø** Open **X** External	**Z** No Device	**Z** No Qualifier
K Hymen ♀	**Ø** Open **4** Percutaneous Endoscopic **7** Via Natural or Artificial Opening **8** Via Natural or Artificial Opening Endoscopic **X** External	**Z** No Device	**Z** No Device

♀   All body part, approach, device, and qualifier values

See Appendix L for Procedure Combinations
⊞   ØUT[2,7]ØZZ
⊞   ØUT[4,C][Ø,4,7,8]ZZ
⊞   ØUTGØZZ
⊞   ØUT9[Ø,4,7,8,F]ZZ
⊞   ØUTM[Ø,X]ZZ

Female Reproductive System

ØUT–ØUT

LC Limited Coverage   **NC** Noncovered   ⊞ Combination Member   HAC associated procedure   Combination Only   DRG Non-OR   Non-OR   New/Revised in GREEN
630   ICD-10-PCS 2019

Ø   Medical and Surgical
U   Female Reproductive System
U   Supplement   Definition: Putting in or on biological or synthetic material that physically reinforces and/or augments the function of a portion of a body part

Explanation: The biological material is non-living, or is living and from the same individual. The body part may have been previously replaced, and the SUPPLEMENT procedure is performed to physically reinforce and/or augment the function of the replaced body part.

Body Part Character 4	Approach Character 5	Device Character 6	Qualifier Character 7
4 Uterine Supporting Structure ♀ Broad ligament Infundibulopelvic ligament Ovarian ligament Round ligament of uterus	**Ø** Open **4** Percutaneous Endoscopic	**7** Autologous Tissue Substitute **J** Synthetic Substitute **K** Nonautologous Tissue Substitute	**Z** No Qualifier
5 Fallopian Tube, Right ♀ Oviduct Salpinx Uterine tube **6** Fallopian Tube, Left ♀ *See 5 Fallopian Tube, Right* **7** Fallopian Tubes, Bilateral ♀ **F** Cul-de-sac ♀	**Ø** Open **4** Percutaneous Endoscopic **7** Via Natural or Artificial Opening **8** Via Natural or Artificial Opening Endoscopic	**7** Autologous Tissue Substitute **J** Synthetic Substitute **K** Nonautologous Tissue Substitute	**Z** No Qualifier
G Vagina ♀ **K** Hymen ♀	**Ø** Open **4** Percutaneous Endoscopic **7** Via Natural or Artificial Opening **8** Via Natural or Artificial Opening Endoscopic **X** External	**7** Autologous Tissue Substitute **J** Synthetic Substitute **K** Nonautologous Tissue Substitute	**Z** No Qualifier
J Clitoris ♀ **M** Vulva ♀ Labia majora Labia minora	**Ø** Open **X** External	**7** Autologous Tissue Substitute **J** Synthetic Substitute **K** Nonautologous Tissue Substitute	**Z** No Qualifier

♀   All body part, approach, device, and qualifier values

Ø   Medical and Surgical
U   Female Reproductive System
V   Restriction   Definition: Partially closing an orifice or the lumen of a tubular body part

Explanation: The orifice can be a natural orifice or an artificially created orifice

Body Part Character 4	Approach Character 5	Device Character 6	Qualifier Character 7
C Cervix ♀	**Ø** Open **3** Percutaneous **4** Percutaneous Endoscopic	**C** Extraluminal Device **D** Intraluminal Device **Z** No Device	**Z** No Qualifier
C Cervix ♀	**7** Via Natural or Artificial Opening **8** Via Natural or Artificial Opening Endoscopic	**D** Intraluminal Device **Z** No Device	**Z** No Qualifier

♀   All body part, approach, device, and qualifier values

LC Limited Coverage   NC Noncovered   ⊞ Combination Member   HAC associated procedure   Combination Only   DRG Non-OR   Non-OR   New/Revised in GREEN

ICD-10-PCS 2019   631

Ø   Medical and Surgical
U   Female Reproductive System
W   Revision   Definition: Correcting, to the extent possible, a portion of a malfunctioning device or the position of a displaced device
                           Explanation: Revision can include correcting a malfunctioning or displaced device by taking out or putting in components of the device such as a screw or pin

Body Part Character 4		Approach Character 5	Device Character 6	Qualifier Character 7
3 Ovary ♀		Ø Open 3 Percutaneous 4 Percutaneous Endoscopic	Ø Drainage Device 3 Infusion Device Y Other Device	Z No Qualifier
3 Ovary ♀		7 Via Natural or Artificial Opening 8 Via Natural or Artificial Opening Endoscopic	Y Other Device	Z No Qualifier
3 Ovary ♀		X External	Ø Drainage Device 3 Infusion Device	Z No Qualifier
8 Fallopian Tube ♀		Ø Open 3 Percutaneous 4 Percutaneous Endoscopic 7 Via Natural or Artificial Opening 8 Via Natural or Artificial Opening Endoscopic	Ø Drainage Device 3 Infusion Device 7 Autologous Tissue Substitute C Extraluminal Device D Intraluminal Device J Synthetic Substitute K Nonautologous Tissue Substitute Y Other Device	Z No Qualifier
8 Fallopian Tube ♀		X External	Ø Drainage Device 3 Infusion Device 7 Autologous Tissue Substitute C Extraluminal Device D Intraluminal Device J Synthetic Substitute K Nonautologous Tissue Substitute	Z No Qualifier
D Uterus and Cervix ♀		Ø Open 3 Percutaneous 4 Percutaneous Endoscopic 7 Via Natural or Artificial Opening 8 Via Natural or Artificial Opening Endoscopic	Ø Drainage Device 1 Radioactive Element 3 Infusion Device 7 Autologous Tissue Substitute C Extraluminal Device D Intraluminal Device H Contraceptive Device J Synthetic Substitute K Nonautologous Tissue Substitute Y Other Device	Z No Qualifier
D Uterus and Cervix ♀		X External	Ø Drainage Device 3 Infusion Device 7 Autologous Tissue Substitute C Extraluminal Device D Intraluminal Device H Contraceptive Device J Synthetic Substitute K Nonautologous Tissue Substitute	Z No Qualifier
H Vagina and Cul-de-sac ♀		Ø Open 3 Percutaneous 4 Percutaneous Endoscopic 7 Via Natural or Artificial Opening 8 Via Natural or Artificial Opening Endoscopic	Ø Drainage Device 1 Radioactive Element 3 Infusion Device 7 Autologous Tissue Substitute D Intraluminal Device J Synthetic Substitute K Nonautologous Tissue Substitute Y Other Device	Z No Qualifier
H Vagina and Cul-de-sac ♀		X External	Ø Drainage Device 3 Infusion Device 7 Autologous Tissue Substitute D Intraluminal Device J Synthetic Substitute K Nonautologous Tissue Substitute	Z No Qualifier

M Vulva
   Labia majora
   Labia minora ♀
		Ø Open
		X External
			Ø Drainage Device
			7 Autologous Tissue Substitute
			J Synthetic Substitute
			K Nonautologous Tissue Substitute
				Z No Qualifier

Non-OR	ØUW3[3,4]YZ	
Non-OR	ØUW3[7,8]YZ	
Non-OR	ØUW3X[Ø,3]Z	
Non-OR	ØUW8[3,4,7,8]YZ	
Non-OR	ØUW8X[Ø,3,7,C,D,J,K]Z	
Non-OR	ØUWD[3,4,7,8]YZ	

Non-OR	ØUWDX[Ø,3,7,C,D,H,J,K]Z
Non-OR	ØUWH[3,4,7,8]YZ
Non-OR	ØUWHX[Ø,3,7,D,J,K]Z
Non-OR	ØUWMX[Ø,7,J,K]Z
♀	All body part, approach, device, and qualifier values

LC Limited Coverage   NC Noncovered   ⊞ Combination Member   HAC associated procedure   Combination Only   DRG Non-OR   Non-OR   New/Revised in GREEN

632   ICD-10-PCS 2019

Ø   **Medical and Surgical**
U   **Female Reproductive System**
Y   **Transplantation**   Definition: Putting in or on all or a portion of a living body part taken from another individual or animal to physically take the place and/or function of all or a portion of a similar body part

Explanation: The native body part may or may not be taken out, and the transplanted body part may take over all or a portion of its function

Body Part Character 4		Approach Character 5	Device Character 6	Qualifier Character 7
Ø Ovary, Right	♀	**Ø** Open	**Z** No Device	**Ø** Allogeneic
1 Ovary, Left	♀			**1** Syngeneic
9 Uterus	♀			**2** Zooplastic
♀	All body part, approach, device, and qualifier values			

Male Reproductive System ØV1–ØVX

Character Meanings

This Character Meaning table is provided as a guide to assist the user in the identification of character members that may be found in this section of code tables. It **SHOULD NOT** be used to build a PCS code.

Operation–Character 3		Body Part–Character 4		Approach–Character 5		Device–Character 6		Qualifier–Character 7	
1	Bypass	Ø	Prostate	Ø	Open	Ø	Drainage Device	D	Urethra
2	Change	1	Seminal Vesicle, Right	3	Percutaneous	1	Radioactive Element	J	Epididymis, Right
5	Destruction	2	Seminal Vesicle, Left	4	Percutaneous Endoscopic	3	Infusion Device	K	Epididymis, Left
7	Dilation	3	Seminal Vesicles, Bilateral	7	Via Natural or Artificial Opening	7	Autologous Tissue Substitute	N	Vas Deferens, Right
9	Drainage	4	Prostate and Seminal Vesicles	8	Via Natural or Artificial Opening Endoscopic	C	Extraluminal Device	P	Vas Deferens, Left
B	Excision	5	Scrotum	X	External	D	Intraluminal Device	S	Penis
C	Extirpation	6	Tunica Vaginalis, Right			J	Synthetic Substitute	X	Diagnostic
H	Insertion	7	Tunica Vaginalis, Left			K	Nonautologous Tissue Substitute	Z	No Qualifier
J	Inspection	8	Scrotum and Tunica Vaginalis			Y	Other Device		
L	Occlusion	9	Testis, Right			Z	No Device		
M	Reattachment	B	Testis, Left						
N	Release	C	Testes, Bilateral						
P	Removal	D	Testis						
Q	Repair	F	Spermatic Cord, Right						
R	Replacement	G	Spermatic Cord, Left						
S	Reposition	H	Spermatic Cords, Bilateral						
T	Resection	J	Epididymis, Right						
U	Supplement	K	Epididymis, Left						
W	Revision	L	Epididymis, Bilateral						
X	Transfer	M	Epididymis and Spermatic Cord						
		N	Vas Deferens, Right						
		P	Vas Deferens, Left						
		Q	Vas Deferens, Bilateral						
		R	Vas Deferens						
		S	Penis						
		T	Prepuce						

AHA Coding Clinic for table ØVB
2016, 1Q, 23   Transurethral resection of ejaculatory ducts
2014, 4Q, 33   Radical prostatectomy

AHA Coding Clinic for table ØVP
2016, 2Q, 28   Removal of multi-component inflatable penile prosthesis with placement of new malleable device

AHA Coding Clinic for table ØVT
2014, 4Q, 33   Radical prostatectomy

AHA Coding Clinic for table ØVU
2016, 2Q, 28   Removal of multi-component inflatable penile prosthesis with placement of new malleable device
2015, 3Q, 25   Placement of inflatable penile prosthesis

Male Reproductive System

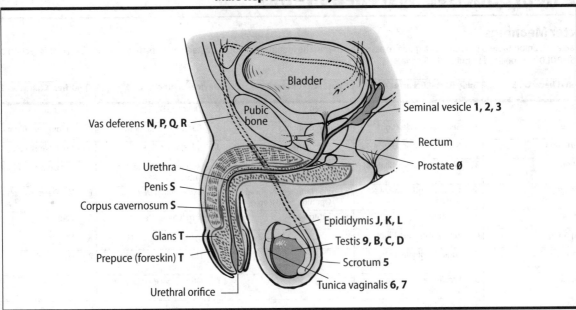

Penis

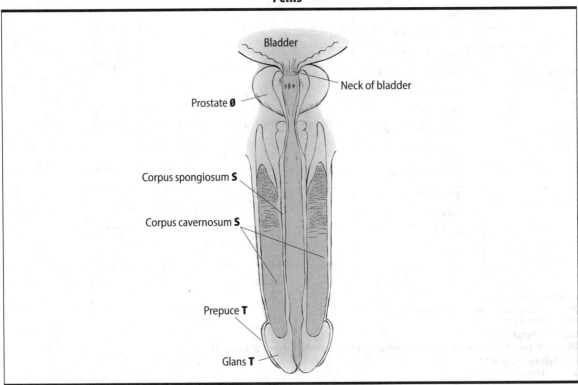

Ø   Medical and Surgical
V   Male Reproductive System
1   Bypass   Definition: Altering the route of passage of the contents of a tubular body part

                Explanation: Rerouting contents of a body part to a downstream area of the normal route, to a similar route and body part, or to an abnormal route and dissimilar body part. Includes one or more anastomoses, with or without the use of a device.

Body Part Character 4	Approach Character 5	Device Character 6	Qualifier Character 7

N Vas Deferens, Right ♂
   Ductus deferens
   Ejaculatory duct
P Vas Deferens, Left ♂
   See N Vas Deferens, Right
Q Vas Deferens, Bilateral ♂
   See N Vas Deferens, Right
	Ø Open
	4 Percutaneous Endoscopic
		7 Autologous Tissue Substitute
		J Synthetic Substitute
		K Nonautologous Tissue Substitute
		Z No Device
			J Epididymis, Right
			K Epididymis, Left
			N Vas Deferens, Right
			P Vas Deferens, Left

     ♂   All body part, approach, device, and qualifier values

Ø   Medical and Surgical
V   Male Reproductive System
2   Change   Definition: Taking out or off a device from a body part and putting back an identical or similar device in or on the same body part without cutting or puncturing the skin or a mucous membrane

                Explanation: All CHANGE procedures are coded using the approach EXTERNAL

Body Part Character 4	Approach Character 5	Device Character 6	Qualifier Character 7

4 Prostate and Seminal Vesicles ♂
8 Scrotum and Tunica Vaginalis ♂
D Testis ♂
M Epididymis and Spermatic Cord ♂
R Vas Deferens ♂
   Ductus deferens
   Ejaculatory duct
S Penis ♂
   Corpus cavernosum
   Corpus spongiosum
	X External	**Ø Drainage Device**
		Y Other Device
			Z No Qualifier

    Non-OR   All body part, approach, device, and qualifier values   ♂   All body part, approach, device, and qualifier values

Ø   Medical and Surgical
V   Male Reproductive System
5   Destruction   Definition: Physical eradication of all or a portion of a body part by the direct use of energy, force, or a destructive agent

                Explanation: None of the body part is physically taken out

Body Part Character 4	Approach Character 5	Device Character 6	Qualifier Character 7
Ø Prostate ♂	**Ø Open** **3 Percutaneous** **4 Percutaneous Endoscopic** **7 Via Natural or Artificial Opening** **8 Via Natural or Artificial Opening Endoscopic**	**Z No Device**	**Z No Qualifier**
1 Seminal Vesicle, Right ♂ **2 Seminal Vesicle, Left** ♂ **3 Seminal Vesicles, Bilateral** ♂ **6 Tunica Vaginalis, Right** ♂ **7 Tunica Vaginalis, Left** ♂ **9 Testis, Right** ♂ **B Testis, Left** ♂ **C Testes, Bilateral** ♂	**Ø Open** **3 Percutaneous** **4 Percutaneous Endoscopic**	**Z No Device**	**Z No Qualifier**

5 Scrotum ♂
S Penis ♂
   Corpus cavernosum
   Corpus spongiosum
T Prepuce ♂
   Foreskin
   Glans penis
	Ø Open
	3 Percutaneous
	4 Percutaneous Endoscopic
	X External
		Z No Device	**Z No Qualifier**

F Spermatic Cord, Right ♂
G Spermatic Cord, Left ♂
H Spermatic Cords, Bilateral ♂
J Epididymis, Right ♂
K Epididymis, Left ♂
L Epididymis, Bilateral ♂
N Vas Deferens, Right NC ♂
   Ductus deferens
   Ejaculatory duct
P Vas Deferens, Left NC ♂
   See N Vas Deferens, Right
Q Vas Deferens, Bilateral NC ♂
   See N Vas Deferens, Right
	Ø Open
	3 Percutaneous
	4 Percutaneous Endoscopic
	8 Via Natural or Artificial Opening Endoscopic
		Z No Device	**Z No Qualifier**

    Non-OR   ØV55[Ø,3,4,X]ZZ   NC   ØV5[N,P,Q][Ø,3,4]ZZ with principal or secondary diagnosis of Z3Ø.2
    Non-OR   ØV5[N,P,Q][Ø,3,4,8]ZZ   ♂   All body part, approach, device, and qualifier values

LC Limited Coverage   **NC** Noncovered   ⊞ Combination Member   HAC associated procedure   Combination Only   DRG Non-OR   Non-OR   New/Revised in GREEN

ICD-10-PCS 2019   **637**

ØV1–ØV5

Ø Medical and Surgical
V Male Reproductive System
7 Dilation   Definition: Expanding an orifice or the lumen of a tubular body part

Explanation: The orifice can be a natural orifice or an artificially created orifice. Accomplished by stretching a tubular body part using intraluminal pressure or by cutting part of the orifice or wall of the tubular body part.

Body Part Character 4		Approach Character 5	Device Character 6	Qualifier Character 7

N Vas Deferens, Right ♂
    Ductus deferens
    Ejaculatory duct
 P Vas Deferens, Left ♂
    See N Vas Deferens, Right
 Q Vas Deferens, Bilateral ♂
    See N Vas Deferens, Right
	Ø Open
	 3 Percutaneous
	 4 Percutaneous Endoscopic
			D Intraluminal Device
			 Z No Device
				Z No Qualifier

♂   All body part, approach, device, and qualifier values

Ø Medical and Surgical
V Male Reproductive System
9 Drainage   Definition: Taking or letting out fluids and/or gases from a body part

Explanation: The qualifier DIAGNOSTIC is used to identify drainage procedures that are biopsies

Body Part Character 4		Approach Character 5	Device Character 6	Qualifier Character 7
Ø Prostate ♂		Ø Open 3 Percutaneous 4 Percutaneous Endoscopic 7 Via Natural or Artificial Opening 8 Via Natural or Artificial Opening Endoscopic	Ø Drainage Device	Z No Qualifier
Ø Prostate ♂		Ø Open 3 Percutaneous 4 Percutaneous Endoscopic 7 Via Natural or Artificial Opening 8 Via Natural or Artificial Opening Endoscopic	Z No Device	X Diagnostic Z No Qualifier

1 Seminal Vesicle, Right ♂
 2 Seminal Vesicle, Left ♂
 3 Seminal Vesicles, Bilateral ♂
 6 Tunica Vaginalis, Right ♂
 7 Tunica Vaginalis, Left ♂
 9 Testis, Right ♂
 B Testis, Left ♂
 C Testes, Bilateral ♂
 F Spermatic Cord, Right ♂
 G Spermatic Cord, Left ♂
 H Spermatic Cords, Bilateral ♂
 J Epididymis, Right ♂
 K Epididymis, Left ♂
 L Epididymis, Bilateral ♂
 N Vas Deferens, Right ♂
    Ductus deferens
    Ejaculatory duct
 P Vas Deferens, Left ♂
    See N Vas Deferens, Right
 Q Vas Deferens, Bilateral ♂
    See N Vas Deferens, Right
		Ø Open
		 3 Percutaneous
		 4 Percutaneous Endoscopic
			Ø Drainage Device	Z No Qualifier

ØV9 Continued on next page

Non-OR	ØV9Ø[3,4]ØZ		**Non-OR**	ØV9[6,7,F,G,H,N,P,Q][Ø,3,4]ØZ
Non-OR	ØV9Ø[3,4]Z[X,Z]		**Non-OR**	ØV9[J,K,L]3ØZ
Non-OR	ØV9Ø[7,8]ZX		♂	All body part, approach, device, and qualifier values
Non-OR	ØV9[1,2,3,9,B,C][3,4]ØZ			

0 **Medical and Surgical**

V **Male Reproductive System**
9 **Drainage**　　　　Definition: Taking or letting out fluids and/or gases from a body part
　　　　　　　　　　　Explanation: The qualifier DIAGNOSTIC is used to identify drainage procedures that are biopsies

Body Part Character 4		Approach Character 5	Device Character 6	Qualifier Character 7
1 **Seminal Vesicle, Right** ♂ **2** **Seminal Vesicle, Left** ♂ **3** **Seminal Vesicles, Bilateral** ♂ **6** **Tunica Vaginalis, Right** ♂ **7** **Tunica Vaginalis, Left** ♂ **9** **Testis, Right** ♂ **B** **Testis, Left** ♂ **C** **Testes, Bilateral** ♂ **F** **Spermatic Cord, Right** ♂ **G** **Spermatic Cord, Left** ♂ **H** **Spermatic Cords, Bilateral** ♂ **J** **Epididymis, Right** ♂ **K** **Epididymis, Left** ♂ **L** **Epididymis, Bilateral** ♂ **N** **Vas Deferens, Right** ♂ 　　Ductus deferens 　　Ejaculatory duct **P** **Vas Deferens, Left** ♂ 　　*See N Vas Deferens, Right* **Q** **Vas Deferens, Bilateral** ♂ 　　*See N Vas Deferens, Right*		**0** Open **3** Percutaneous **4** Percutaneous Endoscopic	**Z** No Device	**X** Diagnostic **Z** No Qualifier
5 **Scrotum** ♂ **S** **Penis** ♂ 　　Corpus cavernosum 　　Corpus spongiosum **T** **Prepuce** ♂ 　　Foreskin 　　Glans penis		**0** Open **3** Percutaneous **4** Percutaneous Endoscopic **X** External	**0** Drainage Device	**Z** No Qualifier
5 **Scrotum** ♂ **S** **Penis** ♂ 　　Corpus cavernosum 　　Corpus spongiosum **T** **Prepuce** ♂ 　　Foreskin 　　Glans penis		**0** Open **3** Percutaneous **4** Percutaneous Endoscopic **X** External	**Z** No Device	**X** Diagnostic **Z** No Qualifier

Non-OR　0V9[1,2,3,9,B,C][3,4]Z[X,Z]
Non-OR　0V9[6,7,F,G,H,J,K,L,N,P,Q][0,3,4]ZX
Non-OR　0V9[6,7,F,G,H,N,P,Q][0,3,4]ZZ
Non-OR　0V9[J,K,L]3ZZ
Non-OR　0V95[0,3,4,X]0Z

Non-OR　0V9[S,T]30Z
Non-OR　0V95[0,3,4,X]Z[X,Z]
Non-OR　0V9[S,T]3ZZ
♂　　All body part, approach, device, and qualifier values

Ø **Medical and Surgical**
V **Male Reproductive System**
B **Excision**   Definition: Cutting out or off, without replacement, a portion of a body part
Explanation: The qualifier DIAGNOSTIC is used to identify excision procedures that are biopsies

Body Part Character 4		Approach Character 5	Device Character 6	Qualifier Character 7
Ø Prostate	♂	**Ø** Open **3** Percutaneous **4** Percutaneous Endoscopic **7** Via Natural or Artificial Opening **8** Via Natural or Artificial Opening Endoscopic	**Z** No Device	**X** Diagnostic **Z** No Qualifier
1 Seminal Vesicle, Right **2** Seminal Vesicle, Left **3** Seminal Vesicles, Bilateral **6** Tunica Vaginalis, Right **7** Tunica Vaginalis, Left **9** Testis, Right **B** Testis, Left **C** Testes, Bilateral	♂ ♂ ♂ ♂ ♂ ♂ ♂ ♂	**Ø** Open **3** Percutaneous **4** Percutaneous Endoscopic	**Z** No Device	**X** Diagnostic **Z** No Qualifier
5 Scrotum **S** Penis Corpus cavernosum Corpus spongiosum **T** Prepuce Foreskin Glans penis	♂ ♂ ♂	**Ø** Open **3** Percutaneous **4** Percutaneous Endoscopic **X** External	**Z** No Device	**X** Diagnostic **Z** No Qualifier
F Spermatic Cord, Right **G** Spermatic Cord, Left **H** Spermatic Cords, Bilateral **J** Epididymis, Right **K** Epididymis, Left **L** Epididymis, Bilateral **N** Vas Deferens, Right Ductus deferens Ejaculatory duct **P** Vas Deferens, Left *See N Vas Deferens, Right* **Q** Vas Deferens, Bilateral *See N Vas Deferens, Right*	♂ ♂ ♂ ♂ ♂ ♂ NC ♂ NC ♂ NC ♂	**Ø** Open **3** Percutaneous **4** Percutaneous Endoscopic **8** Via Natural or Artificial Opening Endoscopic	**Z** No Device	**X** Diagnostic **Z** No Qualifier

Non-OR	ØVBØ[3,4,7,8]ZX	Non-OR	ØVB[F,G,H,J,K,L][Ø,3,4,8]ZX
Non-OR	ØVB[1,2,3,9,B,C][3,4]ZX	Non-OR	ØVB[N,P,Q][Ø,3,4,8]Z[X,Z]
Non-OR	ØVB[6,7][Ø,3,4]ZX	NC	ØVB[N,P,Q][Ø,3,4]ZZ with principal or secondary diagnosis of Z3Ø.2
Non-OR	ØVB5[Ø,3,4,X]Z[X,Z]	♂	All body part, approach, device, and qualifier values

Ø   Medical and Surgical
V   Male Reproductive System
C   Extirpation   Definition: Taking or cutting out solid matter from a body part

Explanation: The solid matter may be an abnormal byproduct of a biological function or a foreign body; it may be imbedded in a body part or in the lumen of a tubular body part. The solid matter may or may not have been previously broken into pieces.

Body Part Character 4		Approach Character 5	Device Character 6	Qualifier Character 7
Ø Prostate	♂	**Ø** Open **3** Percutaneous **4** Percutaneous Endoscopic **7** Via Natural or Artificial Opening **8** Via Natural or Artificial Opening Endoscopic	**Z** No Device	**Z** No Qualifier
1 Seminal Vesicle, Right	♂	**Ø** Open	**Z** No Device	**Z** No Qualifier
2 Seminal Vesicle, Left	♂	**3** Percutaneous		
3 Seminal Vesicles, Bilateral	♂	**4** Percutaneous Endoscopic		
6 Tunica Vaginalis, Right	♂			
7 Tunica Vaginalis, Left	♂			
9 Testis, Right	♂			
B Testis, Left	♂			
C Testes, Bilateral	♂			
F Spermatic Cord, Right	♂			
G Spermatic Cord, Left	♂			
H Spermatic Cords, Bilateral	♂			
J Epididymis, Right	♂			
K Epididymis, Left	♂			
L Epididymis, Bilateral	♂			

N   Vas Deferens, Right
     Ductus deferens
     Ejaculatory duct
	♂			

P Vas Deferens, Left *See N Vas Deferens, Right*	♂			
Q Vas Deferens, Bilateral *See N Vas Deferens, Right*	♂			
5 Scrotum	♂	**Ø** Open	**Z** No Device	**Z** No Qualifier

S   Penis
     Corpus cavernosum
     Corpus spongiosum
	♂	**3** Percutaneous
		4 Percutaneous Endoscopic
		X External		

T   Prepuce
     Foreskin
     Glans penis
	♂			

Non-OR   ØVC[6,7,N,P,Q][Ø,3,4]ZZ
Non-OR   ØVC5[Ø,3,4,X]ZZ

Non-OR   ØVCSXZZ
♂   All body part, approach, device, and qualifier values

Male Reproductive System *(left margin)*

Ø　**Medical and Surgical**
V　**Male Reproductive System**
H　**Insertion**　Definition: Putting in a nonbiological appliance that monitors, assists, performs, or prevents a physiological function but does not physically take the place of a body part
　　　　　　　Explanation: None

Body Part Character 4	Approach Character 5	Device Character 6	Qualifier Character 7
Ø Prostate ♂	Ø Open 3 Percutaneous 4 Percutaneous Endoscopic 7 Via Natural or Artificial Opening 8 Via Natural or Artificial Opening Endoscopic	1 Radioactive Element	Z No Qualifier
4 Prostate and Seminal Vesicles ♂ 8 Scrotum and Tunica Vaginalis ♂ D Testis ♂ M Epididymis and Spermatic Cord ♂ R Vas Deferens ♂ 　Ductus deferens 　Ejaculatory duct	Ø Open 3 Percutaneous 4 Percutaneous Endoscopic 7 Via Natural or Artificial Opening 8 Via Natural or Artificial Opening Endoscopic	3 Infusion Device Y Other Device	Z No Qualifier
S Penis ♂ 　Corpus cavernosum 　Corpus spongiosum	Ø Open 3 Percutaneous 4 Percutaneous Endoscopic	3 Infusion Device Y Other Device	Z No Qualifier
S Penis ♂ 　Corpus cavernosum 　Corpus spongiosum	7 Via Natural or Artificial Opening 8 Via Natural or Artificial Opening Endoscopic	Y Other Device	Z No Qualifier
S Penis ♂ 　Corpus cavernosum 　Corpus spongiosum	X External	3 Infusion Device	Z No Qualifier

Non-OR　ØVH[4,8,D,M,R][Ø,3,4,7,8][3,Y]Z
Non-OR　ØVHS[Ø,3,4][3,Y]Z
Non-OR　ØVHS[7,8]YZ

Non-OR　ØVHSX3Z
♂　　　All body part, approach, device, and qualifier values

Ø　**Medical and Surgical**
V　**Male Reproductive System**
J　**Inspection**　Definition: Visually and/or manually exploring a body part
　　　　　　　Explanation: Visual exploration may be performed with or without optical instrumentation. Manual exploration may be performed directly or through intervening body layers.

Body Part Character 4	Approach Character 5	Device Character 6	Qualifier Character 7
4 Prostate and Seminal Vesicles ♂ 8 Scrotum and Tunica Vaginalis ♂ D Testis ♂ M Epididymis and Spermatic Cord ♂ R Vas Deferens ♂ 　Ductus deferens 　Ejaculatory duct S Penis ♂ 　Corpus cavernosum 　Corpus spongiosum	Ø Open 3 Percutaneous 4 Percutaneous Endoscopic X External	Z No Device	Z No Qualifier

Non-OR　ØVJ[4,D,M,R][3,X]ZZ
Non-OR　ØVJ[8,S][Ø,3,4,X]ZZ

♂　　　All body part, approach, device, and qualifier values

Ø　**Medical and Surgical**
V　**Male Reproductive System**
L　**Occlusion**　Definition: Completely closing an orifice or the lumen of a tubular body part
　　　　　　　Explanation: The orifice can be a natural orifice or an artificially created orifice

Body Part Character 4	Approach Character 5	Device Character 6	Qualifier Character 7
F Spermatic Cord, Right NC ♂ G Spermatic Cord, Left NC ♂ H Spermatic Cords, Bilateral NC ♂ N Vas Deferens, Right NC ♂ 　Ductus deferens 　Ejaculatory duct P Vas Deferens, Left NC ♂ 　See N Vas Deferens, Right Q Vas Deferens, Bilateral NC ♂ 　See N Vas Deferens, Right	Ø Open 3 Percutaneous 4 Percutaneous Endoscopic 8 Via Natural or Artificial Opening Endoscopic	C Extraluminal Device D Intraluminal Device Z No Device	Z No Qualifier

Non-OR　ØVL[F,G,H][Ø,3,4,8][C,D,Z]Z
Non-OR　ØVL[N,P,Q][Ø,3,4,8][C,Z]Z

NC　ØVL[F,G,H][Ø,3,4][C,D,Z]Z with principal or secondary diagnosis of Z3Ø.2
NC　ØVL[N,P,Q][Ø,3,4][C,Z]Z with principal or secondary diagnosis of Z3Ø.2
♂　All body part, approach, device, and qualifier values

Ø   **Medical and Surgical**
V   **Male Reproductive System**
M   **Reattachment**   Definition: Putting back in or on all or a portion of a separated body part to its normal location or other suitable location
           Explanation: Vascular circulation and nervous pathways may or may not be reestablished

Body Part Character 4	Approach Character 5	Device Character 6	Qualifier Character 7

5   Scrotum   ♂
S   Penis   ♂
    Corpus cavernosum
    Corpus spongiosum
	X External	**Z** No Device	**Z** No Qualifier

6 Tunica Vaginalis, Right ♂ **7** Tunica Vaginalis, Left ♂ **9** Testis, Right ♂ **B** Testis, Left ♂ **C** Testes, Bilateral ♂ **F** Spermatic Cord, Right ♂ **G** Spermatic Cord, Left ♂ **H** Spermatic Cords, Bilateral ♂	**Ø** Open **4** Percutaneous Endoscopic	**Z** No Device	**Z** No Qualifier

♂   All body part, approach, device, and qualifier values

Ø   **Medical and Surgical**
V   **Male Reproductive System**
N   **Release**   Definition: Freeing a body part from an abnormal physical constraint by cutting or by the use of force
           Explanation: Some of the restraining tissue may be taken out but none of the body part is taken out

Body Part Character 4	Approach Character 5	Device Character 6	Qualifier Character 7
Ø Prostate ♂	**Ø** Open **3** Percutaneous **4** Percutaneous Endoscopic **7** Via Natural or Artificial Opening **8** Via Natural or Artificial Opening Endoscopic	**Z** No Device	**Z** No Qualifier
1 Seminal Vesicle, Right ♂ **2** Seminal Vesicle, Left ♂ **3** Seminal Vesicles, Bilateral ♂ **6** Tunica Vaginalis, Right ♂ **7** Tunica Vaginalis, Left ♂ **9** Testis, Right ♂ **B** Testis, Left ♂ **C** Testes, Bilateral ♂	**Ø** Open **3** Percutaneous **4** Percutaneous Endoscopic	**Z** No Device	**Z** No Qualifier

5   Scrotum   ♂
S   Penis   ♂
    Corpus cavernosum
    Corpus spongiosum
T   Prepuce   ♂
    Foreskin
    Glans penis
	Ø Open
	3 Percutaneous
	4 Percutaneous Endoscopic
	X External
		Z No Device	**Z** No Qualifier

F   Spermatic Cord, Right   ♂
G   Spermatic Cord, Left   ♂
H   Spermatic Cords, Bilateral   ♂
J   Epididymis, Right   ♂
K   Epididymis, Left   ♂
L   Epididymis, Bilateral   ♂
N   Vas Deferens, Right   ♂
    Ductus deferens
    Ejaculatory duct
P   Vas Deferens, Left   ♂
    See N Vas Deferens, Right
Q   Vas Deferens, Bilateral   ♂
    See N Vas Deferens, Right
	Ø Open
	3 Percutaneous
	4 Percutaneous Endoscopic
	8 Via Natural or Artificial Opening
	    Endoscopic
		Z No Device	**Z** No Qualifier

Non-OR   ØVN[9,B,C][Ø,3,4]ZZ
Non-OR   ØVNT[Ø,3,4,X]ZZ   ♂   All body part, approach, device, and qualifier values

Ø   **Medical and Surgical**
V   **Male Reproductive System**
P   **Removal**   Definition: Taking out or off a device from a body part

Explanation: If a device is taken out and a similar device put in without cutting or puncturing the skin or mucous membrane, the procedure is coded to the root operation CHANGE. Otherwise, the procedure for taking out the device is coded to the root operation REMOVAL.

Body Part Character 4	Approach Character 5	Device Character 6	Qualifier Character 7
4 Prostate and Seminal Vesicles ♂	**Ø** Open **3** Percutaneous **4** Percutaneous Endoscopic **7** Via Natural or Artificial Opening **8** Via Natural or Artificial Opening Endoscopic	**Ø** Drainage Device **1** Radioactive Element **3** Infusion Device **7** Autologous Tissue Substitute **J** Synthetic Substitute **K** Nonautologous Tissue Substitute **Y** Other Device	**Z** No Qualifier
4 Prostate and Seminal Vesicles ♂	**X** External	**Ø** Drainage Device **1** Radioactive Element **3** Infusion Device	**Z** No Qualifier

8 Scrotum and Tunica Vaginalis ♂
D Testis ♂
S Penis ♂
   Corpus cavernosum
   Corpus spongiosum
	Ø Open
	3 Percutaneous
	4 Percutaneous Endoscopic
	7 Via Natural or Artificial Opening
	8 Via Natural or Artificial Opening Endoscopic
		Ø Drainage Device
		3 Infusion Device
		7 Autologous Tissue Substitute
		J Synthetic Substitute
		K Nonautologous Tissue Substitute
		Y Other Device
			Z No Qualifier

8 Scrotum and Tunica Vaginalis ♂
D Testis ♂
S Penis ♂
   Corpus cavernosum
   Corpus spongiosum
	X External	**Ø** Drainage Device
		3 Infusion Device
			Z No Qualifier

M Epididymis and Spermatic Cord ♂	**Ø** Open **3** Percutaneous **4** Percutaneous Endoscopic **7** Via Natural or Artificial Opening **8** Via Natural or Artificial Opening Endoscopic	**Ø** Drainage Device **3** Infusion Device **7** Autologous Tissue Substitute **C** Extraluminal Device **J** Synthetic Substitute **K** Nonautologous Tissue Substitute **Y** Other Device	**Z** No Qualifier
M Epididymis and Spermatic Cord ♂	**X** External	**Ø** Drainage Device **3** Infusion Device	**Z** No Qualifier

R Vas Deferens ♂
   Ductus deferens
   Ejaculatory duct
	Ø Open
	3 Percutaneous
	4 Percutaneous Endoscopic
	7 Via Natural or Artificial Opening
	8 Via Natural or Artificial Opening Endoscopic
		Ø Drainage Device
		3 Infusion Device
		7 Autologous Tissue Substitute
		C Extraluminal Device
		D Intraluminal Device
		J Synthetic Substitute
		K Nonautologous Tissue Substitute
		Y Other Device
			Z No Qualifier

R Vas Deferens ♂
   Ductus deferens
   Ejaculatory duct
	X External	**Ø** Drainage Device
		3 Infusion Device
		D Intraluminal Device
			Z No Qualifier

Non-OR ØVP4[3,4]YZ		**Non-OR** ØVPM[3,4]YZ	
Non-OR ØVP4[7,8][Ø,3,Y]Z		**Non-OR** ØVPM[7,8][Ø,3,Y]Z	
Non-OR ØVP4X[Ø,1,3]Z		**Non-OR** ØVPMX[Ø,3]Z	
Non-OR ØVP8[Ø,3,4,7,8][Ø,3,7,J,K,Y]Z		**Non-OR** ØVPR[Ø,3,4][Ø,3,7,C,J,K,Y]Z	
Non-OR ØVP[D,S][3,4]YZ		**Non-OR** ØVPR[7,8][Ø,3,7,C,D,J,K,Y]Z	
Non-OR ØVP[D,S][7,8][Ø,3,Y]Z		**Non-OR** ØVPRX[Ø,3,D]Z	
Non-OR ØVP[8,D,S]X[Ø,3]Z		♂ All body part, approach, device, and qualifier values	

LC Limited Coverage   **NC** Noncovered   ⊞ Combination Member   HAC associated procedure   Combination Only   DRG Non-OR   Non-OR   New/Revised in GREEN

644   ICD-10-PCS 2019

0   **Medical and Surgical**
V   **Male Reproductive System**
Q   **Repair**   Definition: Restoring, to the extent possible, a body part to its normal anatomic structure and function
                  Explanation: Used only when the method to accomplish the repair is not one of the other root operations

Body Part Character 4	Approach Character 5	Device Character 6	Qualifier Character 7
0 Prostate ♂	**0** Open **3** Percutaneous **4** Percutaneous Endoscopic **7** Via Natural or Artificial Opening **8** Via Natural or Artificial Opening Endoscopic	**Z** No Device	**Z** No Qualifier
1 Seminal Vesicle, Right ♂ **2** Seminal Vesicle, Left ♂ **3** Seminal Vesicles, Bilateral ♂ **6** Tunica Vaginalis, Right ♂ **7** Tunica Vaginalis, Left ♂ **9** Testis, Right ♂ **B** Testis, Left ♂ **C** Testes, Bilateral ♂	**0** Open **3** Percutaneous **4** Percutaneous Endoscopic	**Z** No Device	**Z** No Qualifier

5 Scrotum ♂
S Penis ♂
    Corpus cavernosum
    Corpus spongiosum
T Prepuce ♂
    Foreskin
    Glans penis
	0 Open
	3 Percutaneous
	4 Percutaneous Endoscopic
	X External
		Z No Device	**Z** No Qualifier

F Spermatic Cord, Right ♂
G Spermatic Cord, Left ♂
H Spermatic Cords, Bilateral ♂
J Epididymis, Right ♂
K Epididymis, Left ♂
L Epididymis, Bilateral ♂
N Vas Deferens, Right ♂
    Ductus deferens
    Ejaculatory duct
P Vas Deferens, Left ♂
    See N Vas Deferens, Right
Q Vas Deferens, Bilateral ♂
    See N Vas Deferens, Right
	0 Open
	3 Percutaneous
	4 Percutaneous Endoscopic
	8 Via Natural or Artificial Opening Endoscopic
		Z No Device	**Z** No Qualifier

Non-OR   0VQ[6,7][0,3,4]ZZ
Non-OR   0VQ5[0,3,4,X]ZZ   ♂   All body part, approach, device, and qualifier values

0   **Medical and Surgical**
V   **Male Reproductive System**
R   **Replacement**   Definition: Putting in or on biological or synthetic material that physically takes the place and/or function of all or a portion of a body part
                       Explanation: The body part may have been taken out or replaced, or may be taken out, physically eradicated, or rendered nonfunctional during the REPLACEMENT procedure. A REMOVAL procedure is coded for taking out the device used in a previous replacement procedure.

Body Part Character 4	Approach Character 5	Device Character 6	Qualifier Character 7
9 Testis, Right ♂ **B** Testis, Left ♂ **C** Testes, Bilateral ♂	**0** Open	**J** Synthetic Substitute	**Z** No Qualifier

     ♂   All body part, approach, device, and qualifier values

0   **Medical and Surgical**
V   **Male Reproductive System**
S   **Reposition**   Definition: Moving to its normal location, or other suitable location, all or a portion of a body part
                   Explanation: The body part is moved to a new location from an abnormal location, or from a normal location where it is not functioning correctly. The body part may or may not be cut out or off to be moved to the new location.

Body Part Character 4	Approach Character 5	Device Character 6	Qualifier Character 7
9 Testis, Right ♂ **B** Testis, Left ♂ **C** Testes, Bilateral ♂ **F** Spermatic Cord, Right ♂ **G** Spermatic Cord, Left ♂ **H** Spermatic Cords, Bilateral ♂	**0** Open **3** Percutaneous **4** Percutaneous Endoscopic **8** Via Natural or Artificial Opening Endoscopic	**Z** No Device	**Z** No Qualifier

     ♂   All body part, approach, device, and qualifier values

Male Reproductive System

Ø   **Medical and Surgical**
V   **Male Reproductive System**
T   **Resection**   Definition: Cutting out or off, without replacement, all of a body part
                 Explanation: None

Body Part Character 4	Approach Character 5	Device Character 6	Qualifier Character 7
Ø Prostate ⊞♂	Ø Open 4 Percutaneous Endoscopic 7 Via Natural or Artificial Opening 8 Via Natural or Artificial Opening Endoscopic	Z No Device	Z No Qualifier

1   Seminal Vesicle, Right   ♂
2   Seminal Vesicle, Left   ♂
3   Seminal Vesicles, Bilateral   ⊞♂
6   Tunica Vaginalis, Right   ♂
7   Tunica Vaginalis, Left   ♂
9   Testis, Right   ♂
B   Testis, Left   ♂
C   Testes, Bilateral   ♂
F   Spermatic Cord, Right   ♂
G   Spermatic Cord, Left   ♂
H   Spermatic Cords, Bilateral   ♂
J   Epididymis, Right   ♂
K   Epididymis, Left   ♂
L   Epididymis, Bilateral   ♂
N   Vas Deferens, Right   NC♂
     Ductus deferens
     Ejaculatory duct
P   Vas Deferens, Left   NC♂
     See N Vas Deferens, Right
Q   Vas Deferens, Bilateral   NC♂
     See N Vas Deferens, Right
	Ø Open
	4 Percutaneous Endoscopic
		Z No Device	Z No Qualifier

5   Scrotum   ♂
S   Penis   ♂
     Corpus cavernosum
     Corpus spongiosum
T   Prepuce   ♂
     Foreskin
     Glans penis
	Ø Open
	4 Percutaneous Endoscopic
	X External
		Z No Device	Z No Qualifier

Non-OR ØVT[N,P,Q][Ø,4]ZZ	**See Appendix L for Procedure Combinations**
Non-OR ØVT[5,T][Ø,4,X]ZZ	⊞ ØVTØ[Ø,4,7,8]ZZ
NC ØVT[N,P,Q][Ø,4]ZZ with principal or secondary diagnosis of Z30.2	⊞ ØVT3[Ø,4]ZZ
♂ All body part, approach, device, and qualifier values	

LC Limited Coverage   NC Noncovered   ⊞ Combination Member   HAC associated procedure   Combination Only   DRG Non-OR   Non-OR   New/Revised in GREEN

646   ICD-10-PCS 2019

Ø   Medical and Surgical
V   Male Reproductive System
U   Supplement   Definition: Putting in or on biological or synthetic material that physically reinforces and/or augments the function of a portion of a body part

Explanation: The biological material is non-living, or is living and from the same individual. The body part may have been previously replaced, and the SUPPLEMENT procedure is performed to physically reinforce and/or augment the function of the replaced body part.

Body Part Character 4		Approach Character 5	Device Character 6	Qualifier Character 7
1 Seminal Vesicle, Right ♂	Ø Open	7 Autologous Tissue Substitute	Z No Qualifier
2 Seminal Vesicle, Left ♂	4 Percutaneous Endoscopic	J Synthetic Substitute	
3 Seminal Vesicles, Bilateral ♂	8 Via Natural or Artificial Opening Endoscopic	K Nonautologous Tissue Substitute	
6 Tunica Vaginalis, Right ♂			
7 Tunica Vaginalis, Left ♂			
F Spermatic Cord, Right ♂			
G Spermatic Cord, Left ♂			
H Spermatic Cords, Bilateral ♂			
J Epididymis, Right ♂			
K Epididymis, Left ♂			
L Epididymis, Bilateral ♂			
N Vas Deferens, Right ♂ Ductus deferens Ejaculatory duct			
P Vas Deferens, Left ♂ *See N Vas Deferens, Right*			
Q Vas Deferens, Bilateral ♂ *See N Vas Deferens, Right*			
5 Scrotum ♂	Ø Open	7 Autologous Tissue Substitute	Z No Qualifier
S Penis ♂ Corpus cavernosum Corpus spongiosum	4 Percutaneous Endoscopic X External	J Synthetic Substitute K Nonautologous Tissue Substitute	
T Prepuce ♂ Foreskin Glans penis			
9 Testis, Right ♂	Ø Open	7 Autologous Tissue Substitute	Z No Qualifier
B Testis, Left ♂		J Synthetic Substitute	
C Testes, Bilateral ♂		K Nonautologous Tissue Substitute	

Non-OR   ØVUSX[7,J,K]Z   ♂   All body part, approach, device, and qualifier values

Ø   **Medical and Surgical**
V   **Male Reproductive System**
W   **Revision**   Definition: Correcting, to the extent possible, a portion of a malfunctioning device or the position of a displaced device

                  Explanation: Revision can include correcting a malfunctioning or displaced device by taking out or putting in components of the device such as a screw or pin

Body Part Character 4	Approach Character 5	Device Character 6	Qualifier Character 7

4 Prostate and Seminal Vesicles ♂
8 Scrotum and Tunica Vaginalis ♂
D Testis ♂
S Penis ♂
    Corpus cavernosum
    Corpus spongiosum
	Ø Open
	3 Percutaneous
	4 Percutaneous Endoscopic
	7 Via Natural or Artificial Opening
	8 Via Natural or Artificial Opening Endoscopic
		Ø Drainage Device
		3 Infusion Device
		7 Autologous Tissue Substitute
		J Synthetic Substitute
		K Nonautologous Tissue Substitute
		Y Other Device
			Z No Qualifier

4 Prostate and Seminal Vesicles ♂
8 Scrotum and Tunica Vaginalis ♂
D Testis ♂
S Penis ♂
    Corpus cavernosum
    Corpus spongiosum
	X External	**Ø** Drainage Device
		3 Infusion Device
		7 Autologous Tissue Substitute
		J Synthetic Substitute
		K Nonautologous Tissue Substitute
			Z No Qualifier

M Epididymis and Spermatic Cord ♂	**Ø** Open **3** Percutaneous **4** Percutaneous Endoscopic **7** Via Natural or Artificial Opening **8** Via Natural or Artificial Opening Endoscopic	**Ø** Drainage Device **3** Infusion Device **7** Autologous Tissue Substitute **C** Extraluminal Device **J** Synthetic Substitute **K** Nonautologous Tissue Substitute **Y** Other Device	**Z** No Qualifier
M Epididymis and Spermatic Cord ♂	**X** External	**Ø** Drainage Device **3** Infusion Device **7** Autologous Tissue Substitute **C** Extraluminal Device **J** Synthetic Substitute **K** Nonautologous Tissue Substitute	**Z** No Qualifier

R Vas Deferens ♂
    Ductus deferens
    Ejaculatory duct
	Ø Open
	3 Percutaneous
	4 Percutaneous Endoscopic
	7 Via Natural or Artificial Opening
	8 Via Natural or Artificial Opening Endoscopic
		Ø Drainage Device
		3 Infusion Device
		7 Autologous Tissue Substitute
		C Extraluminal Device
		D Intraluminal Device
		J Synthetic Substitute
		K Nonautologous Tissue Substitute
		Y Other Device
			Z No Qualifier

R Vas Deferens ♂
    Ductus deferens
    Ejaculatory duct
	X External	**Ø** Drainage Device
		3 Infusion Device
		7 Autologous Tissue Substitute
		C Extraluminal Device
		D Intraluminal Device
		J Synthetic Substitute
		K Nonautologous Tissue Substitute
			Z No Qualifier

Non-OR	ØVW[4,D,S][3,4,7,8]YZ	Non-OR	ØVWMX[Ø,3,7,C,J,K]Z
Non-OR	ØVW8[Ø,3,4,7,8][Ø,3,7,J,K,Y]Z	Non-OR	ØVWR[Ø,3,4,7,8][Ø,3,7,C,D,J,K,Y]Z
Non-OR	ØVW[4,8,D,S]X[Ø,3,7,J,K]Z	Non-OR	ØVWRX[Ø,3,7,C,D,J,K]Z
Non-OR	ØVWM[3,4,7,8]YZ	♂	All body part, approach, device, and qualifier values

Ø   **Medical and Surgical**
V   **Male Reproductive System**
X   **Transfer**   Definition: Moving, without taking out, all or a portion of a body part to another location to take over the function of all or a portion of a body part

                  Explanation: The body part transferred remains connected to its vascular and nervous supply

Body Part Character 4	Approach Character 5	Device Character 6	Qualifier Character 7

T Prepuce ♂
    Foreskin
    Glans penis
	Ø Open
	X External
		Z No Device	**D** Urethra
			S Penis

♂	All body part, approach, device, and qualifier values

LC Limited Coverage   **NC** Noncovered   ⊞ Combination Member   HAC associated procedure   Combination Only   DRG Non-OR   Non-OR   New/Revised in GREEN

648   ICD-10-PCS 2019

ØVW–ØVX

Anatomical Regions, General ØWØ–ØWY

Character Meanings

This Character Meaning table is provided as a guide to assist the user in the identification of character members that may be found in this section of code tables. It **SHOULD NOT** be used to build a PCS code.

Operation–Character 3	Body Region–Character 4	Approach–Character 5	Device–Character 6	Qualifier–Character 7
Ø Alteration	Ø Head	Ø Open	Ø Drainage Device	Ø Vagina OR Allogeneic
1 Bypass	1 Cranial Cavity	3 Percutaneous	1 Radioactive Element	1 Penis OR Syngeneic
2 Change	2 Face	4 Percutaneous Endoscopic	3 Infusion Device	2 Stoma
3 Control	3 Oral Cavity and Throat	7 Via Natural or Artificial Opening	7 Autologous Tissue Substitute	4 Cutaneous
4 Creation	4 Upper Jaw	8 Via Natural or Artificial Opening Endoscopic	J Synthetic Substitute	9 Pleural Cavity, Right
8 Division	5 Lower Jaw	X External	K Nonautologous Tissue Substitute	B Pleural Cavity, Left
9 Drainage	6 Neck		Y Other Device	G Peritoneal Cavity
B Excision	8 Chest Wall		Z No Device	J Pelvic Cavity
C Extirpation	9 Pleural Cavity, Right			W Upper Vein
F Fragmentation	B Pleural Cavity, Left			X Diagnostic
H Insertion	C Mediastinum			Y Lower Vein
J Inspection	D Pericardial Cavity			Z No Qualifier
M Reattachment	F Abdominal Wall			
P Removal	G Peritoneal Cavity			
Q Repair	H Retroperitoneum			
U Supplement	J Pelvic Cavity			
W Revision	K Upper Back			
Y Transplantation	L Lower Back			
	M Perineum, Male			
	N Perineum, Female			
	P Gastrointestinal Tract			
	Q Respiratory Tract			
	R Genitourinary Tract			

AHA Coding Clinic for table ØWØ
2015, 1Q, 31   Bilateral browpexy

AHA Coding Clinic for table ØW1
2015, 2Q, 36   Insertion of infusion device into peritoneal cavity
2013, 4Q, 126-127 Creation of percutaneous cutaneoperitoneal fistula

AHA Coding Clinic for table ØW3
2018, 1Q, 19   Argon plasma coagulation of duodenal arteriovenous malformation
2018, 1Q, 19   Control of epistaxis via silver nitrate cauterization
2017, 4Q, 57-58   Added approach values - Transorifice esophageal vein banding
2017, 4Q, 105   Control of gastrointestinal bleeding
2017, 4Q, 106   Control of bleeding of external naris using suture
2017, 4Q, 106   Nasal packing for epistaxis
2016, 4Q, 99-100 Root operation Control
2014, 4Q, 44   Bakri balloon for control of postpartum hemorrhage
2013, 3Q, 23   Control of intraoperative bleeding

AHA Coding Clinic for table ØW4
2016, 4Q, 101   Root operation Creation

AHA Coding Clinic for table ØW9
2017, 3Q, 12   Therapeutic and diagnostic paracentesis
2017, 2Q, 16   Incision and drainage of floor of mouth

AHA Coding Clinic for table ØWB
2017, 2Q, 16   Excision of floor of mouth
2016, 1Q, 21   Excision of urachal mass
2013, 4Q, 119   Excision of inclusion cyst of perineum

AHA Coding Clinic for table ØWC
2017, 2Q, 16   Excision of floor of mouth

AHA Coding Clinic for table ØWH
2018, 1Q, 25   Intrauterine brachytherapy & placement of tandems & ovoids
2017, 4Q, 104   Intrauterine brachytherapy & placement of tandems & ovoids
2016, 2Q, 14   Insertion of peritoneal totally implantable venous access device
2015, 2Q, 36   Insertion of infusion device into peritoneal cavity

AHA Coding Clinic for table ØWJ
2016, 4Q, 58   Longitudinal vaginal septum
2013, 2Q, 36   Insertion of ventriculoperitoneal shunt with laparoscopic assistance

AHA Coding Clinic for table ØWQ
2017, 4Q, 106   Control of bleeding of external naris using suture
2017, 3Q, 8   Removal of silo and closure of gastroschisis
2016, 2Q, 14   Stoma creation & takedown procedures
2014, 4Q, 38   Abdominoplasty and abdominal wall plication for hernia repair
2014, 3Q, 28   Ileostomy takedown and parastomal hernia repair

AHA Coding Clinic for table ØWU
2017, 3Q, 8   First stage of gastroschisis repair with silo placement
2016, 3Q, 40   Omentoplasty
2015, 2Q, 29   Placement of Ioban™ antimicrobial drape over surgical wound
2014, 4Q, 39   Abdominal component release with placement of mesh for hernia repair
2012, 4Q, 101   Rib resection with reconstruction of anterior chest wall

AHA Coding Clinic for table ØWW
2015, 2Q, 9   Revision of ventriculoperitoneal (VP) shunt

AHA Coding Clinic for table ØWY
2016, 4Q, 112-113 Transplantation

Anatomical Regions, General

Ø   **Medical and Surgical**
W   **Anatomical Regions, General**
Ø   **Alteration**   Definition: Modifying the anatomic structure of a body part without affecting the function of the body part
                      Explanation: Principal purpose is to improve appearance

Body Part Character 4	Approach Character 5	Device Character 6	Qualifier Character 7
Ø Head **2** Face **4** Upper Jaw **5** Lower Jaw **6** Neck **8** Chest Wall **F** Abdominal Wall **K** Upper Back **L** Lower Back **M** Perineum, Male ♂ **N** Perineum, Female ♀	**Ø** Open **3** Percutaneous **4** Percutaneous Endoscopic	**7** Autologous Tissue Substitute **J** Synthetic Substitute **K** Nonautologous Tissue Substitute **Z** No Device	**Z** No Qualifier

     ♂   ØWØM[Ø,3,4][7,J,K,Z]Z
     ♀   ØWØN[Ø,3,4][7,J,K,Z]Z

Ø   **Medical and Surgical**
W   **Anatomical Regions, General**
1   **Bypass**   Definition: Altering the route of passage of the contents of a tubular body part
                      Explanation: Rerouting contents of a body part to a downstream area of the normal route, to a similar route and body part, or to an abnormal route and dissimilar body part. Includes one or more anastomoses, with or without the use of a device.

Body Part Character 4	Approach Character 5	Device Character 6	Qualifier Character 7
1 Cranial Cavity	**Ø** Open	**J** Synthetic Substitute	**9** Pleural Cavity, Right **B** Pleural Cavity, Left **G** Peritoneal Cavity **J** Pelvic Cavity
9 Pleural Cavity, Right **B** Pleural Cavity, Left **G** Peritoneal Cavity **J** Pelvic Cavity Retropubic space	**Ø** Open **3** Percutaneous **4** Percutaneous Endoscopic	**J** Synthetic Substitute	**4** Cutaneous **9** Pleural Cavity, Right **B** Pleural Cavity, Left **G** Peritoneal Cavity **J** Pelvic Cavity **W** Upper Vein **Y** Lower Vein

   Non-OR   ØW1[9,B][Ø,4]J[4,G,Y]   **Non-OR**   ØW1J[Ø,4]J[4,Y]
   Non-OR   ØW1G[Ø,4]J[9,B,G,J]   **Non-OR**   ØW1[9,B,J]3J4

Ø   **Medical and Surgical**
W   **Anatomical Regions, General**
2   **Change**   Definition: Taking out or off a device from a body part and putting back an identical or similar device in or on the same body part without cutting or puncturing the skin or a mucous membrane
                      Explanation: All CHANGE procedures are coded using the approach EXTERNAL

Body Part Character 4	Approach Character 5	Device Character 6	Qualifier Character 7

Ø Head
1 Cranial Cavity
2 Face
4 Upper Jaw
5 Lower Jaw
6 Neck
8 Chest Wall
9 Pleural Cavity, Right
B Pleural Cavity, Left
C Mediastinum
     Mediastinal cavity
     Mediastinal space
D Pericardial Cavity
F Abdominal Wall
G Peritoneal Cavity
H Retroperitoneum
     Retroperitoneal cavity
     Retroperitoneal space
J Pelvic Cavity
     Retropubic space
K Upper Back
L Lower Back
M Perineum, Male   ♂
N Perineum, Female   ♀
	X External	**Ø** Drainage Device
		Y Other Device
			Z No Qualifier

   Non-OR   All body part, approach, device, and qualifier values   ♂   ØW2MX[Ø,Y]Z
                                                        ♀   ØW2NX[Ø,Y]Z

Ø   **Medical and Surgical**
W   **Anatomical Regions, General**
3   **Control**   Definition: Stopping, or attempting to stop, postprocedural or other acute bleeding
                   Explanation: The site of the bleeding is coded as an anatomical region and not to a specific body part

Body Part Character 4	Approach Character 5	Device Character 6	Qualifier Character 7

Ø Head
1 Cranial Cavity
2 Face
4 Upper Jaw
5 Lower Jaw
6 Neck
8 Chest Wall
9 Pleural Cavity, Right
B Pleural Cavity, Left
C Mediastinum
    Mediastinal cavity
    Mediastinal space
D Pericardial Cavity
F Abdominal Wall
G Peritoneal Cavity
H Retroperitoneum
    Retroperitoneal cavity
    Retroperitoneal space
J Pelvic Cavity
    Retropubic space
K Upper Back
L Lower Back
M Perineum, Male ♂
N Perineum, Female ♀
	Ø Open
	3 Percutaneous
	4 Percutaneous Endoscopic
		Z No Device	**Z** No Qualifier

3 Oral Cavity and Throat	**Ø** Open **3** Percutaneous **4** Percutaneous Endoscopic **7** Via Natural or Artificial Opening **8** Via Natural or Artificial Opening Endoscopic **X** External	**Z** No Device	**Z** No Qualifier
P Gastrointestinal Tract **Q** Respiratory Tract **R** Genitourinary Tract	**Ø** Open **3** Percutaneous **4** Percutaneous Endoscopic **7** Via Natural or Artificial Opening **8** Via Natural or Artificial Opening Endoscopic	**Z** No Device	**Z** No Qualifier

    Non-OR   ØW3GØZZ
    Non-OR   ØW3P8ZZ
                                              ♂   ØW3M[Ø,3,4]ZZ
                                               ♀   ØW3N[Ø,3,4]ZZ

Ø   **Medical and Surgical**
W   **Anatomical Regions, General**
4   **Creation**   Definition: Putting in or on biological or synthetic material to form a new body part that to the extent possible replicates the anatomic structure or function of an absent body part
                   Explanation: Used for gender reassignment surgery and corrective procedures in individuals with congenital anomalies

Body Part Character 4	Approach Character 5	Device Character 6	Qualifier Character 7
M Perineum, Male ♂	**Ø** Open	**7** Autologous Tissue Substitute **J** Synthetic Substitute **K** Nonautologous Tissue Substitute	**Ø** Vagina
N Perineum, Female ♀	**Ø** Open	**7** Autologous Tissue Substitute **J** Synthetic Substitute **K** Nonautologous Tissue Substitute	**1** Penis

    ♂   ØW4MØ[7,J,K]Ø
    ♀   ØW4NØ[7,J,K]1

Ø   **Medical and Surgical**
W   **Anatomical Regions, General**
8   **Division**   Definition: Cutting into a body part, without draining fluids and/or gases from the body part, in order to separate or transect a body part
               Explanation: All or a portion of the body part is separated into two or more portions

Body Part Character 4	Approach Character 5	Device Character 6	Qualifier Character 7
N Perineum, Female ♀	**X** External	**Z** No Device	**Z** No Qualifier

    Non-OR   ØW8NXZZ   ♀   ØW8NXZZ

LC Limited Coverage   NC Noncovered   ⊞ Combination Member   HAC associated procedure   Combination Only   DRG Non-OR   Non-OR   New/Revised in GREEN

ICD-10-PCS 2019   651

ØW3–ØW8

Ø   Medical and Surgical
W   Anatomical Regions, General
9   Drainage   Definition: Taking or letting out fluids and/or gases from a body part
                 Explanation: The qualifier DIAGNOSTIC is used to identify drainage procedures that are biopsies

Body Part Character 4	Approach Character 5	Device Character 6	Qualifier Character 7

Ø Head
1 Cranial Cavity
2 Face
3 Oral Cavity and Throat
4 Upper Jaw
5 Lower Jaw
6 Neck
8 Chest Wall
9 Pleural Cavity, Right
B Pleural Cavity, Left
C Mediastinum
     Mediastinal cavity
     Mediastinal space
D Pericardial Cavity
F Abdominal Wall
G Peritoneal Cavity
H Retroperitoneum
     Retroperitoneal cavity
     Retroperitoneal space
J Pelvic Cavity
     Retropubic space
K Upper Back
L Lower Back
M Perineum, Male   ♂
N Perineum, Female   ♀
	Ø Open
	3 Percutaneous
	4 Percutaneous Endoscopic
		Ø Drainage Device	Z No Qualifier

Ø Head
1 Cranial Cavity
2 Face
3 Oral Cavity and Throat
4 Upper Jaw
5 Lower Jaw
6 Neck
8 Chest Wall
9 Pleural Cavity, Right
B Pleural Cavity, Left
C Mediastinum
     Mediastinal cavity
     Mediastinal space
D Pericardial Cavity
F Abdominal Wall
G Peritoneal Cavity
H Retroperitoneum
     Retroperitoneal cavity
     Retroperitoneal space
J Pelvic Cavity
     Retropubic space
K Upper Back
L Lower Back
M Perineum, Male   ♂
N Perineum, Female   ♀
	Ø Open
	3 Percutaneous
	4 Percutaneous Endoscopic
		Z No Device	X Diagnostic
			Z No Qualifier

Non-OR	ØW9[Ø,8,9,B,K,L,M]ØØZ	♂	ØW9M[Ø,3,4]ØZ
Non-OR	ØW9[Ø,1,2,3,4,5,6,8,9,B,C,D,F,G,H,J,K,L,M,N]3ØZ	♂	ØW9M[Ø,3,4]Z[X,Z]
Non-OR	ØW9[Ø,1,8,D,F,G,K,L,M]4ØZ	♀	ØW9N[Ø,3,4]ØZ
Non-OR	ØW9[Ø,2,3,4,5,6,8,9,B,K,L,M,N]ØZX	♀	ØW9N[Ø,3]Z[X,Z]
Non-OR	ØW9[Ø,1,2,3,4,5,6,8,9,B,C,D,G,K,L,M,N]3ZX	♀	ØW9N4ZZ
Non-OR	ØW9[Ø,1,2,3,4,5,6,8,9,B,C,D,K,L,M,N]4ZX		
Non-OR	ØW9[Ø,8,9,B,K,L,M]ØZZ		
Non-OR	ØW9[Ø,1,2,3,4,5,6,8,9,B,C,D,F,G,H,J,K,L,M,N]3ZZ		
Non-OR	ØW9[Ø,1,8,D,F,G,K,L,M]4ZZ		

0   Medical and Surgical
W   Anatomical Regions, General
B   Excision   Definition: Cutting out or off, without replacement, a portion of a body part

Explanation: The qualifier DIAGNOSTIC is used to identify excision procedures that are biopsies

Body Part Character 4	Approach Character 5	Device Character 6	Qualifier Character 7
0 Head 2 Face 3 Oral Cavity and Throat 4 Upper Jaw 5 Lower Jaw 8 Chest Wall K Upper Back L Lower Back M Perineum, Male ♂ N Perineum, Female ♀	0 Open 3 Percutaneous 4 Percutaneous Endoscopic X External	Z No Device	X Diagnostic Z No Qualifier
6 Neck F Abdominal Wall	0 Open 3 Percutaneous 4 Percutaneous Endoscopic	Z No Device	X Diagnostic Z No Qualifier
6 Neck F Abdominal Wall	X External	Z No Device	2 Stoma X Diagnostic Z No Qualifier

C   Mediastinum
     Mediastinal cavity
     Mediastinal space
H   Retroperitoneum
     Retroperitoneal cavity
     Retroperitoneal space
	0 Open
	3 Percutaneous
	4 Percutaneous Endoscopic
		Z No Device	X Diagnostic
			Z No Qualifier

Non-OR 0WB[0,2,4,5,8,K,L,M][0,3,4,X]ZX		♂	0WBM[0,3,4,X]Z[X,Z]
Non-OR 0WB6[0,3,4]ZX		♀	0WBN[0,3,4,X]Z[X,Z]
Non-OR 0WB6XZX			
Non-OR 0WB[C,H][3,4]ZX			

0   Medical and Surgical
W   Anatomical Regions, General
C   Extirpation   Definition: Taking or cutting out solid matter from a body part

Explanation: The solid matter may be an abnormal byproduct of a biological function or a foreign body; it may be imbedded in a body part or in the lumen of a tubular body part. The solid matter may or may not have been previously broken into pieces.

Body Part Character 4	Approach Character 5	Device Character 6	Qualifier Character 7

1   Cranial Cavity
3   Oral Cavity and Throat
9   Pleural Cavity, Right
B   Pleural Cavity, Left
C   Mediastinum
     Mediastinal cavity
     Mediastinal space
D   Pericardial Cavity
G   Peritoneal Cavity
H   Retroperitoneum
     Retroperitoneal cavity
     Retroperitoneal space
J   Pelvic Cavity
     Retropubic space
	0 Open
	3 Percutaneous
	4 Percutaneous Endoscopic
	X External
		Z No Device	Z No Qualifier

P Gastrointestinal Tract Q Respiratory Tract R Genitourinary Tract	0 Open 3 Percutaneous 4 Percutaneous Endoscopic 7 Via Natural or Artificial Opening 8 Via Natural or Artificial Opening Endoscopic X External	Z No Device	Z No Qualifier

Non-OR   0WC[1,3]XZZ
Non-OR   0WC[9,B][0,3,4,X]ZZ
Non-OR   0WC[C,D,G,H,J]XZZ
Non-OR   0WC[P,R][7,8,X]ZZ
Non-OR   0WCQ[0,3,4,X]ZZ

Ø   Medical and Surgical
W   Anatomical Regions, General
F   Fragmentation   Definition: Breaking solid matter in a body part into pieces

                Explanation: Physical force (e.g., manual, ultrasonic) applied directly or indirectly is used to break the solid matter into pieces. The solid matter may be an abnormal byproduct of a biological function or a foreign body. The pieces of solid matter are not taken out.

Body Part Character 4	Approach Character 5	Device Character 6	Qualifier Character 7

1   Cranial Cavity   NC
3   Oral Cavity and Throat   NC
9   Pleural Cavity, Right   NC
B   Pleural Cavity, Left   NC
C   Mediastinum   NC
     Mediastinal cavity
     Mediastinal space
D   Pericardial Cavity
G   Peritoneal Cavity   NC
J   Pelvic Cavity   NC
     Retropubic space
	Ø Open
	3 Percutaneous
	4 Percutaneous Endoscopic
	X External
		Z No Device	Z No Qualifier

P Gastrointestinal Tract NC Q Respiratory Tract NC R Genitourinary Tract	Ø Open 3 Percutaneous 4 Percutaneous Endoscopic 7 Via Natural or Artificial Opening 8 Via Natural or Artificial Opening Endoscopic X External	Z No Device	Z No Qualifier

DRG Non-OR	ØWFRXZZ	NC	ØWF[1,3,9,B,C,G,J]XZZ
Non-OR	ØWF[1,3,9,B,C,G]XZZ	NC	ØWF[P,Q]XZZ
Non-OR	ØWFJ[Ø,3,4,X]ZZ		
Non-OR	ØWFP[Ø,3,4,7,8,X]ZZ		
Non-OR	ØWFQXZZ		
Non-OR	ØWFR[Ø,3,4,7,8]ZZ		

Ø   Medical and Surgical
W   Anatomical Regions, General
H   Insertion   Definition: Putting in a nonbiological appliance that monitors, assists, performs, or prevents a physiological function but does not physically take the place of a body part

                Explanation: None

Body Part Character 4	Approach Character 5	Device Character 6	Qualifier Character 7

Ø   Head
1   Cranial Cavity
2   Face
3   Oral Cavity and Throat
4   Upper Jaw
5   Lower Jaw
6   Neck
8   Chest Wall
9   Pleural Cavity, Right
B   Pleural Cavity, Left
C   Mediastinum
     Mediastinal cavity
     Mediastinal space
D   Pericardial Cavity
F   Abdominal Wall
G   Peritoneal Cavity
H   Retroperitoneum
     Retroperitoneal cavity
     Retroperitoneal space
J   Pelvic Cavity
     Retropubic space
K   Upper Back
L   Lower Back
M   Perineum, Male
N   Perineum, Female   ♀
	Ø Open
	3 Percutaneous
	4 Percutaneous Endoscopic
		1 Radioactive Element
		3 Infusion Device
		Y Other Device
			Z No Qualifier

P Gastrointestinal Tract Q Respiratory Tract R Genitourinary Tract	Ø Open 3 Percutaneous 4 Percutaneous Endoscopic 7 Via Natural or Artificial Opening 8 Via Natural or Artificial Opening Endoscopic	1 Radioactive Element 3 Infusion Device Y Other Device	Z No Qualifier

DRG Non-OR	ØWH[Ø,2,4,5,6,K,L,M][Ø,3,4][3,Y]Z	Non-OR	ØWHP[3,4,7,8][3,Y]Z
Non-OR	ØWH1[Ø,3,4]3Z	Non-OR	ØWHQ[Ø,7,8][3,Y]Z
Non-OR	ØWH[8,9,B][Ø,3,4][3,Y]Z	Non-OR	ØWHR[Ø,3,4,7,8][3,Y]Z
Non-OR	ØWHPØYZ	♀	ØWHN[Ø,3,4][3,Y]Z

LC Limited Coverage   NC Noncovered   ⊞ Combination Member   HAC associated procedure   Combination Only   DRG Non-OR   Non-OR   New/Revised in GREEN

654   ICD-10-PCS 2019

Ø **Medical and Surgical**
W **Anatomical Regions, General**
J **Inspection**   Definition: Visually and/or manually exploring a body part
     Explanation: Visual exploration may be performed with or without optical instrumentation. Manual exploration may be performed directly or through intervening body layers.

Body Part Character 4	Approach Character 5	Device Character 6	Qualifier Character 7
Ø Head 2 Face 3 Oral Cavity and Throat 4 Upper Jaw 5 Lower Jaw 6 Neck 8 Chest Wall F Abdominal Wall K Upper Back L Lower Back M Perineum, Male ♂ N Perineum, Female ♀	Ø Open 3 Percutaneous 4 Percutaneous Endoscopic X External	Z No Device	Z No Qualifier

1 Cranial Cavity
9 Pleural Cavity, Right
B Pleural Cavity, Left
C Mediastinum
  Mediastinal cavity
  Mediastinal space
D Pericardial Cavity
G Peritoneal Cavity
H Retroperitoneum
  Retroperitoneal cavity
  Retroperitoneal space
J Pelvic Cavity
  Retropubic space
	Ø Open
	3 Percutaneous
	4 Percutaneous Endoscopic
		Z No Device	Z No Qualifier

P Gastrointestinal Tract Q Respiratory Tract R Genitourinary Tract	Ø Open 3 Percutaneous 4 Percutaneous Endoscopic 7 Via Natural or Artificial Opening 8 Via Natural or Artificial Opening Endoscopic	Z No Device	Z No Qualifier

DRG Non-OR	ØWJ[Ø,2,4,5,K,L]ØZZ	♂ ØWJM[Ø,3,4,X]ZZ
DRG Non-OR	ØWJM[Ø,4]ZZ	♀ ØWJN[Ø,3,4,X]ZZ
Non-OR	ØWJ3ØZZ	
Non-OR	ØWJ[Ø,2,3,4,5,6,8,F,K,L,M,N][3,X]ZZ	
Non-OR	ØWJ[Ø,2,3,4,5,K,L]4ZZ	
Non-OR	ØWJDØZZ	
Non-OR	ØWJ[1,9,B,C,D,G,H,J]3ZZ	
Non-OR	ØWJ[P,Q,R][3,7,8]ZZ	

Ø **Medical and Surgical**
W **Anatomical Regions, General**
M **Reattachment**   Definition: Putting back in or on all or a portion of a separated body part to its normal location or other suitable location
     Explanation: Vascular circulation and nervous pathways may or may not be reestablished

Body Part Character 4	Approach Character 5	Device Character 6	Qualifier Character 7
2 Face 4 Upper Jaw 5 Lower Jaw 6 Neck 8 Chest Wall F Abdominal Wall K Upper Back L Lower Back M Perineum, Male ♂ N Perineum, Female ♀	Ø Open	Z No Device	Z No Qualifier

♂ ØWMMØZZ
♀ ØWMNØZZ

LC Limited Coverage   NC Noncovered   ⊞ Combination Member   HAC associated procedure   Combination Only   DRG Non-OR   Non-OR   New/Revised in GREEN
ICD-10-PCS 2019   655

ØWJ–ØWM

Anatomical Regions, General

0   **Medical and Surgical**
W   **Anatomical Regions, General**
P   **Removal**   Definition: Taking out or off a device from a body part

Explanation: If a device is taken out and a similar device put in without cutting or puncturing the skin or mucous membrane, the procedure is coded to the root operation CHANGE. Otherwise, the procedure for taking out the device is coded to the root operation REMOVAL.

Body Part Character 4		Approach Character 5	Device Character 6	Qualifier Character 7

0 Head
2 Face
4 Upper Jaw
5 Lower Jaw
6 Neck
8 Chest Wall
C Mediastinum
   Mediastinal cavity
   Mediastinal space
F Abdominal Wall
K Upper Back
L Lower Back
M Perineum, Male
N Perineum, Female
	♂
	♀
		0 Open
		3 Percutaneous
		4 Percutaneous Endoscopic
		X External
			0 Drainage Device
			1 Radioactive Element
			3 Infusion Device
			7 Autologous Tissue Substitute
			J Synthetic Substitute
			K Nonautologous Tissue Substitute
			Y Other Device
				Z No Qualifier

1 Cranial Cavity **9** Pleural Cavity, Right **B** Pleural Cavity, Left **G** Peritoneal Cavity **J** Pelvic Cavity Retropubic space		**0** Open **3** Percutaneous **4** Percutaneous Endoscopic	**0** Drainage Device **1** Radioactive Element **3** Infusion Device **J** Synthetic Substitute **Y** Other Device	**Z** No Qualifier
1 Cranial Cavity **9** Pleural Cavity, Right **B** Pleural Cavity, Left **G** Peritoneal Cavity **J** Pelvic Cavity Retropubic space		**X** External	**0** Drainage Device **1** Radioactive Element **3** Infusion Device	**Z** No Qualifier

D Pericardial Cavity
H Retroperitoneum
   Retroperitoneal cavity
   Retroperitoneal space
		0 Open
		3 Percutaneous
		4 Percutaneous Endoscopic
			0 Drainage Device
			1 Radioactive Element
			3 Infusion Device
			Y Other Device
				Z No Qualifier

D Pericardial Cavity
H Retroperitoneum
   Retroperitoneal cavity
   Retroperitoneal space
		X External	**0** Drainage Device
			1 Radioactive Element
			3 Infusion Device
				Z No Qualifier

P Gastrointestinal Tract **Q** Respiratory Tract **R** Genitourinary Tract		**0** Open **3** Percutaneous **4** Percutaneous Endoscopic **7** Via Natural or Artificial Opening **8** Via Natural or Artificial Opening Endoscopic **X** External	**1** Radioactive Element **3** Infusion Device **Y** Other Device	**Z** No Qualifier

Non-OR	0WP[0,2,4,5,6,8][0,3,4,X][0,1,3,7,J,K,Y]Z	♂ 0WPM[0,3,4,X][0,1,3,7,J,K,Y]Z
Non-OR	0WP[C,F]X[0,1,3,7,J,K,Y]Z	♀ 0WPN[0,3,4,X][0,1,3,7,J,K,Y]Z
Non-OR	0WP[K,L][0,3,4,X][0,1,3,7,J,K,Y]Z	
Non-OR	0WPM[0,3,4][0,1,3,J,Y]Z	
Non-OR	0WPMX[0,1,3,Y]Z	
Non-OR	0WPNX[0,1,3,7,J,K,Y]Z	
Non-OR	0WP1[0,3,4]3Z	
Non-OR	0WP[9,B,J][0,3,4][0,1,3,J,Y]Z	
Non-OR	0WP[1,9,B,G,J]X[0,1,3]Z	
Non-OR	0WP[D,H]X[0,1,3]Z	
Non-OR	0WPP[3,4,7,8,X][1,3,Y]Z	
Non-OR	0WPQ73Z	
Non-OR	0WPQ8[3,Y]Z	
Non-OR	0WPQ[0,X][1,3,Y]Z	
Non-OR	0WPR[0,3,4,7,8,X][1,3,Y]Z	

🅛🅒 Limited Coverage   🅝🅒 Noncovered   ⊞ Combination Member   HAC associated procedure   Combination Only   DRG Non-OR   Non-OR   New/Revised in GREEN

656   ICD-10-PCS 2019

Ø   **Medical and Surgical**
W   **Anatomical Regions, General**
Q   **Repair**   Definition: Restoring, to the extent possible, a body part to its normal anatomic structure and function
                      Explanation: Used only when the method to accomplish the repair is not one of the other root operations

Body Part Character 4	Approach Character 5	Device Character 6	Qualifier Character 7
Ø Head **2** Face **3** Oral Cavity and Throat **4** Upper Jaw **5** Lower Jaw **8** Chest Wall **K** Upper Back **L** Lower Back **M** Perineum, Male ♂ **N** Perineum, Female ♀	**Ø** Open **3** Percutaneous **4** Percutaneous Endoscopic **X** External	**Z** No Device	**Z** No Qualifier
6 Neck **F** Abdominal Wall	**Ø** Open **3** Percutaneous **4** Percutaneous Endoscopic	**Z** No Device	**Z** No Qualifier
6 Neck **F** Abdominal Wall ⊞	**X** External	**Z** No Device	**2** Stoma **Z** No Qualifier

C Mediastinum
    Mediastinal cavity
    Mediastinal space
	Ø Open
	3 Percutaneous
	4 Percutaneous Endoscopic
		Z No Device	**Z** No Qualifier

Non-OR   ØWQNXZZ
♂   ØWQM[Ø,3,4,X]ZZ
♀   ØWQN[Ø,3,4,X]ZZ

See Appendix L for Procedure Combinations
    ⊞   ØWQFXZ[2,Z]

Ø   **Medical and Surgical**
W   **Anatomical Regions, General**
U   **Supplement**   Definition: Putting in or on biological or synthetic material that physically reinforces and/or augments the function of a portion of a body part
                      Explanation: The biological material is non-living, or is living and from the same individual. The body part may have been previously replaced, and the SUPPLEMENT procedure is performed to physically reinforce and/or augment the function of the replaced body part.

Body Part Character 4	Approach Character 5	Device Character 6	Qualifier Character 7

Ø Head
2 Face
4 Upper Jaw
5 Lower Jaw
6 Neck
8 Chest Wall
C Mediastinum
    Mediastinal cavity
    Mediastinal space
F Abdominal Wall
K Upper Back
L Lower Back
M Perineum, Male   ♂
N Perineum, Female   ♀
	Ø Open
	4 Percutaneous Endoscopic
		7 Autologous Tissue Substitute
		J Synthetic Substitute
		K Nonautologous Tissue Substitute
			Z No Qualifier

♂   ØWUM[Ø,4][7,J,K]Z
♀   ØWUN[Ø,4][7,J,K]Z

LC Limited Coverage   **NC** Noncovered   ⊞ Combination Member   HAC associated procedure   Combination Only   DRG Non-OR   Non-OR   New/Revised in GREEN

Anatomical Regions, General

Ø   Medical and Surgical
W   Anatomical Regions, General
W   Revision   Definition: Correcting, to the extent possible, a portion of a malfunctioning device or the position of a displaced device

Explanation: Revision can include correcting a malfunctioning or displaced device by taking out or putting in components of the device such as a screw or pin

Body Part Character 4	Approach Character 5	Device Character 6	Qualifier Character 7

Ø Head
2 Face
4 Upper Jaw
5 Lower Jaw
6 Neck
8 Chest Wall
C Mediastinum
    Mediastinal cavity
    Mediastinal space
F Abdominal Wall
K Upper Back
L Lower Back
M Perineum, Male   ♂
N Perineum, Female ♀
	Ø Open
	3 Percutaneous
	4 Percutaneous Endoscopic
	X External
		Ø Drainage Device
		1 Radioactive Element
		3 Infusion Device
		7 Autologous Tissue Substitute
		J Synthetic Substitute
		K Nonautologous Tissue Substitute
		Y Other Device
			Z No Qualifier

1 Cranial Cavity 9 Pleural Cavity, Right B Pleural Cavity, Left G Peritoneal Cavity J Pelvic Cavity Retropubic space	Ø Open 3 Percutaneous 4 Percutaneous Endoscopic X External	Ø Drainage Device 1 Radioactive Element 3 Infusion Device J Synthetic Substitute Y Other Device	Z No Qualifier

D Pericardial Cavity
H Retroperitoneum
    Retroperitoneal cavity
    Retroperitoneal space
	Ø Open
	3 Percutaneous
	4 Percutaneous Endoscopic
	X External
		Ø Drainage Device
		1 Radioactive Element
		3 Infusion Device
		Y Other Device
			Z No Qualifier

P Gastrointestinal Tract Q Respiratory Tract R Genitourinary Tract	Ø Open 3 Percutaneous 4 Percutaneous Endoscopic 7 Via Natural or Artificial Opening 8 Via Natural or Artificial Opening Endoscopic X External	1 Radioactive Element 3 Infusion Device Y Other Device	Z No Qualifier

DRG Non-OR	ØWW[Ø,2,4,5,6,K,L][Ø,3,4][Ø,1,3,7,J,K,Y]Z	♂	ØWWM[Ø,3,4,X][Ø,1,3,7,K,Y]Z
DRG Non-OR	ØWWM[Ø,3,4][Ø,1,3,J,Y]Z	♀	ØWWN[Ø,3,4,X][Ø,1,3,7,K,Y]Z
Non-OR	ØWW[Ø,2,4,5,6,C,F,K,L,M,N]X[Ø,1,3,7,J,K,Y]Z		
Non-OR	ØWW8[Ø,3,4,X][Ø,1,3,7,J,K,Y]Z		
Non-OR	ØWW[1,G,J]X[Ø,1,3,J,Y]Z		
Non-OR	ØWW[9,B][Ø,3,4,X][Ø,1,3,J,Y]Z		
Non-OR	ØWW[D,H]X[Ø,1,3,Y]Z		
Non-OR	ØWWP[3,4,7,8,X][1,3,Y]Z		
Non-OR	ØWWQ[Ø,X][1,3,Y]Z		
Non-OR	ØWWR[Ø,3,4,7,8,X][1,3,Y]Z		

Ø   Medical and Surgical
W   Anatomical Regions, General
Y   Transplantation   Definition: Putting in or on all or a portion of a living body part taken from another individual or animal to physically take the place and/or function of all or a portion of a similar body part

Explanation: The native body part may or may not be taken out, and the transplanted body part may take over all or a portion of its function

Body Part Character 4	Approach Character 5	Device Character 6	Qualifier Character 7
2 Face	Ø Open	Z No Device	Ø Allogeneic 1 Syngeneic

LC Limited Coverage   NC Noncovered   ⊞ Combination Member   HAC associated procedure   Combination Only   DRG Non-OR   Non-OR   New/Revised in GREEN

658   ICD-10-PCS 2019

ØWW–ØWY

Anatomical Regions, Upper Extremities ØXØ–ØXY

Character Meanings

This Character Meaning table is provided as a guide to assist the user in the identification of character members that may be found in this section of code tables. It **SHOULD NOT** be used to build a PCS code.

Operation–Character 3		Body Part–Character 4		Approach–Character 5		Device–Character 6		Qualifier–Character 7	
Ø	Alteration	Ø	Forequarter, Right	Ø	Open	Ø	Drainage Device	Ø	Complete OR Allogeneic
2	Change	1	Forequarter, Left	3	Percutaneous	1	Radioactive Element	1	High OR Syngeneic
3	Control	2	Shoulder Region, Right	4	Percutaneous Endoscopic	3	Infusion Device	2	Mid
6	Detachment	3	Shoulder Region, Left	X	External	7	Autologous Tissue Substitute	3	Low
9	Drainage	4	Axilla, Right			J	Synthetic Substitute	4	Complete 1st Ray
B	Excision	5	Axilla, Left			K	Nonautologous Tissue Substitute	5	Complete 2nd Ray
H	Insertion	6	Upper Extremity, Right			Y	Other Device	6	Complete 3rd Ray
J	Inspection	7	Upper Extremity, Left			Z	No Device	7	Complete 4th Ray
M	Reattachment	8	Upper Arm, Right					8	Complete 5th Ray
P	Removal	9	Upper Arm, Left					9	Partial 1st Ray
Q	Repair	B	Elbow Region, Right					B	Partial 2nd Ray
R	Replacement	C	Elbow Region, Left					C	Partial 3rd Ray
U	Supplement	D	Lower Arm, Right					D	Partial 4th Ray
W	Revision	F	Lower Arm, Left					F	Partial 5th Ray
X	Transfer	G	Wrist Region, Right					L	Thumb, Right
Y	Transplantation	H	Wrist Region, Left					M	Thumb, Left
		J	Hand, Right					N	Toe, Right
		K	Hand, Left					P	Toe, Left
		L	Thumb, Right					X	Diagnostic
		M	Thumb, Left					Z	No Qualifier
		N	Index Finger, Right						
		P	Index Finger, Left						
		Q	Middle Finger, Right						
		R	Middle Finger, Left						
		S	Ring Finger, Right						
		T	Ring Finger, Left						
		V	Little Finger, Right						
		W	Little Finger, Left						

AHA Coding Clinic for table ØX3

2016, 4Q, 99	Root operation Control
2015, 1Q, 35	Evacuation of hematoma for control of postprocedural bleeding
2013, 3Q, 23	Control of intraoperative bleeding

AHA Coding Clinic for table ØX6

2017, 2Q, 3-4	Qualifiers for the root operation detachment
2017, 2Q, 18	Removal of polydactyl digits
2017, 1Q, 52	Further distal phalangeal amputation
2016, 3Q, 33	Traumatic amputation of fingers with further revision amputation

AHA Coding Clinic for table ØXH

2017, 2Q, 20	Exchange of intramedullary antibiotic impregnated spacer

AHA Coding Clinic for table ØXP

2017, 2Q, 20	Exchange of intramedullary antibiotic impregnated spacer

AHA Coding Clinic for table ØXY

2016, 4Q, 112-113 Transplantation

Detachment Qualifier Descriptions

Qualifier Definition	Upper Arm	Lower Arm
1 **High:** Amputation at the proximal portion of the shaft of the:	Humerus	Radius/Ulna
2 **Mid:** Amputation at the middle portion of the shaft of the:	Humerus	Radius/Ulna
3 **Low:** Amputation at the distal portion of the shaft of the:	Humerus	Radius/Ulna

Qualifier Definition	Hand
Ø Complete 1st through 5th Rays Ray: digit of hand or foot with corresponding metacarpus or metatarsus	Through carpo-metacarpal joint, **Wrist**
4 Complete 1st Ray	Through carpo-metacarpal joint, **Thumb**
5 Complete 2nd Ray	Through carpo-metacarpal joint, **Index Finger**
6 Complete 3rd Ray	Through carpo-metacarpal joint, **Middle Finger**
7 Complete 4th Ray	Through carpo-metacarpal joint, **Ring Finger**
8 Complete 5th Ray	Through carpo-metacarpal joint, **Little Finger**
9 Partial 1st Ray	Anywhere along shaft or head of metacarpal bone, **Thumb**
B Partial 2nd Ray	Anywhere along shaft or head of metacarpal bone, **Index Finger**
C Partial 3rd Ray	Anywhere along shaft or head of metacarpal bone, **Middle Finger**
D Partial 4th Ray	Anywhere along shaft or head of metacarpal bone, **Ring Finger**
F Partial 5th Ray	Anywhere along shaft or head of metacarpal bone, **Little Finger**

Qualifier Definition	Thumb/Finger
Ø Complete	At the metacarpophalangeal joint
1 High	Anywhere along the proximal phalanx
2 Mid	Through the proximal interphalangeal joint or anywhere along the middle phalanx
3 Low	Through the distal interphalangeal joint or anywhere along the distal phalanx

0   **Medical and Surgical**
X   **Anatomical Regions, Upper Extremities**
0   **Alteration**   Definition: Modifying the anatomic structure of a body part without affecting the function of the body part
           Explanation: Principal purpose is to improve appearance

Body Part Character 4	Approach Character 5	Device Character 6	Qualifier Character 7
2 Shoulder Region, Right 3 Shoulder Region, Left 4 Axilla, Right 5 Axilla, Left 6 Upper Extremity, Right 7 Upper Extremity, Left 8 Upper Arm, Right 9 Upper Arm, Left B Elbow Region, Right C Elbow Region, Left D Lower Arm, Right F Lower Arm, Left G Wrist Region, Right H Wrist Region, Left	0 Open 3 Percutaneous 4 Percutaneous Endoscopic	7 Autologous Tissue Substitute J Synthetic Substitute K Nonautologous Tissue Substitute Z No Device	Z No Qualifier

0   **Medical and Surgical**
X   **Anatomical Regions, Upper Extremities**
2   **Change**   Definition: Taking out or off a device from a body part and putting back an identical or similar device in or on the same body part without cutting or puncturing the skin or a mucous membrane
           Explanation: All CHANGE procedures are coded using the approach EXTERNAL

Body Part Character 4	Approach Character 5	Device Character 6	Qualifier Character 7
6 Upper Extremity, Right 7 Upper Extremity, Left	X External	0 Drainage Device Y Other Device	Z No Qualifier

Non-OR   All body part, approach, device, and qualifier values

0   **Medical and Surgical**
X   **Anatomical Regions, Upper Extremities**
3   **Control**   Definition: Stopping, or attempting to stop, postprocedural or other acute bleeding
           Explanation: The site of the bleeding is coded as an anatomical region and not to a specific body part

Body Part Character 4	Approach Character 5	Device Character 6	Qualifier Character 7
2 Shoulder Region, Right 3 Shoulder Region, Left 4 Axilla, Right 5 Axilla, Left 6 Upper Extremity, Right 7 Upper Extremity, Left 8 Upper Arm, Right 9 Upper Arm, Left B Elbow Region, Right C Elbow Region, Left D Lower Arm, Right F Lower Arm, Left G Wrist Region, Right H Wrist Region, Left J Hand, Right K Hand, Left	0 Open 3 Percutaneous 4 Percutaneous Endoscopic	Z No Device	Z No Qualifier

Anatomical Regions, Upper Extremities *(side margin)*

Ø   **Medical and Surgical**
X   **Anatomical Regions, Upper Extremities**
6   **Detachment**   Definition: Cutting off all or a portion of the upper or lower extremities

                     Explanation: The body part value is the site of the detachment, with a qualifier if applicable to further specify the level where the extremity was detached

Body Part Character 4	Approach Character 5	Device Character 6	Qualifier Character 7
Ø Forequarter, Right 1 Forequarter, Left 2 Shoulder Region, Right 3 Shoulder Region, Left B Elbow Region, Right C Elbow Region, Left	Ø Open	Z No Device	Z No Qualifier
8 Upper Arm, Right 9 Upper Arm, Left D Lower Arm, Right F Lower Arm, Left	Ø Open	Z No Device	1 High 2 Mid 3 Low
J Hand, Right K Hand, Left	Ø Open	Z No Device	Ø Complete 4 Complete 1st Ray 5 Complete 2nd Ray 6 Complete 3rd Ray 7 Complete 4th Ray 8 Complete 5th Ray 9 Partial 1st Ray B Partial 2nd Ray C Partial 3rd Ray D Partial 4th Ray F Partial 5th Ray
L Thumb, Right M Thumb, Left N Index Finger, Right P Index Finger, Left Q Middle Finger, Right R Middle Finger, Left S Ring Finger, Right T Ring Finger, Left V Little Finger, Right W Little Finger, Left	Ø Open	Z No Device	Ø Complete 1 High 2 Mid 3 Low

LC Limited Coverage   NC Noncovered   ⊞ Combination Member   HAC associated procedure   Combination Only   DRG Non-OR   Non-OR   New/Revised in GREEN

662   ICD-10-PCS 2019

ØX6–ØX6 *(side margin, bottom)*

0   **Medical and Surgical**
X   **Anatomical Regions, Upper Extremities**
9   **Drainage**   Definition: Taking or letting out fluids and/or gases from a body part

             Explanation: The qualifier DIAGNOSTIC is used to identify drainage procedures that are biopsies

Body Part Character 4	Approach Character 5	Device Character 6	Qualifier Character 7
2 Shoulder Region, Right **3** Shoulder Region, Left **4** Axilla, Right **5** Axilla, Left **6** Upper Extremity, Right **7** Upper Extremity, Left **8** Upper Arm, Right **9** Upper Arm, Left **B** Elbow Region, Right **C** Elbow Region, Left **D** Lower Arm, Right **F** Lower Arm, Left **G** Wrist Region, Right **H** Wrist Region, Left **J** Hand, Right **K** Hand, Left	**0** Open **3** Percutaneous **4** Percutaneous Endoscopic	**0** Drainage Device	**Z** No Qualifier
2 Shoulder Region, Right **3** Shoulder Region, Left **4** Axilla, Right **5** Axilla, Left **6** Upper Extremity, Right **7** Upper Extremity, Left **8** Upper Arm, Right **9** Upper Arm, Left **B** Elbow Region, Right **C** Elbow Region, Left **D** Lower Arm, Right **F** Lower Arm, Left **G** Wrist Region, Right **H** Wrist Region, Left **J** Hand, Right **K** Hand, Left	**0** Open **3** Percutaneous **4** Percutaneous Endoscopic	**Z** No Device	**X** Diagnostic **Z** No Qualifier

Non-OR   All body part, approach, device, and qualifier values

0   **Medical and Surgical**
X   **Anatomical Regions, Upper Extremities**
B   **Excision**   Definition: Cutting out or off, without replacement, a portion of a body part

             Explanation: The qualifier DIAGNOSTIC is used to identify excision procedures that are biopsies

Body Part Character 4	Approach Character 5	Device Character 6	Qualifier Character 7
2 Shoulder Region, Right **3** Shoulder Region, Left **4** Axilla, Right **5** Axilla, Left **6** Upper Extremity, Right **7** Upper Extremity, Left **8** Upper Arm, Right **9** Upper Arm, Left **B** Elbow Region, Right **C** Elbow Region, Left **D** Lower Arm, Right **F** Lower Arm, Left **G** Wrist Region, Right **H** Wrist Region, Left **J** Hand, Right **K** Hand, Left	**0** Open **3** Percutaneous **4** Percutaneous Endoscopic	**Z** No Device	**X** Diagnostic **Z** No Qualifier

Non-OR   0XB[2,3,4,5,6,7,8,9,B,C,D,F,G,H,J,K][0,3,4]ZX

 LC Limited Coverage   NC Noncovered   ⊞ Combination Member   HAC associated procedure   Combination Only   DRG Non-OR   Non-OR   New/Revised in GREEN

ICD-10-PCS 2019   **663**

0X9–0XB

Anatomical Regions, Upper Extremities *(left margin)*

Ø **Medical and Surgical**
X **Anatomical Regions, Upper Extremities**
H **Insertion**   Definition: Putting in a nonbiological appliance that monitors, assists, performs, or prevents a physiological function but does not physically take the place of a body part

         Explanation: None

Body Part Character 4	Approach Character 5	Device Character 6	Qualifier Character 7
2 Shoulder Region, Right	Ø Open	1 Radioactive Element	Z No Qualifier
3 Shoulder Region, Left	3 Percutaneous	3 Infusion Device	
4 Axilla, Right	4 Percutaneous Endoscopic	Y Other Device	
5 Axilla, Left			
6 Upper Extremity, Right			
7 Upper Extremity, Left			
8 Upper Arm, Right			
9 Upper Arm, Left			
B Elbow Region, Right			
C Elbow Region, Left			
D Lower Arm, Right			
F Lower Arm, Left			
G Wrist Region, Right			
H Wrist Region, Left			
J Hand, Right			
K Hand, Left			

DRG Non-OR   ØXH[2,3,4,5,6,7,8,9,B,C,D,F,G,H,J,K][Ø,3,4][3,Y]Z

Ø **Medical and Surgical**
X **Anatomical Regions, Upper Extremities**
J **Inspection**   Definition: Visually and/or manually exploring a body part

         Explanation: Visual exploration may be performed with or without optical instrumentation. Manual exploration may be performed directly or through intervening body layers.

Body Part Character 4	Approach Character 5	Device Character 6	Qualifier Character 7
2 Shoulder Region, Right	Ø Open	Z No Device	Z No Qualifier
3 Shoulder Region, Left	3 Percutaneous		
4 Axilla, Right	4 Percutaneous Endoscopic		
5 Axilla, Left	X External		
6 Upper Extremity, Right			
7 Upper Extremity, Left			
8 Upper Arm, Right			
9 Upper Arm, Left			
B Elbow Region, Right			
C Elbow Region, Left			
D Lower Arm, Right			
F Lower Arm, Left			
G Wrist Region, Right			
H Wrist Region, Left			
J Hand, Right			
K Hand, Left			

DRG Non-OR   ØXJ[2,3,4,5,6,7,8,9,B,C,D,F,G,H,J,K]ØZZ
Non-OR   ØXJ[2,3,4,5,6,7,8,9,B,C,D,F,G,H][3,4,X]ZZ
Non-OR   ØXJ[J,K][3,X]ZZ

LC Limited Coverage   NC Noncovered   ⊞ Combination Member   HAC associated procedure   Combination Only   DRG Non-OR   Non-OR   New/Revised in GREEN

Ø   Medical and Surgical
X   Anatomical Regions, Upper Extremities
M   Reattachment   Definition: Putting back in or on all or a portion of a separated body part to its normal location or other suitable location

Explanation: Vascular circulation and nervous pathways may or may not be reestablished

Body Part Character 4	Approach Character 5	Device Character 6	Qualifier Character 7
Ø Forequarter, Right	Ø Open	Z No Device	Z No Qualifier
1 Forequarter, Left			
2 Shoulder Region, Right			
3 Shoulder Region, Left			
4 Axilla, Right			
5 Axilla, Left			
6 Upper Extremity, Right			
7 Upper Extremity, Left			
8 Upper Arm, Right			
9 Upper Arm, Left			
B Elbow Region, Right			
C Elbow Region, Left			
D Lower Arm, Right			
F Lower Arm, Left			
G Wrist Region, Right			
H Wrist Region, Left			
J Hand, Right			
K Hand, Left			
L Thumb, Right			
M Thumb, Left			
N Index Finger, Right			
P Index Finger, Left			
Q Middle Finger, Right			
R Middle Finger, Left			
S Ring Finger, Right			
T Ring Finger, Left			
V Little Finger, Right			
W Little Finger, Left			

Ø   Medical and Surgical
X   Anatomical Regions, Upper Extremities
P   Removal   Definition: Taking out or off a device from a body part

Explanation: If a device is taken out and a similar device put in without cutting or puncturing the skin or mucous membrane, the procedure is coded to the root operation CHANGE. Otherwise, the procedure for taking out the device is coded to the root operation REMOVAL.

Body Part Character 4	Approach Character 5	Device Character 6	Qualifier Character 7
6 Upper Extremity, Right	Ø Open	Ø Drainage Device	Z No Qualifier
7 Upper Extremity, Left	3 Percutaneous	1 Radioactive Element	
	4 Percutaneous Endoscopic	3 Infusion Device	
	X External	7 Autologous Tissue Substitute	
		J Synthetic Substitute	
		K Nonautologous Tissue Substitute	
		Y Other Device	

Non-OR   All body part, approach, device, and qualifier values

LC Limited Coverage   NC Noncovered   ⊞ Combination Member   HAC associated procedure   Combination Only   DRG Non-OR   Non-OR   New/Revised in GREEN

ICD-10-PCS 2019   665

Ø   **Medical and Surgical**
X   **Anatomical Regions, Upper Extremities**
Q   **Repair**   Definition: Restoring, to the extent possible, a body part to its normal anatomic structure and function
         Explanation: Used only when the method to accomplish the repair is not one of the other root operations

Body Part Character 4	Approach Character 5	Device Character 6	Qualifier Character 7
2 Shoulder Region, Right	Ø Open	Z No Device	Z No Qualifier
3 Shoulder Region, Left	3 Percutaneous		
4 Axilla, Right	4 Percutaneous Endoscopic		
5 Axilla, Left	X External		
6 Upper Extremity, Right			
7 Upper Extremity, Left			
8 Upper Arm, Right			
9 Upper Arm, Left			
B Elbow Region, Right			
C Elbow Region, Left			
D Lower Arm, Right			
F Lower Arm, Left			
G Wrist Region, Right			
H Wrist Region, Left			
J Hand, Right			
K Hand, Left			
L Thumb, Right			
M Thumb, Left			
N Index Finger, Right			
P Index Finger, Left			
Q Middle Finger, Right			
R Middle Finger, Left			
S Ring Finger, Right			
T Ring Finger, Left			
V Little Finger, Right			
W Little Finger, Left			

Ø   **Medical and Surgical**
X   **Anatomical Regions, Upper Extremities**
R   **Replacement**   Definition: Putting in or on biological or synthetic material that physically takes the place and/or function of all or a portion of a body part
         Explanation: The body part may have been taken out or replaced, or may be taken out, physically eradicated, or rendered nonfunctional during the REPLACEMENT procedure. A REMOVAL procedure is coded for taking out the device used in a previous replacement procedure.

Body Part Character 4	Approach Character 5	Device Character 6	Qualifier Character 7
L Thumb, Right	Ø Open	7 Autologous Tissue Substitute	N Toe, Right
M Thumb, Left	4 Percutaneous Endoscopic		P Toe, Left

Ø   **Medical and Surgical**
X   **Anatomical Regions, Upper Extremities**
U   **Supplement**   Definition: Putting in or on biological or synthetic material that physically reinforces and/or augments the function of a portion of a body part

           Explanation: The biological material is non-living, or is living and from the same individual. The body part may have been previously replaced, and the SUPPLEMENT procedure is performed to physically reinforce and/or augment the function of the replaced body part.

Body Part Character 4	Approach Character 5	Device Character 6	Qualifier Character 7
2 Shoulder Region, Right 3 Shoulder Region, Left 4 Axilla, Right 5 Axilla, Left 6 Upper Extremity, Right 7 Upper Extremity, Left 8 Upper Arm, Right 9 Upper Arm, Left B Elbow Region, Right C Elbow Region, Left D Lower Arm, Right F Lower Arm, Left G Wrist Region, Right H Wrist Region, Left J Hand, Right K Hand, Left L Thumb, Right M Thumb, Left N Index Finger, Right P Index Finger, Left Q Middle Finger, Right R Middle Finger, Left S Ring Finger, Right T Ring Finger, Left V Little Finger, Right W Little Finger, Left	Ø Open 4 Percutaneous Endoscopic	7 Autologous Tissue Substitute J Synthetic Substitute K Nonautologous Tissue Substitute	Z No Qualifier

Ø   **Medical and Surgical**
X   **Anatomical Regions, Upper Extremities**
W   **Revision**   Definition: Correcting, to the extent possible, a portion of a malfunctioning device or the position of a displaced device

           Explanation: Revision can include correcting a malfunctioning or displaced device by taking out or putting in components of the device such as a screw or pin

Body Part Character 4	Approach Character 5	Device Character 6	Qualifier Character 7
6 Upper Extremity, Right 7 Upper Extremity, Left	Ø Open 3 Percutaneous 4 Percutaneous Endoscopic X External	Ø Drainage Device 3 Infusion Device 7 Autologous Tissue Substitute J Synthetic Substitute K Nonautologous Tissue Substitute Y Other Device	Z No Qualifier

DRG Non-OR	ØXW[6,7][Ø,3,4][Ø,3,7,J,K,Y]Z
Non-OR	ØXW[6,7]X[Ø,3,7,J,K,Y]Z

Ø   **Medical and Surgical**
X   **Anatomical Regions, Upper Extremities**
X   **Transfer**   Definition: Moving, without taking out, all or a portion of a body part to another location to take over the function of all or a portion of a body part

           Explanation: The body part transferred remains connected to its vascular and nervous supply

Body Part Character 4	Approach Character 5	Device Character 6	Qualifier Character 7
N Index Finger, Right	Ø Open	Z No Device	L Thumb, Right
P Index Finger, Left	Ø Open	Z No Device	M Thumb, Left

Ø   **Medical and Surgical**
X   **Anatomical Regions, Upper Extremities**
Y   **Transplantation**   Definition: Putting in or on all or a portion of a living body part taken from another individual or animal to physically take the place and/or function of all or a portion of a similar body part

           Explanation: The native body part may or may not be taken out, and the transplanted body part may take over all or a portion of its function

Body Part Character 4	Approach Character 5	Device Character 6	Qualifier Character 7
J Hand, Right K Hand, Left	Ø Open	Z No Device	Ø Allogeneic 1 Syngeneic

🔲 Limited Coverage   🔲 Noncovered   ⊞ Combination Member   HAC associated procedure   Combination Only   DRG Non-OR   Non-OR   New/Revised in GREEN

ICD-10-PCS 2019   667

Anatomical Regions, Lower Extremities ØYØ–ØYW

Character Meanings

This Character Meaning table is provided as a guide to assist the user in the identification of character members that may be found in this section of code tables. It **SHOULD NOT** be used to build a PCS code.

Operation–Character 3		Body Part–Character 4		Approach–Character 5		Device–Character 6		Qualifier–Character 7	
Ø	Alteration	Ø	Buttock, Right	Ø	Open	Ø	Drainage Device	Ø	Complete
2	Change	1	Buttock, Left	3	Percutaneous	1	Radioactive Element	1	High
3	Control	2	Hindquarter, Right	4	Percutaneous Endoscopic	3	Infusion Device	2	Mid
6	Detachment	3	Hindquarter, Left	X	External	7	Autologous Tissue Substitute	3	Low
9	Drainage	4	Hindquarter, Bilateral			J	Synthetic Substitute	4	Complete 1st Ray
B	Excision	5	Inguinal Region, Right			K	Nonautologous Tissue Substitute	5	Complete 2nd Ray
H	Insertion	6	Inguinal Region, Left			Y	Other Device	6	Complete 3rd Ray
J	Inspection	7	Femoral Region, Right			Z	No Device	7	Complete 4th Ray
M	Reattachment	8	Femoral Region, Left					8	Complete 5th Ray
P	Removal	9	Lower Extremity, Right					9	Partial 1st Ray
Q	Repair	A	Inguinal Region, Bilateral					B	Partial 2nd Ray
U	Supplement	B	Lower Extremity, Left					C	Partial 3rd Ray
W	Revision	C	Upper Leg, Right					D	Partial 4th Ray
		D	Upper Leg, Left					F	Partial 5th Ray
		E	Femoral Region, Bilateral					X	Diagnostic
		F	Knee Region, Right					Z	No Qualifier
		G	Knee Region, Left						
		H	Lower Leg, Right						
		J	Lower Leg, Left						
		K	Ankle Region, Right						
		L	Ankle Region, Left						
		M	Foot, Right						
		N	Foot, Left						
		P	1st Toe, Right						
		Q	1st Toe, Left						
		R	2nd Toe, Right						
		S	2nd Toe, Left						
		T	3rd Toe, Right						
		U	3rd Toe, Left						
		V	4th Toe, Right						
		W	4th Toe, Left						
		X	5th Toe, Right						
		Y	5th Toe, Left						

AHA Coding Clinic for table ØY3
2016, 4Q, 99   Root operation Control
2013, 3Q, 23   Control of intraoperative bleeding

AHA Coding Clinic for table ØY6
2017, 2Q, 3-4   Qualifiers for the root operation detachment
2017, 1Q, 22   Chopart amputation of foot
2015, 2Q, 28   Partial amputation of hallux at interphalangeal Joint
2015, 1Q, 28   Mid-foot amputation

AHA Coding Clinic for table ØY9
2015, 1Q, 22   Incision and drainage of abscess of femoropopliteal bypass site
2015, 1Q, 22   Incision and drainage of groin abscess

Detachment Qualifier Descriptions

Qualifier Definition	Upper Leg	Lower Leg
1 **High:** Amputation at the proximal portion of the shaft of the:	Femur	Tibia/Fibula
2 **Mid:** Amputation at the middle portion of the shaft of the:	Femur	Tibia/Fibula
3 **Low:** Amputation at the distal portion of the shaft of the:	Femur	Tibia/Fibula

Qualifier Definition	Foot
Ø Complete 1st through 5th Rays Ray: digit of hand or foot with corresponding metacarpus or metatarsus	Through tarso-metatarsal Joint, **Ankle**
4 Complete 1st Ray	Through tarso-metatarsal joint, **Great Toe**
5 Complete 2nd Ray	Through tarso-metatarsal joint, **2nd Toe**
6 Complete 3rd Ray	Through tarso-metatarsal joint, **3rd Toe**
7 Complete 4th Ray	Through tarso-metatarsal joint, **4th Toe**
8 Complete 5th Ray	Through tarso-metatarsal joint, **Little Toe**
9 Partial 1st Ray	Anywhere along shaft or head of metatarsal bone, **Great Toe**
B Partial 2nd Ray	Anywhere along shaft or head of metatarsal bone, **2nd Toe**
C Partial 3rd Ray	Anywhere along shaft or head of metatarsal bone, **3rd Toe**
D Partial 4th Ray	Anywhere along shaft or head of metatarsal bone, **4th Toe**
F Partial 5th Ray	Anywhere along shaft or head of metatarsal bone, **Little Toe**

Qualifier Definition	Toe
Ø Complete	At the metatarsal-phalangeal joint
1 High	Anywhere along the proximal phalanx
2 Mid	Through the proximal interphalangeal joint or anywhere along the middle phalanx
3 Low	Through the distal interphalangeal joint or anywhere along the distal phalanx

Ø   **Medical and Surgical**
Y   **Anatomical Regions, Lower Extremities**
Ø   **Alteration**   Definition: Modifying the anatomic structure of a body part without affecting the function of the body part
                   Explanation: Principal purpose is to improve appearance

Body Part Character 4	Approach Character 5	Device Character 6	Qualifier Character 7
Ø Buttock, Right	**Ø** Open	**7** Autologous Tissue Substitute	**Z** No Qualifier
1 Buttock, Left	**3** Percutaneous	**J** Synthetic Substitute	
9 Lower Extremity, Right	**4** Percutaneous Endoscopic	**K** Nonautologous Tissue Substitute	
B Lower Extremity, Left		**Z** No Device	
C Upper Leg, Right			
D Upper Leg, Left			
F Knee Region, Right			
G Knee Region, Left			
H Lower Leg, Right			
J Lower Leg, Left			
K Ankle Region, Right			
L Ankle Region, Left			

Ø   **Medical and Surgical**
Y   **Anatomical Regions, Lower Extremities**
2   **Change**   Definition: Taking out or off a device from a body part and putting back an identical or similar device in or on the same body part without cutting or puncturing the skin or a mucous membrane
                   Explanation: All CHANGE procedures are coded using the approach EXTERNAL

Body Part Character 4	Approach Character 5	Device Character 6	Qualifier Character 7
9 Lower Extremity, Right	**X** External	**Ø** Drainage Device	**Z** No Qualifier
B Lower Extremity, Left		**Y** Other Device	

Non-OR   All body part, approach, device, and qualifier values

Ø   **Medical and Surgical**
Y   **Anatomical Regions, Lower Extremities**
3   **Control**   Definition: Stopping, or attempting to stop, postprocedural or other acute bleeding
                   Explanation: The site of the bleeding is coded as an anatomical region and not to a specific body part

Body Part Character 4	Approach Character 5	Device Character 6	Qualifier Character 7
Ø Buttock, Right	**Ø** Open	**Z** No Device	**Z** No Qualifier
1 Buttock, Left	**3** Percutaneous		
5 Inguinal Region, Right	**4** Percutaneous Endoscopic		
Inguinal canal			
Inguinal triangle			
6 Inguinal Region, Left			
See 5 Inguinal Region, Right			
7 Femoral Region, Right			
8 Femoral Region, Left			
9 Lower Extremity, Right			
B Lower Extremity, Left			
C Upper Leg, Right			
D Upper Leg, Left			
F Knee Region, Right			
G Knee Region, Left			
H Lower Leg, Right			
J Lower Leg, Left			
K Ankle Region, Right			
L Ankle Region, Left			
M Foot, Right			
N Foot, Left			

LC Limited Coverage   **NC** Noncovered   ⊞ Combination Member   HAC associated procedure   Combination Only   DRG Non-OR   Non-OR   New/Revised in GREEN

ICD-10-PCS 2019   **671**

Ø   Medical and Surgical
Y   Anatomical Regions, Lower Extremities
6   Detachment   Definition: Cutting off all or a portion of the upper or lower extremities

Explanation: The body part value is the site of the detachment, with a qualifier if applicable to further specify the level where the extremity was detached

Body Part Character 4	Approach Character 5	Device Character 6	Qualifier Character 7
2 Hindquarter, Right **3** Hindquarter, Left **4** Hindquarter, Bilateral **7** Femoral Region, Right **8** Femoral Region, Left **F** Knee Region, Right **G** Knee Region, Left	**Ø** Open	**Z** No Device	**Z** No Qualifier
C Upper Leg, Right **D** Upper Leg, Left **H** Lower Leg, Right **J** Lower Leg, Left	**Ø** Open	**Z** No Device	**1** High **2** Mid **3** Low
M Foot, Right **N** Foot, Left	**Ø** Open	**Z** No Device	**Ø** Complete **4** Complete 1st Ray **5** Complete 2nd Ray **6** Complete 3rd Ray **7** Complete 4th Ray **8** Complete 5th Ray **9** Partial 1st Ray **B** Partial 2nd Ray **C** Partial 3rd Ray **D** Partial 4th Ray **F** Partial 5th Ray

P 1st Toe, Right
   Hallux
Q 1st Toe, Left
   See 1st Toe, Right
R 2nd Toe, Right
S 2nd Toe, Left
T 3rd Toe, Right
U 3rd Toe, Left
V 4th Toe, Right
W 4th Toe, Left
X 5th Toe, Right
Y 5th Toe, Left
	Ø Open	**Z** No Device	**Ø** Complete
			1 High
			2 Mid
			3 Low

LC Limited Coverage   NC Noncovered   ⊞ Combination Member   HAC associated procedure   Combination Only   DRG Non-OR   Non-OR   New/Revised in GREEN

672   ICD-10-PCS 2019

Ø   **Medical and Surgical**
Y   **Anatomical Regions, Lower Extremities**
9   **Drainage**   Definition: Taking or letting out fluids and/or gases from a body part
                     Explanation: The qualifier DIAGNOSTIC is used to identify drainage procedures that are biopsies

Body Part Character 4	Approach Character 5	Device Character 6	Qualifier Character 7

Ø Buttock, Right
1 Buttock, Left
5 Inguinal Region, Right
    Inguinal canal
    Inguinal triangle
6 Inguinal Region, Left
    See 5 Inguinal Region, Right
7 Femoral Region, Right
8 Femoral Region, Left
9 Lower Extremity, Right
B Lower Extremity, Left
C Upper Leg, Right
D Upper Leg, Left
F Knee Region, Right
G Knee Region, Left
H Lower Leg, Right
J Lower Leg, Left
K Ankle Region, Right
L Ankle Region, Left
M Foot, Right
N Foot, Left
	Ø Open
	3 Percutaneous
	4 Percutaneous Endoscopic
		Ø Drainage Device	Z No Qualifier

Ø Buttock, Right
1 Buttock, Left
5 Inguinal Region, Right
    Inguinal canal
    Inguinal triangle
6 Inguinal Region, Left
    See 5 Inguinal Region, Right
7 Femoral Region, Right
8 Femoral Region, Left
9 Lower Extremity, Right
B Lower Extremity, Left
C Upper Leg, Right
D Upper Leg, Left
F Knee Region, Right
G Knee Region, Left
H Lower Leg, Right
J Lower Leg, Left
K Ankle Region, Right
L Ankle Region, Left
M Foot, Right
N Foot, Left
	Ø Open
	3 Percutaneous
	4 Percutaneous Endoscopic
		Z No Device	X Diagnostic
			Z No Qualifier

Non-OR   ØY9[Ø,1,7,8,9,B,C,D,F,G,H,J,K,L,M,N][Ø,3,4]ØZ
Non-OR   ØY9[5,6]3ØZ
Non-OR   ØY9[Ø,1,7,8,9,B,C,D,F,G,H,J,K,L,M,N][Ø,3,4]Z[X,Z]
Non-OR   ØY9[5,6]3ZZ

Ø **Medical and Surgical**
Y **Anatomical Regions, Lower Extremities**
B **Excision** Definition: Cutting out or off, without replacement, a portion of a body part
Explanation: The qualifier DIAGNOSTIC is used to identify excision procedures that are biopsies

Body Part Character 4	Approach Character 5	Device Character 6	Qualifier Character 7
Ø Buttock, Right	Ø Open	Z No Device	X Diagnostic
1 Buttock, Left	3 Percutaneous		Z No Qualifier
5 Inguinal Region, Right	4 Percutaneous Endoscopic		
Inguinal canal			
Inguinal triangle			
6 Inguinal Region, Left			
See 5 Inguinal Region, Right			
7 Femoral Region, Right			
8 Femoral Region, Left			
9 Lower Extremity, Right			
B Lower Extremity, Left			
C Upper Leg, Right			
D Upper Leg, Left			
F Knee Region, Right			
G Knee Region, Left			
H Lower Leg, Right			
J Lower Leg, Left			
K Ankle Region, Right			
L Ankle Region, Left			
M Foot, Right			
N Foot, Left			

Non-OR ØYB[Ø,1,9,B,C,D,F,G,H,J,K,L,M,N][Ø,3,4]ZX

Ø **Medical and Surgical**
Y **Anatomical Regions, Lower Extremities**
H **Insertion** Definition: Putting in a nonbiological appliance that monitors, assists, performs, or prevents a physiological function but does not physically take the place of a body part
Explanation: None

Body Part Character 4	Approach Character 5	Device Character 6	Qualifier Character 7
Ø Buttock, Right	Ø Open	1 Radioactive Element	Z No Qualifier
1 Buttock, Left	3 Percutaneous	3 Infusion Device	
5 Inguinal Region, Right	4 Percutaneous Endoscopic	Y Other Device	
Inguinal canal			
Inguinal triangle			
6 Inguinal Region, Left			
See 5 Inguinal Region, Right			
7 Femoral Region, Right			
8 Femoral Region, Left			
9 Lower Extremity, Right			
B Lower Extremity, Left			
C Upper Leg, Right			
D Upper Leg, Left			
F Knee Region, Right			
G Knee Region, Left			
H Lower Leg, Right			
J Lower Leg, Left			
K Ankle Region, Right			
L Ankle Region, Left			
M Foot, Right			
N Foot, Left			

DRG Non-OR ØYH[Ø,1,5,6,7,8,9,B,C,D,F,G,H,J,K,L,M,N][Ø,3,4][3,Y]Z

Ø   Medical and Surgical
Y   Anatomical Regions, Lower Extremities
J   Inspection   Definition: Visually and/or manually exploring a body part

                Explanation: Visual exploration may be performed with or without optical instrumentation. Manual exploration may be performed directly or through intervening body layers.

Body Part Character 4	Approach Character 5	Device Character 6	Qualifier Character 7

Ø Buttock, Right
1 Buttock, Left
5 Inguinal Region, Right
    Inguinal canal
    Inguinal triangle
6 Inguinal Region, Left
    See 5 Inguinal Region, Right
7 Femoral Region, Right
8 Femoral Region, Left
9 Lower Extremity, Right
A Inguinal Region, Bilateral
    See 5 Inguinal Region, Right
B Lower Extremity, Left
C Upper Leg, Right
D Upper Leg, Left
E Femoral Region, Bilateral
F Knee Region, Right
G Knee Region, Left
H Lower Leg, Right
J Lower Leg, Left
K Ankle Region, Right
L Ankle Region, Left
M Foot, Right
N Foot, Left
	Ø Open
	3 Percutaneous
	4 Percutaneous Endoscopic
	X External
		Z No Device	**Z** No Qualifier

DRG Non-OR	ØYJ[Ø,1,8,9,B,C,D,E,F,G,H,J,K,L,M,N]ØZZ
Non-OR	ØYJ[Ø,1,9,B,C,D,F,G,H,J,K,L,M,N][3,4,X]ZZ
Non-OR	ØYJ[5,6,7,8,A,E][3,X]ZZ

LC Limited Coverage **NC** Noncovered ⊞ Combination Member HAC associated procedure Combination Only DRG Non-OR Non-OR New/Revised in GREEN

ICD-10-PCS 2019   675

Anatomical Regions, Lower Extremities

Ø　Medical and Surgical
Y　Anatomical Regions, Lower Extremities
M　Reattachment　　Definition: Putting back in or on all or a portion of a separated body part to its normal location or other suitable location
　　　　　　　　　　Explanation: Vascular circulation and nervous pathways may or may not be reestablished

Body Part Character 4	Approach Character 5	Device Character 6	Qualifier Character 7
Ø　Buttock, Right	Ø　Open	Z　No Device	Z　No Qualifier
1　Buttock, Left			
2　Hindquarter, Right			
3　Hindquarter, Left			
4　Hindquarter, Bilateral			
5　Inguinal Region, Right 　　Inguinal canal 　　Inguinal triangle			
6　Inguinal Region, Left 　　See 5 Inguinal Region, Right			
7　Femoral Region, Right			
8　Femoral Region, Left			
9　Lower Extremity, Right			
B　Lower Extremity, Left			
C　Upper Leg, Right			
D　Upper Leg, Left			
F　Knee Region, Right			
G　Knee Region, Left			
H　Lower Leg, Right			
J　Lower Leg, Left			
K　Ankle Region, Right			
L　Ankle Region, Left			
M　Foot, Right			
N　Foot, Left			
P　1st Toe, Right 　　Hallux			
Q　1st Toe, Left 　　See 1st Toe, Right			
R　2nd Toe, Right			
S　2nd Toe, Left			
T　3rd Toe, Right			
U　3rd Toe, Left			
V　4th Toe, Right			
W　4th Toe, Left			
X　5th Toe, Right			
Y　5th Toe, Left			

Ø　Medical and Surgical
Y　Anatomical Regions, Lower Extremities
P　Removal　　Definition: Taking out or off a device from a body part
　　　　　　　Explanation: If a device is taken out and a similar device put in without cutting or puncturing the skin or mucous membrane, the procedure is coded to the root operation CHANGE. Otherwise, the procedure for taking out the device is coded to the root operation REMOVAL.

Body Part Character 4	Approach Character 5	Device Character 6	Qualifier Character 7
9　Lower Extremity, Right	Ø　Open	Ø　Drainage Device	Z　No Qualifier
B　Lower Extremity, Left	3　Percutaneous	1　Radioactive Element	
	4　Percutaneous Endoscopic	3　Infusion Device	
	X　External	7　Autologous Tissue Substitute	
		J　Synthetic Substitute	
		K　Nonautologous Tissue Substitute	
		Y　Other Device	

Non-OR　All body part, approach, device, and qualifier values

Ø   Medical and Surgical
Y   Anatomical Regions, Lower Extremities
Q   Repair   Definition: Restoring, to the extent possible, a body part to its normal anatomic structure and function
                       Explanation: Used only when the method to accomplish the repair is not one of the other root operations

Body Part Character 4	Approach Character 5	Device Character 6	Qualifier Character 7
Ø Buttock, Right	Ø Open	Z No Device	Z No Qualifier
1 Buttock, Left	3 Percutaneous		
5 Inguinal Region, Right	4 Percutaneous Endoscopic		
Inguinal canal	X External		
Inguinal triangle			
6 Inguinal Region, Left			
See 5 Inguinal Region, Right			
7 Femoral Region, Right			
8 Femoral Region, Left			
9 Lower Extremity, Right			
A Inguinal Region, Bilateral			
See 5 Inguinal Region, Right			
B Lower Extremity, Left			
C Upper Leg, Right			
D Upper Leg, Left			
E Femoral Region, Bilateral			
F Knee Region, Right			
G Knee Region, Left			
H Lower Leg, Right			
J Lower Leg, Left			
K Ankle Region, Right			
L Ankle Region, Left			
M Foot, Right			
N Foot, Left			
P 1st Toe, Right			
Hallux			
Q 1st Toe, Left			
See 1st Toe, Right			
R 2nd Toe, Right			
S 2nd Toe, Left			
T 3rd Toe, Right			
U 3rd Toe, Left			
V 4th Toe, Right			
W 4th Toe, Left			
X 5th Toe, Right			
Y 5th Toe, Left			

Non-OR   ØYQ[5,6,7,8,A,E]XZZ

Ø Medical and Surgical
Y Anatomical Regions, Lower Extremities
U Supplement   Definition: Putting in or on biological or synthetic material that physically reinforces and/or augments the function of a portion of a body part

                  Explanation: The biological material is non-living, or is living and from the same individual. The body part may have been previously replaced, and the SUPPLEMENT procedure is performed to physically reinforce and/or augment the function of the replaced body part.

Body Part Character 4	Approach Character 5	Device Character 6	Qualifier Character 7
Ø Buttock, Right	Ø Open	7 Autologous Tissue Substitute	Z No Qualifier
1 Buttock, Left	4 Percutaneous Endoscopic	J Synthetic Substitute	
5 Inguinal Region, Right Inguinal canal Inguinal triangle		K Nonautologous Tissue Substitute	
6 Inguinal Region, Left *See 5 Inguinal Region, Right*			
7 Femoral Region, Right			
8 Femoral Region, Left			
9 Lower Extremity, Right			
A Inguinal Region, Bilateral *See 5 Inguinal Region, Right*			
B Lower Extremity, Left			
C Upper Leg, Right			
D Upper Leg, Left			
E Femoral Region, Bilateral			
F Knee Region, Right			
G Knee Region, Left			
H Lower Leg, Right			
J Lower Leg, Left			
K Ankle Region, Right			
L Ankle Region, Left			
M Foot, Right			
N Foot, Left			
P 1st Toe, Right Hallux			
Q 1st Toe, Left *See 1st Toe, Right*			
R 2nd Toe, Right			
S 2nd Toe, Left			
T 3rd Toe, Right			
U 3rd Toe, Left			
V 4th Toe, Right			
W 4th Toe, Left			
X 5th Toe, Right			
Y 5th Toe, Left			

Ø Medical and Surgical
Y Anatomical Regions, Lower Extremities
W Revision   Definition: Correcting, to the extent possible, a portion of a malfunctioning device or the position of a displaced device

                  Explanation: Revision can include correcting a malfunctioning or displaced device by taking out or putting in components of the device such as a screw or pin

Body Part Character 4	Approach Character 5	Device Character 6	Qualifier Character 7
9 Lower Extremity, Right	Ø Open	Ø Drainage Device	Z No Qualifier
B Lower Extremity, Left	3 Percutaneous	3 Infusion Device	
	4 Percutaneous Endoscopic	7 Autologous Tissue Substitute	
	X External	J Synthetic Substitute	
		K Nonautologous Tissue Substitute	
		Y Other Device	

DRG Non-OR   ØYW[9,B][Ø,3,4][Ø,3,7,J,K,Y]Z
Non-OR   ØYW[9,B]X[Ø,3,7,J,K,Y]Z

Obstetrics 102–10Y

Character Meanings

This Character Meaning table is provided as a guide to assist the user in the identification of character members that may be found in this section of code tables. It **SHOULD NOT** be used to build a PCS code.

0: Pregnancy

Operation–Character 3	Body Part–Character 4	Approach–Character 5	Device–Character 6	Qualifier–Character 7
2 Change	0 Products of Conception	0 Open	3 Monitoring Electrode	0 High
9 Drainage	1 Products of Conception, Retained	3 Percutaneous	Y Other Device	1 Low
A Abortion	2 Products of Conception, Ectopic	4 Percutaneous Endoscopic	Z No Device	2 Extraperitoneal
D Extraction		7 Via Natural or Artificial Opening		3 Low Forceps
E Delivery		8 Via Natural or Artificial Opening Endoscopic		4 Mid Forceps
H Insertion		X External		5 High Forceps
J Inspection				6 Vacuum
P Removal				7 Internal Version
Q Repair				8 Other
S Reposition				9 Fetal Blood OR Manual
T Resection				A Fetal Cerebrospinal Fluid
Y Transplantation				B Fetal Fluid, Other
				C Amniotic Fluid, Therapeutic
				D Fluid, Other
				E Nervous System
				F Cardiovascular System
				G Lymphatics & Hemic
				H Eye
				J Ear, Nose & Sinus
				K Respiratory System
				L Mouth & Throat
				M Gastrointestinal System
				N Hepatobiliary & Pancreas
				P Endocrine System
				Q Skin
				R Musculoskeletal System
				S Urinary System
				T Female Reproductive System
				U Amniotic Fluid, Diagnostic
				V Male Reproductive System
				W Laminaria
				X Abortifacient
				Y Other Body System
				Z No Qualifier

AHA Coding Clinic for table 109
2014, 3Q, 12   Fetoscopic laser photocoagulation and laser microseptostomy for twin-twin transfusion syndrome
2014, 2Q, 9   Pitocin administration to augment labor

AHA Coding Clinic for table 10D
2018, 2Q, 17   High transverse cesarean section
2016, 1Q, 9   Vaginal delivery assisted by vacuum and low forceps extraction
2014, 4Q, 43   Cesarean delivery assisted by vacuum extraction
2014, 4Q, 43   Vacuum dilation and curettage for blighted ovum

AHA Coding Clinic for table 10E
2017, 3Q, 5   Delivery of placenta
2016, 2Q, 34   Assisted vaginal delivery
2014, 4Q, 17   RH (D) alloimmunization (sensitization)
2014, 2Q, 9   Pitocin administration to augment labor

AHA Coding Clinic for table 10H
2013, 2Q, 36   Intrauterine pressure monitor

AHA Coding Clinic for table 10Q
2014, 3Q, 12   Fetoscopic laser photocoagulation and laser microseptostomy for twin-twin transfusion syndrome

AHA Coding Clinic for table 10T
2015, 3Q, 31   Laparoscopic partial salpingectomy for ectopic pregnancy

1   **Obstetrics**
Ø   **Pregnancy**
2   **Change**   Definition: Taking out or off a device from a body part and putting back an identical or similar device in or on the same body part without cutting or puncturing the skin or a mucous membrane
                   Explanation: None

Body Part Character 4	Approach Character 5	Device Character 6	Qualifier Character 7
Ø Products of Conception ♀	7 Via Natural or Artificial Opening	3 Monitoring Electrode Y Other Device	Z No Qualifier

Non-OR	All body part, approach, device, and qualifier values	♀	All body part, approach, device, and qualifier values

1   **Obstetrics**
Ø   **Pregnancy**
9   **Drainage**   Definition: Taking or letting out fluids and/or gases from a body part
                   Explanation: None

Body Part Character 4	Approach Character 5	Device Character 6	Qualifier Character 7
Ø Products of Conception ♀	Ø Open 3 Percutaneous 4 Percutaneous Endoscopic 7 Via Natural or Artificial Opening 8 Via Natural or Artificial Opening Endoscopic	Z No Device	9 Fetal Blood A Fetal Cerebrospinal Fluid B Fetal Fluid, Other C Amniotic Fluid, Therapeutic D Fluid, Other U Amniotic Fluid, Diagnostic

Non-OR	All body part, approach, device, and qualifier values	♀	All body part, approach, device, and qualifier values

1   **Obstetrics**
Ø   **Pregnancy**
A   **Abortion**   Definition: Artificially terminating a pregnancy
                   Explanation: None

Body Part Character 4	Approach Character 5	Device Character 6	Qualifier Character 7
Ø Products of Conception ♀	Ø Open 3 Percutaneous 4 Percutaneous Endoscopic 8 Via Natural or Artificial Opening Endoscopic	Z No Device	Z No Qualifier
Ø Products of Conception ♀	7 Via Natural or Artificial Opening	Z No Device	6 Vacuum W Laminaria X Abortifacient Z No Qualifier

DRG Non-OR	10A07Z6	♀	All body part, approach, device, and qualifier values
Non-OR	10A07Z[W,X]		

1   **Obstetrics**
Ø   **Pregnancy**
D   **Extraction**   Definition: Pulling or stripping out or off all or a portion of a body part by the use of force
                   Explanation: None

Body Part Character 4	Approach Character 5	Device Character 6	Qualifier Character 7
Ø Products of Conception ♀	Ø Open	Z No Device	Ø High 1 Low 2 Extraperitoneal
Ø Products of Conception ♀	7 Via Natural or Artificial Opening	Z No Device	3 Low Forceps 4 Mid Forceps 5 High Forceps 6 Vacuum 7 Internal Version 8 Other
1 Products of Conception, Retained ♀	7 Via Natural or Artificial Opening 8 Via Natural or Artificial Opening Endoscopic	Z No Device	9 Manual Z No Qualifier
2 Products of Conception, Ectopic ♀	7 Via Natural or Artificial Opening 8 Via Natural or Artificial Opening Endoscopic	Z No Device	Z No Qualifier

DRG Non-OR	10D07Z[3,4,5,6,7,8]	♀	All body part, approach, device, and qualifier values

1 Obstetrics
0 Pregnancy
E Delivery   Definition: Assisting the passage of the products of conception from the genital canal
Explanation: None

Body Part Character 4	Approach Character 5	Device Character 6	Qualifier Character 7
0 Products of Conception ♀	X External	Z No Device	Z No Qualifier

DRG Non-OR 10E0XZZ ♀ All body part, approach, device, and qualifier values

1 Obstetrics
0 Pregnancy
H Insertion   Definition: Putting in a nonbiological appliance that monitors, assists, performs, or prevents a physiological function but does not physically take the place of a body part
Explanation: None

Body Part Character 4	Approach Character 5	Device Character 6	Qualifier Character 7
0 Products of Conception ♀	0 Open 7 Via Natural or Artificial Opening	3 Monitoring Electrode Y Other Device	Z No Qualifier

Non-OR 10H07[3,Y]Z ♀ All body part, approach, device, and qualifier values

1 Obstetrics
0 Pregnancy
J Inspection   Definition: Visually and/or manually exploring a body part
Explanation: Visual exploration may be performed with or without optical instrumentation. Manual exploration may be performed directly or through intervening body layers.

Body Part Character 4	Approach Character 5	Device Character 6	Qualifier Character 7
0 Products of Conception ♀ 1 Products of Conception, Retained ♀ 2 Products of Conception, Ectopic ♀	0 Open 3 Percutaneous 4 Percutaneous Endoscopic 7 Via Natural or Artificial Opening 8 Via Natural or Artificial Opening Endoscopic X External	Z No Device	Z No Qualifier

Non-OR All body part, approach, device, and qualifier values ♀ All body part, approach, device, and qualifier values

1 Obstetrics
0 Pregnancy
P Removal   Definition: Taking out or off a device from a body part, region or orifice
Explanation: If a device is taken out and a similar device put in without cutting or puncturing the skin or mucous membrane, the procedure is coded to the root operation CHANGE. Otherwise, the procedure for taking out a device is coded to the root operation REMOVAL.

Body Part Character 4	Approach Character 5	Device Character 6	Qualifier Character 7
0 Products of Conception ♀	0 Open 7 Via Natural or Artificial Opening	3 Monitoring Electrode Y Other Device	Z No Qualifier

♀ All body part, approach, device, and qualifier values

1 Obstetrics
0 Pregnancy
Q Repair   Definition: Restoring, to the extent possible, a body part to its normal anatomic structure and function
Explanation: Used only when the method to accomplish the repair is not one of the other root operations

Body Part Character 4	Approach Character 5	Device Character 6	Qualifier Character 7
0 Products of Conception ♀	0 Open 3 Percutaneous 4 Percutaneous Endoscopic 7 Via Natural or Artificial Opening 8 Via Natural or Artificial Opening Endoscopic	Y Other Device Z No Device	E Nervous System F Cardiovascular System G Lymphatics and Hemic H Eye J Ear, Nose and Sinus K Respiratory System L Mouth and Throat M Gastrointestinal System N Hepatobiliary and Pancreas P Endocrine System Q Skin R Musculoskeletal System S Urinary System T Female Reproductive System V Male Reproductive System Y Other Body System

♀ All body part, approach, device, and qualifier values

LC Limited Coverage NC Noncovered ⊞ Combination Member HAC associated procedure Combination Only DRG Non-OR Non-OR New/Revised in GREEN

Obstetrics

1 Obstetrics
Ø Pregnancy
S Reposition

Definition: Moving to its normal location, or other suitable location, all or a portion of a body part

Explanation: The body part is moved to a new location from an abnormal location, or from a normal location where it is not functioning correctly. The body part may or may not be cut out or off to be moved to the new location.

Body Part Character 4	Approach Character 5	Device Character 6	Qualifier Character 7
Ø Products of Conception ♀	7 Via Natural or Artificial Opening X External	Z No Device	Z No Qualifier
2 Products of Conception, Ectopic ♀	Ø Open 3 Percutaneous 4 Percutaneous Endoscopic 7 Via Natural or Artificial Opening 8 Via Natural or Artificial Opening Endoscopic	Z No Device	Z No Qualifier

DRG Non-OR   10S07ZZ
Non-OR   10S0XZZ

♀ All body part, approach, device, and qualifier values

1 Obstetrics
Ø Pregnancy
T Resection

Definition: Cutting out or off, without replacement, all of a body part

Explanation: None

Body Part Character 4	Approach Character 5	Device Character 6	Qualifier Character 7
2 Products of Conception, Ectopic ♀	Ø Open 3 Percutaneous 4 Percutaneous Endoscopic 7 Via Natural or Artificial Opening 8 Via Natural or Artificial Opening Endoscopic	Z No Device	Z No Qualifier

♀ All body part, approach, device, and qualifier values

1 Obstetrics
Ø Pregnancy
Y Transplantation

Definition: Putting in or on all or a portion of a living body part taken from another individual or animal to physically take the place and/or function of all or a portion of a similar body part

Explanation: The native body part may or may not be taken out, and the transplanted body part may take over all or a portion of its function

Body Part Character 4	Approach Character 5	Device Character 6	Qualifier Character 7
Ø Products of Conception ♀	3 Percutaneous 4 Percutaneous Endoscopic 7 Via Natural or Artificial Opening	Z No Device	E Nervous System F Cardiovascular System G Lymphatics and Hemic H Eye J Ear, Nose and Sinus K Respiratory System L Mouth and Throat M Gastrointestinal System N Hepatobiliary and Pancreas P Endocrine System Q Skin R Musculoskeletal System S Urinary System T Female Reproductive System V Male Reproductive System Y Other Body System

♀ All body part, approach, device, and qualifier values

LG Limited Coverage   NC Noncovered   ⊞ Combination Member   HAC associated procedure   Combination Only   DRG Non-OR   Non-OR   New/Revised in GREEN

682   ICD-10-PCS 2019

Placement 2WØ–2Y5

Character Meanings

This Character Meaning table is provided as a guide to assist the user in the identification of character members that may be found in this section of code tables. It **SHOULD NOT** be used to build a PCS code.

W: Anatomical Regions

Operation–Character 3	Body Region–Character 4	Approach–Character 5	Device–Character 6	Qualifier–Character 7
Ø Change	Ø Head	X External	Ø Traction Apparatus	Z No Qualifier
1 Compression	1 Face		1 Splint	
2 Dressing	2 Neck		2 Cast	
3 Immobilization	3 Abdominal Wall		3 Brace	
4 Packing	4 Chest Wall		4 Bandage	
5 Removal	5 Back		5 Packing Material	
6 Traction	6 Inguinal Region, Right		6 Pressure Dressing	
	7 Inguinal Region, Left		7 Intermittent Pressure Device	
	8 Upper Extremity, Right		9 Wire	
	9 Upper Extremity, Left		Y Other Device	
	A Upper Arm, Right		Z No Device	
	B Upper Arm, Left			
	C Lower Arm, Right			
	D Lower Arm, Left			
	E Hand, Right			
	F Hand, Left			
	G Thumb, Right			
	H Thumb, Left			
	J Finger, Right			
	K Finger, Left			
	L Lower Extremity, Right			
	M Lower Extremity, Left			
	N Upper Leg, Right			
	P Upper Leg, Left			
	Q Lower Leg, Right			
	R Lower Leg, Left			
	S Foot, Right			
	T Foot, Left			
	U Toe, Right			
	V Toe, Left			

Y: Anatomical Orifices

Operation–Character 3	Body Orifice–Character 4	Approach–Character 5	Device–Character 6	Qualifier–Character 7
Ø Change	Ø Mouth and Pharynx	X External	5 Packing Material	Z No Qualifier
4 Packing	1 Nasal			
5 Removal	2 Ear			
	3 Anorectal			
	4 Female Genital Tract			
	5 Urethra			

AHA Coding Clinic for table 2W6
2015, 2Q, 35   Application of tongs to reduce and stabilize cervical fracture
2013, 2Q, 39   Application of cervical tongs for reduction of cervical fracture

AHA Coding Clinic for table 2Y4
2017, 4Q, 106   Nasal packing for epistaxis

Placement

2W0–2W0

2   **Placement**
W **Anatomical Regions**
0   **Change**   Definition: Taking out or off a device from a body part and putting back an identical or similar device in or on the same body part without cutting or puncturing the skin or a mucous membrane

Body Region Character 4	Approach Character 5	Device Character 6	Qualifier Character 7
0 Head 2 Neck 3 Abdominal Wall 4 Chest Wall 5 Back 6 Inguinal Region, Right 7 Inguinal Region, Left 8 Upper Extremity, Right 9 Upper Extremity, Left A Upper Arm, Right B Upper Arm, Left C Lower Arm, Right D Lower Arm, Left E Hand, Right F Hand, Left G Thumb, Right H Thumb, Left J Finger, Right K Finger, Left L Lower Extremity, Right M Lower Extremity, Left N Upper Leg, Right P Upper Leg, Left Q Lower Leg, Right R Lower Leg, Left S Foot, Right T Foot, Left U Toe, Right V Toe, Left	X External	0 Traction Apparatus 1 Splint 2 Cast 3 Brace 4 Bandage 5 Packing Material 6 Pressure Dressing 7 Intermittent Pressure Device Y Other Device	Z No Qualifier
1 Face	X External	0 Traction Apparatus 1 Splint 2 Cast 3 Brace 4 Bandage 5 Packing Material 6 Pressure Dressing 7 Intermittent Pressure Device 9 Wire Y Other Device	Z No Qualifier

2   Placement
W   Anatomical Regions
1   Compression   Definition: Putting pressure on a body region

Body Region Character 4	Approach Character 5	Device Character 6	Qualifier Character 7
0 Head	X External	6 Pressure Dressing	Z No Qualifier
1 Face		7 Intermittent Pressure Device	
2 Neck			
3 Abdominal Wall			
4 Chest Wall			
5 Back			
6 Inguinal Region, Right			
7 Inguinal Region, Left			
8 Upper Extremity, Right			
9 Upper Extremity, Left			
A Upper Arm, Right			
B Upper Arm, Left			
C Lower Arm, Right			
D Lower Arm, Left			
E Hand, Right			
F Hand, Left			
G Thumb, Right			
H Thumb, Left			
J Finger, Right			
K Finger, Left			
L Lower Extremity, Right			
M Lower Extremity, Left			
N Upper Leg, Right			
P Upper Leg, Left			
Q Lower Leg, Right			
R Lower Leg, Left			
S Foot, Right			
T Foot, Left			
U Toe, Right			
V Toe, Left			

2   Placement
W   Anatomical Regions
2   Dressing   Definition: Putting material on a body region for protection

Body Region Character 4	Approach Character 5	Device Character 6	Qualifier Character 7
0 Head	X External	4 Bandage	Z No Qualifier
1 Face			
2 Neck			
3 Abdominal Wall			
4 Chest Wall			
5 Back			
6 Inguinal Region, Right			
7 Inguinal Region, Left			
8 Upper Extremity, Right			
9 Upper Extremity, Left			
A Upper Arm, Right			
B Upper Arm, Left			
C Lower Arm, Right			
D Lower Arm, Left			
E Hand, Right			
F Hand, Left			
G Thumb, Right			
H Thumb, Left			
J Finger, Right			
K Finger, Left			
L Lower Extremity, Right			
M Lower Extremity, Left			
N Upper Leg, Right			
P Upper Leg, Left			
Q Lower Leg, Right			
R Lower Leg, Left			
S Foot, Right			
T Foot, Left			
U Toe, Right			
V Toe, Left			

2 Placement
W Anatomical Regions
3 Immobilization Definition: Limiting or preventing motion of a body region

Body Region Character 4	Approach Character 5	Device Character 6	Qualifier Character 7
Ø Head	X External	1 Splint	Z No Qualifier
2 Neck		2 Cast	
3 Abdominal Wall		3 Brace	
4 Chest Wall		Y Other Device	
5 Back			
6 Inguinal Region, Right			
7 Inguinal Region, Left			
8 Upper Extremity, Right			
9 Upper Extremity, Left			
A Upper Arm, Right			
B Upper Arm, Left			
C Lower Arm, Right			
D Lower Arm, Left			
E Hand, Right			
F Hand, Left			
G Thumb, Right			
H Thumb, Left			
J Finger, Right			
K Finger, Left			
L Lower Extremity, Right			
M Lower Extremity, Left			
N Upper Leg, Right			
P Upper Leg, Left			
Q Lower Leg, Right			
R Lower Leg, Left			
S Foot, Right			
T Foot, Left			
U Toe, Right			
V Toe, Left			
1 Face	X External	1 Splint	Z No Qualifier
		2 Cast	
		3 Brace	
		9 Wire	
		Y Other Device	

2 Placement
W Anatomical Regions
4 Packing Definition: Putting material in a body region or orifice

Body Region Character 4	Approach Character 5	Device Character 6	Qualifier Character 7
Ø Head	X External	5 Packing Material	Z No Qualifier
1 Face			
2 Neck			
3 Abdominal Wall			
4 Chest Wall			
5 Back			
6 Inguinal Region, Right			
7 Inguinal Region, Left			
8 Upper Extremity, Right			
9 Upper Extremity, Left			
A Upper Arm, Right			
B Upper Arm, Left			
C Lower Arm, Right			
D Lower Arm, Left			
E Hand, Right			
F Hand, Left			
G Thumb, Right			
H Thumb, Left			
J Finger, Right			
K Finger, Left			
L Lower Extremity, Right			
M Lower Extremity, Left			
N Upper Leg, Right			
P Upper Leg, Left			
Q Lower Leg, Right			
R Lower Leg, Left			
S Foot, Right			
T Foot, Left			
U Toe, Right			
V Toe, Left			

LC Limited Coverage   **NC** Noncovered   ⊞ Combination Member   HAC   Valid OR   Combination Only   DRG Non-OR   New/Revised in GREEN

686   ICD-10-PCS 2019

2   Placement
W   Anatomical Regions
5   Removal   Definition: Taking out or off a device from a body part

Body Region Character 4	Approach Character 5	Device Character 6	Qualifier Character 7
Ø Head 2 Neck 3 Abdominal Wall 4 Chest Wall 5 Back 6 Inguinal Region, Right 7 Inguinal Region, Left 8 Upper Extremity, Right 9 Upper Extremity, Left A Upper Arm, Right B Upper Arm, Left C Lower Arm, Right D Lower Arm, Left E Hand, Right F Hand, Left G Thumb, Right H Thumb, Left J Finger, Right K Finger, Left L Lower Extremity, Right M Lower Extremity, Left N Upper Leg, Right P Upper Leg, Left Q Lower Leg, Right R Lower Leg, Left S Foot, Right T Foot, Left U Toe, Right V Toe, Left	X External	Ø Traction Apparatus 1 Splint 2 Cast 3 Brace 4 Bandage 5 Packing Material 6 Pressure Dressing 7 Intermittent Pressure Device Y Other Device	Z No Qualifier
1 Face	X External	Ø Traction Apparatus 1 Splint 2 Cast 3 Brace 4 Bandage 5 Packing Material 6 Pressure Dressing 7 Intermittent Pressure Device 9 Wire Y Other Device	Z No Qualifier

2   Placement
W   Anatomical Regions
6   Traction   Definition: Exerting a pulling force on a body region in a distal direction

Body Region Character 4	Approach Character 5	Device Character 6	Qualifier Character 7
Ø Head 1 Face 2 Neck 3 Abdominal Wall 4 Chest Wall 5 Back 6 Inguinal Region, Right 7 Inguinal Region, Left 8 Upper Extremity, Right 9 Upper Extremity, Left A Upper Arm, Right B Upper Arm, Left C Lower Arm, Right D Lower Arm, Left E Hand, Right F Hand, Left G Thumb, Right H Thumb, Left J Finger, Right K Finger, Left L Lower Extremity, Right M Lower Extremity, Left N Upper Leg, Right P Upper Leg, Left Q Lower Leg, Right R Lower Leg, Left S Foot, Right T Foot, Left U Toe, Right V Toe, Left	X External	Ø Traction Apparatus Z No Device	Z No Qualifier

2   Placement
Y   Anatomical Orifices
Ø   Change   Definition: Taking out or off a device from a body part and putting back an identical or similar device in or on the same body part without cutting or puncturing the skin or a mucous membrane

Body Region Character 4	Approach Character 5	Device Character 6	Qualifier Character 7
Ø Mouth and Pharynx 1 Nasal 2 Ear 3 Anorectal 4 Female Genital Tract ♀ 5 Urethra	X External	5 Packing Material	Z No Qualifier

♀   2YØ4X5Z

2   Placement
Y   Anatomical Orifices
4   Packing   Definition: Putting material in a body region or orifice

Body Region Character 4	Approach Character 5	Device Character 6	Qualifier Character 7
Ø Mouth and Pharynx 1 Nasal 2 Ear 3 Anorectal 4 Female Genital Tract ♀ 5 Urethra	X External	5 Packing Material	Z No Qualifier

♀   2Y44X5Z

2   Placement
Y   Anatomical Orifices
5   Removal   Definition: Taking out or off a device from a body part

Body Region Character 4	Approach Character 5	Device Character 6	Qualifier Character 7
Ø Mouth and Pharynx 1 Nasal 2 Ear 3 Anorectal 4 Female Genital Tract ♀ 5 Urethra	X External	5 Packing Material	Z No Qualifier

♀   2Y54X5Z

Administration 3Ø2–3E1

Character Meanings

This Character Meaning table is provided as a guide to assist the user in the identification of character members that may be found in this section of code tables. It **SHOULD NOT** be used to build a PCS code.

Ø: Circulatory

Operation–Character 3	Body System/Region – Character 4	Approach–Character 5	Substance–Character 6	Qualifier–Character 7
2　Transfusion	3　Peripheral Vein	Ø　Open	A　Stem Cells, Embryonic	Ø　Autologous
	4　Central Vein	3　Percutaneous	B　4-Factor Prothrombin Complex Concentrate	1　Nonautologous
	5　Peripheral Artery	7　Via Natural or Artificial Opening	G　Bone Marrow	2　Allogeneic, Related
	6　Central Artery		H　Whole Blood	3　Allogeneic, Unrelated
	7　Products of Conception, Circulatory		J　Serum Albumin	4　Allogeneic, Unspecified
	8　Vein		K　Frozen Plasma	Z　No Qualifier
			L　Fresh Plasma	
			M　Plasma Cryoprecipitate	
			N　Red Blood Cells	
			P　Frozen Red Cells	
			Q　White Cells	
			R　Platelets	
			S　Globulin	
			T　Fibrinogen	
			V　Antihemophilic Factors	
			W　Factor IX	
			X　Stem Cells, Cord Blood	
			Y　Stem Cells, Hematopoietic	

C: Indwelling Device

Operation–Character 3	Body System/Region – Character 4	Approach–Character 5	Substance–Character 6	Qualifier–Character 7
1　Irrigation	Z　None	X　External	8　Irrigating Substance	Z　No Qualifier

Continued on next page

E: Physiological Systems and Anatomical Regions

Administration Character Meanings Continued

Operation–Character 3	Body System/Region–Character 4	Approach–Character 5	Substance–Character 6	Qualifier–Character 7
Ø Introduction	Ø Skin and Mucous Membranes	Ø Open	Ø Antineoplastic	Ø Autologous OR Influenza Vaccine
1 Irrigation	1 Subcutaneous Tissue	3 Percutaneous	1 Thrombolytic	1 Nonautologous
	2 Muscle	4 Percutaneous Endoscopic	2 Anti-infective	2 High-dose Interleukin-2
	3 Peripheral Vein	7 Via Natural or Artificial Opening	3 Anti-inflammatory	3 Low-dose Interleukin-2
	4 Central Vein	8 Via Natural or Artificial Opening Endoscopic	4 Serum, Toxoid and Vaccine	4 Liquid Brachytherapy Radioisotope
	5 Peripheral Artery	X External	5 Adhesion Barrier	5 Other Antineoplastic
	6 Central Artery		6 Nutritional Substance	6 Recombinant Human-activated Protein C
	7 Coronary Artery		7 Electrolytic and Water Balance Substance	7 Other Thrombolytic
	8 Heart		8 Irrigating Substance	8 Oxazolidinones
	9 Nose		9 Dialysate	9 Other Anti-infective
	A Bone Marrow		A Stem Cells, Embryonic	A Anti-infective Envelope
	B Ear		B Anesthetic Agent	B Recombinant Bone Morphogenetic Protein
	C Eye		E Stem Cells, Somatic	C Other Substance
	D Mouth and Pharynx		F Intracirculatory Anesthetic	D Nitric Oxide
	E Products of Conception		G Other Therapeutic Substance	F Other Gas
	F Respiratory Tract		H Radioactive Substance	G Insulin
	G Upper GI		K Other Diagnostic Substance	H Human B-type Natriuretic Peptide
	H Lower GI		L Sperm	J Other Hormone
	J Biliary and Pancreatic Tract		M Pigment	K Immunostimulator
	K Genitourinary Tract		N Analgesics, Hypnotics, Sedatives	L Immunosuppressive
	L Pleural Cavity		P Platelet Inhibitor	M Monoclonal Antibody
	M Peritoneal Cavity		Q Fertilized Ovum	N Blood Brain Barrier Disruption
	N Male Reproductive		R Antiarrhythmic	P Clofarabine
	P Female Reproductive		S Gas	Q Glucarpidase
	Q Cranial Cavity and Brain		T Destructive Agent	X Diagnostic
	R Spinal Canal		U Pancreatic Islet Cells	Z No Qualifier
	S Epidural Space		V Hormone	
	T Peripheral Nerves and Plexi		W Immunotherapeutic	
	U Joints		X Vasopressor	
	V Bones			
	W Lymphatics			
	X Cranial Nerves			
	Y Pericardial Cavity			

AHA Coding Clinic for table 3Ø2

2016, 4Q, 113   Bone marrow and stem cell transfusion (Transplantation)

AHA Coding Clinic for table 3EØ

2018, 1Q, 8   Placement of bone morphogenetic protein & spinal fusion surgery
2017, 2Q, 14   Infusion of tPA into pleural cavity
2017, 1Q, 37   Injection of glue into enteric fistula tract
2016, 4Q, 113-114 Substances applied to cranial cavity and brain
2016, 3Q, 29   Closure of bilateral alveolar clefts
2016, 1Q, 20   Metatarsophalangeal joint resection arthroplasty
2015, 3Q, 24   Esophagogastroduodenoscopy with epinephrine injection for control of bleeding
2015, 3Q, 29   Placement of adhesion barrier
2015, 2Q, 29   Insertion of nasogastric tube for drainage and feeding
2015, 2Q, 31   Thoracoscopic talc pleurodesis
2015, 1Q, 31   Intrathecal chemotherapy
2015, 1Q, 38   Chemoembolization of the hepatic artery
2014, 4Q, 16   Administration of RH (D) immunoglobulin
2014, 4Q, 17   RH (D) alloimmunization (sensitization)
2014, 4Q, 19   Ultrasound accelerated thrombolysis
2014, 4Q, 34   Resection of brain malignancy with implantation of chemotherapeutic wafer
2014, 4Q, 38   Placement of saline and seprafilm solution into abdominal cavity
2014, 3Q, 26   Coil embolization of gastroduodenal artery with chemoembolization of hepatic artery
2014, 2Q, 8   Medical induction of labor with Cervidil tampon insertion
2014, 2Q, 10   Prophylactic Neulasta injection for infection prevention
2013, 4Q, 124   Administration of tPA for stroke treatment prior to transfer
2013, 1Q, 27   Injection of sclerosing agent into an esophageal varix

AHA Coding Clinic for table 3E1

2017, 3Q, 14   Bronchoscopy with suctioning and washings for removal of mucus plug

3   **Administration**
Ø   **Circulatory**
2   **Transfusion**   Definition: Putting in blood or blood products

Body System/Region Character 4	Approach Character 5	Substance Character 6	Qualifier Character 7
3 Peripheral Vein NC **4** Central Vein NC	**Ø** Open **3** Percutaneous	**A** Stem Cells, Embryonic	**Z** No Qualifier
3 Peripheral Vein NC **4** Central Vein NC	**Ø** Open **3** Percutaneous	**G** Bone Marrow **X** Stem Cells, Cord Blood **Y** Stem Cells, Hematopoietic	**Ø** Autologous **2** Allogeneic, Related **3** Allogeneic, Unrelated **4** Allogeneic, Unspecified
3 Peripheral Vein **4** Central Vein	**Ø** Open **3** Percutaneous	**H** Whole Blood **J** Serum Albumin **K** Frozen Plasma **L** Fresh Plasma **M** Plasma Cryoprecipitate **N** Red Blood Cells **P** Frozen Red Cells **Q** White Cells **R** Platelets **S** Globulin **T** Fibrinogen **V** Antihemophilic Factors **W** Factor IX	**Ø** Autologous **1** Nonautologous
5 Peripheral Artery NC **6** Central Artery NC	**Ø** Open **3** Percutaneous	**G** Bone Marrow **H** Whole Blood **J** Serum Albumin **K** Frozen Plasma **L** Fresh Plasma **M** Plasma Cryoprecipitate **N** Red Blood Cells **P** Frozen Red Cells **Q** White Cells **R** Platelets **S** Globulin **T** Fibrinogen **V** Antihemophilic Factors **W** Factor IX **X** Stem Cells, Cord Blood **Y** Stem Cells, Hematopoietic	**Ø** Autologous **1** Nonautologous
7 Products of Conception, ♀ Circulatory	**3** Percutaneous **7** Via Natural or Artificial Opening	**H** Whole Blood **J** Serum Albumin **K** Frozen Plasma **L** Fresh Plasma **M** Plasma Cryoprecipitate **N** Red Blood Cells **P** Frozen Red Cells **Q** White Cells **R** Platelets **S** Globulin **T** Fibrinogen **V** Antihemophilic Factors **W** Factor IX	**1** Nonautologous
8 Vein	**Ø** Open **3** Percutaneous	**B** 4-Factor Prothrombin Complex Concentrate	**1** Nonautologous

Valid OR	3Ø2[3,4]ØAZ
Valid OR	3Ø2[3,4]Ø[G,X,Y][Ø,2,3,4]
Valid OR	3Ø2[3,4]3[G,X,Y][2,3,4]
Valid OR	3Ø2[5,6]Ø[G,X,Y][Ø,1]
DRG-Non-OR	3Ø2[3,4]3AZ
DRG-Non-OR	3Ø2[3,4]3[G,X,Y]Ø
DRG-Non-OR	3Ø2[5,6]3[G,X,Y][Ø,1]
NC	3Ø2[3,4][Ø,3]AZ Only when reported with PDx or SDx of C91.ØØ, C92.ØØ, C92.1Ø, C92.11, C92.4Ø, C92.5Ø, C92.6Ø, C92.AØ, C93.ØØ, C94.ØØ, C95.ØØ
NC	3Ø2[3,4][Ø,3][G,Y]Ø Only when reported with PDx or SDx of C91.ØØ, C92.ØØ, C92.1Ø, C92.11, C92.4Ø, C92.5Ø, C92.6Ø, C92.AØ, C93.ØØ, C94.ØØ, C95.ØØ
NC	3Ø2[3,4][Ø,3][G,Y][2,3,4]
NC	3Ø2[5,6][Ø,3][G,Y]Ø Only when reported with PDx or SDx of C91.ØØ, C92.ØØ, C92.1Ø, C92.11, C92.4Ø, C92.5Ø, C92.6Ø, C92.AØ, C93.ØØ, C94.ØØ, C95.ØØ
NC	3Ø2[5,6][Ø,3][G,Y]1 Only when reported with PDx or SDx of C9Ø.ØØ or C9Ø.Ø1
♀	3Ø27[3,7][H,J,K,L,M,N,P,Q,R,S,T,V,W]1

3   **Administration**
C   **Indwelling Device**
1   **Irrigation**   Definition: Putting in or on a cleansing substance

Body System/Region Character 4	Approach Character 5	Substance Character 6	Qualifier Character 7
Z None	**X** External	**8** Irrigating Substance	**Z** No Qualifier

3   Administration
E   Physiological Systems and Anatomical Regions
0   Introduction   Definition: Putting in or on a therapeutic, diagnostic, nutritional, physiological, or prophylactic substance except blood or blood products

Body System/Region Character 4	Approach Character 5	Substance Character 6	Qualifier Character 7
0 Skin and Mucous Membranes	X External	0 Antineoplastic	5 Other Antineoplastic M Monoclonal Antibody
0 Skin and Mucous Membranes	X External	2 Anti-infective	8 Oxazolidinones 9 Other Anti-infective
0 Skin and Mucous Membranes	X External	3 Anti-inflammatory 4 Serum, Toxoid and Vaccine B Anesthetic Agent K Other Diagnostic Substance M Pigment N Analgesics, Hypnotics, Sedatives T Destructive Agent	Z No Qualifier
0 Skin and Mucous Membranes	X External	G Other Therapeutic Substance	C Other Substance
1 Subcutaneous Tissue	0 Open	2 Anti-infective	A Anti-Infective Envelope
1 Subcutaneous Tissue	3 Percutaneous	0 Antineoplastic	5 Other Antineoplastic M Monoclonal Antibody
1 Subcutaneous Tissue	3 Percutaneous	2 Anti-infective	8 Oxazolidinones 9 Other Anti-infective A Anti-Infective Envelope
1 Subcutaneous Tissue	3 Percutaneous	3 Anti-inflammatory 6 Nutritional Substance 7 Electrolytic and Water Balance Substance B Anesthetic Agent H Radioactive Substance K Other Diagnostic Substance N Analgesics, Hypnotics, Sedatives T Destructive Agent	Z No Qualifier
1 Subcutaneous Tissue	3 Percutaneous	4 Serum, Toxoid and Vaccine	0 Influenza Vaccine Z No Qualifier
1 Subcutaneous Tissue	3 Percutaneous	G Other Therapeutic Substance	C Other Substance
1 Subcutaneous Tissue	3 Percutaneous	V Hormone	G Insulin J Other Hormone
2 Muscle	3 Percutaneous	0 Antineoplastic	5 Other Antineoplastic M Monoclonal Antibody
2 Muscle	3 Percutaneous	2 Anti-infective	8 Oxazolidinones 9 Other Anti-infective
2 Muscle	3 Percutaneous	3 Anti-inflammatory 6 Nutritional Substance 7 Electrolytic and Water Balance Substance B Anesthetic Agent H Radioactive Substance K Other Diagnostic Substance N Analgesics, Hypnotics, Sedatives T Destructive Agent	Z No Qualifier
2 Muscle	3 Percutaneous	4 Serum, Toxoid and Vaccine	0 Influenza Vaccine Z No Qualifier
2 Muscle	3 Percutaneous	G Other Therapeutic Substance	C Other Substance
3 Peripheral Vein	0 Open	0 Antineoplastic	2 High-dose Interleukin-2 3 Low-dose Interleukin-2 5 Other Antineoplastic M Monoclonal Antibody P Clofarabine
3 Peripheral Vein	0 Open	1 Thrombolytic	6 Recombinant Human- activated Protein C 7 Other Thrombolytic
3 Peripheral Vein	0 Open	2 Anti-infective	8 Oxazolidinones 9 Other Anti-infective

3E0 Continued on next page

DRG Non-OR	3E03002
DRG Non-OR	3E03017

3 Administration
E Physiological Systems and Anatomical Regions
0 Introduction   Definition: Putting in or on a therapeutic, diagnostic, nutritional, physiological, or prophylactic substance except blood or blood products

3E0 Continued

Body System/Region Character 4	Approach Character 5	Substance Character 6	Qualifier Character 7
3 Peripheral Vein	0 Open	3 Anti-inflammatory 4 Serum, Toxoid and Vaccine 6 Nutritional Substance 7 Electrolytic and Water Balance Substance F Intracirculatory Anesthetic H Radioactive Substance K Other Diagnostic Substance N Analgesics, Hypnotics, Sedatives P Platelet Inhibitor R Antiarrhythmic T Destructive Agent X Vasopressor	Z No Qualifier
3 Peripheral Vein	0 Open	G Other Therapeutic Substance	C Other Substance N Blood Brain Barrier Disruption
3 Peripheral Vein	0 Open	U Pancreatic Islet Cells	0 Autologous 1 Nonautologous
3 Peripheral Vein	0 Open	V Hormone	G Insulin H Human B-type Natriuretic Peptide J Other Hormone
3 Peripheral Vein	0 Open	W Immunotherapeutic	K Immunostimulator L Immunosuppressive
3 Peripheral Vein	3 Percutaneous	0 Antineoplastic	2 High-dose Interleukin-2 3 Low-dose Interleukin-2 5 Other Antineoplastic M Monoclonal Antibody P Clofarabine
3 Peripheral Vein	3 Percutaneous	1 Thrombolytic	6 Recombinant Human- activated Protein C 7 Other Thrombolytic
3 Peripheral Vein	3 Percutaneous	2 Anti-infective	8 Oxazolidinones 9 Other Anti-infective
3 Peripheral Vein	3 Percutaneous	3 Anti-inflammatory 4 Serum, Toxoid and Vaccine 6 Nutritional Substance 7 Electrolytic and Water Balance Substance F Intracirculatory Anesthetic H Radioactive Substance K Other Diagnostic Substance N Analgesics, Hypnotics, Sedatives P Platelet Inhibitor R Antiarrhythmic T Destructive Agent X Vasopressor	Z No Qualifier
3 Peripheral Vein	3 Percutaneous	G Other Therapeutic Substance	C Other Substance N Blood Brain Barrier Disruption Q Glucarpidase
3 Peripheral Vein	3 Percutaneous	U Pancreatic Islet Cells	0 Autologous 1 Nonautologous
3 Peripheral Vein	3 Percutaneous	V Hormone	G Insulin H Human B-type Natriuretic Peptide J Other Hormone
3 Peripheral Vein	3 Percutaneous	W Immunotherapeutic	K Immunostimulator L Immunosuppressive
4 Central Vein	0 Open	0 Antineoplastic	2 High-dose Interleukin-2 3 Low-dose Interleukin-2 5 Other Antineoplastic M Monoclonal Antibody P Clofarabine

3E0 Continued on next page

Valid OR	3E030TZ	DRG Non-OR	3E03317
DRG Non-OR	3E030U[0,1]	DRG Non-OR	3E033U[0,1]
DRG Non-OR	3E03302	DRG Non-OR	3E04002

LC Limited Coverage   NC Noncovered   ⊞ Combination Member   HAC   Valid OR   Combination Only   DRG Non-OR   New/Revised in GREEN

3E0 Continued

3   **Administration**
E   **Physiological Systems and Anatomical Regions**
0   **Introduction**   Definition: Putting in or on a therapeutic, diagnostic, nutritional, physiological, or prophylactic substance except blood or blood products

Body System/Region Character 4	Approach Character 5	Substance Character 6	Qualifier Character 7
4 Central Vein	0 Open	1 Thrombolytic	6 Recombinant Human- activated Protein C 7 Other Thrombolytic
4 Central Vein	0 Open	2 Anti-infective	8 Oxazolidinones 9 Other Anti-infective
4 Central Vein	0 Open	3 Anti-inflammatory 4 Serum, Toxoid and Vaccine 6 Nutritional Substance 7 Electrolytic and Water Balance Substance F Intracirculatory Anesthetic H Radioactive Substance K Other Diagnostic Substance N Analgesics, Hypnotics, Sedatives P Platelet Inhibitor R Antiarrhythmic T Destructive Agent X Vasopressor	Z No Qualifier
4 Central Vein	0 Open	G Other Therapeutic Substance	C Other Substance N Blood Brain Barrier Disruption
4 Central Vein	0 Open	V Hormone	G Insulin H Human B-type Natriuretic Peptide J Other Hormone
4 Central Vein	0 Open	W Immunotherapeutic	K Immunostimulator L Immunosuppressive
4 Central Vein	3 Percutaneous	0 Antineoplastic	2 High-dose Interleukin-2 3 Low-dose Interleukin-2 5 Other Antineoplastic M Monoclonal Antibody P Clofarabine
4 Central Vein	3 Percutaneous	1 Thrombolytic	6 Recombinant Human- activated Protein C 7 Other Thrombolytic
4 Central Vein	3 Percutaneous	2 Anti-infective	8 Oxazolidinones 9 Other Anti-infective
4 Central Vein	3 Percutaneous	3 Anti-inflammatory 4 Serum, Toxoid and Vaccine 6 Nutritional Substance 7 Electrolytic and Water Balance Substance F Intracirculatory Anesthetic H Radioactive Substance K Other Diagnostic Substance N Analgesics, Hypnotics, Sedatives P Platelet Inhibitor R Antiarrhythmic T Destructive Agent X Vasopressor	Z No Qualifier
4 Central Vein	3 Percutaneous	G Other Therapeutic Substance	C Other Substance N Blood Brain Barrier Disruption Q Glucarpidase
4 Central Vein	3 Percutaneous	V Hormone	G Insulin H Human B-type Natriuretic Peptide J Other Hormone
4 Central Vein	3 Percutaneous	W Immunotherapeutic	K Immunostimulator L Immunosuppressive
5 Peripheral Artery 6 Central Artery	0 Open 3 Percutaneous	0 Antineoplastic	2 High-dose Interleukin-2 3 Low-dose Interleukin-2 5 Other Antineoplastic M Monoclonal Antibody P Clofarabine

3E0 Continued on next page

Valid OR	3E040TZ	DRG Non-OR	3E04317
DRG Non-OR	3E04017	DRG Non-OR	3E0[5,6][0,3]02
DRG Non-OR	3E04302		

3   **Administration**
E   **Physiological Systems and Anatomical Regions**
Ø   **Introduction**   Definition: Putting in or on a therapeutic, diagnostic, nutritional, physiological, or prophylactic substance except blood or blood products

3EØ Continued

Body System/Region Character 4	Approach Character 5	Substance Character 6	Qualifier Character 7
5 Peripheral Artery 6 Central Artery	Ø Open 3 Percutaneous	1 Thrombolytic	6 Recombinant Human- activated Protein C 7 Other Thrombolytic
5 Peripheral Artery 6 Central Artery	Ø Open 3 Percutaneous	2 Anti-infective	8 Oxazolidinones 9 Other Anti-infective
5 Peripheral Artery 6 Central Artery	Ø Open 3 Percutaneous	3 Anti-inflammatory 4 Serum, Toxoid and Vaccine 6 Nutritional Substance 7 Electrolytic and Water Balance Substance F Intracirculatory Anesthetic H Radioactive Substance K Other Diagnostic Substance N Analgesics, Hypnotics, Sedatives P Platelet Inhibitor R Antiarrhythmic T Destructive Agent X Vasopressor	Z No Qualifier
5 Peripheral Artery 6 Central Artery	Ø Open 3 Percutaneous	G Other Therapeutic Substance	C Other Substance N Blood Brain Barrier Disruption
5 Peripheral Artery 6 Central Artery	Ø Open 3 Percutaneous	V Hormone	G Insulin H Human B-type Natriuretic Peptide J Other Hormone
5 Peripheral Artery 6 Central Artery	Ø Open 3 Percutaneous	W Immunotherapeutic	K Immunostimulator L Immunosuppressive
7 Coronary Artery 8 Heart	Ø Open 3 Percutaneous	1 Thrombolytic	6 Recombinant Human- activated Protein C 7 Other Thrombolytic
7 Coronary Artery 8 Heart	Ø Open 3 Percutaneous	G Other Therapeutic Substance	C Other Substance
7 Coronary Artery 8 Heart	Ø Open 3 Percutaneous	K Other Diagnostic Substance P Platelet Inhibitor	Z No Qualifier
7 Coronary Artery 8 Heart	4 Percutaneous Endoscopic	G Other Therapeutic Substance	C Other Substance
9 Nose	3 Percutaneous 7 Via Natural or Artificial Opening X External	Ø Antineoplastic	5 Other Antineoplastic M Monoclonal Antibody
9 Nose	3 Percutaneous 7 Via Natural or Artificial Opening X External	2 Anti-infective	8 Oxazolidinones 9 Other Anti-infective
9 Nose	3 Percutaneous 7 Via Natural or Artificial Opening X External	3 Anti-inflammatory 4 Serum, Toxoid and Vaccine B Anesthetic Agent H Radioactive Substance K Other Diagnostic Substance N Analgesics, Hypnotics, Sedatives T Destructive Agent	Z No Qualifier
9 Nose	3 Percutaneous 7 Via Natural or Artificial Opening X External	G Other Therapeutic Substance	C Other Substance
A Bone Marrow	3 Percutaneous	Ø Antineoplastic	5 Other Antineoplastic M Monoclonal Antibody
A Bone Marrow	3 Percutaneous	G Other Therapeutic Substance	C Other Substance
B Ear	3 Percutaneous 7 Via Natural or Artificial Opening X External	Ø Antineoplastic	4 Liquid Brachytherapy Radioisotope 5 Other Antineoplastic M Monoclonal Antibody
B Ear	3 Percutaneous 7 Via Natural or Artificial Opening X External	2 Anti-infective	8 Oxazolidinones 9 Other Anti-infective

3EØ Continued on next page

DRG Non-OR   3EØ[5,6][Ø,3]17
DRG Non-OR   3EØ8[Ø,3]17

Administration

3E0 Continued

3   **Administration**
E   **Physiological Systems and Anatomical Regions**
Ø   **Introduction**   Definition: Putting in or on a therapeutic, diagnostic, nutritional, physiological, or prophylactic substance except blood or blood products

Body System/Region Character 4	Approach Character 5	Substance Character 6	Qualifier Character 7
B Ear	3 Percutaneous 7 Via Natural or Artificial Opening X External	3 Anti-inflammatory B Anesthetic Agent H Radioactive Substance K Other Diagnostic Substance N Analgesics, Hypnotics, Sedatives T Destructive Agent	Z No Qualifier
B Ear	3 Percutaneous 7 Via Natural or Artificial Opening X External	G Other Therapeutic Substance	C Other Substance
C Eye	3 Percutaneous 7 Via Natural or Artificial Opening X External	Ø Antineoplastic	4 Liquid Brachytherapy Radioisotope 5 Other Antineoplastic M Monoclonal Antibody
C Eye	3 Percutaneous 7 Via Natural or Artificial Opening X External	2 Anti-infective	8 Oxazolidinones 9 Other Anti-infective
C Eye	3 Percutaneous 7 Via Natural or Artificial Opening X External	3 Anti-inflammatory B Anesthetic Agent H Radioactive Substance K Other Diagnostic Substance M Pigment N Analgesics, Hypnotics, Sedatives T Destructive Agent	Z No Qualifier
C Eye	3 Percutaneous 7 Via Natural or Artificial Opening X External	G Other Therapeutic Substance	C Other Substance
C Eye	3 Percutaneous 7 Via Natural or Artificial Opening X External	S Gas	F Other Gas
D Mouth and Pharynx	3 Percutaneous 7 Via Natural or Artificial Opening X External	Ø Antineoplastic	4 Liquid Brachytherapy Radioisotope 5 Other Antineoplastic M Monoclonal Antibody
D Mouth and Pharynx	3 Percutaneous 7 Via Natural or Artificial Opening X External	2 Anti-infective	8 Oxazolidinones 9 Other Anti-infective
D Mouth and Pharynx	3 Percutaneous 7 Via Natural or Artificial Opening X External	3 Anti-inflammatory 4 Serum, Toxoid and Vaccine 6 Nutritional Substance 7 Electrolytic and Water Balance Substance B Anesthetic Agent H Radioactive Substance K Other Diagnostic Substance N Analgesics, Hypnotics, Sedatives R Antiarrhythmic T Destructive Agent	Z No Qualifier
D Mouth and Pharynx	3 Percutaneous 7 Via Natural or Artificial Opening X External	G Other Therapeutic Substance	C Other Substance
E Products of Conception ♀ G Upper GI H Lower GI K Genitourinary Tract N Male Reproductive ♂	3 Percutaneous 7 Via Natural or Artificial Opening 8 Via Natural or Artificial Opening Endoscopic	Ø Antineoplastic	4 Liquid Brachytherapy Radioisotope 5 Other Antineoplastic M Monoclonal Antibody
E Products of Conception ♀ G Upper GI H Lower GI K Genitourinary Tract N Male Reproductive ♂	3 Percutaneous 7 Via Natural or Artificial Opening 8 Via Natural or Artificial Opening Endoscopic	2 Anti-infective	8 Oxazolidinones 9 Other Anti-infective

3EØ Continued on next page

♂   All approach, substance, and qualifier values for body system/region (character 4) with this icon
♀   All approach, substance, and qualifier values for body system/region (character 4) with this icon

[LC] Limited Coverage   [NC] Noncovered   ⊞ Combination Member   HAC   Valid OR   Combination Only   DRG Non-OR   New/Revised in GREEN

696   ICD-10-PCS 2019

3   Administration
E   Physiological Systems and Anatomical Regions
Ø   Introduction   Definition: Putting in or on a therapeutic, diagnostic, nutritional, physiological, or prophylactic substance except blood or blood products

3EØ Continued

Body System/Region Character 4	Approach Character 5	Substance Character 6	Qualifier Character 7
E Products of Conception ♀ G Upper GI H Lower GI K Genitourinary Tract N Male Reproductive ♂	3 Percutaneous 7 Via Natural or Artificial Opening 8 Via Natural or Artificial Opening Endoscopic	3 Anti-inflammatory 6 Nutritional Substance 7 Electrolytic and Water Balance Substance B Anesthetic Agent H Radioactive Substance K Other Diagnostic Substance N Analgesics, Hypnotics, Sedatives T Destructive Agent	Z No Qualifier
E Products of Conception ♀ G Upper GI H Lower GI K Genitourinary Tract N Male Reproductive ♂	3 Percutaneous 7 Via Natural or Artificial Opening 8 Via Natural or Artificial Opening Endoscopic	G Other Therapeutic Substance	C Other Substance
E Products of Conception ♀ G Upper GI H Lower GI K Genitourinary Tract N Male Reproductive ♂	3 Percutaneous 7 Via Natural or Artificial Opening 8 Via Natural or Artificial Opening Endoscopic	S Gas	F Other Gas
E Products of Conception ♀ G Upper GI H Lower GI K Genitourinary Tract N Male Reproductive ♂	4 Percutaneous Endoscopic	G Other Therapeutic Substance	C Other Substance
F Respiratory Tract	3 Percutaneous 7 Via Natural or Artificial Opening 8 Via Natural or Artificial Opening Endoscopic	Ø Antineoplastic	4 Liquid Brachytherapy Radioisotope 5 Other Antineoplastic M Monoclonal Antibody
F Respiratory Tract	3 Percutaneous 7 Via Natural or Artificial Opening 8 Via Natural or Artificial Opening Endoscopic	2 Anti-infective	8 Oxazolidinones 9 Other Anti-infective
F Respiratory Tract	3 Percutaneous 7 Via Natural or Artificial Opening 8 Via Natural or Artificial Opening Endoscopic	3 Anti-inflammatory 6 Nutritional Substance 7 Electrolytic and Water Balance Substance B Anesthetic Agent H Radioactive Substance K Other Diagnostic Substance N Analgesics, Hypnotics, Sedatives T Destructive Agent	Z No Qualifier
F Respiratory Tract	3 Percutaneous 7 Via Natural or Artificial Opening 8 Via Natural or Artificial Opening Endoscopic	G Other Therapeutic Substance	C Other Substance
F Respiratory Tract	3 Percutaneous 7 Via Natural or Artificial Opening 8 Via Natural or Artificial Opening Endoscopic	S Gas	D Nitric Oxide F Other Gas
F Respiratory Tract	4 Percutaneous Endoscopic	G Other Therapeutic Substance	C Other Substance
J Biliary and Pancreatic Tract	3 Percutaneous 7 Via Natural or Artificial Opening 8 Via Natural or Artificial Opening Endoscopic	Ø Antineoplastic	4 Liquid Brachytherapy Radioisotope 5 Other Antineoplastic M Monoclonal Antibody

3EØ Continued on next page

♂   All approach, substance, and qualifier values for body system/region (character 4) with this icon
♀   All approach, substance, and qualifier values for body system/region (character 4) with this icon

3E0 Continued

Administration

3   **Administration**
E   **Physiological Systems and Anatomical Regions**
0   **Introduction**   Definition: Putting in or on a therapeutic, diagnostic, nutritional, physiological, or prophylactic substance except blood or blood products

Body System/Region Character 4	Approach Character 5	Substance Character 6	Qualifier Character 7
J Biliary and Pancreatic Tract	3 Percutaneous 7 Via Natural or Artificial Opening 8 Via Natural or Artificial Opening Endoscopic	2 Anti-infective	8 Oxazolidinones 9 Other Anti-infective
J Biliary and Pancreatic Tract	3 Percutaneous 7 Via Natural or Artificial Opening 8 Via Natural or Artificial Opening Endoscopic	3 Anti-inflammatory 6 Nutritional Substance 7 Electrolytic and Water Balance Substance B Anesthetic Agent H Radioactive Substance K Other Diagnostic Substance N Analgesics, Hypnotics, Sedatives T Destructive Agent	Z No Qualifier
J Biliary and Pancreatic Tract	3 Percutaneous 7 Via Natural or Artificial Opening 8 Via Natural or Artificial Opening Endoscopic	G Other Therapeutic Substance	C Other Substance
J Biliary and Pancreatic Tract	3 Percutaneous 7 Via Natural or Artificial Opening 8 Via Natural or Artificial Opening Endoscopic	S Gas	F Other Gas
J Biliary and Pancreatic Tract	3 Percutaneous 7 Via Natural or Artificial Opening 8 Via Natural or Artificial Opening Endoscopic	U Pancreatic Islet Cells	0 Autologous 1 Nonautologous
J Biliary and Pancreatic Tract	4 Percutaneous Endoscopic	G Other Therapeutic Substance	C Other Substance
L Pleural Cavity M Peritoneal Cavity	0 Open	5 Adhesion Barrier	Z No Qualifier
L Pleural Cavity M Peritoneal Cavity	3 Percutaneous	0 Antineoplastic	4 Liquid Brachytherapy Radioisotope 5 Other Antineoplastic M Monoclonal Antibody
L Pleural Cavity M Peritoneal Cavity	3 Percutaneous	2 Anti-infective	8 Oxazolidinones 9 Other Anti-infective
L Pleural Cavity M Peritoneal Cavity	3 Percutaneous	3 Anti-inflammatory 5 Adhesion Barrier 6 Nutritional Substance 7 Electrolytic and Water Balance Substance B Anesthetic Agent H Radioactive Substance K Other Diagnostic Substance N Analgesics, Hypnotics, Sedatives T Destructive Agent	Z No Qualifier
L Pleural Cavity M Peritoneal Cavity	3 Percutaneous	G Other Therapeutic Substance	C Other Substance
L Pleural Cavity M Peritoneal Cavity	3 Percutaneous	S Gas	F Other Gas
L Pleural Cavity M Peritoneal Cavity	4 Percutaneous Endoscopic	5 Adhesion Barrier	Z No Qualifier
L Pleural Cavity M Peritoneal Cavity	4 Percutaneous Endoscopic	G Other Therapeutic Substance	C Other Substance
L Pleural Cavity M Peritoneal Cavity	7 Via Natural or Artificial Opening	0 Antineoplastic	4 Liquid Brachytherapy Radioisotope 5 Other Antineoplastic M Monoclonal Antibody
L Pleural Cavity M Peritoneal Cavity	7 Via Natural or Artificial Opening	S Gas	F Other Gas
P Female Reproductive ♀	0 Open	5 Adhesion Barrier	Z No Qualifier
P Female Reproductive ♀	3 Percutaneous	0 Antineoplastic	4 Liquid Brachytherapy Radioisotope 5 Other Antineoplastic M Monoclonal Antibody
P Female Reproductive ♀	3 Percutaneous	2 Anti-infective	8 Oxazolidinones 9 Other Anti-infective

3E0 Continued on next page

DRG Non-OR   3E0J[3,7,8]U[0,1]
♀   All approach, substance, and qualifier values for body system/region (character 4) with this icon

3   **Administration**
E   **Physiological Systems and Anatomical Regions**
Ø   **Introduction**   Definition: Putting in or on a therapeutic, diagnostic, nutritional, physiological, or prophylactic substance except blood or blood products

3EØ Continued

Body System/Region Character 4		Approach Character 5	Substance Character 6	Qualifier Character 7
P	Female Reproductive ♀	3 Percutaneous	3 Anti-inflammatory 5 Adhesion Barrier 6 Nutritional Substance 7 Electrolytic and Water Balance Substance B Anesthetic Agent H Radioactive Substance K Other Diagnostic Substance L Sperm N Analgesics, Hypnotics, Sedatives T Destructive Agent V Hormone	Z No Qualifier
P	Female Reproductive ♀	3 Percutaneous	G Other Therapeutic Substance	C Other Substance
P	Female Reproductive ♀	3 Percutaneous	Q Fertilized Ovum	Ø Autologous 1 Nonautologous
P	Female Reproductive ♀	3 Percutaneous	S Gas	F Other Gas
P	Female Reproductive ♀	4 Percutaneous Endoscopic	5 Adhesion Barrier	Z No Qualifier
P	Female Reproductive ♀	4 Percutaneous Endoscopic	G Other Therapeutic Substance	C Other Substance
P	Female Reproductive ♀	7 Via Natural or Artificial Opening	Ø Antineoplastic	4 Liquid Brachytherapy Radioisotope 5 Other Antineoplastic M Monoclonal Antibody
P	Female Reproductive ♀	7 Via Natural or Artificial Opening	2 Anti-infective	8 Oxazolidinones 9 Other Anti-infective
P	Female Reproductive ♀	7 Via Natural or Artificial Opening	3 Anti-inflammatory 6 Nutritional Substance 7 Electrolytic and Water Balance Substance B Anesthetic Agent H Radioactive Substance K Other Diagnostic Substance L Sperm N Analgesics, Hypnotics, Sedatives T Destructive Agent V Hormone	Z No Qualifier
P	Female Reproductive ♀	7 Via Natural or Artificial Opening	G Other Therapeutic Substance	C Other Substance
P	Female Reproductive ♀	7 Via Natural or Artificial Opening	Q Fertilized Ovum	Ø Autologous 1 Nonautologous
P	Female Reproductive ♀	7 Via Natural or Artificial Opening	S Gas	F Other Gas
P	Female Reproductive ♀	8 Via Natural or Artificial Opening Endoscopic	Ø Antineoplastic	4 Liquid Brachytherapy Radioisotope 5 Other Antineoplastic M Monoclonal Antibody
P	Female Reproductive ♀	8 Via Natural or Artificial Opening Endoscopic	2 Anti-infective	8 Oxazolidinones 9 Other Anit-infection
P	Female Reproductive ♀	8 Via Natural or Artificial Opening Endoscopic	3 Anti-inflammatory 6 Nutritional Substance 7 Electrolytic and Water Balance Substance B Anesthetic Agent H Radioactive Substance K Other Diagnostic Substance N Analgesics, Hypnotics, Sedative T Destructive Agent	Z No Qualifier
P	Female Reproductive ♀	8 Via Natural or Artificial Opening Endoscopic	G Other Therapeutic Substance	C Other Substance
P	Female Reproductive ♀	8 Via Natural or Artificial Opening Endoscopic	S Gas	F Other Gas
Q	Cranial Cavity and Brain	Ø Open 3 Percutaneous	Ø Antineoplastic	4 Liquid Brachytherapy Radioisotope 5 Other Antineoplastic M Monoclonal Antibody
Q	Cranial Cavity and Brain	Ø Open 3 Percutaneous	2 Anti-infective	8 Oxazolidinones 9 Other Anti-infective

3EØ Continued on next page

Valid OR	3E0P3Q[Ø,1]	
Valid OR	3E0P7Q[Ø,1]	
DRG Non-OR	3E0Q[Ø,3]Ø5	
♀	All approach, substance, and qualifier values for body system/region (character 4) with this icon	

LC Limited Coverage   NC Noncovered   ⊞ Combination Member   HAC   Valid OR   Combination Only   DRG Non-OR   New/Revised in GREEN

Administration

3   **Administration**
E   **Physiological Systems and Anatomical Regions**
Ø   **Introduction**   Definition: Putting in or on a therapeutic, diagnostic, nutritional, physiological, or prophylactic substance except blood or blood products

Body System/Region Character 4	Approach Character 5	Substance Character 6	Qualifier Character 7
Q Cranial Cavity and Brain	Ø Open 3 Percutaneous	3 Anti-inflammatory 6 Nutritional Substance 7 Electrolytic and Water Balance Substance A Stem Cells, Embryonic B Anesthetic Agent H Radioactive Substance K Other Diagnostic Substance N Analgesics, Hypnotics, Sedatives T Destructive Agent	Z No Qualifier
Q Cranial Cavity and Brain	Ø Open 3 Percutaneous	E Stem Cells, Somatic	Ø Autologous 1 Nonautologous
Q Cranial Cavity and Brain	Ø Open 3 Percutaneous	G Other Therapeutic Substance	C Other Substance
Q Cranial Cavity and Brain	Ø Open 3 Percutaneous	S Gas	F Other Gas
Q Cranial Cavity and Brain	7 Via Natural or Artificial Opening	Ø Antineoplastic	4 Liquid Brachytherapy Radioisotope 5 Other Antineoplastic M Monoclonal Antibody
Q Cranial Cavity and Brain	7 Via Natural or Artificial Opening	S Gas	F Other Gas
R Spinal Canal	Ø Open	A Stem Cells, Embryonic	Z No Qualifier
R Spinal Canal	Ø Open	E Stem Cells, Somatic	Ø Autologous 1 Nonautologous
R Spinal Canal	3 Percutaneous	Ø Antineoplastic	2 High-dose Interleukin-2 3 Low-dose Interleukin-2 4 Liquid Brachytherapy Radioisotope 5 Other Antineoplastic M Monoclonal Antibody
R Spinal Canal	3 Percutaneous	2 Anti-infective	8 Oxazolidinones 9 Other Anti-infective
R Spinal Canal	3 Percutaneous	3 Anti-inflammatory 6 Nutritional Substance 7 Electrolytic and Water Balance Substance A Stem Cells, Embryonic B Anesthetic Agent H Radioactive Substance K Other Diagnostic Substance N Analgesics, Hypnotics, Sedatives T Destructive Agent	Z No Qualifier
R Spinal Canal	3 Percutaneous	E Stem Cells, Somatic	Ø Autologous 1 Nonautologous
R Spinal Canal	3 Percutaneous	G Other Therapeutic Substance	C Other Substance
R Spinal Canal	3 Percutaneous	S Gas	F Other Gas
R Spinal Canal	7 Via Natural or Artificial Opening	S Gas	F Other Gas
S Epidural Space	3 Percutaneous	Ø Antineoplastic	2 High-dose Interleukin-2 3 Low-dose Interleukin-2 4 Liquid Brachytherapy Radioisotope 5 Other Antineoplastic M Monoclonal Antibody
S Epidural Space	3 Percutaneous	2 Anti-infective	8 Oxazolidinones 9 Other Anti-infective
S Epidural Space	3 Percutaneous	3 Anti-inflammatory 6 Nutritional Substance 7 Electrolytic and Water Balance Substance B Anesthetic Agent H Radioactive Substance K Other Diagnostic Substance N Analgesics, Hypnotics, Sedatives T Destructive Agent	Z No Qualifier

3EØ Continued on next page

DRG Non-OR	3EØQ7Ø5
DRG Non-OR	3EØR3Ø2
DRG Non-OR	3EØS3Ø2

LC Limited Coverage   **NC** Noncovered   ⊞ Combination Member   HAC   Valid OR   Combination Only   DRG Non-OR   New/Revised in GREEN

3   **Administration**
E   **Physiological Systems and Anatomical Regions**
Ø   **Introduction**   Definition: Putting in or on a therapeutic, diagnostic, nutritional, physiological, or prophylactic substance except blood or blood products

3EØ Continued

Body System/Region Character 4	Approach Character 5	Substance Character 6	Qualifier Character 7
S Epidural Space	**3** Percutaneous	**G** Other Therapeutic Substance	**C** Other Substance
S Epidural Space	**3** Percutaneous	**S** Gas	**F** Other Gas
S Epidural Space	**7** Via Natural or Artificial Opening	**S** Gas	**F** Other Gas
T Peripheral Nerves and Plexi **X** Cranial Nerves	**3** Percutaneous	**3** Anti-inflammatory **B** Anesthetic Agent **T** Destructive Agent	**Z** No Qualifier
T Peripheral Nerves and Plexi **X** Cranial Nerves	**3** Percutaneous	**G** Other Therapeutic Substance	**C** Other Substance
U Joints	**Ø** Open	**2** Anti-infective	**8** Oxazolidinones **9** Other Anti-infective
U Joints	**Ø** Open	**G** Other Therapeutic Substance	**B** Recombinant Bone Morphogenetic Protein
U Joints	**3** Percutaneous	**Ø** Antineoplastic	**4** Liquid Brachytherapy Radioisotope **5** Other Antineoplastic **M** Monoclonal Antibody
U Joints	**3** Percutaneous	**2** Anti-infective	**8** Oxazolidinones **9** Other Anti-infective
U Joints	**3** Percutaneous	**3** Anti-inflammatory **6** Nutritional Substance **7** Electrolytic and Water Balance Substance **B** Anesthetic Agent **H** Radioactive Substance **K** Other Diagnostic Substance **N** Analgesics, Hypnotics, Sedatives **T** Destructive Agent	**Z** No Qualifier
U Joints	**3** Percutaneous	**G** Other Therapeutic Substance	**B** Recombinant Bone Morphogenetic Protein **C** Other Substance
U Joints	**3** Percutaneous	**S** Gas	**F** Other Gas
U Joints	**4** Percutaneous Endoscopic	**G** Other Therapeutic Substance	**C** Other Substance
V Bones	**Ø** Open	**G** Other Therapeutic Substance	**B** Recombinant Bone Morphogenetic Protein
V Bones	**3** Percutaneous	**Ø** Antineoplastic	**5** Other Antineoplastic **M** Monoclonal Antibody
V Bones	**3** Percutaneous	**2** Anti-infective	**8** Oxazolidinones **9** Other Anti-infective
V Bones	**3** Percutaneous	**3** Anti-inflammatory **6** Nutritional Substance **7** Electrolytic and Water Balance Substance **B** Anesthetic Agent **H** Radioactive Substance **K** Other Diagnostic Substance **N** Analgesics, Hypnotics, Sedatives **T** Destructive Agent	**Z** No Qualifier
V Bones	**3** Percutaneous	**G** Other Therapeutic Substance	**B** Recombinant Bone Morphogenetic Protein **C** Other Substance
W Lymphatics	**3** Percutaneous	**Ø** Antineoplastic	**5** Other Antineoplastic **M** Monoclonal Antibody
W Lymphatics	**3** Percutaneous	**2** Anti-infective	**8** Oxazolidinones **9** Other Anti-infective
W Lymphatics	**3** Percutaneous	**3** Anti-inflammatory **6** Nutritional Substance **7** Electrolytic and Water Balance Substance **B** Anesthetic Agent **H** Radioactive Substance **K** Other Diagnostic Substance **N** Analgesics, Hypnotics, Sedatives **T** Destructive Agent	**Z** No Qualifier

3EØ Continued on next page

LC Limited Coverage   NC Noncovered   ⊞ Combination Member   HAC   Valid OR   Combination Only   DRG Non-OR   New/Revised in GREEN

Administration

3EØ Continued

3　**Administration**
E　**Physiological Systems and Anatomical Regions**
Ø　**Introduction**　　Definition: Putting in or on a therapeutic, diagnostic, nutritional, physiological, or prophylactic substance except blood or blood products

Body System/Region Character 4	Approach Character 5	Substance Character 6	Qualifier Character 7
W Lymphatics	3 Percutaneous	G Other Therapeutic Substance	C Other Substance
Y Pericardial Cavity	3 Percutaneous	Ø Antineoplastic	4 Liquid Brachytherapy Radioisotope 5 Other Antineoplastic M Monoclonal Antibody
Y Pericardial Cavity	3 Percutaneous	2 Anti-infective	8 Oxazolidinones 9 Other Anti-infective
Y Pericardial Cavity	3 Percutaneous	3 Anti-inflammatory 6 Nutritional Substance 7 Electrolytic and Water Balance Substance B Anesthetic Agent H Radioactive Substance K Other Diagnostic Substance N Analgesics, Hypnotics, Sedatives T Destructive Agent	Z No Qualifier
Y Pericardial Cavity	3 Percutaneous	G Other Therapeutic Substance	C Other Substance
Y Pericardial Cavity	3 Percutaneous	S Gas	F Other Gas
Y Pericardial Cavity	4 Percutaneous Endoscopic	G Other Therapeutic Substance	C Other Substance
Y Pericardial Cavity	7 Via Natural or Artificial Opening	Ø Antineoplastic	4 Liquid Brachytherapy Radioisotope 5 Other Antineoplastic M Monoclonal Antibody
Y Pericardial Cavity	7 Via Natural or Artificial Opening	S Gas	F Other Gas

3　**Administration**
E　**Physiological Systems and Anatomical Regions**
1　**Irrigation**　　Definition: Putting in or on a cleansing substance

Body System/Region Character 4	Approach Character 5	Substance Character 6	Qualifier Character 7
Ø Skin and Mucous Membranes C Eye	3 Percutaneous X External	8 Irrigating Substance	X Diagnostic Z No Qualifier
9 Nose B Ear F Respiratory Tract G Upper GI H Lower GI J Biliary and Pancreatic Tract K Genitourinary Tract N Male Reproductive ♂ P Female Reproductive ♀	3 Percutaneous 7 Via Natural or Artificial Opening 8 Via Natural or Artificial Opening Endoscopic	8 Irrigating Substance	X Diagnostic Z No Qualifier
L Pleural Cavity Q Cranial Cavity and Brain R Spinal Canal S Epidural Space U Joints Y Pericardial Cavity	3 Percutaneous	8 Irrigating Substance	X Diagnostic Z No Qualifier
M Peritoneal Cavity	3 Percutaneous	8 Irrigating Substance	X Diagnostic Z No Qualifier
M Peritoneal Cavity	3 Percutaneous	9 Dialysate	Z No Qualifier

♂　3E1N[3,7,8]8[X,Z]
♀　3E1P[3,7,8]8[X,Z]

Measurement and Monitoring 4A0–4B0

Character Meanings

This Character Meaning table is provided as a guide to assist the user in the identification of character members that may be found in this section of code tables. It **SHOULD NOT** be used to build a PCS code.

A: Physiological Systems

Operation–Character 3	Body System–Character 4	Approach–Character 5	Function/Device–Character 6	Qualifier–Character 7
0 Measurement	0 Central Nervous	0 Open	0 Acuity	0 Central
1 Monitoring	1 Peripheral Nervous	3 Percutaneous	1 Capacity	1 Peripheral
	2 Cardiac	4 Percutaneous Endoscopic	2 Conductivity	2 Portal
	3 Arterial	7 Via Natural or Artificial Opening	3 Contractility	3 Pulmonary
	4 Venous	8 Via Natural or Artificial Opening Endoscopic	4 Electrical Activity	4 Stress
	5 Circulatory	X External	5 Flow	5 Ambulatory
	6 Lymphatic		6 Metabolism	6 Right Heart
	7 Visual		7 Mobility	7 Left Heart
	8 Olfactory		8 Motility	8 Bilateral
	9 Respiratory		9 Output	9 Sensory
	B Gastrointestinal		B Pressure	A Guidance
	C Biliary		C Rate	B Motor
	D Urinary		D Resistance	C Coronary
	F Musculoskeletal		F Rhythm	D Intracranial
	G Skin and Breast		G Secretion	F Other Thoracic
	H Products of Conception, Cardiac		H Sound	G Intraoperative
	J Products of Conception, Nervous		J Pulse	H Indocyanine Green Dye
	Z None		K Temperature	Z No Qualifier
			L Volume	
			M Total Activity	
			N Sampling and Pressure	
			P Action Currents	
			Q Sleep	
			R Saturation	
			S Vascular Perfusion	

B: Physiological Devices

Operation–Character 3	Body System–Character 4	Approach–Character 5	Function/Device–Character 6	Qualifier–Character 7
0 Measurement	0 Central Nervous	X External	S Pacemaker	Z No Qualifier
	1 Peripheral Nervous		T Defibrillator	
	2 Cardiac		V Stimulator	
	9 Respiratory			
	F Musculoskeletal			

AHA Coding Clinic for table 4A0

2018, 1Q, 12	Percutaneous balloon valvuloplasty & cardiac catheterization with ventriculogram
2016, 3Q, 37	Fractional flow reserve
2015, 3Q, 29	Approach value for esophageal electrophysiology study

AHA Coding Clinic for table 4A1

2016, 4Q, 114	Fluorescence vascular angiography
2016, 2Q, 29	Decompressive craniectomy with cryopreservation and storage of bone flap
2016, 2Q, 33	Monitoring of arterial pressure & pulse
2015, 3Q, 35	Swan Ganz catheterization
2015, 2Q, 14	Intraoperative EMG monitoring via endotracheal tube
2015, 1Q, 26	Intraoperative monitoring using Sentio MMG®
2014, 4Q, 28	Removal and replacement of displaced growing rods

4   Measurement and Monitoring
A   Physiological Systems
0   Measurement   Definition: Determining the level of a physiological or physical function at a point in time

Body System Character 4	Approach Character 5	Function/Device Character 6	Qualifier Character 7
0 Central Nervous	0 Open	2 Conductivity 4 Electrical Activity B Pressure	Z No Qualifier
0 Central Nervous	3 Percutaneous 7 Via Natural or Artificial Opening 8 Via Natural or Artificial Opening Endoscopic	4 Electrical Activity	Z No Qualifier
0 Central Nervous	3 Percutaneous 7 Via Natural or Artificial Opening 8 Via Natural or Artificial Opening Endoscopic	B Pressure K Temperature R Saturation	D Intracranial
0 Central Nervous	X External	2 Conductivity 4 Electrical Activity	Z No Qualifier
1 Peripheral Nervous	0 Open 3 Percutaneous 7 Via Natural or Artificial Opening 8 Via Natural or Artificial Opening Endoscopic X External	2 Conductivity	9 Sensory B Motor
1 Peripheral Nervous	0 Open 3 Percutaneous 7 Via Natural or Artificial Opening 8 Via Natural or Artificial Opening Endoscopic X External	4 Electrical Activity	Z No Qualifier
2 Cardiac	0 Open 3 Percutaneous 7 Via Natural or Artificial Opening 8 Via Natural or Artificial Opening Endoscopic	4 Electrical Activity 9 Output C Rate F Rhythm H Sound P Action Currents	Z No Qualifier
2 Cardiac	0 Open 3 Percutaneous 7 Via Natural or Artificial Opening 8 Via Natural or Artificial Opening Endoscopic	N Sampling and Pressure	6 Right Heart 7 Left Heart 8 Bilateral
2 Cardiac	X External	4 Electrical Activity	A Guidance Z No Qualifier
2 Cardiac	X External	9 Output C Rate F Rhythm H Sound P Action Currents	Z No Qualifier
2 Cardiac	X External	M Total Activity	4 Stress
3 Arterial	0 Open 3 Percutaneous	5 Flow J Pulse	1 Peripheral 3 Pulmonary C Coronary
3 Arterial	0 Open 3 Percutaneous	B Pressure	1 Peripheral 3 Pulmonary C Coronary F Other Thoracic
3 Arterial	0 Open 3 Percutaneous	H Sound R Saturation	1 Peripheral
3 Arterial	X External	5 Flow B Pressure H Sound J Pulse R Saturation	1 Peripheral

4A0 Continued on next page

DRG Non-OR   4A02[3,7,8]FZ
DRG Non-OR   4A02[0,3,7,8]N[6,7,8]

4   Measurement and Monitoring
A   Physiological Systems
Ø   Measurement   Definition: Determining the level of a physiological or physical function at a point in time

4AØ Continued

Body System Character 4	Approach Character 5	Function/Device Character 6	Qualifier Character 7
4 Venous	Ø Open 3 Percutaneous	5 Flow B Pressure J Pulse	Ø Central 1 Peripheral 2 Portal 3 Pulmonary
4 Venous	Ø Open 3 Percutaneous	R Saturation	1 Peripheral
4 Venous	X External	5 Flow B Pressure J Pulse R Saturation	1 Peripheral
5 Circulatory	X External	L Volume	Z No Qualifier
6 Lymphatic	Ø Open 3 Percutaneous 7 Via Natural or Artificial Opening 8 Via Natural or Artificial Opening Endoscopic	5 Flow B Pressure	Z No Qualifier
7 Visual	X External	Ø Acuity 7 Mobility B Pressure	Z No Qualifier
8 Olfactory	X External	Ø Acuity	Z No Qualifier
9 Respiratory	7 Via Natural or Artificial Opening 8 Via Natural or Artificial Opening Endoscopic X External	1 Capacity 5 Flow C Rate D Resistance L Volume M Total Activity	Z No Qualifier
B Gastrointestinal	7 Via Natural or Artificial Opening 8 Via Natural or Artificial Opening Endoscopic	8 Motility B Pressure G Secretion	Z No Qualifier
C Biliary	3 Percutaneous 4 Percutaneous Endoscopic 7 Via Natural or Artificial Opening 8 Via Natural or Artificial Opening Endoscopic	5 Flow B Pressure	Z No Qualifier
D Urinary	7 Via Natural or Artificial Opening 8 Via Natural or Artificial Opening Endoscopic	3 Contractility 5 Flow B Pressure D Resistance L Volume	Z No Qualifier
F Musculoskeletal	3 Percutaneous X External	3 Contractility	Z No Qualifier
H Products of Conception, Cardiac ♀	7 Via Natural or Artificial Opening 8 Via Natural or Artificial Opening Endoscopic X External	4 Electrical Activity C Rate F Rhythm H Sound	Z No Qualifier
J Products of Conception, Nervous ♀	7 Via Natural or Artificial Opening 8 Via Natural or Artificial Opening Endoscopic X External	2 Conductivity 4 Electrical Activity B Pressure	Z No Qualifier
Z None	7 Via Natural or Artificial Opening	6 Metabolism K Temperature	Z No Qualifier
Z None	X External	6 Metabolism K Temperature Q Sleep	Z No Qualifier

Valid OR   4AØ6Ø[5,B]Z   ♀   4AØH[7,8,X][4,C,F,H]Z
Valid OR   4AØC4[5,B]Z   ♀   4AØJ[7,8,X][2,4,B]Z

4   Measurement and Monitoring
A   Physiological Systems
1   Monitoring   Definition: Determining the level of a physiological or physical function repetitively over a period of time

Body System Character 4	Approach Character 5	Function/Device Character 6	Qualifier Character 7
Ø Central Nervous	Ø Open	2 Conductivity B Pressure	Z No Qualifier
Ø Central Nervous	Ø Open	4 Electrical Activity	G Intraoperative Z No Qualifier
Ø Central Nervous	3 Percutaneous 7 Via Natural or Artificial Opening 8 Via Natural or Artificial Opening Endoscopic	4 Electrical Activity	G Intraoperative Z No Qualifier
Ø Central Nervous	3 Percutaneous 7 Via Natural or Artificial Opening 8 Via Natural or Artificial Opening Endoscopic	B Pressure K Temperature R Saturation	D Intracranial
Ø Central Nervous	X External	2 Conductivity	Z No Qualifier
Ø Central Nervous	X External	4 Electrical Activity	G Intraoperative Z No Qualifier
1 Peripheral Nervous	Ø Open 3 Percutaneous 7 Via Natural or Artificial Opening 8 Via Natural or Artificial Opening Endoscopic X External	2 Conductivity	9 Sensory B Motor
1 Peripheral Nervous	Ø Open 3 Percutaneous 7 Via Natural or Artificial Opening 8 Via Natural or Artificial Opening Endoscopic X External	4 Electrical Activity	G Intraoperative Z No Qualifier
2 Cardiac	Ø Open 3 Percutaneous 7 Via Natural or Artificial Opening 8 Via Natural or Artificial Opening Endoscopic	4 Electrical Activity 9 Output C Rate F Rhythm H Sound	Z No Qualifier
2 Cardiac	X External	4 Electrical Activity	5 Ambulatory Z No Qualifier
2 Cardiac	X External	9 Output C Rate F Rhythm H Sound	Z No Qualifier
2 Cardiac	X External	M Total Activity	4 Stress
2 Cardiac	X External	S Vascular Perfusion	H Indocyanine Green Dye
3 Arterial	Ø Open 3 Percutaneous	5 Flow B Pressure J Pulse	1 Peripheral 3 Pulmonary C Coronary
3 Arterial	Ø Open 3 Percutaneous	H Sound R Saturation	1 Peripheral
3 Arterial	X External	5 Flow B Pressure H Sound J Pulse R Saturation	1 Peripheral
4 Venous	Ø Open 3 Percutaneous	5 Flow B Pressure J Pulse	Ø Central 1 Peripheral 2 Portal 3 Pulmonary
4 Venous	Ø Open 3 Percutaneous	R Saturation	Ø Central 2 Portal 3 Pulmonary
4 Venous	X External	5 Flow B Pressure J Pulse	1 Peripheral
6 Lymphatic	Ø Open 3 Percutaneous 7 Via Natural or Artificial Opening 8 Via Natural or Artificial Opening Endoscopic	5 Flow B Pressure	Z No Qualifier

4A1 Continued on next page

Valid OR   4A16Ø[5,B]Z

4   Measurement and Monitoring
A   Physiological Systems
1   Monitoring   Definition: Determining the level of a physiological or physical function repetitively over a period of time

Body System Character 4	Approach Character 5	Function/Device Character 6	Qualifier Character 7
9 Respiratory	**7** Via Natural or Artificial Opening **X** External	**1** Capacity **5** Flow **C** Rate **D** Resistance **L** Volume	**Z** No Qualifier
B Gastrointestinal	**7** Via Natural or Artificial Opening **8** Via Natural or Artificial Opening Endoscopic	**8** Motility **B** Pressure **G** Secretion	**Z** No Qualifier
B Gastrointestinal	**X** External	**S** Vascular Perfusion	**H** Indocyanine Green Dye
D Urinary	**7** Via Natural or Artificial Opening **8** Via Natural or Artificial Opening Endoscopic	**3** Contractility **5** Flow **B** Pressure **D** Resistance **L** Volume	**Z** No Qualifier
G Skin and Breast	**X** External	**S** Vascular Perfusion	**H** Indocyanine Green Dye
H Products of Conception, Cardiac ♀	**7** Via Natural or Artificial Opening **8** Via Natural or Artificial Opening Endoscopic **X** External	**4** Electrical Activity **C** Rate **F** Rhythm **H** Sound	**Z** No Qualifier
J Products of Conception, Nervous ♀	**7** Via Natural or Artificial Opening **8** Via Natural or Artificial Opening Endoscopic **X** External	**2** Conductivity **4** Electrical Activity **B** Pressure	**Z** No Qualifier
Z None	**7** Via Natural or Artificial Opening	**K** Temperature	**Z** No Qualifier
Z None	**X** External	**K** Temperature **Q** Sleep	**Z** No Qualifier

♀   4A1H[7,8,X][4,C,F,H]Z
♀   4A1J[7,8,X][2,4,B]Z

4   Measurement and Monitoring
B   Physiological Devices
Ø   Measurement   Definition: Determining the level of a physiological or physical function at a point in time

Body System Character 4	Approach Character 5	Function/Device Character 6	Qualifier Character 7
Ø Central Nervous **1** Peripheral Nervous **F** Musculoskeletal	**X** External	**V** Stimulator	**Z** No Qualifier
2 Cardiac	**X** External	**S** Pacemaker **T** Defibrillator	**Z** No Qualifier
9 Respiratory	**X** External	**S** Pacemaker	**Z** No Qualifier

Extracorporeal or Systemic Assistance and Performance 5A0–5A2

Character Meanings

This Character Meaning table is provided as a guide to assist the user in the identification of character members that may be found in this section of code tables. It **SHOULD NOT** be used to build a PCS code.

A: Physiological Systems

Operation–Character 3		Body System–Character 4		Duration–Character 5		Function–Character 6		Qualifier–Character 7	
0	Assistance	2	Cardiac	0	Single	0	Filtration	0	Balloon Pump
1	Performance	5	Circulatory	1	Intermittent	1	Output	1	Hyperbaric
2	Restoration	9	Respiratory	2	Continuous	2	Oxygenation	2	Manual
		C	Biliary	3	Less than 24 Consecutive Hours	3	Pacing	4	Nonmechanical
		D	Urinary	4	24-96 Consecutive Hours	4	Rhythm	5	Pulsatile Compression
				5	Greater than 96 Consecutive Hours	5	Ventilation	6	Other Pump
				6	Multiple			7	Continuous Positive Airway Pressure
				7	Intermittent, Less than 6 Hours per Day			8	Intermittent Positive Airway Pressure
				8	Prolonged Intermittent, 6-18 hours per Day			9	Continuous Negative Airway Pressure
				9	Continuous, Greater than 18 hours per Day			B	Intermittent Negative Airway Pressure
								C	Supersaturated
								D	Impeller Pump
								F	Membrane, Central
								G	Membrane, Peripheral Veno-arterial
								H	Membrane, Peripheral Veno-venous
								Z	No Qualifier

AHA Coding Clinic for table 5A0

2018, 2Q, 3-5	Intra-aortic balloon pump
2017, 4Q, 43-44	Insertion of external heart assist devices
2017, 3Q, 18	Intra-aortic balloon pump removal
2017, 1Q, 10-11	External heart assist device
2017, 1Q, 29	Newborn resuscitation using positive pressure ventilation
2017, 1Q, 29	Newborn noninvasive ventilation
2016, 4Q, 137-139	Heart assist device systems
2014, 4Q, 9	Mechanical ventilation
2014, 3Q, 19	Ablation of ventricular tachycardia with Impella® support
2013, 3Q, 18	Heart transplant surgery

AHA Coding Clinic for table 5A1

2018, 1Q, 13	Mechanical ventilation using patient's equipment
2017, 4Q, 71-73	Hemodialysis and renal replacement therapy
2017, 3Q, 7	Senning procedure (arterial switch)
2017, 1Q, 19	Norwood Sano procedure
2016, 1Q, 27	Aortocoronary bypass graft utilizing Y-graft
2016, 1Q, 28	Extracorporeal liver assist device
2016, 1Q, 29	Duration of hemodialysis
2015, 4Q, 22-24	Congenital heart corrective procedures
2014, 4Q, 3-10	Mechanical ventilation
2014, 4Q, 11-15	Sequencing of mechanical ventilation with other procedures
2014, 3Q, 16	Repair of Tetralogy of Fallot
2014, 3Q, 20	MAZE procedure performed with coronary artery bypass graft
2014, 1Q, 10	Repair of thoracic aortic aneurysm & coronary artery bypass graft
2013, 3Q, 18	Heart transplant surgery

5   Extracorporeal or Systemic Assistance and Performance
A   Physiological Systems
0   Assistance   Definition: Taking over a portion of a physiological function by extracorporeal means

Body System Character 4	Duration Character 5	Function Character 6	Qualifier Character 7
2 Cardiac	1 Intermittent 2 Continuous	1 Output	0 Balloon Pump 5 Pulsatile Compression 6 Other Pump D Impeller Pump
5 Circulatory	1 Intermittent 2 Continuous	2 Oxygenation	1 Hyperbaric C Supersaturated
9 Respiratory	2 Continuous	0 Filtration	Z No Qualifier
9 Respiratory	3 Less than 24 Consecutive Hours 4 24-96 Consecutive Hours 5 Greater than 96 Consecutive Hours	5 Ventilation	7 Continuous Positive Airway Pressure 8 Intermittent Positive Airway Pressure 9 Continuous Negative Airway Pressure B Intermittent Negative Airway Pressure Z No Qualifier

Valid OR   5A02[1,2]1[0,6,D]

5   Extracorporeal or Systemic Assistance and Performance
A   Physiological Systems
1   Performance   Definition: Completely taking over a physiological function by extracorporeal means

Body System Character 4	Duration Character 5	Function Character 6	Qualifier Character 7
2 Cardiac	0 Single	1 Output	2 Manual
2 Cardiac	1 Intermittent	3 Pacing	Z No Qualifier
2 Cardiac	2 Continuous	1 Output 3 Pacing	Z No Qualifier
5 Circulatory	2 Continuous	2 Oxygenation	F Membrane, Central G Membrane, Peripheral Veno-arterial H Membrane, Peripheral Veno-venous
9 Respiratory	0 Single	5 Ventilation	4 Nonmechanical
9 Respiratory	3 Less than 24 Consecutive Hours 4 24-96 Consecutive Hours 5 Greater than 96 Consecutive Hours	5 Ventilation	Z No Qualifier
C Biliary	0 Single 6 Multiple	0 Filtration	Z No Qualifier
D Urinary	7 Intermittent, Less than 6 Hours per day 8 Prolonged Intermittent, 6-18 Hours per day 9 Continuous, Greater than 18 Hours per day	0 Filtration	Z No Qualifier

Valid OR   5A1522[F,G,H]
DRG Non-OR   5A19[3,4,5]5Z
Note: For code 5A1955Z, length of stay must be > 4 consecutive days.

5   Extracorporeal or Systemic Assistance and Performance
A   Physiological Systems
2   Restoration   Definition: Returning, or attempting to return, a physiological function to its original state by extracorporeal means.

Body System Character 4	Duration Character 5	Function Character 6	Qualifier Character 7
2 Cardiac	0 Single	4 Rhythm	Z No Qualifier

Extracorporeal or Systemic Therapies 6A0–6AB

Character Meanings

This Character Meaning table is provided as a guide to assist the user in the identification of character members that may be found in this section of code tables. It **SHOULD NOT** be used to build a PCS code.

A: Physiological Systems

Operation–Character 3	Body System–Character 4	Duration–Character 5	Qualifier–Character 6	Qualifier–Character 7
0 Atmospheric Control	0 Skin	0 Single	B Donor Organ	0 Erythrocytes
1 Decompression	1 Urinary	1 Multiple	Z No Qualifier	1 Leukocytes
2 Electromagnetic Therapy	2 Central Nervous			2 Platelets
3 Hyperthermia	3 Musculoskeletal			3 Plasma
4 Hypothermia	5 Circulatory			4 Head and Neck Vessels
5 Pheresis	B Respiratory System			5 Heart
6 Phototherapy	F Hepatobiliary System and Pancreas			6 Peripheral Vessels
7 Ultrasound Therapy	T Urinary System			7 Other Vessels
8 Ultraviolet Light Therapy	Z None			T Stem Cells, Cord Blood
9 Shock Wave Therapy				V Stem Cells, Hematopoietic
B Perfusion				Z No Qualifier

AHA Coding Clinic for table 6A7
2014, 4Q, 19   Ultrasound accelerated thrombolysis

AHA Coding Clinic for table 6AB
2016, 4Q, 115   Donor organ perfusion

6   **Extracorporeal or Systemic Therapies**
A   **Physiological Systems**
0   **Atmospheric Control**   Definition: Extracorporeal control of atmospheric pressure and composition

Body System Character 4	Duration Character 5	Qualifier Character 6	Qualifier Character 7
Z None	0 Single 1 Multiple	Z No Qualifier	Z No Qualifier

6   **Extracorporeal or Systemic Therapies**
A   **Physiological Systems**
1   **Decompression**   Definition: Extracorporeal elimination of undissolved gas from body fluids

Body System Character 4	Duration Character 5	Qualifier Character 6	Qualifier Character 7
5 Circulatory	0 Single 1 Multiple	Z No Qualifier	Z No Qualifier

6   **Extracorporeal or Systemic Therapies**
A   **Physiological Systems**
2   **Electromagnetic Therapy**   Definition: Extracorporeal treatment by electromagnetic rays

Body System Character 4	Duration Character 5	Qualifier Character 6	Qualifier Character 7
1 Urinary 2 Central Nervous	0 Single 1 Multiple	Z No Qualifier	Z No Qualifier

6   **Extracorporeal or Systemic Therapies**
A   **Physiological Systems**
3   **Hyperthermia**   Definition: Extracorporeal raising of body temperature

Body System Character 4	Duration Character 5	Qualifier Character 6	Qualifier Character 7
Z None	0 Single 1 Multiple	Z No Qualifier	Z No Qualifier

6   **Extracorporeal or Systemic Therapies**
A   **Physiological Systems**
4   **Hypothermia**   Definition: Extracorporeal lowering of body temperature

Body System Character 4	Duration Character 5	Qualifier Character 6	Qualifier Character 7
Z None	0 Single 1 Multiple	Z No Qualifier	Z No Qualifier

6   **Extracorporeal or Systemic Therapies**
A   **Physiological Systems**
5   **Pheresis**   Definition: Extracorporeal separation of blood products

Body System Character 4	Duration Character 5	Qualifier Character 6	Qualifier Character 7
5 Circulatory	0 Single 1 Multiple	Z No Qualifier	0 Erythrocytes 1 Leukocytes 2 Platelets 3 Plasma T Stem Cells, Cord Blood V Stem Cells, Hematopoietic

6   **Extracorporeal or Systemic Therapies**
A   **Physiological Systems**
6   **Phototherapy**   Definition: Extracorporeal treatment by light rays

Body System Character 4	Duration Character 5	Qualifier Character 6	Qualifier Character 7
0 Skin 5 Circulatory	0 Single 1 Multiple	Z No Qualifier	Z No Qualifier

6   **Extracorporeal or Systemic Therapies**
A   **Physiological Systems**
7   **Ultrasound Therapy**   Definition: Extracorporeal treatment by ultrasound

Body System Character 4	Duration Character 5	Qualifier Character 6	Qualifier Character 7
5 Circulatory	0 Single 1 Multiple	Z No Qualifier	4 Head and Neck Vessels 5 Heart 6 Peripheral Vessels 7 Other Vessels Z No Qualifier

6   Extracorporeal or Systemic Therapies
A   Physiological Systems
8   Ultraviolet Light Therapy   Definition: Extracorporeal treatment by ultraviolet light

Body System Character 4	Duration Character 5	Qualifier Character 6	Qualifier Character 7
Ø Skin	Ø Single 1 Multiple	Z No Qualifier	Z No Qualifier

6   Extracorporeal or Systemic Therapies
A   Physiological Systems
9   Shock Wave Therapy   Definition: Extracorporeal treatment by shock waves

Body System Character 4	Duration Character 5	Qualifier Character 6	Qualifier Character 7
3 Musculoskeletal	Ø Single 1 Multiple	Z No Qualifier	Z No Qualifier

6   Extracorporeal or Systemic Therapies
A   Physiological Systems
B   Perfusion   Definition: Extracorporeal treatment by diffusion of therapeutic fluid

Body System Character 4	Duration Character 5	Qualifier Character 6	Qualifier Character 7
5 Circulatory B Respiratory System F Hepatobiliary System and Pancreas T Urinary System	Ø Single	B Donor Organ	Z No Qualifier

Osteopathic 7W0

Character Meanings

This Character Meaning table is provided as a guide to assist the user in the identification of character members that may be found in this section of code tables. It **SHOULD NOT** be used to build a PCS code.

W: Anatomical Regions

Operation–Character 3	Body Region–Character 4	Approach–Character 5	Method–Character 6	Qualifier–Character 7
0 Treatment	0 Head	X External	0 Articulatory-Raising	Z None
	1 Cervical		1 Fascial Release	
	2 Thoracic		2 General Mobilization	
	3 Lumbar		3 High Velocity-Low Amplitude	
	4 Sacrum		4 Indirect	
	5 Pelvis		5 Low Velocity-High Amplitude	
	6 Lower Extremities		6 Lymphatic Pump	
	7 Upper Extremities		7 Muscle Energy-Isometric	
	8 Rib Cage		8 Muscle Energy-Isotonic	
	9 Abdomen		9 Other Method	

Osteopathic

7WØ–7WØ

7   **Osteopathic**
W   **Anatomical Regions**
Ø   **Treatment**   Definition: Manual treatment to eliminate or alleviate somatic dysfunction and related disorders

Body Region Character 4	Approach Character 5	Method Character 6	Qualifier Character 7
Ø Head	X External	Ø Articulatory-Raising	Z None
1 Cervical		1 Fascial Release	
2 Thoracic		2 General Mobilization	
3 Lumbar		3 High Velocity-Low Amplitude	
4 Sacrum		4 Indirect	
5 Pelvis		5 Low Velocity-High Amplitude	
6 Lower Extremities		6 Lymphatic Pump	
7 Upper Extremities		7 Muscle Energy-Isometric	
8 Rib Cage		8 Muscle Energy-Isotonic	
9 Abdomen		9 Other Method	

Other Procedures 8C0–8E0

Character Meanings

This Character Meaning table is provided as a guide to assist the user in the identification of character members that may be found in this section of code tables. It **SHOULD NOT** be used to build a PCS code.

C: Indwelling Devices

Operation–Character 3	Body Region–Character 4	Approach–Character 5	Method–Character 6	Qualifier–Character 7
0 Other procedures	1 Nervous System	X External	6 Collection	J Cerebrospinal Fluid
	2 Circulatory System			K Blood
				L Other Fluid

E: Physiological Systems and Anatomical Regions

Operation–Character 3	Body Region–Character 4	Approach–Character 5	Method–Character 6	Qualifier–Character 7
0 Other Procedures	1 Nervous System	0 Open	0 Acupuncture	0 Anesthesia
	2 Circulatory System	3 Percutaneous	1 Therapeutic Massage	1 In Vitro Fertilization
	9 Head and Neck Region	4 Percutaneous Endoscopic	6 Collection	2 Breast Milk
	H Integumentary System and Breast	7 Via Natural or Artificial Opening	B Computer Assisted Procedure	3 Sperm
	K Musculoskeletal System	8 Via Natural or Artificial Opening Endoscopic	C Robotic Assisted Procedure	4 Yoga Therapy
	U Female Reproductive System	X External	D Near Infrared Spectroscopy	5 Meditation
	V Male Reproductive System		Y Other Method	6 Isolation
	W Trunk Region			7 Examination
	X Upper Extremity			8 Suture Removal
	Y Lower Extremity			9 Piercing
	Z None			C Prostate
				D Rectum
				F With Fluoroscopy
				G With Computerized Tomography
				H With Magnetic Resonance Imaging
				Z No Qualifier

AHA Coding Clinic for table 8E0

2015, 1Q, 33	Robotic-assisted laparoscopic hysterectomy converted to open procedure
2014, 4Q, 33	Radical prostatectomy

Other Procedures

8   Other Procedures
C   Indwelling Device
0   Other Procedures   Definition: Methodologies which attempt to remediate or cure a disorder or disease

Body Region Character 4	Approach Character 5	Method Character 6	Qualifier Character 7
1 Nervous System	X External	6 Collection	J Cerebrospinal Fluid L Other Fluid
2 Circulatory System	X External	6 Collection	K Blood L Other Fluid

8   Other Procedures
E   Physiological Systems and Anatomical Regions
0   Other Procedures   Definition: Methodologies which attempt to remediate or cure a disorder or disease

Body Region Character 4	Approach Character 5	Method Character 6	Qualifier Character 7
1 Nervous System U Female Reproductive System ♀	X External	Y Other Method	7 Examination
2 Circulatory System	3 Percutaneous	D Near Infrared Spectroscopy	Z No Qualifier
9 Head and Neck Region W Trunk Region	0 Open 3 Percutaneous 4 Percutaneous Endoscopic 7 Via Natural or Artificial Opening 8 Via Natural or Artificial Opening Endoscopic	C Robotic Assisted Procedure	Z No Qualifier
9 Head and Neck Region W Trunk Region	X External	B Computer Assisted Procedure	F With Fluoroscopy G With Computerized Tomography H With Magnetic Resonance Imaging Z No Qualifier
9 Head and Neck Region W Trunk Region	X External	C Robotic Assisted Procedure	Z No Qualifier
9 Head and Neck Region W Trunk Region	X External	Y Other Method	8 Suture Removal
H Integumentary System and Breast	3 Percutaneous	0 Acupuncture	0 Anesthesia Z No Qualifier
H Integumentary System and Breast ♀	X External	6 Collection	2 Breast Milk
H Integumentary System and Breast	X External	Y Other Method	9 Piercing
K Musculoskeletal System	X External	1 Therapeutic Massage	Z No Qualifier
K Musculoskeletal System	X External	Y Other Method	7 Examination
V Male Reproductive System ♂	X External	1 Therapeutic Massage	C Prostate D Rectum
V Male Reproductive System ♂	X External	6 Collection	3 Sperm
X Upper Extremity Y Lower Extremity	0 Open 3 Percutaneous 4 Percutaneous Endoscopic	C Robotic Assisted Procedure	Z No Qualifier
X Upper Extremity Y Lower Extremity	X External	B Computer Assisted Procedure	F With Fluoroscopy G With Computerized Tomography H With Magnetic Resonance Imaging Z No Qualifier
X Upper Extremity Y Lower Extremity	X External	C Robotic Assisted Procedure	Z No Qualifier
X Upper Extremity Y Lower Extremity	X External	Y Other Method	8 Suture Removal
Z None	X External	Y Other Method	1 In Vitro Fertilization 4 Yoga Therapy 5 Meditation 6 Isolation

♂   8E0VX1C
♂   8E0VX63
♀   8E0UXY7
♀   8E0HX62

Chiropractic 9WB

Character Meanings

This Character Meaning table is provided as a guide to assist the user in the identification of character members that may be found in this section of code tables. It **SHOULD NOT** be used to build a PCS code.

W: Anatomical Regions

Operation–Character 3	Body Region–Character 4	Approach–Character 5	Method–Character 6	Qualifier–Character 7
B Manipulation	Ø Head	X External	B Non-Manual	Z None
	1 Cervical		C Indirect Visceral	
	2 Thoracic		D Extra-Articular	
	3 Lumbar		F Direct Visceral	
	4 Sacrum		G Long Lever Specific Contact	
	5 Pelvis		H Short Lever Specific Contact	
	6 Lower Extremities		J Long and Short Lever Specific Contact	
	7 Upper Extremities		K Mechanically Assisted	
	8 Rib Cage		L Other Method	
	9 Abdomen			

9 Chiropractic
W Anatomical Regions
B Manipulation Definition: Manual procedure that involves a directed thrust to move a joint past the physiological range of motion, without exceeding the anatomical limit

Body Region Character 4	Approach Character 5	Method Character 6	Qualifier Character 7
Ø Head	X External	B Non-Manual	Z None
1 Cervical		C Indirect Visceral	
2 Thoracic		D Extra-Articular	
3 Lumbar		F Direct Visceral	
4 Sacrum		G Long Lever Specific Contact	
5 Pelvis		H Short Lever Specific Contact	
6 Lower Extremities		J Long and Short Lever Specific	
7 Upper Extremities		Contact	
8 Rib Cage		K Mechanically Assisted	
9 Abdomen		L Other Method	

Imaging BØØ–BY4

Character Meanings

This Character Meaning table is provided as a guide to assist the user in the identification of character members that may be found in this section of code tables. It **SHOULD NOT** be used to build a PCS code.

Body System–Character 2	Type–Character 3	Body Part–Character 4	Contrast–Character 5	Qualifier–Character 6	Qualifier–Character 7
Ø Central Nervous System	Ø Plain Radiography	See next page	Ø High Osmolar	Ø Unenhanced and Enhanced	Ø Intraoperative
2 Heart	1 Fluoroscopy		1 Low Osmolar	1 Laser	1 Densitometry
3 Upper Arteries	2 Computerized Tomography (CT Scan)		Y Other Contrast	2 Intravascular Optical Coherence	3 Intravascular
4 Lower Arteries	3 Magnetic Resonance Imaging (MRI)		Z None	Z None	4 Transesophageal
5 Veins	4 Ultrasonography				A Guidance
7 Lymphatic System					Z None
8 Eye					
9 Ear, Nose, Mouth and Throat					
B Respiratory System					
D Gastrointestinal System					
F Hepatobiliary System and Pancreas					
G Endocrine System					
H Skin, Subcutaneous Tissue and Breast					
L Connective Tissue					
N Skull and Facial Bones					
P Non-Axial Upper Bones					
Q Non-Axial Lower Bones					
R Axial Skeleton, Except Skull and Facial Bones					
T Urinary System					
U Female Reproductive System					
V Male Reproductive System					
W Anatomical Regions					
Y Fetus and Obstetrical					

Continued on next page

Body Part—Character 4 Meanings

Continued from previous page

Body System–Character 2	Body Part– Character 4		
Ø Central Nervous System	Ø Brain	9	Sella Turcica/Pituitary Gland
	7 Cisterna	B	Spinal Cord
	8 Cerebral Ventricle(s)	C	Acoustic Nerves
2 Heart	Ø Coronary Artery, Single	7	Internal Mammary Bypass Graft, Right
	1 Coronary Arteries, Multiple	8	Internal Mammary Bypass Graft, Left
	2 Coronary Artery Bypass Graft, Single	B	Heart with Aorta
	3 Coronary Artery Bypass Grafts, Multiple	C	Pericardium
	4 Heart, Right	D	Pediatric Heart
	5 Heart, Left	F	Bypass Graft, Other
	6 Heart, Right and Left		
3 Upper Arteries	Ø Thoracic Aorta	G	Vertebral Arteries, Bilateral
	1 Brachiocephalic-Subclavian Artery, Right	H	Upper Extremity Arteries, Right
	2 Subclavian Artery, Left	J	Upper Extremity Arteries, Left
	3 Common Carotid Artery, Right	K	Upper Extremity Arteries, Bilateral
	4 Common Carotid Artery, Left	L	Intercostal and Bronchial Arteries
	5 Common Carotid Arteries, Bilateral	M	Spinal Arteries
	6 Internal Carotid Artery, Right	N	Upper Arteries, Other
	7 Internal Carotid Artery, Left	P	Thoraco-Abdominal Aorta
	8 Internal Carotid Arteries, Bilateral	Q	Cervico-Cerebral Arch
	9 External Carotid Artery, Right	R	Intracranial Arteries
	B External Carotid Artery, Left	S	Pulmonary Artery, Right
	C External Carotid Arteries, Bilateral	T	Pulmonary Artery, Left
	D Vertebral Artery, Right	U	Pulmonary Trunk
	F Vertebral Artery, Left	V	Ophthalmic Arteries
4 Lower Arteries	Ø Abdominal Aorta	C	Pelvic Arteries
	1 Celiac Artery	D	Aorta and Bilateral Lower Extremity Arteries
	2 Hepatic Artery	F	Lower Extremity Arteries, Right
	3 Splenic Arteries	G	Lower Extremity Arteries, Left
	4 Superior Mesenteric Artery	H	Lower Extremity Arteries, Bilateral
	5 Inferior Mesenteric Artery	J	Lower Arteries, Other
	6 Renal Artery, Right	K	Celiac and Mesenteric Arteries
	7 Renal Artery, Left	L	Femoral Artery
	8 Renal Arteries, Bilateral	M	Renal Artery Transplant
	9 Lumbar Arteries	N	Penile Arteries
	B Intra-Abdominal Arteries, Other		
5 Veins	Ø Epidural Veins	G	Pelvic (Iliac) Veins, Left
	1 Cerebral and Cerebellar Veins	H	Pelvic (Iliac) Veins, Bilateral
	2 Intracranial Sinuses	J	Renal Vein, Right
	3 Jugular Veins, Right	K	Renal Vein, Left
	4 Jugular Veins, Left	L	Renal Veins, Bilateral
	5 Jugular Veins, Bilateral	M	Upper Extremity Veins, Right
	6 Subclavian Vein, Right	N	Upper Extremity Veins, Left
	7 Subclavian Vein, Left	P	Upper Extremity Veins, Bilateral
	8 Superior Vena Cava	Q	Pulmonary Vein, Right
	9 Inferior Vena Cava	R	Pulmonary Vein, Left
	B Lower Extremity Veins, Right	S	Pulmonary Veins, Bilateral
	C Lower Extremity Veins, Left	T	Portal and Splanchnic Veins
	D Lower Extremity Veins, Bilateral	V	Veins, Other
	F Pelvic (Iliac) Veins, Right	W	Dialysis Shunt/Fistula
7 Lymphatic System	Ø Abdominal/Retroperitoneal Lymphatics, Unilateral	7	Upper Extremity Lymphatics, Bilateral
	1 Abdominal/Retroperitoneal Lymphatics, Bilateral	8	Lower Extremity Lymphatics, Right
	4 Lymphatics, Head and Neck	9	Lower Extremity Lymphatics, Left
	5 Upper Extremity Lymphatics, Right	B	Lower Extremity Lymphatics, Bilateral
	6 Upper Extremity Lymphatics, Left	C	Lymphatics, Pelvic
8 Eye	Ø Lacrimal Duct, Right	4	Optic Foramina, Left
	1 Lacrimal Duct, Left	5	Eye, Right
	2 Lacrimal Ducts, Bilateral	6	Eye, Left
	3 Optic Foramina, Right	7	Eyes, Bilateral
9 Ear, Nose, Mouth and Throat	Ø Ear	B	Salivary Gland, Right
	2 Paranasal Sinuses	C	Salivary Gland, Left
	4 Parotid Gland, Right	D	Salivary Glands, Bilateral
	5 Parotid Gland, Left	F	Nasopharynx/Oropharynx
	6 Parotid Glands, Bilateral	G	Pharynx and Epiglottis
	7 Submandibular Gland, Right	H	Mastoids
	8 Submandibular Gland, Left	J	Larynx
	9 Submandibular Glands, Bilateral		
B Respiratory System	2 Lung, Right	9	Tracheobronchial Trees, Bilateral
	3 Lung, Left	B	Pleura
	4 Lungs, Bilateral	C	Mediastinum
	6 Diaphragm	D	Upper Airways
	7 Tracheobronchial Tree, Right	F	Trachea/Airways
	8 Tracheobronchial Tree, Left	G	Lung Apices

Continued on next page

Continued from previous page

Body System–Character 2	Body Part– Character 4	
D Gastrointestinal System	1 Esophagus 2 Stomach 3 Small Bowel 4 Colon 5 Upper GI 6 Upper GI and Small Bowel	7 Gastrointestinal Tract 8 Appendix 9 Duodenum B Mouth/Oropharynx C Rectum
F Hepatobiliary System and Pancreas	Ø Bile Ducts 1 Biliary and Pancreatic Ducts 2 Gallbladder 3 Gallbladder and Bile Ducts 4 Gallbladder, Bile Ducts and Pancreatic Ducts	5 Liver 6 Liver and Spleen 7 Pancreas 8 Pancreatic Ducts C Hepatobiliary System, All
G Endocrine System	Ø Adrenal Gland, Right 1 Adrenal Gland, Left 2 Adrenal Glands, Bilateral	3 Parathyroid Glands 4 Thyroid Gland
H Skin, Subcutaneous Tissue and Breast	Ø Breast, Right 1 Breast, Left 2 Breasts, Bilateral 3 Single Mammary Duct, Right 4 Single Mammary Duct, Left 5 Multiple Mammary Ducts, Right 6 Multiple Mammary Ducts, Left 7 Extremity, Upper 8 Extremity, Lower	9 Abdominal Wall B Chest Wall C Head and Neck D Subcutaneous Tissue, Head/Neck F Subcutaneous Tissue, Upper Extremity G Subcutaneous Tissue, Thorax H Subcutaneous Tissue, Abdomen and Pelvis J Subcutaneous Tissue, Lower Extremity
L Connective Tissue	Ø Connective Tissue, Upper Extremity 1 Connective Tissue, Lower Extremity	2 Tendons, Upper Extremity 3 Tendons, Lower Extremity
N Skull and Facial Bones	Ø Skull 1 Orbit, Right 2 Orbit, Left 3 Orbits, Bilateral 4 Nasal Bones 5 Facial Bones 6 Mandible 7 Temporomandibular Joint, Right 8 Temporomandibular Joint, Left	9 Temporomandibular Joints, Bilateral B Zygomatic Arch, Right C Zygomatic Arch, Left D Zygomatic Arches, Bilateral F Temporal Bones G Tooth, Single H Teeth, Multiple J Teeth, All
P Non-Axial Upper Bones	Ø Sternoclavicular Joint, Right 1 Sternoclavicular Joint, Left 2 Sternoclavicular Joints, Bilateral 3 Acromioclavicular Joints, Bilateral 4 Clavicle, Right 5 Clavicle, Left 6 Scapula, Right 7 Scapula, Left 8 Shoulder, Right 9 Shoulder, Left A Humerus, Right B Humerus, Left C Hand/Finger Joint, Right D Hand/Finger Joint, Left E Upper Arm, Right F Upper Arm, Left G Elbow, Right	H Elbow, Left J Forearm, Right K Forearm, Left L Wrist, Right M Wrist, Left N Hand, Right P Hand, Left Q Hands and Wrists, Bilateral R Finger(s), Right S Finger(s), Left T Upper Extremity, Right U Upper Extremity, Left V Upper Extremities, Bilateral W Thorax X Ribs, Right Y Ribs, Left
Q Non-Axial Lower Bones	Ø Hip, Right 1 Hip, Left 2 Hips, Bilateral 3 Femur, Right 4 Femur, Left 7 Knee, Right 8 Knee, Left 9 Knees, Bilateral B Tibia/Fibula, Right C Tibia/Fibula, Left D Lower Leg, Right F Lower Leg, Left G Ankle, Right	H Ankle, Left J Calcaneus, Right K Calcaneus, Left L Foot, Right M Foot, Left P Toe(s), Right Q Toe(s), Left R Lower Extremity, Right S Lower Extremity, Left V Patella, Right W Patella, Left X Foot/Toe Joint, Right Y Foot/Toe Joint, Left
R Axial Skeleton, Except Skull and Facial Bones	Ø Cervical Spine 1 Cervical Disc(s) 2 Thoracic Disc(s) 3 Lumbar Disc(s) 4 Cervical Facet Joint(s) 5 Thoracic Facet Joint(s) 6 Lumbar Facet Joint(s) 7 Thoracic Spine	8 Thoracolumbar Joint 9 Lumbar Spine B Lumbosacral Joint C Pelvis D Sacroiliac Joints F Sacrum and Coccyx G Whole Spine H Sternum

Continued on next page

Continued from previous page

Body System–Character 2	Body Part– Character 4	
T Urinary System	Ø Bladder 1 Kidney, Right 2 Kidney, Left 3 Kidneys, Bilateral 4 Kidneys, Ureters and Bladder 5 Urethra 6 Ureter, Right 7 Ureter, Left	8 Ureters, Bilateral 9 Kidney Transplant B Bladder and Urethra C Ileal Diversion Loop D Kidney, Ureter and Bladder, Right F Kidney, Ureter and Bladder, Left G Ileal Loop, Ureters and Kidneys J Kidneys and Bladder
U Female Reproductive System	Ø Fallopian Tube, Right 1 Fallopian Tube, Left 2 Fallopian Tubes, Bilateral 3 Ovary, Right 4 Ovary, Left 5 Ovaries, Bilateral	6 Uterus 8 Uterus and Fallopian Tubes 9 Vagina B Pregnant Uterus C Uterus and Ovaries
V Male Reproductive System	Ø Corpora Cavernosa 1 Epididymis, Right 2 Epididymis, Left 3 Prostate 4 Scrotum 5 Testicle, Right	6 Testicle, Left 7 Testicles, Bilateral 8 Vasa Vasorum 9 Prostate and Seminal Vesicles B Penis
W Anatomical Regions	Ø Abdomen 1 Abdomen and Pelvis 3 Chest 4 Chest and Abdomen 5 Chest, Abdomen and Pelvis 8 Head 9 Head and Neck B Long Bones, All C Lower Extremity	F Neck G Pelvic Region H Retroperitoneum J Upper Extremity K Whole Body L Whole Skeleton M Whole Body, Infant P Brachial Plexus
Y Fetus and Obstetrical	Ø Fetal Head 1 Fetal Heart 2 Fetal Thorax 3 Fetal Abdomen 4 Fetal Spine 5 Fetal Extremities 6 Whole Fetus 7 Fetal Umbilical Cord	8 Placenta 9 First Trimester, Single Fetus B First Trimester, Multiple Gestation C Second Trimester, Single Fetus D Second Trimester, Multiple Gestation F Third Trimester, Single Fetus G Third Trimester, Multiple Gestation

AHA Coding Clinic for table B21

2018, 1Q, 12	Percutaneous balloon valvuloplasty & cardiac catheterization with ventriculogram
2016, 3Q, 36	Type of contrast medium for angiography (high osmolar, low osmolar, and other)

AHA Coding Clinic for table B41

2015, 3Q, 9	Aborted endovascular stenting of superficial femoral artery

AHA Coding Clinic for table B51

2015, 4Q, 30	Vascular access devices

AHA Coding Clinic for table BF4

2014, 3Q, 15	Drainage of pancreatic pseudocyst

B   **Imaging**
0   **Central Nervous System**
0   **Plain Radiography**   Definition: Planar display of an image developed from the capture of external ionizing radiation on photographic or photoconductive plate

Body Part Character 4	Contrast Character 5	Qualifier Character 6	Qualifier Character 7
B Spinal Cord	**0** High Osmolar **1** Low Osmolar **Y** Other Contrast **Z** None	**Z** None	**Z** None

B   **Imaging**
0   **Central Nervous System**
1   **Fluoroscopy**   Definition: Single plane or bi-plane real time display of an image developed from the capture of external ionizing radioation on a fluorescent screen. The image may also be stored by either digital or analog means.

Body Part Character 4	Contrast Character 5	Qualifier Character 6	Qualifier Character 7
B Spinal Cord	**0** High Osmolar **1** Low Osmolar **Y** Other Contrast **Z** None	**Z** None	**Z** None

B   **Imaging**
0   **Central Nervous System**
2   **Computerized Tomography (CT Scan)**   Definition: Computer reformatted digital display of multiplanar images developed from the capture of multiple exposures of external ionizing radiation

Body Part Character 4	Contrast Character 5	Qualifier Character 6	Qualifier Character 7
0 Brain **7** Cisterna **8** Cerebral Ventricle(s) **9** Sella Turcica/Pituitary Gland **B** Spinal Cord	**0** High Osmolar **1** Low Osmolar **Y** Other Contrast	**0** Unenhanced and Enhanced **Z** None	**Z** None
0 Brain **7** Cisterna **8** Cerebral Ventricle(s) **9** Sella Turcica/Pituitary Gland **B** Spinal Cord	**Z** None	**Z** None	**Z** None

B   **Imaging**
0   **Central Nervous System**
3   **Magnetic Resonance Imaging (MRI)**   Definition: Computer reformatted digital display of multiplanar images developed from the capture of radio-frequency signals emitted by nuclei in a body site excited within a magnetic field

Body Part Character 4	Contrast Character 5	Qualifier Character 6	Qualifier Character 7
0 Brain **9** Sella Turcica/Pituitary Gland **B** Spinal Cord **C** Acoustic Nerves	**Y** Other Contrast	**0** Unenhanced and Enhanced **Z** None	**Z** None
0 Brain **9** Sella Turcica/Pituitary Gland **B** Spinal Cord **C** Acoustic Nerves	**Z** None	**Z** None	**Z** None

B   **Imaging**
0   **Central Nervous System**
4   **Ultrasonography**   Definition: Real time display of images of anatomy or flow information developed from the capture of relected and attenuated high frequency sound waves

Body Part Character 4	Contrast Character 5	Qualifier Character 6	Qualifier Character 7
0 Brain **B** Spinal Cord	**Z** None	**Z** None	**Z** None

B   Imaging
2   Heart
Ø   Plain Radiography   Definition: Planar display of an image developed from the capture of external ionizing radiation on photographic or photoconductive plate

Body Part Character 4	Contrast Character 5	Qualifier Character 6	Qualifier Character 7
Ø Coronary Artery, Single 1 Coronary Arteries, Multiple 2 Coronary Artery Bypass Graft, Single 3 Coronary Artery Bypass Grafts, Multiple 4 Heart, Right 5 Heart, Left 6 Heart, Right and Left 7 Internal Mammary Bypass Graft, Right 8 Internal Mammary Bypass Graft, Left F Bypass Graft, Other	Ø High Osmolar 1 Low Osmolar Y Other Contrast	Z None	Z None

DRG Non-OR   All body part, contrast, and qualifier values

B   Imaging
2   Heart
1   Fluoroscopy   Definition: Single plane or bi-plane real time display of an image developed from the capture of external ionizing radioation on a fluorescent screen. The image may also be stored by either digital or analog means.

Body Part Character 4	Contrast Character 5	Qualifier Character 6	Qualifier Character 7
Ø Coronary Artery, Single 1 Coronary Arteries, Multiple 2 Coronary Artery Bypass Graft, Single 3 Coronary Artery Bypass Grafts, Multiple	Ø High Osmolar 1 Low Osmolar Y Other Contrast	1 Laser	Ø Intraoperative
Ø Coronary Artery, Single 1 Coronary Arteries, Multiple 2 Coronary Artery Bypass Graft, Single 3 Coronary Artery Bypass Grafts, Multiple	Ø High Osmolar 1 Low Osmolar Y Other Contrast	Z None	Z None
4 Heart, Right 5 Heart, Left 6 Heart, Right and Left 7 Internal Mammary Bypass Graft, Right 8 Internal Mammary Bypass Graft, Left F Bypass Graft, Other	Ø High Osmolar 1 Low Osmolar Y Other Contrast	Z None	Z None

DRG Non-OR   All body part, contrast, and qualifier values

B   Imaging
2   Heart
2   Computerized Tomography (CT Scan)   Definition: Computer reformatted digital display of multiplanar images developed from the capture of multiple exposures of external ionizing radiation

Body Part Character 4	Contrast Character 5	Qualifier Character 6	Qualifier Character 7
1 Coronary Arteries, Multiple 3 Coronary Artery Bypass Grafts, Multiple 6 Heart, Right and Left	Ø High Osmolar 1 Low Osmolar Y Other Contrast	Ø Unenhanced and Enhanced Z None	Z None
1 Coronary Arteries, Multiple 3 Coronary Artery Bypass Grafts, Multiple 6 Heart, Right and Left	Z None	2 Intravascular Optical Coherence Z None	Z None

B   Imaging
2   Heart
3   Magnetic Resonance Imaging (MRI)   Definition: Computer reformatted digital display of multiplanar images developed from the capture of radio-frequency signals emitted by nuclei in a body site excited within a magnetic field

Body Part Character 4	Contrast Character 5	Qualifier Character 6	Qualifier Character 7
1 Coronary Arteries, Multiple 3 Coronary Artery Bypass Grafts, Multiple 6 Heart, Right and Left	Y Other Contrast	Ø Unenhanced and Enhanced Z None	Z None
1 Coronary Arteries, Multiple 3 Coronary Artery Bypass Grafts, Multiple 6 Heart, Right and Left	Z None	Z None	Z None

B   Imaging
2   Heart
4   Ultrasonography   Definition: Real time display of images of anatomy or flow information developed from the capture of relected and attenuated high frequency sound waves

Body Part Character 4	Contrast Character 5	Qualifier Character 6	Qualifier Character 7
Ø Coronary Artery, Single 1 Coronary Arteries, Multiple 4 Heart, Right 5 Heart, Left 6 Heart, Right and Left B Heart with Aorta C Pericardium D Pediatric Heart	Y Other Contrast	Z None	Z None
Ø Coronary Artery, Single 1 Coronary Arteries, Multiple 4 Heart, Right 5 Heart, Left 6 Heart, Right and Left B Heart with Aorta C Pericardium D Pediatric Heart	Z None	Z None	3 Intravascular 4 Transesophageal Z None

B   Imaging
3   Upper Arteries
Ø   Plain Radiography   Definition: Planar display of an image developed from the capture of external ionizing radiation on photographic or photoconductive plate

Body Part Character 4	Contrast Character 5	Qualifier Character 6	Qualifier Character 7
Ø Thoracic Aorta 1 Brachiocephalic-Subclavian Artery, Right 2 Subclavian Artery, Left 3 Common Carotid Artery, Right 4 Common Carotid Artery, Left 5 Common Carotid Arteries, Bilateral 6 Internal Carotid Artery, Right 7 Internal Carotid Artery, Left 8 Internal Carotid Arteries, Bilateral 9 External Carotid Artery, Right B External Carotid Artery, Left C External Carotid Arteries, Bilateral D Vertebral Artery, Right F Vertebral Artery, Left G Vertebral Arteries, Bilateral H Upper Extremity Arteries, Right J Upper Extremity Arteries, Left K Upper Extremity Arteries, Bilateral L Intercostal and Bronchial Arteries M Spinal Arteries N Upper Arteries, Other P Thoraco-Abdominal Aorta Q Cervico-Cerebral Arch R Intracranial Arteries S Pulmonary Artery, Right T Pulmonary Artery, Left	Ø High Osmolar 1 Low Osmolar Y Other Contrast Z None	Z None	Z None

B　Imaging
3　Upper Arteries
1　Fluoroscopy　Definition: Single plane or bi-plane real time display of an image developed from the capture of external ionizing radiation on a fluorescent screen. The image may also be stored by either digital or analog means.

Body Part Character 4	Contrast Character 5	Qualifier Character 6	Qualifier Character 7
Ø Thoracic Aorta 1 Brachiocephalic-Subclavian Artery, Right 2 Subclavian Artery, Left 3 Common Carotid Artery, Right 4 Common Carotid Artery, Left 5 Common Carotid Arteries, Bilateral 6 Internal Carotid Artery, Right 7 Internal Carotid Artery, Left 8 Internal Carotid Arteries, Bilateral 9 External Carotid Artery, Right B External Carotid Artery, Left C External Carotid Arteries, Bilateral D Vertebral Artery, Right F Vertebral Artery, Left G Vertebral Arteries, Bilateral H Upper Extremity Arteries, Right J Upper Extremity Arteries, Left K Upper Extremity Arteries, Bilateral L Intercostal and Bronchial Arteries M Spinal Arteries N Upper Arteries, Other P Thoraco-Abdominal Aorta Q Cervico-Cerebral Arch R Intracranial Arteries S Pulmonary Artery, Right T Pulmonary Artery, Left U Pulmonary Trunk	Ø High Osmolar 1 Low Osmolar Y Other Contrast	1 Laser	Ø Intraoperative
Ø Thoracic Aorta 1 Brachiocephalic-Subclavian Artery, Right 2 Subclavian Artery, Left 3 Common Carotid Artery, Right 4 Common Carotid Artery, Left 5 Common Carotid Arteries, Bilateral 6 Internal Carotid Artery, Right 7 Internal Carotid Artery, Left 8 Internal Carotid Arteries, Bilateral 9 External Carotid Artery, Right B External Carotid Artery, Left C External Carotid Arteries, Bilateral D Vertebral Artery, Right F Vertebral Artery, Left G Vertebral Arteries, Bilateral H Upper Extremity Arteries, Right J Upper Extremity Arteries, Left K Upper Extremity Arteries, Bilateral L Intercostal and Bronchial Arteries M Spinal Arteries N Upper Arteries, Other P Thoraco-Abdominal Aorta Q Cervico-Cerebral Arch R Intracranial Arteries S Pulmonary Artery, Right T Pulmonary Artery, Left U Pulmonary Trunk	Ø High Osmolar 1 Low Osmolar Y Other Contrast	Z None	Z None

B31 Continued on next page

LC Limited Coverage　　NC Noncovered　　⊞ Combination Member　　HAC　　Valid OR　　Combination Only　　DRG Non-OR　　New/Revised in GREEN

B   **Imaging**
3   **Upper Arteries**
1   **Fluoroscopy**   Definition: Single plane or bi-plane real time display of an image developed from the capture of external ionizing radiation on a fluorescent screen. The image may also be stored by either digital or analog means.

Body Part Character 4	Contrast Character 5	Qualifier Character 6	Qualifier Character 7
Ø Thoracic Aorta	**Z** None	**Z** None	**Z** None
1 Brachiocephalic-Subclavian Artery, Right			
2 Subclavian Artery, Left			
3 Common Carotid Artery, Right			
4 Common Carotid Artery, Left			
5 Common Carotid Arteries, Bilateral			
6 Internal Carotid Artery, Right			
7 Internal Carotid Artery, Left			
8 Internal Carotid Arteries, Bilateral			
9 External Carotid Artery, Right			
B External Carotid Artery, Left			
C External Carotid Arteries, Bilateral			
D Vertebral Artery, Right			
F Vertebral Artery, Left			
G Vertebral Arteries, Bilateral			
H Upper Extremity Arteries, Right			
J Upper Extremity Arteries, Left			
K Upper Extremity Arteries, Bilateral			
L Intercostal and Bronchial Arteries			
M Spinal Arteries			
N Upper Arteries, Other			
P Thoraco-Abdominal Aorta			
Q Cervico-Cerebral Arch			
R Intracranial Arteries			
S Pulmonary Artery, Right			
T Pulmonary Artery, Left			
U Pulmonary Trunk			

B   **Imaging**
3   **Upper Arteries**
2   **Computerized Tomography (CT Scan)**   Definition: Computer reformatted digital display of multiplanar images developed from the capture of multiple exposures of external ionizing radiation

Body Part Character 4	Contrast Character 5	Qualifier Character 6	Qualifier Character 7
Ø Thoracic Aorta	**Ø** High Osmolar	**Z** None	**Z** None
5 Common Carotid Arteries, Bilateral	**1** Low Osmolar		
8 Internal Carotid Arteries, Bilateral	**Y** Other Contrast		
G Vertebral Arteries, Bilateral			
R Intracranial Arteries			
S Pulmonary Artery, Right			
T Pulmonary Artery, Left			
Ø Thoracic Aorta	**Z** None	**2** Intravascular Optical Coherence	**Z** None
5 Common Carotid Arteries, Bilateral		**Z** None	
8 Internal Carotid Arteries, Bilateral			
G Vertebral Arteries, Bilateral			
R Intracranial Arteries			
S Pulmonary Artery, Right			
T Pulmonary Artery, Left			

LC Limited Coverage   **NC** Noncovered   ⊞ Combination Member   HAC   Valid OR   Combination Only   DRG Non-OR   New/Revised in GREEN

ICD-10-PCS 2019   729

B31–B32

Imaging

B Imaging
3 Upper Arteries
3 Magnetic Resonance Imaging (MRI) Definition: Computer reformatted digital display of multiplanar images developed from the capture of radio-frequency signals emitted by nuclei in a body site excited within a magnetic field

Body Part Character 4	Contrast Character 5	Qualifier Character 6	Qualifier Character 7
Ø Thoracic Aorta **5** Common Carotid Arteries, Bilateral **8** Internal Carotid Arteries, Bilateral **G** Vertebral Arteries, Bilateral **H** Upper Extremity Arteries, Right **J** Upper Extremity Arteries, Left **K** Upper Extremity Arteries, Bilateral **M** Spinal Arteries **Q** Cervico-Cerebral Arch **R** Intracranial Arteries	**Y** Other Contrast	**Ø** Unenhanced and Enhanced **Z** None	**Z** None
Ø Thoracic Aorta **5** Common Carotid Arteries, Bilateral **8** Internal Carotid Arteries, Bilateral **G** Vertebral Arteries, Bilateral **H** Upper Extremity Arteries, Right **J** Upper Extremity Arteries, Left **K** Upper Extremity Arteries, Bilateral **M** Spinal Arteries **Q** Cervico-Cerebral Arch **R** Intracranial Arteries	**Z** None	**Z** None	**Z** None

B Imaging
3 Upper Arteries
4 Ultrasonography Definition: Real time display of images of anatomy or flow information developed from the capture of relected and attenuated high frequency sound waves

Body Part Character 4	Contrast Character 5	Qualifier Character 6	Qualifier Character 7
Ø Thoracic Aorta **1** Brachiocephalic-Subclavian Artery, Right **2** Subclavian Artery, Left **3** Common Carotid Artery, Right **4** Common Carotid Artery, Left **5** Common Carotid Arteries, Bilateral **6** Internal Carotid Artery, Right **7** Internal Carotid Artery, Left **8** Internal Carotid Arteries, Bilateral **H** Upper Extremity Arteries, Right **J** Upper Extremity Arteries, Left **K** Upper Extremity Arteries, Bilateral **R** Intracranial Arteries **S** Pulmonary Artery, Right **T** Pulmonary Artery, Left **V** Ophthalmic Arteries	**Z** None	**Z** None	**3** Intravascular **Z** None

B Imaging
4 Lower Arteries
Ø Plain Radiography Definition: Planar display of an image developed from the capture of external ionizing radiation on photographic or photoconductive plate

Body Part Character 4	Contrast Character 5	Qualifier Character 6	Qualifier Character 7
Ø Abdominal Aorta **2** Hepatic Artery **3** Splenic Arteries **4** Superior Mesenteric Artery **5** Inferior Mesenteric Artery **6** Renal Artery, Right **7** Renal Artery, Left **8** Renal Arteries, Bilateral **9** Lumbar Arteries **B** Intra-Abdominal Arteries, Other **C** Pelvic Arteries **D** Aorta and Bilateral Lower Extremity Arteries **F** Lower Extremity Arteries, Right **G** Lower Extremity Arteries, Left **J** Lower Arteries, Other **M** Renal Artery Transplant	**Ø** High Osmolar **1** Low Osmolar **Y** Other Contrast	**Z** None	**Z** None

B   **Imaging**
4   **Lower Arteries**
1   **Fluoroscopy**   Definition: Single plane or bi-plane real time display of an image developed from the capture of external ionizing radiation on a fluorescent screen. The image may also be stored by either digital or analog means.

Body Part Character 4	Contrast Character 5	Qualifier Character 6	Qualifier Character 7
Ø Abdominal Aorta **2** Hepatic Artery **3** Splenic Arteries **4** Superior Mesenteric Artery **5** Inferior Mesenteric Artery **6** Renal Artery, Right **7** Renal Artery, Left **8** Renal Arteries, Bilateral **9** Lumbar Arteries **B** Intra-Abdominal Arteries, Other **C** Pelvic Arteries **D** Aorta and Bilateral Lower Extremity Arteries **F** Lower Extremity Arteries, Right **G** Lower Extremity Arteries, Left **J** Lower Arteries, Other	**Ø** High Osmolar **1** Low Osmolar **Y** Other Contrast	**1** Laser	**Ø** Intraoperative
Ø Abdominal Aorta **2** Hepatic Artery **3** Splenic Arteries **4** Superior Mesenteric Artery **5** Inferior Mesenteric Artery **6** Renal Artery, Right **7** Renal Artery, Left **8** Renal Arteries, Bilateral **9** Lumbar Arteries **B** Intra-Abdominal Arteries, Other **C** Pelvic Arteries **D** Aorta and Bilateral Lower Extremity Arteries **F** Lower Extremity Arteries, Right **G** Lower Extremity Arteries, Left **J** Lower Arteries, Other	**Ø** High Osmolar **1** Low Osmolar **Y** Other Contrast	**Z** None	**Z** None
Ø Abdominal Aorta **2** Hepatic Artery **3** Splenic Arteries **4** Superior Mesenteric Artery **5** Inferior Mesenteric Artery **6** Renal Artery, Right **7** Renal Artery, Left **8** Renal Arteries, Bilateral **9** Lumbar Arteries **B** Intra-Abdominal Arteries, Other **C** Pelvic Arteries **D** Aorta and Bilateral Lower Extremity Arteries **F** Lower Extremity Arteries, Right **G** Lower Extremity Arteries, Left **J** Lower Arteries, Other	**Z** None	**Z** None	**Z** None

Imaging

B   **Imaging**
4   **Lower Arteries**
2   **Computerized Tomography (CT Scan)**   Definition: Computer reformatted digital display of multiplanar images developed from the capture of multiple exposures of external ionizing radiation

Body Part Character 4	Contrast Character 5	Qualifier Character 6	Qualifier Character 7
Ø Abdominal Aorta 1 Celiac Artery 4 Superior Mesenteric Artery 8 Renal Arteries, Bilateral C Pelvic Arteries F Lower Extremity Arteries, Right G Lower Extremity Arteries, Left H Lower Extremity Arteries, Bilateral M Renal Artery Transplant	Ø High Osmolar 1 Low Osmolar Y Other Contrast	Z None	Z None
Ø Abdominal Aorta 1 Celiac Artery 4 Superior Mesenteric Artery 8 Renal Arteries, Bilateral C Pelvic Arteries F Lower Extremity Arteries, Right G Lower Extremity Arteries, Left H Lower Extremity Arteries, Bilateral M Renal Artery Transplant	Z None	2 Intravascular Optical Coherence Z None	Z None

B   **Imaging**
4   **Lower Arteries**
3   **Magnetic Resonance Imaging (MRI)**   Definition: Computer reformatted digital display of multiplanar images developed from the capture of radio-frequency signals emitted by nuclei in a body site excited within a magnetic field

Body Part Character 4	Contrast Character 5	Qualifier Character 6	Qualifier Character 7
Ø Abdominal Aorta 1 Celiac Artery 4 Superior Mesenteric Artery 8 Renal Arteries, Bilateral C Pelvic Arteries F Lower Extremity Arteries, Right G Lower Extremity Arteries, Left H Lower Extremity Arteries, Bilateral	Y Other Contrast	Ø Unenhanced and Enhanced Z None	Z None
Ø Abdominal Aorta 1 Celiac Artery 4 Superior Mesenteric Artery 8 Renal Arteries, Bilateral C Pelvic Arteries F Lower Extremity Arteries, Right G Lower Extremity Arteries, Left H Lower Extremity Arteries, Bilateral	Z None	Z None	Z None

B   **Imaging**
4   **Lower Arteries**
4   **Ultrasonography**   Definition: Real time display of images of anatomy or flow information developed from the capture of relected and attenuated high frequency sound waves

Body Part Character 4	Contrast Character 5	Qualifier Character 6	Qualifier Character 7
Ø Abdominal Aorta 4 Superior Mesenteric Artery 5 Inferior Mesenteric Artery 6 Renal Artery, Right 7 Renal Artery, Left 8 Renal Arteries, Bilateral B Intra-Abdominal Arteries, Other F Lower Extremity Arteries, Right G Lower Extremity Arteries, Left H Lower Extremity Arteries, Bilateral K Celiac and Mesenteric Arteries L Femoral Artery N Penile Arteries	Z None	Z None	3 Intravascular Z None

B   **Imaging**
5   **Veins**
Ø   **Plain Radiography**   Definition: Planar display of an image developed from the capture of external ionizing radiation on photographic or photoconductive plate

Body Part Character 4	Contrast Character 5	Qualifier Character 6	Qualifier Character 7
Ø Epidural Veins	Ø High Osmolar	Z None	Z None
1 Cerebral and Cerebellar Veins	1 Low Osmolar		
2 Intracranial Sinuses	Y Other Contrast		
3 Jugular Veins, Right			
4 Jugular Veins, Left			
5 Jugular Veins, Bilateral			
6 Subclavian Vein, Right			
7 Subclavian Vein, Left			
8 Superior Vena Cava			
9 Inferior Vena Cava			
B Lower Extremity Veins, Right			
C Lower Extremity Veins, Left			
D Lower Extremity Veins, Bilateral			
F Pelvic (Iliac) Veins, Right			
G Pelvic (Iliac) Veins, Left			
H Pelvic (Iliac) Veins, Bilateral			
J Renal Vein, Right			
K Renal Vein, Left			
L Renal Veins, Bilateral			
M Upper Extremity Veins, Right			
N Upper Extremity Veins, Left			
P Upper Extremity Veins, Bilateral			
Q Pulmonary Vein, Right			
R Pulmonary Vein, Left			
S Pulmonary Veins, Bilateral			
T Portal and Splanchnic Veins			
V Veins, Other			
W Dialysis Shunt/Fistula			

B   **Imaging**
5   **Veins**
1   **Fluoroscopy**   Definition: Single plane or bi-plane real time display of an image developed from the capture of external ionizing radioation on a fluorescent screen. The image may also be stored by either digital or analog means.

Body Part Character 4	Contrast Character 5	Qualifier Character 6	Qualifier Character 7
Ø Epidural Veins	Ø High Osmolar	Z None	A Guidance
1 Cerebral and Cerebellar Veins	1 Low Osmolar		Z None
2 Intracranial Sinuses	Y Other Contrast		
3 Jugular Veins, Right	Z None		
4 Jugular Veins, Left			
5 Jugular Veins, Bilateral			
6 Subclavian Vein, Right			
7 Subclavian Vein, Left			
8 Superior Vena Cava			
9 Inferior Vena Cava			
B Lower Extremity Veins, Right			
C Lower Extremity Veins, Left			
D Lower Extremity Veins, Bilateral			
F Pelvic (Iliac) Veins, Right			
G Pelvic (Iliac) Veins, Left			
H Pelvic (Iliac) Veins, Bilateral			
J Renal Vein, Right			
K Renal Vein, Left			
L Renal Veins, Bilateral			
M Upper Extremity Veins, Right			
N Upper Extremity Veins, Left			
P Upper Extremity Veins, Bilateral			
Q Pulmonary Vein, Right			
R Pulmonary Vein, Left			
S Pulmonary Veins, Bilateral			
T Portal and Splanchnic Veins			
V Veins, Other			
W Dialysis Shunt/Fistula			

LC Limited Coverage   **NC** Noncovered   ⊞ Combination Member   HAC   Valid OR   Combination Only   DRG Non-OR   New/Revised in GREEN

ICD-10-PCS 2019   733

B5Ø–B51

B Imaging
5 Veins
2 Computerized Tomography (CT Scan) Definition: Computer reformatted digital display of multiplanar images developed from the capture of multiple exposures of external ionizing radiation

Body Part Character 4	Contrast Character 5	Qualifier Character 6	Qualifier Character 7
2 Intracranial Sinuses 8 Superior Vena Cava 9 Inferior Vena Cava F Pelvic (Iliac) Veins, Right G Pelvic (Iliac) Veins, Left H Pelvic (Iliac) Veins, Bilateral J Renal Vein, Right K Renal Vein, Left L Renal Veins, Bilateral Q Pulmonary Vein, Right R Pulmonary Vein, Left S Pulmonary Veins, Bilateral T Portal and Splanchnic Veins	Ø High Osmolar 1 Low Osmolar Y Other Contrast	Ø Unenhanced and Enhanced Z None	Z None
2 Intracranial Sinuses 8 Superior Vena Cava 9 Inferior Vena Cava F Pelvic (Iliac) Veins, Right G Pelvic (Iliac) Veins, Left H Pelvic (Iliac) Veins, Bilateral J Renal Vein, Right K Renal Vein, Left L Renal Veins, Bilateral Q Pulmonary Vein, Right R Pulmonary Vein, Left S Pulmonary Veins, Bilateral T Portal and Splanchnic Veins	Z None	2 Intravascular Optical Coherence Z None	Z None

B Imaging
5 Veins
3 Magnetic Resonance Imaging (MRI) Definition: Computer reformatted digital display of multiplanar images developed from the capture of radio-frequency signals emitted by nuclei in a body site excited within a magnetic field

Body Part Character 4	Contrast Character 5	Qualifier Character 6	Qualifier Character 7
1 Cerebral and Cerebellar Veins 2 Intracranial Sinuses 5 Jugular Veins, Bilateral 8 Superior Vena Cava 9 Inferior Vena Cava B Lower Extremity Veins, Right C Lower Extremity Veins, Left D Lower Extremity Veins, Bilateral H Pelvic (Iliac) Veins, Bilateral L Renal Veins, Bilateral M Upper Extremity Veins, Right N Upper Extremity Veins, Left P Upper Extremity Veins, Bilateral S Pulmonary Veins, Bilateral T Portal and Splanchnic Veins V Veins, Other	Y Other Contrast	Ø Unenhanced and Enhanced Z None	Z None
1 Cerebral and Cerebellar Veins 2 Intracranial Sinuses 5 Jugular Veins, Bilateral 8 Superior Vena Cava 9 Inferior Vena Cava B Lower Extremity Veins, Right C Lower Extremity Veins, Left D Lower Extremity Veins, Bilateral H Pelvic (Iliac) Veins, Bilateral L Renal Veins, Bilateral M Upper Extremity Veins, Right N Upper Extremity Veins, Left P Upper Extremity Veins, Bilateral S Pulmonary Veins, Bilateral T Portal and Splanchnic Veins V Veins, Other	Z None	Z None	Z None

B   Imaging
5   Veins
4   Ultrasonography   Definition: Real time display of images of anatomy or flow information developed from the capture of relected and attenuated high frequency sound waves

Body Part Character 4	Contrast Character 5	Qualifier Character 6	Qualifier Character 7
3 Jugular Veins, Right **4** Jugular Veins, Left **6** Subclavian Vein, Right **7** Subclavian Vein, Left **8** Superior Vena Cava **9** Inferior Vena Cava **B** Lower Extremity Veins, Right **C** Lower Extremity Veins, Left **D** Lower Extremity Veins, Bilateral **J** Renal Vein, Right **K** Renal Vein, Left **L** Renal Veins, Bilateral **M** Upper Extremity Veins, Right **N** Upper Extremity Veins, Left **P** Upper Extremity Veins, Bilateral **T** Portal and Splanchnic Veins	**Z** None	**Z** None	**3** Intravascular **A** Guidance **Z** None

B   Imaging
7   Lymphatic System
Ø   Plain Radiography   Definition: Planar display of an image developed from the capture of external ionizing radiation on photographic or photoconductive plate

Body Part Character 4	Contrast Character 5	Qualifier Character 6	Qualifier Character 7
Ø Abdominal/Retroperitoneal Lymphatics, Unilateral **1** Abdominal/Retroperitoneal Lymphatics, Bilateral **4** Lymphatics, Head and Neck **5** Upper Extremity Lymphatics, Right **6** Upper Extremity Lymphatics, Left **7** Upper Extremity Lymphatics, Bilateral **8** Lower Extremity Lymphatics, Right **9** Lower Extremity Lymphatics, Left **B** Lower Extremity Lymphatics, Bilateral **C** Lymphatics, Pelvic	**Ø** High Osmolar **1** Low Osmolar **Y** Other Contrast	**Z** None	**Z** None

B   Imaging
8   Eye
Ø   Plain Radiography   Definition: Planar display of an image developed from the capture of external ionizing radiation on photographic or photoconductive plate

Body Part Character 4	Contrast Character 5	Qualifier Character 6	Qualifier Character 7
Ø Lacrimal Duct, Right **1** Lacrimal Duct, Left **2** Lacrimal Ducts, Bilateral	**Ø** High Osmolar **1** Low Osmolar **Y** Other Contrast	**Z** None	**Z** None
3 Optic Foramina, Right **4** Optic Foramina, Left **5** Eye, Right **6** Eye, Left **7** Eyes, Bilateral	**Z** None	**Z** None	**Z** None

B   Imaging
8   Eye
2   Computerized Tomography (CT Scan)   Definition: Computer reformatted digital display of multiplanar images developed from the capture of multiple exposures of external ionizing radiation

Body Part Character 4	Contrast Character 5	Qualifier Character 6	Qualifier Character 7
5 Eye, Right **6** Eye, Left **7** Eyes, Bilateral	**Ø** High Osmolar **1** Low Osmolar **Y** Other Contrast	**Ø** Unenhanced and Enhanced **Z** None	**Z** None
5 Eye, Right **6** Eye, Left **7** Eyes, Bilateral	**Z** None	**Z** None	**Z** None

B Imaging
8 Eye
3 Magnetic Resonance Imaging (MRI)   Definition: Computer reformatted digital display of multiplanar images developed from the capture of radio-frequency signals emitted by nuclei in a body site excited within a magnetic field

Body Part Character 4	Contrast Character 5	Qualifier Character 6	Qualifier Character 7
5 Eye, Right 6 Eye, Left 7 Eyes, Bilateral	Y Other Contrast	Ø Unenhanced and Enhanced Z None	Z None
5 Eye, Right 6 Eye, Left 7 Eyes, Bilateral	Z None	Z None	Z None

B Imaging
8 Eye
4 Ultrasonography   Definition: Real time display of images of anatomy or flow information developed from the capture of relected and attenuated high frequency sound waves

Body Part Character 4	Contrast Character 5	Qualifier Character 6	Qualifier Character 7
5 Eye, Right 6 Eye, Left 7 Eyes, Bilateral	Z None	Z None	Z None

B Imaging
9 Ear, Nose, Mouth and Throat
Ø Plain Radiography   Definition: Planar display of an image developed from the capture of external ionizing radiation on photographic or photoconductive plate

Body Part Character 4	Contrast Character 5	Qualifier Character 6	Qualifier Character 7
2 Paranasal Sinuses F Nasopharynx/Oropharynx H Mastoids	Z None	Z None	Z None
4 Parotid Gland, Right 5 Parotid Gland, Left 6 Parotid Glands, Bilateral 7 Submandibular Gland, Right 8 Submandibular Gland, Left 9 Submandibular Glands, Bilateral B Salivary Gland, Right C Salivary Gland, Left D Salivary Glands, Bilateral	Ø High Osmolar 1 Low Osmolar Y Other Contrast	Z None	Z None

B Imaging
9 Ear, Nose, Mouth and Throat
1 Fluoroscopy   Definition: Single plane or bi-plane real time display of an image developed from the capture of external ionizing radioation on a fluorescent screen. The image may also be stored by either digital or analog means.

Body Part Character 4	Contrast Character 5	Qualifier Character 6	Qualifier Character 7
G Pharynx and Epiglottis J Larynx	Y Other Contrast Z None	Z None	Z None

B Imaging
9 Ear, Nose, Mouth and Throat
2 Computerized Tomography (CT Scan)   Definition: Computer reformatted digital display of multiplanar images developed from the capture of multiple exposures of external ionizing radiation

Body Part Character 4	Contrast Character 5	Qualifier Character 6	Qualifier Character 7
Ø Ear 2 Paranasal Sinuses 6 Parotid Glands, Bilateral 9 Submandibular Glands, Bilateral D Salivary Glands, Bilateral F Nasopharynx/Oropharynx J Larynx	Ø High Osmolar 1 Low Osmolar Y Other Contrast	Ø Unenhanced and Enhanced Z None	Z None
Ø Ear 2 Paranasal Sinuses 6 Parotid Glands, Bilateral 9 Submandibular Glands, Bilateral D Salivary Glands, Bilateral F Nasopharynx/Oropharynx J Larynx	Z None	Z None	Z None

B   Imaging
9   Ear, Nose, Mouth and Throat
3   Magnetic Resonance Imaging (MRI)   Definition: Computer reformatted digital display of multiplanar images developed from the capture of radio-frequency signals emitted by nuclei in a body site excited within a magnetic field

Body Part Character 4	Contrast Character 5	Qualifier Character 6	Qualifier Character 7
Ø Ear **2** Paranasal Sinuses **6** Parotid Glands, Bilateral **9** Submandibular Glands, Bilateral **D** Salivary Glands, Bilateral **F** Nasopharynx/Oropharynx **J** Larynx	**Y** Other Contrast	**Ø** Unenhanced and Enhanced **Z** None	**Z** None
Ø Ear **2** Paranasal Sinuses **6** Parotid Glands, Bilateral **9** Submandibular Glands, Bilateral **D** Salivary Glands, Bilateral **F** Nasopharynx/Oropharynx **J** Larynx	**Z** None	**Z** None	**Z** None

B   Imaging
B   Respiratory System
Ø   Plain Radiography   Definition: Planar display of an image developed from the capture of external ionizing radiation on photographic or photoconductive plate

Body Part Character 4	Contrast Character 5	Qualifier Character 6	Qualifier Character 7
7 Tracheobronchial Tree, Right **8** Tracheobronchial Tree, Left **9** Tracheobronchial Trees, Bilateral	**Y** Other Contrast	**Z** None	**Z** None
D Upper Airways	**Z** None	**Z** None	**Z** None

B   Imaging
B   Respiratory System
1   Fluoroscopy   Definition: Single plane or bi-plane real time display of an image developed from the capture of external ionizing radioation on a fluorescent screen. The image may also be stored by either digital or analog means.

Body Part Character 4	Contrast Character 5	Qualifier Character 6	Qualifier Character 7
2 Lung, Right **3** Lung, Left **4** Lungs, Bilateral **6** Diaphragm **C** Mediastinum **D** Upper Airways	**Z** None	**Z** None	**Z** None
7 Tracheobronchial Tree, Right **8** Tracheobronchial Tree, Left **9** Tracheobronchial Trees, Bilateral	**Y** Other Contrast	**Z** None	**Z** None

B   Imaging
B   Respiratory System
2   Computerized Tomography (CT Scan)   Definition: Computer reformatted digital display of multiplanar images developed from the capture of multiple exposures of external ionizing radiation

Body Part Character 4	Contrast Character 5	Qualifier Character 6	Qualifier Character 7
4 Lungs, Bilateral **7** Tracheobronchial Tree, Right **8** Tracheobronchial Tree, Left **9** Tracheobronchial Trees, Bilateral **F** Trachea/Airways	**Ø** High Osmolar **1** Low Osmolar **Y** Other Contrast	**Ø** Unenhanced and Enhanced **Z** None	**Z** None
4 Lungs, Bilateral **7** Tracheobronchial Tree, Right **8** Tracheobronchial Tree, Left **9** Tracheobronchial Trees, Bilateral **F** Trachea/Airways	**Z** None	**Z** None	**Z** None

B   **Imaging**
B   **Respiratory System**
3   **Magnetic Resonance Imaging (MRI)**   Definition: Computer reformatted digital display of multiplanar images developed from the capture of radio-frequency signals emitted by nuclei in a body site excited within a magnetic field

Body Part Character 4	Contrast Character 5	Qualifier Character 6	Qualifier Character 7
G Lung Apices	Y Other Contrast	Ø Unenhanced and Enhanced Z None	Z None
G Lung Apices	Z None	Z None	Z None

B   **Imaging**
B   **Respiratory System**
4   **Ultrasonography**   Definition: Real time display of images of anatomy or flow information developed from the capture of relected and attenuated high frequency sound waves

Body Part Character 4	Contrast Character 5	Qualifier Character 6	Qualifier Character 7
B Pleura C Mediastinum	Z None	Z None	Z None

B   **Imaging**
D   **Gastrointestinal System**
1   **Fluoroscopy**   Definition: Single plane or bi-plane real time display of an image developed from the capture of external ionizing radioation on a fluorescent screen. The image may also be stored by either digital or analog means.

Body Part Character 4	Contrast Character 5	Qualifier Character 6	Qualifier Character 7
1 Esophagus 2 Stomach 3 Small Bowel 4 Colon 5 Upper GI 6 Upper GI and Small Bowel 9 Duodenum B Mouth/Oropharynx	Y Other Contrast Z None	Z None	Z None

B   **Imaging**
D   **Gastrointestinal System**
2   **Computerized Tomography (CT Scan)**   Definition: Computer reformatted digital display of multiplanar images developed from the capture of multiple exposures of external ionizing radiation

Body Part Character 4	Contrast Character 5	Qualifier Character 6	Qualifier Character 7
4 Colon	Ø High Osmolar 1 Low Osmolar Y Other Contrast	Ø Unenhanced and Enhanced Z None	Z None
4 Colon	Z None	Z None	Z None

B   **Imaging**
D   **Gastrointestinal System**
4   **Ultrasonography**   Definition: Real time display of images of anatomy or flow information developed from the capture of relected and attenuated high frequency sound waves

Body Part Character 4	Contrast Character 5	Qualifier Character 6	Qualifier Character 7
1 Esophagus 2 Stomach 7 Gastrointestinal Tract 8 Appendix 9 Duodenum C Rectum	Z None	Z None	Z None

B   **Imaging**
F   **Hepatobiliary System and Pancreas**
Ø   **Plain Radiography**   Definition: Planar display of an image developed from the capture of external ionizing radiation on photographic or photoconductive plate

Body Part Character 4	Contrast Character 5	Qualifier Character 6	Qualifier Character 7
Ø Bile Ducts 3 Gallbladder and Bile Ducts C Hepatobiliary System, All	Ø High Osmolar 1 Low Osmolar Y Other Contrast	Z None	Z None

B   **Imaging**
F   **Hepatobiliary System and Pancreas**
1   **Fluoroscopy**   Definition: Single plane or bi-plane real time display of an image developed from the capture of external ionizing radioation on a fluorescent screen. The image may also be stored by either digital or analog means.

Body Part Character 4	Contrast Character 5	Qualifier Character 6	Qualifier Character 7
Ø Bile Ducts 1 Biliary and Pancreatic Ducts 2 Gallbladder 3 Gallbladder and Bile Ducts 4 Gallbladder, Bile Ducts and Pancreatic Ducts 8 Pancreatic Ducts	Ø High Osmolar 1 Low Osmolar Y Other Contrast	Z None	Z None

B   **Imaging**
F   **Hepatobiliary System and Pancreas**
2   **Computerized Tomography (CT Scan)**   Definition: Computer reformatted digital display of multiplanar images developed from the capture of multiple exposures of external ionizing radiation

Body Part Character 4	Contrast Character 5	Qualifier Character 6	Qualifier Character 7
5 Liver 6 Liver and Spleen 7 Pancreas C Hepatobiliary System, All	Ø High Osmolar 1 Low Osmolar Y Other Contrast	Ø Unenhanced and Enhanced Z None	Z None
5 Liver 6 Liver and Spleen 7 Pancreas C Hepatobiliary System, All	Z None	Z None	Z None

B   **Imaging**
F   **Hepatobiliary System and Pancreas**
3   **Magnetic Resonance Imaging (MRI)**   Definition: Computer reformatted digital display of multiplanar images developed from the capture of radio-frequency signals emitted by nuclei in a body site excited within a magnetic field

Body Part Character 4	Contrast Character 5	Qualifier Character 6	Qualifier Character 7
5 Liver 6 Liver and Spleen 7 Pancreas	Y Other Contrast	Ø Unenhanced and Enhanced Z None	Z None
5 Liver 6 Liver and Spleen 7 Pancreas	Z None	Z None	Z None

B   **Imaging**
F   **Hepatobiliary System and Pancreas**
4   **Ultrasonography**   Definition: Real time display of images of anatomy or flow information developed from the capture of relected and attenuated high frequency sound waves

Body Part Character 4	Contrast Character 5	Qualifier Character 6	Qualifier Character 7
Ø Bile Ducts 2 Gallbladder 3 Gallbladder and Bile Ducts 5 Liver 6 Liver and Spleen 7 Pancreas C Hepatobiliary System, All	Z None	Z None	Z None

B   **Imaging**
G   **Endocrine System**
2   **Computerized Tomography (CT Scan)**   Definition: Computer reformatted digital display of multiplanar images developed from the capture of multiple exposures of external ionizing radiation

Body Part Character 4	Contrast Character 5	Qualifier Character 6	Qualifier Character 7
2 Adrenal Glands, Bilateral 3 Parathyroid Glands 4 Thyroid Gland	Ø High Osmolar 1 Low Osmolar Y Other Contrast	Ø Unenhanced and Enhanced Z None	Z None
2 Adrenal Glands, Bilateral 3 Parathyroid Glands 4 Thyroid Gland	Z None	Z None	Z None

B Imaging
G Endocrine System
3 Magnetic Resonance Imaging (MRI) Definition: Computer reformatted digital display of multiplanar images developed from the capture of radio-frequency signals emitted by nuclei in a body site excited within a magnetic field

Body Part Character 4	Contrast Character 5	Qualifier Character 6	Qualifier Character 7
2 Adrenal Glands, Bilateral 3 Parathyroid Glands 4 Thyroid Gland	Y Other Contrast	Ø Unenhanced and Enhanced Z None	Z None
2 Adrenal Glands, Bilateral 3 Parathyroid Glands 4 Thyroid Gland	Z None	Z None	Z None

B Imaging
G Endocrine System
4 Ultrasonography Definition: Real time display of images of anatomy or flow information developed from the capture of reflected and attenuated high frequency sound waves

Body Part Character 4	Contrast Character 5	Qualifier Character 6	Qualifier Character 7
Ø Adrenal Gland, Right 1 Adrenal Gland, Left 2 Adrenal Glands, Bilateral 3 Parathyroid Glands 4 Thyroid Gland	Z None	Z None	Z None

B Imaging
H Skin, Subcutaneous Tissue and Breast
Ø Plain Radiography Definition: Planar display of an image developed from the capture of external ionizing radiation on photographic or photoconductive plate

Body Part Character 4	Contrast Character 5	Qualifier Character 6	Qualifier Character 7
Ø Breast, Right 1 Breast, Left 2 Breasts, Bilateral	Z None	Z None	Z None
3 Single Mammary Duct, Right 4 Single Mammary Duct, Left 5 Multiple Mammary Ducts, Right 6 Multiple Mammary Ducts, Left	Ø High Osmolar 1 Low Osmolar Y Other Contrast Z None	Z None	Z None

B Imaging
H Skin, Subcutaneous Tissue and Breast
3 Magnetic Resonance Imaging (MRI) Definition: Computer reformatted digital display of multiplanar images developed from the capture of radio-frequency signals emitted by nuclei in a body site excited within a magnetic field

Body Part Character 4	Contrast Character 5	Qualifier Character 6	Qualifier Character 7
Ø Breast, Right 1 Breast, Left 2 Breasts, Bilateral D Subcutaneous Tissue, Head/Neck F Subcutaneous Tissue, Upper Extremity G Subcutaneous Tissue, Thorax H Subcutaneous Tissue, Abdomen and Pelvis J Subcutaneous Tissue, Lower Extremity	Y Other Contrast	Ø Unenhanced and Enhanced Z None	Z None
Ø Breast, Right 1 Breast, Left 2 Breasts, Bilateral D Subcutaneous Tissue, Head/Neck F Subcutaneous Tissue, Upper Extremity G Subcutaneous Tissue, Thorax H Subcutaneous Tissue, Abdomen and Pelvis J Subcutaneous Tissue, Lower Extremity	Z None	Z None	Z None

B   **Imaging**
H   **Skin, Subcutaneous Tissue and Breast**
4   **Ultrasonography**   Definition: Real time display of images of anatomy or flow information developed from the capture of relected and attenuated high frequency sound waves

Body Part Character 4	Contrast Character 5	Qualifier Character 6	Qualifier Character 7
Ø Breast, Right 1 Breast, Left 2 Breasts, Bilateral 7 Extremity, Upper 8 Extremity, Lower 9 Abdominal Wall B Chest Wall C Head and Neck	Z None	Z None	Z None

B   **Imaging**
L   **Connective Tissue**
3   **Magnetic Resonance Imaging (MRI)**   Definition: Computer reformatted digital display of multiplanar images developed from the capture of radio-frequency signals emitted by nuclei in a body site excited within a magnetic field

Body Part Character 4	Contrast Character 5	Qualifier Character 6	Qualifier Character 7
Ø Connective Tissue, Upper Extremity 1 Connective Tissue, Lower Extremity 2 Tendons, Upper Extremity 3 Tendons, Lower Extremity	Y Other Contrast	Ø Unenhanced and Enhanced Z None	Z None
Ø Connective Tissue, Upper Extremity 1 Connective Tissue, Lower Extremity 2 Tendons, Upper Extremity 3 Tendons, Lower Extremity	Z None	Z None	Z None

B   **Imaging**
L   **Connective Tissue**
4   **Ultrasonography**   Definition: Real time display of images of anatomy or flow information developed from the capture of relected and attenuated high frequency sound waves

Body Part Character 4	Contrast Character 5	Qualifier Character 6	Qualifier Character 7
Ø Connective Tissue, Upper Extremity 1 Connective Tissue, Lower Extremity 2 Tendons, Upper Extremity 3 Tendons, Lower Extremity	Z None	Z None	Z None

B   **Imaging**
N   **Skull and Facial Bones**
Ø   **Plain Radiography**   Definition: Planar display of an image developed from the capture of external ionizing radiation on photographic or photoconductive plate

Body Part Character 4	Contrast Character 5	Qualifier Character 6	Qualifier Character 7
Ø Skull 1 Orbit, Right 2 Orbit, Left 3 Orbits, Bilateral 4 Nasal Bones 5 Facial Bones 6 Mandible B Zygomatic Arch, Right C Zygomatic Arch, Left D Zygomatic Arches, Bilateral G Tooth, Single H Teeth, Multiple J Teeth, All	Z None	Z None	Z None
7 Temporomandibular Joint, Right 8 Temporomandibular Joint, Left 9 Temporomandibular Joints, Bilateral	Ø High Osmolar 1 Low Osmolar Y Other Contrast Z None	Z None	Z None

LC Limited Coverage   **NC** Noncovered   ⊞ Combination Member   HAC   Valid OR   Combination Only   DRG Non-OR   New/Revised in GREEN
ICD-10-PCS 2019

741

BH4–BNØ

B Imaging
N Skull and Facial Bones
1 Fluoroscopy   Definition: Single plane or bi-plane real time display of an image developed from the capture of external ionizing radioation on a fluorescent screen. The image may also be stored by either digital or analog means.

Body Part Character 4	Contrast Character 5	Qualifier Character 6	Qualifier Character 7
7 Temporomandibular Joint, Right 8 Temporomandibular Joint, Left 9 Temporomandibular Joints, Bilateral	Ø High Osmolar 1 Low Osmolar Y Other Contrast Z None	Z None	Z None

B Imaging
N Skull and Facial Bones
2 Computerized Tomography (CT Scan)   Definition: Computer reformatted digital display of multiplanar images developed from the capture of multiple exposures of external ionizing radiation

Body Part Character 4	Contrast Character 5	Qualifier Character 6	Qualifier Character 7
Ø Skull 3 Orbits, Bilateral 5 Facial Bones 6 Mandible 9 Temporomandibular Joints, Bilateral F Temporal Bones	Ø High Osmolar 1 Low Osmolar Y Other Contrast Z None	Z None	Z None

B Imaging
N Skull and Facial Bones
3 Magnetic Resonance Imaging (MRI)   Definition: Computer reformatted digital display of multiplanar images developed from the capture of radio-frequency signals emitted by nuclei in a body site excited within a magnetic field

Body Part Character 4	Contrast Character 5	Qualifier Character 6	Qualifier Character 7
9 Temporomandibular Joints, Bilateral	Y Other Contrast Z None	Z None	Z None

B Imaging
P Non-Axial Upper Bones
Ø Plain Radiography   Definition: Planar display of an image developed from the capture of external ionizing radiation on photographic or photoconductive plate

Body Part Character 4	Contrast Character 5	Qualifier Character 6	Qualifier Character 7
Ø Sternoclavicular Joint, Right 1 Sternoclavicular Joint, Left 2 Sternoclavicular Joints, Bilateral 3 Acromioclavicular Joints, Bilateral 4 Clavicle, Right 5 Clavicle, Left 6 Scapula, Right 7 Scapula, Left A Humerus, Right B Humerus, Left E Upper Arm, Right F Upper Arm, Left J Forearm, Right K Forearm, Left N Hand, Right P Hand, Left R Finger(s), Right S Finger(s), Left X Ribs, Right Y Ribs, Left	Z None	Z None	Z None
8 Shoulder, Right 9 Shoulder, Left C Hand/Finger Joint, Right D Hand/Finger Joint, Left G Elbow, Right H Elbow, Left L Wrist, Right M Wrist, Left	Ø High Osmolar 1 Low Osmolar Y Other Contrast Z None	Z None	Z None

B   Imaging
P   Non-Axial Upper Bones
1   Fluoroscopy   Definition: Single plane or bi-plane real time display of an image developed from the capture of external ionizing radioation on a fluorescent screen. The image may also be stored by either digital or analog means.

Body Part Character 4	Contrast Character 5	Qualifier Character 6	Qualifier Character 7
Ø Sternoclavicular Joint, Right 1 Sternoclavicular Joint, Left 2 Sternoclavicular Joints, Bilateral 3 Acromioclavicular Joints, Bilateral 4 Clavicle, Right 5 Clavicle, Left 6 Scapula, Right 7 Scapula, Left A Humerus, Right B Humerus, Left E Upper Arm, Right F Upper Arm, Left J Forearm, Right K Forearm, Left N Hand, Right P Hand, Left R Finger(s), Right S Finger(s), Left X Ribs, Right Y Ribs, Left	Z None	Z None	Z None
8 Shoulder, Right 9 Shoulder, Left L Wrist, Right M Wrist, Left	Ø High Osmolar 1 Low Osmolar Y Other Contrast Z None	Z None	Z None
C Hand/Finger Joint, Right D Hand/Finger Joint, Left G Elbow, Right H Elbow, Left	Ø High Osmolar 1 Low Osmolar Y Other Contrast	Z None	Z None

B   Imaging
P   Non-Axial Upper Bones
2   Computerized Tomography (CT Scan)   Definition: Computer reformatted digital display of multiplanar images developed from the capture of multiple exposures of external ionizing radiation

Body Part Character 4	Contrast Character 5	Qualifier Character 6	Qualifier Character 7
Ø Sternoclavicular Joint, Right 1 Sternoclavicular Joint, Left W Thorax	Ø High Osmolar 1 Low Osmolar Y Other Contrast	Z None	Z None
2 Sternoclavicular Joints, Bilateral 3 Acromioclavicular Joints, Bilateral 4 Clavicle, Right 5 Clavicle, Left 6 Scapula, Right 7 Scapula, Left 8 Shoulder, Right 9 Shoulder, Left A Humerus, Right B Humerus, Left E Upper Arm, Right F Upper Arm, Left G Elbow, Right H Elbow, Left J Forearm, Right K Forearm, Left L Wrist, Right M Wrist, Left N Hand, Right P Hand, Left Q Hands and Wrists, Bilateral R Finger(s), Right S Finger(s), Left T Upper Extremity, Right U Upper Extremity, Left V Upper Extremities, Bilateral X Ribs, Right Y Ribs, Left	Ø High Osmolar 1 Low Osmolar Y Other Contrast Z None	Z None	Z None
C Hand/Finger Joint, Right D Hand/Finger Joint, Left	Z None	Z None	Z None

B Imaging
P Non-Axial Upper Bones
3 Magnetic Resonance Imaging (MRI) · Definition: Computer reformatted digital display of multiplanar images developed from the capture of radio-frequency signals emitted by nuclei in a body site excited within a magnetic field

Body Part Character 4	Contrast Character 5	Qualifier Character 6	Qualifier Character 7
8 Shoulder, Right 9 Shoulder, Left C Hand/Finger Joint, Right D Hand/Finger Joint, Left E Upper Arm, Right F Upper Arm, Left G Elbow, Right H Elbow, Left J Forearm, Right K Forearm, Left L Wrist, Right M Wrist, Left	Y Other Contrast	Ø Unenhanced and Enhanced Z None	Z None
8 Shoulder, Right 9 Shoulder, Left C Hand/Finger Joint, Right D Hand/Finger Joint, Left E Upper Arm, Right F Upper Arm, Left G Elbow, Right H Elbow, Left J Forearm, Right K Forearm, Left L Wrist, Right M Wrist, Left	Z None	Z None	Z None

B Imaging
P Non-Axial Upper Bones
4 Ultrasonography Definition: Real time display of images of anatomy or flow information developed from the capture of relected and attenuated high frequency sound waves

Body Part Character 4	Contrast Character 5	Qualifier Character 6	Qualifier Character 7
8 Shoulder, Right 9 Shoulder, Left G Elbow, Right H Elbow, Left L Wrist, Right M Wrist, Left N Hand, Right P Hand, Left	Z None	Z None	1 Densitometry Z None

B Imaging
Q Non-Axial Lower Bones
Ø Plain Radiography Definition: Planar display of an image developed from the capture of external ionizing radiation on photographic or photoconductive plate

Body Part Character 4	Contrast Character 5	Qualifier Character 6	Qualifier Character 7
Ø Hip, Right 1 Hip, Left	Ø High Osmolar 1 Low Osmolar Y Other Contrast	Z None	Z None
Ø Hip, Right 1 Hip, Left	Z None	Z None	1 Densitometry Z None
3 Femur, Right 4 Femur, Left	Z None	Z None	1 Densitometry Z None
7 Knee, Right 8 Knee, Left G Ankle, Right H Ankle, Left	Ø High Osmolar 1 Low Osmolar Y Other Contrast Z None	Z None	Z None
D Lower Leg, Right F Lower Leg, Left J Calcaneus, Right K Calcaneus, Left L Foot, Right M Foot, Left P Toe(s), Right Q Toe(s), Left V Patella, Right W Patella, Left	Z None	Z None	Z None
X Foot/Toe Joint, Right Y Foot/Toe Joint, Left	Ø High Osmolar 1 Low Osmolar Y Other Contrast	Z None	Z None

B   **Imaging**
Q   **Non-Axial Lower Bones**
1   **Fluoroscopy**   Definition: Single plane or bi-plane real time display of an image developed from the capture of external ionizing radioation on a fluorescent screen. The image may also be stored by either digital or analog means.

Body Part Character 4	Contrast Character 5	Qualifier Character 6	Qualifier Character 7
Ø Hip, Right 1 Hip, Left 7 Knee, Right 8 Knee, Left G Ankle, Right H Ankle, Left X Foot/Toe Joint, Right Y Foot/Toe Joint, Left	Ø High Osmolar 1 Low Osmolar Y Other Contrast Z None	Z None	Z None
3 Femur, Right 4 Femur, Left D Lower Leg, Right F Lower Leg, Left J Calcaneus, Right K Calcaneus, Left L Foot, Right M Foot, Left P Toe(s), Right Q Toe(s), Left V Patella, Right W Patella, Left	Z None	Z None	Z None

B   **Imaging**
Q   **Non-Axial Lower Bones**
2   **Computerized Tomography (CT Scan)**   Definition: Computer reformatted digital display of multiplanar images developed from the capture of multiple exposures of external ionizing radiation

Body Part Character 4	Contrast Character 5	Qualifier Character 6	Qualifier Character 7
Ø Hip, Right 1 Hip, Left 3 Femur, Right 4 Femur, Left 7 Knee, Right 8 Knee, Left D Lower Leg, Right F Lower Leg, Left G Ankle, Right H Ankle, Left J Calcaneus, Right K Calcaneus, Left L Foot, Right M Foot, Left P Toe(s), Right Q Toe(s), Left R Lower Extremity, Right S Lower Extremity, Left V Patella, Right W Patella, Left X Foot/Toe Joint, Right Y Foot/Toe Joint, Left	Ø High Osmolar 1 Low Osmolar Y Other Contrast Z None	Z None	Z None
B Tibia/Fibula, Right C Tibia/Fibula, Left	Ø High Osmolar 1 Low Osmolar Y Other Contrast	Z None	Z None

B   Imaging
Q   Non-Axial Lower Bones
3   Magnetic Resonance Imaging (MRI)   Definition: Computer reformatted digital display of multiplanar images developed from the capture of radio-frequency signals emitted by nuclei in a body site excited within a magnetic field

Body Part Character 4	Contrast Character 5	Qualifier Character 6	Qualifier Character 7
Ø Hip, Right 1 Hip, Left 3 Femur, Right 4 Femur, Left 7 Knee, Right 8 Knee, Left D Lower Leg, Right F Lower Leg, Left G Ankle, Right H Ankle, Left J Calcaneus, Right K Calcaneus, Left L Foot, Right M Foot, Left P Toe(s), Right Q Toe(s), Left V Patella, Right W Patella, Left	Y Other Contrast	Ø Unenhanced and Enhanced Z None	Z None
Ø Hip, Right 1 Hip, Left 3 Femur, Right 4 Femur, Left 7 Knee, Right 8 Knee, Left D Lower Leg, Right F Lower Leg, Left G Ankle, Right H Ankle, Left J Calcaneus, Right K Calcaneus, Left L Foot, Right M Foot, Left P Toe(s), Right Q Toe(s), Left V Patella, Right W Patella, Left	Z None	Z None	Z None

B   Imaging
Q   Non-Axial Lower Bones
4   Ultrasonography   Definition: Real time display of images of anatomy or flow information developed from the capture of relected and attenuated high frequency sound waves

Body Part Character 4	Contrast Character 5	Qualifier Character 6	Qualifier Character 7
Ø Hip, Right 1 Hip, Left 2 Hips, Bilateral 7 Knee, Right 8 Knee, Left 9 Knees, Bilateral	Z None	Z None	Z None

B   **Imaging**
R   **Axial Skeleton, Except Skull and Facial Bones**
Ø   **Plain Radiography**   Definition: Planar display of an image developed from the capture of external ionizing radiation on photographic or photoconductive plate

Body Part Character 4	Contrast Character 5	Qualifier Character 6	Qualifier Character 7
Ø Cervical Spine 7 Thoracic Spine 9 Lumbar Spine G Whole Spine	Z None	Z None	1 Densitometry Z None
1 Cervical Disc(s) 2 Thoracic Disc(s) 3 Lumbar Disc(s) 4 Cervical Facet Joint(s) 5 Thoracic Facet Joint(s) 6 Lumbar Facet Joint(s) D Sacroiliac Joints	Ø High Osmolar 1 Low Osmolar Y Other Contrast Z None	Z None	Z None
8 Thoracolumbar Joint B Lumbosacral Joint C Pelvis F Sacrum and Coccyx H Sternum	Z None	Z None	Z None

B   **Imaging**
R   **Axial Skeleton, Except Skull and Facial Bones**
1   **Fluoroscopy**   Definition: Single plane or bi-plane real time display of an image developed from the capture of external ionizing radioation on a fluorescent screen. The image may also be stored by either digital or analog means.

Body Part Character 4	Contrast Character 5	Qualifier Character 6	Qualifier Character 7
Ø Cervical Spine 1 Cervical Disc(s) 2 Thoracic Disc(s) 3 Lumbar Disc(s) 4 Cervical Facet Joint(s) 5 Thoracic Facet Joint(s) 6 Lumbar Facet Joint(s) 7 Thoracic Spine 8 Thoracolumbar Joint 9 Lumbar Spine B Lumbosacral Joint C Pelvis D Sacroiliac Joints F Sacrum and Coccyx G Whole Spine H Sternum	Ø High Osmolar 1 Low Osmolar Y Other Contrast Z None	Z None	Z None

B   **Imaging**
R   **Axial Skeleton, Except Skull and Facial Bones**
2   **Computerized Tomography (CT Scan)**   Definition: Computer reformatted digital display of multiplanar images developed from the capture of multiple exposures of external ionizing radiation

Body Part Character 4	Contrast Character 5	Qualifier Character 6	Qualifier Character 7
Ø Cervical Spine 7 Thoracic Spine 9 Lumbar Spine C Pelvis D Sacroiliac Joints F Sacrum and Coccyx	Ø High Osmolar 1 Low Osmolar Y Other Contrast Z None	Z None	Z None

B   Imaging
R   Axial Skeleton, Except Skull and Facial Bones
3   Magnetic Resonance Imaging (MRI)   Definition: Computer reformatted digital display of multiplanar images developed from the capture of radio-frequency signals emitted by nuclei in a body site excited within a magnetic field

Body Part Character 4	Contrast Character 5	Qualifier Character 6	Qualifier Character 7
Ø Cervical Spine 1 Cervical Disc(s) 2 Thoracic Disc(s) 3 Lumbar Disc(s) 7 Thoracic Spine 9 Lumbar Spine C Pelvis F Sacrum and Coccyx	Y Other Contrast	Ø Unenhanced and Enhanced Z None	Z None
Ø Cervical Spine 1 Cervical Disc(s) 2 Thoracic Disc(s) 3 Lumbar Disc(s) 7 Thoracic Spine 9 Lumbar Spine C Pelvis F Sacrum and Coccyx	Z None	Z None	Z None

B   Imaging
R   Axial Skeleton, Except Skull and Facial Bones
4   Ultrasonography   Definition: Real time display of images of anatomy or flow information developed from the capture of relected and attenuated high frequency sound waves

Body Part Character 4	Contrast Character 5	Qualifier Character 6	Qualifier Character 7
Ø Cervical Spine 7 Thoracic Spine 9 Lumbar Spine F Sacrum and Coccyx	Z None	Z None	Z None

B   Imaging
T   Urinary System
Ø   Plain Radiography   Definition: Planar display of an image developed from the capture of external ionizing radiation on photographic or photoconductive plate

Body Part Character 4	Contrast Character 5	Qualifier Character 6	Qualifier Character 7
Ø Bladder 1 Kidney, Right 2 Kidney, Left 3 Kidneys, Bilateral 4 Kidneys, Ureters and Bladder 5 Urethra 6 Ureter, Right 7 Ureter, Left 8 Ureters, Bilateral B Bladder and Urethra C Ileal Diversion Loop	Ø High Osmolar 1 Low Osmolar Y Other Contrast Z None	Z None	Z None

B   Imaging
T   Urinary System
1   Fluoroscopy   Definition: Single plane or bi-plane real time display of an image developed from the capture of external ionizing radioation on a fluorescent screen. The image may also be stored by either digital or analog means.

Body Part Character 4	Contrast Character 5	Qualifier Character 6	Qualifier Character 7
Ø Bladder 1 Kidney, Right 2 Kidney, Left 3 Kidneys, Bilateral 4 Kidneys, Ureters and Bladder 5 Urethra 6 Ureter, Right 7 Ureter, Left B Bladder and Urethra C Ileal Diversion Loop D Kidney, Ureter and Bladder, Right F Kidney, Ureter and Bladder, Left G Ileal Loop, Ureters and Kidneys	Ø High Osmolar 1 Low Osmolar Y Other Contrast Z None	Z None	Z None

B   **Imaging**
T   **Urinary System**
2   **Computerized Tomography (CT Scan)**   Definition: Computer reformatted digital display of multiplanar images developed from the capture of multiple exposures of external ionizing radiation

Body Part Character 4	Contrast Character 5	Qualifier Character 6	Qualifier Character 7
Ø Bladder 1 Kidney, Right 2 Kidney, Left 3 Kidneys, Bilateral 9 Kidney Transplant	Ø High Osmolar 1 Low Osmolar Y Other Contrast	Ø Unenhanced and Enhanced Z None	Z None
Ø Bladder 1 Kidney, Right 2 Kidney, Left 3 Kidneys, Bilateral 9 Kidney Transplant	Z None	Z None	Z None

B   **Imaging**
T   **Urinary System**
3   **Magnetic Resonance Imaging (MRI)**   Definition: Computer reformatted digital display of multiplanar images developed from the capture of radio-frequency signals emitted by nuclei in a body site excited within a magnetic field

Body Part Character 4	Contrast Character 5	Qualifier Character 6	Qualifier Character 7
Ø Bladder 1 Kidney, Right 2 Kidney, Left 3 Kidneys, Bilateral 9 Kidney Transplant	Y Other Contrast	Ø Unenhanced and Enhanced Z None	Z None
Ø Bladder 1 Kidney, Right 2 Kidney, Left 3 Kidneys, Bilateral 9 Kidney Transplant	Z None	Z None	Z None

B   **Imaging**
T   **Urinary System**
4   **Ultrasonography**   Definition: Real time display of images of anatomy or flow information developed from the capture of relected and attenuated high frequency sound waves

Body Part Character 4	Contrast Character 5	Qualifier Character 6	Qualifier Character 7
Ø Bladder 1 Kidney, Right 2 Kidney, Left 3 Kidneys, Bilateral 5 Urethra 6 Ureter, Right 7 Ureter, Left 8 Ureters, Bilateral 9 Kidney Transplant J Kidneys and Bladder	Z None	Z None	Z None

B   **Imaging**
U   **Female Reproductive System**
Ø   **Plain Radiography**   Definition: Planar display of an image developed from the capture of external ionizing radiation on photographic or photoconductive plate

Body Part Character 4	Contrast Character 5	Qualifier Character 6	Qualifier Character 7
Ø Fallopian Tube, Right ♀ 1 Fallopian Tube, Left ♀ 2 Fallopian Tubes, Bilateral ♀ 6 Uterus ♀ 8 Uterus and Fallopian Tubes ♀ 9 Vagina ♀	Ø High Osmolar 1 Low Osmolar Y Other Contrast	Z None	Z None

♀   All body part, contrast, and qualifier values

Imaging (side tab)

B Imaging
U Female Reproductive System
1 Fluoroscopy   Definition: Single plane or bi-plane real time display of an image developed from the capture of external ionizing radioation on a fluorescent screen. The image may also be stored by either digital or analog means.

Body Part Character 4	Contrast Character 5	Qualifier Character 6	Qualifier Character 7
Ø Fallopian Tube, Right ♀ 1 Fallopian Tube, Left ♀ 2 Fallopian Tubes, Bilateral ♀ 6 Uterus ♀ 8 Uterus and Fallopian Tubes ♀ 9 Vagina ♀	Ø High Osmolar 1 Low Osmolar Y Other Contrast Z None	Z None	Z None

♀ All body part, contrast, and qualifier values

B Imaging
U Female Reproductive System
3 Magnetic Resonance Imaging (MRI)   Definition: Computer reformatted digital display of multiplanar images developed from the capture of radio-frequency signals emitted by nuclei in a body site excited within a magnetic field

Body Part Character 4	Contrast Character 5	Qualifier Character 6	Qualifier Character 7
3 Ovary, Right ♀ 4 Ovary, Left ♀ 5 Ovaries, Bilateral ♀ 6 Uterus ♀ 9 Vagina ♀ B Pregnant Uterus ♀ C Uterus and Ovaries ♀	Y Other Contrast	Ø Unenhanced and Enhanced Z None	Z None
3 Ovary, Right ♀ 4 Ovary, Left ♀ 5 Ovaries, Bilateral ♀ 6 Uterus ♀ 9 Vagina ♀ B Pregnant Uterus ♀ C Uterus and Ovaries ♀	Z None	Z None	Z None

♀ All body part, contrast, and qualifier values

B Imaging
U Female Reproductive System
4 Ultrasonography   Definition: Real time display of images of anatomy or flow information developed from the capture of relected and attenuated high frequency sound waves

Body Part Character 4	Contrast Character 5	Qualifier Character 6	Qualifier Character 7
Ø Fallopian Tube, Right ♀ 1 Fallopian Tube, Left ♀ 2 Fallopian Tubes, Bilateral ♀ 3 Ovary, Right ♀ 4 Ovary, Left ♀ 5 Ovaries, Bilateral ♀ 6 Uterus ♀ C Uterus and Ovaries ♀	Y Other Contrast Z None	Z None	Z None

♀ All body part, contrast, and qualifier values

B Imaging
V Male Reproductive System
Ø Plain Radiography   Definition: Planar display of an image developed from the capture of external ionizing radiation on photographic or photoconductive plate

Body Part Character 4	Contrast Character 5	Qualifier Character 6	Qualifier Character 7
Ø Corpora Cavernosa ♂ 1 Epididymis, Right ♂ 2 Epididymis, Left ♂ 3 Prostate ♂ 5 Testicle, Right ♂ 6 Testicle, Left ♂ 8 Vasa Vasorum ♂	Ø High Osmolar 1 Low Osmolar Y Other Contrast	Z None	Z None

♂ All body part, contrast, and qualifier values

B   **Imaging**
V   **Male Reproductive System**
1   **Fluoroscopy**   Definition: Single plane or bi-plane real time display of an image developed from the capture of external ionizing radioation on a fluorescent screen. The image may also be stored by either digital or analog means.

Body Part Character 4	Contrast Character 5	Qualifier Character 6	Qualifier Character 7
Ø Corpora Cavernosa ♂ 8 Vasa Vasorum ♂	Ø High Osmolar 1 Low Osmolar Y Other Contrast Z None	Z None	Z None

♂   All body part, contrast, and qualifier values

B   **Imaging**
V   **Male Reproductive System**
2   **Computerized Tomography (CT Scan)**   Definition: Computer reformatted digital display of multiplanar images developed from the capture of multiple exposures of external ionizing radiation

Body Part Character 4	Contrast Character 5	Qualifier Character 6	Qualifier Character 7
3 Prostate ♂	Ø High Osmolar 1 Low Osmolar Y Other Contrast	Ø Unenhanced and Enhanced Z None	Z None
3 Prostate ♂	Z None	Z None	Z None

♂ BV23[Ø,Y][Ø,Z]Z   ♂ BV23ZZZ
♂ BV231ØZ

B   **Imaging**
V   **Male Reproductive System**
3   **Magnetic Resonance Imaging (MRI)**   Definition: Computer reformatted digital display of multiplanar images developed from the capture of radio-frequency signals emitted by nuclei in a body site excited within a magnetic field

Body Part Character 4	Contrast Character 5	Qualifier Character 6	Qualifier Character 7
Ø Corpora Cavernosa ♂ 3 Prostate ♂ 4 Scrotum ♂ 5 Testicle, Right ♂ 6 Testicle, Left ♂ 7 Testicles, Bilateral ♂	Y Other Contrast	Ø Unenhanced and Enhanced Z None	Z None
Ø Corpora Cavernosa ♂ 3 Prostate ♂ 4 Scrotum ♂ 5 Testicle, Right ♂ 6 Testicle, Left ♂ 7 Testicles, Bilateral ♂	Z None	Z None	Z None

♂   All body part, contrast, and qualifier values

B   **Imaging**
V   **Male Reproductive System**
4   **Ultrasonography**   Definition: Real time display of images of anatomy or flow information developed from the capture of relected and attenuated high frequency sound waves

Body Part Character 4	Contrast Character 5	Qualifier Character 6	Qualifier Character 7
4 Scrotum ♂ 9 Prostate and Seminal Vesicles ♂ B Penis ♂	Z None	Z None	Z None

♂   All body part, contrast, and qualifier values

B   **Imaging**
W   **Anatomical Regions**
Ø   **Plain Radiography**   Definition: Planar display of an image developed from the capture of external ionizing radiation on photographic or photoconductive plate

Body Part Character 4	Contrast Character 5	Qualifier Character 6	Qualifier Character 7
Ø Abdomen 1 Abdomen and Pelvis 3 Chest B Long Bones, All C Lower Extremity J Upper Extremity K Whole Body L Whole Skeleton M Whole Body, Infant	Z None	Z None	Z None

B Imaging
W Anatomical Regions
1 Fluoroscopy Definition: Single plane or bi-plane real time display of an image developed from the capture of external ionizing radioation on a fluorescent screen. The image may also be stored by either digital or analog means.

Body Part Character 4	Contrast Character 5	Qualifier Character 6	Qualifier Character 7
1 Abdomen and Pelvis	Ø High Osmolar	Z None	Z None
9 Head and Neck	1 Low Osmolar		
C Lower Extremity	Y Other Contrast		
J Upper Extremity	Z None		

B Imaging
W Anatomical Regions
2 Computerized Tomography (CT Scan) Definition: Computer reformatted digital display of multiplanar images developed from the capture of multiple exposures of external ionizing radiation

Body Part Character 4	Contrast Character 5	Qualifier Character 6	Qualifier Character 7
Ø Abdomen	Ø High Osmolar	Ø Unenhanced and Enhanced	Z None
1 Abdomen and Pelvis	1 Low Osmolar	Z None	
4 Chest and Abdomen	Y Other Contrast		
5 Chest, Abdomen and Pelvis			
8 Head			
9 Head and Neck			
F Neck			
G Pelvic Region			
Ø Abdomen	Z None	Z None	Z None
1 Abdomen and Pelvis			
4 Chest and Abdomen			
5 Chest, Abdomen and Pelvis			
8 Head			
9 Head and Neck			
F Neck			
G Pelvic Region			

B Imaging
W Anatomical Regions
3 Magnetic Resonance Imaging (MRI) Definition: Computer reformatted digital display of multiplanar images developed from the capture of radio-frequency signals emitted by nuclei in a body site excited within a magnetic field

Body Part Character 4	Contrast Character 5	Qualifier Character 6	Qualifier Character 7
Ø Abdomen	Y Other Contrast	Ø Unenhanced and Enhanced	Z None
8 Head		Z None	
F Neck			
G Pelvic Region			
H Retroperitoneum			
P Brachial Plexus			
Ø Abdomen	Z None	Z None	Z None
8 Head			
F Neck			
G Pelvic Region			
H Retroperitoneum			
P Brachial Plexus			
3 Chest	Y Other Contrast	Ø Unenhanced and Enhanced	Z None
		Z None	

B Imaging
W Anatomical Regions
4 Ultrasonography Definition: Real time display of images of anatomy or flow information developed from the capture of relected and attenuated high frequency sound waves

Body Part Character 4	Contrast Character 5	Qualifier Character 6	Qualifier Character 7
Ø Abdomen	Z None	Z None	Z None
1 Abdomen and Pelvis			
F Neck			
G Pelvic Region			

B   **Imaging**
Y   **Fetus and Obstetrical**
3   **Magnetic Resonance Imaging (MRI)**   Definition: Computer reformatted digital display of multiplanar images developed from the capture of radio-frequency signals emitted by nuclei in a body site excited within a magnetic field

Body Part Character 4		Contrast Character 5	Qualifier Character 6	Qualifier Character 7
Ø Fetal Head ♀ **1** Fetal Heart ♀ **2** Fetal Thorax ♀ **3** Fetal Abdomen ♀ **4** Fetal Spine ♀ **5** Fetal Extremities ♀ **6** Whole Fetus ♀		**Y** Other Contrast	**Ø** Unenhanced and Enhanced **Z** None	**Z** None
Ø Fetal Head ♀ **1** Fetal Heart ♀ **2** Fetal Thorax ♀ **3** Fetal Abdomen ♀ **4** Fetal Spine ♀ **5** Fetal Extremities ♀ **6** Whole Fetus ♀		**Z** None	**Z** None	**Z** None

  ♀ BY3[Ø,1,2,3,5,6]Y[Ø,Z]Z
  ♀ BY34YZZ
  ♀ BY3[Ø,1,2,3,4,5,6]ZZZ

B   **Imaging**
Y   **Fetus and Obstetrical**
4   **Ultrasonography**   Definition: Real time display of images of anatomy or flow information developed from the capture of relected and attenuated high frequency sound-waves

Body Part Character 4		Contrast Character 5	Qualifier Character 6	Qualifier Character 7
7 Fetal Umbilical Cord ♀ **8** Placenta ♀ **9** First Trimester, Single Fetus ♀ **B** First Trimester, Multiple Gestation ♀ **C** Second Trimester, Single Fetus ♀ **D** Second Trimester, Multiple Gestation ♀ **F** Third Trimester, Single Fetus ♀ **G** Third Trimester, Multiple Gestation ♀		**Z** None	**Z** None	**Z** None

  ♀   All body part, contrast, and qualifier values

LC Limited Coverage   NC Noncovered   ⊞ Combination Member   HAC   Valid OR   Combination Only   DRG Non-OR   New/Revised in GREEN
ICD-10-PCS 2019   **753**

BY3–BY4

Nuclear Medicine CØ1–CW7

Character Meanings

This Character Meaning table is provided as a guide to assist the user in the identification of character members that may be found in this section of code tables. It **SHOULD NOT** be used to build a PCS code.

Body System–Character 2	Type–Character 3	Body Part–Character 4	Radionuclide–Character 5	Qualifier–Character 6	Qualifier–Character 7
Ø Central Nervous System	1 Planar Nuclear Medicine Imaging	See below	1 Technetium 99m (Tc-99m)	Z None	Z None
2 Heart	2 Tomographic (Tomo) Nuclear Medicine Imaging		7 Cobalt 58 (Co-58)		
5 Veins	3 Positron Emission Tomographic (PET) Imaging		8 Samarium 153 (Sm-153)		
7 Lymphatic and Hematologic System	4 Nonimaging Nuclear Medicine Uptake		9 Krypton (Kr-81m)		
8 Eye	5 Nonimaging Nuclear Medicine Probe		B Carbon 11 (C-11)		
9 Ear, Nose, Mouth and Throat	6 Nonimaging Nuclear Medicine Assay		C Cobalt 57 (Co-57)		
B Respiratory System	7 Systemic Nuclear Medicine Therapy		D Indium 111 (In-111)		
D Gastrointestinal System			F Iodine 123 (I-123)		
F Hepatobiliary System and Pancreas			G Iodine 131 (I-131)		
G Endocrine System			H Iodine 125 (I-125)		
H Skin, Subcutaneous Tissue and Breast			K Fluorine 18 (F-18)		
P Musculoskeletal System			L Gallium 67 (Ga-67)		
T Urinary System			M Oxygen 15 (O-15)		
V Male Reproductive System			N Phosphorus 32 (P-32)		
W Anatomical Regions			P Strontium 89 (Sr-89)		
			Q Rubidium 82 (Rb-82)		
			R Nitrogen 13 (N-13)		
			S Thallium 2Ø1 (Tl-2Ø1)		
			T Xenon 127 (Xe-127)		
			V Xenon 133 (Xe-133)		
			W Chromium (Cr-51)		
			Y Other Radionuclide		
			Z None		

Body Part—Character 4 Meanings

Body System– Character 2	Body Part– Character 4
Ø Central Nervous System	Ø Brain 5 Cerebrospinal Fluid Y Central Nervous System
2 Heart	6 Heart, Right and Left G Myocardium Y Heart
5 Veins	B Lower Extremity Veins, Right C Lower Extremity Veins, Left D Lower Extremity Veins, Bilateral N Upper Extremity Veins, Right P Upper Extremity Veins, Left Q Upper Extremity Veins, Bilateral R Central Veins Y Veins

Continued on next page

Continued from previous page

Body System– Character 2	Body Part– Character 4
7 Lymphatic and Hematologic System	Ø Bone Marrow 2 Spleen 3 Blood 5 Lymphatics, Head and Neck D Lymphatics, Pelvic J Lymphatics, Head K Lymphatics, Neck L Lymphatics, Upper Chest M Lymphatics, Trunk N Lymphatics, Upper Extremity P Lymphatics, Lower Extremity Y Lymphatic and Hematologic System
8 Eye	9 Lacrimal Ducts, Bilateral Y Eye
9 Ear, Nose, Mouth and Throat	B Salivary Glands, Bilateral Y Ear, Nose, Mouth and Throat
B Respiratory System	2 Lungs and Bronchi Y Respiratory System
D Gastrointestinal System	5 Upper Gastrointestinal Tract 7 Gastrointestinal Tract Y Digestive System
F Hepatobiliary System and Pancreas	4 Gallbladder 5 Liver 6 Liver and Spleen C Hepatobiliary System, All Y Hepatobiliary System and Pancreas
G Endocrine System	1 Parathyroid Glands 2 Thyroid Gland 4 Adrenal Glands, Bilateral Y Endocrine System
H Skin, Subcutaneous Tissue and Breast	Ø Breast, Right 1 Breast, Left 2 Breasts, Bilateral Y Skin, Subcutaneous Tissue and Breast
P Musculoskeletal System	1 Skull 2 Cervical Spine 3 Skull and Cervical Spine 4 Thorax 5 Spine 6 Pelvis 7 Spine and Pelvis 8 Upper Extremity, Right 9 Upper Extremity, Left B Upper Extremities, Bilateral C Lower Extremity, Right D Lower Extremity, Left F Lower Extremities, Bilateral G Thoracic Spine H Lumbar Spine J Thoracolumbar Spine N Upper Extremities P Lower Extremities Y Musculoskeletal System, Other Z Musculoskeletal System, All
T Urinary System	3 Kidneys, Ureters and Bladder H Bladder and Ureters Y Urinary System
V Male Reproductive System	9 Testicles, Bilateral Y Male Reproductive System
W Anatomical Regions	Ø Abdomen 1 Abdomen and Pelvis 3 Chest 4 Chest and Abdomen 6 Chest and Neck B Head and Neck D Lower Extremity G Thyroid J Pelvic Region M Upper Extremity N Whole Body Y Anatomical Regions, Multiple Z Anatomical Region, Other

C   **Nuclear Medicine**
Ø   **Central Nervous System**
1   **Planar Nuclear Medicine Imaging**   Definition: Introduction of radioactive materials into the body for single plane display of images developed from the capture of radioactive emissions

Body Part Character 4	Radionuclide Character 5	Qualifier Character 6	Qualifier Character 7
Ø Brain	**1** Technetium 99m (Tc-99m) **Y** Other Radionuclide	**Z** None	**Z** None
5 Cerebrospinal Fluid	**D** Indium 111 (In-111) **Y** Other Radionuclide	**Z** None	**Z** None
Y Central Nervous System	**Y** Other Radionuclide	**Z** None	**Z** None

C   **Nuclear Medicine**
Ø   **Central Nervous System**
2   **Tomographic (Tomo) Nuclear Medicine Imaging**   Definition: Introduction of radioactive materials into the body for three dimensional display of images developed from the capture of radioactive emissions

Body Part Character 4	Radionuclide Character 5	Qualifier Character 6	Qualifier Character 7
Ø Brain	**1** Technetium 99m (Tc-99m) **F** Iodine 123 (I-123) **S** Thallium 201 (Tl-201) **Y** Other Radionuclide	**Z** None	**Z** None
5 Cerebrospinal Fluid	**D** Indium 111 (In-111) **Y** Other Radionuclide	**Z** None	**Z** None
Y Central Nervous System	**Y** Other Radionuclide	**Z** None	**Z** None

C   **Nuclear Medicine**
Ø   **Central Nervous System**
3   **Positron Emission Tomographic (PET) Imaging**   Definition: Introduction of radioactive materials into the body for three dimensional display of images developed from the simultaneous capture, 180 degrees apart, of radioactive emissions

Body Part Character 4	Radionuclide Character 5	Qualifier Character 6	Qualifier Character 7
Ø Brain	**B** Carbon 11 (C-11) **K** Fluorine 18 (F-18) **M** Oxygen 15 (O-15) **Y** Other Radionuclide	**Z** None	**Z** None
Y Central Nervous System	**Y** Other Radionuclide	**Z** None	**Z** None

C   **Nuclear Medicine**
Ø   **Central Nervous System**
5   **Nonimaging Nuclear Medicine Probe**   Definition: Introduction of radioactive materials into the body for the study of distribution and fate of certain substances by the detection of radioactive emissions; or, alternatively, measurement of absorption of radioactive emissions from an external source

Body Part Character 4	Radionuclide Character 5	Qualifier Character 6	Qualifier Character 7
Ø Brain	**V** Xenon 133 (Xe-133) **Y** Other Radionuclide	**Z** None	**Z** None
Y Central Nervous System	**Y** Other Radionuclide	**Z** None	**Z** None

C   **Nuclear Medicine**
2   **Heart**
1   **Planar Nuclear Medicine Imaging**   Definition: Introduction of radioactive materials into the body for single plane display of images developed from the capture of radioactive emissions

Body Part Character 4	Radionuclide Character 5	Qualifier Character 6	Qualifier Character 7
6 Heart, Right and Left	**1** Technetium 99m (Tc-99m) **Y** Other Radionuclide	**Z** None	**Z** None
G Myocardium	**1** Technetium 99m (Tc-99m) **D** Indium 111 (In-111) **S** Thallium 201 (Tl-201) **Y** Other Radionuclide **Z** None	**Z** None	**Z** None
Y Heart	**Y** Other Radionuclide	**Z** None	**Z** None

C Nuclear Medicine
2 Heart
2 Tomographic (Tomo) Nuclear Medicine Imaging   Definition: Introduction of radioactive materials into the body for three dimensional display of images developed from the capture of radioactive emissions

Body Part Character 4	Radionuclide Character 5	Qualifier Character 6	Qualifier Character 7
6 Heart, Right and Left	1 Technetium 99m (Tc-99m) Y Other Radionuclide	Z None	Z None
G Myocardium	1 Technetium 99m (Tc-99m) D Indium 111 (In-111) K Fluorine 18 (F-18) S Thallium 201 (TI-201) Y Other Radionuclide Z None	Z None	Z None
Y Heart	Y Other Radionuclide	Z None	Z None

C Nuclear Medicine
2 Heart
3 Positron Emission Tomographic (PET) Imaging   Definition: Introduction of radioactive materials into the body for three dimensional display of images developed from the simultaneous capture, 180 degrees apart, of radioactive emissions

Body Part Character 4	Radionuclide Character 5	Qualifier Character 6	Qualifier Character 7
G Myocardium	K Fluorine 18 (F-18) M Oxygen 15 (O-15) Q Rubidium 82 (Rb-82) R Nitrogen 13 (N-13) Y Other Radionuclide	Z None	Z None
Y Heart	Y Other Radionuclide	Z None	Z None

C Nuclear Medicine
2 Heart
5 Nonimaging Nuclear Medicine Probe   Definition: Introduction of radioactive materials into the body for the study of distribution and fate of certain substances by the detection of radioactive emissions; or, alternatively, measurement of absorption of radioactive emissions from an external source

Body Part Character 4	Radionuclide Character 5	Qualifier Character 6	Qualifier Character 7
6 Heart, Right and Left	1 Technetium 99m (Tc-99m) Y Other Radionuclide	Z None	Z None
Y Heart	Y Other Radionuclide	Z None	Z None

C Nuclear Medicine
5 Veins
1 Planar Nuclear Medicine Imaging   Definition: Introduction of radioactive materials into the body for single plane display of images developed from the capture of radioactive emissions

Body Part Character 4	Radionuclide Character 5	Qualifier Character 6	Qualifier Character 7
B Lower Extremity Veins, Right C Lower Extremity Veins, Left D Lower Extremity Veins, Bilateral N Upper Extremity Veins, Right P Upper Extremity Veins, Left Q Upper Extremity Veins, Bilateral R Central Veins	1 Technetium 99m (Tc-99m) Y Other Radionuclide	Z None	Z None
Y Veins	Y Other Radionuclide	Z None	Z None

[LC] Limited Coverage   [NC] Noncovered   ⊞ Combination Member   HAC   Valid OR   Combination Only   DRG Non-OR   New/Revised in GREEN

758   ICD-10-PCS 2019

C   **Nuclear Medicine**
7   **Lymphatic and Hematologic System**
1   **Planar Nuclear Medicine Imaging**   Definition: Introduction of radioactive materials into the body for single plane display of images developed from the capture of radioactive emissions

Body Part Character 4	Radionuclide Character 5	Qualifier Character 6	Qualifier Character 7
Ø Bone Marrow	**1** Technetium 99m (Tc-99m) **D** Indium 111 (In-111) **Y** Other Radionuclide	**Z** None	**Z** None
2 Spleen **5** Lymphatics, Head and Neck **D** Lymphatics, Pelvic **J** Lymphatics, Head **K** Lymphatics, Neck **L** Lymphatics, Upper Chest **M** Lymphatics, Trunk **N** Lymphatics, Upper Extremity **P** Lymphatics, Lower Extremity	**1** Technetium 99m (Tc-99m) **Y** Other Radionuclide	**Z** None	**Z** None
3 Blood	**D** Indium 111 (In-111) **Y** Other Radionuclide	**Z** None	**Z** None
Y Lymphatic and Hematologic System	**Y** Other Radionuclide	**Z** None	**Z** None

C   **Nuclear Medicine**
7   **Lymphatic and Hematologic System**
2   **Tomographic (Tomo) Nuclear Medicine Imaging**   Definition: Introduction of radioactive materials into the body for three dimensional display of images developed from the capture of radioactive emissions

Body Part Character 4	Radionuclide Character 5	Qualifier Character 6	Qualifier Character 7
2 Spleen	**1** Technetium 99m (Tc-99m) **Y** Other Radionuclide	**Z** None	**Z** None
Y Lymphatic and Hematologic System	**Y** Other Radionuclide	**Z** None	**Z** None

C   **Nuclear Medicine**
7   **Lymphatic and Hematologic System**
5   **Nonimaging Nuclear Medicine Probe**   Definition: Introduction of radioactive materials into the body for the study of distribution and fate of certain substances by the detection of radioactive emissions; or, alternatively, measurement of absorption of radioactive emissions from an external source

Body Part Character 4	Radionuclide Character 5	Qualifier Character 6	Qualifier Character 7
5 Lymphatics, Head and Neck **D** Lymphatics, Pelvic **J** Lymphatics, Head **K** Lymphatics, Neck **L** Lymphatics, Upper Chest **M** Lymphatics, Trunk **N** Lymphatics, Upper Extremity **P** Lymphatics, Lower Extremity	**1** Technetium 99m (Tc-99m) **Y** Other Radionuclide	**Z** None	**Z** None
Y Lymphatic and Hematologic System	**Y** Other Radionuclide	**Z** None	**Z** None

C   **Nuclear Medicine**
7   **Lymphatic and Hematologic System**
6   **Nonimaging Nuclear Medicine Assay**   Definition: Introduction of radioactive materials into the body for the study of body fluids and blood elements, by the detection of radioactive emissions

Body Part Character 4	Radionuclide Character 5	Qualifier Character 6	Qualifier Character 7
3 Blood	**1** Technetium 99m (Tc-99m) **7** Cobalt 58 (Co-58) **C** Cobalt 57 (Co-57) **D** Indium 111 (In-111) **H** Iodine 125 (I-125) **W** Chromium (Cr-51) **Y** Other Radionuclide	**Z** None	**Z** None
Y Lymphatic and Hematologic System	**Y** Other Radionuclide	**Z** None	**Z** None

C   **Nuclear Medicine**
8   **Eye**
1   **Planar Nuclear Medicine Imaging**   Definition: Introduction of radioactive materials into the body for single plane display of images developed from the capture of radioactive emissions

Body Part Character 4	Radionuclide Character 5	Qualifier Character 6	Qualifier Character 7
9 Lacrimal Ducts, Bilateral	**1** Technetium 99m (Tc-99m) **Y** Other Radionuclide	**Z** None	**Z** None
Y Eye	**Y** Other Radionuclide	**Z** None	**Z** None

C   **Nuclear Medicine**
9   **Ear, Nose, Mouth and Throat**
1   **Planar Nuclear Medicine Imaging**   Definition: Introduction of radioactive materials into the body for single plane display of images developed from the capture of radioactive emissions

Body Part Character 4	Radionuclide Character 5	Qualifier Character 6	Qualifier Character 7
B Salivary Glands, Bilateral	**1** Technetium 99m (Tc-99m) **Y** Other Radionuclide	**Z** None	**Z** None
Y Ear, Nose, Mouth and Throat	**Y** Other Radionuclide	**Z** None	**Z** None

C   **Nuclear Medicine**
B   **Respiratory System**
1   **Planar Nuclear Medicine Imaging**   Definition: Introduction of radioactive materials into the body for single plane display of images developed from the capture of radioactive emissions

Body Part Character 4	Radionuclide Character 5	Qualifier Character 6	Qualifier Character 7
2 Lungs and Bronchi	**1** Technetium 99m (Tc-99m) **9** Krypton (Kr-81m) **T** Xenon 127 (Xe-127) **V** Xenon 133 (Xe-133) **Y** Other Radionuclide	**Z** None	**Z** None
Y Respiratory System	**Y** Other Radionuclide	**Z** None	**Z** None

C   **Nuclear Medicine**
B   **Respiratory System**
2   **Tomographic (Tomo) Nuclear Medicine Imaging**   Definition: Introduction of radioactive materials into the body for three dimensional display of images developed from the capture of radioactive emissions

Body Part Character 4	Radionuclide Character 5	Qualifier Character 6	Qualifier Character 7
2 Lungs and Bronchi	**1** Technetium 99m (Tc-99m) **9** Krypton (Kr-81m) **Y** Other Radionuclide	**Z** None	**Z** None
Y Respiratory System	**Y** Other Radionuclide	**Z** None	**Z** None

C   **Nuclear Medicine**
B   **Respiratory System**
3   **Positron Emission Tomographic (PET) Imaging**   Definition: Introduction of radioactive materials into the body for three dimensional display of images developed from the simultaneous capture, 180 degrees apart, of radioactive emissions

Body Part Character 4	Radionuclide Character 5	Qualifier Character 6	Qualifier Character 7
2 Lungs and Bronchi	**K** Fluorine 18 (F-18) **Y** Other Radionuclide	**Z** None	**Z** None
Y Respiratory System	**Y** Other Radionuclide	**Z** None	**Z** None

C   **Nuclear Medicine**
D   **Gastrointestinal System**
1   **Planar Nuclear Medicine Imaging**   Definition: Introduction of radioactive materials into the body for single plane display of images developed from the capture of radioactive emissions

Body Part Character 4	Radionuclide Character 5	Qualifier Character 6	Qualifier Character 7
5 Upper Gastrointestinal Tract **7** Gastrointestinal Tract	**1** Technetium 99m (Tc-99m) **D** Indium 111 (In-111) **Y** Other Radionuclide	**Z** None	**Z** None
Y Digestive System	**Y** Other Radionuclide	**Z** None	**Z** None

C   **Nuclear Medicine**
D   **Gastrointestinal System**
2   **Tomographic (Tomo) Nuclear Medicine Imaging**   Definition: Introduction of radioactive materials into the body for three dimensional display of images developed from the capture of radioactive emissions

Body Part Character 4	Radionuclide Character 5	Qualifier Character 6	Qualifier Character 7
7 Gastrointestinal Tract	**1** Technetium 99m (Tc-99m) **D** Indium 111 (In-111) **Y** Other Radionuclide	**Z** None	**Z** None
Y Digestive System	**Y** Other Radionuclide	**Z** None	**Z** None

C   **Nuclear Medicine**
F   **Hepatobiliary System and Pancreas**
1   **Planar Nuclear Medicine Imaging**   Definition: Introduction of radioactive materials into the body for single plane display of images developed from the capture of radioactive emissions

Body Part Character 4	Radionuclide Character 5	Qualifier Character 6	Qualifier Character 7
4 Gallbladder **5** Liver **6** Liver and Spleen **C** Hepatobiliary System, All	**1** Technetium 99m (Tc-99m) **Y** Other Radionuclide	**Z** None	**Z** None
Y Hepatobiliary System and Pancreas	**Y** Other Radionuclide	**Z** None	**Z** None

C   **Nuclear Medicine**
F   **Hepatobiliary System and Pancreas**
2   **Tomographic (Tomo) Nuclear Medicine Imaging**   Definition: Introduction of radioactive materials into the body for three dimensional display of images developed from the capture of radioactive emissions

Body Part Character 4	Radionuclide Character 5	Qualifier Character 6	Qualifier Character 7
4 Gallbladder **5** Liver **6** Liver and Spleen	**1** Technetium 99m (Tc-99m) **Y** Other Radionuclide	**Z** None	**Z** None
Y Hepatobiliary System and Pancreas	**Y** Other Radionuclide	**Z** None	**Z** None

C   **Nuclear Medicine**
G   **Endocrine System**
1   **Planar Nuclear Medicine Imaging**   Definition: Introduction of radioactive materials into the body for single plane display of images developed from the capture of radioactive emissions

Body Part Character 4	Radionuclide Character 5	Qualifier Character 6	Qualifier Character 7
1 Parathyroid Glands	**1** Technetium 99m (Tc-99m) **S** Thallium 201 (Tl-201) **Y** Other Radionuclide	**Z** None	**Z** None
2 Thyroid Gland	**1** Technetium 99m (Tc-99m) **F** Iodine 123 (I-123) **G** Iodine 131 (I-131) **Y** Other Radionuclide	**Z** None	**Z** None
4 Adrenal Glands, Bilateral	**G** Iodine 131 (I-131) **Y** Other Radionuclide	**Z** None	**Z** None
Y Endocrine System	**Y** Other Radionuclide	**Z** None	**Z** None

C   **Nuclear Medicine**
G   **Endocrine System**
2   **Tomographic (Tomo) Nuclear Medicine Imaging**   Definition: Introduction of radioactive materials into the body for three dimensional display of images developed from the capture of radioactive emissions

Body Part Character 4	Radionuclide Character 5	Qualifier Character 6	Qualifier Character 7
1 Parathyroid Glands	**1** Technetium 99m (Tc-99m) **S** Thallium 201 (Tl-201) **Y** Other Radionuclide	**Z** None	**Z** None
Y Endocrine System	**Y** Other Radionuclide	**Z** None	**Z** None

Nuclear Medicine

C   **Nuclear Medicine**
G   **Endocrine System**
4   **Nonimaging Nuclear Medicine Uptake**   Definition: Introduction of radioactive materials into the body for measurements of organ function, from the detection of radioactive emmissions

Body Part Character 4	Radionuclide Character 5	Qualifier Character 6	Qualifier Character 7
2 Thyroid Gland	1 Technetium 99m (Tc-99m) F Iodine 123 (I-123) G Iodine 131 (I-131) Y Other Radionuclide	Z None	Z None
Y Endocrine System	Y Other Radionuclide	Z None	Z None

C   **Nuclear Medicine**
H   **Skin, Subcutaneous Tissue and Breast**
1   **Planar Nuclear Medicine Imaging**   Definition: Introduction of radioactive materials into the body for single plane display of images developed from the capture of radioactive emissions

Body Part Character 4	Radionuclide Character 5	Qualifier Character 6	Qualifier Character 7
Ø Breast, Right 1 Breast, Left 2 Breasts, Bilateral	1 Technetium 99m (Tc-99m) S Thallium 201 (Tl-201) Y Other Radionuclide	Z None	Z None
Y Skin, Subcutaneous Tissue and Breast	Y Other Radionuclide	Z None	Z None

C   **Nuclear Medicine**
H   **Skin, Subcutaneous Tissue and Breast**
2   **Tomographic (Tomo) Nuclear Medicine Imaging**   Definition: Introduction of radioactive materials into the body for three dimensional display of images developed from the capture of radioactive emissions

Body Part Character 4	Radionuclide Character 5	Qualifier Character 6	Qualifier Character 7
Ø Breast, Right 1 Breast, Left 2 Breasts, Bilateral	1 Technetium 99m (Tc-99m) S Thallium 201 (Tl-201) Y Other Radionuclide	Z None	Z None
Y Skin, Subcutaneous Tissue and Breast	Y Other Radionuclide	Z None	Z None

C   **Nuclear Medicine**
P   **Musculoskeletal System**
1   **Planar Nuclear Medicine Imaging**   Definition: Introduction of radioactive materials into the body for single plane display of images developed from the capture of radioactive emissions

Body Part Character 4	Radionuclide Character 5	Qualifier Character 6	Qualifier Character 7
1 Skull 4 Thorax 5 Spine 6 Pelvis 7 Spine and Pelvis 8 Upper Extremity, Right 9 Upper Extremity, Left B Upper Extremities, Bilateral C Lower Extremity, Right D Lower Extremity, Left F Lower Extremities, Bilateral Z Musculoskeletal System, All	1 Technetium 99m (Tc-99m) Y Other Radionuclide	Z None	Z None
Y Musculoskeletal System, Other	Y Other Radionuclide	Z None	Z None

C   **Nuclear Medicine**
P   **Musculoskeletal System**
2   **Tomographic (Tomo) Nuclear Medicine Imaging**   Definition: Introduction of radioactive materials into the body for three dimensional display of images developed from the capture of radioactive emissions

Body Part Character 4	Radionuclide Character 5	Qualifier Character 6	Qualifier Character 7
1 Skull 2 Cervical Spine 3 Skull and Cervical Spine 4 Thorax 6 Pelvis 7 Spine and Pelvis 8 Upper Extremity, Right 9 Upper Extremity, Left B Upper Extremities, Bilateral C Lower Extremity, Right D Lower Extremity, Left F Lower Extremities, Bilateral G Thoracic Spine H Lumbar Spine J Thoracolumbar Spine	1 Technetium 99m (Tc-99m) Y Other Radionuclide	Z None	Z None
Y Musculoskeletal System, Other	Y Other Radionuclide	Z None	Z None

C   **Nuclear Medicine**
P   **Musculoskeletal System**
5   **Nonimaging Nuclear Medicine Probe**   Definition: Introduction of radioactive materials into the body for the study of distribution and fate of certain substances by the detection of radioactive emissions; or, alternatively, measurement of absorption of radioactive emissions from an external source

Body Part Character 4	Radionuclide Character 5	Qualifier Character 6	Qualifier Character 7
5 Spine N Upper Extremities P Lower Extremities	Z None	Z None	Z None
Y Musculoskeletal System, Other	Y Other Radionuclide	Z None	Z None

C   **Nuclear Medicine**
T   **Urinary System**
1   **Planar Nuclear Medicine Imaging**   Definition: Introduction of radioactive materials into the body for single plane display of images developed from the capture of radioactive emissions

Body Part Character 4	Radionuclide Character 5	Qualifier Character 6	Qualifier Character 7
3 Kidneys, Ureters and Bladder	1 Technetium 99m (Tc-99m) F Iodine 123 (I-123) G Iodine 131 (I-131) Y Other Radionuclide	Z None	Z None
H Bladder and Ureters	1 Technetium 99m (Tc-99m) Y Other Radionuclide	Z None	Z None
Y Urinary System	Y Other Radionuclide	Z None	Z None

C   **Nuclear Medicine**
T   **Urinary System**
2   **Tomographic (Tomo) Nuclear Medicine Imaging**   Definition: Introduction of radioactive materials into the body for three dimensional display of images developed from the capture of radioactive emissions

Body Part Character 4	Radionuclide Character 5	Qualifier Character 6	Qualifier Character 7
3 Kidneys, Ureters and Bladder	1 Technetium 99m (Tc-99m) Y Other Radionuclide	Z None	Z None
Y Urinary System	Y Other Radionuclide	Z None	Z None

C   **Nuclear Medicine**
T   **Urinary System**
6   **Nonimaging Nuclear Medicine Assay**   Definition: Introduction of radioactive materials into the body for the study of body fluids and blood elements, by the detection of radioactive emissions

Body Part Character 4	Radionuclide Character 5	Qualifier Character 6	Qualifier Character 7
3 Kidneys, Ureters and Bladder	1 Technetium 99m (Tc-99m) F Iodine 123 (I-123) G Iodine 131 (I-131) H Iodine 125 (I-125) Y Other Radionuclide	Z None	Z None
Y Urinary System	Y Other Radionuclide	Z None	Z None

C   **Nuclear Medicine**
V   **Male Reproductive System**
1   **Planar Nuclear Medicine Imaging**   Definition: Introduction of radioactive materials into the body for single plane display of images developed from the capture of radioactive emissions

Body Part Character 4	Radionuclide Character 5	Qualifier Character 6	Qualifier Character 7
9 Testicles, Bilateral ♂	1 Technetium 99m (Tc-99m) Y Other Radionuclide	Z None	Z None
Y Male Reproductive System ♂	Y Other Radionuclide	Z None	Z None

♂   All body part, radionuclide, and qualifier values

C   **Nuclear Medicine**
W   **Anatomical Regions**
1   **Planar Nuclear Medicine Imaging**   Definition: Introduction of radioactive materials into the body for single plane display of images developed from the capture of radioactive emissions

Body Part Character 4	Radionuclide Character 5	Qualifier Character 6	Qualifier Character 7
Ø Abdomen 1 Abdomen and Pelvis 4 Chest and Abdomen 6 Chest and Neck B Head and Neck D Lower Extremity J Pelvic Region M Upper Extremity N Whole Body	1 Technetium 99m (Tc-99m) D Indium 111 (In-111) F Iodine 123 (I-123) G Iodine 131 (I-131) L Gallium 67 (Ga-67) S Thallium 201 (Tl-201) Y Other Radionuclide	Z None	Z None
3 Chest	1 Technetium 99m (Tc-99m) D Indium 111 (In-111) F Iodine 123 (I-123) G Iodine 131 (I-131) K Fluorine 18 (F-18) L Gallium 67 (Ga-67) S Thallium 201 (Tl-201) Y Other Radionuclide	Z None	Z None
Y Anatomical Regions, Multiple	Y Other Radionuclide	Z None	Z None
Z Anatomical Region, Other	Z None	Z None	Z None

C   **Nuclear Medicine**
W   **Anatomical Regions**
2   **Tomographic (Tomo) Nuclear Medicine Imaging**   Definition: Introduction of radioactive materials into the body for three dimensional display of images developed from the capture of radioactive emissions

Body Part Character 4	Radionuclide Character 5	Qualifier Character 6	Qualifier Character 7
Ø Abdomen 1 Abdomen and Pelvis 3 Chest 4 Chest and Abdomen 6 Chest and Neck B Head and Neck D Lower Extremity J Pelvic Region M Upper Extremity	1 Technetium 99m (Tc-99m) D Indium 111 (In-111) F Iodine 123 (I-123) G Iodine 131 (I-131) K Fluorine 18 (F-18) L Gallium 67 (Ga-67) S Thallium 201 (Tl-201) Y Other Radionuclide	Z None	Z None
Y Anatomical Regions, Multiple	Y Other Radionuclide	Z None	Z None

C   **Nuclear Medicine**
W   **Anatomical Regions**
3   **Positron Emission Tomographic (PET) Imaging**   Definition: Introduction of radioactive materials into the body for three dimensional display of images developed from the simultaneous capture, 180 degrees apart, of radioactive emissions

Body Part Character 4	Radionuclide Character 5	Qualifier Character 6	Qualifier Character 7
N Whole Body	Y Other Radionuclide	Z None	Z None

C   **Nuclear Medicine**
W   **Anatomical Regions**
5   **Nonimaging Nuclear Medicine Probe**   Definition: Introduction of radioactive materials into the body for the study of distribution and fate of certain substances by the detection of radioactive emissions; or, alternatively, measurement of absorption of radioactive emissions from an external source

Body Part Character 4	Radionuclide Character 5	Qualifier Character 6	Qualifier Character 7
Ø Abdomen 1 Abdomen and Pelvis 3 Chest 4 Chest and Abdomen 6 Chest and Neck B Head and Neck D Lower Extremity J Pelvic Region M Upper Extremity	1 Technetium 99m (Tc-99m) D Indium 111 (In-111) Y Other Radionuclide	Z None	Z None

C   **Nuclear Medicine**
W   **Anatomical Regions**
7   **Systemic Nuclear Medicine Therapy**   Definition: Introduction of unsealed radioactive materials into the body for treatment

Body Part Character 4	Radionuclide Character 5	Qualifier Character 6	Qualifier Character 7
Ø Abdomen 3 Chest	N Phosphorus 32 (P-32) Y Other Radionuclide	Z None	Z None
G Thyroid	G Iodine 131 (I-131) Y Other Radionuclide	Z None	Z None
N Whole Body	8 Samarium 153 (Sm-153) G Iodine 131 (I-131) N Phosphorus 32 (P-32) P Strontium 89 (Sr-89) Y Other Radionuclide	Z None	Z None
Y Anatomical Regions, Multiple	Y Other Radionuclide	Z None	Z None

Radiation Therapy DØØ–DWY

Character Meanings

This Character Meaning table is provided as a guide to assist the user in the identification of character members that may be found in this section of code tables. It **SHOULD NOT** be used to build a PCS code.

Body System– Character 2	Modality– Character 3	Treatment Site– Character 4	Modality Qualifier– Character 5	Isotope– Character 6	Qualifier– Character 7
Ø Central and Peripheral Nervous System	Ø Beam Radiation	See next page	Ø Photons <1 MeV	7 Cesium 137 (Cs-137)	Ø Intraoperative
7 Lymphatic and Hematologic System	1 Brachytherapy		1 Photons 1 - 1Ø MeV	8 Iridium 192 (Ir-192)	Z None
8 Eye	2 Stereotactic Radiosurgery		2 Photons >1Ø MeV	9 Iodine 125 (I-125)	
9 Ear, Nose, Mouth and Throat	Y Other Radiation		3 Electrons	B Palladium 1Ø3 (Pd-1Ø3)	
B Respiratory System			4 Heavy Particles (Protons, Ions)	C Californium 252 (Cf-252)	
D Gastrointestinal System			5 Neutrons	D Iodine 131 (I-131)	
F Hepatobiliary System and Pancreas			6 Neutron Capture	F Phosphorus 32 (P-32)	
G Endocrine System			7 Contact Radiation	G Strontium 89 (Sr-89)	
H Skin			8 Hyperthermia	H Strontium 9Ø (Sr-9Ø)	
M Breast			9 High Dose Rate (HDR)	Y Other Isotope	
P Musculoskeletal System			B Low Dose Rate (LDR)	Z None	
T Urinary System			C Intraoperative Radiation Therapy (IORT)		
U Female Reproductive System			D Stereotactic Other Photon Radiosurgery		
V Male Reproductive System			F Plaque Radiation		
W Anatomical Regions			G Isotope Administration		
			H Stereotactic Particulate Radiosurgery		
			J Stereotactic Gamma Beam Radiosurgery		
			K Laser Interstitial Thermal Therapy		

Treatment Site—Character 4 Meanings

Body System– Character 2	Treatment Site– Character 4			
Ø　Central and Peripheral Nervous System	Ø　Brain 1　Brain Stem 6　Spinal Cord 7　Peripheral Nerve			
7　Lymphatic and Hematologic System	Ø　Bone Marrow 1　Thymus 2　Spleen 3　Lymphatics, Neck 4　Lymphatics, Axillary	5　Lymphatics, Thorax 6　Lymphatics, Abdomen 7　Lymphatics, Pelvis 8　Lymphatics, Inguinal		
8　Eye	Ø　Eye			
9　Ear, Nose, Mouth and Throat	Ø　Ear 1　Nose 3　Hypopharynx 4　Mouth 5　Tongue 6　Salivary Glands 7　Sinuses	8　Hard Palate 9　Soft Palate B　Larynx C　Pharynx D　Nasopharynx F　Oropharynx		
B　Respiratory System	Ø　Trachea 1　Bronchus 2　Lung 5　Pleura	6　Mediastinum 7　Chest Wall 8　Diaphragm		
D　Gastrointestinal System	Ø　Esophagus 1　Stomach 2　Duodenum 3　Jejunum	4　Ileum 5　Colon 7　Rectum 8　Anus		
F　Hepatobiliary System and Pancreas	Ø　Liver 1　Gallbladder	2　Bile Ducts 3　Pancreas		
G　Endocrine System	Ø　Pituitary Gland 1　Pineal Body 2　Adrenal Glands	4　Parathyroid Glands 5　Thyroid		
H　Skin	2　Skin, Face 3　Skin, Neck 4　Skin, Arm 5　Skin, Hand 6　Skin, Chest	7　Skin, Back 8　Skin, Abdomen 9　Skin, Buttock B　Skin, Leg C　Skin, Foot		
M　Breast	Ø　Breast, Left 1　Breast, Right			
P　Musculoskeletal System	Ø　Skull 2　Maxilla 3　Mandible 4　Sternum 5　Rib(s) 6　Humerus	7　Radius/Ulna 8　Pelvic Bones 9　Femur B　Tibia/Fibula C　Other Bone		
T　Urinary System	Ø　Kidney 1　Ureter	2　Bladder 3　Urethra		
U　Female Reproductive System	Ø　Ovary 1　Cervix 2　Uterus			
V　Male Reproductive System	Ø　Prostate 1　Testis			
W　Anatomical Regions	1　Head and Neck 2　Chest 3　Abdomen	4　Hemibody 5　Whole Body 6　Pelvic Region		

AHA Coding Clinic for table DU1
2017, 4Q, 104　　　Intrauterine brachytherapy & placement of tandems & ovoids

D   **Radiation Therapy**
Ø   **Central and Peripheral Nervous System**
Ø   **Beam Radiation**

Treatment Site Character 4	Modality Qualifier Character 5	Isotope Character 6	Qualifier Character 7
Ø Brain 1 Brain Stem 6 Spinal Cord 7 Peripheral Nerve	Ø Photons <1 MeV 1 Photons 1- 10 MeV 2 Photons >10 MeV 4 Heavy Particles (Protons, Ions) 5 Neutrons 6 Neutron Capture	Z None	Z None
Ø Brain 1 Brain Stem 6 Spinal Cord 7 Peripheral Nerve	3 Electrons	Z None	Ø Intraoperative Z None

D   **Radiation Therapy**
Ø   **Central and Peripheral Nervous System**
1   **Brachytherapy**

Treatment Site Character 4	Modality Qualifier Character 5	Isotope Character 6	Qualifier Character 7
Ø Brain 1 Brain Stem 6 Spinal Cord 7 Peripheral Nerve	9 High Dose Rate (HDR) B Low Dose Rate (LDR)	7 Cesium 137 (Cs-137) 8 Iridium 192 (Ir-192) 9 Iodine 125 (I-125) B Palladium 103 (Pd-103) C Californium 252 (Cf-252) Y Other Isotope	Z None

D   **Radiation Therapy**
Ø   **Central and Peripheral Nervous System**
2   **Stereotactic Radiosurgery**

Treatment Site Character 4	Modality Qualifier Character 5	Isotope Character 6	Qualifier Character 7
Ø Brain 1 Brain Stem 6 Spinal Cord 7 Peripheral Nerve	D Stereotactic Other Photon Radiosurgery H Stereotactic Particulate Radiosurgery J Stereotactic Gamma Beam Radiosurgery	Z None	Z None

DRG Non-OR   All treatment site, modality, isotope, and qualifier values

D   **Radiation Therapy**
Ø   **Central and Peripheral Nervous System**
Y   **Other Radiation**

Treatment Site Character 4	Modality Qualifier Character 5	Isotope Character 6	Qualifier Character 7
Ø Brain 1 Brain Stem 6 Spinal Cord 7 Peripheral Nerve	7 Contact Radiation 8 Hyperthermia F Plaque Radiation K Laser Interstitial Thermal Therapy	Z None	Z None

Valid OR   DØY[Ø,1,6,7]KZZ

D   Radiation Therapy
7   Lymphatic and Hematologic System
Ø   Beam Radiation

Treatment Site Character 4	Modality Qualifier Character 5	Isotope Character 6	Qualifier Character 7
Ø Bone Marrow 1 Thymus 2 Spleen 3 Lymphatics, Neck 4 Lymphatics, Axillary 5 Lymphatics, Thorax 6 Lymphatics, Abdomen 7 Lymphatics, Pelvis 8 Lymphatics, Inguinal	Ø Photons <1 MeV 1 Photons 1- 10 MeV 2 Photons >10 MeV 4 Heavy Particles (Protons, Ions) 5 Neutrons 6 Neutron Capture	Z None	Z None
Ø Bone Marrow 1 Thymus 2 Spleen 3 Lymphatics, Neck 4 Lymphatics, Axillary 5 Lymphatics, Thorax 6 Lymphatics, Abdomen 7 Lymphatics, Pelvis 8 Lymphatics, Inguinal	3 Electrons	Z None	Ø Intraoperative Z None

D   Radiation Therapy
7   Lymphatic and Hematologic System
1   Brachytherapy

Treatment Site Character 4	Modality Qualifier Character 5	Isotope Character 6	Qualifier Character 7
Ø Bone Marrow 1 Thymus 2 Spleen 3 Lymphatics, Neck 4 Lymphatics, Axillary 5 Lymphatics, Thorax 6 Lymphatics, Abdomen 7 Lymphatics, Pelvis 8 Lymphatics, Inguinal	9 High Dose Rate (HDR) B Low Dose Rate (LDR)	7 Cesium 137 (Cs-137) 8 Iridium 192 (Ir-192) 9 Iodine 125 (I-125) B Palladium 103 (Pd-103) C Californium 252 (Cf-252) Y Other Isotope	Z None

D   Radiation Therapy
7   Lymphatic and Hematologic System
2   Stereotactic Radiosurgery

Treatment Site Character 4	Modality Qualifier Character 5	Isotope Character 6	Qualifier Character 7

Ø Bone Marrow
1 Thymus
2 Spleen
3 Lymphatics, Neck
4 Lymphatics, Axillary
5 Lymphatics, Thorax
6 Lymphatics, Abdomen
7 Lymphatics, Pelvis
8 Lymphatics, Inguinal
	D Stereotactic Other Photon
	   Radiosurgery
	H Stereotactic Particulate
	   Radiosurgery
	J Stereotactic Gamma Beam
	   Radiosurgery
		Z None	Z None

DRG Non-OR All treatment site, modality, isotope, and qualifier values

D   Radiation Therapy
7   Lymphatic and Hematologic System
Y   Other Radiation

Treatment Site Character 4	Modality Qualifier Character 5	Isotope Character 6	Qualifier Character 7
Ø Bone Marrow 1 Thymus 2 Spleen 3 Lymphatics, Neck 4 Lymphatics, Axillary 5 Lymphatics, Thorax 6 Lymphatics, Abdomen 7 Lymphatics, Pelvis 8 Lymphatics, Inguinal	8 Hyperthermia F Plaque Radiation	Z None	Z None

D Radiation Therapy
8 Eye
0 Beam Radiation

Treatment Site Character 4	Modality Qualifier Character 5	Isotope Character 6	Qualifier Character 7
0 Eye	0 Photons <1 MeV 1 Photons 1- 10 MeV 2 Photons >10 MeV 4 Heavy Particles (Protons, Ions) 5 Neutrons 6 Neutron Capture	Z None	Z None
0 Eye	3 Electrons	Z None	0 Intraoperative Z None

D Radiation Therapy
8 Eye
1 Brachytherapy

Treatment Site Character 4	Modality Qualifier Character 5	Isotope Character 6	Qualifier Character 7
0 Eye	9 High Dose Rate (HDR) B Low Dose Rate (LDR)	7 Cesium 137 (Cs-137) 8 Iridium 192 (Ir-192) 9 Iodine 125 (I-125) B Palladium 103 (Pd-103) C Californium 252 (Cf-252) Y Other Isotope	Z None

D Radiation Therapy
8 Eye
2 Stereotactic Radiosurgery

Treatment Site Character 4	Modality Qualifier Character 5	Isotope Character 6	Qualifier Character 7
0 Eye	D Stereotactic Other Photon 　　Radiosurgery H Stereotactic Particulate 　　Radiosurgery J Stereotactic Gamma Beam 　　Radiosurgery	Z None	Z None

DRG Non-OR　All treatment site, modality, isotope, and qualifier values

D Radiation Therapy
8 Eye
Y Other Radiation

Treatment Site Character 4	Modality Qualifier Character 5	Isotope Character 6	Qualifier Character 7
0 Eye	7 Contact Radiation 8 Hyperthermia F Plaque Radiation	Z None	Z None

Radiation Therapy

D   **Radiation Therapy**
9   **Ear, Nose, Mouth and Throat**
Ø   **Beam Radiation**

Treatment Site Character 4	Modality Qualifier Character 5	Isotope Character 6	Qualifier Character 7
Ø Ear	Ø Photons <1 MeV	Z None	Z None
1 Nose	1 Photons 1- 10 MeV		
3 Hypopharynx	2 Photons >10 MeV		
4 Mouth	4 Heavy Particles (Protons, Ions)		
5 Tongue	5 Neutrons		
6 Salivary Glands	6 Neutron Capture		
7 Sinuses			
8 Hard Palate			
9 Soft Palate			
B Larynx			
D Nasopharynx			
F Oropharynx			
Ø Ear	3 Electrons	Z None	Ø Intraoperative
1 Nose			Z None
3 Hypopharynx			
4 Mouth			
5 Tongue			
6 Salivary Glands			
7 Sinuses			
8 Hard Palate			
9 Soft Palate			
B Larynx			
D Nasopharynx			
F Oropharynx			

D   **Radiation Therapy**
9   **Ear, Nose, Mouth and Throat**
1   **Brachytherapy**

Treatment Site Character 4	Modality Qualifier Character 5	Isotope Character 6	Qualifier Character 7
Ø Ear	9 High Dose Rate (HDR)	7 Cesium 137 (Cs-137)	Z None
1 Nose	B Low Dose Rate (LDR)	8 Iridium 192 (Ir-192)	
3 Hypopharynx		9 Iodine 125 (I-125)	
4 Mouth		B Palladium 103 (Pd-103)	
5 Tongue		C Californium 252 (Cf-252)	
6 Salivary Glands		Y Other Isotope	
7 Sinuses			
8 Hard Palate			
9 Soft Palate			
B Larynx			
D Nasopharynx			
F Oropharynx			

D   **Radiation Therapy**
9   **Ear, Nose, Mouth and Throat**
2   **Stereotactic Radiosurgery**

Treatment Site Character 4	Modality Qualifier Character 5	Isotope Character 6	Qualifier Character 7
Ø Ear	D Stereotactic Other Photon Radiosurgery	Z None	Z None
1 Nose	H Stereotactic Particulate Radiosurgery		
4 Mouth	J Stereotactic Gamma Beam Radiosurgery		
5 Tongue			
6 Salivary Glands			
7 Sinuses			
8 Hard Palate			
9 Soft Palate			
B Larynx			
C Pharynx			
D Nasopharynx			

DRG Non-OR All treatment site, modality, isotope, and qualifier values

D   Radiation Therapy
9   Ear, Nose, Mouth and Throat
Y   Other Radiation

Treatment Site Character 4	Modality Qualifier Character 5	Isotope Character 6	Qualifier Character 7
0 Ear 1 Nose 5 Tongue 6 Salivary Glands 7 Sinuses 8 Hard Palate 9 Soft Palate	7 Contact Radiation 8 Hyperthermia F Plaque Radiation	Z None	Z None
3 Hypopharynx F Oropharynx	7 Contact Radiation 8 Hyperthermia	Z None	Z None
4 Mouth B Larynx D Nasopharynx	7 Contact Radiation 8 Hyperthermia C Intraoperative Radiation Therapy (IORT) F Plaque Radiation	Z None	Z None
C Pharynx	C Intraoperative Radiation Therapy (IORT) F Plaque Radiation	Z None	Z None

D   Radiation Therapy
B   Respiratory System
0   Beam Radiation

Treatment Site Character 4	Modality Qualifier Character 5	Isotope Character 6	Qualifier Character 7
0 Trachea 1 Bronchus 2 Lung 5 Pleura 6 Mediastinum 7 Chest Wall 8 Diaphragm	0 Photons <1 MeV 1 Photons 1- 10 MeV 2 Photons >10 MeV 4 Heavy Particles (Protons, Ions) 5 Neutrons 6 Neutron Capture	Z None	Z None
0 Trachea 1 Bronchus 2 Lung 5 Pleura 6 Mediastinum 7 Chest Wall 8 Diaphragm	3 Electrons	Z None	0 Intraoperative Z None

D   Radiation Therapy
B   Respiratory System
1   Brachytherapy

Treatment Site Character 4	Modality Qualifier Character 5	Isotope Character 6	Qualifier Character 7
0 Trachea 1 Bronchus 2 Lung 5 Pleura 6 Mediastinum 7 Chest Wall 8 Diaphragm	9 High Dose Rate (HDR) B Low Dose Rate (LDR)	7 Cesium 137 (Cs-137) 8 Iridium 192 (Ir-192) 9 Iodine 125 (I-125) B Palladium 103 (Pd-103) C Californium 252 (Cf-252) Y Other Isotope	Z None

D   Radiation Therapy
B   Respiratory System
2   Stereotactic Radiosurgery

Treatment Site Character 4	Modality Qualifier Character 5	Isotope Character 6	Qualifier Character 7
0 Trachea 1 Bronchus 2 Lung 5 Pleura 6 Mediastinum 7 Chest Wall 8 Diaphragm	D Stereotactic Other Photon Radiosurgery H Stereotactic Particulate Radiosurgery J Stereotactic Gamma Beam Radiosurgery	Z None	Z None

DRG Non-OR   All treatment site, modality, isotope, and qualifier values

Radiation Therapy

D Radiation Therapy
B Respiratory System
Y Other Radiation

Treatment Site Character 4	Modality Qualifier Character 5	Isotope Character 6	Qualifier Character 7
0 Trachea 1 Bronchus 2 Lung 5 Pleura 6 Mediastinum 7 Chest Wall 8 Diaphragm	7 Contact Radiation 8 Hyperthermia F Plaque Radiation K Laser Interstitial Thermal Therapy	Z None	Z None

Valid OR   DBY[0,1,2,5,6,7,8]KZZ

D Radiation Therapy
D Gastrointestinal System
0 Beam Radiation

Treatment Site Character 4	Modality Qualifier Character 5	Isotope Character 6	Qualifier Character 7
0 Esophagus 1 Stomach 2 Duodenum 3 Jejunum 4 Ileum 5 Colon 7 Rectum	0 Photons <1 MeV 1 Photons 1- 10 MeV 2 Photons >10 MeV 4 Heavy Particles (Protons, Ions) 5 Neutrons 6 Neutron Capture	Z None	Z None
0 Esophagus 1 Stomach 2 Duodenum 3 Jejunum 4 Ileum 5 Colon 7 Rectum	3 Electrons	Z None	0 Intraoperative Z None

D Radiation Therapy
D Gastrointestinal System
1 Brachytherapy

Treatment Site Character 4	Modality Qualifier Character 5	Isotope Character 6	Qualifier Character 7
0 Esophagus 1 Stomach 2 Duodenum 3 Jejunum 4 Ileum 5 Colon 7 Rectum	9 High Dose Rate (HDR) B Low Dose Rate (LDR)	7 Cesium 137 (Cs-137) 8 Iridium 192 (Ir-192) 9 Iodine 125 (I-125) B Palladium 103 (Pd-103) C Californium 252 (Cf-252) Y Other Isotope	Z None

D Radiation Therapy
D Gastrointestinal System
2 Stereotactic Radiosurgery

Treatment Site Character 4	Modality Qualifier Character 5	Isotope Character 6	Qualifier Character 7
0 Esophagus 1 Stomach 2 Duodenum 3 Jejunum 4 Ileum 5 Colon 7 Rectum	D Stereotactic Other Photon Radiosurgery H Stereotactic Particulate Radiosurgery J Stereotactic Gamma Beam Radiosurgery	Z None	Z None

DRG Non-OR   All treatment site, modality, isotope, and qualifier values

D   **Radiation therapy**
D   **Gastrointestinal System**
Y   **Other Radiation**

Treatment Site Character 4	Modality Qualifier Character 5	Isotope Character 6	Qualifier Character 7
Ø Esophagus	**7** Contact Radiation **8** Hyperthermia **F** Plaque Radiation **K** Laser Interstitial Thermal Therapy	**Z** None	**Z** None
1 Stomach **2** Duodenum **3** Jejunum **4** Ileum **5** Colon **7** Rectum	**7** Contact Radiation **8** Hyperthermia **C** Intraoperative Radiation Therapy (IORT) **F** Plaque Radiation **K** Laser Interstitial Thermal Therapy	**Z** None	**Z** None
8 Anus	**C** Intraoperative Radiation Therapy (IORT) **F** Plaque Radiation **K** Laser Interstitial Thermal Therapy	**Z** None	**Z** None

Valid OR	DDYØKZZ	
Valid OR	DDY[1,2,3,4,5,7]KZZ	
Valid OR	DDY8KZZ	

D   **Radiation Therapy**
F   **Hepatobiliary System and Pancreas**
Ø   **Beam Radiation**

Treatment Site Character 4	Modality Qualifier Character 5	Isotope Character 6	Qualifier Character 7
Ø Liver **1** Gallbladder **2** Bile Ducts **3** Pancreas	**Ø** Photons <1 MeV **1** Photons 1- 10 MeV **2** Photons >10 MeV **4** Heavy Particles (Protons, Ions) **5** Neutrons **6** Neutron Capture	**Z** None	**Z** None
Ø Liver **1** Gallbladder **2** Bile Ducts **3** Pancreas	**3** Electrons	**Z** None	**Ø** Intraoperative **Z** None

D   **Radiation Therapy**
F   **Hepatobiliary System and Pancreas**
1   **Brachytherapy**

Treatment Site Character 4	Modality Qualifier Character 5	Isotope Character 6	Qualifier Character 7
Ø Liver **1** Gallbladder **2** Bile Ducts **3** Pancreas	**9** High Dose Rate (HDR) **B** Low Dose Rate (LDR)	**7** Cesium 137 (Cs-137) **8** Iridium 192 (Ir-192) **9** Iodine 125 (I-125) **B** Palladium 103 (Pd-103) **C** Californium 252 (Cf-252) **Y** Other Isotope	**Z** None

D   **Radiation Therapy**
F   **Hepatobiliary System and Pancreas**
2   **Stereotactic Radiosurgery**

Treatment Site Character 4	Modality Qualifier Character 5	Isotope Character 6	Qualifier Character 7
Ø Liver **1** Gallbladder **2** Bile Ducts **3** Pancreas	**D** Stereotactic Other Photon Radiosurgery **H** Stereotactic Particulate Radiosurgery **J** Stereotactic Gamma Beam Radiosurgery	**Z** None	**Z** None

DRG Non-OR   All treatment site, modality, isotope, and qualifier values

LC Limited Coverage   **NC** Noncovered   ⊞ Combination Member   HAC   Valid OR   Combination Only   DRG Non-OR   New/Revised in GREEN

ICD-10-PCS 2019   775

Radiation Therapy *(side tab)*

D Radiation Therapy
F Hepatobiliary System and Pancreas
Y Other Radiation

Treatment Site Character 4	Modality Qualifier Character 5	Isotope Character 6	Qualifier Character 7
Ø Liver 1 Gallbladder 2 Bile Ducts 3 Pancreas	7 Contact Radiation 8 Hyperthermia C Intraoperative Radiation Therapy (IORT) F Plaque Radiation K Laser Interstitial Thermal Therapy	Z None	Z None

Valid OR DFY[Ø,1,2,3]KZZ

D Radiation Therapy
G Endocrine System
Ø Beam Radiation

Treatment Site Character 4	Modality Qualifier Character 5	Isotope Character 6	Qualifier Character 7
Ø Pituitary Gland 1 Pineal Body 2 Adrenal Glands 4 Parathyroid Glands 5 Thyroid	Ø Photons <1 MeV 1 Photons 1- 10 MeV 2 Photons >10 MeV 5 Neutrons 6 Neutron Capture	Z None	Z None
Ø Pituitary Gland 1 Pineal Body 2 Adrenal Glands 4 Parathyroid Glands 5 Thyroid	3 Electrons	Z None	Ø Intraoperative Z None

D Radiation Therapy
G Endocrine System
1 Brachytherapy

Treatment Site Character 4	Modality Qualifier Character 5	Isotope Character 6	Qualifier Character 7
Ø Pituitary Gland 1 Pineal Body 2 Adrenal Glands 4 Parathyroid Glands 5 Thyroid	9 High Dose Rate (HDR) B Low Dose Rate (LDR)	7 Cesium 137 (Cs-137) 8 Iridium 192 (Ir-192) 9 Iodine 125 (I-125) B Palladium 103 (Pd-103) C Californium 252 (Cf-252) Y Other Isotope	Z None

D Radiation Therapy
G Endocrine System
2 Stereotactic Radiosurgery

Treatment Site Character 4	Modality Qualifier Character 5	Isotope Character 6	Qualifier Character 7
Ø Pituitary Gland 1 Pineal Body 2 Adrenal Glands 4 Parathyroid Glands 5 Thyroid	D Stereotactic Other Photon Radiosurgery H Stereotactic Particulate Radiosurgery J Stereotactic Gamma Beam Radiosurgery	Z None	Z None

DRG Non-OR All treatment site, modality, isotope, and qualifier values

D Radiation therapy
G Endocrine System
Y Other Radiation

Treatment Site Character 4	Modality Qualifier Character 5	Isotope Character 6	Qualifier Character 7
Ø Pituitary Gland 1 Pineal Body 2 Adrenal Glands 4 Parathyroid Glands 5 Thyroid	7 Contact Radiation 8 Hyperthermia F Plaque Radiation K Laser Interstitial Thermal Therapy	Z None	Z None

Valid OR DGY[Ø,1,2,4,5]KZZ

LC Limited Coverage   NC Noncovered   ⊞ Combination Member   HAC   Valid OR   Combination Only   DRG Non-OR   New/Revised in GREEN

D   Radiation Therapy
H   Skin
Ø   Beam Radiation

Treatment Site Character 4	Modality Qualifier Character 5	Isotope Character 6	Qualifier Character 7
2 Skin, Face 3 Skin, Neck 4 Skin, Arm 6 Skin, Chest 7 Skin, Back 8 Skin, Abdomen 9 Skin, Buttock B Skin, Leg	Ø Photons <1 MeV 1 Photons 1- 10 MeV 2 Photons >10 MeV 4 Heavy Particles (Protons, Ions) 5 Neutrons 6 Neutron Capture	Z None	Z None
2 Skin, Face 3 Skin, Neck 4 Skin, Arm 6 Skin, Chest 7 Skin, Back 8 Skin, Abdomen 9 Skin, Buttock B Skin, Leg	3 Electrons	Z None	Ø Intraoperative Z None

D   Radiation Therapy
H   Skin
Y   Other Radiation

Treatment Site Character 4	Modality Qualifier Character 5	Isotope Character 6	Qualifier Character 7
2 Skin, Face 3 Skin, Neck 4 Skin, Arm 6 Skin, Chest 7 Skin, Back 8 Skin, Abdomen 9 Skin, Buttock B Skin, Leg	7 Contact Radiation 8 Hyperthermia F Plaque Radiation	Z None	Z None
5 Skin, Hand C Skin, Foot	F Plaque Radiation	Z None	Z None

D   Radiation Therapy
M   Breast
Ø   Beam Radiation

Treatment Site Character 4	Modality Qualifier Character 5	Isotope Character 6	Qualifier Character 7
Ø Breast, Left 1 Breast, Right	Ø Photons <1 MeV 1 Photons 1- 10 MeV 2 Photons >10 MeV 4 Heavy Particles (Protons, Ions) 5 Neutrons 6 Neutron Capture	Z None	Z None
Ø Breast, Left 1 Breast, Right	3 Electrons	Z None	Ø Intraoperative Z None

D   Radiation Therapy
M   Breast
1   Brachytherapy

Treatment Site Character 4	Modality Qualifier Character 5	Isotope Character 6	Qualifier Character 7
Ø Breast, Left 1 Breast, Right	9 High Dose Rate (HDR) B Low Dose Rate (LDR)	7 Cesium 137 (Cs-137) 8 Iridium 192 (Ir-192) 9 Iodine 125 (I-125) B Palladium 103 (Pd-103) C Californium 252 (Cf-252) Y Other Isotope	Z None

Radiation Therapy

D   **Radiation Therapy**
M   **Breast**
2   **Stereotactic Radiosurgery**

Treatment Site Character 4	Modality Qualifier Character 5	Isotope Character 6	Qualifier Character 7

Ø Breast, Left
1 Breast, Right
	D Stereotactic Other Photon
	    Radiosurgery
	H Stereotactic Particulate
	    Radiosurgery
	J Stereotactic Gamma Beam
	   Radiosurgery
		Z None	Z None

DRG Non-OR   All treatment site, modality, isotope, and qualifier values

D   **Radiation Therapy**
M   **Breast**
Y   **Other Radiation**

Treatment Site Character 4	Modality Qualifier Character 5	Isotope Character 6	Qualifier Character 7
Ø Breast, Left 1 Breast, Right	7 Contact Radiation 8 Hyperthermia F Plaque Radiation K Laser Interstitial Thermal Therapy	Z None	Z None

Valid OR   DMY[Ø,1]KZZ

D   **Radiation Therapy**
P   **Musculoskeletal System**
Ø   **Beam Radiation**

Treatment Site Character 4	Modality Qualifier Character 5	Isotope Character 6	Qualifier Character 7
Ø Skull 2 Maxilla 3 Mandible 4 Sternum 5 Rib(s) 6 Humerus 7 Radius/Ulna 8 Pelvic Bones 9 Femur B Tibia/Fibula C Other Bone	Ø Photons <1 MeV 1 Photons 1- 10 MeV 2 Photons >10 MeV 4 Heavy Particles (Protons, Ions) 5 Neutrons 6 Neutron Capture	Z None	Z None
Ø Skull 2 Maxilla 3 Mandible 4 Sternum 5 Rib(s) 6 Humerus 7 Radius/Ulna 8 Pelvic Bones 9 Femur B Tibia/Fibula C Other Bone	3 Electrons	Z None	Ø Intraoperative Z None

D   **Radiation Therapy**
P   **Musculoskeletal System**
Y   **Other Radiation**

Treatment Site Character 4	Modality Qualifier Character 5	Isotope Character 6	Qualifier Character 7
Ø Skull 2 Maxilla 3 Mandible 4 Sternum 5 Rib(s) 6 Humerus 7 Radius/Ulna 8 Pelvic Bones 9 Femur B Tibia/Fibula C Other Bone	7 Contact Radiation 8 Hyperthermia F Plaque Radiation	Z None	Z None

D　Radiation Therapy
T　Urinary System
Ø　Beam Radiation

Treatment Site Character 4	Modality Qualifier Character 5	Isotope Character 6	Qualifier Character 7
Ø　Kidney 1　Ureter 2　Bladder 3　Urethra	Ø　Photons <1 MeV 1　Photons 1- 10 MeV 2　Photons >10 MeV 4　Heavy Particles (Protons, Ions) 5　Neutrons 6　Neutron Capture	Z　None	Z　None
Ø　Kidney 1　Ureter 2　Bladder 3　Urethra	3　Electrons	Z　None	Ø　Intraoperative Z　None

D　Radiation Therapy
T　Urinary System
1　Brachytherapy

Treatment Site Character 4	Modality Qualifier Character 5	Isotope Character 6	Qualifier Character 7
Ø　Kidney 1　Ureter 2　Bladder 3　Urethra	9　High Dose Rate (HDR) B　Low Dose Rate (LDR)	7　Cesium 137 (Cs-137) 8　Iridium 192 (Ir-192) 9　Iodine 125 (I-125) B　Palladium 103 (Pd-103) C　Californium 252 (Cf-252) Y　Other Isotope	Z　None

D　Radiation Therapy
T　Urinary System
2　Stereotactic Radiosurgery

Treatment Site Character 4	Modality Qualifier Character 5	Isotope Character 6	Qualifier Character 7
Ø　Kidney 1　Ureter 2　Bladder 3　Urethra	D　Stereotactic Other Photon Radiosurgery H　Stereotactic Particulate Radiosurgery J　Stereotactic Gamma Beam Radiosurgery	Z　None	Z　None

DRG Non-OR All treatment site, modality, isotope, and qualifier values

D　Radiation Therapy
T　Urinary System
Y　Other Radiation

Treatment Site Character 4	Modality Qualifier Character 5	Isotope Character 6	Qualifier Character 7
Ø　Kidney 1　Ureter 2　Bladder 3　Urethra	7　Contact Radiation 8　Hyperthermia C　Intraoperative Radiation Therapy (IORT) F　Plaque Radiation	Z　None	Z　None

D　Radiation Therapy
U　Female Reproductive System
Ø　Beam Radiation

Treatment Site Character 4	Modality Qualifier Character 5	Isotope Character 6	Qualifier Character 7
Ø　Ovary　♀ 1　Cervix　♀ 2　Uterus　♀	Ø　Photons <1 MeV 1　Photons 1- 10 MeV 2　Photons >10 MeV 4　Heavy Particles (Protons, Ions) 5　Neutrons 6　Neutron Capture	Z　None	Z　None
Ø　Ovary　♀ 1　Cervix　♀ 2　Uterus　♀	3　Electrons	Z　None	Ø　Intraoperative Z　None

♀　　All treatment site, modality, isotope, and qualifier values

Radiation Therapy

D Radiation Therapy
U Female Reproductive System
1 Brachytherapy

Treatment Site Character 4		Modality Qualifier Character 5	Isotope Character 6	Qualifier Character 7
Ø Ovary	♀	9 High Dose Rate (HDR)	7 Cesium 137 (Cs-137)	Z None
1 Cervix	♀	B Low Dose Rate (LDR)	8 Iridium 192 (Ir-192)	
2 Uterus	♀		9 Iodine 125 (I-125)	
			B Palladium 103 (Pd-103)	
			C Californium 252 (Cf-252)	
			Y Other Isotope	

♀   All treatment site, modality, isotope, and qualifier values

D Radiation Therapy
U Female Reproductive System
2 Stereotactic Radiosurgery

Treatment Site Character 4		Modality Qualifier Character 5	Isotope Character 6	Qualifier Character 7
Ø Ovary	♀	D Stereotactic Other Photon Radiosurgery	Z None	Z None
1 Cervix	♀	H Stereotactic Particulate Radiosurgery		
2 Uterus	♀	J Stereotactic Gamma Beam Radiosurgery		

DRG Non-OR   All treatment site, modality, isotope, and qualifier values
♀   All treatment site, modality, isotope, and qualifier values

D Radiation Therapy
U Female Reproductive System
Y Other Radiation

Treatment Site Character 4		Modality Qualifier Character 5	Isotope Character 6	Qualifier Character 7
Ø Ovary	♀	7 Contact Radiation	Z None	Z None
1 Cervix	♀	8 Hyperthermia		
2 Uterus	♀	C Intraoperative Radiation Therapy (IORT)		
		F Plaque Radiation		

♀   All treatment site, modality, isotope, and qualifier values

D Radiation Therapy
V Male Reproductive System
Ø Beam Radiation

Treatment Site Character 4		Modality Qualifier Character 5	Isotope Character 6	Qualifier Character 7
Ø Prostate	♂	Ø Photons <1 MeV	Z None	Z None
1 Testis	♂	1 Photons 1- 10 MeV		
		2 Photons >10 MeV		
		4 Heavy Particles (Protons, Ions)		
		5 Neutrons		
		6 Neutron Capture		
Ø Prostate	♂	3 Electrons	Z None	Ø Intraoperative
1 Testis	♂			Z None

♂   All treatment site, modality, isotope, and qualifier values

D Radiation Therapy
V Male Reproductive System
1 Brachytherapy

Treatment Site Character 4		Modality Qualifier Character 5	Isotope Character 6	Qualifier Character 7
Ø Prostate	♂	9 High Dose Rate (HDR)	7 Cesium 137 (Cs-137)	Z None
1 Testis	♂	B Low Dose Rate (LDR)	8 Iridium 192 (Ir-192)	
			9 Iodine 125 (I-125)	
			B Palladium 103 (Pd-103)	
			C Californium 252 (Cf-252)	
			Y Other Isotope	

♂   All treatment site, modality, isotope, and qualifier values

DU1–DV1

D Radiation Therapy
V Male Reproductive System
2 Stereotactic Radiosurgery

Treatment Site Character 4		Modality Qualifier Character 5	Isotope Character 6	Qualifier Character 7
Ø Prostate	♂	D Stereotactic Other Photon Radiosurgery	Z None	Z None
1 Testis	♂	H Stereotactic Particulate Radiosurgery		
		J Stereotactic Gamma Beam Radiosurgery		

DRG Non-OR	All treatment site, modality, isotope, and qualifier values
♂	All treatment site, modality, isotope, and qualifier values

D Radiation Therapy
V Male Reproductive System
Y Other Radiation

Treatment Site Character 4		Modality Qualifier Character 5	Isotope Character 6	Qualifier Character 7
Ø Prostate	♂	7 Contact Radiation	Z None	Z None
		8 Hyperthermia		
		C Intraoperative Radiation Therapy (IORT)		
		F Plaque Radiation		
		K Laser Interstitial Thermal Therapy		
1 Testis	♂	7 Contact Radiation	Z None	Z None
		8 Hyperthermia		
		F Plaque Radiation		

Valid OR	DVYØKZZ
♂	All treatment site, modality, isotope, and qualifier values

D Radiation Therapy
W Anatomical Regions
Ø Beam Radiation

Treatment Site Character 4	Modality Qualifier Character 5	Isotope Character 6	Qualifier Character 7
1 Head and Neck	Ø Photons <1 MeV	Z None	Z None
2 Chest	1 Photons 1- 10 MeV		
3 Abdomen	2 Photons >10 MeV		
4 Hemibody	4 Heavy Particles (Protons, Ions)		
5 Whole Body	5 Neutrons		
6 Pelvic Region	6 Neutron Capture		
1 Head and Neck	3 Electrons	Z None	Ø Intraoperative
2 Chest			Z None
3 Abdomen			
4 Hemibody			
5 Whole Body			
6 Pelvic Region			

D Radiation Therapy
W Anatomical Regions
1 Brachytherapy

Treatment Site Character 4	Modality Qualifier Character 5	Isotope Character 6	Qualifier Character 7
1 Head and Neck	9 High Dose Rate (HDR)	7 Cesium 137 (Cs-137)	Z None
2 Chest	B Low Dose Rate (LDR)	8 Iridium 192 (Ir-192)	
3 Abdomen		9 Iodine 125 (I-125)	
6 Pelvic Region		B Palladium 103 (Pd-103)	
		C Californium 252 (Cf-252)	
		Y Other Isotope	

Radiation Therapy

D   Radiation Therapy
W   Anatomical Regions
2   Stereotactic Radiosurgery

Treatment Site Character 4	Modality Qualifier Character 5	Isotope Character 6	Qualifier Character 7

1   Head and Neck
2   Chest
3   Abdomen
6   Pelvic Region
	D Stereotactic Other Photon
	     Radiosurgery
	H Stereotactic Particulate
	     Radiosurgery
	J Stereotactic Gamma Beam
	     Radiosurgery
		Z None	Z None

DRG Non-OR   All treatment site, modality, isotope, and qualifier values

D   Radiation Therapy
W   Anatomical Regions
Y   Other Radiation

Treatment Site Character 4	Modality Qualifier Character 5	Isotope Character 6	Qualifier Character 7
1 Head and Neck 2 Chest 3 Abdomen 4 Hemibody 6 Pelvic Region	7 Contact Radiation 8 Hyperthermia F Plaque Radiation	Z None	Z None
5 Whole Body	7 Contact Radiation 8 Hyperthermia F Plaque Radiation	Z None	Z None
5 Whole Body	G Isotope Administration	D Iodine 131 (I-131) F Phosphorus 32 (P-32) G Strontium 89 (Sr-89) H Strontium 90 (Sr-90) Y Other Isotope	Z None

Physical Rehabilitation and Diagnostic Audiology F00–F15

Character Meanings

This Character Meaning table is provided as a guide to assist the user in the identification of character members that may be found in this section of code tables. It **SHOULD NOT** be used to build a PCS code.

0: Rehabilitation

Type–Character 3		Body System/Region–Character 4		Type Qualifier–Character 5	Equipment –Character 6		Qualifier–Character 7	
0	Speech Assessment	0	Neurological System - Head and Neck	See next page	1	Audiometer	Z	None
1	Motor and/or Nerve Function Assessment	1	Neurological System - Upper Back / Upper Extremity		2	Sound Field / Booth		
2	Activities of Daily Living Assessment	2	Neurological System - Lower Back / Lower Extremity		4	Electroacoustic Immitance/ Acoustic Reflex		
6	Speech Treatment	3	Neurological System - Whole Body		5	Hearing Aid Selection / Fitting / Test		
7	Motor Treatment	4	Circulatory System - Head and Neck		7	Electrophysiologic		
8	Activities of Daily Living Treatment	5	Circulatory System - Upper Back / Upper Extremity		8	Vestibular / Balance		
9	Hearing Treatment	6	Circulatory System - Lower Back / Lower Extremity		9	Cochlear Implant		
B	Cochlear Implant Treatment	7	Circulatory System - Whole Body		B	Physical Agents		
C	Vestibular Treatment	8	Respiratory System - Head and Neck		C	Mechanical		
D	Device Fitting	9	Respiratory System - Upper Back / Upper Extremity		D	Electrotherapeutic		
F	Caregiver Training	B	Respiratory System - Lower Back / Lower Extremity		E	Orthosis		
		C	Respiratory System - Whole Body		F	Assistive, Adaptive, Supportive or Protective		
		D	Integumentary System - Head and Neck		G	Aerobic Endurance and Conditioning		
		F	Integumentary System - Upper Back / Upper Extremity		H	Mechanical or Electromechanical		
		G	Integumentary System - Lower Back / Lower Extremity		J	Somatosensory		
		H	Integumentary System - Whole Body		K	Audiovisual		
		J	Musculoskeletal System - Head and Neck		L	Assistive Listening		
		K	Musculoskeletal System - Upper Back / Upper Extremity		M	Augmentative / Alternative Communication		
		L	Musculoskeletal System - Lower Back / Lower Extremity		N	Biosensory Feedback		
		M	Musculoskeletal System - Whole Body		P	Computer		
		N	Genitourinary System		Q	Speech Analysis		
		Z	None		S	Voice Analysis		
					T	Aerodynamic Function		
					U	Prosthesis		
					V	Speech Prosthesis		
					W	Swallowing		
					X	Cerumen Management		
					Y	Other Equipment		
					Z	None		

Continued on next page

Ø: Rehabilitation
Type Qualifier—Character 5 Meanings

Continued from previous page

Type–Character 3	Type Qualifier–Character 5
Ø Speech Assessment	Ø Filtered Speech 1 Speech Threshold 2 Speech/Word Recognition 3 Staggered Spondaic Word 4 Sensorineural Acuity Level 5 Synthetic Sentence Identification 6 Speech and/or Language Screening 7 Nonspoken Language 8 Receptive/Expressive Language 9 Articulation/Phonology B Motor Speech C Aphasia D Fluency F Voice G Communicative/Cognitive Integration Skills H Bedside Swallowing and Oral Function	J Instrumental Swallowing and Oral Function K Orofacial Myofunctional L Augmentative/Alternative Communication System M Voice Prosthetic N Non-invasive Instrumental Status P Oral Peripheral Mechanism Q Performance Intensity Phonetically Balanced Speech Discrimination R Brief Tone Stimuli S Distorted Speech T Dichotic Stimuli V Temporal Ordering of Stimuli W Masking Patterns X Other Specified Central Auditory Processing
1 Motor and/or Nerve Function Assessment	Ø Muscle Performance 1 Integumentary Integrity 2 Visual Motor Integration 3 Coordination/Dexterity 4 Motor Function 5 Range of Motion and Joint Integrity 6 Sensory Awareness/Processing/Integrity	7 Facial Nerve Function 9 Somatosensory Evoked Potentials B Bed Mobility C Transfer D Gait and/or Balance F Wheelchair Mobility G Reflex Integrity
2 Activities of Daily Living Assessment	Ø Bathing/Showering 1 Dressing 2 Feeding/Eating 3 Grooming/Personal Hygiene 4 Home Management 5 Perceptual Processing 6 Psychosocial Skills 7 Aerobic Capacity and Endurance 8 Anthropometric Characteristics	9 Cranial Nerve Integrity B Environmental, Home and Work Barriers C Ergonomics and Body Mechanics D Neuromotor Development F Pain G Ventilation, Respiration and Circulation H Vocational Activities and Functional Community or Work Reintegration Skills

6 Speech Treatment	Ø Nonspoken Language
	1 Speech-Language Pathology and Related Disorders
	   Counseling
	2 Speech-Language Pathology and Related Disorders
	   Prevention
	3 Aphasia
	4 Articulation/Phonology
	5 Aural Rehabilitation
		6 Communicative/Cognitive Integration Skills
		7 Fluency
		8 Motor Speech
		9 Orofacial Myofunctional
		B Receptive/Expressive Language
		C Voice
		D Swallowing Dysfunction

7 Motor Treatment	Ø Range of Motion and Joint Mobility 1 Muscle Performance 2 Coordination/Dexterity 3 Motor Function 4 Wheelchair Mobility	5 Bed Mobility 6 Therapeutic Exercise 7 Manual Therapy Techniques 8 Transfer Training 9 Gait Training/Functional Ambulation
8 Activities of Daily Living Treatment	Ø Bathing/Showering Techniques 1 Dressing Techniques 2 Grooming/Personal Hygiene 3 Feeding/Eating 4 Home Management	5 Wound Management 6 Psychosocial Skills 7 Vocational Activities and Functional Community or Work Reintegration Skills
9 Hearing Treatment	Ø Hearing and Related Disorders Counseling 1 Hearing and Related Disorders Prevention 2 Auditory Processing 3 Cerumen Management	
B Cochlear Implant Treatment	Ø Cochlear Implant Rehabilitation	
C Vestibular Treatment	Ø Vestibular 1 Perceptual Processing	2 Visual Motor Integration 3 Postural Control
D Device Fitting	Ø Tinnitus Masker 1 Monaural Hearing Aid 2 Binaural Hearing Aid 3 Augmentative/Alternative Communication System 4 Voice Prosthetic	5 Assistive Listening Device 6 Dynamic Orthosis 7 Static Orthosis 8 Prosthesis 9 Assistive, Adaptive, Supportive or Protective Devices

F Caregiver Training	Ø Bathing/Showering Technique
	1 Dressing
	2 Feeding and Eating
	3 Grooming/Personal Hygiene
	4 Bed Mobility
	5 Transfer
	6 Wheelchair Mobility
	7 Therapeutic Exercise
	8 Airway Clearance Techniques
	9 Wound Management
		B Vocational Activities and Functional Community or
		   Work Reintegration Skills
		C Gait Training/Functional Ambulation
		D Application, Proper Use and Care of Assistive,
		   Adaptive, Supportive or Protective Devices
		F Application, Proper Use and Care of Orthoses
		G Application, Proper Use and Care of Prosthesis
		H Home Management
		J Communication Skills

1: Diagnostic Audiology

Type– Character 3	Body System/Region– Character 4	Type Qualifier– Character 5	Equipment– Character 6	Qualifer– Character 7
3 Hearing Assessment	Z None	See below	Ø Occupational Hearing	Z None
4 Hearing Aid Assessment			1 Audiometer	
5 Vestibular Assessment			2 Sound Field / Booth	
			3 Tympanometer	
			4 Electroacoustic Immitance / Acoustic Reflex	
			5 Hearing Aid Selection / Fitting / Test	
			6 Otoacoustic Emission (OAE)	
			7 Electrophysiologic	
			8 Vestibular / Balance	
			9 Cochlear Implant	
			K Audiovisual	
			L Assistive Listening	
			P Computer	
			Y Other Equipment	
			Z None	

1: Diagnostic Audiology
Type Qualifier—Character 5 Meanings

Type–Character 3	Type Qualifier–Character 5
3 Hearing Assessment	Ø Hearing Screening 1 Pure Tone Audiometry, Air 2 Pure Tone Audiometry, Air and Bone 3 Bekesy Audiometry 4 Conditioned Play Audiometry 5 Select Picture Audiometry 6 Visual Reinforcement Audiometry 7 Alternate Binaural or Monaural Loudness Balance 8 Tone Decay 9 Short Increment Sensitivity Index B Stenger C Pure Tone Stenger D Tympanometry F Eustachian Tube Function G Acoustic Reflex Patterns H Acoustic Reflex Threshold J Acoustic Reflex Decay K Electrocochleography L Auditory Evoked Potentials M Evoked Otoacoustic Emissions, Screening N Evoked Otoacoustic Emissions, Diagnostic P Aural Rehabilitation Status Q Auditory Processing
4 Hearing Aid Assessment	Ø Cochlear Implant 1 Ear Canal Probe Microphone 2 Monaural Hearing Aid 3 Binaural Hearing Aid 4 Assistive Listening System/Device Selection 5 Sensory Aids 6 Binaural Electroacoustic Hearing Aid Check 7 Ear Protector Attentuation 8 Monaural Electroacoustic Hearing Aid Check
5 Vestibular Assessment	Ø Bithermal, Bionaural Caloric Irrigation 1 Bithermal, Monaural Caloric Irrigation 2 Unithermal Binaural Screen 3 Oscillating Tracking 4 Sinusoidal Vertical Axis Rotational 5 Dix-Hallpike Dynamic 6 Computerized Dynamic Posturography 7 Tinnitus Masker

F   Physical Rehabilitation and Diagnostic Audiology
0   Rehabilitation
0   Speech Assessment   Definition: Measurement of speech and related functions

Body System/Region Character 4	Type Qualifier Character 5	Equipment Character 6	Qualifier Character 7

3 Neurological System - Whole Body	G Communicative/Cognitive
	     Integration Skills
		K Audiovisual
		M Augmentative / Alternative
		     Communication
		P Computer
		Y Other Equipment
		Z None
			Z None

Z None	0 Filtered Speech 3 Staggered Spondaic Word Q Performance Intensity Phonetically Balanced Speech Discrimination R Brief Tone Stimuli S Distorted Speech T Dichotic Stimuli V Temporal Ordering of Stimuli W Masking Patterns	1 Audiometer 2 Sound Field / Booth K Audiovisual Z None	Z None
Z None	1 Speech Threshold 2 Speech/Word Recognition	1 Audiometer 2 Sound Field / Booth 9 Cochlear Implant K Audiovisual Z None	Z None
Z None	4 Sensorineural Acuity Level	1 Audiometer 2 Sound Field / Booth Z None	Z None
Z None	5 Synthetic Sentence Identification	1 Audiometer 2 Sound Field / Booth 9 Cochlear Implant K Audiovisual	Z None

Z None	6 Speech and/or Language Screening
	7 Nonspoken Language
	8 Receptive/Expressive Language
	C Aphasia
	G Communicative/Cognitive
	     Integration Skills
	L Augmentative/Alternative
	     Communication System
		K Audiovisual
		M Augmentative / Alternative
		     Communication
		P Computer
		Y Other Equipment
		Z None
			Z None

Z None	9 Articulation/Phonology	K Audiovisual P Computer Q Speech Analysis Y Other Equipment Z None	Z None
Z None	B Motor Speech	K Audiovisual N Biosensory Feedback P Computer Q Speech Analysis T Aerodynamic Function Y Other Equipment Z None	Z None
Z None	D Fluency	K Audiovisual N Biosensory Feedback P Computer Q Speech Analysis S Voice Analysis T Aerodynamic Function Y Other Equipment Z None	Z None
Z None	F Voice	K Audiovisual N Biosensory Feedback P Computer S Voice Analysis T Aerodynamic Function Y Other Equipment Z None	Z None

F00 Continued on next page

DRG Non-OR   All body system/region, type qualifier, equipment, and qualifier values

LC Limited Coverage   NC Noncovered   ⊞ Combination Member   HAC   Valid OR   Combination Only   DRG Non-OR   New/Revised in GREEN

F   Physical Rehabilitation and Diagnostic Audiology
Ø   Rehabilitation
Ø   Speech Assessment   Definition: Measurement of speech and related functions

F0Ø Continued

Body System/Region Character 4	Type Qualifier Character 5	Equipment Character 6	Qualifier Character 7
Z None	H Bedside Swallowing and Oral Function P Oral Peripheral Mechanism	Y Other Equipment Z None	Z None
Z None	J Instrumental Swallowing and Oral Function	T Aerodynamic Function W Swallowing Y Other Equipment	Z None
Z None	K Orofacial Myofunctional	K Audiovisual P Computer Y Other Equipment Z None	Z None
Z None	M Voice Prosthetic	K Audiovisual P Computer S Voice Analysis V Speech Prosthesis Y Other Equipment Z None	Z None
Z None	N Non-invasive Instrumental Status	N Biosensory Feedback P Computer Q Speech Analysis S Voice Analysis T Aerodynamic Function Y Other Equipment	Z None
Z None	X Other Specified Central Auditory Processing	Z None	Z None

DRG Non-OR   All body system/region, type qualifier, equipment, and qualifier values

---

F   Physical Rehabilitation and Diagnostic Audiology
Ø   Rehabilitation
1   Motor and/or Nerve Function Assessment   Definition: Measurement of motor, nerve, and related functions

Body System/Region Character 4	Type Qualifier Character 5	Equipment Character 6	Qualifier Character 7
Ø Neurological System - Head and Neck 1 Neurological System - Upper Back/ Upper Extremity 2 Neurological System - Lower Back/ Lower Extremity 3 Neurological System - Whole Body	Ø Muscle Performance	E Orthosis F Assistive, Adaptive, Supportive or Protective U Prosthesis Y Other Equipment Z None	Z None
Ø Neurological System - Head and Neck 1 Neurological System - Upper Back/ Upper Extremity 2 Neurological System - Lower Back/ Lower Extremity 3 Neurological System - Whole Body	1 Integumentary Integrity 3 Coordination/Dexterity 4 Motor Function G Reflex Integrity	Z None	Z None
Ø Neurological System - Head and Neck 1 Neurological System - Upper Back/ Upper Extremity 2 Neurological System - Lower Back/ Lower Extremity 3 Neurological System - Whole Body	5 Range of Motion and Joint Integrity 6 Sensory Awareness/Processing/ Integrity	Y Other Equipment Z None	Z None
D Integumentary System - Head and Neck F Integumentary System - Upper Back/ Upper Extremity G Integumentary System - Lower Back/ Lower Extremity H Integumentary System - Whole Body J Musculoskeletal System - Head and Neck K Musculoskeletal System - Upper Back/ Upper Extremity L Musculoskeletal System - Lower Back/ Lower Extremity M Musculoskeletal System - Whole Body	Ø Muscle Performance	E Orthosis F Assistive, Adaptive, Supportive or Protective U Prosthesis Y Other Equipment Z None	Z None

F01 Continued on next page

DRG Non-OR   All body system/region, type qualifier, equipment, and qualifier values

---

LC Limited Coverage   NC Noncovered   ⊞ Combination Member   HAC   Valid OR   Combination Only   DRG Non-OR   New/Revised in GREEN

F   Physical Rehabilitation and Diagnostic Audiology
Ø   Rehabilitation
1   Motor and/or Nerve Function Assessment   Definition: Measurement of motor, nerve, and related functions

Body System/Region Character 4	Type Qualifier Character 5	Equipment Character 6	Qualifier Character 7
D Integumentary System - Head and Neck **F** Integumentary System - Upper Back/ Upper Extremity **G** Integumentary System - Lower Back/ Lower Extremity **H** Integumentary System - Whole Body **J** Musculoskeletal System - Head and Neck **K** Musculoskeletal System - Upper Back/ Upper Extremity **L** Musculoskeletal System - Lower Back/ Lower Extremity **M** Musculoskeletal System - Whole Body	**1** Integumentary Integrity	**Z** None	**Z** None
D Integumentary System - Head and Neck **F** Integumentary System - Upper Back/ Upper Extremity **G** Integumentary System - Lower Back/ Lower Extremity **H** Integumentary System - Whole Body **J** Musculoskeletal System - Head and Neck **K** Musculoskeletal System - Upper Back/ Upper Extremity **L** Musculoskeletal System - Lower Back/ Lower Extremity **M** Musculoskeletal System - Whole Body	**5** Range of Motion and Joint Integrity **6** Sensory Awareness/Processing/ Integrity	**Y** Other Equipment **Z** None	**Z** None
N Genitourinary System	**Ø** Muscle Performance	**E** Orthosis **F** Assistive, Adaptive, Supportive or Protective **U** Prosthesis **Y** Other Equipment **Z** None	**Z** None
Z None	**2** Visual Motor Integration	**K** Audiovisual **M** Augmentative / Alternative Communication **N** Biosensory Feedback **P** Computer **Q** Speech Analysis **S** Voice Analysis **Y** Other Equipment **Z** None	**Z** None
Z None	**7** Facial Nerve Function	**7** Electrophysiologic	**Z** None
Z None	**9** Somatosensory Evoked Potentials	**J** Somatosensory	**Z** None
Z None	**B** Bed Mobility **C** Transfer **F** Wheelchair Mobility	**E** Orthosis **F** Assistive, Adaptive, Supportive or Protective **U** Prosthesis **Z** None	**Z** None
Z None	**D** Gait and/or Balance	**E** Orthosis **F** Assistive, Adaptive, Supportive or Protective **U** Prosthesis **Y** Other Equipment **Z** None	**Z** None

DRG Non-OR   All body system/region, type qualifier, equipment, and qualifier values

F   **Physical Rehabilitation and Diagnostic Audiology**
Ø   **Rehabilitation**
2   **Activities of Daily Living Assessment**   Definition: Measurement of functional level for activities of daily living

Body System/Region Character 4	Type Qualifier Character 5	Equipment Character 6	Qualifier Character 7
Ø Neurological System - Head and Neck	**9** Cranial Nerve Integrity **D** Neuromotor Development	**Y** Other Equipment **Z** None	**Z** None
1 Neurological System - Upper Back/ Upper Extremity **2** Neurological System - Lower Back/ Lower Extremity **3** Neurological System - Whole Body	**D** Neuromotor Development	**Y** Other Equipment **Z** None	**Z** None
4 Circulatory System - Head and Neck **5** Circulatory System - Upper Back/ Upper Extremity **6** Circulatory System - Lower Back/ Lower Extremity **8** Respiratory System - Head and Neck **9** Respiratory System - Upper Back/ Upper Extremity **B** Respiratory System - Lower Back/ Lower Extremity	**G** Ventilation, Respiration and Circulation	**C** Mechanical **G** Aerobic Endurance and Conditioning **Y** Other Equipment **Z** None	**Z** None
7 Circulatory System - Whole Body **C** Respiratory System - Whole Body	**7** Aerobic Capacity and Endurance	**E** Orthosis **G** Aerobic Endurance and Conditioning **U** Prosthesis **Y** Other Equipment **Z** None	**Z** None
7 Circulatory System - Whole Body **C** Respiratory System - Whole Body	**G** Ventilation, Respiration and Circulation	**C** Mechanical **G** Aerobic Endurance and Conditioning **Y** Other Equipment **Z** None	**Z** None
Z None	**Ø** Bathing/Showering **1** Dressing **3** Grooming/Personal Hygiene **4** Home Management	**E** Orthosis **F** Assistive, Adaptive, Supportive or Protective **U** Prosthesis **Z** None	**Z** None
Z None	**2** Feeding/Eating **8** Anthropometric Characteristics **F** Pain	**Y** Other Equipment **Z** None	**Z** None
Z None	**5** Perceptual Processing	**K** Audiovisual **M** Augmentative / Alternative Communication **N** Biosensory Feedback **P** Computer **Q** Speech Analysis **S** Voice Analysis **Y** Other Equipment **Z** None	**Z** None
Z None	**6** Psychosocial Skills	**Z** None	**Z** None
Z None	**B** Environmental, Home and Work Barriers **C** Ergonomics and Body Mechanics	**E** Orthosis **F** Assistive, Adaptive, Supportive or Protective **U** Prosthesis **Y** Other Equipment **Z** None	**Z** None
Z None	**H** Vocational Activities and Functional Community or Work Reintegration Skills	**E** Orthosis **F** Assistive, Adaptive, Supportive or Protective **G** Aerobic Endurance and Conditioning **U** Prosthesis **Y** Other Equipment **Z** None	**Z** None

DRG Non-OR   All body system/region, type qualifier, equipment, and qualifier values

LC Limited Coverage   **NC** Noncovered   ⊞ Combination Member   **HAC**   Valid OR   Combination Only   DRG Non-OR   New/Revised in **GREEN**

ICD-10-PCS 2019   **789**

Physical Rehabilitation and Diagnostic Audiology

F   Physical Rehabilitation and Diagnostic Audiology
Ø   Rehabilitation
6   Speech Treatment   Definition: Application of techniques to improve, augment, or compensate for speech and related functional impairment

Body System/Region Character 4	Type Qualifier Character 5	Equipment Character 6	Qualifier Character 7
3 Neurological System - Whole Body	6 Communicative/Cognitive Integration Skills	K Audiovisual M Augmentative / Alternative Communication P Computer Y Other Equipment Z None	Z None
Z None	Ø Nonspoken Language 3 Aphasia 6 Communicative/Cognitive Integration Skills	K Audiovisual M Augmentative / Alternative Communication P Computer Y Other Equipment Z None	Z None
Z None	1 Speech-Language Pathology and Related Disorders Counseling 2 Speech-Language Pathology and Related Disorders Prevention	K Audiovisual Z None	Z None
Z None	4 Articulation/Phonology	K Audiovisual P Computer Q Speech Analysis T Aerodynamic Function Y Other Equipment Z None	Z None
Z None	5 Aural Rehabilitation	K Audiovisual L Assistive Listening M Augmentative / Alternative Communication N Biosensory Feedback P Computer Q Speech Analysis S Voice Analysis Y Other Equipment Z None	Z None
Z None	7 Fluency	4 Electroacoustic Immitance / Acoustic Reflex K Audiovisual N Biosensory Feedback Q Speech Analysis S Voice Analysis T Aerodynamic Function Y Other Equipment Z None	Z None
Z None	8 Motor Speech	K Audiovisual N Biosensory Feedback P Computer Q Speech Analysis S Voice Analysis T Aerodynamic Function Y Other Equipment Z None	Z None
Z None	9 Orofacial Myofunctional	K Audiovisual P Computer Y Other Equipment Z None	Z None
Z None	B Receptive/Expressive Language	K Audiovisual L Assistive Listening M Augmentative / Alternative Communication P Computer Y Other Equipment Z None	Z None

F06 Continued on next page

DRG Non-OR All body system/region, type qualifier, equipment, and qualifier values

F   Physical Rehabilitation and Diagnostic Audiology   *F06 Continued*
Ø   Rehabilitation
6   Speech Treatment   Definition: Application of techniques to improve, augment, or compensate for speech and related functional impairment

Body System/Region Character 4	Type Qualifier Character 5	Equipment Character 6	Qualifier Character 7
Z None	**C** Voice	**K** Audiovisual **N** Biosensory Feedback **P** Computer **S** Voice Analysis **T** Aerodynamic Function **V** Speech Prosthesis **Y** Other Equipment **Z** None	**Z** None
Z None	**D** Swallowing Dysfunction	**M** Augmentative / Alternative Communication **T** Aerodynamic Function **V** Speech Prosthesis **Y** Other Equipment **Z** None	**Z** None

DRG Non-OR All body system/region, type qualifier, equipment, and qualifier values

🔒 Limited Coverage   🚫 Noncovered   ⊞ Combination Member   HAC   Valid OR   Combination Only   DRG Non-OR   New/Revised in GREEN

Physical Rehabilitation and Diagnostic Audiology *(side margin)*

F   **Physical Rehabilitation and Diagnostic Audiology**
Ø   **Rehabilitation**
7   **Motor Treatment**   Definition: Exercise or activities to increase or facilitate motor function

Body System/Region Character 4	Type Qualifier Character 5	Equipment Character 6	Qualifier Character 7
Ø Neurological System - Head and Neck 1 Neurological System - Upper Back/ Upper Extremity 2 Neurological System - Lower Back/ Lower Extremity 3 Neurological System - Whole Body D Integumentary System - Head and Neck F Integumentary System - Upper Back/Upper Extremity G Integumentary System - Lower Back/Lower Extremity H Integumentary System - Whole Body J Musculoskeletal System - Head and Neck K Musculoskeletal System - Upper Back/Upper Extremity L Musculoskeletal System - Lower Back/Lower Extremity M Musculoskeletal System - Whole Body	Ø Range of Motion and Joint Mobility 1 Muscle Performance 2 Coordination/Dexterity 3 Motor Function	E Orthosis F Assistive, Adaptive, Supportive or Protective U Prosthesis Y Other Equipment Z None	Z None
Ø Neurological System - Head and Neck 1 Neurological System - Upper Back/ Upper Extremity 2 Neurological System - Lower Back/ Lower Extremity 3 Neurological System - Whole Body D Integumentary System - Head and Neck F Integumentary System - Upper Back/Upper Extremity G Integumentary System - Lower Back/Lower Extremity H Integumentary System - Whole Body J Musculoskeletal System - Head and Neck K Musculoskeletal System - Upper Back/Upper Extremity L Musculoskeletal System - Lower Back/Lower Extremity M Musculoskeletal System - Whole Body	6 Therapeutic Exercise	B Physical Agents C Mechanical D Electrotherapeutic E Orthosis F Assistive, Adaptive, Supportive or Protective G Aerobic Endurance and Conditioning H Mechanical or Electromechanical U Prosthesis Y Other Equipment Z None	Z None
Ø Neurological System - Head and Neck 1 Neurological System - Upper Back/ Upper Extremity 2 Neurological System - Lower Back/ Lower Extremity 3 Neurological System - Whole Body D Integumentary System - Head and Neck F Integumentary System - Upper Back/Upper Extremity G Integumentary System - Lower Back/Lower Extremity H Integumentary System - Whole Body J Musculoskeletal System - Head and Neck K Musculoskeletal System - Upper Back/Upper Extremity L Musculoskeletal System - Lower Back/Lower Extremity M Musculoskeletal System - Whole Body	7 Manual Therapy Techniques	Z None	Z None

F07 Continued on next page

DRG Non-OR   All body system/region, type qualifier, equipment, and qualifier values

---

LC Limited Coverage   **NC** Noncovered   ⊞ Combination Member   HAC   Valid OR   Combination Only   DRG Non-OR   New/Revised in GREEN

792   ICD-10-PCS 2019

F Physical Rehabilitation and Diagnostic Audiology
0 Rehabilitation
7 Motor Treatment   Definition: Exercise or activities to increase or facilitate motor function

F07 Continued

Body System/Region Character 4	Type Qualifier Character 5	Equipment Character 6	Qualifier Character 7
4 Circulatory System - Head and Neck 5 Circulatory System - Upper Back / Upper Extremity 6 Circulatory System - Lower Back / Lower Extremity 7 Circulatory System - Whole Body 8 Respiratory System - Head and Neck 9 Respiratory System - Upper Back / Upper Extremity B Respiratory System -Lower Back / Lower Extremity C Respiratory System -Whole Body	6 Therapeutic Exercise	B Physical Agents C Mechanical D Electrotherapeutic E Orthosis F Assistive, Adaptive, Supportive or Protective G Aerobic Endurance and Conditioning H Mechanical or Electromechanical U Prosthesis Y Other Equipment Z None	Z None
N Genitourinary System	1 Muscle Performance	E Orthosis F Assistive, Adaptive, Supportive or Protective U Prosthesis Y Other Equipment Z None	Z None
N Genitourinary System	6 Therapeutic Exercise	B Physical Agents C Mechanical D Electrotherapeutic E Orthosis F Assistive, Adaptive, Supportive or Protective G Aerobic Endurance and Conditioning H Mechanical or Electromechanical U Prosthesis Y Other Equipment Z None	Z None
Z None	4 Wheelchair Mobility	D Electrotherapeutic E Orthosis F Assistive, Adaptive, Supportive or Protective U Prosthesis Y Other Equipment Z None	Z None
Z None	5 Bed Mobility	C Mechanical E Orthosis F Assistive, Adaptive, Supportive or Protective U Prosthesis Y Other Equipment Z None	Z None
Z None	8 Transfer Training	C Mechanical D Electrotherapeutic E Orthosis F Assistive, Adaptive, Supportive or Protective U Prosthesis Y Other Equipment Z None	Z None
Z None	9 Gait Training/Functional Ambulation	C Mechanical D Electrotherapeutic E Orthosis F Assistive, Adaptive, Supportive or Protective G Aerobic Endurance and Conditioning U Prosthesis Y Other Equipment Z None	Z None

DRG Non-OR All body system/region, type qualifier, equipment, and qualifier values

Physical Rehabilitation and Diagnostic Audiology (sidebar)

F   **Physical Rehabilitation and Diagnostic Audiology**
Ø   **Rehabilitation**
8   **Activities of Daily Living Treatment**   Definition: Exercise or activities to facilitate functional competence for activities of daily living

Body System/Region Character 4	Type Qualifier Character 5	Equipment Character 6	Qualifier Character 7
D Integumentary System - Head and Neck F Integumentary System - Upper Back/Upper Extremity G Integumentary System - Lower Back/Lower Extremity H Integumentary System - Whole Body J Musculoskeletal System - Head and Neck K Musculoskeletal System - Upper Back/Upper Extremity L Musculoskeletal System - Lower Back/Lower Extremity M Musculoskeletal System - Whole Body	5 Wound Management	B Physical Agents C Mechanical D Electrotherapeutic E Orthosis F Assistive, Adaptive, Supportive or Protective U Prosthesis Y Other Equipment Z None	Z None
Z None	Ø Bathing/Showering Techniques 1 Dressing Techniques 2 Grooming/Personal Hygiene	E Orthosis F Assistive, Adaptive, Supportive or Protective U Prosthesis Y Other Equipment Z None	Z None
Z None	3 Feeding/Eating	C Mechanical D Electrotherapeutic E Orthosis F Assistive, Adaptive, Supportive or Protective U Prosthesis Y Other Equipment Z None	Z None
Z None	4 Home Management	D Electrotherapeutic E Orthosis F Assistive, Adaptive, Supportive or Protective U Prosthesis Y Other Equipment Z None	Z None
Z None	6 Psychosocial Skills	Z None	Z None
Z None	7 Vocational Activities and Functional Community or Work Reintegration Skills	B Physical Agents C Mechanical D Electrotherapeutic E Orthosis F Assistive, Adaptive, Supportive or Protective G Aerobic Endurance and Conditioning U Prosthesis Y Other Equipment Z None	Z None

DRG Non-OR   All body system/region, type qualifier, equipment, and qualifier values

F   **Physical Rehabilitation and Diagnostic Audiology**
Ø   **Rehabilitation**
9   **Hearing Treatment**   Definition: Application of techniques to improve, augment, or compensate for hearing and related functional impairment

Body System/Region Character 4	Type Qualifier Character 5	Equipment Character 6	Qualifier Character 7
Z None	Ø Hearing and Related Disorders Counseling 1 Hearing and Related Disorders Prevention	K Audiovisual Z None	Z None
Z None	2 Auditory Processing	K Audiovisual L Assistive Listening P Computer Y Other Equipment Z None	Z None
Z None	3 Cerumen Management	X Cerumen Management Z None	Z None

DRG Non-OR   All body system/region, type qualifier, equipment, and qualifier values

F   Physical Rehabilitation and Diagnostic Audiology
Ø   Rehabilitation
B   Cochlear Implant Treatment   Definition: Application of techniques to improve the communication abilities of individuals with cochlear implant

Body System/Region Character 4	Type Qualifier Character 5	Equipment Character 6	Qualifier Character 7
Z None	Ø Cochlear Implant Rehabilitation	1 Audiometer 2 Sound Field / Booth 9 Cochlear Implant K Audiovisual P Computer Y Other Equipment	Z None

DRG Non-OR   All body system/region, type qualifier, equipment, and qualifier values

---

F   Physical Rehabilitation and Diagnostic Audiology
Ø   Rehabilitation
C   Vestibular Treatment   Definition: Application of techniques to improve, augment, or compensate for vestibular and related functional impairment

Body System/Region Character 4	Type Qualifier Character 5	Equipment Character 6	Qualifier Character 7
3 Neurological System - Whole Body H Integumentary System - Whole Body M Musculoskeletal System - Whole Body	3 Postural Control	E Orthosis F Assistive, Adaptive, Supportive or Protective U Prosthesis Y Other Equipment Z None	Z None
Z None	Ø Vestibular	8 Vestibular / Balance Z None	Z None
Z None	1 Perceptual Processing 2 Visual Motor Integration	K Audiovisual L Assistive Listening N Biosensory Feedback P Computer Q Speech Analysis S Voice Analysis T Aerodynamic Function Y Other Equipment Z None	Z None

DRG Non-OR   All body system/region, type qualifier, equipment, and qualifier values

---

F   Physical Rehabilitation and Diagnostic Audiology
Ø   Rehabilitation
D   Device Fitting   Definition: Fitting of a device designed to facilitate or support achievement of a higher level of function

Body System/Region Character 4	Type Qualifier Character 5	Equipment Character 6	Qualifier Character 7
Z None	Ø Tinnitus Masker	5 Hearing Aid Selection / Fitting / Test Z None	Z None
Z None	1 Monaural Hearing Aid 2 Binaural Hearing Aid 5 Assistive Listening Device	1 Audiometer 2 Sound Field / Booth 5 Hearing Aid Selection / Fitting / Test K Audiovisual L Assistive Listening Z None	Z None
Z None	3 Augmentative/Alternative Communication System	M Augmentative / Alternative Communication	Z None
Z None	4 Voice Prosthetic	S Voice Analysis V Speech Prosthesis	Z None
Z None	6 Dynamic Orthosis 7 Static Orthosis 8 Prosthesis 9 Assistive, Adaptive, Supportive or Protective Devices	E Orthosis F Assistive, Adaptive, Supportive or Protective U Prosthesis Z None	Z None

DRG Non-OR   FØDZØ[5,Z]Z
DRG Non-OR   FØDZ[1, 2,5][1,2,5, K,L,Z]Z
DRG Non-OR   FØDZ3MZ
DRG Non-OR   FØDZ4[S,V]Z
DRG Non-OR   FØDZ[6,7][E,F,U,Z]Z
DRG Non-OR   FØDZ8[E,F,U]Z

LC Limited Coverage   NC Noncovered   ⊞ Combination Member   HAC   Valid OR   Combination Only   DRG Non-OR   New/Revised in GREEN

F Physical Rehabilitation and Diagnostic Audiology
0 Rehabilitation
F Caregiver Training   Definition: Training in activities to support patient's optimal level of function

Body System/Region Character 4	Type Qualifier Character 5	Equipment Character 6	Qualifier Character 7
Z None	0 Bathing/Showering Technique 1 Dressing 2 Feeding and Eating 3 Grooming/Personal Hygiene 4 Bed Mobility 5 Transfer 6 Wheelchair Mobility 7 Therapeutic Exercise 8 Airway Clearance Techniques 9 Wound Management B Vocational Activities and Functional Community or Work Reintegration Skills C Gait Training/Functional Ambulation D Application, Proper Use and Care of Devices F Application, Proper Use and Care of Orthoses G Application, Proper Use and Care of Prosthesis H Home Management	E Orthosis F Assistive, Adaptive, Supportive or Protective U Prosthesis Z None	Z None
Z None	J Communication Skills	K Audiovisual L Assistive Listening M Augmentative / Alternative Communication P Computer Z None	Z None

DRG Non-OR All body system/region, type qualifier, equipment, and qualifier values

F   **Physical Rehabilitation and Diagnostic Audiology**
1   **Diagnostic Audiology**
3   **Hearing Assessment**   Definition: Measurement of hearing and related functions

Body System/Region Character 4	Type Qualifier Character 5	Equipment Character 6	Qualifier Character 7
Z None	**Ø** Hearing Screening	**Ø** Occupational Hearing **1** Audiometer **2** Sound Field / Booth **3** Tympanometer **8** Vestibular / Balance **9** Cochlear Implant **Z** None	**Z** None
Z None	**1** Pure Tone Audiometry, Air **2** Pure Tone Audiometry, Air and Bone	**Ø** Occupational Hearing **1** Audiometer **2** Sound Field / Booth **Z** None	**Z** None
Z None	**3** Bekesy Audiometry **6** Visual Reinforcement Audiometry **9** Short Increment Sensitivity Index **B** Stenger **C** Pure Tone Stenger	**1** Audiometer **2** Sound Field / Booth **Z** None	**Z** None
Z None	**4** Conditioned Play Audiometry **5** Select Picture Audiometry	**1** Audiometer **2** Sound Field / Booth **K** Audiovisual **Z** None	**Z** None
Z None	**7** Alternate Binaural or Monaural Loudness Balance	**1** Audiometer **K** Audiovisual **Z** None	**Z** None
Z None	**8** Tone Decay **D** Tympanometry **F** Eustachian Tube Function **G** Acoustic Reflex Patterns **H** Acoustic Reflex Threshold **J** Acoustic Reflex Decay	**3** Tympanometer **4** Electroacoustic Immitance / Acoustic Reflex **Z** None	**Z** None
Z None	**K** Electrocochleography **L** Auditory Evoked Potentials	**7** Electrophysiologic **Z** None	**Z** None
Z None	**M** Evoked Otoacoustic Emissions, Screening **N** Evoked Otoacoustic Emissions, Diagnostic	**6** Otoacoustic Emission (OAE) **Z** None	**Z** None
Z None	**P** Aural Rehabilitation Status	**1** Audiometer **2** Sound Field / Booth **4** Electroacoustic Immitance / Acoustic Reflex **9** Cochlear Implant **K** Audiovisual **L** Assistive Listening **P** Computer **Z** None	**Z** None
Z None	**Q** Auditory Processing	**K** Audiovisual **P** Computer **Y** Other Equipment **Z** None	**Z** None

Physical Rehabilitation and Diagnostic Audiology

F   Physical Rehabilitation and Diagnostic Audiology
1   Diagnostic Audiology
4   Hearing Aid Assessment   Definition: Measurement of the appropriateness and/or effectiveness of a hearing device

Body System/Region Character 4	Type Qualifier Character 5	Equipment Character 6	Qualifier Character 7
Z None	Ø Cochlear Implant	1 Audiometer 2 Sound Field / Booth 3 Tympanometer 4 Electroacoustic Immitance / Acoustic Reflex 5 Hearing Aid Selection / Fitting / Test 7 Electrophysiologic 9 Cochlear Implant K Audiovisual L Assistive Listening P Computer Y Other Equipment Z None	Z None

Z None	1 Ear Canal Probe Microphone
	6 Binaural Electroacoustic Hearing
	    Aid Check
	8 Monaural Electroacoustic Hearing
	    Aid Check
		5 Hearing Aid Selection / Fitting / Test
		Z None
			Z None

Z None	2 Monaural Hearing Aid 3 Binaural Hearing Aid	1 Audiometer 2 Sound Field / Booth 3 Tympanometer 4 Electroacoustic Immitance / Acoustic Reflex 5 Hearing Aid Selection / Fitting / Test K Audiovisual L Assistive Listening P Computer Z None	Z None

Z None	4 Assistive Listening System/Device
	    Selection
		1 Audiometer
		2 Sound Field / Booth
		3 Tympanometer
		4 Electroacoustic Immitance /
		    Acoustic Reflex
		K Audiovisual
		L Assistive Listening
		Z None
			Z None

Z None	5 Sensory Aids	1 Audiometer 2 Sound Field / Booth 3 Tympanometer 4 Electroacoustic Immitance / Acoustic Reflex 5 Hearing Aid Selection / Fitting / Test K Audiovisual L Assistive Listening Z None	Z None
Z None	7 Ear Protector Attentuation	Ø Occupational Hearing Z None	Z None

F   Physical Rehabilitation and Diagnostic Audiology
1   Diagnostic Audiology
5   Vestibular Assessment   Definition: Measurement of the vestibular system and related functions

Body System/Region Character 4	Type Qualifier Character 5	Equipment Character 6	Qualifier Character 7

Z None	Ø Bithermal, Binaural Caloric
	    Irrigation
	1 Bithermal, Monaural Caloric
	    Irrigation
	2 Unithermal Binaural Screen
	3 Oscillating Tracking
	4 Sinusoidal Vertical Axis Rotational
	5 Dix-Hallpike Dynamic
	6 Computerized Dynamic
	    Posturography
		8 Vestibular / Balance
		Z None
			Z None

Z None	7 Tinnitus Masker	5 Hearing Aid Selection / Fitting / Test Z None	Z None

Mental Health GZ1–GZJ

Character Meanings

This Character Meaning table is provided as a guide to assist the user in the identification of character members that may be found in this section of code tables. It **SHOULD NOT** be used to build a PCS code.

Z: None

Type–Character 3	Qualifier –Character 4	Qualifier–Character 5	Qualifier–Character 6	Qualifier–Character 7
1 Psychological Tests	0 Developmental	Z None	Z None	Z None
	1 Personality and Behavioral			
	2 Intellectual and Psychoeducational			
	3 Neuropsychological			
	4 Neurobehavioral and Cognitive Status			
2 Crisis Intervention	Z None			
3 Medication Management	Z None			
5 Individual Psychotherapy	0 Interactive			
	1 Behavioral			
	2 Cognitive			
	3 Interpersonal			
	4 Psychoanalysis			
	5 Psychodynamic			
	6 Supportive			
	8 Cognitive-Behavioral			
	9 Psychophysiological			
6 Counseling	0 Educational ·			
	1 Vocational			
	3 Other Counseling			
7 Family Psychotherapy	2 Other Family Psychotherapy			
B Electroconvulsive Therapy	0 Unilateral-Single Seizure			
	1 Unilateral-Multiple Seizure			
	2 Bilateral-Single Seizure			
	3 Bilateral-Multiple Seizure			
	4 Other Electroconvulsive Therapy			
C Biofeedback	9 Other Biofeedback			
F Hypnosis	Z None			
G Narcosynthesis	Z None			
H Group Psychotherapy	Z None			
J Light Therapy	Z None			

Mental Health

G   **Mental Health**
Z   **None**
1   **Psychological Tests**   Definition: The administration and interpretation of standardized psychological tests and measurement instruments for the assessment of psychological function

Qualifier Character 4	Qualifier Character 5	Qualifier Character 6	Qualifier Character 7
Ø Developmental **1** Personality and Behavioral **2** Intellectual and Psychoeducational **3** Neuropsychological **4** Neurobehavioral and Cognitive Status	**Z** None	**Z** None	**Z** None

G   **Mental Health**
Z   **None**
2   **Crisis Intervention**   Definition: Treatment of a traumatized, acutely disturbed or distressed individual for the purpose of short-term stabilization

Qualifier Character 4	Qualifier Character 5	Qualifier Character 6	Qualifier Character 7
Z None	**Z** None	**Z** None	**Z** None

G   **Mental Health**
Z   **None**
3   **Medication Management**   Definition: Monitoring and adjusting the use of medications for the treatment of a mental health disorder

Qualifier Character 4	Qualifier Character 5	Qualifier Character 6	Qualifier Character 7
Z None	**Z** None	**Z** None	**Z** None

G   **Mental Health**
Z   **None**
5   **Individual Psychotherapy**   Definition: Treatment of an individual with a mental health disorder by behavioral, cognitive, psychoanalytic, psychodynamic or psychophysiological means to improve functioning or well-being

Qualifier Character 4	Qualifier Character 5	Qualifier Character 6	Qualifier Character 7
Ø Interactive **1** Behavioral **2** Cognitive **3** Interpersonal **4** Psychoanalysis **5** Psychodynamic **6** Supportive **8** Cognitive-Behavioral **9** Psychophysiological	**Z** None	**Z** None	**Z** None

G   **Mental Health**
Z   **None**
6   **Counseling**   Definition: The application of psychological methods to treat an individual with normal developmental issues and psychological problems in order to increase function, improve well-being, alleviate distress, maladjustment or resolve crises

Qualifier Character 4	Qualifier Character 5	Qualifier Character 6	Qualifier Character 7
Ø Educational **1** Vocational **3** Other Counseling	**Z** None	**Z** None	**Z** None

G   **Mental Health**
Z   **None**
7   **Family Psychotherapy**   Definition: Treatment that includes one or more family members of an individual with a mental health disorder by behavioral, cognitive, psychoanalytic, psychodynamic or psychophysiological means to improve functioning or well-being

     Explanation: Remediation of emotional or behavioral problems presented by one or more family members in cases where psychotherapy with more than one family member is indicated

Qualifier Character 4	Qualifier Character 5	Qualifier Character 6	Qualifier Character 7
2 Other Family Psychotherapy	**Z** None	**Z** None	**Z** None

LC Limited Coverage   **NC** Noncovered   ⊞ Combination Member   HAC   Valid OR   Combination Only   DRG Non-OR   New/Revised in GREEN

800   ICD-10-PCS 2019

G   **Mental Health**
Z   **None**
B   **Electroconvulsive Therapy**   Definition: The application of controlled electrical voltages to treat a mental health disorder

Qualifier Character 4	Qualifier Character 5	Qualifier Character 6	Qualifier Character 7
Ø Unilateral-Single Seizure 1 Unilateral-Multiple Seizure 2 Bilateral-Single Seizure 3 Bilateral-Multiple Seizure 4 Other Electroconvulsive Therapy	Z None	Z None	Z None

G   **Mental Health**
Z   **None**
C   **Biofeedback**   Definition: Provision of information from the monitoring and regulating of physiological processes in conjunction with cognitive-behavioral techniques to improve patient functioning or well-being

Qualifier Character 4	Qualifier Character 5	Qualifier Character 6	Qualifier Character 7
9 Other Biofeedback	Z None	Z None	Z None

G   **Mental Health**
Z   **None**
F   **Hypnosis**   Definition: Induction of a state of heightened suggestibility by auditory, visual and tactile techniques to elicit an emotional or behavioral response

Qualifier Character 4	Qualifier Character 5	Qualifier Character 6	Qualifier Character 7
Z None	Z None	Z None	Z None

G   **Mental Health**
Z   **None**
G   **Narcosynthesis**   Definition: Administration of intravenous barbiturates in order to release suppressed or repressed thoughts

Qualifier Character 4	Qualifier Character 5	Qualifier Character 6	Qualifier Character 7
Z None	Z None	Z None	Z None

G   **Mental Health**
Z   **None**
H   **Group Psychotherapy**   Definition: Treatment of two or more individuals with a mental health disorder by behavioral, cognitive, psychoanalytic, psychodynamic or psychophysiological means to improve functioning or well-being

Qualifier Character 4	Qualifier Character 5	Qualifier Character 6	Qualifier Character 7
Z None	Z None	Z None	Z None

G   **Mental Health**
Z   **None**
J   **Light Therapy**   Definition: Application of specialized light treatments to improve functioning or well-being

Qualifier Character 4	Qualifier Character 5	Qualifier Character 6	Qualifier Character 7
Z None	Z None	Z None	Z None

Substance Abuse Treatment HZ2–HZ9

Character Meanings

This Character Meaning table is provided as a guide to assist the user in the identification of character members that may be found in this section of code tables. It **SHOULD NOT** be used to build a PCS code.

Z: None

Type–Character 3	Qualifier–Character 4	Qualifier–Character 5	Qualifier–Character 6	Qualifier–Character 7
2 Detoxification Services	Z None	Z None	Z None	Z None
3 Individual Counseling	Ø Cognitive 1 Behavioral 2 Cognitive-Behavioral 3 12-Step 4 Interpersonal 5 Vocational 6 Psychoeducation 7 Motivational Enhancement 8 Confrontational 9 Continuing Care B Spiritual C Pre/Post-Test Infectious Disease			
4 Group Counseling	Ø Cognitive 1 Behavioral 2 Cognitive-Behavioral 3 12-Step 4 Interpersonal 5 Vocational 6 Psychoeducation 7 Motivational Enhancement 8 Confrontational 9 Continuing Care B Spiritual C Pre/Post-Test Infectious Disease			
5 Individual Psychotherapy	Ø Cognitive 1 Behavioral 2 Cognitive-Behavioral 3 12-Step 4 Interpersonal 5 Interactive 6 Psychoeducation 7 Motivational Enhancement 8 Confrontational 9 Supportive B Psychoanalysis C Psychodynamic D Psychophysiological			
6 Family Counseling	3 Other Family Counseling			
8 Medication Management	Ø Nicotine Replacement 1 Methadone Maintenance 2 Levo-alpha-acetyl-methadol (LAAM) 3 Antabuse 4 Naltrexone 5 Naloxone 6 Clonidine 7 Bupropion 8 Psychiatric Medication 9 Other Replacement Medication			
9 Pharmacotherapy	Ø Nicotine Replacement 1 Methadone Maintenance 2 Levo-alpha-acetyl-methadol (LAAM) 3 Antabuse 4 Naltrexone 5 Naloxone 6 Clonidine 7 Bupropion 8 Psychiatric Medication 9 Other Replacement Medication			

Substance Abuse Treatment *(side tab)*

H   **Substance Abuse Treatment**
Z   **None**
2   **Detoxification Services**   Definition: Detoxification from alcohol and/or drugs

Explanation: Not a treatment modality, but helps the patient stabilize physically and psychologically until the body becomes free of drugs and the effects of alcohol

Qualifier Character 4	Qualifier Character 5	Qualifier Character 6	Qualifier Character 7
Z None	Z None	Z None	Z None

H   **Substance Abuse Treatment**
Z   **None**
3   **Individual Counseling**   Definition: The application of psychological methods to treat an individual with addictive behavior

Explanation: Comprised of several different techniques, which apply various strategies to address drug addiction

Qualifier Character 4	Qualifier Character 5	Qualifier Character 6	Qualifier Character 7
Ø Cognitive 1 Behavioral 2 Cognitive-Behavioral 3 12-Step 4 Interpersonal 5 Vocational 6 Psychoeducation 7 Motivational Enhancement 8 Confrontational 9 Continuing Care B Spiritual C Pre/Post-Test Infectious Disease	Z None	Z None	Z None

DRG Non-OR   HZ3[Ø,1,2,3,4,5,6,7,8,9,B]ZZZ

H   **Substance Abuse Treatment**
Z   **None**
4   **Group Counseling**   Definition: The application of psychological methods to treat two or more individuals with addictive behavior

Explanation: Provides structured group counseling sessions and healing power through the connection with others

Qualifier Character 4	Qualifier Character 5	Qualifier Character 6	Qualifier Character 7
Ø Cognitive 1 Behavioral 2 Cognitive-Behavioral 3 12-Step 4 Interpersonal 5 Vocational 6 Psychoeducation 7 Motivational Enhancement 8 Confrontational 9 Continuing Care B Spiritual C Pre/Post-Test Infectious Disease	Z None	Z None	Z None

DRG Non-OR   HZ4[Ø,1,2,3,4,5,6,7,8,9,B]ZZZ

H   **Substance Abuse Treatment**
Z   **None**
5   **Individual Psychotherapy**   Definition: Treatment of an individual with addictive behavior by behavioral, cognitive, psychoanalytic, psychodynamic or psychophysiological means

Qualifier Character 4	Qualifier Character 5	Qualifier Character 6	Qualifier Character 7
Ø Cognitive 1 Behavioral 2 Cognitive-Behavioral 3 12-Step 4 Interpersonal 5 Interactive 6 Psychoeducation 7 Motivational Enhancement 8 Confrontational 9 Supportive B Psychoanalysis C Psychodynamic D Psychophysiological	Z None	Z None	Z None

DRG Non-OR   For all qualifier values

H   **Substance Abuse Treatment**
Z   **None**
6   **Family Counseling**   Definition: The application of psychological methods that includes one or more family members to treat an individual with addictive behavior

Explanation: Provides support and education for family members of addicted individuals. Family member participation is seen as a critical area of substance abuse treatment

Qualifier Character 4	Qualifier Character 5	Qualifier Character 6	Qualifier Character 7
3 Other Family Counseling	Z None	Z None	Z None

H   **Substance Abuse Treatment**
Z   **None**
8   **Medication Management**   Definition: Monitoring or adjusting the use of replacement medications for the treatment of addiction

Qualifier Character 4	Qualifier Character 5	Qualifier Character 6	Qualifier Character 7
Ø Nicotine Replacement 1 Methadone Maintenance 2 Levo-alpha-acetyl-methadol (LAAM) 3 Antabuse 4 Naltrexone 5 Naloxone 6 Clonidine 7 Bupropion 8 Psychiatric Medication 9 Other Replacement Medication	Z None	Z None	Z None

H   **Substance Abuse Treatment**
Z   **None**
9   **Pharmacotherapy**   Definition: The use of replacement medications for the treatment of addiction

Qualifier Character 4	Qualifier Character 5	Qualifier Character 6	Qualifier Character 7
Ø Nicotine Replacement 1 Methadone Maintenance 2 Levo-alpha-acetyl-methadol (LAAM) 3 Antabuse 4 Naltrexone 5 Naloxone 6 Clonidine 7 Bupropion 8 Psychiatric Medication 9 Other Replacement Medication	Z None	Z None	Z None

New Technology X2A–XYØ

AHA Coding Clinic for all tables in the New Technology Section
2015, 4Q, 8-11

AHA Coding Clinic for table X2A
2016, 4Q, 115-116 Cerebral embolic filtration

AHA Coding Clinic for table X2C
2016, 4Q, 82-83   Coronary artery, number of arteries
2015, 4Q, 8-14   New Section X codes—New Technology procedures

AHA Coding Clinic for table X2R
2016, 4Q, 116   Aortic valve rapid deployment
2015, 4Q, 8-12   New Section X codes—New Technology procedures

AHA Coding Clinic for table XHR
2016, 4Q, 116   Application of wound matrix

AHA Coding Clinic for table XKØ
2017, 4Q, 74   Intramuscular autologous bone marrow cell therapy

AHA Coding Clinic for table XNS
2017, 4Q, 74-75   Magnetic growth rods
2016, 4Q, 117   Placement of magnetic growth rods

AHA Coding Clinic for table XRG
2017, 4Q, 76   Radiolucent porous interbody fusion device

AHA Coding Clinic for table XWØ
2015, 4Q, 8-15   New Section X codes—New Technology procedures

AHA Coding Clinic for table XYØ
2017, 4Q, 78   Intraoperative treatment of vascular grafts

New Technology

X New Technology
2 Cardiovascular System
A Assistance   Definition: Taking over a portion of a physiological function by extracorporeal means
Explanation: None

Body Part Character 4	Approach Character 5	Device/Substance/Technology Character 6	Qualifier Character 7
5 Innominate Artery and Left Common Carotid Artery	3 Percutaneous	1 Cerebral Embolic Filtration, Dual Filter	2 New Technology Group 2

X New Technology
2 Cardiovascular System
C Extirpation   Definition: Taking or cutting out solid matter from a body part
Explanation: The solid matter may be an abnormal byproduct of a biological function or a foreign body; it may be imbedded in a body part or in the lumen of a tubular body part. The solid matter may or may not have been previously broken into pieces.

Body Part Character 4	Approach Character 5	Device/Substance/Technology Character 6	Qualifier Character 7
Ø Coronary Artery, One Artery 1 Coronary Artery, Two Arteries 2 Coronary Artery, Three Arteries 3 Coronary Artery, Four or More Arteries	3 Percutaneous	6 Orbital Atherectomy Technology	1 New Technology Group 1

Valid OR   All body part, approach, device/substance/technology, and qualifier values

X New Technology
2 Cardiovascular System
R Replacement   Definition: Putting in or on biological or synthetic material that physically takes the place and/or function of all or a portion of a body part
Explanation: The body part may have been taken out or replaced, or may be taken out, physically eradicated, or rendered nonfunctional during the REPLACEMENT procedure. A REMOVAL procedure is coded for taking out the device used in a previous replacement procedure

Body Part Character 4	Approach Character 5	Device/Substance/Technology Character 6	Qualifier Character 7
F Aortic Valve	Ø Open 3 Percutaneous 4 Percutaneous Endoscopic	3 Zooplastic Tissue, Rapid Deployment Technique	2 New Technology Group 2

Valid OR   All body part, approach, device/substance/technology, and qualifier values

X New Technology
H Skin, Subcutaneous Tissue, Fascia and Breast
R Replacement   Definition: Putting in or on biological or synthetic material that physically takes the place and/or function of all or a portion of a body part
Explanation: The body part may have been taken out or replaced, or may be taken out, physically eradicated, or rendered nonfunctional during the REPLACEMENT procedure. A REMOVAL procedure is coded for taking out the device used in a previous replacement procedure

Body Part Character 4	Approach Character 5	Device/Substance/Technology Character 6	Qualifier Character 7
P Skin	X External	L Skin Substitute, Porcine Liver Derived	2 New Technology Group 2

Valid OR   All body part, approach, device/substance/technology, and qualifier values

X New Technology
K Muscles, Tendons, Bursae and Ligaments
Ø Introduction   Definition: Putting in or on a therapeutic, diagnostic, nutritional, physiological, or prophylactic substance except blood or blood products
Explanation: None

Body Part Character 4	Approach Character 5	Device/Substance/Technology Character 6	Qualifier Character 7
2 Muscle	3 Percutaneous	Ø Concentrated Bone Marrow Aspirate	3 New Technology Group 3

X New Technology
N Bones
S Reposition   Definition: Moving to its normal location, or other suitable location, all or a portion of a body part
Explanation: The body part is moved to a new location from an abnormal location, or from a normal location where it is not functioning correctly. The body part may or may not be cut out or off to be moved to the new location.

Body Part Character 4	Approach Character 5	Device/Substance/Technology Character 6	Qualifier Character 7
Ø Lumbar Vertebra 3 Cervical Vertebra 4 Thoracic Vertebra	Ø Open 3 Percutaneous	3 Magnetically Controlled Growth Rod(s)	2 New Technology Group 2

Valid OR   All body part, approach, device/substance/technology, and qualifier values

X   New Technology
R   Joints
2   Monitoring   Definition: Determining the level of a physiological or physical function repetitively over a period of time
Explanation: None

Body Part Character 4	Approach Character 5	Device/Substance/Technology Character 6	Qualifier Character 7
G Knee Joint, Right H Knee Joint, Left	Ø Open	2 Intraoperative Knee Replacement Sensor	1 New Technology Group 1

Valid OR	All body part, approach, device/substance/technology, and qualifier values

X   New Technology
R   Joints
G   Fusion   Definition: Joining together portions of an articular body part rendering the articular body part immobile
Explanation: The body part is joined together by fixation device, bone graft, or other means

Body Part Character 4	Approach Character 5	Device/Substance/Technology Character 6	Qualifier Character 7
Ø Occipital-cervical Joint	Ø Open	9 Interbody Fusion Device, Nanotextured Surface	2 New Technology Group 2
Ø Occipital-cervical Joint	Ø Open	F Interbody Fusion Device, Radiolucent Porous	3 New Technology Group 3
1 Cervical Vertebral Joint	Ø Open	9 Interbody Fusion Device, Nanotextured Surface	2 New Technology Group 2
1 Cervical Vertebral Joint	Ø Open	F Interbody Fusion Device, Radiolucent Porous	3 New Technology Group 3
2 Cervical Vertebral Joints, 2 or more	Ø Open	9 Interbody Fusion Device, Nanotextured Surface	2 New Technology Group 2
2 Cervical Vertebral Joints, 2 or more	Ø Open	F Interbody Fusion Device, Radiolucent Porous	3 New Technology Group 3
4 Cervicothoracic Vertebral Joint	Ø Open	9 Interbody Fusion Device, Nanotextured Surface	2 New Technology Group 2
4 Cervicothoracic Vertebral Joint	Ø Open	F Interbody Fusion Device, Radiolucent Porous	3 New Technology Group 3
6 Thoracic Vertebral Joint	Ø Open	9 Interbody Fusion Device, Nanotextured Surface	2 New Technology Group 2
6 Thoracic Vertebral Joint	Ø Open	F Interbody Fusion Device, Radiolucent Porous	3 New Technology Group 3
7 Thoracic Vertebral Joints, 2 to 7 ⊞	Ø Open	9 Interbody Fusion Device, Nanotextured Surface	2 New Technology Group 2
7 Thoracic Vertebral Joints, 2 to 7 ⊞	Ø Open	F Interbody Fusion Device, Radiolucent Porous	3 New Technology Group 3
8 Thoracic Vertebral Joints, 8 or more	Ø Open	9 Interbody Fusion Device, Nanotextured Surface	2 New Technology Group 2
8 Thoracic Vertebral Joints, 8 or more	Ø Open	F Interbody Fusion Device, Radiolucent Porous	3 New Technology Group 3
A Thoracolumbar Vertebral Joint	Ø Open	9 Interbody Fusion Device, Nanotextured Surface	2 New Technology Group 2
A Thoracolumbar Vertebral Joint	Ø Open	F Interbody Fusion Device, Radiolucent Porous	3 New Technology Group 3
B Lumbar Vertebral Joint	Ø Open	9 Interbody Fusion Device, Nanotextured Surface	2 New Technology Group 2
B Lumbar Vertebral Joint	Ø Open	F Interbody Fusion Device, Radiolucent Porous	3 New Technology Group 3
C Lumbar Vertebral Joints, 2 or more ⊞	Ø Open	9 Interbody Fusion Device, Nanotextured Surface	2 New Technology Group 2
C Lumbar Vertebral Joints, 2 or more ⊞	Ø Open	F Interbody Fusion Device, Radiolucent Porous	3 New Technology Group 3
D Lumbosacral Joint	Ø Open	9 Interbody Fusion Device, Nanotextured Surface	2 New Technology Group 2
D Lumbosacral Joint	Ø Open	F Interbody Fusion Device, Radiolucent Porous	3 New Technology Group 3

Valid OR	All body part, approach, device/substance/technology, and qualifier values	**See Appendix L for Procedure Combinations**
HAC	XRG[Ø,1,2,4,6,7,8,A,B,C,D]Ø92 when reported with SDx K68.11 or T81.4XXA or T84.60-T84.619, T84.63-T84.7 with 7th character A	⊞ XRG7Ø92 ⊞ XRG7ØF3
HAC	XRG[Ø,1,2,4,6,7,8,A,B,C,D]ØF3 when reported with SDx K68.11 or T81.4XXA or T84.60-T84.619, T84.63-T84.7 with 7th character A	⊞ XRGCØ92 ⊞ XRGCØF3

X New Technology
V Male Reproductive System
5 Destruction — Definition: Physical eradication of all or a portion of a body part by the direct use of energy, force, or a destructive agent
Explanation: None of the body part is physically taken out

Body Part Character 4	Approach Character 5	Device/Substance/Technology Character 6	Qualifier Character 7
Ø Prostate	8 Via Natural or Artificial Opening Endoscopic	A Robotic Waterjet Ablation	4 New Technology Group 4

X New Technology
W Anatomical Regions
Ø Introduction — Definition: Putting in or on a therapeutic, diagnostic, nutritional, physiological, or prophylactic substance except blood or blood products
Explanation: None

Body Part Character 4	Approach Character 5	Device/Substance/Technology Character 6	Qualifier Character 7
3 Peripheral Vein	3 Percutaneous	2 Ceftazidime-Avibactam Anti-infective 3 Idarucizumab, Dabigatran Reversal Agent 4 Isavuconazole Anti- infective 5 Blinatumomab Antineoplastic Immunotherapy	1 New Technology Group 1
3 Peripheral Vein	3 Percutaneous	7 Andexanet Alfa, Factor Xa Inhibitor Reversal Agent 9 Defibrotide Sodium Anticoagulant	2 New Technology Group 2
3 Peripheral Vein	3 Percutaneous	A Bezlotoxumab Monoclonal Antibody B Cytarabine and Daunorubicin Liposome Antineoplastic C Engineered Autologous Chimeric Antigen Receptor T-cell Immunotherapy F Other New Technology Therapeutic Substance	3 New Technology Group 3
3 Peripheral Vein	3 Percutaneous	G Plazomicin Anti-infective H Synthetic Human Angiotensin II	4 New Technology Group 4
4 Central Vein	3 Percutaneous	2 Ceftazidime-Avibactam Anti-infective 3 Idarucizumab, Dabigatran Reversal Agent 4 Isavuconazole Anti- infective 5 Blinatumomab Antineoplastic Immunotherapy	1 New Technology Group 1
4 Central Vein	3 Percutaneous	7 Andexanet Alfa, Factor Xa Inhibitor Reversal Agent 9 Defibrotide Sodium Anticoagulant	2 New Technology Group 2
4 Central Vein	3 Percutaneous	A Bezlotoxumab Monoclonal Antibody B Cytarabine and Daunorubicin Liposome Antineoplastic C Engineered Autologous Chimeric Antigen Receptor T-cell Immunotherapy F Other New Technology Therapeutic Substance	3 New Technology Group 3
4 Central Vein	3 Percutaneous	G Plazomicin Anti-infective H Synthetic Human Angiotensin II	4 New Technology Group 4
D Mouth and Pharynx	X External	8 Uridine Triacetate	2 New Technology Group 2

X New Technology
Y Extracorporeal
Ø Introduction — Definition: Putting in or on a therapeutic, diagnostic, nutritional, physiological, or prophylactic substance except blood or blood products
Explanation: None

Body Part Character 4	Approach Character 5	Device/Substance/Technology Character 6	Qualifier Character 7
V Vein Graft	X External	8 Endothelial Damage Inhibitor	3 New Technology Group 3

LC Limited Coverage   NC Noncovered   ⊞ Combination Member   HAC   Valid OR   Combination Only   DRG Non-OR   New/Revised in GREEN

Appendixes

Appendix A: Components of the Medical and Surgical Approach Definitions

ICD-10-PCS Value	Definition	Access Location	Method	Type of Instrumentation	Example
Open (Ø)	Cutting through the skin or mucous membrane and any other body layers necessary to expose the site of the procedure	Skin or mucous membrane, any other body layers	Cutting	None	Abdominal hysterectomy
Percutaneous (3)	Entry, by puncture or minor incision, of instrumentation through the skin or mucous membrane and any other body layers necessary to reach the site of the procedure	Skin or mucous membrane, any other body layers	Puncture or minor incision	Without visualization	Needle biopsy of liver, Liposuction
Percutaneous endoscopic (4)	Entry, by puncture or minor incision, of instrumentation through the skin or mucous membrane and any other body layers necessary to reach and visualize the site of the procedure	Skin or mucous membrane, any other body layers	Puncture or minor incision	With visualization	Arthroscopy, Laparoscopic cholecystectomy
Via natural or artificial opening (7)	Entry of instrumentation through a natural or artificial external opening to reach the site of the procedure	Natural or artificial external opening	Direct entry	Without visualization	Endotracheal tube insertion, Foley catheter placement
Via natural or artificial opening endoscopic (8)	Entry of instrumentation through a natural or artificial external opening to reach and visualize the site of the procedure	Natural or artificial external opening	Direct entry	With visualization	Sigmoidoscopy, EGD, ERCP
Via natural or artificial opening with percutaneous endoscopic assistance (F)	Entry of instrumentation through a natural or artificial external opening and entry, by puncture or minor incision, of instrumentation through the skin or mucous membrane and any other body layers necessary to aid in the performance of the procedure	Skin or mucous membrane, any other body layers	Direct entry with puncture or minor incision for instrumentation only	With visualization	Laparoscopic-assisted vaginal hysterectomy
External (X)	Procedures performed directly on the skin or mucous membrane and procedures performed indirectly by the application of external force through the skin or mucous membrane	Skin or mucous membrane	Direct or indirect application	None	Closed fracture reduction, Resection of tonsils

Open (Ø)

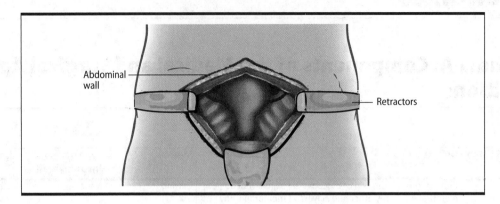

Percutaneous (3)

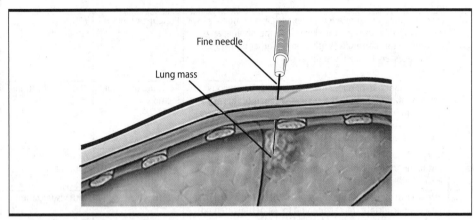

Percutaneous Endoscopic (4)

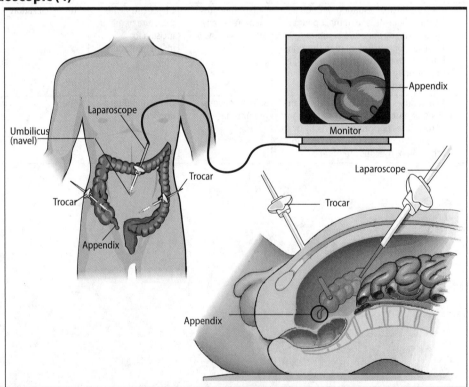

Via Natural or Artificial Opening (7)

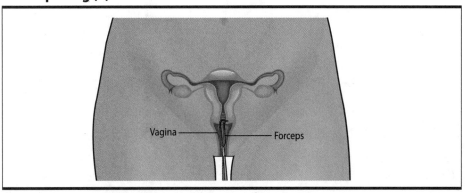

Via Natural or Artificial Opening, Endoscopic (8)

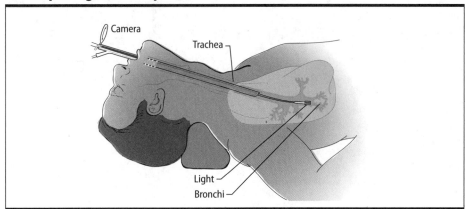

Via Natural or Artificial Opening with Percutaneous Endoscopic Assistance (F)

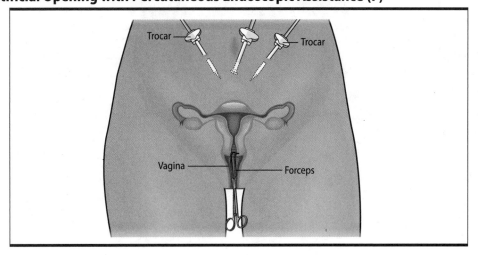

External (X)

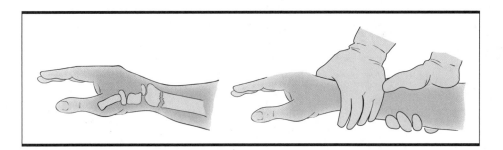

Appendix B: Root Operation Definitions

Ø	Medical and Surgical		
ICD-10-PCS Value		**Definition**	
Ø	Alteration	Definition:	Modifying the anatomic structure of a body part without affecting the function of the body part
		Explanation:	Principal purpose is to improve appearance
		Examples:	Face lift, breast augmentation
1	Bypass	Definition:	Altering the route of passage of the contents of a tubular body part
		Explanation:	Rerouting contents of a body part to a downstream area of the normal route, to a similar route and body part, or to an abnormal route and dissimilar body part. Includes one or more anastomoses, with or without the use of a device.
		Examples:	Coronary artery bypass, colostomy formation
2	Change	Definition:	Taking out or off a device from a body part and putting back an identical or similar device in or on the same body part without cutting or puncturing the skin or a mucous membrane
		Explanation:	All CHANGE procedures are coded using the approach EXTERNAL
		Example:	Urinary catheter change, gastrostomy tube change
3	Control	Definition:	Stopping, or attempting to stop, postprocedural or other acute bleeding
		Explanation:	The site of the bleeding is coded as an anatomical region and not to a specific body part
		Examples:	Control of post-prostatectomy hemorrhage, control of intracranial subdural hemorrhage, control of bleeding duodenal ulcer, control of retroperitoneal hemorrhage
4	Creation	Definition:	Putting in or on biological or synthetic material to form a new body part that to the extent possible replicates the anatomic structure or function of an absent body part
		Explanation:	Used for gender reassignment surgery and corrective procedures in individuals with congenital anomalies
		Examples:	Creation of vagina in a male, creation of right and left atrioventricular valve from common atrioventricular valve
5	Destruction	Definition:	Physical eradication of all or a portion of a body part by the direct use of energy, force, or a destructive agent
		Explanation:	None of the body part is physically taken out
		Examples:	Fulguration of rectal polyp, cautery of skin lesion
6	Detachment	Definition:	Cutting off all or a portion of the upper or lower extremities
		Explanation:	The body part value is the site of the detachment, with a qualifier if applicable to further specify the level where the extremity was detached
		Examples:	Below knee amputation, disarticulation of shoulder
7	Dilation	Definition:	Expanding an orifice or the lumen of a tubular body part
		Explanation:	The orifice can be a natural orifice or an artificially created orifice. Accomplished by stretching a tubular body part using intraluminal pressure or by cutting part of the orifice or wall of the tubular body part.
		Examples:	Percutaneous transluminal angioplasty, internal urethrotomy
8	Division	Definition:	Cutting into a body part, without draining fluids and/or gases from the body part, in order to separate or transect a body part
		Explanation:	All or a portion of the body part is separated into two or more portions
		Examples:	Spinal cordotomy, osteotomy
9	Drainage	Definition:	Taking or letting out fluids and/or gases from a body part
		Explanation:	The qualifier DIAGNOSTIC is used to identify drainage procedures that are biopsies
		Examples:	Thoracentesis, incision and drainage
B	Excision	Definition:	Cutting out or off, without replacement, a portion of a body part
		Explanation:	The qualifier DIAGNOSTIC is used to identify excision procedures that are biopsies
		Examples:	Partial nephrectomy, liver biopsy
C	Extirpation	Definition:	Taking or cutting out solid matter from a body part
		Explanation:	The solid matter may be an abnormal byproduct of a biological function or a foreign body; it may be imbedded in a body part or in the lumen of a tubular body part. The solid matter may or may not have been previously broken into pieces.
		Examples:	Thrombectomy, choledocholithotomy

Continued on next page

Ø	Medical and Surgical		*Continued from previous page*

ICD-10-PCS Value		Definition	
D	Extraction	Definition:	Pulling or stripping out or off all or a portion of a body part by the use of force
		Explanation:	The qualifier DIAGNOSTIC is used to identify extractions that are biopsies
		Examples:	Dilation and curettage, vein stripping
F	Fragmentation	Definition:	Breaking solid matter in a body part into pieces
		Explanation:	Physical force (e.g., manual, ultrasonic) applied directly or indirectly is used to break the solid matter into pieces. The solid matter may be an abnormal byproduct of a biological function or a foreign body. The pieces of solid matter are not taken out.
		Examples:	Extracorporeal shockwave lithotripsy, transurethral lithotripsy
G	Fusion	Definition:	Joining together portions of an articular body part rendering the articular body part immobile
		Explanation:	The body part is joined together by fixation device, bone graft, or other means
		Examples:	Spinal fusion, ankle arthrodesis
H	Insertion	Definition:	Putting in a nonbiological appliance that monitors, assists, performs, or prevents a physiological function but does not physically take the place of a body part
		Explanation:	None
		Examples:	Insertion of radioactive implant, insertion of central venous catheter
J	Inspection	Definition:	Visually and/or manually exploring a body part
		Explanation:	Visual exploration may be performed with or without optical instrumentation. Manual exploration may be performed directly or through intervening body layers.
		Examples:	Diagnostic arthroscopy, exploratory laparotomy
K	Map	Definition:	Locating the route of passage of electrical impulses and/or locating functional areas in a body part
		Explanation:	Applicable only to the cardiac conduction mechanism and the central nervous system
		Examples:	Cardiac mapping, cortical mapping
L	Occlusion	Definition:	Completely closing an orifice or lumen of a tubular body part
		Explanation:	The orifice can be a natural orifice or an artificially created orifice
		Examples:	Fallopian tube ligation, ligation of inferior vena cava
M	Reattachment	Definition:	Putting back in or on all or a portion of a separated body part to its normal location or other suitable location
		Explanation:	Vascular circulation and nervous pathways may or may not be reestablished
		Examples:	Reattachment of hand, reattachment of avulsed kidney
N	Release	Definition:	Freeing a body part from an abnormal physical constraint by cutting or by use of force
		Explanation:	Some of the restraining tissue may be taken out but none of the body part is taken out
		Examples:	Adhesiolysis, carpal tunnel release
P	Removal	Definition:	Taking out or off a device from a body part
		Explanation:	If a device is taken out and a similar device put in without cutting or puncturing the skin or mucous membrane, the procedure is coded to the root operation CHANGE. Otherwise, the procedure for taking out a device is coded to the root operation REMOVAL.
		Examples:	Drainage tube removal, cardiac pacemaker removal
Q	Repair	Definition:	Restoring, to the extent possible, a body part to its normal anatomic structure and function
		Explanation:	Used only when the method to accomplish the repair is not one of the other root operations
		Examples:	Colostomy takedown, suture of laceration
R	Replacement	Definition:	Putting in or on biological or synthetic material that physically takes the place and/or function of all or a portion of a body part
		Explanation:	The body part may have been taken out or replaced, or may be taken out, physically eradicated, or rendered nonfunctional during the REPLACEMENT procedure. A REMOVAL procedure is coded for taking out the device used in a previous replacement procedure.
		Examples:	Total hip replacement, bone graft, free skin graft
S	Reposition	Definition:	Moving to its normal location, or other suitable location, all or a portion of a body part
		Explanation:	The body part is moved to a new location from an abnormal location, or from a normal location where it is not functioning correctly. The body part may or may not be cut out or off to be moved to the new location.
		Examples:	Reposition of undescended testicle, fracture reduction

Continued on next page

Ø	**Medical and Surgical**		*Continued from previous page*

ICD-10-PCS Value			Definition
T	Resection	Definition:	Cutting out or off, without replacement, all of a body part
		Explanation:	None
		Examples:	Total nephrectomy, total lobectomy of lung
V	Restriction	Definition:	Partially closing an orifice or the lumen of a tubular body part
		Explanation:	The orifice can be a natural orifice or an artificially created orifice
		Examples:	Esophagogastric fundoplication, cervical cerclage
W	Revision	Definition:	Correcting, to the extent possible, a portion of a malfunctioning device or the position of a displaced device
		Explanation:	Revision can include correcting a malfunctioning or displaced device by taking out or putting in components of the device such as a screw or pin
		Examples:	Adjustment of position of pacemaker lead, recementing of hip prosthesis
U	Supplement	Definition:	Putting in or on biological or synthetic material that physically reinforces and/or augments the function of a portion of a body part
		Explanation:	The biological material is non-living, or is living and from the same individual. The body part may have been previously replaced, and the SUPPLEMENT procedure is performed to physically reinforce and/or augment the function of the replaced body part.
		Examples:	Herniorrhaphy using mesh, free nerve graft, mitral valve ring annuloplasty, put a new acetabular liner in a previous hip replacement
X	Transfer	Definition:	Moving, without taking out, all or a portion of a body part to another location to take over the function of all or a portion of a body part
		Explanation:	The body part transferred remains connected to its vascular and nervous supply
		Examples:	Tendon transfer, skin pedicle flap transfer
Y	Transplantation	Definition:	Putting in or on all or a portion of a living body part taken from another individual or animal to physically take the place and/or function of all or a portion of a similar body part
		Explanation:	The native body part may or may not be taken out, and the transplanted body part may take over all or a portion of its function
		Examples:	Kidney transplant, heart transplant

Root Operation Definitions for Other Sections

1	**Obstetrics**		

ICD-10-PCS Value			Definition
2	Change	Definition:	Taking out or off a device from a body part and putting back an identical or similar device in or on the same body part without cutting or puncturing the skin or a mucous membrane
		Explanation:	None
		Examples:	Replacement of fetal scalp electrode
9	Drainage	Definition:	Taking or letting out fluids and/or gases from a body part
		Explanation:	None
		Examples:	Biopsy of amniotic fluid
A	Abortion	Definition:	Artificially terminating a pregnancy
		Explanation:	None
		Examples:	Transvaginal abortion using vacuum aspiration technique
D	Extraction	Definition:	Pulling or stripping out or off all or a portion of a body part by the use of force
		Explanation:	None
		Examples:	Low-transverse C-section
E	Delivery	Definition:	Assisting the passage of the products of conception from the genital canal
		Explanation:	None
		Examples:	Manually-assisted delivery
H	Insertion	Definition:	Putting in a nonbiological appliance that monitors, assists, performs, or prevents a physiological function but does not physically take the place of a body part
		Explanation:	None
		Examples:	Placement of fetal scalp electrode

Continued on next page

1   Obstetrics

Continued from previous page

ICD-10-PCS Value			Definition
J	Inspection	Definition:	Visually and/or manually exploring a body part
		Explanation:	Visual exploration may be performed with or without optical instrumentation. Manual exploration may be performed directly or through intervening body layers.
		Examples:	Bimanual pregnancy exam
P	Removal	Definition:	Taking out or off a device from a body part, region or orifice
		Explanation:	If a device is taken out and a similar device put in without cutting or puncturing the skin or mucous membrane, the procedure is coded to the root operation CHANGE. Otherwise, the procedure for taking out a device is coded to the root operation REMOVAL.
		Examples:	Removal of fetal monitoring electrode
Q	Repair	Definition:	Restoring, to the extent possible, a body part to its normal anatomic structure and function
		Explanation:	Used only when the method to accomplish the repair is not one of the other root operations
		Examples:	In utero repair of congenital diaphragmatic hernia
S	Reposition	Definition:	Moving to its normal location, or other suitable location, all or a portion of a body part
		Explanation:	The body part is moved to a new location from an abnormal location, or from a normal location where it is not functioning correctly. The body part may or may not be cut out or off to be moved to the new location.
		Examples:	External version of fetus
T	Resection	Definition:	Cutting out or off, without replacement, all of a body part
		Explanation:	None
		Examples:	Total excision of tubal pregnancy
Y	Transplantation	Definition:	Putting in or on all or a portion of a living body part taken from another individual or animal to physically take the place and/or function of all or a portion of a similar body part
		Explanation:	The native body part may or may not be taken out, and the transplanted body part may take over all or a portion of its function
		Examples:	In utero fetal kidney transplant

2   Placement

ICD-10-PCS Value			Definition
Ø	Change	Definition:	Taking out or off a device from a body part and putting back an identical or similar device in or on the same body part without cutting or puncturing the skin or a mucous membrane
		Examples:	Change of vaginal packing
1	Compression	Definition:	Putting pressure on a body region
		Examples:	Placement of pressure dressing on abdominal wall
2	Dressing	Definition:	Putting material on a body region for protection
		Examples:	Application of sterile dressing to head wound
3	Immobilization	Definition:	Limiting or preventing motion of a body region
		Examples:	Placement of splint on left finger
4	Packing	Definition:	Putting material in a body region or orifice
		Examples:	Placement of nasal packing
5	Removal	Definition:	Taking out or off a device from a body part
		Examples:	Removal of stereotactic head frame
6	Traction	Definition:	Exerting a pulling force on a body region in a distal direction
		Examples:	Lumbar traction using motorized split-traction table

3   Administration

ICD-10-PCS Value			Definition
Ø	Introduction	Definition:	Putting in or on a therapeutic, diagnostic, nutritional, physiological, or prophylactic substance except blood or blood products
		Examples:	Nerve block injection to median nerve
1	Irrigation	Definition:	Putting in or on a cleansing substance
		Examples:	Flushing of eye
2	Transfusion	Definition:	Putting in blood or blood products
		Examples:	Transfusion of cell saver red cells into central venous line

4   Measurement and Monitoring

ICD-10-PCS Value			Definition
Ø	Measurement	Definition:	Determining the level of a physiological or physical function at a point in time
		Examples:	External electrocardiogram(EKG), single reading
1	Monitoring	Definition:	Determining the level of a physiological or physical function repetitively over a period of time
		Examples:	Urinary pressure monitoring

5   Extracorporeal or Systemic Assistance and Performance

ICD-10-PCS Value			Definition
Ø	Assistance	Definition:	Taking over a portion of a physiological function by extracorporeal means
		Examples:	Hyperbaric oxygenation of wound
1	Performance	Definition:	Completely taking over a physiological function by extracorporeal means
		Examples:	Cardiopulmonary bypass in conjunction with CABG
2	Restoration	Definition:	Returning, or attempting to return, a physiological function to its original state by extracorporeal means
		Examples:	Attempted cardiac defibrillation, unsuccessful

6   Extracorporeal or Systemic Therapies

ICD-10-PCS Value			Definition
Ø	Atmospheric Control	Definition:	Extracorporeal control of atmospheric pressure and composition
		Examples:	Antigen-free air conditioning, series treatment
1	Decompression	Definition:	Extracorporeal elimination of undissolved gas from body fluids
		Examples:	Hyperbaric decompression treatment, single
2	Electromagnetic Therapy	Definition:	Extracorporeal treatment by electromagnetic rays
		Examples:	TMS (transcranial magnetic stimulation), series treatment
3	Hyperthermia	Definition:	Extracorporeal raising of body temperature
		Examples:	None
4	Hypothermia	Definition:	Extracorporeal lowering of body temperature
		Examples:	Whole body hypothermia treatment for temperature imbalances, series
5	Pheresis	Definition:	Extracorporeal separation of blood products
		Examples:	Therapeutic leukopheresis, single treatment
6	Phototherapy	Definition:	Extracorporeal treatment by light rays
		Examples:	Phototherapy of circulatory system, series treatment
7	Ultrasound Therapy	Definition:	Extracorporeal treatment by ultrasound
		Examples:	Therapeutic ultrasound of peripheral vessels, single treatment
8	Ultraviolet Light Therapy	Definition:	Extracorporeal treatment by ultraviolet light
		Examples:	Ultraviolet light phototherapy, series treatment
9	Shock Wave Therapy	Definition:	Extracorporeal treatment by shock waves
		Examples:	Shockwave therapy of plantar fascia, single treatment
B	Perfusion	Definition:	Extracorporeal treatment by diffusion of therapeutic fluid
		Examples:	Perfusion of donor liver while preparing transplant patient

7		Osteopathic	
ICD-10-PCS Value			**Definition**
Ø	Treatment	Definition:	Manual treatment to eliminate or alleviate somatic dysfunction and related disorders
		Examples:	Fascial release of abdomen, osteopathic treatment

8		Other Procedures	
ICD-10-PCS Value			**Definition**
Ø	Other Procedures	Definition:	Methodologies which attempt to remediate or cure a disorder or disease
		Examples:	Acupuncture, yoga therapy

9		Chiropractic	
ICD-10-PCS Value			**Definition**
B	Manipulation	Definition:	Manual procedure that involves a directed thrust to move a joint past the physiological range of motion, without exceeding the anatomical limit
		Examples:	Chiropractic treatment of cervical spine, short lever specific contact

Note: Sections B-H (Imaging through Substance Abuse Treatment) do not include root operations. The character 3 position represents type of procedure, therefore those definitions are not included in this appendix. See appendix I for definitions of the type (character 3) or type qualifiers (character 5) that provide details of the procedures performed.

Appendix C: Comparison of Medical and Surgical Root Operations

Note: the character associated with each operation appears in parentheses after its title.

Procedures That Take Out Some or All of a Body Part

Root Operation	Objective of Procedure	Site of Procedure	Example
Destruction (5)	Eradicating without taking out or replacement	Some/all of a body part	Fulguration of endometrium
Detachment (6)	Cutting out/off without replacement	Extremity only, any level	Amputation above elbow
Excision (B)	Cutting out/off without replacement	Some of a body part	Breast lumpectomy
Extraction (D)	Pulling out or off without replacement	Some/all of a body part	Suction D&C
Resection (T)	Cutting out/off without replacement	All of a body part	Total mastectomy

Procedures That Put in/Put Back or Move Some/All of a Body Part

Root Operation	Objective of Procedure	Site of Procedure	Example
Reattachment (M)	Putting back a detached body part	Some/all of a body part	Reattach finger
Reposition (S)	Moving a body part to normal or other suitable location	Some/all of a body part	Move undescended testicle
Transfer (X)	Moving a body part to function for a similar body part	Some/all of a body part	Skin pedicle transfer flap
Transplantation (Y)	Putting in a living body part from a person/animal	Some/all of a body part	Kidney transplant

Procedures That Take Out or Eliminate Solid Matter, Fluids, or Gases From a Body Part

Root Operation	Objective of Procedure	Site of Procedure	Example
Drainage (9)	Taking or letting out	Fluids and/or gases from a body part	Incision and drainage
Extirpation (C)	Taking or cutting out	Solid matter in a body part	Thrombectomy
Fragmentation (F)	Breaking into pieces	Solid matter within a body part	Lithotripsy

Procedures That Involve Only Examination of Body Parts and Regions

Root Operation	Objective of Procedure	Site of Procedure	Example
Inspection (J)	Visual/manual exploration	Some/all of a body part	Diagnostic cystoscopy Exploratory laparoscopy
Map (K)	Locating electrical impulse route/functional areas	Brain/cardiac conduction mechanism	Cardiac mapping

Procedures That Alter the Diameter/Route of a Tubular Body Part

Root Operation	Objective of Procedure	Site of Procedure	Example
Bypass (1)	Altering route of passage of contents	Tubular body part	Coronary artery bypass graft (CABG)
Dilation (7)	Expanding natural or artificially created orifice/lumen	Tubular body part	Percutaneous transluminal coronary angioplasty (PTCA)
Occlusion (L)	Completely closing natural or artificially created orifice/lumen	Tubular body part	Fallopian tube ligation
Restriction (V)	Partially closing natural or artificially created orifice/lumen	Tubular body part	Gastroesophageal fundoplication

Procedures That Always Involve Devices

Root Operation		Objective of Procedure	Site of Procedure	Example
Change (2)	DVC	Exchanging device w/out cutting/puncturing	In/on a body part	Gastrostomy tube change
Insertion (H)	DVC	Putting in nonbiological device	In/on a body part	Central line insertion
Removal (P)	DVC	Taking out device	In/on a body part	Central line removal
Replacement (R)	DVC	Putting in device that replaces a body part	Some/all of a body part	Total hip replacement
Revision (W)	DVC	Correcting a malfunctioning/displaced device	In/on a body part	Revision of pacemaker
Supplement (U)	DVC	Putting in device that reinforces or augments a body part	In/on a body part	Abdominal wall herniorrhaphy using mesh

DVC = Device involved in root operation

Procedures Involving Cutting or Separation Only

Root Operation	Objective of Procedure	Site of Procedure	Example
Division (8)	Cutting into/separating	A body part	Neurotomy
Release (N)	Freeing a body part from constraint	Around a body part	Adhesiolysis

Procedures That Define Other Repairs

Root Operation	Objective of Procedure	Site of Procedure	Example
Control (3)	Stopping/attempting to stop postprocedural or other acute bleeding	Anatomical region	Post-prostatectomy bleeding control, control subdural hemorrhage, bleeding ulcer, retroperitoneal hemorrhage
Repair (Q)	Restoring body part to its normal structure/function	Some/all of a body part	Suture laceration

Procedures That Define Other Objectives

Root Operation	Objective of Procedure	Site of Procedure	Example
Alteration (Ø)	Modifying body part for cosmetic purposes without affecting function	Some/all of a body part	Face lift
Creation (4)	Using biological or synthetic material to form a new body part that replicates the anatomic structure or function of a missing body part	Perineum, valve	Sex change/artificial vagina/penis, atrioventricular valve creation
Fusion (G)	Unification or immobilization	Joint or articular body part	Spinal fusion

Appendix D: Body Part Key

Term	ICD-10-PCS Value
Abdominal aortic plexus	Abdominal Sympathetic Nerve
Abdominal esophagus	Esophagus, Lower
Abductor hallucis muscle	Foot Muscle, Right
	Foot Muscle, Left
Accessory cephalic vein	Cephalic Vein, Right
	Cephalic Vein, Left
Accessory obturator nerve	Lumbar Plexus
Accessory phrenic nerve	Phrenic nerve
Accessory spleen	Spleen
Acetabulofemoral joint	Hip Joint, Right
	Hip Joint, Left
Achilles tendon	Lower Leg Tendon, Right
	Lower Leg Tendon, Left
Acromioclavicular ligament	Shoulder Bursa and Ligament, Right
	Shoulder Bursa and Ligament, Left
Acromion (process)	Scapula, Right
	Scapula, Left
Adductor brevis muscle	Upper Leg Muscle, Right
	Upper Leg Muscle, Left
Adductor hallucis muscle	Foot Muscle, Right
	Foot Muscle, Left
Adductor longus muscle	Upper Leg Muscle, Right
	Upper Leg Muscle, Left
Adductor magnus muscle	Upper Leg Muscle, Right
	Upper Leg Muscle, Left
Adenohypophysis	Pituitary Gland
Alar ligament of axis	Head and Neck Bursa and Ligament
Alveolar process of mandible	Mandible, Right
	Mandible, Left
Alveolar process of maxilla	Maxilla
Anal orifice	Anus
Anatomical snuffbox	Lower Arm and Wrist Muscle, Right
	Lower Arm and Wrist Muscle, Left
Angular artery	Face Artery
Angular vein	Face Vein, Right
	Face Vein, Left
Annular ligament	Elbow Bursa and Ligament, Right
	Elbow Bursa and Ligament, Left
Anorectal junction	Rectum
Ansa cervicalis	Cervical Plexus
Antebrachial fascia	Subcutaneous Tissue and Fascia, Right Lower Arm
	Subcutaneous Tissue and Fascia, Left Lower Arm
Anterior (pectoral) lymph node	Lymphatic, Right Axillary
	Lymphatic, Left Axillary
Anterior cerebral artery	Intracranial Artery
Anterior cerebral vein	Intracranial Vein
Anterior choroidal artery	Intracranial Artery
Anterior circumflex humeral artery	Axillary Artery, Right
	Axillary Artery, Left
Anterior communicating artery	Intracranial Artery

Term	ICD-10-PCS Value
Anterior cruciate ligament (ACL)	Knee Bursa and Ligament, Right
	Knee Bursa and Ligament, Left
Anterior crural nerve	Femoral Nerve
Anterior facial vein	Face Vein, Right
	Face Vein, Left
Anterior intercostal artery	Internal Mammary Artery, Right
	Internal Mammary Artery, Left
Anterior interosseous nerve	Median Nerve
Anterior lateral malleolar artery	Anterior Tibial Artery, Right
	Anterior Tibial Artery, Left
Anterior lingual gland	Minor Salivary Gland
Anterior medial malleolar artery	Anterior Tibial Artery, Right
	Anterior Tibial Artery, Left
Anterior spinal artery	Vertebral Artery, Right
	Vertebral Artery, Left
Anterior tibial recurrent artery	Anterior Tibial Artery, Right
	Anterior Tibial Artery, Left
Anterior ulnar recurrent artery	Ulnar Artery, Right
	Ulnar Artery, Left
Anterior vagal trunk	Vagus Nerve
Anterior vertebral muscle	Neck Muscle, Right
	Neck Muscle, Left
Antihelix	External Ear, Right
	External Ear, Left
	External Ear, Bilateral
Antitragus	External Ear, Right
	External Ear, Left
	External Ear, Bilateral
Antrum of Highmore	Maxillary Sinus, Right
	Maxillary Sinus, Left
Aortic annulus	Aortic Valve
Aortic arch	Thoracic Aorta, Ascending/Arch
Aortic intercostal artery	Upper Artery
Apical (subclavicular) lymph node	Lymphatic, Right Axillary
	Lymphatic, Left Axillary
Apneustic center	Pons
Aqueduct of Sylvius	Cerebral Ventricle
Aqueous humour	Anterior Chamber, Right
	Anterior Chamber, Left
Arachnoid mater, intracranial	Cerebral Meninges
Arachnoid mater, spinal	Spinal Meninges
Arcuate artery	Foot Artery, Right
	Foot Artery, Left
Areola	Nipple, Right
	Nipple, Left
Arterial canal (duct)	Pulmonary Artery, Left
Aryepiglottic fold	Larynx
Arytenoid cartilage	Larynx
Arytenoid muscle	Neck Muscle, Right
	Neck Muscle, Left
Ascending aorta	Thoracic Aorta, Ascending/Arch

Term	ICD-10-PCS Value
Ascending palatine artery	Face Artery
Ascending pharyngeal artery	External Carotid Artery, Right
	External Carotid Artery, Left
Atlantoaxial joint	Cervical Vertebral Joint
Atrioventricular node	Conduction Mechanism
Atrium dextrum cordis	Atrium, Right
Atrium pulmonale	Atrium, Left
Auditory tube	Eustachian Tube, Right
	Eustachian Tube, Left
Auerbach's (myenteric)plexus	Abdominal Sympathetic Nerve
Auricle	External Ear, Right
	External Ear, Left
	External Ear, Bilateral
Auricularis muscle	Head Muscle
Axillary fascia	Subcutaneous Tissue and Fascia, Right Upper Arm
	Subcutaneous Tissue and Fascia, Left Upper Arm
Axillary nerve	Brachial Plexus
Bartholin's (greater vestibular) gland	Vestibular Gland
Basal (internal) cerebral vein	Intracranial Vein
Basal nuclei	Basal Ganglia
Base of tongue	Pharynx
Basilar artery	Intracranial Artery
Basis pontis	Pons
Biceps brachii muscle	Upper Arm Muscle, Right
	Upper Arm Muscle, Left
Biceps femoris muscle	Upper Leg Muscle, Right
	Upper Leg Muscle, Left
Bicipital aponeurosis	Subcutaneous Tissue and Fascia, Right Lower Arm
	Subcutaneous Tissue and Fascia, Left Lower Arm
Bicuspid valve	Mitral Valve
Body of femur	Femoral Shaft, Right
	Femoral Shaft, Left
Body of fibula	Fibula, Right
	Fibula, Left
Bony labyrinth	Inner Ear, Right
	Inner Ear, Left
Bony orbit	Orbit, Right
	Orbit, Left
Bony vestibule	Inner Ear, Right
	Inner Ear, Left
Botallo's duct	Pulmonary Artery, Left
Brachial (lateral) lymph node	Lymphatic, Right Axillary
	Lymphatic, Left Axillary
Brachialis muscle	Upper Arm Muscle, Right
	Upper Arm Muscle, Left
Brachiocephalic artery	Innominate Artery
Brachiocephalic trunk	Innominate Artery
Brachiocephalic vein	Innominate Vein, Right
	Innominate Vein, Left

Term	ICD-10-PCS Value
Brachioradialis muscle	Lower Arm and Wrist Muscle, Right
	Lower Arm and Wrist Muscle, Left
Broad ligament	Uterine Supporting Structure
Bronchial artery	Upper Artery
Bronchus intermedius	Main Bronchus, Right
Buccal gland	Buccal Mucosa
Buccinator lymph node	Lymphatic, Head
Buccinator muscle	Facial Muscle
Bulbospongiosus muscle	Perineum Muscle
Bulbourethral (Cowper's) gland	Urethra
Bundle of His	Conduction Mechanism
Bundle of Kent	Conduction Mechanism
Calcaneocuboid joint	Tarsal Joint, Right
	Tarsal Joint, Left
Calcaneocuboid ligament	Foot Bursa and Ligament, Right
	Foot Bursa and Ligament, Left
Calcaneofibular ligament	Ankle Bursa and Ligament, Right
	Ankle Bursa and Ligament, Left
Calcaneus	Tarsal, Right
	Tarsal, Left
Capitate bone	Carpal, Right
	Carpal, Left
Cardia	Esophagogastric Junction
Cardiac plexus	Thoracic Sympathetic Nerve
Cardioesophageal junction	Esophagogastric Junction
Caroticotympanic artery	Internal Carotid Artery, Right
	Internal Carotid Artery, Left
Carotid glomus	Carotid Body, Right
	Carotid Body, Left
	Carotid Bodies, Bilateral
Carotid sinus	Internal Carotid Artery, Right
	Internal Carotid Artery, Left
Carotid sinus nerve	Glossopharyngeal Nerve
Carpometacarpal ligament	Hand Bursa and Ligament, Right
	Hand Bursa and Ligament, Left
Cauda equina	Lumbar Spinal Cord
Cavernous plexus	Head and Neck Sympathetic Nerve
Celiac ganglion	Abdominal Sympathetic Nerve
Celiac (solar) plexus	Abdominal Sympathetic Nerve
Celiac lymph node	Lymphatic, Aortic
Celiac trunk	Celiac Artery
Central axillary lymph node	Lymphatic, Right Axillary
	Lymphatic, Left Axillary
Cerebral aqueduct (Sylvius)	Cerebral Ventricle
Cerebrum	Brain
Cervical esophagus	Esophagus, Upper
Cervical facet joint	Cervical Vertebral Joint
	Cervical Vertebral Joints, 2 or more
Cervical ganglion	Head and Neck Sympathetic Nerve
Cervical interspinous ligament	Head and Neck Bursa and Ligament
Cervical intertransverse ligament	Head and Neck Bursa and Ligament

Term	ICD-10-PCS Value
Cervical ligamentum flavum	Head and Neck Bursa and Ligament
Cervical lymph node	Lymphatic, Right Neck
	Lymphatic, Left Neck
Cervicothoracic facet joint	Cervicothoracic Vertebral Joint
Choana	Nasopharynx
Chondroglossus muscle	Tongue, Palate, Pharynx Muscle
Chorda tympani	Facial Nerve
Choroid plexus	Cerebral Ventricle
Ciliary body	Eye, Right
	Eye, Left
Ciliary ganglion	Head and Neck Sympathetic Nerve
Circle of Willis	Intracranial Artery
Circumflex illiac artery	Femoral Artery, Right
	Femoral Artery, Left
Claustrum	Basal Ganglia
Coccygeal body	Coccygeal Glomus
Coccygeus muscle	Trunk Muscle, Right
	Trunk Muscle, Left
Cochlea	Inner Ear, Right
	Inner Ear, Left
Cochlear nerve	Acoustic Nerve
Columella	Nasal Mucosa and Soft Tissue
Common digital vein	Foot Vein, Right
	Foot Vein, Left
Common facial vein	Face Vein, Right
	Face Vein, Left
Common fibular nerve	Peroneal Nerve
Common hepatic artery	Hepatic Artery
Common iliac (subaortic) lymph node	Lymphatic, Pelvis
Common interosseous artery	Ulnar Artery, Right
	Ulnar Artery, Left
Common peroneal nerve	Peroneal Nerve
Condyloid process	Mandible, Right
	Mandible, Left
Conus arteriosus	Ventricle, Right
Conus medullaris	Lumbar Spinal Cord
Coracoacromial ligament	Shoulder Bursa and Ligament, Right
	Shoulder Bursa and Ligament, Left
Coracobrachialis muscle	Upper Arm Muscle, Right
	Upper Arm Muscle, Left
Coracoclavicular ligament	Shoulder Bursa and Ligament, Right
	Shoulder Bursa and Ligament, Left
Coracohumeral ligament	Shoulder Bursa and Ligament, Right
	Shoulder Bursa and Ligament, Left
Coracoid process	Scapula, Right
	Scapula, Left
Corniculate cartilage	Larynx
Corpus callosum	Brain
Corpus cavernosum	Penis
Corpus spongiosum	Penis
Corpus striatum	Basal Ganglia
Corrugator supercilii muscle	Facial Muscle

Term	ICD-10-PCS Value
Costocervical trunk	Subclavian Artery, Right
	Subclavian Artery, Left
Costoclavicular ligament	Shoulder Bursa and Ligament, Right
	Shoulder Bursa and Ligament, Left
Costotransverse joint	Thoracic Vertebral Joint
Costotransverse ligament	Rib(s) Bursa and Ligament
Costovertebral joint	Thoracic Vertebral Joint
Costoxiphoid ligament	Sternum Bursa and Ligament
Cowper's (bulbourethral) gland	Urethra
Cremaster muscle	Perineum Muscle
Cribriform plate	Ethmoid Bone, Right
	Ethmoid Bone, Left
Cricoid cartilage	Trachea
Cricothyroid artery	Thyroid Artery, Right
	Thyroid Artery, Left
Cricothyroid muscle	Neck Muscle, Right
	Neck Muscle, Left
Crural fascia	Subcutaneous Tissue and Fascia, Right Upper Leg
	Subcutaneous Tissue and Fascia, Left Upper Leg
Cubital lymph node	Lymphatic, Right Upper Extremity
	Lymphatic, Left Upper Extremity
Cubital nerve	Ulnar Nerve
Cuboid bone	Tarsal, Right
	Tarsal, Left
Cuboideonavicular joint	Tarsal Joint, Right
	Tarsal Joint, Left
Culmen	Cerebellum
Cuneiform cartilage	Larynx
Cuneonavicular joint	Tarsal Joint, Right
	Tarsal Joint, Left
Cuneonavicular ligament	Foot Bursa and Ligament, Right
	Foot Bursa and Ligament, Left
Cutaneous (transverse) cervical nerve	Cervical Plexus
Deep cervical fascia	Subcutaneous Tissue and Fascia, Right Neck
	Subcutaneous Tissue and Fascia, Left Neck
Deep cervical vein	Vertebral Vein, Right
	Vertebral Vein, Left
Deep circumflex iliac artery	External Iliac Artery, Right
	External Iliac Artery, Left
Deep facial vein	Face Vein, Right
	Face Vein, Left
Deep femoral artery	Femoral Artery, Right
	Femoral Artery, Left
Deep femoral (profunda femoris) vein	Femoral Vein, Right
	Femoral Vein, Left
Deep palmar arch	Hand Artery, Right
	Hand Artery, Left
Deep transverse perineal muscle	Perineum Muscle
Deferential artery	Internal Iliac Artery, Right
	Internal Iliac Artery, Left

Term	ICD-10-PCS Value
Deltoid fascia	Subcutaneous Tissue and Fascia, Right Upper Arm
	Subcutaneous Tissue and Fascia, Left Upper Arm
Deltoid ligament	Ankle Bursa and Ligament, Right
	Ankle Bursa and Ligament, Left
Deltoid muscle	Shoulder Muscle, Right
	Shoulder Muscle, Left
Deltopectoral (infraclavicular) lymph node	Lymphatic, Right Upper Extremity
	Lymphatic, Left Upper Extremity
Dens	Cervical Vertebra
Denticulate (dentate) ligament	Spinal Meninges
Depressor anguli oris muscle	Facial Muscle
Depressor labii inferioris muscle	Facial Muscle
Depressor septi nasi muscle	Facial Muscle
Depressor supercilii muscle	Facial Muscle
Dermis	Skin
Descending genicular artery	Femoral Artery, Right
	Femoral Artery, Left
Diaphragma sellae	Dura Mater
Distal humerus	Humeral Shaft, Right
	Humeral Shaft, Left
Distal humerus, involving joint	Elbow Joint, Right
	Elbow Joint, Left
Distal radioulnar joint	Wrist Joint, Right
	Wrist Joint, Left
Dorsal digital nerve	Radial Nerve
Dorsal metacarpal vein	Hand Vein, Right
	Hand Vein, Left
Dorsal metatarsal artery	Foot Artery, Right
	Foot Artery, Left
Dorsal metatarsal vein	Foot Vein, Right
	Foot Vein, Left
Dorsal scapular artery	Subclavian Artery, Right
	Subclavian Artery, Left
Dorsal scapular nerve	Brachial Plexus
Dorsal venous arch	Foot Vein, Right
	Foot Vein, Left
Dorsalis pedis artery	Anterior Tibial Artery, Right
	Anterior Tibial Artery, Left
Duct of Santorini	Pancreatic Duct, Accessory
Duct of Wirsung	Pancreatic Duct
Ductus deferens	Vas Deferens, Right
	Vas Deferens, Left
	Vas Deferens, Bilateral
	Vas Deferens
Duodenal ampulla	Ampulla of Vater
Duodenojejunal flexure	Jejunum
Dura mater, intracranial	Dura Mater
Dura mater, spinal	Spinal Meninges
Dural venous sinus	Intracranial Vein

Term	ICD-10-PCS Value
Earlobe	External Ear, Right
	External Ear, Left
	External Ear, Bilateral
Eighth cranial nerve	Acoustic Nerve
Ejaculatory duct	Vas Deferens, Right
	Vas Deferens, Left
	Vas Deferens, Bilateral
	Vas Deferens
Eleventh cranial nerve	Accessory Nerve
Encephalon	Brain
Ependyma	Cerebral Ventricle
Epidermis	Skin
Epidural space, spinal	Spinal Canal
Epiploic foramen	Peritoneum
Epithalamus	Thalamus
Epitroclear lymph node	Lymphatic, Right Upper Extremity
	Lymphatic, Left Upper Extremity
Erector spinae muscle	Trunk Muscle, Right
	Trunk Muscle, Left
Esophageal artery	Upper Artery
Esophageal plexus	Thoracic Sympathetic Nerve
Ethmoidal air cell	Ethmoid Sinus, Right
	Ethmoid Sinus, Left
Extensor carpi radialis muscle	Lower Arm and Wrist Muscle, Right
Extensor carpi ulnaris muscle	Lower Arm and Wrist Muscle, Left
Extensor digitorum brevis muscle	Foot Muscle, Right
	Foot Muscle, Left
Extensor digitorum longus muscle	Lower Leg Muscle, Right
	Lower Leg Muscle, Left
Extensor hallucis brevis muscle	Foot Muscle, Right
	Foot Muscle, Left
Extensor hallucis longus muscle	Lower Leg Muscle, Right
	Lower Leg Muscle, Left
External anal sphincter	Anal Sphincter
External auditory meatus	External Auditory Canal, Right
	External Auditory Canal, Left
External maxillary artery	Face Artery
External naris	Nasal Mucosa and Soft Tissue
External oblique aponeurosis	Subcutaneous Tissue and Fascia, Trunk
External oblique muscle	Abdomen Muscle, Right
	Abdomen Muscle, Left
External popliteal nerve	Peroneal Nerve
External pudendal artery	Femoral Artery, Right
	Femoral Artery, Left
External pudenal vein	Saphenous Vein, Right
	Saphenous Vein, Left
External urethral sphincter	Urethra
Extradural space, intracranial	Epidural Space, Intracranial
Extradural space, spinal	Spinal Canal
Facial artery	Face Artery
False vocal cord	Larynx
Falx cerebri	Dura Mater

Term	ICD-10-PCS Value
Fascia lata	Subcutaneous Tissue and Fascia, Right Upper Leg
	Subcutaneous Tissue and Fascia, Left Upper Leg
Femoral head	Upper Femur, Right
	Upper Femur, Left
Femoral lymph node	Lymphatic, Right Lower Extremity
	Lymphatic, Left Lower Extremity
Femoropatellar joint	Knee Joint, Right
	Knee Joint, Left
	Knee Joint, Femoral Surface, Right
	Knee Joint, Femoral Surface, Left
Femorotibial joint	Knee Joint, Right
	Knee Joint, Left
	Knee Joint, Tibial Surface, Right
	Knee Joint, Tibial Surface, Left
Fibular artery	Peroneal Artery, Right
	Peroneal Artery, Left
Fibularis brevis muscle	Lower Leg Muscle, Right
	Lower Leg Muscle, Left
Fibularis longus muscle	Lower Leg Muscle, Right
	Lower Leg Muscle, Left
Fifth cranial nerve	Trigeminal Nerve
Filum terminale	Spinal Meninges
First cranial nerve	Olfactory Nerve
First intercostal nerve	Brachial Plexus
Flexor carpi radialis muscle	Lower Arm and Wrist Muscle, Right
	Lower Arm and Wrist Muscle, Left
Flexor carpi ulnaris muscle	Lower Arm and Wrist Muscle, Right
	Lower Arm and Wrist Muscle, Left
Flexor digitorum brevis muscle	Foot Muscle, Right
	Foot Muscle, Left
Flexor digitorum longus muscle	Lower Leg Muscle, Right
	Lower Leg Muscle, Left
Flexor hallucis brevis muscle	Foot Muscle, Right
	Foot Muscle, Left
Flexor hallucis longus muscle	Lower Leg Muscle, Right
	Lower Leg Muscle, Left
Flexor pollicis longus muscle	Lower Arm and Wrist Muscle, Right
	Lower Arm and Wrist Muscle, Left
Foramen magnum	Occipital Bone
Foramen of Monro (intraventricular)	Cerebral Ventricle
Foreskin	Prepuce
Fossa of Rosenmuller	Nasopharynx
Fourth cranial nerve	Trochlear Nerve
Fourth ventricle	Cerebral Ventricle
Fovea	Retina, Right
	Retina, Left
Frenulum labii inferioris	Lower Lip
Frenulum labii superioris	Upper Lip
Frenulum linguae	Tongue
Frontal lobe	Cerebral Hemisphere
Frontal vein	Face Vein, Right
	Face Vein, Left

Term	ICD-10-PCS Value
Fundus uteri	Uterus
Galea aponeurotica	Subcutaneous Tissue and Fascia, Scalp
Ganglion impar (ganglion of Walther)	Sacral Sympathetic Nerve
Gasserian ganglion	Trigeminal Nerve
Gastric lymph node	Lymphatic, Aortic
Gastric plexus	Abdominal Sympathetic Nerve
Gastrocnemius muscle	Lower Leg Muscle, Right
	Lower Leg Muscle, Left
Gastrocolic ligament	Omentum
Gastrocolic omentum	Omentum
Gastroduodenal artery	Hepatic Artery
Gastroesophageal (GE) junction	Esophagogastric Junction
Gastrohepatic omentum	Omentum
Gastrophrenic ligament	Omentum
Gastrosplenic ligament	Omentum
Gemellus muscle	Hip Muscle, Right
	Hip Muscle, Left
Geniculate ganglion	Facial Nerve
Geniculate nucleus	Thalamus
Genioglossus muscle	Tongue, Palate, Pharynx Muscle
Genitofemoral nerve	Lumbar Plexus
Glans penis	Prepuce
Glenohumeral joint	Shoulder Joint, Right
	Shoulder Joint, Left
Glenohumeral ligament	Shoulder Bursa and Ligament, Right
	Shoulder Bursa and Ligament, Left
Glenoid fossa (of scapula)	Glenoid Cavity, Right
	Glenoid Cavity, Left
Glenoid ligament (labrum)	Shoulder Joint, Right
	Shoulder Joint, Left
Globus pallidus	Basal Ganglia
Glossoepiglottic fold	Epiglottis
Glottis	Larynx
Gluteal lymph node	Lymphatic, Pelvis
Gluteal vein	Hypogastric Vein, Right
	Hypogastric Vein, Left
Gluteus maximus muscle	Hip Muscle, Right
	Hip Muscle, Left
Gluteus medius muscle	Hip Muscle, Right
	Hip Muscle, Left
Gluteus minimus muscle	Hip Muscle, Right
	Hip Muscle, Left
Gracilis muscle	Upper Leg Muscle, Right
	Upper Leg Muscle, Left
Great auricular nerve	Cervical Plexus
Great cerebral vein	Intracranial Vein
Great(er) saphenous vein	Saphenous Vein, Right
	Saphenous Vein, Left
Greater alar cartilage	Nasal Mucosa and Soft Tissue
Greater occipital nerve	Cervical Nerve
Greater omentum	Omentum
Greater splanchnic nerve	Thoracic Sympathetic Nerve

Term	ICD-10-PCS Value
Greater superficial petrosal nerve	Facial Nerve
Greater trochanter	Upper Femur, Right
	Upper Femur, Left
Greater tuberosity	Humeral Head, Right
	Humeral Head, Left
Greater vestibular (Bartholin's) gland	Vestibular Gland
Greater wing	Sphenoid Bone
Hallux	1st Toe, Right
	1st Toe, Left
Hamate bone	Carpal, Right
	Carpal, Left
Head of fibula	Fibula, Right
	Fibula, Left
Helix	External Ear, Right
	External Ear, Left
	External Ear, Bilateral
Hepatic artery proper	Hepatic Artery
Hepatic flexure	Transverse Colon
Hepatic lymph node	Lymphatic, Aortic
Hepatic plexus	Abdominal Sympathetic Nerve
Hepatic portal vein	Portal Vein
Hepatogastric ligament	Omentum
Hepatopancreatic ampulla	Ampulla of Vater
Humeroradial joint	Elbow Joint, Right
	Elbow Joint, Left
Humeroulnar joint	Elbow Joint, Right
	Elbow Joint, Left
Humerus, distal	Humeral Shaft, Right
	Humeral Shaft, Left
Hyoglossus muscle	Tongue, Palate, Pharynx Muscle
Hyoid artery	Thyroid Artery, Right
	Thyroid Artery, Left
Hypogastric artery	Internal Iliac Artery, Right
	Internal Iliac Artery, Left
Hypopharynx	Pharynx
Hypophysis	Pituitary Gland
Hypothenar muscle	Hand Muscle, Right
	Hand Muscle, Left
Ileal artery	Superior Mesenteric Artery
Ileocolic artery	Superior Mesenteric Artery
Ileocolic vein	Colic Vein
Iliac crest	Pelvic Bone, Right
	Pelvic Bone, Left
Iliac fascia	Subcutaneous Tissue and Fascia, Right Upper Leg
	Subcutaneous Tissue and Fascia, Left Upper Leg
Iliac lymph node	Lymphatic, Pelvis
Iliacus muscle	Hip Muscle, Right
	Hip Muscle, Left
Iliofemoral ligament	Hip Bursa and Ligament, Right
	Hip Bursa and Ligament, Left
Iliohypogastric nerve	Lumbar Plexus
Ilioinguinal nerve	Lumbar Plexus

Term	ICD-10-PCS Value
Iliolumbar artery	Internal Iliac Artery, Right
	Internal Iliac Artery, Left
Iliolumbar ligament	Lower Spine Bursa and Ligament
Iliotibial tract (band)	Subcutaneous Tissue and Fascia, Right Upper Leg
	Subcutaneous Tissue and Fascia, Left Upper Leg
Ilium	Pelvic Bone, Right
	Pelvic Bone, Left
Incus	Auditory Ossicle, Right
	Auditory Ossicle, Left
Inferior cardiac nerve	Thoracic Sympathetic Nerve
Inferior cerebellar vein	Intracranial Vein
Inferior cerebral vein	Intracranial Vein
Inferior epigastric artery	External Iliac Artery, Right
	External Iliac Artery, Left
Inferior epigastric lymph node	Lymphatic, Pelvis
Inferior genicular artery	Popliteal Artery, Right
	Popliteal Artery, Left
Inferior gluteal artery	Internal Iliac Artery, Right
	Internal Iliac Artery, Left
Inferior gluteal nerve	Sacral Plexus
Inferior hypogastric plexus	Abdominal Sympathetic Nerve
Inferior labial artery	Face Artery
Inferior longitudinal muscle	Tongue, Palate, Pharynx Muscle
Inferior mesenteric ganglion	Abdominal Sympathetic Nerve
Inferior mesenteric lymph node	Lymphatic, Mesenteric
Inferior mesenteric plexus	Abdominal Sympathetic Nerve
Inferior oblique muscle	Extraocular Muscle, Right
	Extraocular Muscle, Left
Inferior pancreaticoduo-denal artery	Superior Mesenteric Artery
Inferior phrenic artery	Abdominal Aorta
Inferior rectus muscle	Extraocular Muscle, Right
	Extraocular Muscle, Left
Inferior suprarenal artery	Renal Artery, Right
	Renal Artery, Left
Inferior tarsal plate	Lower Eyelid, Right
	Lower Eyelid, Left
Inferior thyroid vein	Innominate Vein, Right
	Innominate Vein, Left
Inferior tibiofibular joint	Ankle Joint, Right
	Ankle Joint, Left
Inferior turbinate	Nasal Turbinate
Inferior ulnar collateral artery	Brachial Artery, Right
	Brachial Artery, Left
Inferior vesical artery	Internal Iliac Artery, Right
	Internal Iliac Artery, Left
Infraauricular lymph node	Lymphatic, Head
Infraclavicular (deltopectoral) lymph node	Lymphatic, Right Upper Extremity
	Lymphatic, Left Upper Extremity

Term	ICD-10-PCS Value
Infrahyoid muscle	Neck Muscle, Right
	Neck Muscle, Left
Infraparotid lymph node	Lymphatic, Head
Infraspinatus fascia	Subcutaneous Tissue and Fascia, Right Upper Arm
	Subcutaneous Tissue and Fascia, Left Upper Arm
Infraspinatus muscle	Shoulder Muscle, Right
	Shoulder Muscle, Left
Infundibulopelvic ligament	Uterine Supporting Structure
Inguinal canal	Inguinal Region, Right
	Inguinal Region, Left
	Inguinal Region, Bilateral
Inguinal triangle	Inguinal Region, Right
	Inguinal Region, Left
	Inguinal Region, Bilateral
Interatrial septum	Atrial Septum
Intercarpal joint	Carpal Joint, Right
	Carpal Joint, Left
Intercarpal ligament	Hand Bursa and Ligament, Right
	Hand Bursa and Ligament, Left
Interclavicular ligament	Shoulder Bursa and Ligament, Right
	Shoulder Bursa and Ligament, Left
Intercostal lymph node	Lymphatic, Thorax
Intercostal muscle	Thorax Muscle, Right
	Thorax Muscle, Left
Intercostal nerve	Thoracic Nerve
Intercostobrachial nerve	Thoracic Nerve
Intercuneiform joint	Tarsal Joint, Right
	Tarsal Joint, Left
Intercuneiform ligament	Foot Bursa and Ligament, Right
	Foot Bursa and Ligament, Left
Intermediate bronchus	Main Bronchus, Right
Intermediate cuneiform bone	Tarsal, Right
	Tarsal, Left
Internal anal sphincter	Anal Sphincter
Internal (basal) cerebral vein	Intracranial Vein
Internal carotid artery, intracranial portion	Intracranial Artery
Internal carotid plexus	Head and Neck Sympathetic Nerve
Internal iliac vein	Hypogastric Vein, Right
	Hypogastric Vein, Left
Internal maxillary artery	External Carotid Artery, Right
	External Carotid Artery, Left
Internal naris	Nasal Mucosa and Soft Tissue
Internal oblique muscle	Abdomen Muscle, Right
	Abdomen Muscle, Left
Internal pudendal artery	Internal Iliac Artery, Right
	Internal Iliac Artery, Left
Internal pudendal vein	Hypogastric Vein, Right
	Hypogastric Vein, Left

Term	ICD-10-PCS Value
Internal thoracic artery	Internal Mammary Artery, Right
	Internal Mammary Artery, Left
	Subclavian Artery, Right
	Subclavian Artery, Left
Internal urethral sphincter	Urethra
Interphalangeal (IP) joint	Finger Phalangeal Joint, Right
	Finger Phalangeal Joint, Left
	Toe Phalangeal Joint, Right
	Toe Phalangeal Joint, Left
Interphalangeal ligament	Foot Bursa and Ligament, Right
	Foot Bursa and Ligament, Left
	Hand Bursa and Ligament, Right
	Hand Bursa and Ligament, Left
Interspinalis muscle	Trunk Muscle, Right
	Trunk Muscle, Left
Interspinous ligament, cervical	Head and Neck Bursa and Ligament
Interspinous ligament, lumbar	Lower Spine Bursa and Ligament
Interspinous ligament, thoracic	Upper Spine Bursa and Ligament
Intertransversarius muscle	Trunk Muscle, Right
	Trunk Muscle, Left
Intertransverse ligament, cervical	Head and Neck Bursa and Ligament
Intertransverse ligament, lumbar	Lower Spine Bursa and Ligament
Intertransverse ligament, thoracic	Upper Spine Bursa and Ligament
Interventricular foramen (Monro)	Cerebral Ventricle
Interventricular septum	Ventricular Septum
Intestinal lymphatic trunk	Cisterna Chyli
Ischiatic nerve	Sciatic Nerve
Ischiocavernosus muscle	Perineum Muscle
Ischiofemoral ligament	Hip Bursa and Ligament, Right
	Hip Bursa and Ligament, Left
Ischium	Pelvic Bone, Right
	Pelvic Bone, Left
Jejunal artery	Superior Mesenteric Artery
Jugular body	Glomus Jugulare
Jugular lymph node	Lymphatic, Right Neck
	Lymphatic, Left Neck
Labia majora	Vulva
Labia minora	Vulva
Labial gland	Upper Lip
	Lower Lip
Lacrimal canaliculus	Lacrimal Duct, Right
	Lacrimal Duct, Left
Lacrimal punctum	Lacrimal Duct, Right
	Lacrimal Duct, Left
Lacrimal sac	Lacrimal Duct, Right
	Lacrimal Duct, Left
Laryngopharynx	Pharynx
Lateral (brachial) lymph node	Lymphatic, Right Axillary
	Lymphatic, Left Axillary

Term	ICD-10-PCS Value
Lateral canthus	Upper Eyelid, Right
	Upper Eyelid, Left
Lateral collateral ligament (LCL)	Knee Bursa and Ligament, Right
	Knee Bursa and Ligament, Left
Lateral condyle of femur	Lower Femur, Right
	Lower Femur, Left
Lateral condyle of tibia	Tibia, Right
	Tibia, Left
Lateral cuneiform bone	Tarsal, Right
	Tarsal, Left
Lateral epicondyle of femur	Lower Femur, Right
	Lower Femur, Left
Lateral epicondyle of humerus	Humeral Shaft, Right
	Humeral Shaft, Left
Lateral femoral cutaneous nerve	Lumbar Plexus
Lateral malleolus	Fibula, Right
	Fibula, Left
Lateral meniscus	Knee Joint, Right
	Knee Joint, Left
Lateral nasal cartilage	Nasal Mucosa and Soft Tissue
Lateral plantar artery	Foot Artery, Right
	Foot Artery, Left
Lateral plantar nerve	Tibial Nerve
Lateral rectus muscle	Extraocular Muscle, Right
	Extraocular Muscle, Left
Lateral sacral artery	Internal Iliac Artery, Right
	Internal Iliac Artery, Left
Lateral sacral vein	Hypogastric Vein, Right
	Hypogastric Vein, Left
Lateral sural cutaneous nerve	Peroneal Nerve
Lateral tarsal artery	Foot Artery, Right
	Foot Artery, Left
Lateral temporo-mandibular ligament	Head and Neck Bursa and Ligament
Lateral thoracic artery	Axillary Artery, Right
	Axillary Artery, Left
Latissimus dorsi muscle	Trunk Muscle, Right
	Trunk Muscle, Left
Least splanchnic nerve	Thoracic Sympathetic Nerve
Left ascending lumbar vein	Hemiazygos Vein
Left atrioventricular valve	Mitral Valve
Left auricular appendix	Atrium, Left
Left colic vein	Colic Vein
Left coronary sulcus	Heart, Left
Left gastric artery	Gastric Artery
Left gastroepiploic artery	Splenic Artery
Left gastroepiploic vein	Splenic Vein
Left inferior phrenic vein	Renal Vein, Left
Left inferior pulmonary vein	Pulmonary Vein, Left
Left jugular trunk	Thoracic Duct
Left lateral ventricle	Cerebral Ventricle
Left ovarian vein	Renal Vein, Left
Left second lumbar vein	Renal Vein, Left

Term	ICD-10-PCS Value
Left subclavian trunk	Thoracic Duct
Left subcostal vein	Hemiazygos Vein
Left superior pulmonary vein	Pulmonary Vein, Left
Left suprarenal vein	Renal Vein, Left
Left testicular vein	Renal Vein, Left
Leptomeninges, intracranial	Cerebral Meninges
Leptomeninges, spinal	Spinal Meninges
Lesser alar cartilage	Nasal Mucosa and Soft Tissue
Lesser occipital nerve	Cervical Plexus
Lesser omentum	Omentum
Lesser saphenous vein	Saphenous Vein, Right
	Saphenous Vein, Left
Lesser splanchnic nerve	Thoracic Sympathetic Nerve
Lesser trochanter	Upper Femur, Right
	Upper Femur, Left
Lesser tuberosity	Humeral Head, Right
	Humeral Head, Left
Lesser wing	Sphenoid Bone
Levator anguli oris muscle	Facial Muscle
Levator ani muscle	Perineum Muscle
Levator labii superioris alaeque nasi muscle	Facial Muscle
Levator labii superioris muscle	Facial Muscle
Levator palpebrae superioris muscle	Upper Eyelid, Right
	Upper Eyelid, Left
Levator scapulae muscle	Neck Muscle, Right
	Neck Muscle, Left
Levator veli palatini muscle	Tongue, Palate, Pharynx Muscle
Levatores costarum muscle	Thorax Muscle, Right
	Thorax Muscle, Left
Ligament of head of fibula	Knee Bursa and Ligament, Right
	Knee Bursa and Ligament, Left
Ligament of the lateral malleolus	Ankle Bursa and Ligament, Right
	Ankle Bursa and Ligament, Left
Ligamentum flavum, cervical	Head and Neck Bursa and Ligament
Ligamentum flavum, lumbar	Lower Spine Bursa and Ligament
Ligamentum flavum, thoracic	Upper Spine Bursa and Ligament
Lingual artery	External Carotid Artery, Right
	External Carotid Artery, Left
Lingual tonsil	Pharynx
Locus ceruleus	Pons
Long thoracic nerve	Brachial Plexus
Lumbar artery	Abdominal Aorta
Lumbar facet joint	Lumbar Vertebral Joint
Lumbar ganglion	Lumbar Sympathetic Nerve
Lumbar lymph node	Lymphatic, Aortic
Lumbar lymphatic trunk	Cisterna Chyli
Lumbar splanchnic nerve	Lumbar Sympathetic Nerve
Lumbosacral facet joint	Lumbosacral Joint
Lumbosacral trunk	Lumbar Nerve

Term	ICD-10-PCS Value
Lunate bone	Carpal, Right
	Carpal, Left
Lunotriquetral ligament	Hand Bursa and Ligament, Right
	Hand Bursa and Ligament, Left
Macula	Retina, Right
	Retina, Left
Malleus	Auditory Ossicle, Right
	Auditory Ossicle, Left
Mammary duct	Breast, Right
	Breast, Left
	Breast, Bilateral
Mammary gland	Breast, Right
	Breast, Left
	Breast, Bilateral
Mammillary body	Hypothalamus
Mandibular nerve	Trigeminal Nerve
Mandibular notch	Mandible, Right
	Mandible, Left
Manubrium	Sternum
Masseter muscle	Head Muscle
Masseteric fascia	Subcutaneous Tissue and Fascia, Face
Mastoid (postauricular) lymph node	Lymphatic, Right Neck
	Lymphatic, Left Neck
Mastoid air cells	Mastoid Sinus, Right
	Mastoid Sinus, Left
Mastoid process	Temporal Bone, Right
	Temporal Bone, Left
Maxillary artery	External Carotid Artery, Right
	External Carotid Artery, Left
Maxillary nerve	Trigeminal Nerve
Medial canthus	Lower Eyelid, Right
	Lower Eyelid, Left
Medial collateral ligament (MCL)	Knee Bursa and Ligament, Right
	Knee Bursa and Ligament, Left
Medial condyle of femur	Lower Femur, Right
	Lower Femur, Left
Medial condyle of tibia	Tibia, Right
	Tibia, Left
Medial cuneiform bone	Tarsal, Right
	Tarsal, Left
Medial epicondyle of femur	Lower Femur, Right
	Lower Femur, Left
Medial epicondyle of humerus	Humeral Shaft, Right
	Humeral Shaft, Left
Medial malleolus	Tibia, Right
	Tibia, Left
Medial meniscus	Knee Joint, Right
	Knee Joint, Left
Medial plantar artery	Foot Artery, Right
	Foot Artery, Left
Medial plantar nerve	Tibial Nerve
Medial popliteal nerve	Tibial Nerve
Medial rectus muscle	Extraocular Muscle, Right
	Extraocular Muscle, Left

Term	ICD-10-PCS Value
Medial sural cutaneous nerve	Tibial Nerve
Median antebrachial vein	Basilic Vein, Right
	Basilic Vein, Left
Median cubital vein	Basilic Vein, Right
	Basilic Vein, Left
Median sacral artery	Abdominal Aorta
Mediastinal cavity	Mediastinum
Mediastinal lymph node	Lymphatic, Thorax
Mediastinal space	Mediastinum
Meissner's (submucous) plexus	Abdominal Sympathetic Nerve
Membranous urethra	Urethra
Mental foramen	Mandible, Right
	Mandible, Left
Mentalis muscle	Facial Muscle
Mesoappendix	Mesentery
Mesocolon	Mesentery
Metacarpal ligament	Hand Bursa and Ligament, Right
	Hand Bursa and Ligament, Left
Metacarpophalangeal ligament	Hand Bursa and Ligament, Right
	Hand Bursa and Ligament, Left
Metatarsal ligament	Foot Bursa and Ligament, Right
	Foot Bursa and Ligament, Left
Metatarsophalangeal ligament	Foot Bursa and Ligament, Right
	Foot Bursa and Ligament, Left
Metatarsophalangeal (MTP) joint	Metatarsal-Phalangeal Joint, Right
	Metatarsal-Phalangeal Joint, Left
Metathalamus	Thalamus
Midcarpal joint	Carpal Joint, Right
	Carpal Joint, Left
Middle cardiac nerve	Thoracic Sympathetic Nerve
Middle cerebral artery	Intracranial Artery
Middle cerebral vein	Intracranial Vein
Middle colic vein	Colic Vein
Middle genicular artery	Popliteal Artery, Right
	Popliteal Artery, Left
Middle hemorrhoidal vein	Hypogastric Vein, Right
	Hypogastric Vein, Left
Middle rectal artery	Internal Iliac Artery, Right
	Internal Iliac Artery, Left
Middle suprarenal artery	Abdominal Aorta
Middle temporal artery	Temporal Artery, Right
	Temporal Artery, Left
Middle turbinate	Nasal Turbinate
Mitral annulus	Mitral Valve
Molar gland	Buccal Mucosa
Musculocutaneous nerve	Brachial Plexus
Musculophrenic artery	Internal Mammary Artery, Right
	Internal Mammary Artery, Left
Musculospiral nerve	Radial Nerve
Myelencephalon	Medulla Oblongata
Myenteric (Auerbach's) plexus	Abdominal Sympathetic Nerve
Myometrium	Uterus

Term	ICD-10-PCS Value
Nail bed	Finger Nail
	Toe Nail
Nail plate	Finger Nail
	Toe Nail
Nasal cavity	Nasal Mucosa and Soft Tissue
Nasal concha	Nasal Turbinate
Nasalis muscle	Facial Muscle
Nasolacrimal duct	Lacrimal Duct, Right
	Lacrimal Duct, Left
Navicular bone	Tarsal, Right
	Tarsal, Left
Neck of femur	Upper Femur, Right
	Upper Femur, Left
Neck of humerus (anatomical) (surgical)	Humeral Head, Right
	Humeral Head, Left
Nerve to the stapedius	Facial Nerve
Neurohypophysis	Pituitary Gland
Ninth cranial nerve	Glossopharyngeal Nerve
Nostril	Nasal Mucosa and Soft Tissue
Obturator artery	Internal Iliac Artery, Right
	Internal Iliac Artery, Left
Obturator lymph node	Lymphatic, Pelvis
Obturator muscle	Hip Muscle, Right
	Hip Muscle, Left
Obturator nerve	Lumbar Plexus
Obturator vein	Hypogastric Vein, Right
	Hypogastric Vein, Left
Obtuse margin	Heart, Left
Occipital artery	External Carotid Artery, Right
	External Carotid Artery, Left
Occipital lobe	Cerebral Hemisphere
Occipital lymph node	Lymphatic, Right Neck
	Lymphatic, Left Neck
Occipitofrontalis muscle	Facial Muscle
Odontoid process	Cervical Vertebra
Olecranon bursa	Elbow Bursa and Ligament, Right
	Elbow Bursa and Ligament, Left
Olecranon process	Ulna, Right
	Ulna, Left
Olfactory bulb	Olfactory Nerve
Ophthalmic artery	Intracranial Artery
Ophthalmic nerve	Trigeminal Nerve
Ophthalmic vein	Intracranial Vein
Optic chiasma	Optic Nerve
Optic disc	Retina, Right
	Retina, Left
Optic foramen	Sphenoid Bone
Orbicularis oculi muscle	Upper Eyelid, Right
	Upper Eyelid, Left
Orbicularis oris muscle	Facial Muscle
Orbital fascia	Subcutaneous Tissue and Fascia, Face
Orbital portion of ethmoid bone	Orbit, Right
	Orbit, Left

Term	ICD-10-PCS Value
Orbital portion of frontal bone	Orbit, Right
	Orbit, Left
Orbital portion of lacrimal bone	Orbit, Right
	Orbit, Left
Orbital portion of maxilla	Orbit, Right
	Orbit, Left
Orbital portion of palatine bone	Orbit, Right
	Orbit, Left
Orbital portion of sphenoid bone	Orbit, Right
	Orbit, Left
Orbital portion of zygomatic bone	Orbit, Right
	Orbit, Left
Oropharynx	Pharynx
Otic ganglion	Head and Neck Sympathetic Nerve
Oval window	Middle Ear, Right
	Middle Ear, Left
Ovarian artery	Abdominal Aorta
Ovarian ligament	Uterine Supporting Structure
Oviduct	Fallopian Tube, Right
	Fallopian Tube, Left
Palatine gland	Buccal Mucosa
Palatine tonsil	Tonsils
Palatine uvula	Uvula
Palatoglossal muscle	Tongue, Palate, Pharynx Muscle
Palatopharyngeal muscle	Tongue, Palate, Pharynx Muscle
Palmar (volar) digital vein	Hand Vein, Right
	Hand Vein, Left
Palmar (volar) metacarpal vein	Hand Vein, Right
	Hand Vein, Left
Palmar cutaneous nerve	Median Nerve
	Radial Nerve
Palmar fascia (aponeurosis)	Subcutaneous Tissue and Fascia, Right Hand
	Subcutaneous Tissue and Fascia, Left Hand
Palmar interosseous muscle	Hand Muscle, Right
	Hand Muscle, Left
Palmar ulnocarpal ligament	Wrist Bursa and Ligament, Right
	Wrist Bursa and Ligament, Left
Palmaris longus muscle	Lower Arm and Wrist Muscle, Right
	Lower Arm and Wrist Muscle, Left
Pancreatic artery	Splenic Artery
Pancreatic plexus	Abdominal Sympathetic Nerve
Pancreatic vein	Splenic Vein
Pancreaticosplenic lymph node	Lymphatic, Aortic
Paraaortic lymph node	Lymphatic, Aortic
Pararectal lymph node	Lymphatic, Mesenteric
Parasternal lymph node	Lymphatic, Thorax
Paratracheal lymph node	Lymphatic, Thorax
Paraurethral (Skene's) gland	Vestibular Gland
Parietal lobe	Cerebral Hemisphere
Parotid lymph node	Lymphatic, Head
Parotid plexus	Facial Nerve

Term	ICD-10-PCS Value
Pars flaccida	Tympanic Membrane, Right
	Tympanic Membrane, Left
Patellar ligament	Knee Bursa and Ligament, Right
	Knee Bursa and Ligament, Left
Patellar tendon	Knee Tendon, Right
	Knee Tendon, Left
Patellofemoral joint	Knee Joint, Right
	Knee Joint, Left
	Knee Joint, Femoral Surface, Right
	Knee Joint, Femoral Surface, Left
Pectineus muscle	Upper Leg Muscle, Right
	Upper Leg Muscle, Left
Pectoral (anterior) lymph node	Lymphatic, Right Axillary
	Lymphatic, Left Axillary
Pectoral fascia	Subcutaneous Tissue and Fascia, Chest
Pectoralis major muscle	Thorax Muscle, Right
	Thorax Muscle, Left
Pectoralis minor muscle	Thorax Muscle, Right
	Thorax Muscle, Left
Pelvic splanchnic nerve	Abdominal Sympathetic Nerve
	Sacral Sympathetic Nerve
Penile urethra	Urethra
Pericardiophrenic artery	Internal Mammary Artery, Right
	Internal Mammary Artery, Left
Perimetrium	Uterus
Peroneus brevis muscle	Lower Leg Muscle, Right
	Lower Leg Muscle, Left
Peroneus longus muscle	Lower Leg Muscle, Right
	Lower Leg Muscle, Left
Petrous part of temporal bone	Temporal Bone, Right
	Temporal Bone, Left
Pharyngeal constrictor muscle	Tongue, Palate, Pharynx Muscle
Pharyngeal plexus	Vagus Nerve
Pharyngeal recess	Nasopharynx
Pharyngeal tonsil	Adenoids
Pharyngotympanic tube	Eustachian Tube, Right
	Eustachian Tube, Left
Pia mater, intracranial	Cerebral Meninges
Pia mater, spinal	Spinal Meninges
Pinna	External Ear, Right
	External Ear, Left
	External Ear, Bilateral
Piriform recess (sinus)	Pharynx
Piriformis muscle	Hip Muscle, Right
	Hip Muscle, Left
Pisiform bone	Carpal, Right
	Carpal, Left
Pisohamate ligament	Hand Bursa and Ligament, Right
	Hand Bursa and Ligament, Left
Pisometacarpal ligament	Hand Bursa and Ligament, Right
	Hand Bursa and Ligament, Left
Plantar digital vein	Foot Vein, Right
	Foot Vein, Left

Term	ICD-10-PCS Value
Plantar fascia (aponeurosis)	Subcutaneous Tissue and Fascia, Right Foot
	Subcutaneous Tissue and Fascia, Left Foot
Plantar metatarsal vein	Foot Vein, Right
	Foot Vein, Left
Plantar venous arch	Foot Vein, Right
	Foot Vein, Left
Platysma muscle	Neck Muscle, Right
	Neck Muscle, Left
Plica semilunaris	Conjunctiva, Right
	Conjunctiva, Left
Pneumogastric nerve	Vagus Nerve
Pneumotaxic center	Pons
Pontine tegmentum	Pons
Popliteal ligament	Knee Bursa and Ligament, Right
	Knee Bursa and Ligament, Left
Popliteal lymph node	Lymphatic, Left Lower Extremity
	Lymphatic, Right Lower Extremity
Popliteal vein	Femoral Vein, Right
	Femoral Vein, Left
Popliteus muscle	Lower Leg Muscle, Right
	Lower Leg Muscle, Left
Postauricular (mastoid) lymph node	Lymphatic, Right Neck
	Lymphatic, Left Neck
Postcava	Inferior Vena Cava
Posterior (subscapular) lymph node	Lymphatic, Right Axillary
	Lymphatic, Left Axillary
Posterior auricular artery	External Carotid Artery, Right
	External Carotid Artery, Left
Posterior auricular nerve	Facial Nerve
Posterior auricular vein	External Jugular Vein, Right
	External Jugular Vein, Left
Posterior cerebral artery	Intracranial Artery
Posterior chamber	Eye, Right
	Eye, Left
Posterior circumflex humeral artery	Axillary Artery, Right
	Axillary Artery, Left
Posterior communicating artery	Intracranial Artery
Posterior cruciate ligament (PCL)	Knee Bursa and Ligament, Right
	Knee Bursa and Ligament, Left
Posterior facial (retromandibular) vein	Face Vein, Right
	Face Vein, Left
Posterior femoral cutaneous nerve	Sacral Plexus
Posterior inferior cerebellar artery (PICA)	Intracranial Artery
Posterior interosseous nerve	Radial Nerve
Posterior labial nerve	Pudendal Nerve
Posterior scrotal nerve	Pudendal Nerve
Posterior spinal artery	Vertebral Artery, Right
	Vertebral Artery, Left
Posterior tibial recurrent artery	Anterior Tibial Artery, Right
	Anterior Tibial Artery, Left
Posterior ulnar recurrent artery	Ulnar Artery, Right
	Ulnar Artery, Left

Term	ICD-10-PCS Value
Posterior vagal trunk	Vagus Nerve
Preauricular lymph node	Lymphatic, Head
Precava	Superior Vena Cava
Prepatellar bursa	Knee Bursa and Ligament, Right
	Knee Bursa and Ligament, Left
Pretracheal fascia	Subcutaneous Tissue and Fascia, Right Neck
	Subcutaneous Tissue and Fascia, Left Neck
Prevertebral fascia	Subcutaneous Tissue and Fascia, Right Neck
	Subcutaneous Tissue and Fascia, Left Neck
Princeps pollicis artery	Hand Artery, Right
	Hand Artery, Left
Procerus muscle	Facial Muscle
Profunda brachii	Brachial Artery, Right
	Brachial Artery, Left
Profunda femoris (deep femoral) vein	Femoral Vein, Right
	Femoral Vein, Left
Pronator quadratus muscle	Lower Arm and Wrist Muscle, Right
	Lower Arm and Wrist Muscle, Left
Pronator teres muscle	Lower Arm and Wrist Muscle, Right
	Lower Arm and Wrist Muscle, Left
Prostatic urethra	Urethra
Proximal radioulnar joint	Elbow Joint, Right
	Elbow Joint, Left
Psoas muscle	Hip Muscle, Right
	Hip Muscle, Left
Pterygoid muscle	Head Muscle
Pterygoid process	Sphenoid Bone
Pterygopalatine (sphenopalatine) ganglion	Head and Neck Sympathetic Nerve
Pubis	Pelvic Bone, Right
	Pelvic Bone, Left
Pubofemoral ligament	Hip Bursa and Ligament, Right
	Hip Bursa and Ligament, Left
Pudendal nerve	Sacral Plexus
Pulmoaortic canal	Pulmonary Artery, Left
Pulmonary annulus	Pulmonary Valve
Pulmonary plexus	Thoracic Sympathetic Nerve
	Vagus Nerve
Pulmonic valve	Pulmonary Valve
Pulvinar	Thalamus
Pyloric antrum	Stomach, Pylorus
Pyloric canal	Stomach, Pylorus
Pyloric sphincter	Stomach, Pylorus
Pyramidalis muscle	Abdomen Muscle, Right
	Abdomen Muscle, Left
Quadrangular cartilage	Nasal Septum
Quadrate lobe	Liver
Quadratus femoris muscle	Hip Muscle, Right
	Hip Muscle, Left
Quadratus lumborum muscle	Trunk Muscle, Right
	Trunk Muscle, Left
Quadratus plantae muscle	Foot Muscle, Right
	Foot Muscle, Left

Term	ICD-10-PCS Value
Quadriceps (femoris)	Upper Leg Muscle, Right
	Upper Leg Muscle, Left
Radial collateral carpal ligament	Wrist Bursa and Ligament, Right
	Wrist Bursa and Ligament, Left
Radial collateral ligament	Elbow Bursa and Ligament, Right
	Elbow Bursa and Ligament, Left
Radial notch	Ulna, Right
	Ulna, Left
Radial recurrent artery	Radial Artery, Right
	Radial Artery, Left
Radial vein	Brachial Vein, Right
	Brachial Vein, Left
Radialis indicis	Hand Artery, Right
	Hand Artery, Left
Radiocarpal joint	Wrist Joint, Right
	Wrist Joint, Left
Radiocarpal ligament	Wrist Bursa and Ligament, Right
	Wrist Bursa and Ligament, Left
Radioulnar ligament	Wrist Bursa and Ligament, Right
	Wrist Bursa and Ligament, Left
Rectosigmoid junction	Sigmoid Colon
Rectus abdominis muscle	Abdomen Muscle, Right
	Abdomen Muscle, Left
Rectus femoris muscle	Upper Leg Muscle, Right
	Upper Leg Muscle, Left
Recurrent laryngeal nerve	Vagus Nerve
Renal calyx	Kidney, Right
	Kidney, Left
	Kidneys, Bilateral
	Kidney
Renal capsule	Kidney, Right
	Kidney, Left
	Kidneys, Bilateral
	Kidney
Renal cortex	Kidney, Right
	Kidney, Left
	Kidneys, Bilateral
	Kidney
Renal plexus	Abdominal Sympathetic Nerve
Renal segment	Kidney, Right
	Kidney, Left
	Kidneys, Bilateral
	Kidney
Renal segmental artery	Renal Artery, Right
	Renal Artery, Left
Retroperitoneal cavity	Retroperitoneum
Retroperitoneal lymph node	Lymphatic, Aortic
Retroperitoneal space	Retroperitoneum
Retropharyngeal lymph node	Lymphatic, Right Neck
	Lymphatic, Left Neck
Retropubic space	Pelvic Cavity
Rhinopharynx	Nasopharynx
Rhomboid major muscle	Trunk Muscle, Right
	Trunk Muscle, Left

Term	ICD-10-PCS Value
Rhomboid minor muscle	Trunk Muscle, Right
	Trunk Muscle, Left
Right ascending lumbar vein	Azygos Vein
Right atrioventricular valve	Tricuspid Valve
Right auricular appendix	Atrium, Right
Right colic vein	Colic Vein
Right coronary sulcus	Heart, Right
Right gastric artery	Gastric Artery
Right gastroepiploic vein	Superior Mesenteric Vein
Right inferior phrenic vein	Inferior Vena Cava
Right inferior pulmonary vein	Pulmonary Vein, Right
Right jugular trunk	Lymphatic, Right Neck
Right lateral ventricle	Cerebral Ventricle
Right lymphatic duct	Lymphatic, Right Neck
Right ovarian vein	Inferior Vena Cava
Right second lumbar vein	Inferior Vena Cava
Right subclavian trunk	Lymphatic, Right Neck
Right subcostal vein	Azygos Vein
Right superior pulmonary vein	Pulmonary Vein, Right
Right suprarenal vein	Inferior Vena Cava
Right testicular vein	Inferior Vena Cava
Rima glottidis	Larynx
Risorius muscle	Facial Muscle
Round ligament of uterus	Uterine Supporting Structure
Round window	Inner Ear, Right
	Inner Ear, Left
Sacral ganglion	Sacral Sympathetic Nerve
Sacral lymph node	Lymphatic, Pelvis
Sacral splanchnic nerve	Sacral Sympathetic Nerve
Sacrococcygeal ligament	Lower Spine Bursa and Ligament
Sacrococcygeal symphysis	Sacrococcygeal Joint
Sacroiliac ligament	Lower Spine Bursa and Ligament
Sacrospinous ligament	Lower Spine Bursa and Ligament
Sacrotuberous ligament	Lower Spine Bursa and Ligament
Salpingopharyngeus muscle	Tongue, Palate, Pharynx Muscle
Salpinx	Fallopian Tube, Right
	Fallopian Tube, Left
Saphenous nerve	Femoral Nerve
Sartorius muscle	Upper Leg Muscle, Right
	Upper Leg Muscle, Left
Scalene muscle	Neck Muscle, Right
	Neck Muscle, Left
Scaphoid bone	Carpal, Right
	Carpal, Left
Scapholunate ligament	Hand Bursa and Ligament, Right
	Hand Bursa and Ligament, Left
Scaphotrapezium ligament	Hand Bursa and Ligament, Right
	Hand Bursa and Ligament, Left
Scarpa's (vestibular) ganglion	Acoustic Nerve
Sebaceous gland	Skin

Term	ICD-10-PCS Value
Second cranial nerve	Optic Nerve
Sella turcica	Sphenoid Bone
Semicircular canal	Inner Ear, Right
	Inner Ear, Left
Semimembranosus muscle	Upper Leg Muscle, Right
	Upper Leg Muscle, Left
Semitendinosus muscle	Upper Leg Muscle, Right
	Upper Leg Muscle, Left
Septal cartilage	Nasal Septum
Serratus anterior muscle	Thorax Muscle, Right
	Thorax Muscle, Left
Serratus posterior muscle	Trunk Muscle, Right
	Trunk Muscle, Left
Seventh cranial nerve	Facial Nerve
Short gastric artery	Splenic Artery
Sigmoid artery	Inferior Mesenteric Artery
Sigmoid flexure	Sigmoid Colon
Sigmoid vein	Inferior Mesenteric Vein
Sinoatrial node	Conduction Mechanism
Sinus venosus	Atrium, Right
Sixth cranial nerve	Abducens Nerve
Skene's (paraurethral) gland	Vestibular Gland
Small saphenous vein	Saphenous Vein, Right
	Saphenous Vein, Left
Solar (celiac) plexus	Abdominal Sympathetic Nerve
Soleus muscle	Lower Leg Muscle, Right
	Lower Leg Muscle, Left
Sphenomandibular ligament	Head and Neck Bursa and Ligament
Sphenopalatine (pterygopalatine) ganglion	Head and Neck Sympathetic Nerve
Spinal nerve, cervical	Cervical Nerve
Spinal nerve, lumbar	Lumbar Nerve
Spinal nerve, sacral	Sacral Nerve
Spinal nerve, thoracic	Thoracic Nerve
Spinous process	Cervical Vertebra
	Lumbar Vertebra
	Thoracic Vertebra
Spiral ganglion	Acoustic Nerve
Splenic flexure	Transverse Colon
Splenic plexus	Abdominal Sympathetic Nerve
Splenius capitis muscle	Head Muscle
Splenius cervicis muscle	Neck Muscle, Right
	Neck Muscle, Left
Stapes	Auditory Ossicle, Right
	Auditory Ossicle, Left
Stellate ganglion	Head and Neck Sympathetic Nerve
Stensen's duct	Parotid Duct, Right
	Parotid Duct, Left
Sternoclavicular ligament	Shoulder Bursa and Ligament, Right
	Shoulder Bursa and Ligament, Left
Sternocleidomastoid artery	Thyroid Artery, Right
	Thyroid Artery, Left

Appendix D: Body Part Key

Term	ICD-10-PCS Value
Sternocleidomastoid muscle	Neck Muscle, Right
	Neck Muscle, Left
Sternocostal ligament	Sternum Bursa and Ligament
Styloglossus muscle	Tongue, Palate, Pharynx Muscle
Stylomandibular ligament	Head and Neck Bursa and Ligament
Stylopharyngeus muscle	Tongue, Palate, Pharynx Muscle
Subacromial bursa	Shoulder Bursa and Ligament, Right
	Shoulder Bursa and Ligament, Left
Subaortic (common iliac) lymph node	Lymphatic, Pelvis
Subarachnoid space, spinal	Spinal Canal
Subclavicular (apical) lymph node	Lymphatic, Right Axillary
	Lymphatic, Left Axillary
Subclavius muscle	Thorax Muscle, Right
	Thorax Muscle, Left
Subclavius nerve	Brachial Plexus
Subcostal artery	Upper Artery
Subcostal muscle	Thorax Muscle, Right
	Thorax Muscle, Left
Subcostal nerve	Thoracic Nerve
Subdural space, spinal	Spinal Canal
Submandibular ganglion	Facial Nerve
	Head and Neck Sympathetic Nerve
Submandibular gland	Submaxillary Gland, Right
	Submaxillary Gland, Left
Submandibular lymph node	Lymphatic, Head
Submaxillary ganglion	Head and Neck Sympathetic Nerve
Submaxillary lymph node	Lymphatic, Head
Submental artery	Face Artery
Submental lymph node	Lymphatic, Head
Submucous (Meissner's) plexus	Abdominal Sympathetic Nerve
Suboccipital nerve	Cervical Nerve
Suboccipital venous plexus	Vertebral Vein, Right
	Vertebral Vein, Left
Subparotid lymph node	Lymphatic, Head
Subscapular aponeurosis	Subcutaneous Tissue and Fascia, Right Upper Arm
	Subcutaneous Tissue and Fascia, Left Upper Arm
Subscapular artery	Axillary Artery, Right
	Axillary Artery, Left
Subscapular (posterior) lymph node	Lymphatic, Right Axillary
	Lymphatic, Left Axillary
Subscapularis muscle	Shoulder Muscle, Right
	Shoulder Muscle, Left
Substantia nigra	Basal Ganglia
Subtalar (talocalcaneal) joint	Tarsal Joint, Right
	Tarsal Joint, Left
Subtalar ligament	Foot Bursa and Ligament, Right
	Foot Bursa and Ligament, Left
Subthalamic nucleus	Basal Ganglia
Superficial circumflex iliac vein	Saphenous Vein, Right
	Saphenous Vein, Left

Term	ICD-10-PCS Value
Superficial epigastric artery	Femoral Artery, Right
	Femoral Artery, Left
Superficial epigastric vein	Saphenous Vein, Right
	Saphenous Vein, Left
Superficial palmar arch	Hand Artery, Right
	Hand Artery, Left
Superficial palmar venous arch	Hand Vein, Right
	Hand Vein, Left
Superficial temporal artery	Temporal Artery, Right
	Temporal Artery, Left
Superficial transverse perineal muscle	Perineum Muscle
Superior cardiac nerve	Thoracic Sympathetic Nerve
Superior cerebellar vein	Intracranial Vein
Superior cerebral vein	Intracranial Vein
Superior clunic (cluneal) nerve	Lumbar Nerve
Superior epigastric artery	Internal Mammary Artery, Right
	Internal Mammary Artery, Left
Superior genicular artery	Popliteal Artery, Right
	Popliteal Artery, Left
Superior gluteal artery	Internal Iliac Artery, Right
	Internal Iliac Artery, Left
Superior gluteal nerve	Lumbar Plexus
Superior hypogastric plexus	Abdominal Sympathetic Nerve
Superior labial artery	Face Artery
Superior laryngeal artery	Thyroid Artery, Right
	Thyroid Artery, Left
Superior laryngeal nerve	Vagus Nerve
Superior longitudinal muscle	Tongue, Palate, Pharynx Muscle
Superior mesenteric ganglion	Abdominal Sympathetic Nerve
Superior mesenteric lymph node	Lymphatic, Mesenteric
Superior mesenteric plexus	Abdominal Sympathetic Nerve
Superior oblique muscle	Extraocular Muscle, Right
	Extraocular Muscle, Left
Superior olivary nucleus	Pons
Superior rectal artery	Inferior Mesenteric Artery
Superior rectal vein	Inferior Mesenteric Vein
Superior rectus muscle	Extraocular Muscle, Right
	Extraocular Muscle, Left
Superior tarsal plate	Upper Eyelid, Right
	Upper Eyelid, Left
Superior thoracic artery	Axillary Artery, Right
	Axillary Artery, Left
Superior thyroid artery	External Carotid Artery, Right
	External Carotid Artery, Left
	Thyroid Artery, Right
	Thyroid Artery, Left
Superior turbinate	Nasal Turbinate
Superior ulnar collateral artery	Brachial Artery, Right
	Brachial Artery, Left
Supraclavicular nerve	Cervical Plexus

Term	ICD-10-PCS Value
Supraclavicular (Virchow's) lymph node	Lymphatic, Right Neck
	Lymphatic, Left Neck
Suprahyoid lymph node	Lymphatic, Head
Suprahyoid muscle	Neck Muscle, Right
	Neck Muscle, Left
Suprainguinal lymph node	Lymphatic, Pelvis
Supraorbital vein	Face Vein, Right
	Face Vein, Left
Suprarenal gland	Adrenal Gland, Right
	Adrenal Gland, Left
	Adrenal Glands, Bilateral
	Adrenal Gland
Suprarenal plexus	Abdominal Sympathetic Nerve
Suprascapular nerve	Brachial Plexus
Supraspinatus fascia	Subcutaneous Tissue and Fascia, Right Upper Arm
	Subcutaneous Tissue and Fascia, Left Upper Arm
Supraspinatus muscle	Shoulder Muscle, Right
	Shoulder Muscle, Left
Supraspinous ligament	Upper Spine Bursa and Ligament
	Lower Spine Bursa and Ligament
Suprasternal notch	Sternum
Supratrochlear lymph node	Lymphatic, Right Upper Extremity
	Lymphatic, Left Upper Extremity
Sural artery	Popliteal Artery, Right
	Popliteal Artery, Left
Sweat gland	Skin
Talocalcaneal ligament	Foot Bursa and Ligament, Right
	Foot Bursa and Ligament, Left
Talocalcaneal (subtalar) joint	Tarsal Joint, Right
	Tarsal Joint, Left
Talocalcaneonavicular joint	Tarsal Joint, Right
	Tarsal Joint, Left
Talocalcaneonavicular ligament	Foot Bursa and Ligament, Right
	Foot Bursa and Ligament, Left
Talocrural joint	Ankle Joint, Right
	Ankle Joint, Left
Talofibular ligament	Ankle Bursa and Ligament, Right
	Ankle Bursa and Ligament, Left
Talus bone	Tarsal, Right
	Tarsal, Left
Tarsometatarsal ligament	Foot Bursa and Ligament, Right
	Foot Bursa and Ligament, Left
Temporal lobe	Cerebral Hemisphere
Temporalis muscle	Head Muscle
Temporoparietalis muscle	Head Muscle
Tensor fasciae latae muscle	Hip Muscle, Right
	Hip Muscle, Left
Tensor veli palatini muscle	Tongue, Palate, Pharynx Muscle
Tenth cranial nerve	Vagus Nerve
Tentorium cerebelli	Dura Mater
Teres major muscle	Shoulder Muscle, Right
	Shoulder Muscle, Left

Term	ICD-10-PCS Value
Teres minor muscle	Shoulder Muscle, Right
	Shoulder Muscle, Left
Testicular artery	Abdominal Aorta
Thenar muscle	Hand Muscle, Right
	Hand Muscle, Left
Third cranial nerve	Oculomotor Nerve
Third occipital nerve	Cervical Nerve
Third ventricle	Cerebral Ventricle
Thoracic aortic plexus	Thoracic Sympathetic Nerve
Thoracic esophagus	Esophagus, Middle
Thoracic facet joint	Thoracic Vertebral Joint
Thoracic ganglion	Thoracic Sympathetic Nerve
Thoracoacromial artery	Axillary Artery, Right
	Axillary Artery, Left
Thoracolumbar facet joint	Thoracolumbar Vertebral Joint
Thymus gland	Thymus
Thyroarytenoid muscle	Neck Muscle, Right
	Neck Muscle, Left
Thyrocervical trunk	Thyroid Artery, Right
	Thyroid Artery, Left
Thyroid cartilage	Larynx
Tibialis anterior muscle	Lower Leg Muscle, Right
	Lower Leg Muscle, Left
Tibialis posterior muscle	Lower Leg Muscle, Right
	Lower Leg Muscle, Left
Tibiofemoral joint	Knee Joint, Right
	Knee Joint, Left
	Knee Joint, Tibial Surface, Right
	Knee Joint, Tibial Surface, Left
Tongue, base of	Pharynx
Tracheobronchial lymph node	Lymphatic, Thorax
Tragus	External Ear, Right
	External Ear, Left
	External Ear, Bilateral
Transversalis fascia	Subcutaneous Tissue and Fascia, Trunk
Transverse acetabular ligament	Hip Bursa and Ligament, Right
	Hip Bursa and Ligament, Left
Transverse (cutaneous) cervical nerve	Cervical Plexus
Transverse facial artery	Temporal Artery, Right
	Temporal Artery, Left
Transverse foramen	Cervical Vertebra
Transverse humeral ligament	Shoulder Bursa and Ligament, Right
	Shoulder Bursa and Ligament, Left
Transverse ligament of atlas	Head and Neck Bursa and Ligament
Transverse process	Cervical Vertebra
	Thoracic Vertebra
	Lumbar Vertebra
Transverse scapular ligament	Shoulder Bursa and Ligament, Right
	Shoulder Bursa and Ligament, Left
Transverse thoracis muscle	Thorax Muscle, Right
	Thorax Muscle, Left

Term	ICD-10-PCS Value
Transversospinalis muscle	Trunk Muscle, Right
	Trunk Muscle, Left
Transversus abdominis muscle	Abdomen Muscle, Right
	Abdomen Muscle, Left
Trapezium bone	Carpal, Right
	Carpal, Left
Trapezius muscle	Trunk Muscle, Right
	Trunk Muscle, Left
Trapezoid bone	Carpal, Right
	Carpal, Left
Triceps brachii muscle	Upper Arm Muscle, Right
	Upper Arm Muscle, Left
Tricuspid annulus	Tricuspid Valve
Trifacial nerve	Trigeminal Nerve
Trigone of bladder	Bladder
Triquetral bone	Carpal, Right
	Carpal, Left
Trochantericbursa	Hip Bursa and Ligament, Right
	Hip Bursa and Ligament, Left
Twelfth cranial nerve	Hypoglossal Nerve
Tympanic cavity	Middle Ear, Right
	Middle Ear, Left
Tympanic nerve	Glossopharyngeal Nerve
Tympanic part of temoporal bone	Temporal Bone, Right
	Temporal Bone, Left
Ulnar collateral carpal ligament	Wrist Bursa and Ligament, Right
	Wrist Bursa and Ligament, Left
Ulnar collateral ligament	Elbow Bursa and Ligament, Right
	Elbow Bursa and Ligament, Left
Ulnar notch	Radius, Right
	Radius, Left
Ulnar vein	Brachial Vein, Right
	Brachial Vein, Left
Umbilical artery	Internal Iliac Artery, Right
	Internal Iliac Artery, Left
	Lower Artery
Ureteral orifice	Ureter, Right
	Ureter, Left
	Ureters, Bilateral
	Ureter
Ureteropelvic junction (UPJ)	Kidney Pelvis, Right
	Kidney Pelvis, Left
Ureterovesical orifice	Ureter, Right
	Ureter, Left
	Ureters, Bilateral
	Ureter
Uterine artery	Internal Iliac Artery, Right
	Internal Iliac Artery, Left
Uterine cornu	Uterus
Uterine tube	Fallopian Tube, Right
	Fallopian Tube, Left
Uterine vein	Hypogastric Vein, Right
	Hypogastric Vein, Left
Vaginal artery	Internal Iliac Artery, Right
	Internal Iliac Artery, Left

Term	ICD-10-PCS Value
Vaginal vein	Hypogastric Vein, Right
	Hypogastric Vein, Left
Vastus intermedius muscle	Upper Leg Muscle, Right
	Upper Leg Muscle, Left
Vastus lateralis muscle	Upper Leg Muscle, Right
	Upper Leg Muscle, Left
Vastus medialis muscle	Upper Leg Muscle, Right
	Upper Leg Muscle, Left
Ventricular fold	Larynx
Vermiform appendix	Appendix
Vermilion border	Upper Lip
	Lower Lip
Vertebral arch	Cervical Vertebra
	Lumbar Vertebra
	Thoracic Vertebra
Vertebral body	Cervical Vertebra
	Lumbar Vertebra
	Thoracic Vertebra
Vertebral canal	Spinal Canal
Vertebral foramen	Cervical Vertebra
	Lumbar Vertebra
	Thoracic Vertebra
Vertebral lamina	Cervical Vertebra
	Lumbar Vertebra
	Thoracic Vertebra
Vertebral pedicle	Cervical Vertebra
	Lumbar Vertebra
	Thoracic Vertebra
Vesical vein	Hypogastric Vein, Right
	Hypogastric Vein, Left
Vestibular (Scarpa's) ganglion	Acoustic Nerve
Vestibular nerve	Acoustic Nerve
Vestibulocochlear nerve	Acoustic Nerve
Virchow's (supraclavicular) lymph node	Lymphatic, Right Neck
	Lymphatic, Left Neck
Vitreous body	Vitreous, Right
	Vitreous, Left
Vocal fold	Vocal Cord, Right
	Vocal Cord, Left
Volar (palmar) digital vein	Hand Vein, Right
	Hand Vein, Left
Volar (palmar) metacarpal vein	Hand Vein, Right
	Hand Vein, Left
Vomer bone	Nasal Septum
Vomer of nasal septum	Nasal Bone
Xiphoid process	Sternum
Zonule of Zinn	Lens, Right
	Lens, Left
Zygomatic process of frontal bone	Frontal Bone
Zygomatic process of temporal bone	Temporal Bone, Right
	Temporal Bone, Left
Zygomaticus muscle	Facial Muscle

Appendix E: Body Part Definitions

ICD-10-PCS Value	Definition
1st Toe, Left 1st Toe, Right	**Includes:** Hallux
Abdomen Muscle, Left Abdomen Muscle, Right	**Includes:** External oblique muscle Internal oblique muscle Pyramidalis muscle Rectus abdominis muscle Transversus abdominis muscle
Abdominal Aorta	**Includes:** Inferior phrenic artery Lumbar artery Median sacral artery Middle suprarenal artery Ovarian artery Testicular artery
Abdominal Sympathetic Nerve	**Includes:** Abdominal aortic plexus Auerbach's (myenteric) plexus Celiac (solar) plexus Celiac ganglion Gastric plexus Hepatic plexus Inferior hypogastric plexus Inferior mesenteric ganglion Inferior mesenteric plexus Meissner's (submucous) plexus Myenteric (Auerbach's) plexus Pancreatic plexus Pelvic splanchnic nerve Renal plexus Solar (celiac) plexus Splenic plexus Submucous (Meissner's) plexus Superior hypogastric plexus Superior mesenteric ganglion Superior mesenteric plexus Suprarenal plexus
Abducens Nerve	**Includes:** Sixth cranial nerve
Accessory Nerve	**Includes:** Eleventh cranial nerve
Acoustic Nerve	**Includes:** Cochlear nerve Eighth cranial nerve Scarpa's (vestibular) ganglion Spiral ganglion Vestibular (Scarpa's) ganglion Vestibular nerve Vestibulocochlear nerve
Adenoids	**Includes:** Pharyngeal tonsil
Adrenal Gland Adrenal Gland, Left Adrenal Gland, Right Adrenal Glands, Bilateral	**Includes:** Suprarenal gland
Ampulla of Vater	**Includes:** Duodenal ampulla Hepatopancreatic ampulla
Anal Sphincter	**Includes:** External anal sphincter Internal anal sphincter

ICD-10-PCS Value	Definition
Ankle Bursa and Ligament, Left Ankle Bursa and Ligament, Right	**Includes:** Calcaneofibular ligament Deltoid ligament Ligament of the lateral malleolus Talofibular ligament
Ankle Joint, Left Ankle Joint, Right	**Includes:** Inferior tibiofibular joint Talocrural joint
Anterior Chamber, Left Anterior Chamber, Right	**Includes:** Aqueous humour
Anterior Tibial Artery, Left Anterior Tibial Artery, Right	**Includes:** Anterior lateral malleolar artery Anterior medial malleolar artery Anterior tibial recurrent artery Dorsalis pedis artery Posterior tibial recurrent artery
Anus	**Includes:** Anal orifice
Aortic Valve	**Includes:** Aortic annulus
Appendix	**Includes:** Vermiform appendix
Atrial Septum	**Includes:** Interatrial septum
Atrium, Left	**Includes:** Atrium pulmonale Left auricular appendix
Atrium, Right	**Includes:** Atrium dextrum cordis Right auricular appendix Sinus venosus
Auditory Ossicle, Left Auditory Ossicle, Right	**Includes:** Incus Malleus Stapes
Axillary Artery, Left Axillary Artery, Right	**Includes:** Anterior circumflex humeral artery Lateral thoracic artery Posterior circumflex humeral artery Subscapular artery Superior thoracic artery Thoracoacromial artery
Azygos Vein	**Includes:** Right ascending lumbar vein Right subcostal vein
Basal Ganglia	**Includes:** Basal nuclei Claustrum Corpus striatum Globus pallidus Substantia nigra Subthalamic nucleus
Basilic Vein, Left Basilic Vein, Right	**Includes:** Median antebrachial vein Median cubital vein
Bladder	**Includes:** Trigone of bladder
Brachial Artery, Left Brachial Artery, Right	**Includes:** Inferior ulnar collateral artery Profunda brachii Superior ulnar collateral artery

ICD-10-PCS Value	Definition
Brachial Plexus	**Includes:** Axillary nerve Dorsal scapular nerve First intercostal nerve Long thoracic nerve Musculocutaneous nerve Subclavius nerve Suprascapular nerve
Brachial Vein, Left **Brachial Vein, Right**	**Includes:** Radial vein Ulnar vein
Brain	**Includes:** Cerebrum Corpus callosum Encephalon
Breast, Bilateral **Breast, Left** **Breast, Right**	**Includes:** Mammary duct Mammary gland
Buccal Mucosa	**Includes:** Buccal gland Molar gland Palatine gland
Carotid Bodies, Bilateral **Carotid Body, Left** **Carotid Body, Right**	**Includes:** Carotid glomus
Carpal Joint, Left **Carpal Joint, Right**	**Includes:** Intercarpal joint Midcarpal joint
Carpal, Left **Carpal, Right**	**Includes:** Capitate bone Hamate bone Lunate bone Pisiform bone Scaphoid bone Trapezium bone Trapezoid bone Triquetral bone
Celiac Artery	**Includes:** Celiac trunk
Cephalic Vein, Left **Cephalic Vein, Right**	**Includes:** Accessory cephalic vein
Cerebellum	**Includes:** Culmen
Cerebral Hemisphere	**Includes:** Frontal lobe Occipital lobe Parietal lobe Temporal lobe
Cerebral Meninges	**Includes:** Arachnoid mater, intracranial Leptomeninges, intracranial Pia mater, intracranial
Cerebral Ventricle	**Includes:** Aqueduct of Sylvius Cerebral aqueduct (Sylvius) Choroid plexus Ependyma Foramen of Monro (intraventricular) Fourth ventricle Interventricular foramen (Monro) Left lateral ventricle Right lateral ventricle Third ventricle

ICD-10-PCS Value	Definition
Cervical Nerve	**Includes:** Greater occipital nerve Spinal nerve, cervical Suboccipital nerve Third occipital nerve
Cervical Plexus	**Includes:** Ansa cervicalis Cutaneous (transverse) cervical nerve Great auricular nerve Lesser occipital nerve Supraclavicular nerve Transverse (cutaneous) cervical nerve
Cervical Vertebra	**Includes:** Dens Odontoid process Spinous process Transverse foramen Transverse process Vertebral arch Vertebral body Vertebral foramen Vertebral lamina Vertebral pedicle
Cervical Vertebral Joint	**Includes:** Atlantoaxial joint Cervical facet joint
Cervical Vertebral Joints, **2 or more**	**Includes:** Cervical facet joint
Cervicothoracic Vertebral **Joint**	**Includes:** Cervicothoracic facet joint
Cisterna Chyli	**Includes:** Intestinal lymphatic trunk Lumbar lymphatic trunk
Coccygeal Glomus	**Includes:** Coccygeal body
Colic Vein	**Includes:** Ileocolic vein Left colic vein Middle colic vein Right colic vein
Conduction Mechanism	**Includes:** Atrioventricular node Bundle of His Bundle of Kent Sinoatrial node
Conjunctiva, Left **Conjunctiva, Right**	**Includes:** Plica semilunaris
Dura Mater	**Includes:** Diaphragma sellae Dura mater, intracranial Falx cerebri Tentorium cerebelli
Elbow Bursa and **Ligament, Left** **Elbow Bursa and** **Ligament, Right**	**Includes:** Annular ligament Olecranon bursa Radial collateral ligament Ulnar collateral ligament
Elbow Joint, Left **Elbow Joint, Right**	**Includes:** Distal humerus, involving joint Humeroradial joint Humeroulnar joint Proximal radioulnar joint
Epidural Space, **Intracranial**	**Includes:** Extradural space, intracranial

ICD-10-PCS Value	Definition
Epiglottis	**Includes:** Glossoepiglottic fold
Esophagogastric Junction	**Includes:** Cardia Cardioesophageal junction Gastroesophageal (GE) junction
Esophagus, Lower	**Includes:** Abdominal esophagus
Esophagus, Middle	**Includes:** Thoracic esophagus
Esophagus, Upper	**Includes:** Cervical esophagus
Ethmoid Bone, Left Ethmoid Bone, Right	**Includes:** Cribriform plate
Ethmoid Sinus, Left Ethmoid Sinus, Right	**Includes:** Ethmoidal air cell
Eustachian Tube, Left Eustachian Tube, Right	**Includes:** Auditory tube Pharyngotympanic tube
External Auditory Canal, Left External Auditory Canal, Right	**Includes:** External auditory meatus
External Carotid Artery, Left External Carotid Artery, Right	**Includes:** Ascending pharyngeal artery Internal maxillary artery Lingual artery Maxillary artery Occipital artery Posterior auricular artery Superior thyroid artery
External Ear, Bilateral External Ear, Left External Ear, Right	**Includes:** Antihelix Antitragus Auricle Earlobe Helix Pinna Tragus
External Iliac Artery, Left External Iliac Artery, Right	**Includes:** Deep circumflex iliac artery Inferior epigastric artery
External Jugular Vein, Left External Jugular Vein, Right	**Includes:** Posterior auricular vein
Extraocular Muscle, Left Extraocular Muscle, Right	**Includes:** Inferior oblique muscle Inferior rectus muscle Lateral rectus muscle Medial rectus muscle Superior oblique muscle Superior rectus muscle
Eye, Left Eye, Right	**Includes:** Ciliary body Posterior chamber
Face Artery	**Includes:** Angular artery Ascending palatine artery External maxillary artery Facial artery Inferior labial artery Submental artery Superior labial artery

ICD-10-PCS Value	Definition
Face Vein, Left Face Vein, Right	**Includes:** Angular vein Anterior facial vein Common facial vein Deep facial vein Frontal vein Posterior facial (retromandibular) vein Supraorbital vein
Facial Muscle	**Includes:** Buccinator muscle Corrugator supercilii muscle Depressor anguli oris muscle Depressor labii inferioris muscle Depressor septi nasi muscle Depressor supercilii muscle Levator anguli oris muscle Levator labii superioris alaeque nasi muscle Levator labii superioris muscle Mentalis muscle Nasalis muscle Occipitofrontalis muscle Orbicularis oris muscle Procerus muscle Risorius muscle Zygomaticus muscle
Facial Nerve	**Includes:** Chorda tympani Geniculate ganglion Greater superficial petrosal nerve Nerve to the stapedius Parotid plexus Posterior auricular nerve Seventh cranial nerve Submandibular ganglion
Fallopian Tube, Left Fallopian Tube, Right	**Includes:** Oviduct Salpinx Uterine tube
Femoral Artery, Left Femoral Artery, Right	**Includes:** Circumflex iliac artery Deep femoral artery Descending genicular artery External pudendal artery Superficial epigastric artery
Femoral Nerve	**Includes:** Anterior crural nerve Saphenous nerve
Femoral Shaft, Left Femoral Shaft, Right	**Includes:** Body of femur
Femoral Vein, Left Femoral Vein, Right	**Includes:** Deep femoral (profunda femoris) vein Popliteal vein Profunda femoris (deep femoral) vein
Fibula, Left Fibula, Right	**Includes:** Body of fibula Head of fibula Lateral malleolus
Finger Nail	**Includes:** Nail bed Nail plate

ICD-10-PCS Value	Definition
Finger Phalangeal Joint, Left **Finger Phalangeal Joint, Right**	**Includes:** Interphalangeal (IP) joint
Foot Artery, Left **Foot Artery, Right**	**Includes:** Arcuate artery Dorsal metatarsal artery Lateral plantar artery Lateral tarsal artery Medial plantar artery
Foot Bursa and Ligament, Left **Foot Bursa and Ligament, Right**	**Includes:** Calcaneocuboid ligament Cuneonavicular ligament Intercuneiform ligament Interphalangeal ligament Metatarsal ligament Metatarsophalangeal ligament Subtalar ligament Talocalcaneal ligament Talocalcaneonavicular ligament Tarsometatarsal ligament
Foot Muscle, Left **Foot Muscle, Right**	**Includes:** Abductor hallucis muscle Adductor hallucis muscle Extensor digitorum brevis muscle Extensor hallucis brevis muscle Flexor digitorum brevis muscle Flexor hallucis brevis muscle Quadratus plantae muscle
Foot Vein, Left **Foot Vein, Right**	**Includes:** Common digital vein Dorsal metatarsal vein Dorsal venous arch Plantar digital vein Plantar metatarsal vein Plantar venous arch
Frontal Bone	**Includes:** Zygomatic process of frontal bone
Gastric Artery	**Includes:** Left gastric artery Right gastric artery
Glenoid Cavity, Left **Glenoid Cavity, Right**	**Includes:** Glenoid fossa (of scapula)
Glomus Jugulare	**Includes:** Jugular body
Glossopharyngeal Nerve	**Includes:** Carotid sinus nerve Ninth cranial nerve Tympanic nerve
Hand Artery, Left **Hand Artery, Right**	**Includes:** Deep palmar arch Princeps pollicis artery Radialis indicis Superficial palmar arch
Hand Bursa and Ligament, Left **Hand Bursa and Ligament, Right**	**Includes:** Carpometacarpal ligament Intercarpal ligament Interphalangeal ligament Lunotriquetral ligament Metacarpal ligament Metacarpophalangeal ligament Pisohamate ligament Pisometacarpal ligament Scapholunate ligament Scaphotrapezium ligament

ICD-10-PCS Value	Definition
Hand Muscle, Left **Hand Muscle, Right**	**Includes:** Hypothenar muscle Palmar interosseous muscle Thenar muscle
Hand Vein, Left **Hand Vein, Right**	**Includes:** Dorsal metacarpal vein Palmar (volar) digital vein Palmar (volar) metacarpal vein Superficial palmar venous arch Volar (palmar) digital vein Volar (palmar) metacarpal vein
Head and Neck Bursa and Ligament	**Includes:** Alar ligament of axis Cervical interspinous ligament Cervical intertransverse ligament Cervical ligamentum flavum Interspinous ligament, cervical Intertransverse ligament, cervical Lateral temporomandibular ligament Ligamentum flavum, cervical Sphenomandibular ligament Stylomandibular ligament Transverse ligament of atlas
Head and Neck Sympathetic Nerve	**Includes:** Cavernous plexus Cervical ganglion Ciliary ganglion Internal carotid plexus Otic ganglion Pterygopalatine (sphenopalatine) ganglion Sphenopalatine (pterygopalatine) ganglion Stellate ganglion Submandibular ganglion Submaxillary ganglion
Head Muscle	**Includes:** Auricularis muscle Masseter muscle Pterygoid muscle Splenius capitis muscle Temporalis muscle Temporoparietalis muscle
Heart, Left	**Includes:** Left coronary sulcus Obtuse margin
Heart, Right	**Includes:** Right coronary sulcus
Hemiazygos Vein	**Includes:** Left ascending lumbar vein Left subcostal vein
Hepatic Artery	**Includes:** Common hepatic artery Gastroduodenal artery Hepatic artery proper
Hip Bursa and Ligament, Left **Hip Bursa and Ligament, Right**	**Includes:** Iliofemoral ligament Ischiofemoral ligament Pubofemoral ligament Transverse acetabular ligament Trochanteric bursa
Hip Joint, Left **Hip Joint, Right**	**Includes:** Acetabulofemoral joint

ICD-10-PCS Value	Definition
Hip Muscle, Left Hip Muscle, Right	Includes: Gemellus muscle Gluteus maximus muscle Gluteus medius muscle Gluteus minimus muscle Iliacus muscle Obturator muscle Piriformis muscle Psoas muscle Quadratus femoris muscle Tensor fasciae latae muscle
Humeral Head, Left Humeral Head, Right	Includes: Greater tuberosity Lesser tuberosity Neck of humerus (anatomical)(surgical)
Humeral Shaft, Left Humeral Shaft, Right	Includes: Distal humerus Humerus, distal Lateral epicondyle of humerus Medial epicondyle of humerus
Hypogastric Vein, Left Hypogastric Vein, Right	Includes: Gluteal vein Internal iliac vein Internal pudendal vein Lateral sacral vein Middle hemorrhoidal vein Obturator vein Uterine vein Vaginal vein Vesical vein
Hypoglossal Nerve	Includes: Twelfth cranial nerve
Hypothalamus	Includes: Mammillary body
Inferior Mesenteric Artery	Includes: Sigmoid artery Superior rectal artery
Inferior Mesenteric Vein	Includes: Sigmoid vein Superior rectal vein
Inferior Vena Cava	Includes: Postcava Right inferior phrenic vein Right ovarian vein Right second lumbar vein Right suprarenal vein Right testicular vein
Inguinal Region, Bilateral Inguinal Region, Left Inguinal Region, Right	Includes: Inguinal canal Inguinal triangle
Inner Ear, Left Inner Ear, Right	Includes: Bony labyrinth Bony vestibule Cochlea Round window Semicircular canal
Innominate Artery	Includes: Brachiocephalic artery Brachiocephalic trunk
Innominate Vein, Left Innominate Vein, Right	Includes: Brachiocephalic vein Inferior thyroid vein
Internal Carotid Artery, Left Internal Carotid Artery, Right	Includes: Caroticotympanic artery Carotid sinus

ICD-10-PCS Value	Definition
Internal Iliac Artery, Left Internal Iliac Artery, Right	Includes: Deferential artery Hypogastric artery Iliolumbar artery Inferior gluteal artery Inferior vesical artery Internal pudendal artery Lateral sacral artery Middle rectal artery Obturator artery Superior gluteal artery Umbilical artery Uterine artery Vaginal artery
Internal Mammary Artery, Left Internal Mammary Artery, Right	Includes: Anterior intercostal artery Internal thoracic artery Musculophrenic artery Pericardiophrenic artery Superior epigastric artery
Intracranial Artery	Includes: Anterior cerebral artery Anterior choroidal artery Anterior communicating artery Basilar artery Circle of Willis Internal carotid artery, intracranial portion Middle cerebral artery Ophthalmic artery Posterior cerebral artery Posterior communicating artery Posterior inferior cerebellar artery (PICA)
Intracranial Vein	Includes: Anterior cerebral vein Basal (internal) cerebral vein Dural venous sinus Great cerebral vein Inferior cerebellar vein Inferior cerebral vein Internal (basal) cerebral vein Middle cerebral vein Ophthalmic vein Superior cerebellar vein Superior cerebral vein
Jejunum	Includes: Duodenojejunal flexure
Kidney	Includes: Renal calyx Renal capsule Renal cortex Renal segment
Kidney Pelvis, Left Kidney Pelvis, Right	Includes: Ureteropelvic junction (UPJ)
Kidney, Left Kidney, Right Kidneys, Bilateral	Includes: Renal calyx Renal capsule Renal cortex Renal segment

ICD-10-PCS Value	Definition
Knee Bursa and Ligament, Left **Knee Bursa and Ligament, Right**	**Includes:** Anterior cruciate ligament (ACL) Lateral collateral ligament (LCL) Ligament of head of fibula Medial collateral ligament (MCL) Patellar ligament Popliteal ligament Posterior cruciate ligament (PCL) Prepatellar bursa
Knee Joint, Femoral Surface, Left **Knee Joint, Femoral Surface, Right**	**Includes:** Femoropatellar joint Patellofemoral joint
Knee Joint, Left **Knee Joint, Right**	**Includes:** Femoropatellar joint Femorotibial joint Lateral meniscus Medial meniscus Patellofemoral joint Tibiofemoral joint
Knee Joint, Tibial Surface, Left **Knee Joint, Tibial Surface, Right**	**Includes:** Femorotibial joint Tibiofemoral joint
Knee Tendon, Left **Knee Tendon, Right**	**Includes:** Patellar tendon
Lacrimal Duct, Left **Lacrimal Duct, Right**	**Includes:** Lacrimal canaliculus Lacrimal punctum Lacrimal sac Nasolacrimal duct
Larynx	**Includes:** Aryepiglottic fold Arytenoid cartilage Corniculate cartilage Cuneiform cartilage False vocal cord Glottis Rima glottidis Thyroid cartilage Ventricular fold
Lens, Left **Lens, Right**	**Includes:** Zonule of Zinn
Liver	**Includes:** Quadrate lobe
Lower Arm and Wrist Muscle, Left **Lower Arm and Wrist Muscle, Right**	**Includes:** Anatomical snuffbox Brachioradialis muscle Extensor carpi radialis muscle Extensor carpi ulnaris muscle Flexor carpi radialis muscle Flexor carpi ulnaris muscle Flexor pollicis longus muscle Palmaris longus muscle Pronator quadratus muscle Pronator teres muscle
Lower Artery	**Includes:** Umbilical artery
Lower Eyelid, Left **Lower Eyelid, Right**	**Includes:** Inferior tarsal plate Medial canthus
Lower Femur, Left **Lower Femur, Right**	**Includes:** Lateral condyle of femur Lateral epicondyle of femur Medial condyle of femur Medial epicondyle of femur

ICD-10-PCS Value	Definition
Lower Leg Muscle, Left **Lower Leg Muscle, Right**	**Includes:** Extensor digitorum longus muscle Extensor hallucis longus muscle Fibularis brevis muscle Fibularis longus muscle Flexor digitorum longus muscle Flexor hallucis longus muscle Gastrocnemius muscle Peroneus brevis muscle Peroneus longus muscle Popliteus muscle Soleus muscle Tibialis anterior muscle Tibialis posterior muscle
Lower Leg Tendon, Left **Lower Leg Tendon, Right**	**Includes:** Achilles tendon
Lower Lip	**Includes:** Frenulum labii inferioris Labial gland Vermilion border
Lower Spine Bursa and Ligament	**Includes:** Iliolumbar ligament Interspinous ligament, lumbar Intertransverse ligament, lumbar Ligamentum flavum, lumbar Sacrococcygeal ligament Sacroiliac ligament Sacrospinous ligament Sacrotuberous ligament Supraspinous ligament
Lumbar Nerve	**Includes:** Lumbosacral trunk Spinal nerve, lumbar Superior clunic (cluneal) nerve
Lumbar Plexus	**Includes:** Accessory obturator nerve Genitofemoral nerve Iliohypogastric nerve Ilioinguinal nerve Lateral femoral cutaneous nerve Obturator nerve Superior gluteal nerve
Lumbar Spinal Cord	**Includes:** Cauda equina Conus medullaris
Lumbar Sympathetic Nerve	**Includes:** Lumbar ganglion Lumbar splanchnic nerve
Lumbar Vertebra	**Includes:** Spinous process Transverse process Vertebral arch Vertebral body Vertebral foramen Vertebral lamina Vertebral pedicle
Lumbar Vertebral Joint	**Includes:** Lumbar facet joint
Lumbosacral Joint	**Includes:** Lumbosacral facet joint

ICD-10-PCS Value	Definition
Lymphatic, Aortic	**Includes:** Celiac lymph node Gastric lymph node Hepatic lymph node Lumbar lymph node Pancreaticosplenic lymph node Paraaortic lymph node Retroperitoneal lymph node
Lymphatic, Head	**Includes:** Buccinator lymph node Infraauricular lymph node Infraparotid lymph node Parotid lymph node Preauricular lymph node Submandibular lymph node Submaxillary lymph node Submental lymph node Subparotid lymph node Suprahyoid lymph node
Lymphatic, Left Axillary	**Includes:** Anterior (pectoral) lymph node Apical (subclavicular) lymph node Brachial (lateral) lymph node Central axillary lymph node Lateral (brachial) lymph node Pectoral (anterior) lymph node Posterior (subscapular) lymph node Subclavicular (apical) lymph node Subscapular (posterior) lymph node
Lymphatic, Left Lower Extremity	**Includes:** Femoral lymph node Popliteal lymph node
Lymphatic, Left Neck	**Includes:** Cervical lymph node Jugular lymph node Mastoid (postauricular) lymph node Occipital lymph node Postauricular (mastoid) lymph node Retropharyngeal lymph node Supraclavicular (Virchow's) lymph node Virchow's (supraclavicular) lymph node
Lymphatic, Left Upper Extremity	**Includes:** Cubital lymph node Deltopectoral (infraclavicular) lymph node Epitrochlear lymph node Infraclavicular (deltopectoral) lymph node Supratrochlear lymph node
Lymphatic, Mesenteric	**Includes:** Inferior mesenteric lymph node Pararectal lymph node Superior mesenteric lymph node
Lymphatic, Pelvis	**Includes:** Common iliac (subaortic) lymph node Gluteal lymph node Iliac lymph node Inferior epigastric lymph node Obturator lymph node Sacral lymph node Subaortic (common iliac) lymph node Suprainguinal lymph node
Lymphatic, Right Axillary	**Includes:** Anterior (pectoral) lymph node Apical (subclavicular) lymph node Brachial (lateral) lymph node Central axillary lymph node Lateral (brachial) lymph node Pectoral (anterior) lymph node Posterior (subscapular) lymph node Subclavicular (apical) lymph node Subscapular (posterior) lymph node
Lymphatic, Right Lower Extremity	**Includes:** Femoral lymph node Popliteal lymph node
Lymphatic, Right Neck	**Includes:** Cervical lymph node Jugular lymph node Mastoid (postauricular) lymph node Occipital lymph node Postauricular (mastoid) lymph node Retropharyngeal lymph node Right jugular trunk Right lymphatic duct Right subclavian trunk Supraclavicular (Virchow's) lymph node Virchow's (supraclavicular) lymph node
Lymphatic, Right Upper Extremity	**Includes:** Cubital lymph node Deltopectoral (infraclavicular) lymph node Epitrochlear lymph node Infraclavicular (deltopectoral) lymph node Supratrochlear lymph node
Lymphatic, Thorax	**Includes:** Intercostal lymph node Mediastinal lymph node Parasternal lymph node Paratracheal lymph node Tracheobronchial lymph node
Main Bronchus, Right	**Includes:** Bronchus intermedius Intermediate bronchus
Mandible, Left Mandible, Right	**Includes:** Alveolar process of mandible Condyloid process Mandibular notch Mental foramen
Mastoid Sinus, Left Mastoid Sinus, Right	**Includes:** Mastoid air cells
Maxilla	**Includes:** Alveolar process of maxilla
Maxillary Sinus, Left Maxillary Sinus, Right	**Includes:** Antrum of Highmore
Median Nerve	**Includes:** Anterior interosseous nerve Palmar cutaneous nerve
Mediastinum	**Includes:** Mediastinal cavity Mediastinal space
Medulla Oblongata	**Includes:** Myelencephalon
Mesentery	**Includes:** Mesoappendix Mesocolon

ICD-10-PCS Value	Definition
Metatarsal-Phalangeal Joint, Left Metatarsal-Phalangeal Joint, Right	**Includes:** Metatarsophalangeal (MTP) joint
Middle Ear, Left Middle Ear, Right	**Includes:** Oval window Tympanic cavity
Minor Salivary Gland	**Includes:** Anterior lingual gland
Mitral Valve	**Includes:** Bicuspid valve Left atrioventricular valve Mitral annulus
Nasal Bone	**Includes:** Vomer of nasal septum
Nasal Mucosa and Soft Tissue	**Includes:** Columella External naris Greater alar cartilage Internal naris Lateral nasal cartilage Lesser alar cartilage Nasal cavity Nostril
Nasal Septum	**Includes:** Quadrangular cartilage Septal cartilage Vomer bone
Nasal Turbinate	**Includes:** Inferior turbinate Middle turbinate Nasal concha Superior turbinate
Nasopharynx	**Includes:** Choana Fossa of Rosenmuller Pharyngeal recess Rhinopharynx
Neck Muscle, Left Neck Muscle, Right	**Includes:** Anterior vertebral muscle Arytenoid muscle Cricothyroid muscle Infrahyoid muscle Levator scapulae muscle Platysma muscle Scalene muscle Splenius cervicis muscle Sternocleidomastoid muscle Suprahyoid muscle Thyroarytenoid muscle
Nipple, Left Nipple, Right	**Includes:** Areola
Occipital Bone	**Includes:** Foramen magnum
Oculomotor Nerve	**Includes:** Third cranial nerve
Olfactory Nerve	**Includes:** First cranial nerve Olfactory bulb

ICD-10-PCS Value	Definition
Omentum	**Includes:** Gastrocolic ligament Gastrocolic omentum Gastrohepatic omentum Gastrophrenic ligament Gastrosplenic ligament Greater Omentum Hepatogastric ligament Lesser Omentum
Optic Nerve	**Includes:** Optic chiasma Second cranial nerve
Orbit, Left Orbit, Right	**Includes:** Bony orbit Orbital portion of ethmoid bone Orbital portion of frontal bone Orbital portion of lacrimal bone Orbital portion of maxilla Orbital portion of palatine bone Orbital portion of sphenoid bone Orbital portion of zygomatic bone
Pancreatic Duct	**Includes:** Duct of Wirsung
Pancreatic Duct, Accessory	**Includes:** Duct of Santorini
Parotid Duct, Left Parotid Duct, Right	**Includes:** Stensen's duct
Pelvic Bone, Left Pelvic Bone, Right	**Includes:** Iliac crest Ilium Ischium Pubis
Pelvic Cavity	**Includes:** Retropubic space
Penis	**Includes:** Corpus cavernosum Corpus spongiosum
Perineum Muscle	**Includes:** Bulbospongiosus muscle Cremaster muscle Deep transverse perineal muscle Ischiocavernosus muscle Levator ani muscle Superficial transverse perineal muscle
Peritoneum	**Includes:** Epiploic foramen
Peroneal Artery, Left Peroneal Artery, Right	**Includes:** Fibular artery
Peroneal Nerve	**Includes:** Common fibular nerve Common peroneal nerve External popliteal nerve Lateral sural cutaneous nerve
Pharynx	**Includes:** Base of Tongue Hypopharynx Laryngopharynx Lingual tonsil Oropharynx Piriform recess (sinus) Tongue, base of
Phrenic Nerve	**Includes:** Accessory phrenic nerve

ICD-10-PCS Value	Definition
Pituitary Gland	**Includes:** Adenohypophysis Hypophysis Neurohypophysis
Pons	**Includes:** Apneustic center Basis pontis Locus ceruleus Pneumotaxic center Pontine tegmentum Superior olivary nucleus
Popliteal Artery, Left Popliteal Artery, Right	**Includes:** Inferior genicular artery Middle genicular artery Superior genicular artery Sural artery
Portal Vein	**Includes:** Hepatic portal vein
Prepuce	**Includes:** Foreskin Glans penis
Pudendal Nerve	**Includes:** Posterior labial nerve Posterior scrotal nerve
Pulmonary Artery, Left	**Includes:** Arterial canal (duct) Botallo's duct Pulmoaortic canal
Pulmonary Valve	**Includes:** Pulmonary annulus Pulmonic valve
Pulmonary Vein, Left	**Includes:** Left inferior pulmonary vein Left superior pulmonary vein
Pulmonary Vein, Right	**Includes:** Right inferior pulmonary vein Right superior pulmonary vein
Radial Artery, Left Radial Artery, Right	**Includes:** Radial recurrent artery
Radial Nerve	**Includes:** Dorsal digital nerve Musculospiral nerve Palmar cutaneous nerve Posterior interosseous nerve
Radius, Left Radius, Right	**Includes:** Ulnar notch
Rectum	**Includes:** Anorectal junction
Renal Artery, Left Renal Artery, Right	**Includes:** Inferior suprarenal artery Renal segmental artery
Renal Vein, Left	**Includes:** Left inferior phrenic vein Left ovarian vein Left second lumbar vein Left suprarenal vein Left testicular vein
Retina, Left Retina, Right	**Includes:** Fovea Macula Optic disc
Retroperitoneum	**Includes:** Retroperitoneal cavity Retroperitoneal space

ICD-10-PCS Value	Definition
Rib(s) Bursa and Ligament	**Includes:** Costotransverse ligament
Sacral Nerve	**Includes:** Spinal nerve, sacral
Sacral Plexus	**Includes:** Inferior gluteal nerve Posterior femoral cutaneous nerve Pudendal nerve
Sacral Sympathetic Nerve	**Includes:** Ganglion impar (ganglion of Walther) Pelvic splanchnic nerve Sacral ganglion Sacral splanchnic nerve
Sacrococcygeal Joint	**Includes:** Sacrococcygeal symphysis
Saphenous Vein, Left Saphenous Vein, Right	**Includes:** External pudendal vein Great(er) saphenous vein Lesser saphenous vein Small saphenous vein Superficial circumflex iliac vein Superficial epigastric vein
Scapula, Left Scapula, Right	**Includes:** Acromion (process) Coracoid process
Sciatic Nerve	**Includes:** Ischiatic nerve
Shoulder Bursa and Ligament, Left Shoulder Bursa and Ligament, Right	**Includes:** Acromioclavicular ligament Coracoacromial ligament Coracoclavicular ligament Coracohumeral ligament Costoclavicular ligament Glenohumeral ligament Interclavicular ligament Sternoclavicular ligament Subacromial bursa Transverse humeral ligament Transverse scapular ligament
Shoulder Joint, Left Shoulder Joint, Right	**Includes:** Glenohumeral joint Glenoid ligament (labrum)
Shoulder Muscle, Left Shoulder Muscle, Right	**Includes:** Deltoid muscle Infraspinatus muscle Subscapularis muscle Supraspinatus muscle Teres major muscle Teres minor muscle
Sigmoid Colon	**Includes:** Rectosigmoid junction Sigmoid flexure
Skin	**Includes:** Dermis Epidermis Sebaceous gland Sweat gland
Sphenoid Bone	**Includes:** Greater wing Lesser wing Optic foramen Pterygoid process Sella turcica

ICD-10-PCS Value	Definition
Spinal Canal	**Includes:** Epidural space, spinal Extradural space, spinal Subarachnoid space, spinal Subdural space, spinal Vertebral canal
Spinal Meninges	**Includes:** Arachnoid mater, spinal Denticulate (dentate) ligament Dura mater, spinal Filum terminale Leptomeninges, spinal Pia mater, spinal
Spleen	**Includes:** Accessory spleen
Splenic Artery	**Includes:** Left gastroepiploic artery Pancreatic artery Short gastric artery
Splenic Vein	**Includes:** Left gastroepiploic vein Pancreatic vein
Sternum	**Includes:** Manubrium Suprasternal notch Xiphoid process
Sternum Bursa and Ligament	**Includes:** Costoxiphoid ligament Sternocostal ligament
Stomach, Pylorus	**Includes:** Pyloric antrum Pyloric canal Pyloric sphincter
Subclavian Artery, Left Subclavian Artery, Right	**Includes:** Costocervical trunk Dorsal scapular artery Internal thoracic artery
Subcutaneous Tissue and Fascia, Chest	**Includes:** Pectoral fascia
Subcutaneous Tissue and Fascia, Face	**Includes:** Masseteric fascia Orbital fascia
Subcutaneous Tissue and Fascia, Left Foot	**Includes:** Plantar fascia (aponeurosis)
Subcutaneous Tissue and Fascia, Left Hand	**Includes:** Palmar fascia (aponeurosis)
Subcutaneous Tissue and Fascia, Left Lower Arm	**Includes:** Antebrachial fascia Bicipital aponeurosis
Subcutaneous Tissue and Fascia, Left Neck	**Includes:** Deep cervical fascia Pretracheal fascia Prevertebral fascia
Subcutaneous Tissue and Fascia, Left Upper Arm	**Includes:** Axillary fascia Deltoid fascia Infraspinatus fascia Subscapular aponeurosis Supraspinatus fascia
Subcutaneous Tissue and Fascia, Left Upper Leg	**Includes:** Crural fascia Fascia lata Iliac fascia Iliotibial tract (band)

ICD-10-PCS Value	Definition
Subcutaneous Tissue and Fascia, Right Foot	**Includes:** Plantar fascia (aponeurosis)
Subcutaneous Tissue and Fascia, Right Hand	**Includes:** Palmar fascia (aponeurosis)
Subcutaneous Tissue and Fascia, Right Lower Arm	**Includes:** Antebrachial fascia Bicipital aponeurosis
Subcutaneous Tissue and Fascia, Right Neck	**Includes:** Deep cervical fascia Pretracheal fascia Prevertebral fascia
Subcutaneous Tissue and Fascia, Right Upper Arm	**Includes:** Axillary fascia Deltoid fascia Infraspinatus fascia Subscapular aponeurosis Supraspinatus fascia
Subcutaneous Tissue and Fascia, Right Upper Leg	**Includes:** Crural fascia Fascia lata Iliac fascia Iliotibial tract (band)
Subcutaneous Tissue and Fascia, Scalp	**Includes:** Galea aponeurotica
Subcutaneous Tissue and Fascia, Trunk	**Includes:** External oblique aponeurosis Transversalis fascia
Submaxillary Gland, Left Submaxillary Gland, Right	**Includes:** Submandibular gland
Superior Mesenteric Artery	**Includes:** Ileal artery Ileocolic artery Inferior pancreaticoduodenal artery Jejunal artery
Superior Mesenteric Vein	**Includes:** Right gastroepiploic vein
Superior Vena Cava	**Includes:** Precava
Tarsal Joint, Left Tarsal Joint, Right	**Includes:** Calcaneocuboid joint Cuboideonavicular joint Cuneonavicular joint Intercuneiform joint Subtalar (talocalcaneal) joint Talocalcaneal (subtalar) joint Talocalcaneonavicular joint
Tarsal, Left Tarsal, Right	**Includes:** Calcaneus Cuboid bone Intermediate cuneiform bone Lateral cuneiform bone Medial cuneiform bone Navicular bone Talus bone
Temporal Artery, Left Temporal Artery, Right	**Includes:** Middle temporal artery Superficial temporal artery Transverse facial artery
Temporal Bone, Left Temporal Bone, Right	**Includes:** Mastoid process Petrous part of temporal bone Tympanic part of temporal bone Zygomatic process of temporal bone

ICD-10-PCS Value	Definition
Thalamus	**Includes:** Epithalamus Geniculate nucleus Metathalamus Pulvinar
Thoracic Aorta, Ascending/Arch	**Includes:** Aortic arch Ascending aorta
Thoracic Duct	**Includes:** Left jugular trunk Left subclavian trunk
Thoracic Nerve	**Includes:** Intercostal nerve Intercostobrachial nerve Spinal nerve, thoracic Subcostal nerve
Thoracic Sympathetic Nerve	**Includes:** Cardiac plexus Esophageal plexus Greater splanchnic nerve Inferior cardiac nerve Least splanchnic nerve Lesser splanchnic nerve Middle cardiac nerve Pulmonary plexus Superior cardiac nerve Thoracic aortic plexus Thoracic ganglion
Thoracic Vertebra	**Includes:** Spinous process Transverse process Vertebral arch Vertebral body Vertebral foramen Vertebral lamina Vertebral pedicle
Thoracic Vertebral Joint	**Includes:** Costotransverse joint Costovertebral joint Thoracic facet joint
Thoracolumbar Vertebral Joint	**Includes:** Thoracolumbar facet joint
Thorax Muscle, Left Thorax Muscle, Right	**Includes:** Intercostal muscle Levatores costarum muscle Pectoralis major muscle Pectoralis minor muscle Serratus anterior muscle Subclavius muscle Subcostal muscle Transverse thoracis muscle
Thymus	**Includes:** Thymus gland
Thyroid Artery, Left Thyroid Artery, Right	**Includes:** Cricothyroid artery Hyoid artery Sternocleidomastoid artery Superior laryngeal artery Superior thyroid artery Thyrocervical trunk
Tibia, Left Tibia, Right	**Includes:** Lateral condyle of tibia Medial condyle of tibia Medial malleolus

ICD-10-PCS Value	Definition
Tibial Nerve	**Includes:** Lateral plantar nerve Medial plantar nerve Medial popliteal nerve Medial sural cutaneous nerve
Toe Nail	**Includes:** Nail bed Nail plate
Toe Phalangeal Joint, Left Toe Phalangeal Joint, Right	**Includes:** Interphalangeal (IP) joint
Tongue	**Includes:** Frenulum linguae
Tongue, Palate, Pharynx Muscle	**Includes:** Chondroglossus muscle Genioglossus muscle Hyoglossus muscle Inferior longitudinal muscle Levator veli palatini muscle Palatoglossal muscle Palatopharyngeal muscle Pharyngeal constrictor muscle Salpingopharyngeus muscle Styloglossus muscle Stylopharyngeus muscle Superior longitudinal muscle Tensor veli palatini muscle
Tonsils	**Includes:** Palatine tonsil
Trachea	**Includes:** Cricoid cartilage
Transverse Colon	**Includes:** Hepatic flexure Splenic flexure
Tricuspid Valve	**Includes:** Right atrioventricular valve Tricuspid annulus
Trigeminal Nerve	**Includes:** Fifth cranial nerve Gasserian ganglion Mandibular nerve Maxillary nerve Ophthalmic nerve Trifacial nerve
Trochlear Nerve	**Includes:** Fourth cranial nerve
Trunk Muscle, Left Trunk Muscle, Right	**Includes:** Coccygeus muscle Erector spinae muscle Interspinalis muscle Intertransversarius muscle Latissimus dorsi muscle Quadratus lumborum muscle Rhomboid major muscle Rhomboid minor muscle Serratus posterior muscle Transversospinalis muscle Trapezius muscle
Tympanic Membrane, Left Tympanic Membrane, Right	**Includes:** Pars flaccida
Ulna, Left Ulna, Right	**Includes:** Olecranon process Radial notch

ICD-10-PCS Value	Definition
Ulnar Artery, Left Ulnar Artery, Right	**Includes:** Anterior ulnar recurrent artery Common interosseous artery Posterior ulnar recurrent artery
Ulnar Nerve	**Includes:** Cubital nerve
Upper Arm Muscle, Left Upper Arm Muscle, Right	**Includes:** Biceps brachii muscle Brachialis muscle Coracobrachialis muscle Triceps brachii muscle
Upper Artery	**Includes:** Aortic intercostal artery Bronchial artery Esophageal artery Subcostal artery
Upper Eyelid, Left Upper Eyelid, Right	**Includes:** Lateral canthus Levator palpebrae superioris muscle Orbicularis oculi muscle Superior tarsal plate
Upper Femur, Left Upper Femur, Right	**Includes:** Femoral head Greater trochanter Lesser trochanter Neck of femur
Upper Leg Muscle, Left Upper Leg Muscle, Right	**Includes:** Adductor brevis muscle Adductor longus muscle Adductor magnus muscle Biceps femoris muscle Gracilis muscle Pectineus muscle Quadriceps (femoris) Rectus femoris muscle Sartorius muscle Semimembranosus muscle Semitendinosus muscle Vastus intermedius muscle Vastus lateralis muscle Vastus medialis muscle
Upper Lip	**Includes:** Frenulum labii superioris Labial gland Vermilion border
Upper Spine Bursa and Ligament	**Includes:** Interspinous ligament, thoracic Intertransverse ligament, thoracic Ligamentum flavum, thoracic Supraspinous ligament
Ureter Ureter, Left Ureter, Right Ureters, Bilateral	**Includes:** Ureteral orifice Ureterovesical orifice
Urethra	**Includes:** Bulbourethral (Cowper's) gland Cowper's (bulbourethral) gland External urethral sphincter Internal urethral sphincter Membranous urethra Penile urethra Prostatic urethra
Uterine Supporting Structure	**Includes:** Broad ligament Infundibulopelvic ligament Ovarian ligament Round ligament of uterus

ICD-10-PCS Value	Definition
Uterus	**Includes:** Fundus uteri Myometrium Perimetrium Uterine cornu
Uvula	**Includes:** Palatine uvula
Vagus Nerve	**Includes:** Anterior vagal trunk Pharyngeal plexus Pneumogastric nerve Posterior vagal trunk Pulmonary plexus Recurrent laryngeal nerve Superior laryngeal nerve Tenth cranial nerve
Vas Deferens Vas Deferens, Bilateral Vas Deferens, Left Vas Deferens, Right	**Includes:** Ductus deferens Ejaculatory duct
Ventricle, Right	**Includes:** Conus arteriosus
Ventricular Septum	**Includes:** Interventricular septum
Vertebral Artery, Left Vertebral Artery, Right	**Includes:** Anterior spinal artery Posterior spinal artery
Vertebral Vein, Left Vertebral Vein, Right	**Includes:** Deep cervical vein Suboccipital venous plexus
Vestibular Gland	**Includes:** Bartholin's (greater vestibular) gland Greater vestibular (Bartholin's) gland Paraurethral (Skene's) gland Skene's (paraurethral) gland
Vitreous, Left Vitreous, Right	**Includes:** Vitreous body
Vocal Cord, Left Vocal Cord, Right	**Includes:** Vocal fold
Vulva	**Includes:** Labia majora Labia minora
Wrist Bursa and Ligament, Left Wrist Bursa and Ligament, Right	**Includes:** Palmar ulnocarpal ligament Radial collateral carpal ligament Radiocarpal ligament Radioulnar ligament Ulnar collateral carpal ligament
Wrist Joint, Left Wrist Joint, Right	**Includes:** Distal radioulnar joint Radiocarpal joint

Appendix F: Device Key and Aggregation Table

Device Key

Term	ICD-10-PCS Value
3f (Aortic) Bioprosthesis valve	Zooplastic Tissue in Heart and Great Vessels
AbioCor® Total Replacement Heart	Synthetic Substitute
Absolute Pro Vascular (OTW) Self-Expanding Stent System	Intraluminal Device
Acculink (RX) Carotid Stent System	Intraluminal Device
Acellular Hydrated Dermis	Nonautologous Tissue Substitute
Acetabular cup	Liner in Lower Joints
Activa PC neurostimulator	Stimulator Generator, Multiple Array for Insertion in Subcutaneous Tissue and Fascia
Activa RC neurostimulator	Stimulator Generator, Multiple Array Rechargeable for Insertion in Subcutaneous Tissue and Fascia
Activa SC neurostimulator	Stimulator Generator, Single Array for Insertion in Subcutaneous Tissue and Fascia
ACUITY™ Steerable Lead	Cardiac Lead, Pacemaker for Insertion in Heart and Great Vessels Cardiac Lead, Defibrillator for Insertion in Heart and Great Vessels
Advisa (MRI)	Pacemaker, Dual Chamber for Insertion in Subcutaneous Tissue and Fascia
AFX® Endovascular AAA System	Intraluminal Device
AMPLATZER® Muscular VSD Occluder	Synthetic Substitute
AMS 800® Urinary Control System	Artificial Sphincter in Urinary System
AneuRx® AAA Advantage®	Intraluminal Device
Annuloplasty ring	Synthetic Substitute
Articulating Spacer (Antibiotic)	Articulating Spacer in Lower Joints
Artificial anal sphincter (AAS)	Artificial Sphincter in Gastrointestinal System
Artificial bowel sphincter (neosphincter)	Artificial Sphincter in Gastrointestinal System
Artificial urinary sphincter (AUS)	Artificial Sphincter in Urinary System
Ascenda Intrathecal Catheter	Infusion Device
Assurant (Cobalt) stent	Intraluminal Device
AtriClip LAA Exclusion System	Extraluminal Device
Attain Ability® Lead	Cardiac Lead, Pacemaker for Insertion in Heart and Great Vessels Cardiac Lead, Defibrillator for Insertion in Heart and Great Vessels
Attain StarFix® (OTW) Lead	Cardiac Lead, Pacemaker for Insertion in Heart and Great Vessels Cardiac Lead, Defibrillator for Insertion in Heart and Great Vessels
Autograft	Autologous Tissue Substitute

Term	ICD-10-PCS Value
Autologous artery graft	Autologous Arterial Tissue in Heart and Great Vessels Autologous Arterial Tissue in Upper Arteries Autologous Arterial Tissue in Lower Arteries Autologous Arterial Tissue in Upper Veins Autologous Arterial Tissue in Lower Veins
Autologous vein graft	Autologous Venous Tissue in Heart and Great Vessels Autologous Venous Tissue in Upper Arteries Autologous Venous Tissue in Lower Arteries Autologous Venous Tissue in Upper Veins Autologous Venous Tissue in Lower Veins
Axial Lumbar Interbody Fusion System	Interbody Fusion Device in Lower Joints
AxiaLIF® System	Interbody Fusion Device in Lower Joints
BAK/C® Interbody Cervical Fusion System	Interbody Fusion Device in Upper Joints
Bard® Composix® (E/X)(LP) mesh	Synthetic Substitute
Bard® Composix® Kugel® patch	Synthetic Substitute
Bard® Dulex™ mesh	Synthetic Substitute
Bard® Ventralex™ hernia patch	Synthetic Substitute
Baroreflex Activation Therapy® (BAT®)	Stimulator Lead in Upper Arteries Stimulator Generator in Subcutaneous Tissue and Fascia
Berlin Heart Ventricular Assist Device	Implantable Heart Assist System in Heart and Great Vessels
Bioactive embolization coil(s)	Intraluminal Device, Bioactive in Upper Arteries
Biventricular external heart assist system	Short-term External Heart Assist System in Heart and Great Vessels
Blood glucose monitoring system	Monitoring Device
Bone anchored hearing device	Hearing Device, Bone Conduction for Insertion in Ear, Nose, Sinus Hearing Device, in Head and Facial Bones
Bone bank bone graft	Nonautologous Tissue Substitute
Bone screw (interlocking)(lag)(pedicle)(recessed)	Internal Fixation Device in Head and Facial Bones Internal Fixation Device in Upper Bones Internal Fixation Device in Lower Bones
Bovine pericardial valve	Zooplastic Tissue in Heart and Great Vessels
Bovine pericardium graft	Zooplastic Tissue in Heart and Great Vessels
Brachytherapy seeds	Radioactive Element
BRYAN® Cervical Disc System	Synthetic Substitute
BVS 5000 Ventricular Assist Device	Short-term External Heart Assist System in Heart and Great Vessels
Cardiac contractility modulation lead	Cardiac Lead in Heart and Great Vessels

Term	ICD-10-PCS Value
Cardiac event recorder	Monitoring Device
Cardiac resynchronization therapy (CRT) lead	Cardiac Lead, Pacemaker for Insertion in Heart and Great Vessels Cardiac Lead, Defibrillator for Insertion in Heart and Great Vessels
CardioMEMS® pressure sensor	Monitoring Device, Pressure Sensor for Insertion in Heart and Great Vessels
Carotid (artery) sinus (baroreceptor) lead	Stimulator Lead in Upper Arteries
Carotid WALLSTENT® Monorail® Endoprosthesis	Intraluminal Device
Centrimag® Blood Pump	Short-term External Heart Assist System in Heart and Great Vessels
Ceramic on ceramic bearing surface	Synthetic Substitute, Ceramic for Replacement in Lower Joints
Cesium-131 Collagen Implant	Radioactive Element, Cesium-131 Collagen Implant for Insertion in Central Nervous System and Cranial Nerves
Clamp and rod internal fixation system (CRIF)	Internal Fixation Device in Upper Bones Internal Fixation Device in Lower Bones
COALESCE® radiolucent interbody fusion device	Interbody Fusion Device, Radiolucent Porous in New Technology
CoAxia NeuroFlo catheter	Intraluminal Device
Cobalt/chromium head and polyethylene socket	Synthetic Substitute, Metal on Polyethylene for Replacement in Lower Joints
Cobalt/chromium head and socket	Synthetic Substitute, Metal for Replacement in Lower Joints
Cochlear implant (CI), multiple channel (electrode)	Hearing Device, Multiple Channel Cochlear Prosthesis for Insertion in Ear, Nose, Sinus
Cochlear implant (CI), single channel (electrode)	Hearing Device, Single Channel Cochlear Prosthesis for Insertion in Ear, Nose, Sinus
COGNIS® CRT-D	Cardiac Resynchronization Defibrillator Pulse Generator for Insertion in Subcutaneous Tissue and Fascia
COHERE® radiolucent interbody fusion device	Interbody Fusion Device, Radiolucent Porous in New Technology
Colonic Z-Stent®	Intraluminal Device
Complete (SE) stent	Intraluminal Device
Concerto II CRT-D	Cardiac Resynchronization Defibrillator Pulse Generator for Insertion in Subcutaneous Tissue and Fascia
CONSERVE® PLUS Total Resurfacing Hip System	Resurfacing Device in Lower Joints
Consulta CRT-D	Cardiac Resynchronization Defibrillator Pulse Generator for Insertion in Subcutaneous Tissue and Fascia
Consulta CRT-P	Cardiac Resynchronization Pacemaker Pulse Generator for Insertion in Subcutaneous Tissue and Fascia
CONTAK RENEWAL® 3 RF (HE) CRT-D	Cardiac Resynchronization Defibrillator Pulse Generator for Insertion in Subcutaneous Tissue and Fascia
Contegra Pulmonary Valved Conduit	Zooplastic Tissue in Heart and Great Vessels
Continuous Glucose Monitoring (CGM) device	Monitoring Device
Cook Biodesign® Fistula Plug(s)	Nonautologous Tissue Substitute

Term	ICD-10-PCS Value
Cook Biodesign® Hernia Graft(s)	Nonautologous Tissue Substitute
Cook Biodesign® Layered Graft(s)	Nonautologous Tissue Substitute
Cook Zenapro™ Layered Graft(s)	Nonautologous Tissue Substitute
Cook Zenith AAA Endovascular Graft	Intraluminal Device Intraluminal Device, Branched or Fenestrated, One or Two Arteries for Restriction in Lower Arteries Intraluminal Device, Branched or Fenestrated, Three or More Arteries for Restriction in Lower Arteries
CoreValve transcatheter aortic valve	Zooplastic Tissue in Heart and Great Vessels
Cormet Hip Resurfacing System	Resurfacing Device in Lower Joints
CoRoent® XL	Interbody Fusion Device in Lower Joints
Corox (OTW) Bipolar Lead	Cardiac Lead, Pacemaker for Insertion in Heart and Great Vessels Cardiac Lead, Defibrillator for Insertion in Heart and Great Vessels
Cortical strip neurostimulator lead	Neurostimulator Lead in Central Nervous System and Cranial Nerves
Cultured epidermal cell autograft	Autologous Tissue Substitute
CYPHER® Stent	Intraluminal Device, Drug-eluting in Heart and Great Vessels
Cystostomy tube	Drainage Device
DBS lead	Neurostimulator Lead in Central Nervous System and Cranial Nerves
DeBakey Left Ventricular Assist Device	Implantable Heart Assist System in Heart and Great Vessels
Deep brain neurostimulator lead	Neurostimulator Lead in Central Nervous System and Cranial Nerves
Delta frame external fixator	External Fixation Device, Hybrid for Insertion in Upper Bones External Fixation Device, Hybrid for Reposition in Upper Bones External Fixation Device, Hybrid for Insertion in Lower Bones External Fixation Device, Hybrid for Reposition in Lower Bones
Delta III Reverse shoulder prosthesis	Synthetic Substitute, Reverse Ball and Socket for Replacement in Upper Joints
Diaphragmatic pacemaker generator	Stimulator Generator in Subcutaneous Tissue and Fascia
Direct Lateral Interbody Fusion (DLIF) device	Interbody Fusion Device in Lower Joints
Driver stent (RX) (OTW)	Intraluminal Device
DuraHeart Left Ventricular Assist System	Implantable Heart Assist System in Heart and Great Vessels
Durata® Defibrillation Lead	Cardiac Lead, Defibrillator for Insertion in Heart and Great Vessels
Dynesys® Dynamic Stabilization System	Spinal Stabilization Device, Pedicle-Based for Insertion in Upper Joints Spinal Stabilization Device, Pedicle-Based for Insertion in Lower Joints
E-Luminexx™ (Biliary)(Vascular) Stent	Intraluminal Device
EDWARDS INTUITY Elite valve system	Zooplastic Tissue, Rapid Deployment Technique in New Technology

Term	ICD-10-PCS Value
Electrical bone growth stimulator (EBGS)	Bone Growth Stimulator in Head and Facial Bones Bone Growth Stimulator in Upper Bones Bone Growth Stimulator in Lower Bones
Electrical muscle stimulation (EMS) lead	Stimulator Lead in Muscles
Electronic muscle stimulator lead	Stimulator Lead in Muscles
Embolization coil(s)	Intraluminal Device
Endeavor® (III)(IV) (Sprint) Zotarolimus-eluting Coronary Stent System	Intraluminal Device, Drug-eluting in Heart and Great Vessels
Endologix AFX® Endovascular AAA System	Intraluminal Device
EndoSure® sensor	Monitoring Device, Pressure Sensor for Insertion in Heart and Great Vessels
ENDOTAK RELIANCE® (G) Defibrillation Lead	Cardiac Lead, Defibrillator for Insertion in Heart and Great Vessels
Endotracheal tube (cuffed)(double-lumen)	Intraluminal Device, Endotracheal Airway in Respiratory System
Endurant® Endovascular Stent Graft	Intraluminal Device
Endurant® II AAA stent graft system	Intraluminal Device
EnRhythm	Pacemaker, Dual Chamber for Insertion in Subcutaneous Tissue and Fascia
Enterra gastric neurostimulator	Stimulator Generator, Multiple Array for Insertion in Subcutaneous Tissue and Fascia
Epic™ Stented Tissue Valve (aortic)	Zooplastic Tissue in Heart and Great Vessels
Epicel® cultured epidermal autograft	Autologous Tissue Substitute
Esophageal obturator airway (EOA)	Intraluminal Device, Airway in Gastrointestinal System
Esteem® implantable hearing system	Hearing Device in Ear, Nose, Sinus
Evera (XT)(S)(DR/VR)	Defibrillator Generator for Insertion in Subcutaneous Tissue and Fascia
Everolimus-eluting coronary stent	Intraluminal Device, Drug-eluting in Heart and Great Vessels
Ex-PRESS™ mini glaucoma shunt	Synthetic Substitute
EXCLUDER® AAA Endoprosthesis	Intraluminal Device Intraluminal Device, Branched or Fenestrated, One or Two Arteries for Restriction in Lower Arteries Intraluminal Device, Branched or Fenestrated, Three or More Arteries for Restriction in Lower Arteries
EXCLUDER® IBE Endoprosthesis	Intraluminal Device, Branched or Fenestrated, One or Two Arteries for Restriction in Lower Arteries
Express® (LD) Premounted Stent System	Intraluminal Device
Express® Biliary SD Monorail® Premounted Stent System	Intraluminal Device
Express® SD Renal Monorail® Premounted Stent System	Intraluminal Device

Term	ICD-10-PCS Value
External fixator	External Fixation Device in Head and Facial Bones External Fixation Device in Upper Bones External Fixation Device in Lower Bones External Fixation Device in Upper Joints External Fixation Device in Lower Joints
EXtreme Lateral Interbody Fusion (XLIF) device	Interbody Fusion Device in Lower Joints
Facet replacement spinal stabilization device	Spinal Stabilization Device, Facet Replacement for Insertion in Upper Joints Spinal Stabilization Device, Facet Replacement for Insertion in Lower Joints
FLAIR® Endovascular Stent Graft	Intraluminal Device
Flexible Composite Mesh	Synthetic Substitute
Foley catheter	Drainage Device
Formula™ Balloon-Expandable Renal Stent System	Intraluminal Device
Freestyle (Stentless) Aortic Root Bioprosthesis	Zooplastic Tissue in Heart and Great Vessels
Fusion screw (compression)(lag)(locking)	Internal Fixation Device in Upper Joints Internal Fixation Device in Lower Joints
GammaTile™	Radioactive Element, Cesium-131 Collagen Implant for Insertion in Central Nervous System and Cranial Nerves
Gastric electrical stimulation (GES) lead	Stimulator Lead in Gastrointestinal System
Gastric pacemaker lead	Stimulator Lead in Gastrointestinal System
GORE EXCLUDER® AAA Endoprosthesis	Intraluminal Device Intraluminal Device, Branched or Fenestrated, One or Two Arteries for Restriction in Lower Arteries Intraluminal Device, Branched or Fenestrated, Three or More Arteries for Restriction in Lower Arteries
GORE EXCLUDER® IBE Endoprosthesis	Intraluminal Device, Branched or Fenestrated, One or Two Arteries for Restriction in Lower Arteries
GORE TAG® Thoracic Endoprosthesis	Intraluminal Device
GORE® DUALMESH®	Synthetic Substitute
Guedel airway	Intraluminal Device, Airway in Mouth and Throat
Hancock Bioprosthesis (aortic)(mitral) valve	Zooplastic Tissue in Heart and Great Vessels
Hancock Bioprosthetic Valved Conduit	Zooplastic Tissue in Heart and Great Vessels
HeartMate 3™ LVAS	Implantable Heart Assist System in Heart and Great Vessels
HeartMate II® Left Ventricular Assist Device (LVAD)	Implantable Heart Assist System in Heart and Great Vessels
HeartMate XVE® Left Ventricular Assist Device (LVAD)	Implantable Heart Assist System in Heart and Great Vessels
Herculink (RX) Elite Renal Stent System	Intraluminal Device

Term	ICD-10-PCS Value
Hip (joint) liner	Liner in Lower Joints
Holter valve ventricular shunt	Synthetic Substitute
Ilizarov external fixator	External Fixation Device, Ring for Insertion in Upper Bones External Fixation Device, Ring for Reposition in Upper Bones External Fixation Device, Ring for Insertion in Lower Bones External Fixation Device, Ring for Reposition in Lower Bones
Ilizarov-Vecklich device	External Fixation Device, Limb Lengthening for Insertion in Upper Bones External Fixation Device, Limb Lengthening for Insertion in Lower Bones
Impella® heart pump	Short-term External Heart Assist System in Heart and Great Vessels
Implantable cardioverter-defibrillator (ICD)	Defibrillator Generator for Insertion in Subcutaneous Tissue and Fascia
Implantable drug infusion pump (anti-spasmodic) (chemotherapy)(pain)	Infusion Device, Pump in Subcutaneous Tissue and Fascia
Implantable glucose monitoring device	Monitoring Device
Implantable hemodynamic monitor (IHM)	Monitoring Device, Hemodynamic for Insertion in Subcutaneous Tissue and Fascia
Implantable hemodynamic monitoring system (IHMS)	Monitoring Device, Hemodynamic for Insertion in Subcutaneous Tissue and Fascia
Implantable Miniature Telescope™ (IMT)	Synthetic Substitute, Intraocular Telescope for Replacement in Eye
Implanted (venous)(access) port	Vascular Access Device, Totally Implantable in Subcutaneous Tissue and Fascia
InDura, intrathecal catheter (1P) (spinal)	Infusion Device
Injection reservoir, port	Vascular Access Device, Totally Implantable in Subcutaneous Tissue and Fascia
Injection reservoir, pump	Infusion Device, Pump in Subcutaneous Tissue and Fascia
Interbody fusion (spine) cage	Interbody Fusion Device in Upper Joints Interbody Fusion Device in Lower Joints
Interspinous process spinal stabilization device	Spinal Stabilization Device, Interspinous Process for Insertion in Upper Joints Spinal Stabilization Device, Interspinous Process for Insertion in Lower Joints
InterStim® Therapy lead	Neurostimulator Lead in Peripheral Nervous System
InterStim® Therapy neurostimulator	Stimulator Generator, Single Array for Insertion in Subcutaneous Tissue and Fascia
Intramedullary (IM) rod (nail)	Internal Fixation Device, Intramedullary in Upper Bones Internal Fixation Device, Intramedullary in Lower Bones

Term	ICD-10-PCS Value
Intramedullary skeletal kinetic distractor (ISKD)	Internal Fixation Device, Intramedullary in Upper Bones Internal Fixation Device, Intramedullary in Lower Bones
Intrauterine Device (IUD)	Contraceptive Device in Female Reproductive System
INTUITY Elite valve system, EDWARDS	Zooplastic Tissue, Rapid Deployment Technique in New Technology
Itrel (3)(4) neurostimulator	Stimulator Generator, Single Array for Insertion in Subcutaneous Tissue and Fascia
Joint fixation plate	Internal Fixation Device in Upper Joints Internal Fixation Device in Lower Joints
Joint liner (insert)	Liner in Lower Joints
Joint spacer (antibiotic)	Spacer in Upper Joints Spacer in Lower Joints
Kappa	Pacemaker, Dual Chamber for Insertion in Subcutaneous Tissue and Fascia
Kirschner wire (K-wire)	Internal Fixation Device in Head and Facial Bones Internal Fixation Device in Upper Bones Internal Fixation Device in Lower Bones Internal Fixation Device in Upper Joints Internal Fixation Device in Lower Joints
Knee (implant) insert	Liner in Lower Joints
Kuntscher nail	Internal Fixation Device, Intramedullary in Upper Bones Internal Fixation Device, Intramedullary in Lower Bones
LAP-BAND® adjustable gastric banding system	Extraluminal Device
LifeStent® (Flexstar)(XL) Vascular Stent System	Intraluminal Device
LIVIAN™ CRT-D	Cardiac Resynchronization Defibrillator Pulse Generator for Insertion in Subcutaneous Tissue and Fascia
Loop recorder, implantable	Monitoring Device
MAGEC® Spinal Bracing and Distraction System	Magnetically Controlled Growth Rod(s) in New Technology
Mark IV Breathing Pacemaker System	Stimulator Generator in Subcutaneous Tissue and Fascia
Maximo II DR (VR)	Defibrillator Generator for Insertion in Subcutaneous Tissue and Fascia
Maximo II DR CRT-D	Cardiac Resynchronization Defibrillator Pulse Generator for Insertion in Subcutaneous Tissue and Fascia
Medtronic Endurant® II AAA stent graft system	Intraluminal Device
Melody® transcatheter pulmonary valve	Zooplastic Tissue in Heart and Great Vessels
Metal on metal bearing surface	Synthetic Substitute, Metal for Replacement in Lower Joints
Micro-Driver stent (RX) (OTW)	Intraluminal Device
MicroMed HeartAssist	Implantable Heart Assist System in Heart and Great Vessels
Micrus CERECYTE microcoil	Intraluminal Device, Bioactive in Upper Arteries
MIRODERM™ Biologic Wound Matrix	Skin Substitute, Porcine Liver Derived in New Technology
MitraClip valve repair system	Synthetic Substitute

Term	ICD-10-PCS Value
Mitroflow® Aortic Pericardial Heart Valve	Zooplastic Tissue in Heart and Great Vessels
Mosaic Bioprosthesis (aortic) (mitral) valve	Zooplastic Tissue in Heart and Great Vessels
MULTI-LINK (VISION)(MINI-VISION)(ULTRA) Coronary Stent System	Intraluminal Device
nanoLOCK™ interbody fusion device	Interbody Fusion Device, Nanotextured Surface in New Technology
Nasopharyngeal airway (NPA)	Intraluminal Device, Airway in Ear, Nose, Sinus
Neuromuscular electrical stimulation (NEMS) lead	Stimulator Lead in Muscles
Neurostimulator generator, multiple channel	Stimulator Generator, Multiple Array for Insertion in Subcutaneous Tissue and Fascia
Neurostimulator generator, multiple channel rechargeable	Stimulator Generator, Multiple Array Rechargeable for Insertion in Subcutaneous Tissue and Fascia
Neurostimulator generator, single channel	Stimulator Generator, Single Array for Insertion in Subcutaneous Tissue and Fascia
Neurostimulator generator, single channel rechargeable	Stimulator Generator, Single Array Rechargeable for Insertion in Subcutaneous Tissue and Fascia
Neutralization plate	Internal Fixation Device in Head and Facial Bones Internal Fixation Device in Upper Bones Internal Fixation Device in Lower Bones
Nitinol framed polymer mesh	Synthetic Substitute
Non-tunneled central venous catheter	Infusion Device
Novacor Left Ventricular Assist Device	Implantable Heart Assist System in Heart and Great Vessels
Novation® Ceramic AHS® (Articulation Hip System)	Synthetic Substitute, Ceramic for Replacement in Lower Joints
Omnilink Elite Vascular Balloon Expandable Stent System	Intraluminal Device
Open Pivot Aortic Valve Graft (AVG)	Synthetic Substitute
Open Pivot (mechanical) Valve	Synthetic Substitute
Optimizer™ III implantable pulse generator	Contractility Modulation Device for Insertion in Subcutaneous Tissue and Fascia
Oropharyngeal airway (OPA)	Intraluminal Device, Airway in Mouth and Throat
Ovatio™ CRT-D	Cardiac Resynchronization Defibrillator Pulse Generator for Insertion in Subcutaneous Tissue and Fascia
OXINIUM	Synthetic Substitute, Oxidized Zirconium on Polyethylene for Replacement in Lower Joints
Paclitaxel-eluting coronary stent	Intraluminal Device, Drug-eluting in Heart and Great Vessels
Paclitaxel-eluting peripheral stent	Intraluminal Device, Drug-eluting in Upper Arteries Intraluminal Device, Drug-eluting in Lower Arteries
Partially absorbable mesh	Synthetic Substitute

Term	ICD-10-PCS Value
Pedicle-based dynamic stabilization device	Spinal Stabilization Device, Pedicle-Based for Insertion in Upper Joints Spinal Stabilization Device, Pedicle-Based for Insertion in Lower Joints
Perceval sutureless valve	Zooplastic Tissue, Rapid Deployment Technique in New Technology
Percutaneous endoscopic gastrojejunostomy (PEG/J) tube	Feeding Device in Gastrointestinal System
Percutaneous endoscopic gastrostomy (PEG) tube	Feeding Device in Gastrointestinal System
Percutaneous nephrostomy catheter	Drainage Device
Peripherally inserted central catheter (PICC)	Infusion Device
Pessary ring	Intraluminal Device, Pessary in Female Reproductive System
Phrenic nerve stimulator generator	Stimulator Generator in Subcutaneous Tissue and Fascia
Phrenic nerve stimulator lead	Diaphragmatic Pacemaker Lead in Respiratory System
PHYSIOMESH™ Flexible Composite Mesh	Synthetic Substitute
Pipeline™ Embolization device (PED)	Intraluminal Device
Polyethylene socket	Synthetic Substitute, Polyethylene for Replacement in Lower Joints
Polymethylmethacrylate (PMMA)	Synthetic Substitute
Polypropylene mesh	Synthetic Substitute
Porcine (bioprosthetic) valve	Zooplastic Tissue in Heart and Great Vessels
PRESTIGE® Cervical Disc	Synthetic Substitute
PrimeAdvanced neurostimulator (SureScan)(MRI Safe)	Stimulator Generator, Multiple Array for Insertion in Subcutaneous Tissue and Fascia
PROCEED™ Ventral Patch	Synthetic Substitute
Prodisc-C	Synthetic Substitute
Prodisc-L	Synthetic Substitute
PROLENE Polypropylene Hernia System (PHS)	Synthetic Substitute
Protecta XT CRT-D	Cardiac Resynchronization Defibrillator Pulse Generator for Insertion in Subcutaneous Tissue and Fascia
Protecta XT DR (XT VR)	Defibrillator Generator for Insertion in Subcutaneous Tissue and Fascia
Protégé® RX Carotid Stent System	Intraluminal Device
Pump reservoir	Infusion Device, Pump in Subcutaneous Tissue and Fascia
REALIZE® Adjustable Gastric Band	Extraluminal Device
Rebound HRD® (Hernia Repair Device)	Synthetic Substitute
RestoreAdvanced neurostimulator (SureScan)(MRI Safe)	Stimulator Generator, Multiple Array Rechargeable for Insertion in Subcutaneous Tissue and Fascia
RestoreSensor neurostimulator (SureScan)(MRI Safe)	Stimulator Generator, Multiple Array Rechargeable for Insertion in Subcutaneous Tissue and Fascia
RestoreUltra neurostimulator (SureScan)(MRI Safe)	Stimulator Generator, Multiple Array Rechargeable for Insertion in Subcutaneous Tissue and Fascia

Term	ICD-10-PCS Value
Reveal (DX)(XT)	Monitoring Device
Reverse® Shoulder Prosthesis	Synthetic Substitute, Reverse Ball and Socket for Replacement in Upper Joints
Revo MRI™ SureScan® pacemaker	Pacemaker, Dual Chamber for Insertion in Subcutaneous Tissue and Fascia
Rheos® System device	Stimulator Generator in Subcutaneous Tissue and Fascia
Rheos® System lead	Stimulator Lead in Upper Arteries
RNS System lead	Neurostimulator Lead in Central Nervous System and Cranial Nerves
RNS system neurostimulator generator	Neurostimulator Generator in Head and Facial Bones
Sacral nerve modulation (SNM) lead	Stimulator Lead in Urinary System
Sacral neuromodulation lead	Stimulator Lead in Urinary System
SAPIEN transcatheter aortic valve	Zooplastic Tissue in Heart and Great Vessels
Secura (DR) (VR)	Defibrillator Generator for Insertion in Subcutaneous Tissue and Fascia
Sheffield hybrid external fixator	External Fixation Device, Hybrid for Insertion in Upper Bones External Fixation Device, Hybrid for Reposition in Upper Bones External Fixation Device, Hybrid for Insertion in Lower Bones External Fixation Device, Hybrid for Reposition in Lower Bones
Sheffield ring external fixator	External Fixation Device, Ring for Insertion in Upper Bones External Fixation Device, Ring for Reposition in Upper Bones External Fixation Device, Ring for Insertion in Lower Bones External Fixation Device, Ring for Reposition in Lower Bones
Single lead pacemaker (atrium)(ventricle)	Pacemaker, Single Chamber for Insertion in Subcutaneous Tissue and Fascia
Single lead rate responsive pacemaker (atrium)(ventricle)	Pacemaker, Single Chamber Rate Responsive for Insertion in Subcutaneous Tissue and Fascia
Sirolimus-eluting coronary stent	Intraluminal Device, Drug-eluting in Heart and Great Vessels
SJM Biocor® Stented Valve System	Zooplastic Tissue in Heart and Great Vessels
Spacer, Articulating (Antibiotic)	Articulating Spacer in Lower Joints
Spacer, Static (Antibiotic)	Spacer in Lower Joints
Spinal cord neurostimulator lead	Neurostimulator Lead in Central Nervous System and Cranial Nerves
Spinal growth rods, magnetically controlled	Magnetically Controlled Growth Rod(s) in New Technology
Spiration IBV™ Valve System	Intraluminal Device, Endobronchial Valve in Respiratory System
Static Spacer (Antibiotic)	Spacer in Lower Joints
Stent, intraluminal (cardiovascular)(gastrointestinal)(hepatobiliary)(urinary)	Intraluminal Device
Stented tissue valve	Zooplastic Tissue in Heart and Great Vessels
Stratos LV	Cardiac Resynchronization Pacemaker Pulse Generator for Insertion in Subcutaneous Tissue and Fascia

Term	ICD-10-PCS Value
Subcutaneous injection reservoir, port	Vascular Access Device, Totally Implantable in Subcutaneous Tissue and Fascia
Subcutaneous injection reservoir, pump	Infusion Device, Pump in Subcutaneous Tissue and Fascia
Subdermal progesterone implant	Contraceptive Device in Subcutaneous Tissue and Fascia
Sutureless valve, Perceval	Zooplastic Tissue, Rapid Deployment Technique in New Technology
SynCardia Total Artificial Heart	Synthetic Substitute
Synchra CRT-P	Cardiac Resynchronization Pacemaker Pulse Generator for Insertion in Subcutaneous Tissue and Fascia
SyncroMed Pump	Infusion Device, Pump in Subcutaneous Tissue and Fascia
Talent® Converter	Intraluminal Device
Talent® Occluder	Intraluminal Device
Talent® Stent Graft (abdominal)(thoracic)	Intraluminal Device
TandemHeart® System	Short-term External Heart Assist System in Heart and Great Vessels
TAXUS® Liberté® Paclitaxel-eluting Coronary Stent System	Intraluminal Device, Drug-eluting in Heart and Great Vessels
Therapeutic occlusion coil(s)	Intraluminal Device
Thoracostomy tube	Drainage Device
Thoratec IVAD (Implantable Ventricular Assist Device)	Implantable Heart Assist System in Heart and Great Vessels
Thoratec Paracorporeal Ventricular Assist Device	Short-term External Heart Assist System in Heart and Great Vessels
Tibial insert	Liner in Lower Joints
Tissue bank graft	Nonautologous Tissue Substitute
Tissue expander (inflatable)(injectable)	Tissue Expander in Skin and Breast Tissue Expander in Subcutaneous Tissue and Fascia
Titanium Sternal Fixation System (TSFS)	Internal Fixation Device, Rigid Plate for Insertion in Upper Bones Internal Fixation Device, Rigid Plate for Reposition in Upper Bones
Total artificial (replacement) heart	Synthetic Substitute
Tracheostomy tube	Tracheostomy Device in Respiratory System
Trifecta™ Valve (aortic)	Zooplastic Tissue in Heart and Great Vessels
Tunneled central venous catheter	Vascular Access Device, Tunneled in Subcutaneous Tissue and Fascia
Tunneled spinal (intrathecal) catheter	Infusion Device
Two lead pacemaker	Pacemaker, Dual Chamber for Insertion in Subcutaneous Tissue and Fascia
Ultraflex™ Precision Colonic Stent System	Intraluminal Device
ULTRAPRO Hernia System (UHS)	Synthetic Substitute
ULTRAPRO Partially Absorbable Lightweight Mesh	Synthetic Substitute
ULTRAPRO Plug	Synthetic Substitute

Term	ICD-10-PCS Value
Ultrasonic osteogenic stimulator	Bone Growth Stimulator in Head and Facial Bones Bone Growth Stimulator in Upper Bones Bone Growth Stimulator in Lower Bones
Ultrasound bone healing system	Bone Growth Stimulator in Head and Facial Bones Bone Growth Stimulator in Upper Bones Bone Growth Stimulator in Lower Bones
Uniplanar external fixator	External Fixation Device, Monoplanar for Insertion in Upper Bones External Fixation Device, Monoplanar for Reposition in Upper Bones External Fixation Device, Monoplanar for Insertion in Lower Bones External Fixation Device, Monoplanar for Reposition in Lower Bones
Urinary incontinence stimulator lead	Stimulator Lead in Urinary System
Vaginal pessary	Intraluminal Device, Pessary in Female Reproductive System
Valiant Thoracic Stent Graft	Intraluminal Device
Vectra® Vascular Access Graft	Vascular Access Device, Tunneled in Subcutaneous Tissue and Fascia
Ventrio™ Hernia Patch	Synthetic Substitute
Versa	Pacemaker, Dual Chamber for Insertion in Subcutaneous Tissue and Fascia
Virtuoso (II) (DR) (VR)	Defibrillator Generator for Insertion in Subcutaneous Tissue and Fascia
Viva(XT)(S)	Cardiac Resynchronization Defibrillator Pulse Generator for Insertion in Subcutaneous Tissue and Fascia
WALLSTENT® Endoprosthesis	Intraluminal Device

Term	ICD-10-PCS Value
X-STOP® Spacer	Spinal Stabilization Device, Interspinous Process for Insertion in Upper Joints Spinal Stabilization Device, Interspinous Process for Insertion in Lower Joints
Xact Carotid Stent System	Intraluminal Device
Xenograft	Zooplastic Tissue in Heart and Great Vessels
XIENCE Everolimus Eluting Coronary Stent System	Intraluminal Device, Drug-eluting in Heart and Great Vessels
XLIF® System	Interbody Fusion Device in Lower Joints
Zenith AAA Endovascular Graft	Intraluminal Device, Branched or Fenestrated, One or Two Arteries for Restriction in Lower Arteries Intraluminal Device, Branched or Fenestrated, Three or More Arteries for Restriction in Lower Arteries Intraluminal Device
Zenith Flex® AAA Endovascular Graft	Intraluminal Device
Zenith TX2® TAA Endovascular Graft	Intraluminal Device
Zenith® Renu™ AAA Ancillary Graft	Intraluminal Device
Zilver® PTX® (paclitaxel) Drug-Eluting Peripheral Stent	Intraluminal Device, Drug-eluting in Upper Arteries Intraluminal Device, Drug-eluting in Lower Arteries
Zimmer® NexGen® LPS Mobile Bearing Knee	Synthetic Substitute
Zimmer® NexGen® LPS-Flex Mobile Knee	Synthetic Substitute
Zotarolimus-eluting coronary stent	Intraluminal Device, Drug-eluting in Heart and Great Vessels

Device Aggregation Table

This table crosswalks specific device character value definitions for specific root operations in a specific body system to the more general device character value to be used when the root operation covers a wide range of body parts and the device character represents an entire family of devices.

Specific Device	for Operation	in Body System	General Device	
Autologous Arterial Tissue (A)	All applicable	Heart and Great Vessels Lower Arteries Lower Veins Upper Arteries Upper Veins	7	Autologous Tissue Substitute
Autologous Venous Tissue (9)	All applicable	Heart and Great Vessels Lower Arteries Lower Veins Upper Arteries Upper Veins	7	Autologous Tissue Substitute
Cardiac Lead, Defibrillator (K)	Insertion	Heart and Great Vessels	M	Cardiac Lead
Cardiac Lead, Pacemaker (J)	Insertion	Heart and Great Vessels	M	Cardiac Lead
Cardiac Resynchronization Defibrillator Pulse Generator (9)	Insertion	Subcutaneous Tissue and Fascia	P	Cardiac Rhythm Related Device
Cardiac Resynchronization Pacemaker Pulse Generator (7)	Insertion	Subcutaneous Tissue and Fascia	P	Cardiac Rhythm Related Device
Contractility Modulation Device (A)	Insertion	Subcutaneous Tissue and Fascia	P	Cardiac Rhythm Related Device
Defibrillator Generator (8)	Insertion	Subcutaneous Tissue and Fascia	P	Cardiac Rhythm Related Device
Epiretinal Visual Prosthesis (5)	All applicable	Eye	J	Synthetic Substitute
External Fixation Device, Hybrid (D)	Insertion	Lower Bones Upper Bones	5	External Fixation Device
External Fixation Device, Hybrid (D)	Reposition	Lower Bones Upper Bones	5	External Fixation Device
External Fixation Device, Limb Lengthening (8)	Insertion	Lower Bones Upper Bones	5	External Fixation Device
External Fixation Device, Monoplanar (B)	Insertion	Lower Bones Upper Bones	5	External Fixation Device
External Fixation Device, Monoplanar (B)	Reposition	Lower Bones Upper Bones	5	External Fixation Device
External Fixation Device, Ring (C)	Insertion	Lower Bones Upper Bones	5	External Fixation Device
External Fixation Device, Ring (C)	Reposition	Lower Bones Upper Bones	5	External Fixation Device
Hearing Device, Bone Conduction (4)	Insertion	Ear, Nose, Sinus	S	Hearing Device
Hearing Device, Multiple Channel Cochlear Prosthesis (6)	Insertion	Ear, Nose, Sinus	S	Hearing Device
Hearing Device, Single Channel Cochlear Prosthesis (5)	Insertion	Ear, Nose, Sinus	S	Hearing Device
Internal Fixation Device, Intramedullary (6)	All applicable	Lower Bones Upper Bones	4	Internal Fixation Device
Internal Fixation Device, Rigid Plate (Ø)	Insertion	Upper Bones	4	Internal Fixation Device
Internal Fixation Device, Rigid Plate (Ø)	Reposition	Upper Bones	4	Internal Fixation Device
Intraluminal Device, Airway (B)	All applicable	Ear, Nose, Sinus Gastrointestinal System Mouth and Throat	D	Intraluminal Device
Intraluminal Device, Bioactive (B)	All applicable	Upper Arteries	D	Intraluminal Device
Intraluminal Device, Branched or Fenestrated, One or Two Arteries (E)	Restriction	Heart and Great Vessels Lower Arteries	D	Intraluminal Device
Intraluminal Device, Branched or Fenestrated, Three or More Arteries (F)	Restriction	Heart and Great Vessels Lower Arteries	D	Intraluminal Device
Intraluminal Device, Drug-eluting (4)	All applicable	Heart and Great Vessels Lower Arteries Upper Arteries	D	Intraluminal Device
Intraluminal Device, Drug-eluting, Four or More (7)	All applicable	Heart and Great Vessels Lower Arteries Upper Arteries	D	Intraluminal Device

Specific Device	for Operation	in Body System	General Device	
Intraluminal Device, Drug-eluting, Three (6)	All applicable	Heart and Great Vessels Lower Arteries Upper Arteries	**D**	Intraluminal Device
Intraluminal Device, Drug-eluting, Two (5)	All applicable	Heart and Great Vessels Lower Arteries Upper Arteries	**D**	Intraluminal Device
Intraluminal Device, Endobronchial Valve (G)	All applicable	Respiratory System	**D**	Intraluminal Device
Intraluminal Device, Endotracheal Airway (E)	All applicable	Respiratory System	**D**	Intraluminal Device
Intraluminal Device, Four or More (G)	All applicable	Heart and Great Vessels Lower Arteries Upper Arteries	**D**	Intraluminal Device
Intraluminal Device, Pessary (G)	All applicable	Female Reproductive System	**D**	Intraluminal Device
Intraluminal Device, Radioactive (T)	All applicable	Heart and Great Vessels	**D**	Intraluminal Device
Intraluminal Device, Three (F)	All applicable	Heart and Great Vessels Lower Arteries Upper Arteries	**D**	Intraluminal Device
Intraluminal Device, Two (E)	All applicable	Heart and Great Vessels Lower Arteries Upper Arteries	**D**	Intraluminal Device
Monitoring Device, Hemodynamic (Ø)	Insertion	Subcutaneous Tissue and Fascia	**2**	Monitoring Device
Monitoring Device, Pressure Sensor (Ø)	Insertion	Heart and Great Vessels	**2**	Monitoring Device
Pacemaker, Dual Chamber (6)	Insertion	Subcutaneous Tissue and Fascia	**P**	Cardiac Rhythm Related Device
Pacemaker, Single Chamber (4)	Insertion	Subcutaneous Tissue and Fascia	**P**	Cardiac Rhythm Related Device
Pacemaker, Single Chamber Rate Responsive (5)	Insertion	Subcutaneous Tissue and Fascia	**P**	Cardiac Rhythm Related Device
Spinal Stabilization Device, Facet Replacement (D)	Insertion	Lower Joints Upper Joints	**4**	Internal Fixation Device
Spinal Stabilization Device, Interspinous Process (B)	Insertion	Lower Joints Upper Joints	**4**	Internal Fixation Device
Spinal Stabilization Device, Pedicle-Based (C)	Insertion	Lower Joints Upper Joints	**4**	Internal Fixation Device
Stimulator Generator, Multiple Array (D)	Insertion	Subcutaneous Tissue and Fascia	**M**	Stimulator Generator
Stimulator Generator, Multiple Array Rechargeable (E)	Insertion	Subcutaneous Tissue and Fascia	**M**	Stimulator Generator
Stimulator Generator, Single Array (B)	Insertion	Subcutaneous Tissue and Fascia	**M**	Stimulator Generator
Stimulator Generator, Single Array Rechargeable (C)	Insertion	Subcutaneous Tissue and Fascia	**M**	Stimulator Generator
Synthetic Substitute, Ceramic (3)	Replacement	Lower Joints	**J**	Synthetic Substitute
Synthetic Substitute, Ceramic on Polyethylene (4)	Replacement	Lower Joints	**J**	Synthetic Substitute
Synthetic Substitute, Intraocular Telescope (Ø)	Replacement	Eye	**J**	Synthetic Substitute
Synthetic Substitute, Metal (1)	Replacement	Lower Joints	**J**	Synthetic Substitute
Synthetic Substitute, Metal on Polyethylene (2)	Replacement	Lower Joints	**J**	Synthetic Substitute
Synthetic Substitute, Oxidized Zirconium on Polyethylene (6)	Replacement	Lower Joints	**J**	Synthetic Substitute
Synthetic Substitute, Polyethylene (Ø)	Replacement	Lower Joints	**J**	Synthetic Substitute
Synthetic Substitute, Reverse Ball and Socket (Ø)	Replacement	Upper Joints	**J**	Synthetic Substitute

Appendix G: Device Definitions

ICD-10-PCS Value	Definition
Articulating Spacer in Lower Joints	**Includes:** Articulating Spacer (Antibiotic) Spacer, Articulating (Antibiotic)
Artificial Sphincter in Gastrointestinal System	**Includes:** Artificial anal sphincter (AAS) Artificial bowel sphincter (neosphincter)
Artificial Sphincter in Urinary System	**Includes:** AMS 800® Urinary Control System Artificial urinary sphincter (AUS)
Autologous Arterial Tissue in Heart and Great Vessels	**Includes:** Autologous artery graft
Autologous Arterial Tissue in Lower Arteries	**Includes:** Autologous artery graft
Autologous Arterial Tissue in Lower Veins	**Includes:** Autologous artery graft
Autologous Arterial Tissue in Upper Arteries	**Includes:** Autologous artery graft
Autologous Arterial Tissue in Upper Veins	**Includes:** Autologous artery graft
Autologous Tissue Substitute	**Includes:** Autograft Cultured epidermal cell autograft Epicel® cultured epidermal autograft
Autologous Venous Tissue in Heart and Great Vessels	**Includes:** Autologous vein graft
Autologous Venous Tissue in Lower Arteries	**Includes:** Autologous vein graft
Autologous Venous Tissue in Lower Veins	**Includes:** Autologous vein graft
Autologous Venous Tissue in Upper Arteries	**Includes:** Autologous vein graft
Autologous Venous Tissue in Upper Veins	**Includes:** Autologous vein graft
Bone Growth Stimulator in Head and Facial Bones	**Includes:** Electrical bone growth stimulator (EBGS) Ultrasonic osteogenic stimulator Ultrasound bone healing system
Bone Growth Stimulator in Lower Bones	**Includes:** Electrical bone growth stimulator (EBGS) Ultrasonic osteogenic stimulator Ultrasound bone healing system
Bone Growth Stimulator in Upper Bones	**Includes:** Electrical bone growth stimulator (EBGS) Ultrasonic osteogenic stimulator Ultrasound bone healing system
Cardiac Lead in Heart and Great Vessels	**Includes:** Cardiac contractility modulation lead

ICD-10-PCS Value	Definition
Cardiac Lead, Defibrillator for Insertion in Heart and Great Vessels	**Includes:** ACUITY™ Steerable Lead Attain Ability® lead Attain StarFix® (OTW) lead Cardiac resynchronization therapy (CRT) lead Corox (OTW) Bipolar Lead Durata® Defibrillation Lead ENDOTAK RELIANCE® (G) Defibrillation Lead
Cardiac Lead, Pacemaker for Insertion in Heart and Great Vessels	**Includes:** ACUITY™ Steerable Lead Attain Ability® lead Attain StarFix® (OTW) lead Cardiac resynchronization therapy (CRT) lead Corox (OTW) Bipolar Lead
Cardiac Resynchronization Defibrillator Pulse Generator for Insertion in Subcutaneous Tissue and Fascia	**Includes:** COGNIS® CRT-D Concerto II CRT-D Consulta CRT-D CONTAK RENEWA® 3 RF (HE) CRT-D LIVIAN™ CRT-D Maximo II DR CRT-D Ovatio™ CRT-D Protecta XT CRT-D Viva (XT)(S)
Cardiac Resynchronization Pacemaker Pulse Generator for Insertion in Subcutaneous Tissue and Fascia	**Includes:** Consulta CRT-P Stratos LV Synchra CRT-P
Contraceptive Device in Female Reproductive System	**Includes:** Intrauterine device (IUD)
Contraceptive Device in Subcutaneous Tissue and Fascia	**Includes:** Subdermal progesterone implant
Contractility Modulation Device for Insertion in Subcutaneous Tissue and Fascia	**Includes:** Optimizer™ III implantable pulse generator
Defibrillator Generator for Insertion in Subcutaneous Tissue and Fascia	**Includes:** Evera (XT)(S)(DR/VR) Implantable cardioverter-defibrillator (ICD) Maximo II DR (VR) Protecta XT DR (XT VR) Secura (DR) (VR) Virtuoso (II) (DR) (VR)
Diaphragmatic Pacemaker Lead in Respiratory System	**Includes:** Phrenic nerve stimulator lead
Drainage Device	**Includes:** Cystostomy tube Foley catheter Percutaneous nephrostomy catheter Thoracostomy tube
External Fixation Device in Head and Facial Bones	**Includes:** External fixator
External Fixation Device in Lower Bones	**Includes:** External fixator
External Fixation Device in Lower Joints	**Includes:** External fixator

ICD-10-PCS Value	Definition
External Fixation Device in Upper Bones	**Includes:** External fixator
External Fixation Device in Upper Joints	**Includes:** External fixator
External Fixation Device, Hybrid for Insertion in Lower Bones	**Includes:** Delta frame external fixator Sheffield hybrid external fixator
External Fixation Device, Hybrid for Insertion in Upper Bones	**Includes:** Delta frame external fixator Sheffield hybrid external fixator
External Fixation Device, Hybrid for Reposition in Lower Bones	**Includes:** Delta frame external fixator Sheffield hybrid external fixator
External Fixation Device, Hybrid for Reposition in Upper Bones	**Includes:** Delta frame external fixator Sheffield hybrid external fixator
External Fixation Device, Limb Lengthening for Insertion in Lower Bones	**Includes:** Ilizarov-Vecklich device
External Fixation Device, Limb Lengthening for Insertion in Upper Bones	**Includes:** Ilizarov-Vecklich device
External Fixation Device, Monoplanar for Insertion in Lower Bones	**Includes:** Uniplanar external fixator
External Fixation Device, Monoplanar for Insertion in Upper Bones	**Includes:** Uniplanar external fixator
External Fixation Device, Monoplanar for Reposition in Lower Bones	**Includes:** Uniplanar external fixator
External Fixation Device, Monoplanar for Reposition in Upper Bones	**Includes:** Uniplanar external fixator
External Fixation Device, Ring for Insertion in Lower Bones	**Includes:** Ilizarov external fixator Sheffield ring external fixator
External Fixation Device, Ring for Insertion in Upper Bones	**Includes:** Ilizarov external fixator Sheffield ring external fixator
External Fixation Device, Ring for Reposition in Lower Bones	**Includes:** Ilizarov external fixator Sheffield ring external fixator
External Fixation Device, Ring for Reposition in Upper Bones	**Includes:** Ilizarov external fixator Sheffield ring external fixator
Extraluminal Device	**Includes:** AtriClip LAA Exclusion System LAP-BAND® adjustable gastric banding system REALIZE® Adjustable Gastric Band
Feeding Device in Gastrointestinal System	**Includes:** Percutaneous endoscopic gastrojejunostomy (PEG/J) tube Percutaneous endoscopic gastrostomy (PEG) tube
Hearing Device in Ear, Nose, Sinus	**Includes:** Esteem® implantable hearing system
Hearing Device in Head and Facial Bones	**Includes:** Bone anchored hearing device

ICD-10-PCS Value	Definition
Hearing Device, Bone Conduction for Insertion in Ear, Nose, Sinus	**Includes:** Bone anchored hearing device
Hearing Device, Multiple Channel Cochlear Prosthesis for Insertion in Ear, Nose, Sinus	**Includes:** Cochlear implant (CI), multiple channel (electrode)
Hearing Device, Single Channel Cochlear Prosthesis for Insertion in Ear, Nose, Sinus	**Includes:** Cochlear implant (CI), single channel (electrode)
Implantable Heart Assist System in Heart and Great Vessels	**Includes:** Berlin Heart Ventricular Assist Device DeBakey Left Ventricular Assist Device DuraHeart Left Ventricular Assist System HeartMate 3™ LVAS HeartMate II® Left Ventricular Assist Device (LVAD) HeartMate XVE® Left Ventricular Assist Device (LVAD) MicroMed HeartAssist Novacor Left Ventricular Assist Device Thoratec IVAD (Implantable Ventricular Assist Device)
Infusion Device	**Includes:** Ascenda Intrathecal Catheter InDura, intrathecal catheter (1P) (spinal) Non-tunneled central venous catheter Peripherally inserted central catheter (PICC) Tunneled spinal (intrathecal) catheter
Infusion Device, Pump in Subcutaneous Tissue and Fascia	**Includes:** Implantable drug infusion pump (anti-spasmodic)(chemotherapy) (pain) Injection reservoir, pump Pump reservoir Subcutaneous injection reservoir, pump SynchroMed pump
Interbody Fusion Device in Lower Joints	**Includes:** Axial Lumbar Interbody Fusion System AxiaLIF® System CoRoent® XL Direct Lateral Interbody Fusion (DLIF) device EXtreme Lateral Interbody Fusion (XLIF) device Interbody fusion (spine) cage XLIF® System
Interbody Fusion Device in Upper Joints	**Includes:** BAK/C® Interbody Cervical Fusion System Interbody fusion (spine) cage
Interbody Fusion Device, Nanotextured Surface in New Technology	**Includes:** nanoLOCK™ interbody fusion device

ICD-10-PCS Value	Definition
Interbody Fusion Device, Radiolucent Porous in New Technology	**Includes:** COALESCE® radiolucent interbody fusion device COHERE® radiolucent interbody fusion device
Internal Fixation Device in Head and Facial Bones	**Includes:** Bone screw (interlocking)(lag)(pedicle)(recessed) Kirschner wire (K-wire) Neutralization plate
Internal Fixation Device in Lower Bones	**Includes:** Bone screw (interlocking)(lag)(pedicle)(recessed) Clamp and rod internal fixation system (CRIF) Kirschner wire (K-wire) Neutralization plate
Internal Fixation Device in Lower Joints	**Includes:** Fusion screw (compression)(lag)(locking) Joint fixation plate Kirschner wire (K-wire)
Internal Fixation Device in Upper Bones	**Includes:** Bone screw (interlocking)(lag)(pedicle)(recessed) Clamp and rod internal fixation system (CRIF) Kirschner wire (K-wire) Neutralization plate
Internal Fixation Device in Upper Joints	**Includes:** Fusion screw (compression)(lag)(locking) Joint fixation plate Kirschner wire (K-wire)
Internal Fixation Device, Intramedullary in Lower Bones	**Includes:** Intramedullary (IM) rod (nail) Intramedullary skeletal kinetic distractor (ISKD) Kuntscher nail
Internal Fixation Device, Intramedullary in Upper Bones	**Includes:** Intramedullary (IM) rod (nail) Intramedullary skeletal kinetic distractor (ISKD) Kuntscher nail
Internal Fixation Device, Rigid Plate for Insertion in Upper Bones	**Includes:** Titanium Sternal Fixation System (TSFS)
Internal Fixation Device, Rigid Plate for Reposition in Upper Bones	**Includes:** Titanium Sternal Fixation System (TSFS)

ICD-10-PCS Value	Definition
Intraluminal Device	**Includes:** Absolute Pro Vascular (OTW) Self-Expanding Stent System Acculink (RX) Carotid Stent System AFX® Endovascular AAA System AneuRx® AAA Advantage® Assurant (Cobalt) stent Carotid WALLSTENT® Monorail® Endoprosthesis CoAxia NeuroFlo catheter Colonic Z-Stent® Complete (SE) stent Cook Zenith AAA Endovascular Graft Driver stent (RX) (OTW) E-Luminexx™ (Biliary)(Vascular) Stent Embolization coil(s) Endologix AFX® Endovascular AAA System Endurant® Endovascular Stent Graft Endurant® II AAA stent graft system EXCLUDER® AAA Endoprosthesis Express® (LD) Premounted Stent System Express® Biliary SD Monorail® Premounted Stent System Express® SD Renal Monorail® Premounted Stent System FLAIR® Endovascular Stent Graft Formula™ Balloon-Expandable Renal Stent System GORE EXCLUDER® AAA Endoprosthesis GORE TAG® Thoracic Endoprosthesis Herculink (RX) Elite Renal Stent System LifeStent® (Flexstar)(XL) Vascular Stent System Medtronic Endurant® II AAA stent graft system Micro-Driver stent (RX) (OTW) MULTI-LINK (VISION)(MINI-VISION)(ULTRA) Coronary Stent System Omnilink Elite Vascular Balloon Expandable Stent System Pipeline™ Embolization device (PED) Protege® RX Carotid Stent System Stent, intraluminal (cardiovascular)(gastrointestinal)(hepatobiliary)(urinary) Talent® Converter Talent® Occluder Talent® Stent Graft (abdominal)(thoracic) Therapeutic occlusion coil(s) Ultraflex™ Precision Colonic Stent System Valiant Thoracic Stent Graft WALLSTENT® Endoprosthesis Xact Carotid Stent System Zenith AAA Endovascular Graft Zenith Flex® AAA Endovascular Graft Zenith TX2® TAA Endovascular Graft Zenith® Renu™ AAA Ancillary Graft
Intraluminal Device, Airway in Ear, Nose, Sinus	**Includes:** Nasopharyngeal airway (NPA)
Intraluminal Device, Airway in Gastrointestinal System	**Includes:** Esophageal obturator airway (EOA)

ICD-10-PCS Value	Definition
Intraluminal Device, Airway in Mouth and Throat	**Includes:** Guedel airway Oropharyngeal airway (OPA)
Intraluminal Device, Bioactive in Upper Arteries	**Includes:** Bioactive embolization coil(s) Micrus CERECYTE microcoil
Intraluminal Device, Branched or Fenestrated, One or Two Arteries for Restriction in Lower Arteries	**Includes:** Cook Zenith AAA Endovascular Graft EXCLUDER® AAA Endoprosthesis EXCLUDER® IBE Endoprosthesis GORE EXCLUDER® AAA Endoprosthesis GORE EXCLUDER®IBE Endoprosthesis Zenith AAA Endovascular Graft
Intraluminal Device, Branched or Fenestrated, Three or More Arteries for Restriction in Lower Arteries	**Includes:** Cook Zenith AAA Endovascular Graft EXCLUDER® AAA Endoprosthesis GORE EXCLUDER® AAA Endoprosthesis Zenith AAA Endovascular Graft

Intraluminal Device, Drug-eluting in Heart and Great Vessels	**Includes:**
	CYPHER® Stent
	Endeavor® (III)(IV) (Sprint)
	  Zotarolimus-eluting Coronary Stent
	  System
	Everolimus-eluting coronary stent
	Paclitaxel-eluting coronary stent
	Sirolimus-eluting coronary stent
	TAXUS® Liberte® Paclitaxel-eluting
	  Coronary Stent System
	XIENCE Everolimus Eluting Coronary
	  Stent System
	Zotarolimus-eluting coronary stent

Intraluminal Device, Drug-eluting in Lower Arteries	**Includes:** Paclitaxel-eluting peripheral stent Zilver® PTX® (paclitaxel) Drug-Eluting Peripheral Stent
Intraluminal Device, Drug-eluting in Upper Arteries	**Includes:** Paclitaxel-eluting peripheral stent Zilver® PTX® (paclitaxel) Drug-Eluting Peripheral Stent
Intraluminal Device, Endobronchial Valve in Respiratory System	**Includes:** Spiration IBV™ Valve System
Intraluminal Device, Endotracheal Airway in Respiratory System	**Includes:** Endotracheal tube (cuffed)(double-lumen)
Intraluminal Device, Pessary in Female Reproductive System	**Includes:** Pessary ring Vaginal pessary
Liner in Lower Joints	**Includes:** Acetabular cup Hip (joint) liner Joint liner (insert) Knee (implant) insert Tibial insert

Magnetically Controlled Growth Rod(s) in New Technology	**Includes:**
	MAGEC® Spinal Bracing and
	  Distraction System
	Spinal growth rods, magnetically
	  controlled

ICD-10-PCS Value	Definition

Monitoring Device	**Includes:**
	Blood glucose monitoring system
	Cardiac event recorder
	Continuous Glucose Monitoring
	  (CGM) device
	Implantable glucose monitoring
	  device
	Loop recorder, implantable
	Reveal (DX)(XT)

Monitoring Device, Hemodynamic for Insertion in Subcutaneous Tissue and Fascia	**Includes:**
	Implantable hemodynamic monitor
	  (IHM)
	Implantable hemodynamic
	  monitoring system (IHMS)

Monitoring Device, Pressure Sensor for Insertion in Heart and Great Vessels	**Includes:** CardioMEMS® pressure sensor EndoSure® sensor
Neurostimulator Generator in Head and Facial Bones	**Includes:** RNS system neurostimulator generator
Neurostimulator Lead in Central Nervous System and Cranial Nerves	**Includes:** Cortical strip neurostimulator lead DBS lead Deep brain neurostimulator lead RNS System lead Spinal cord neurostimulator lead
Neurostimulator Lead in Peripheral Nervous System	**Includes:** InterStim® Therapy lead
Nonautologous Tissue Substitute	**Includes:** Acellular Hydrated Dermis Bone bank bone graft Cook Biodesign® Fistula Plug(s) Cook Biodesign® Hernia Graft(s) Cook Biodesign® Layered Graft(s) Cook Zenapro™ Layered Graft(s) Tissue bank graft
Pacemaker, Dual Chamber for Insertion in Subcutaneous Tissue and Fascia	**Includes:** Advisa (MRI) EnRhythm Kappa Revo MRI™ SureScan® pacemaker Two lead pacemaker Versa
Pacemaker, Single Chamber for Insertion in Subcutaneous Tissue and Fascia	**Includes:** Single lead pacemaker (atrium)(ventricle)
Pacemaker, Single Chamber Rate Responsive for Insertion in Subcutaneous Tissue and Fascia	**Includes:** Single lead rate responsive pacemaker (atrium)(ventricle)
Radioactive Element	**Includes:** Brachytherapy seeds
Radioactive Element, Cesium-131 Collagen Implant for Insertion in Central Nervous System and Cranial Nerves	**Includes:** Cesium-131 Collagen Implant GammaTile™
Resurfacing Device in Lower Joints	**Includes:** CONSERVE® PLUS Total Resurfacing Hip System Cormet Hip Resurfacing System

ICD-10-PCS Value	Definition
Short-term External Heart Assist System in Heart and Great Vessels	**Includes:** Biventricular external heart assist system BVS 5ØØØ Ventricular Assist Device Centrimag® Blood Pump Impella® heart pump TandemHeart® System Thoratec Paracorporeal Ventricular Assist Device
Skin Substitute, Porcine Liver Derived in New Technology	**Includes:** MIRODERM™ Biologic Wound Matrix
Spacer in Lower Joints	**Includes:** Joint spacer (antibiotic) Spacer, Static (Antibiotic) Static Spacer (Antibiotic)
Spacer in Upper Joints	**Includes:** Joint spacer (antibiotic)
Spinal Stabilization Device, Facet Replacement for Insertion in Lower Joints	**Includes:** Facet replacement spinal stabilization device
Spinal Stabilization Device, Facet Replacement for Insertion in Upper Joints	**Includes:** Facet replacement spinal stabilization device
Spinal Stabilization Device, Interspinous Process for Insertion in Lower Joints	**Includes:** Interspinous process spinal stabilization device X-STOP® Spacer
Spinal Stabilization Device, Interspinous Process for Insertion in Upper Joints	**Includes:** Interspinous process spinal stabilization device X-STOP® Spacer
Spinal Stabilization Device, Pedicle- Based for Insertion in Lower Joints	**Includes:** Dynesys® Dynamic Stabilization System Pedicle-based dynamic stabilization device
Spinal Stabilization Device, Pedicle-Based for Insertion in Upper Joints	**Includes:** Dynesys® Dynamic Stabilization System Pedicle-based dynamic stabilization device
Stimulator Generator in Subcutaneous Tissue and Fascia	**Includes:** Baroreflex Activation Therapy® (BAT®) Diaphragmatic pacemaker generator Mark IV Breathing Pacemaker System Phrenic nerve stimulator generator Rheos® System device
Stimulator Generator, Multiple Array for Insertion in Subcutaneous Tissue and Fascia	**Includes:** Activa PC neurostimulator Enterra gastric neurostimulator Neurostimulator generator, multiple channel PrimeAdvanced neurostimulator (SureScan)(MRI Safe)

ICD-10-PCS Value	Definition
Stimulator Generator, Multiple Array Rechargeable for Insertion in Subcutaneous Tissue and Fascia	**Includes:** Activa RC neurostimulator Neurostimulator generator, multiple channel rechargeable RestoreAdvanced neurostimulator (SureScan)(MRI Safe) RestoreSensor neurostimulator (SureScan)(MRI Safe) RestoreUltra neurostimulator (SureScan)(MRI Safe)
Stimulator Generator, Single Array for Insertion in Subcutaneous Tissue and Fascia	**Includes:** Activa SC neurostimulator InterStim® Therapy neurostimulator Itrel (3)(4) neurostimulator Neurostimulator generator, single channel
Stimulator Generator, Single Array Rechargeable for Insertion in Subcutaneous Tissue and Fascia	**Includes:** Neurostimulator generator, single channel rechargeable
Stimulator Lead in Gastrointestinal System	**Includes:** Gastric electrical stimulation (GES) lead Gastric pacemaker lead
Stimulator Lead in Muscles	**Includes:** Electrical muscle stimulation (EMS) lead Electronic muscle stimulator lead Neuromuscular electrical stimulation (NEMS) lead
Stimulator Lead in Upper Arteries	**Includes:** Baroreflex Activation Therapy® (BAT®) Carotid (artery) sinus (baroreceptor) lead Rheos® System lead
Stimulator Lead in Urinary System	**Includes:** Sacral nerve modulation (SNM) lead Sacral neuromodulation lead Urinary incontinence stimulator lead
Synthetic Substitute	**Includes:** AbioCor® Total Replacement Heart AMPLATZER® Muscular VSD Occluder Annuloplasty ring Bard® Composix® (E/X) (LP) mesh Bard® Composix® Kugel® patch Bard® Dulex™ mesh Bard® Ventralex™ hernia patch BRYAN® Cervical Disc System Ex-PRESS™ mini glaucoma shunt Flexible Composite Mesh GORE® DUALMESH® Holter valve ventricular shunt MitraClip valve repair system Nitinol framed polymer mesh Open Pivot (mechanical) valve Open Pivot Aortic Valve Graft (AVG) Partially absorbable mesh PHYSIOMESH™ Flexible Composite Mesh

Continued on next column

Appendix G: Device Definitions

ICD-10-PCS Value	Definition
Synthetic Substitute (continued)	**Includes:** Polymethylmethacrylate (PMMA) Polypropylene mesh PRESTIGE® Cervical Disc PROCEED™ Ventral Patch Prodisc-C Prodisc-L PROLENE Polypropylene Hernia System (PHS) Rebound HRD® (Hernia Repair Device) SynCardia Total Artificial Heart Total artificial (replacement) heart ULTRAPRO Hernia System (UHS) ULTRAPRO Partially Absorbable Lightweight Mesh ULTRAPRO Plug Ventrio™ Hernia Patch Zimmer® NexGen® LPS Mobile Bearing Knee Zimmer® NexGen® LPS-Flex Mobile Knee
Synthetic Substitute, Ceramic for Replacement in Lower Joints	**Includes:** Ceramic on ceramic bearing surface Novation® Ceramic AHS® (Articulation Hip System)
Synthetic Substitute, Intraocular Telescope for Replacement in Eye	**Includes:** Implantable Miniature Telescope™ (IMT)
Synthetic Substitute, Metal for Replacement in Lower Joints	**Includes:** Cobalt/chromium head and socket Metal on metal bearing surface
Synthetic Substitute, Metal on Polyethylene for Replacement in Lower Joints	**Includes:** Cobalt/chromium head and polyethylene socket
Synthetic Substitute, Oxidized Zirconium on Polyethylene for Replacement in Lower Joints	**Includes:** OXINIUM
Synthetic Substitute, Polyethylene for Replacement in Lower Joints	**Includes:** Polyethylene socket
Synthetic Substitute, Reverse Ball and Socket for Replacement in Upper Joints	**Includes:** Delta III Reverse shoulder prosthesis Reverse® Shoulder Prosthesis
Tissue Expander in Skin and Breast	**Includes:** Tissue expander (inflatable) (injectable)

ICD-10-PCS Value	Definition
Tissue Expander in Subcutaneous Tissue and Fascia	**Includes:** Tissue expander (inflatable) (injectable)
Tracheostomy Device in Respiratory System	**Includes:** Tracheostomy tube
Vascular Access Device, Totally Implantable in Subcutaneous Tissue and Fascia	**Includes:** Implanted (venous)(access) port Injection reservoir, port Subcutaneous injection reservoir, port
Vascular Access Device, Tunneled in Subcutaneous Tissue and Fascia	**Includes:** Tunneled central venous catheter Vectra® Vascular Access Graft
Zooplastic Tissue in Heart and Great Vessels	**Includes:** 3f (Aortic) Bioprosthesis valve Bovine pericardial valve Bovine pericardium graft Contegra Pulmonary Valved Conduit CoreValve transcatheter aortic valve Epic™ Stented Tissue Valve (aortic) Freestyle (Stentless) Aortic Root Bioprosthesis Hancock Bioprosthesis (aortic) (mitral) valve Hancock Bioprosthetic Valved Conduit Melody® transcatheter pulmonary valve Mitroflow® Aortic Pericardial Heart Valve Mosaic Bioprosthesis (aortic) (mitral) valve Porcine (bioprosthetic) valve SAPIEN transcatheter aortic valve SJM Biocor® Stented Valve System Stented tissue valve Trifecta™ Valve (aortic) Xenograft
Zooplastic Tissue, Rapid Deployment Technique in New Technology	**Includes:** EDWARDS INTUITY Elite valve system INTUITY Elite valve system, EDWARDS Perceval sutureless valve Sutureless valve, Perceval

Appendix H: Substance Key/Substance Definitions

Substance Key

This table crosswalks a specific substance, listed by trade name or synonym, to the PCS value that would be used to represent that substance in either the Administration or New Technology section. The ICD-10-PCS value may be located in either the 6th-character Substance column or the 7th-character Qualifier column depending on the section/table to which it is classified. The most specific character is listed in the table.

Trade Name or Synonym	ICD-10-PCS Value	PCS Section
AIGISRx Antibacterial Envelope	Anti-Infective Envelope (A)	Administration (3)
Angiotensin II	Synthetic Human Angiotensin II	New technology (X)
Antimicrobial envelope	Anti-Infective Envelope (A)	Administration (3)
Axicabtagene Ciloeucel	Engineered Autologous Chimeric Antigen Receptor T-cell Immunotherapy (C)	New technology (X)
Bone morphogenetic protein 2 (BMP 2)	Recombinant Bone Morphogenetic Protein (B)	Administration (3)
CBMA (Concentrated Bone Marrow Aspirate)	Concentrated Bone Marrow Aspirate (Ø)	New technology (X)
Clolar	Clofarabine (P)	Administration (3)
Defitelio	Defibrotide Sodium Anticoagulant (9)	New technology (X)
DuraGraft® Endothelial Damage Inhibitor	Endothelial Damage Inhibitor (8)	New technology (X)
Factor Xa Inhibitor Reversal Agent, Andexanet Alfa	Andexanet Alfa, Factor Xa Inhibitor Reversal Agent (7)	New technology (X)
GIAPREZA™	Synthetic Human Angiotensin II	New technology (X)
Human angiotensin II, synthetic	Synthetic Human Angiotensin II	New technology (X)
Kcentra	4-Factor Prothrombin Complex Concentrate (B)	Administration (3)
KYMRIAH	Engineered Autologous Chimeric Antigen Receptor T-cell Immunotherapy	New technology (X)
Nesiritide	Human B-type Natriuretic Peptide (H)	Administration (3)
rhBMP-2	Recombinant Bone Morphogenetic Protein (B)	Administration (3)
Seprafilm	Adhesion Barrier (5)	Administration (3)
STELARA®	Other New Technology Therapeutic Substance (F)	New technology (X)
Tisagenlecleucel	Engineered Autologous Chimeric Antigen Receptor T-cell Immunotherapy	New technology (X)
Tissue Plasminogen Activator (tPA)(r- tPA)	Other Thrombolytic (7)	Administration (3)
Ustekinumab	Other New Technology Therapeutic Substance (F)	New technology (X)
Vistogard®	Uridine Triacetate (8)	New technology (X)
Voraxaze	Glucarpidase (Q)	Administration (3)
VYXEOS™	Cytarabine and Daunorubicin Liposome Antineoplastic (B)	New technology (X)
ZINPLAVA™	Bezlotoxumab Monoclonal Antibody (A)	New technology (X)
Zyvox	Oxazolidinones (8)	Administration (3)

Substance Definitions

This table crosswalks a PCS value, used in the Administration or New Technology section, to a specific substance. The specific substances are listed by trade name or synonym. The ICD-10-PCS value may be located in either the 6th-character Substance column or the 7th-character Qualifier column depending on the section/table to which it is classified.

ICD-10-PCS Value	Trade Name or Synonym	PCS Section
4-Factor Prothrombin Complex Concentrate (B)	**Includes:** Kcentra	Administration (3)
Adhesion Barrier (5)	**Includes:** Seprafilm	Administration (3)
Andexanet Alfa, Factor Xa Inhibitor Reversal Agent (7)	**Includes:** Factor Xa Inhibitor Reversal Agent, Andexanet Alfa	New technology (X)
Anti-Infective Envelope (A)	**Includes:** AIGISRx Antibacterial Envelope Antimicrobial envelope	Administration (3)
Bezlotoxumab Monoclonal Antibody (A)	**Includes:** ZINPLAVA™	New technology (X)
Clofarabine (P)	**Includes:** Clolar	Administration (3)
Concentrated Bone Marrow Aspirate (Ø)	**Includes:** CBMA (Concentrated Bone Marrow Aspirate)	New technology (X)
Cytarabine and Daunorubicin Liposome Antineoplastic (B)	**Includes:** VYXEOS™	New technology (X)
Defibrotide Sodium Anticoagulant (9)	**Includes:** Defitelio	New technology (X)
Endothelial Damage Inhibitor (8)	**Includes:** DuraGraft® Endothelial Damage Inhibitor	New technology (X)
Engineered Autologous Chimeric Antigen Receptor T-cell Immunotherapy (C)	**Includes:** Axicabtagene Ciloeucel KYMRIAH Tisagenlecleucel	New technology (X)
Glucarpidase (Q)	**Includes:** Voraxaze	Administration (3)
Human B-type Natriuretic Peptide (H)	**Includes:** Nesiritide	Administration (3)
Other New Technology Therapeutic Substance (F)	**Includes:** STELARA® Ustekinumab	New technology (X)
Other Thrombolytic (7)	**Includes:** Tissue Plasminogen Activator (tPA)(r-tPA)	Administration (3)
Oxazolidinones (8)	**Includes:** Zyvox	Administration (3)
Recombinant Bone Morphogenetic Protein (B)	**Includes:** Bone morphogenetic protein 2 (BMP 2) rhBMP-2	Administration (3)
Synthetic Human Angiotensin II	**Includes:** Angiotensin II GIAPREZA™ Human angiotensin II, synthetic	New technology (X)
Uridine Triacetate (8)	**Includes:** Vistogard®	New technology (X)

Appendix I: Sections B–H Character Definitions

Section B–Imaging

ICD-10-PCS Value (Character 3)	Definition
Computerized Tomography (CT Scan) (2)	Computer reformatted digital display of multiplanar images developed from the capture of multiple exposures of external ionizing radiation
Fluoroscopy (1)	Single plane or bi-plane real time display of an image developed from the capture of external ionizing radiation on a fluorescent screen. The image may also be stored by either digital or analog means.
Magnetic Resonance Imaging (MRI) (3)	Computer reformatted digital display of multiplanar images developed from the capture of radiofrequency signals emitted by nuclei in a body site excited within a magnetic field
Plain Radiography (Ø)	Planar display of an image developed from the capture of external ionizing radiation on photographic or photoconductive plate
Ultrasonography (4)	Real time display of images of anatomy or flow information developed from the capture of reflected and attenuated high frequency sound waves

Section C–Nuclear Medicine

ICD-10-PCS Value (Character 3)	Definition
Nonimaging Nuclear Medicine Assay (6)	Introduction of radioactive materials into the body for the study of body fluids and blood elements, by the detection of radioactive emissions
Nonimaging Nuclear Medicine Probe (5)	Introduction of radioactive materials into the body for the study of distribution and fate of certain substances by the detection of radioactive emissions; or, alternatively, measurement of absorption of radioactive emissions from an external source
Nonimaging Nuclear Medicine Uptake (4)	Introduction of radioactive materials into the body for measurements of organ function, from the detection of radioactive emissions
Planar Nuclear Medicine Imaging (1)	Introduction of radioactive materials into the body for single plane display of images developed from the capture of radioactive emissions
Positron Emission Tomographic (PET) Imaging (3)	Introduction of radioactive materials into the body for three dimensional display of images developed from the simultaneous capture, 18Ø degrees apart, of radioactive emissions
Systemic Nuclear Medicine Therapy (7)	Introduction of unsealed radioactive materials into the body for treatment
Tomographic (Tomo) Nuclear Medicine Imaging (2)	Introduction of radioactive materials into the body for three dimensional display of images developed from the capture of radioactive emissions

Section F–Physical Rehabilitation and Diagnostic Audiology

ICD-10-PCS Value (Character 3)	Definition
Activities of Daily Living Assessment (2)	Measurement of functional level for activities of daily living
Activities of Daily Living Treatment (8)	Exercise or activities to facilitate functional competence for activities of daily living
Caregiver Training (F)	Training in activities to support patient's optimal level of function
Cochlear Implant Treatment (B)	Application of techniques to improve the communication abilities of individuals with cochlear implant
Device Fitting (D)	Fitting of a device designed to facilitate or support achievement of a higher level of function
Hearing Aid Assessment (4)	Measurement of the appropriateness and/or effectiveness of a hearing device
Hearing Assessment (3)	Measurement of hearing and related functions
Hearing Treatment (9)	Application of techniques to improve, augment, or compensate for hearing and related functional impairment
Motor and/or Nerve Function Assessment (1)	Measurement of motor, nerve, and related functions
Motor Treatment (7)	Exercise or activities to increase or facilitate motor function

Continued on next page

Section F–Physical Rehabilitation and Diagnostic Audiology   *Continued from previous page*

ICD-10-PCS Value (Character 3)	Definition
Speech Assessment (Ø)	Measurement of speech and related functions
Speech Treatment (6)	Application of techniques to improve, augment, or compensate for speech and related functional impairment
Vestibular Assessment (5)	Measurement of the vestibular system and related functions
Vestibular Treatment (C)	Application of techniques to improve, augment, or compensate for vestibular and related functional impairment

Section F–Physical Rehabilitation and Diagnostic Audiology

ICD-10-PCS Value Qualifier (Character 5)	Definition
Acoustic Reflex Decay (J)	Measures reduction in size/strength of acoustic reflex over time Includes/Examples: Includes site of lesion test
Acoustic Reflex Patterns (G)	Defines site of lesion based upon presence/absence of acoustic reflexes with ipsilateral vs. contralateral stimulation
Acoustic Reflex Threshold (H)	Determines minimal intensity that acoustic reflex occurs with ipsilateral and/or contralateral stimulation
Aerobic Capacity and Endurance (7)	Measures autonomic responses to positional changes; perceived exertion, dyspnea or angina during activity; performance during exercise protocols; standard vital signs; and blood gas analysis or oxygen consumption
Alternate Binaural or Monaural Loudness Balance (7)	Determines auditory stimulus parameter that yields the same objective sensation Includes/Examples: Sound intensities that yield same loudness perception
Anthropometric Characteristics (B)	Measures edema, body fat composition, height, weight, length and girth
Aphasia (Assessment) (C)	Measures expressive and receptive speech and language function including reading and writing
Aphasia (Treatment) (3)	Applying techniques to improve, augment, or compensate for receptive/ expressive language impairments
Articulation/Phonology (Assessment) (9)	Measures speech production
Articulation/Phonology (Treatment) (4)	Applying techniques to correct, improve, or compensate for speech productive impairment
Assistive Listening Device (5)	Assists in use of effective and appropriate assistive listening device/system
Assistive Listening System/Device Selection (4)	Measures the effectiveness and appropriateness of assistive listening systems/devices
Assistive, Adaptive, Supportive or Protective Devices (9)	Explanation: Devices to facilitate or support achievement of a higher level of function in wheelchair mobility; bed mobility; transfer or ambulation ability; bath and showering ability; dressing; grooming; personal hygiene; play or leisure
Auditory Evoked Potentials (L)	Measures electric responses produced by the VIIIth cranial nerve and brainstem following auditory stimulation
Auditory Processing (Assessment) (Q)	Evaluates ability to receive and process auditory information and comprehension of spoken language
Auditory Processing (Treatment) (2)	Applying techniques to improve the receiving and processing of auditory information and comprehension of spoken language
Augmentative/Alternative Communication System (Assessment) (L)	Determines the appropriateness of aids, techniques, symbols, and/or strategies to augment or replace speech and enhance communication Includes/Examples: Includes the use of telephones, writing equipment, emergency equipment, and TDD
Augmentative/Alternative Communication System (Treatment) (3)	Includes/Examples: Includes augmentative communication devices and aids
Aural Rehabilitation (5)	Applying techniques to improve the communication abilities associated with hearing loss
Aural Rehabilitation Status (P)	Measures impact of a hearing loss including evaluation of receptive and expressive communication skills
Bathing/Showering (Ø)	Includes/Examples: Includes obtaining and using supplies; soaping, rinsing, and drying body parts; maintaining bathing position; and transferring to and from bathing positions

Continued on next page

Section F–Physical Rehabilitation and Diagnostic Audiology

Continued from previous page

ICD-10-PCS Value Qualifier (Character 5)	Definition
Bathing/Showering Techniques (Ø)	Activities to facilitate obtaining and using supplies, soaping, rinsing and drying body parts, maintaining bathing position, and transferring to and from bathing positions
Bed Mobility (Assessment) (B)	Transitional movement within bed
Bed Mobility (Treatment) (5)	Exercise or activities to facilitate transitional movements within bed
Bedside Swallowing and Oral Function (H)	Includes/Examples: Bedside swallowing includes assessment of sucking, masticating, coughing, and swallowing. Oral function includes assessment of musculature for controlled movements, structures, and functions to determine coordination and phonation.
Bekesy Audiometry (3)	Uses an instrument that provides a choice of discrete or continuously varying pure tones; choice of pulsed or continuous signal
Binaural Electroacoustic Hearing Aid Check (6)	Determines mechanical and electroacoustic function of bilateral hearing aids using hearing aid test box
Binaural Hearing Aid (Assessment) (3)	Measures the candidacy, effectiveness, and appropriateness of a hearing aid Explanation: Measures bilateral fit
Binaural Hearing Aid (Treatment) (2)	Explanation: Assists in achieving maximum understanding and performance
Bithermal, Binaural Caloric Irrigation (Ø)	Measures the rhythmic eye movements stimulated by changing the temperature of the vestibular system
Bithermal, Monaural Caloric Irrigation (1)	Measures the rhythmic eye movements stimulated by changing the temperature of the vestibular system in one ear
Brief Tone Stimuli (R)	Measures specific central auditory process
Cerumen Management (3)	Includes examination of external auditory canal and tympanic membrane and removal of cerumen from external ear canal
Cochlear Implant (Ø)	Measures candidacy for cochlear implant
Cochlear Implant Rehabilitation (Ø)	Applying techniques to improve the communication abilities of individuals with cochlear implant; includes programming the device, providing patients/families with information
Communicative/Cognitive Integration Skills (Assessment) (G)	Measures ability to use higher cortical functions Includes/Examples: Includes orientation, recognition, attention span, initiation and termination of activity, memory, sequencing, categorizing, concept formation, spatial operations, judgment, problem solving, generalization and pragmatic communication
Communicative/Cognitive Integration Skills (Treatment) (6)	Activities to facilitate the use of higher cortical functions Includes/Examples: Includes level of arousal, orientation, recognition, attention span, initiation and termination of activity, memory sequencing, judgment and problem solving, learning and generalization, and pragmatic communication
Computerized Dynamic Posturography (6)	Measures the status of the peripheral and central vestibular system and the sensory/motor component of balance; evaluates the efficacy of vestibular rehabilitation
Conditioned Play Audiometry (4)	Behavioral measures using nonspeech and speech stimuli to obtain frequency-specific and ear-specific information on auditory status from the patient Explanation: Obtains speech reception threshold by having patient point to pictures of spondaic words
Coordination/Dexterity (Assessment) (3)	Measures large and small muscle groups for controlled goal-directed movements Explanation: Dexterity includes object manipulation
Coordination/Dexterity (Treatment) (2)	Exercise or activities to facilitate gross coordination and fine coordination
Cranial Nerve Integrity (9)	Measures cranial nerve sensory and motor functions, including tastes, smell and facial expression
Dichotic Stimuli (T)	Measures specific central auditory process
Distorted Speech (S)	Measures specific central auditory process
Dix-Hallpike Dynamic (5)	Measures nystagmus following Dix-Hallpike maneuver
Dressing (1)	Includes/Examples: Includes selecting clothing and accessories, obtaining clothing from storage, dressing, fastening and adjusting clothing and shoes, and applying and removing personal devices, prosthesis or orthosis

Continued on next page

Section F–Physical Rehabilitation and Diagnostic Audiology   *Continued from previous page*

ICD-10-PCS Value Qualifier (Character 5)	Definition
Dressing Techniques (1)	Activities to facilitate selecting clothing and accessories, dressing and undressing, adjusting clothing and shoes, applying and removing devices, prostheses or orthoses
Dynamic Orthosis (6)	Includes/Examples: Includes customized and prefabricated splints, inhibitory casts, spinal and other braces, and protective devices; allows motion through transfer of movement from other body parts or by use of outside forces
Ear Canal Probe Microphone (1)	Real ear measures
Ear Protector Attentuation (7)	Measures ear protector fit and effectiveness
Electrocochleography (K)	Measures the VIIIth cranial nerve action potential
Environmental, Home, Work Barriers (B)	Measures current and potential barriers to optimal function, including safety hazards, access problems and home or office design
Ergonomics and Body Mechanics (C)	Ergonomic measurement of job tasks, work hardening or work conditioning needs; functional capacity; and body mechanics
Eustachian Tube Function (F)	Measures eustachian tube function and patency of eustachian tube
Evoked Otoacoustic Emissions, Diagnostic (N)	Measures auditory evoked potentials in a diagnostic format
Evoked Otoacoustic Emissions, Screening (M)	Measures auditory evoked potentials in a screening format
Facial Nerve Function (7)	Measures electrical activity of the VIIth cranial nerve (facial nerve)
Feeding/Eating (Assessment) (2)	Includes/Examples: Includes setting up food, selecting and using utensils and tableware, bringing food or drink to mouth, cleaning face, hands, and clothing, and management of alternative methods of nourishment
Feeding/Eating (Treatment) (3)	Exercise or activities to facilitate setting up food, selecting and using utensils and tableware, bringing food or drink to mouth, cleaning face, hands, and clothing, and management of alternative methods of nourishment
Filtered Speech (Ø)	Uses high or low pass filtered speech stimuli to assess central auditory processing disorders, site of lesion testing
Fluency (Assessment) (D)	Measures speech fluency or stuttering
Fluency (Treatment) (7)	Applying techniques to improve and augment fluent speech
Gait and/or Balance (D)	Measures biomechanical, arthrokinematic and other spatial and temporal characteristics of gait and balance
Gait Training/Functional Ambulation (9)	Exercise or activities to facilitate ambulation on a variety of surfaces and in a variety of environments
Grooming/Personal Hygiene (Assessment) (3)	Includes/Examples: Includes ability to obtain and use supplies in a sequential fashion, general grooming, oral hygiene, toilet hygiene, personal care devices, including care for artificial airways
Grooming/Personal Hygiene (Treatment) (2)	Activities to facilitate obtaining and using supplies in a sequential fashion: general grooming, oral hygiene, toilet hygiene, cleaning body, and personal care devices, including artificial airways
Hearing and Related Disorders Counseling (Ø)	Provides patients/families/caregivers with information, support, referrals to facilitate recovery from a communication disorder Includes/Examples: Includes strategies for psychosocial adjustment to hearing loss for clients and families/caregivers
Hearing and Related Disorders Prevention (1)	Provides patients/families/caregivers with information and support to prevent communication disorders
Hearing Screening (Ø)	Pass/refer measures designed to identify need for further audiologic assessment
Home Management (Assessment) (4)	Obtaining and maintaining personal and household possessions and environment Includes/Examples: Includes clothing care, cleaning, meal preparation and cleanup, shopping, money management, household maintenance, safety procedures, and childcare/parenting
Home Management (Treatment) (4)	Activities to facilitate obtaining and maintaining personal household possessions and environment Includes/Examples: Includes clothing care, cleaning, meal preparation and clean-up, shopping, money management, household maintenance, safety procedures, childcare/parenting

Continued on next page

Section F–Physical Rehabilitation and Diagnostic Audiology   *Continued from previous page*

ICD-10-PCS Value Qualifier (Character 5)	Definition
Instrumental Swallowing and Oral Function (J)	Measures swallowing function using instrumental diagnostic procedures Explanation: Methods include videofluoroscopy, ultrasound, manometry, endoscopy
Integumentary Integrity (1)	Includes/Examples: Includes burns, skin conditions, ecchymosis, bleeding, blisters, scar tissue, wounds and other traumas, tissue mobility, turgor and texture
Manual Therapy Techniques (7)	Techniques in which the therapist uses his/her hands to administer skilled movements Includes/Examples: Includes connective tissue massage, joint mobilization and manipulation, manual lymph drainage, manual traction, soft tissue mobilization and manipulation
Masking Patterns (W)	Measures central auditory processing status
Monaural Electroacoustic Hearing Aid Check (8)	Determines mechanical and electroacoustic function of one hearing aid using hearing aid test box
Monaural Hearing Aid (Assessment) (2)	Measures the candidacy, effectiveness, and appropriateness of a hearing aid Explanation: Measures unilateral fit
Monaural Hearing Aid (Treatment) (1)	Explanation: Assists in achieving maximum understanding and performance
Motor Function (Assessment) (4)	Measures the body's functional and versatile movement patterns Includes/Examples: Includes motor assessment scales, analysis of head, trunk and limb movement, and assessment of motor learning
Motor Function (Treatment) (3)	Exercise or activities to facilitate crossing midline, laterality, bilateral integration, praxis, neuromuscular relaxation, inhibition, facilitation, motor function and motor learning
Motor Speech (Assessment) (B)	Measures neurological motor aspects of speech production
Motor Speech (Treatment) (8)	Applying techniques to improve and augment the impaired neurological motor aspects of speech production
Muscle Performance (Assessment) (Ø)	Measures muscle strength, power and endurance using manual testing, dynamometry or computer-assisted electromechanical muscle test; functional muscle strength, power and endurance; muscle pain, tone, or soreness; or pelvic-floor musculature Explanation: Muscle endurance refers to the ability to contract a muscle repeatedly over time
Muscle Performance (Treatment) (1)	Exercise or activities to increase the capacity of a muscle to do work in terms of strength, power, and/or endurance Explanation: Muscle strength is the force exerted to overcome resistance in one maximal effort. Muscle power is work produced per unit of time, or the product of strength and speed. Muscle endurance is the ability to contract a muscle repeatedly over time.
Neuromotor Development (D)	Measures motor development, righting and equilibrium reactions, and reflex and equilibrium reactions
Non-invasive Instrumental Status (N)	Instrumental measures of oral, nasal, vocal, and velopharyngeal functions as they pertain to speech production
Nonspoken Language (Assessment) (7)	Measures nonspoken language (print, sign, symbols) for communication
Nonspoken Language (Treatment) (Ø)	Applying techniques that improve, augment, or compensate spoken communication
Oral Peripheral Mechanism (P)	Structural measures of face, jaw, lips, tongue, teeth, hard and soft palate, pharynx as related to speech production
Orofacial Myofunctional (Assessment) (K)	Measures orofacial myofunctional patterns for speech and related functions
Orofacial Myofunctional (Treatment) (9)	Applying techniques to improve, alter, or augment impaired orofacial myofunctional patterns and related speech production errors
Oscillating Tracking (3)	Measures ability to visually track
Pain (F)	Measures muscle soreness, pain and soreness with joint movement, and pain perception Includes/Examples: Includes questionnaires, graphs, symptom magnification scales or visual analog scales
Perceptual Processing (Assessment) (5)	Measures stereognosis, kinesthesia, body schema, right-left discrimination, form constancy, position in space, visual closure, figure-ground, depth perception, spatial relations and topographical orientation

Continued on next page

Section F–Physical Rehabilitation and Diagnostic Audiology

Continued from previous page

ICD-10-PCS Value Qualifier (Character 5)	Definition
Perceptual Processing (Treatment) (1)	Exercise and activities to facilitate perceptual processing Explanation: Includes stereognosis, kinesthesia, body schema, right-left discrimination, form constancy, position in space, visual closure, figure-ground, depth perception, spatial relations, and topographical orientation Includes/Examples: Includes stereognosis, kinesthesia, body schema, right-left discrimination, form constancy, position in space, visual closure, figure-ground, depth perception, spatial relations, and topographical orientation
Performance Intensity Phonetically Balanced Speech Discrimination (Q)	Measures word recognition over varying intensity levels
Postural Control (3)	Exercise or activities to increase postural alignment and control
Prosthesis (8)	Explanation: Artificial substitutes for missing body parts that augment performance or function Includes/Examples: Limb prosthesis, ocular prosthesis
Psychosocial Skills (Assessment) (6)	The ability to interact in society and to process emotions Includes/Examples: Includes psychological (values, interests, self-concept); social (role performance, social conduct, interpersonal skills, self expression); self-management (coping skills, time management, self-control)
Psychosocial Skills (Treatment) (6)	The ability to interact in society and to process emotions Includes/Examples: Includes psychological (values, interests, self-concept); social (role performance, social conduct, interpersonal skills, self expression); self-management (coping skills, time management, self-control)
Pure Tone Audiometry, Air (1)	Air-conduction pure tone threshold measures with appropriate masking
Pure Tone Audiometry, Air and Bone (2)	Air-conduction and bone-conduction pure tone threshold measures with appropriate masking
Pure Tone Stenger (C)	Measures unilateral nonorganic hearing loss based on simultaneous presentation of pure tones of differing volume
Range of Motion and Joint Integrity (5)	Measures quantity, quality, grade, and classification of joint movement and/or mobility Explanation: Range of Motion is the space, distance or angle through which movement occurs at a joint or series of joints. Joint integrity is the conformance of joints to expected anatomic, biomechanical and kinematic norms.
Range of Motion and Joint Mobility (Ø)	Exercise or activities to increase muscle length and joint mobility
Receptive/Expressive Language (Assessment) (8)	Measures receptive and expressive language
Receptive/Expressive Language (Treatment) (B)	Applying techniques to improve and augment receptive/expressive language
Reflex Integrity (G)	Measures the presence, absence, or exaggeration of developmentally appropriate, pathologic or normal reflexes
Select Picture Audiometry (5)	Establishes hearing threshold levels for speech using pictures
Sensorineural Acuity Level (4)	Measures sensorineural acuity masking presented via bone conduction
Sensory Aids (5)	Determines the appropriateness of a sensory prosthetic device, other than a hearing aid or assistive listening system/device
Sensory Awareness/ Processing/ Integrity (6)	Includes/Examples: Includes light touch, pressure, temperature, pain, sharp/dull, proprioception, vestibular, visual, auditory, gustatory, and olfactory
Short Increment Sensitivity Index (9)	Measures the ear's ability to detect small intensity changes; site of lesion test requiring a behavioral response
Sinusoidal Vertical Axis Rotational (4)	Measures nystagmus following rotation
Somatosensory Evoked Potentials (9)	Measures neural activity from sites throughout the body
Speech/Language Screening (6)	Identifies need for further speech and/or language evaluation
Speech Threshold (1)	Measures minimal intensity needed to repeat spondaic words

Continued on next page

Section F–Physical Rehabilitation and Diagnostic Audiology
Continued from previous page

ICD-10-PCS Value Qualifier (Character 5)	Definition
Speech-Language Pathology and Related Disorders Counseling (1)	Provides patients/families with information, support, referrals to facilitate recovery from a communication disorder
Speech-Language Pathology and Related Disorders Prevention (2)	Applying techniques to avoid or minimize onset and/or development of a communication disorder
Speech/Word Recognition (2)	Measures ability to repeat/identify single syllable words; scores given as a percentage; includes word recognition/speech discrimination
Staggered Spondaic Word (3)	Measures central auditory processing site of lesion based upon dichotic presentation of spondaic words
Static Orthosis (7)	Includes/Examples: Includes customized and prefabricated splints, inhibitory casts, spinal and other braces, and protective devices; has no moving parts, maintains joint(s) in desired position
Stenger (B)	Measures unilateral nonorganic hearing loss based on simultaneous presentation of signals of differing volume
Swallowing Dysfunction (D)	Activities to improve swallowing function in coordination with respiratory function Includes/Examples: Includes function and coordination of sucking, mastication, coughing, swallowing
Synthetic Sentence Identification (5)	Measures central auditory dysfunction using identification of third order approximations of sentences and competing messages
Temporal Ordering of Stimuli (V)	Measures specific central auditory process
Therapeutic Exercise (6)	Exercise or activities to facilitate sensory awareness, sensory processing, sensory integration, balance training, conditioning, reconditioning Includes/Examples: Includes developmental activities, breathing exercises, aerobic endurance activities, aquatic exercises, stretching and ventilatory muscle training
Tinnitus Masker (Assessment) (7)	Determines candidacy for tinnitus masker
Tinnitus Masker (Treatment) (Ø)	Explanation: Used to verify physical fit, acoustic appropriateness, and benefit; assists in achieving maximum benefit
Tone Decay (8)	Measures decrease in hearing sensitivity to a tone; site of lesion test requiring a behavioral response
Transfer (C)	Transitional movement from one surface to another
Transfer Training (8)	Exercise or activities to facilitate movement from one surface to another
Tympanometry (D)	Measures the integrity of the middle ear; measures ease at which sound flows through the tympanic membrane while air pressure against the membrane is varied
Unithermal Binaural Screen (2)	Measures the rhythmic eye movements stimulated by changing the temperature of the vestibular system in both ears using warm water, screening format
Ventilation/Respiration/Circulation (G)	Measures ventilatory muscle strength, power and endurance, pulmonary function and ventilatory mechanics Includes/Examples: Includes ability to clear airway, activities that aggravate or relieve edema, pain, dyspnea or other symptoms, chest wall mobility, cardiopulmonary response to performance of ADL and IAD, cough and sputum, standard vital signs
Vestibular (Ø)	Applying techniques to compensate for balance disorders; includes habituation, exercise therapy, and balance retraining
Visual Motor Integration (Assessment) (2)	Coordinating the interaction of information from the eyes with body movement during activity
Visual Motor Integration (Treatment) (2)	Exercise or activities to facilitate coordinating the interaction of information from eyes with body movement during activity
Visual Reinforcement Audiometry (6)	Behavioral measures using nonspeech and speech stimuli to obtain frequency/ear-specific information on auditory status Includes/Examples: Includes a conditioned response of looking toward a visual reinforcer (e.g., lights, animated toy) every time auditory stimuli are heard
Vocational Activities and Functional Community or Work Reintegration Skills (Assessment) (H)	Measures environmental, home, work (job/school/play) barriers that keep patients from functioning optimally in their environment Includes/Examples: Includes assessment of vocational skills and interests, environment of work (job/school/play), injury potential and injury prevention or reduction, ergonomic stressors, transportation skills, and ability to access and use community resources

Continued on next page

Section F–Physical Rehabilitation and Diagnostic Audiology

Continued from previous page

ICD-10-PCS Value Qualifier (Character 5)	Definition
Vocational Activities and Functional Community or Work Reintegration Skills (Treatment) (7)	Activities to facilitate vocational exploration, body mechanics training, job acquisition, and environmental or work (job/school/play) task adaptation Includes/Examples: Includes injury prevention and reduction, ergonomic stressor reduction, job coaching and simulation, work hardening and conditioning, driving training, transportation skills, and use of community resources
Voice (Assessment) (F)	Measures vocal structure, function and production
Voice (Treatment) (C)	Applying techniques to improve voice and vocal function
Voice Prosthetic (Assessment) (M)	Determines the appropriateness of voice prosthetic/adaptive device to enhance or facilitate communication
Voice Prosthetic (Treatment) (4)	Includes/Examples: Includes electrolarynx, and other assistive, adaptive, supportive devices
Wheelchair Mobility (Assessment) (F)	Measures fit and functional abilities within wheelchair in a variety of environments
Wheelchair Mobility (Treatment) (4)	Management, maintenance and controlled operation of a wheelchair, scooter or other device, in and on a variety of surfaces and environments
Wound Management (5)	Includes/Examples: Includes non-selective and selective debridement (enzymes, autolysis, sharp debridement), dressings (wound coverings, hydrogel, vacuum-assisted closure), topical agents, etc.

Section G–Mental Health

ICD-10-PCS Value (Character 3)	Definition
Biofeedback (C)	Provision of information from the monitoring and regulating of physiological processes in conjunction with cognitive-behavioral techniques to improve patient functioning or well-being Includes/Examples: Includes EEG, blood pressure, skin temperature or peripheral blood flow, ECG, electrooculogram, EMG, respirometry or capnometry, GSR/EDR, perineometry to monitor/regulate bowel/bladder activity, electrogastrogram to monitor/regulate gastric motility
Counseling (6)	The application of psychological methods to treat an individual with normal developmental issues and psychological problems in order to increase function, improve well-being, alleviate distress, maladjustment or resolve crises
Crisis Intervention (2)	Treatment of a traumatized, acutely disturbed or distressed individual for the purpose of short-term stabilization Includes/Examples: Includes defusing, debriefing, counseling, psychotherapy and/or coordination of care with other providers or agencies
Electroconvulsive Therapy (B)	The application of controlled electrical voltages to treat a mental health disorder Includes/Examples: Includes appropriate sedation and other preparation of the individual
Family Psychotherapy (7)	Treatment that includes one or more family members of an individual with a mental health disorder by behavioral, cognitive, psychoanalytic, psychodynamic or psychophysiological means to improve functioning or well-being Explanation: Remediation of emotional or behavioral problems presented by one or more family members in cases where psychotherapy with more than one family member is indicated
Group Psychotherapy (H)	Treatment of two or more individuals with a mental health disorder by behavioral, cognitive, psychoanalytic, psychodynamic or psychophysiological means to improve functioning or well-being
Hypnosis (F)	Induction of a state of heightened suggestibility by auditory, visual and tactile techniques to elicit an emotional or behavioral response
Individual Psychotherapy (5)	Treatment of an individual with a mental health disorder by behavioral, cognitive, psychoanalytic, psychodynamic or psychophysiological means to improve functioning or well-being
Light Therapy (J)	Application of specialized light treatments to improve functioning or well-being
Medication Management (3)	Monitoring and adjusting the use of medications for the treatment of a mental health disorder
Narcosynthesis (G)	Administration of intravenous barbiturates in order to release suppressed or repressed thoughts
Psychological Tests (1)	The administration and interpretation of standardized psychological tests and measurement instruments for the assessment of psychological function

Continued on next page

Section G–Mental Health

ICD-10-PCS Value Qualifier (Character 4)	Definition
Behavioral (1)	Primarily to modify behavior Includes/Examples: Includes modeling and role playing, positive reinforcement of target behaviors, response cost, and training of self-management skills
Cognitive (2)	Primarily to correct cognitive distortions and errors
Cognitive-Behavioral (8)	Combining cognitive and behavioral treatment strategies to improve functioning Explanation: Maladaptive responses are examined to determine how cognitions relate to behavior patterns in response to an event. Uses learning principles and information-processing models.
Developmental (Ø)	Age-normed developmental status of cognitive, social and adaptive behavior skills
Intellectual and Psychoeducational (2)	Intellectual abilities, academic achievement and learning capabilities (including behaviors and emotional factors affecting learning)
Interactive (Ø)	Uses primarily physical aids and other forms of non-oral interaction with a patient who is physically, psychologically or developmentally unable to use ordinary language for communication Includes/Examples: Includes the use of toys in symbolic play
Interpersonal (3)	Helps an individual make changes in interpersonal behaviors to reduce psychological dysfunction Includes/Examples: Includes exploratory techniques, encouragement of affective expression, clarification of patient statements, analysis of communication patterns, use of therapy relationship and behavior change techniques
Neurobehavioral and Cognitive Status (4)	Includes neurobehavioral status exam, interview(s), and observation for the clinical assessment of thinking, reasoning and judgment, acquired knowledge, attention, memory, visual spatial abilities, language functions, and planning
Neuropsychological (3)	Thinking, reasoning and judgment, acquired knowledge, attention, memory, visual spatial abilities, language functions, planning
Personality and Behavioral (1)	Mood, emotion, behavior, social functioning, psychopathological conditions, personality traits and characteristics
Psychoanalysis (4)	Methods of obtaining a detailed account of past and present mental and emotional experiences to determine the source and eliminate or diminish the undesirable effects of unconscious conflicts Explanation: Accomplished by making the individual aware of their existence, origin, and inappropriate expression in emotions and behavior
Psychodynamic (5)	Exploration of past and present emotional experiences to understand motives and drives using insight-oriented techniques to reduce the undesirable effects of internal conflicts on emotions and behavior Explanation: Techniques include empathetic listening, clarifying self-defeating behavior patterns, and exploring adaptive alternatives
Psychophysiological (9)	Monitoring and alteration of physiological processes to help the individual associate physiological reactions combined with cognitive and behavioral strategies to gain improved control of these processes to help the individual cope more effectively
Supportive (6)	Formation of therapeutic relationship primarily for providing emotional support to prevent further deterioration in functioning during periods of particular stress Explanation: Often used in conjunction with other therapeutic approaches
Vocational (1)	Exploration of vocational interests, aptitudes and required adaptive behavior skills to develop and carry out a plan for achieving a successful vocational placement Includes/Examples: Includes enhancing work related adjustment and/or pursuing viable options in training education or preparation

Section H - Substance Abuse Treatment

ICD-10-PCS Value (Character 3)	Definition
Detoxification Services (2)	Detoxification from alcohol and/or drugs Explanation: Not a treatment modality, but helps the patient stabilize physically and psychologically until the body becomes free of drugs and the effects of alcohol
Family Counseling (6)	The application of psychological methods that includes one or more family members to treat an individual with addictive behavior Explanation: Provides support and education for family members of addicted individuals. Family member participation is seen as a critical area of substance abuse treatment.
Group Counseling (4)	The application of psychological methods to treat two or more individuals with addictive behavior Explanation: Provides structured group counseling sessions and healing power through the connection with others
Individual Counseling (3)	The application of psychological methods to treat an individual with addictive behavior Explanation: Comprised of several different techniques, which apply various strategies to address drug addiction
Individual Psychotherapy (5)	Treatment of an individual with addictive behavior by behavioral, cognitive, psychoanalytic, psychodynamic or psychophysiological means
Medication Management (8)	Monitoring and adjusting the use of replacement medications for the treatment of addiction
Pharmacotherapy (9)	The use of replacement medications for the treatment of addiction

Appendix J: Hospital Acquired Conditions

Hospital-acquired conditions (HACs) are conditions considered reasonably preventable through the application of evidence-based guidelines. Although it is the ICD-10-CM code that drives a HAC designation, in some cases a specific ICD-10-PCS code must also be present before that ICD-10-CM code can be considered a HAC. For example, the yellow color bar identifies ØJH63XZ as a HAC in the tabular section of this manual. In the annotation box below table ØJH it is noted that when the ICD-10-CM code J95.811 is reported as a secondary diagnosis, not present on admission, AND ØJH63XZ is also reported during that same admission, J95.811 would be considered a hospital-acquired condition. This resource provides all 14 HAC categories, as well as the specific ICD-10-CM codes and, when applicable, the specific ICD-10-PCS codes applicable to each category.

Note: The resource used to compile this list is the fiscal 2018 ICD-10 MS-DRG Definitions Manual Files v35. The most current version, v36, of ICD-10 MS-DRG Definitions Manual was not available at the time this book was printed. For the most current files related to IPPS please refer to the following: https://www.cms.gov/Medicare/Medicare-Fee-for-Service-Payment/AcuteInpatientPPS/IPPS-Regulations-and-Notices.html.

HAC 01: Foreign Object Retained After Surgery
Secondary diagnosis not POA:
T81.500A
T81.501A
T81.502A
T81.503A
T81.504A
T81.505A
T81.506A
T81.507A
T81.508A
T81.509A
T81.510A
T81.511A
T81.512A
T81.513A
T81.514A
T81.515A
T81.516A
T81.517A
T81.518A
T81.519A
T81.520A
T81.521A
T81.522A
T81.523A
T81.524A
T81.525A
T81.526A
T81.527A
T81.528A
T81.529A
T81.530A
T81.531A
T81.532A
T81.533A
T81.534A
T81.535A
T81.536A
T81.537A
T81.538A
T81.539A
T81.590A
T81.591A
T81.592A
T81.593A
T81.594A
T81.595A
T81.596A
T81.597A
T81.598A
T81.599A
T81.60XA
T81.61XA
T81.69XA

HAC 02: Air Embolism
Secondary diagnosis not POA:
T80.0XXA

HAC 03: Blood Incompatibility
Secondary diagnosis not POA:
T80.30XA
T80.310A
T80.311A
T80.319A
T80.39XA

HAC 04: Stage III and IV Pressure Ulcers
Secondary diagnosis not POA:
L89.003
L89.004
L89.013
L89.014
L89.023
L89.024
L89.103
L89.104
L89.113
L89.114
L89.123
L89.124
L89.133
L89.134
L89.143
L89.144
L89.153
L89.154
L89.203
L89.204
L89.213
L89.214
L89.223
L89.224
L89.303
L89.304
L89.313
L89.314
L89.323
L89.324
L89.43
L89.44
L89.503
L89.504
L89.513
L89.514
L89.523
L89.524
L89.603
L89.604

L89.613
L89.614
L89.623
L89.624
L89.813
L89.814
L89.893
L89.894
L89.93
L89.94

HAC 05: Falls and Trauma
Secondary diagnosis not POA:
M99.10
M99.11
M99.18
S02.0XXA
S02.0XXB
S02.101A
S02.101B
S02.102A
S02.102B
S02.109A
S02.109B
S02.110A
S02.110B
S02.111A
S02.111B
S02.112A
S02.112B
S02.113A
S02.113B
S02.118A
S02.118B
S02.119A
S02.119B
S02.11AA
S02.11AB
S02.11BA
S02.11BB
S02.11CA
S02.11CB
S02.11DA
S02.11DB
S02.11EA
S02.11EB
S02.11FA
S02.11FB
S02.11GA
S02.11GB
S02.11HA
S02.11HB
S02.19XA
S02.19XB
S02.2XXB
S02.30XA
S02.30XB

S02.31XA
S02.31XB
S02.32XA
S02.32XB
S02.400A
S02.400B
S02.401A
S02.401B
S02.402A
S02.402B
S02.40AA
S02.40AB
S02.40BA
S02.40BB
S02.40CA
S02.40CB
S02.40DA
S02.40DB
S02.40EA
S02.40EB
S02.40FA
S02.40FB
S02.411A
S02.411B
S02.412A
S02.412B
S02.413A
S02.413B
S02.42XA
S02.42XB
S02.600A
S02.600B
S02.601A
S02.601B
S02.602A
S02.602B
S02.609A
S02.609B
S02.610A
S02.610B
S02.611A
S02.611B
S02.612A
S02.612B
S02.620A
S02.620B
S02.621A
S02.621B
S02.622A
S02.622B
S02.630A
S02.630B
S02.631A
S02.631B
S02.632A
S02.632B
S02.640A
S02.640B
S02.641A

S02.641B
S02.642A
S02.642B
S02.650A
S02.650B
S02.651A
S02.651B
S02.652A
S02.652B
S02.66XA
S02.66XB
S02.670A
S02.670B
S02.671A
S02.671B
S02.672A
S02.672B
S02.69XA
S02.69XB
S02.80XA
S02.80XB
S02.81XA
S02.81XB
S02.82XA
S02.82XB
S02.91XA
S02.91XB
S02.92XA
S02.92XB
S06.0X1A
S06.0X9A
S06.1X1A
S06.1X2A
S06.1X3A
S06.1X4A
S06.1X5A
S06.1X6A
S06.1X7A
S06.1X8A
S06.1X9A
S06.2X1A
S06.2X2A
S06.2X3A
S06.2X4A
S06.2X5A
S06.2X6A
S06.2X7A
S06.2X8A
S06.2X9A
S06.301A
S06.302A
S06.303A
S06.304A
S06.305A
S06.306A
S06.307A
S06.308A
S06.309A
S06.310A

S06.311A
S06.312A
S06.313A
S06.314A
S06.315A
S06.316A
S06.317A
S06.318A
S06.319A
S06.320A
S06.321A
S06.322A
S06.323A
S06.324A
S06.325A
S06.326A
S06.327A
S06.328A
S06.329A
S06.330A
S06.331A
S06.332A
S06.333A
S06.334A
S06.335A
S06.336A
S06.337A
S06.338A
S06.339A
S06.340A
S06.341A
S06.342A
S06.343A
S06.344A
S06.345A
S06.346A
S06.347A
S06.348A
S06.349A
S06.350A
S06.351A
S06.352A
S06.353A
S06.354A
S06.355A
S06.356A
S06.357A
S06.358A
S06.359A
S06.360A
S06.361A
S06.362A
S06.363A
S06.364A
S06.365A
S06.366A
S06.367A
S06.368A
S06.369A

HAC 05: Falls and Trauma (continued)

S06.370A	S06.897A	S12.251A	S12.691A	S22.011B	S22.089B
S06.371A	S06.898A	S12.251B	S12.691B	S22.012A	S22.20XA
S06.372A	S06.899A	S12.290A	S12.8XXA	S22.012B	S22.20XB
S06.373A	S06.9X1A	S12.290B	S12.9XXA	S22.018A	S22.21XA
S06.374A	S06.9X2A	S12.291A	S13.0XXA	S22.018B	S22.21XB
S06.375A	S06.9X3A	S12.291B	S13.100A	S22.019A	S22.22XA
S06.376A	S06.9X4A	S12.300A	S13.101A	S22.019B	S22.22XB
S06.377A	S06.9X5A	S12.300B	S13.110A	S22.020A	S22.23XA
S06.378A	S06.9X6A	S12.301A	S13.111A	S22.020B	S22.23XB
S06.379A	S06.9X7A	S12.301B	S13.120A	S22.021A	S22.24XA
S06.380A	S06.9X8A	S12.330A	S13.121A	S22.021B	S22.24XB
S06.381A	S06.9X9A	S12.330B	S13.130A	S22.022A	S22.31XA
S06.382A	S07.0XXA	S12.331A	S13.131A	S22.022B	S22.31XB
S06.383A	S07.1XXA	S12.331B	S13.140A	S22.028A	S22.32XA
S06.384A	S07.8XXA	S12.34XA	S13.141A	S22.028B	S22.32XB
S06.385A	S07.9XXA	S12.34XB	S13.150A	S22.029A	S22.39XA
S06.386A	S12.000A	S12.350A	S13.151A	S22.029B	S22.39XB
S06.387A	S12.000B	S12.350B	S13.160A	S22.030A	S22.41XA
S06.388A	S12.001A	S12.351A	S13.161A	S22.030B	S22.41XB
S06.389A	S12.001B	S12.351B	S13.170A	S22.031A	S22.42XA
S06.4X0A	S12.01XA	S12.390A	S13.171A	S22.031B	S22.42XB
S06.4X1A	S12.01XB	S12.390B	S13.180A	S22.032A	S22.43XA
S06.4X2A	S12.02XA	S12.391A	S13.181A	S22.032B	S22.43XB
S06.4X3A	S12.02XB	S12.391B	S13.20XA	S22.038A	S22.49XA
S06.4X4A	S12.030A	S12.400A	S13.29XA	S22.038B	S22.49XB
S06.4X5A	S12.030B	S12.400B	S14.101A	S22.039A	S22.5XXA
S06.4X6A	S12.031A	S12.401A	S14.102A	S22.039B	S22.5XXB
S06.4X7A	S12.031B	S12.401B	S14.103A	S22.040A	S22.9XXA
S06.4X8A	S12.040A	S12.430A	S14.104A	S22.040B	S22.9XXB
S06.4X9A	S12.040B	S12.430B	S14.105A	S22.041A	S24.101A
S06.5X0A	S12.041A	S12.431A	S14.106A	S22.041B	S24.102A
S06.5X1A	S12.041B	S12.431B	S14.107A	S22.042A	S24.103A
S06.5X2A	S12.090A	S12.44XA	S14.111A	S22.042B	S24.104A
S06.5X3A	S12.090B	S12.44XB	S14.112A	S22.048A	S24.111A
S06.5X4A	S12.091A	S12.450A	S14.113A	S22.048B	S24.112A
S06.5X5A	S12.091B	S12.450B	S14.114A	S22.049A	S24.113A
S06.5X6A	S12.100A	S12.451A	S14.115A	S22.049B	S24.114A
S06.5X7A	S12.100B	S12.451B	S14.116A	S22.050A	S24.131A
S06.5X8A	S12.101A	S12.490A	S14.117A	S22.050B	S24.132A
S06.5X9A	S12.101B	S12.490B	S14.121A	S22.051A	S24.133A
S06.6X0A	S12.110A	S12.491A	S14.122A	S22.051B	S24.134A
S06.6X1A	S12.110B	S12.491B	S14.123A	S22.052A	S24.151A
S06.6X2A	S12.111A	S12.500A	S14.124A	S22.052B	S24.152A
S06.6X3A	S12.111B	S12.500B	S14.125A	S22.058A	S24.153A
S06.6X4A	S12.112A	S12.501A	S14.126A	S22.058B	S24.154A
S06.6X5A	S12.112B	S12.501B	S14.127A	S22.059A	S32.000A
S06.6X6A	S12.120A	S12.530A	S14.131A	S22.059B	S32.000B
S06.6X7A	S12.120B	S12.530B	S14.132A	S22.060A	S32.001A
S06.6X8A	S12.121A	S12.531A	S14.133A	S22.060B	S32.001B
S06.6X9A	S12.121B	S12.531B	S14.134A	S22.061A	S32.002A
S06.811A	S12.130A	S12.54XA	S14.135A	S22.061B	S32.002B
S06.812A	S12.130B	S12.54XB	S14.136A	S22.062A	S32.008A
S06.813A	S12.131A	S12.550A	S14.137A	S22.062B	S32.008B
S06.814A	S12.131B	S12.550B	S14.151A	S22.068A	S32.009A
S06.815A	S12.14XA	S12.551A	S14.152A	S22.068B	S32.009B
S06.816A	S12.14XB	S12.551B	S14.153A	S22.069A	S32.010A
S06.817A	S12.150A	S12.590A	S14.154A	S22.069B	S32.010B
S06.818A	S12.150B	S12.590B	S14.155A	S22.070A	S32.011A
S06.819A	S12.151A	S12.591A	S14.156A	S22.070B	S32.011B
S06.821A	S12.151B	S12.591B	S14.157A	S22.071A	S32.012A
S06.822A	S12.190A	S12.600A	S17.0XXA	S22.071B	S32.012B
S06.823A	S12.190B	S12.600B	S17.8XXA	S22.072A	S32.018A
S06.824A	S12.191A	S12.601A	S17.9XXA	S22.072B	S32.018B
S06.825A	S12.191B	S12.601B	S22.000A	S22.078A	S32.019A
S06.826A	S12.200A	S12.630A	S22.000B	S22.078B	S32.019B
S06.827A	S12.200B	S12.630B	S22.001A	S22.079A	S32.020A
S06.828A	S12.201A	S12.631A	S22.001B	S22.079B	S32.020B
S06.829A	S12.201B	S12.631B	S22.002A	S22.080A	S32.021A
S06.891A	S12.230A	S12.64XA	S22.002B	S22.080B	S32.021B
S06.892A	S12.230B	S12.64XB	S22.008A	S22.081A	S32.022A
S06.893A	S12.231A	S12.650A	S22.008B	S22.081B	S32.022B
S06.894A	S12.231B	S12.650B	S22.009A	S22.082A	S32.028A
S06.895A	S12.24XA	S12.651A	S22.009B	S22.082B	S32.028B
S06.896A	S12.24XB	S12.651B	S22.010A	S22.088A	S32.029A
	S12.250A	S12.690A	S22.010B	S22.088B	S32.029B
	S12.250B	S12.690B	S22.011A	S22.089A	S32.030A

HAC 05: Falls and Trauma (continued)

S32.030B	S32.311B	S32.453B	S32.612B	S42.113B	S42.252B
S32.031A	S32.312A	S32.454A	S32.613A	S42.114B	S42.253A
S32.031B	S32.312B	S32.454B	S32.613B	S42.115B	S42.253B
S32.032A	S32.313A	S32.455A	S32.614A	S42.116B	S42.254A
S32.032B	S32.313B	S32.455B	S32.614B	S42.121B	S42.254B
S32.038A	S32.314A	S32.456A	S32.615A	S42.122B	S42.255A
S32.038B	S32.314B	S32.456B	S32.615B	S42.123B	S42.255B
S32.039A	S32.315A	S32.461A	S32.616A	S42.124B	S42.256A
S32.039B	S32.315B	S32.461B	S32.616B	S42.125B	S42.256B
S32.040A	S32.316A	S32.462A	S32.691A	S42.126B	S42.261A
S32.040B	S32.316B	S32.462B	S32.691B	S42.131B	S42.261B
S32.041A	S32.391A	S32.463A	S32.692A	S42.132B	S42.262A
S32.041B	S32.391B	S32.463B	S32.692B	S42.133B	S42.262B
S32.042A	S32.392A	S32.464A	S32.699A	S42.134B	S42.263A
S32.042B	S32.392B	S32.464B	S32.699B	S42.135B	S42.263B
S32.048A	S32.399A	S32.465A	S32.810A	S42.136B	S42.264A
S32.048B	S32.399B	S32.465B	S32.810B	S42.141B	S42.264B
S32.049A	S32.401A	S32.466A	S32.811A	S42.142B	S42.265A
S32.049B	S32.401B	S32.466B	S32.811B	S42.143B	S42.265B
S32.050A	S32.402A	S32.471A	S32.82XA	S42.144B	S42.266A
S32.050B	S32.402B	S32.471B	S32.82XB	S42.145B	S42.266B
S32.051A	S32.409A	S32.472A	S32.89XA	S42.146B	S42.271A
S32.051B	S32.409B	S32.472B	S32.89XB	S42.151B	S42.272A
S32.052A	S32.411A	S32.473A	S32.9XXA	S42.152B	S42.279A
S32.052B	S32.411B	S32.473B	S32.9XXB	S42.153B	S42.291A
S32.058A	S32.412A	S32.474A	S34.101A	S42.154B	S42.291B
S32.058B	S32.412B	S32.474B	S34.102A	S42.155B	S42.292A
S32.059A	S32.413A	S32.475A	S34.103A	S42.156B	S42.292B
S32.059B	S32.413B	S32.475B	S34.104A	S42.191B	S42.293A
S32.10XA	S32.414A	S32.476A	S34.105A	S42.192B	S42.293B
S32.10XB	S32.414B	S32.476B	S34.109A	S42.199B	S42.294A
S32.110A	S32.415A	S32.481A	S34.111A	S42.201A	S42.294B
S32.110B	S32.415B	S32.481B	S34.112A	S42.201B	S42.295A
S32.111A	S32.416A	S32.482A	S34.113A	S42.202A	S42.295B
S32.111B	S32.416B	S32.482B	S34.114A	S42.202B	S42.296A
S32.112A	S32.421A	S32.483A	S34.115A	S42.209A	S42.296B
S32.112B	S32.421B	S32.483B	S34.119A	S42.209B	S42.301A
S32.119A	S32.422A	S32.484A	S34.121A	S42.211A	S42.301B
S32.119B	S32.422B	S32.484B	S34.122A	S42.211B	S42.302A
S32.120A	S32.423A	S32.485A	S34.123A	S42.212A	S42.302B
S32.120B	S32.423B	S32.485B	S34.124A	S42.212B	S42.309A
S32.121A	S32.424A	S32.486A	S34.125A	S42.213A	S42.309B
S32.121B	S32.424B	S32.486B	S34.129A	S42.213B	S42.311A
S32.122A	S32.425A	S32.491A	S34.131A	S42.214A	S42.312A
S32.122B	S32.425B	S32.491B	S34.132A	S42.214B	S42.319A
S32.129A	S32.426A	S32.492A	S34.139A	S42.215A	S42.321A
S32.129B	S32.426B	S32.492B	S34.3XXA	S42.215B	S42.321B
S32.130A	S32.431A	S32.499A	S42.001A	S42.216A	S42.322A
S32.130B	S32.431B	S32.499B	S42.002B	S42.216B	S42.322B
S32.131A	S32.432A	S32.501A	S42.009B	S42.221A	S42.323A
S32.131B	S32.432B	S32.501B	S42.011B	S42.221B	S42.323B
S32.132A	S32.433A	S32.502A	S42.012B	S42.222A	S42.324A
S32.132B	S32.433B	S32.502B	S42.013B	S42.222B	S42.324B
S32.139A	S32.434A	S32.509A	S42.014B	S42.223A	S42.325A
S32.139B	S32.434B	S32.509B	S42.015B	S42.223B	S42.325B
S32.14XA	S32.435A	S32.511A	S42.016B	S42.224A	S42.326A
S32.14XB	S32.435B	S32.511B	S42.017B	S42.224B	S42.326B
S32.15XA	S32.436A	S32.512A	S42.018B	S42.225A	S42.331A
S32.15XB	S32.436B	S32.512B	S42.019B	S42.225B	S42.331B
S32.16XA	S32.441A	S32.519A	S42.021B	S42.226A	S42.332A
S32.16XB	S32.441B	S32.519B	S42.022B	S42.226B	S42.332B
S32.17XA	S32.442A	S32.591A	S42.023B	S42.231A	S42.333A
S32.17XB	S32.442B	S32.591B	S42.024B	S42.231B	S42.333B
S32.19XA	S32.443A	S32.592A	S42.025B	S42.232A	S42.334A
S32.19XB	S32.443B	S32.592B	S42.026B	S42.232B	S42.334B
S32.2XXA	S32.444A	S32.599A	S42.031B	S42.239A	S42.335A
S32.2XXB	S32.444B	S32.599B	S42.032B	S42.239B	S42.335B
S32.301A	S32.445A	S32.601A	S42.033B	S42.241A	S42.336A
S32.301B	S32.445B	S32.601B	S42.034B	S42.241B	S42.336B
S32.302A	S32.446A	S32.602A	S42.035B	S42.242A	S42.341A
S32.302B	S32.446B	S32.602B	S42.036B	S42.242B	S42.341B
S32.309A	S32.451A	S32.609A	S42.101B	S42.249A	S42.342A
S32.309B	S32.451B	S32.609B	S42.102B	S42.249B	S42.342B
S32.311A	S32.452A	S32.611A	S42.109B	S42.251A	S42.343A
	S32.452B	S32.611B	S42.111B	S42.251B	S42.343B
	S32.453A	S32.612A	S42.112B	S42.252A	S42.344A

HAC 05: Falls and Trauma (continued)

S42.344B	S42.435B	S42.92XA	S52.026C	S52.209A	S52.256B
S42.345A	S42.436A	S42.92XB	S52.031B	S52.209B	S52.256C
S42.345B	S42.436B	S43.201A	S52.031C	S52.209C	S52.261A
S42.346A	S42.441A	S43.202A	S52.032B	S52.211A	S52.261B
S42.346B	S42.441B	S43.203A	S52.032C	S52.212A	S52.261C
S42.351A	S42.442A	S43.204A	S52.033B	S52.219A	S52.262A
S42.351B	S42.442B	S43.205A	S52.033C	S52.221A	S52.262B
S42.352A	S42.443A	S43.206A	S52.034B	S52.221B	S52.262C
S42.352B	S42.443B	S43.211A	S52.034C	S52.221C	S52.263A
S42.353A	S42.444A	S43.212A	S52.035B	S52.222A	S52.263B
S42.353B	S42.444B	S43.213A	S52.035C	S52.222B	S52.263C
S42.354A	S42.445A	S43.214A	S52.036B	S52.222C	S52.264A
S42.354B	S42.445B	S43.215A	S52.036C	S52.223A	S52.264B
S42.355A	S42.446A	S43.216A	S52.041B	S52.223B	S52.264C
S42.355B	S42.446B	S43.221A	S52.041C	S52.223C	S52.265A
S42.356A	S42.447A	S43.222A	S52.042B	S52.224A	S52.265B
S42.356B	S42.447B	S43.223A	S52.042C	S52.224B	S52.265C
S42.361A	S42.448A	S43.224A	S52.043B	S52.224C	S52.266A
S42.361B	S42.448B	S43.225A	S52.043C	S52.225A	S52.266B
S42.362A	S42.449A	S43.226A	S52.044B	S52.225B	S52.266C
S42.362B	S42.449B	S49.001A	S52.044C	S52.225C	S52.271B
S42.363A	S42.451A	S49.002A	S52.045B	S52.226A	S52.271C
S42.363B	S42.451B	S49.009A	S52.045C	S52.226B	S52.272B
S42.364A	S42.452A	S49.011A	S52.046B	S52.226C	S52.272C
S42.364B	S42.452B	S49.012A	S52.046C	S52.231A	S52.279B
S42.365A	S42.453A	S49.019A	S52.091B	S52.231B	S52.279C
S42.365B	S42.453B	S49.021A	S52.091C	S52.231C	S52.281A
S42.366A	S42.454A	S49.022A	S52.092B	S52.232A	S52.281B
S42.366B	S42.454B	S49.029A	S52.092C	S52.232B	S52.281C
S42.391A	S42.455A	S49.031A	S52.099B	S52.232C	S52.282A
S42.391B	S42.455B	S49.032A	S52.099C	S52.233A	S52.282B
S42.392A	S42.456A	S49.039A	S52.101B	S52.233B	S52.282C
S42.392B	S42.456B	S49.041A	S52.101C	S52.233C	S52.283A
S42.399A	S42.461A	S49.042A	S52.102B	S52.234A	S52.283B
S42.399B	S42.461B	S49.049A	S52.102C	S52.234B	S52.291A
S42.401A	S42.462A	S49.091A	S52.109B	S52.234C	S52.291B
S42.401B	S42.462B	S49.092A	S52.109C	S52.235A	S52.291C
S42.402A	S42.463A	S49.099A	S52.111A	S52.235B	S52.292A
S42.402B	S42.463B	S49.101A	S52.112A	S52.235C	S52.292B
S42.409A	S42.464A	S49.102A	S52.119A	S52.236A	S52.292C
S42.409B	S42.464B	S49.109A	S52.121B	S52.236B	S52.299A
S42.411A	S42.465A	S49.111A	S52.121C	S52.236C	S52.299B
S42.411B	S42.465B	S49.112A	S52.122B	S52.241A	S52.299C
S42.412A	S42.466A	S49.119A	S52.122C	S52.241B	S52.301A
S42.412B	S42.466B	S49.121A	S52.123B	S52.241C	S52.301B
S42.413A	S42.471A	S49.122A	S52.123C	S52.242A	S52.301C
S42.413B	S42.471B	S49.129A	S52.124B	S52.242B	S52.302A
S42.414A	S42.472A	S49.131A	S52.124C	S52.242C	S52.302B
S42.414B	S42.472B	S49.132A	S52.125B	S52.243A	S52.302C
S42.415A	S42.473A	S49.139A	S52.125C	S52.243B	S52.309A
S42.415B	S42.473B	S49.141A	S52.126B	S52.243C	S52.309B
S42.416A	S42.474A	S49.142A	S52.126C	S52.244A	S52.309C
S42.416B	S42.474B	S49.149A	S52.131B	S52.244B	S52.311A
S42.421A	S42.475A	S49.191A	S52.131C	S52.244C	S52.312A
S42.421B	S42.475B	S49.192A	S52.132B	S52.245A	S52.319A
S42.422A	S42.476A	S49.199A	S52.132C	S52.245B	S52.321A
S42.422B	S42.476B	S52.001B	S52.133B	S52.245C	S52.321B
S42.423A	S42.481A	S52.001C	S52.133C	S52.246A	S52.321C
S42.423B	S42.482A	S52.002B	S52.134B	S52.246B	S52.322A
S42.424A	S42.489A	S52.002C	S52.134C	S52.246C	S52.322B
S42.424B	S42.491A	S52.009B	S52.135B	S52.251A	S52.322C
S42.425A	S42.491B	S52.009C	S52.135C	S52.251B	S52.323A
S42.425B	S42.492A	S52.011A	S52.136B	S52.251C	S52.323B
S42.426A	S42.492B	S52.012A	S52.136C	S52.252A	S52.323C
S42.426B	S42.493A	S52.019A	S52.181B	S52.252B	S52.324A
S42.431A	S42.493B	S52.021B	S52.181C	S52.252C	S52.324B
S42.431B	S42.494A	S52.021C	S52.182B	S52.253A	S52.324C
S42.432A	S42.494B	S52.022B	S52.182C	S52.253B	S52.325A
S42.432B	S42.495A	S52.022C	S52.189B	S52.253C	S52.325B
S42.433A	S42.495B	S52.023B	S52.189C	S52.254A	S52.325C
S42.433B	S42.496A	S52.023C	S52.201A	S52.254B	S52.326A
S42.434A	S42.496B	S52.024B	S52.201B	S52.254C	S52.326B
S42.434B	S42.90XA	S52.024C	S52.201C	S52.255A	S52.326C
S42.435A	S42.90XB	S52.025B	S52.202A	S52.255B	S52.331A
	S42.91XA	S52.025C	S52.202B	S52.255C	S52.331B
	S42.91XB	S52.026B	S52.202C	S52.256A	

HAC 05: Falls and Trauma (continued)

S52.331C	S52.372B	S52.552C	S52.92XA	S62.132B	S62.308B
S52.332A	S52.372C	S52.559A	S52.92XB	S62.133B	S62.309B
S52.332B	S52.379A	S52.559B	S52.92XC	S62.134B	S62.310B
S52.332C	S52.379B	S52.559C	S59.001A	S62.135B	S62.311B
S52.333A	S52.379C	S52.561A	S59.002A	S62.136B	S62.312B
S52.333B	S52.381A	S52.561B	S59.009A	S62.141B	S62.313B
S52.333C	S52.381B	S52.561C	S59.011A	S62.142B	S62.314B
S52.334A	S52.381C	S52.562A	S59.012A	S62.143B	S62.315B
S52.334B	S52.382A	S52.562B	S59.019A	S62.144B	S62.316B
S52.334C	S52.382B	S52.562C	S59.021A	S62.145B	S62.317B
S52.335A	S52.382C	S52.569A	S59.022A	S62.146B	S62.318B
S52.335B	S52.389A	S52.569B	S59.029A	S62.151B	S62.319B
S52.335C	S52.389B	S52.569C	S59.031A	S62.152B	S62.320B
S52.336A	S52.389C	S52.571A	S59.032A	S62.153B	S62.321B
S52.336B	S52.391A	S52.571B	S59.039A	S62.154B	S62.322B
S52.336C	S52.391B	S52.571C	S59.041A	S62.155B	S62.323B
S52.341A	S52.391C	S52.572A	S59.042A	S62.156B	S62.324B
S52.341B	S52.392A	S52.572B	S59.049A	S62.161B	S62.325B
S52.341C	S52.392B	S52.572C	S59.091A	S62.162B	S62.326B
S52.342A	S52.392C	S52.579A	S59.092A	S62.163B	S62.327B
S52.342B	S52.399A	S52.579B	S59.099A	S62.164B	S62.328B
S52.342C	S52.399B	S52.579C	S59.201A	S62.165B	S62.329B
S52.343A	S52.399C	S52.591A	S59.202A	S62.166B	S62.330B
S52.343B	S52.501A	S52.591B	S59.209A	S62.171B	S62.331B
S52.343C	S52.501B	S52.591C	S59.211A	S62.172B	S62.332B
S52.344A	S52.501C	S52.592A	S59.212A	S62.173B	S62.333B
S52.344B	S52.502A	S52.592B	S59.219A	S62.174B	S62.334B
S52.344C	S52.502B	S52.592C	S59.221A	S62.175B	S62.335B
S52.345A	S52.502C	S52.599A	S59.222A	S62.176B	S62.336B
S52.345B	S52.509A	S52.599B	S59.229A	S62.181B	S62.337B
S52.345C	S52.509B	S52.599C	S59.231A	S62.182B	S62.338B
S52.346A	S52.509C	S52.601A	S59.232A	S62.183B	S62.339B
S52.346B	S52.511A	S52.601B	S59.239A	S62.184B	S62.340B
S52.346C	S52.511B	S52.601C	S59.241A	S62.185B	S62.341B
S52.351A	S52.511C	S52.602A	S59.242A	S62.186B	S62.342B
S52.351B	S52.512A	S52.602B	S59.249A	S62.201B	S62.343B
S52.351C	S52.512B	S52.602C	S59.291A	S62.202B	S62.344B
S52.352A	S52.512C	S52.609A	S59.292A	S62.209B	S62.345B
S52.352B	S52.513A	S52.609B	S59.299A	S62.211B	S62.346B
S52.352C	S52.513B	S52.609C	S62.001B	S62.212B	S62.347B
S52.353A	S52.513C	S52.611A	S62.002B	S62.213B	S62.348B
S52.353B	S52.514A	S52.611B	S62.009B	S62.221B	S62.349B
S52.353C	S52.514B	S52.611C	S62.011B	S62.222B	S62.350B
S52.354A	S52.514C	S52.612A	S62.012B	S62.223B	S62.351B
S52.354B	S52.515A	S52.612B	S62.013B	S62.224B	S62.352B
S52.354C	S52.515B	S52.612C	S62.014B	S62.225B	S62.353B
S52.355A	S52.515C	S52.613A	S62.015B	S62.226B	S62.354B
S52.355B	S52.516A	S52.613B	S62.016B	S62.231B	S62.355B
S52.355C	S52.516B	S52.613C	S62.021B	S62.232B	S62.356B
S52.356A	S52.516C	S52.614A	S62.022B	S62.233B	S62.357B
S52.356B	S52.521A	S52.614B	S62.023B	S62.234B	S62.358B
S52.356C	S52.522A	S52.614C	S62.024B	S62.235B	S62.359B
S52.361A	S52.529A	S52.615A	S62.025B	S62.236B	S62.360B
S52.361B	S52.531A	S52.615B	S62.026B	S62.241B	S62.361B
S52.361C	S52.531B	S52.615C	S62.031B	S62.242B	S62.362B
S52.362A	S52.531C	S52.616A	S62.032B	S62.243B	S62.363B
S52.362B	S52.532A	S52.616B	S62.033B	S62.244B	S62.364B
S52.362C	S52.532B	S52.616C	S62.034B	S62.245B	S62.365B
S52.363A	S52.532C	S52.621A	S62.035B	S62.246B	S62.366B
S52.363B	S52.539A	S52.622A	S62.036B	S62.251B	S62.367B
S52.363C	S52.539B	S52.629A	S62.101B	S62.252B	S62.368B
S52.364A	S52.539C	S52.691A	S62.102B	S62.253B	S62.369B
S52.364B	S52.541A	S52.691B	S62.109B	S62.254B	S62.390B
S52.364C	S52.541B	S52.691C	S62.111B	S62.255B	S62.391B
S52.365A	S52.541C	S52.692A	S62.112B	S62.256B	S62.392B
S52.365B	S52.542A	S52.692B	S62.113B	S62.291B	S62.393B
S52.365C	S52.542B	S52.692C	S62.114B	S62.292B	S62.394B
S52.366A	S52.542C	S52.699A	S62.115B	S62.299B	S62.395B
S52.366B	S52.549A	S52.699B	S62.116B	S62.300B	S62.396B
S52.366C	S52.549B	S52.699C	S62.121B	S62.301B	S62.397B
S52.371A	S52.549C	S52.90XA	S62.122B	S62.302B	S62.398B
S52.371B	S52.551A	S52.90XB	S62.123B	S62.303B	S62.399B
S52.371C	S52.551B	S52.90XC	S62.124B	S62.304B	S62.501B
S52.372A	S52.551C	S52.91XA	S62.125B	S62.305B	S62.502B
	S52.552A	S52.91XB	S62.126B	S62.306B	S62.509B
	S52.552B	S52.91XC	S62.131B	S62.307B	S62.511B

HAC 05: Falls and Trauma (continued)

S62.512B	S62.663B	S72.045A	S72.123B	S72.321C	S72.363A
S62.513B	S62.664B	S72.045B	S72.123C	S72.322A	S72.363B
S62.514B	S62.665B	S72.045C	S72.124A	S72.322B	S72.363C
S62.515B	S62.666B	S72.046A	S72.124B	S72.322C	S72.364A
S62.516B	S62.667B	S72.046B	S72.124C	S72.323A	S72.364B
S62.521B	S62.668B	S72.046C	S72.125A	S72.323B	S72.364C
S62.522B	S62.669B	S72.051A	S72.125B	S72.323C	S72.365A
S62.523B	S62.90XB	S72.051B	S72.125C	S72.324A	S72.365B
S62.524B	S62.91XB	S72.051C	S72.126A	S72.324B	S72.365C
S62.525B	S62.92XB	S72.052A	S72.126B	S72.324C	S72.366A
S62.526B	S72.001A	S72.052B	S72.126C	S72.325A	S72.366B
S62.600B	S72.001B	S72.052C	S72.131A	S72.325B	S72.366C
S62.601B	S72.001C	S72.059A	S72.131B	S72.325C	S72.391A
S62.602B	S72.002A	S72.059B	S72.131C	S72.326A	S72.391B
S62.603B	S72.002B	S72.059C	S72.132A	S72.326B	S72.391C
S62.604B	S72.002C	S72.061A	S72.132B	S72.326C	S72.392A
S62.605B	S72.009A	S72.061B	S72.132C	S72.331A	S72.392B
S62.606B	S72.009B	S72.061C	S72.133A	S72.331B	S72.392C
S62.607B	S72.009C	S72.062A	S72.133B	S72.331C	S72.399A
S62.608B	S72.011A	S72.062B	S72.133C	S72.332A	S72.399B
S62.609B	S72.011B	S72.062C	S72.134A	S72.332B	S72.399C
S62.610B	S72.011C	S72.063A	S72.134B	S72.332C	S72.401A
S62.611B	S72.012A	S72.063B	S72.134C	S72.333A	S72.401B
S62.612B	S72.012B	S72.063C	S72.135A	S72.333B	S72.401C
S62.613B	S72.012C	S72.064A	S72.135B	S72.333C	S72.402A
S62.614B	S72.019A	S72.064B	S72.135C	S72.334A	S72.402B
S62.615B	S72.019B	S72.064C	S72.136A	S72.334B	S72.402C
S62.616B	S72.019C	S72.065A	S72.136B	S72.334C	S72.409A
S62.617B	S72.021A	S72.065B	S72.136C	S72.335A	S72.409B
S62.618B	S72.021B	S72.065C	S72.141A	S72.335B	S72.409C
S62.619B	S72.021C	S72.066A	S72.141B	S72.335C	S72.411A
S62.620B	S72.022A	S72.066B	S72.141C	S72.336A	S72.411B
S62.621B	S72.022B	S72.066C	S72.142A	S72.336B	S72.411C
S62.622B	S72.022C	S72.091A	S72.142B	S72.336C	S72.412A
S62.623B	S72.023A	S72.091B	S72.142C	S72.341A	S72.412C
S62.624B	S72.023B	S72.091C	S72.143A	S72.341B	S72.413A
S62.625B	S72.023C	S72.092A	S72.143B	S72.341C	S72.413B
S62.626B	S72.024A	S72.092B	S72.143C	S72.342A	S72.413C
S62.627B	S72.024B	S72.092C	S72.144A	S72.342B	S72.414A
S62.628B	S72.024C	S72.099A	S72.144B	S72.342C	S72.414B
S62.629B	S72.025A	S72.099B	S72.144C	S72.343A	S72.414C
S62.630B	S72.025B	S72.099C	S72.145A	S72.343B	S72.415A
S62.631B	S72.025C	S72.101A	S72.145B	S72.343C	S72.415B
S62.632B	S72.026A	S72.101B	S72.145C	S72.344A	S72.415C
S62.633B	S72.026B	S72.101C	S72.146A	S72.344B	S72.416A
S62.634B	S72.026C	S72.102A	S72.146B	S72.344C	S72.416B
S62.635B	S72.031A	S72.102B	S72.146C	S72.345A	S72.416C
S62.636B	S72.031B	S72.102C	S72.21XA	S72.345B	S72.421A
S62.637B	S72.031C	S72.109A	S72.21XB	S72.345C	S72.421B
S62.638B	S72.032A	S72.109B	S72.21XC	S72.346A	S72.421C
S62.639B	S72.032B	S72.109C	S72.22XA	S72.346B	S72.422A
S62.640B	S72.032C	S72.111A	S72.22XB	S72.346C	S72.422B
S62.641B	S72.033A	S72.111B	S72.22XC	S72.351A	S72.422C
S62.642B	S72.033B	S72.111C	S72.23XA	S72.351B	S72.423A
S62.643B	S72.033C	S72.112A	S72.23XB	S72.351C	S72.423B
S62.644B	S72.034A	S72.112B	S72.23XC	S72.352A	S72.423C
S62.645B	S72.034B	S72.112C	S72.24XA	S72.352B	S72.424A
S62.646B	S72.034C	S72.113A	S72.24XB	S72.352C	S72.424B
S62.647B	S72.035A	S72.113B	S72.24XC	S72.353A	S72.424C
S62.648B	S72.035B	S72.113C	S72.25XA	S72.353B	S72.425A
S62.649B	S72.035C	S72.114A	S72.25XB	S72.353C	S72.425B
S62.650B	S72.036A	S72.114B	S72.25XC	S72.354A	S72.425C
S62.651B	S72.036B	S72.114C	S72.26XA	S72.354B	S72.426A
S62.652B	S72.036C	S72.115A	S72.26XB	S72.354C	S72.426B
S62.653B	S72.041A	S72.115B	S72.26XC	S72.355A	S72.426C
S62.654B	S72.041B	S72.115C	S72.301A	S72.355B	S72.431A
S62.655B	S72.041C	S72.116A	S72.301B	S72.355C	S72.431B
S62.656B	S72.042A	S72.116B	S72.301C	S72.356A	S72.431C
S62.657B	S72.042B	S72.116C	S72.302A	S72.356B	S72.432A
S62.658B	S72.042C	S72.121A	S72.302B	S72.356C	S72.432B
S62.659B	S72.043A	S72.121B	S72.302C	S72.361A	S72.432C
S62.660B	S72.043B	S72.121C	S72.309A	S72.361B	S72.433A
S62.661B	S72.043C	S72.122A	S72.309B	S72.361C	S72.433B
S62.662B	S72.044A	S72.122B	S72.309C	S72.362A	S72.433C
	S72.044B	S72.122C	S72.321A	S72.362B	S72.434A
	S72.044C	S72.123A	S72.321B	S72.362C	

HAC 05: Falls and Trauma (continued)					
S72.434B	S72.8X1A	S79.142A	S82.043C	S82.135A	S82.225B
S72.434C	S72.8X1B	S79.149A	S82.044A	S82.135B	S82.225C
S72.435A	S72.8X1C	S79.191A	S82.044B	S82.135C	S82.226A
S72.435B	S72.8X2A	S79.192A	S82.044C	S82.136A	S82.226B
S72.435C	S72.8X2B	S79.199A	S82.045A	S82.136B	S82.226C
S72.436A	S72.8X2C	S82.001A	S82.045B	S82.136C	S82.231A
S72.436B	S72.8X9A	S82.001B	S82.045C	S82.141A	S82.231B
S72.436C	S72.8X9B	S82.001C	S82.046A	S82.141B	S82.231C
S72.441A	S72.8X9C	S82.002A	S82.046B	S82.141C	S82.232A
S72.441B	S72.90XA	S82.002B	S82.046C	S82.142A	S82.232B
S72.441C	S72.90XB	S82.002C	S82.091A	S82.142B	S82.232C
S72.442A	S72.90XC	S82.009A	S82.091B	S82.142C	S82.233A
S72.442B	S72.91XA	S82.009B	S82.091C	S82.143A	S82.233B
S72.442C	S72.91XB	S82.009C	S82.092A	S82.143B	S82.233C
S72.443A	S72.91XC	S82.011A	S82.092B	S82.143C	S82.234A
S72.443B	S72.92XA	S82.011B	S82.092C	S82.144A	S82.234B
S72.443C	S72.92XB	S82.011C	S82.099A	S82.144B	S82.234C
S72.444A	S72.92XC	S82.012A	S82.099B	S82.144C	S82.235A
S72.444B	S73.001A	S82.012B	S82.099C	S82.145A	S82.235B
S72.444C	S73.002A	S82.012C	S82.101A	S82.145B	S82.235C
S72.445A	S73.003A	S82.013A	S82.101B	S82.145C	S82.236A
S72.445B	S73.004A	S82.013B	S82.101C	S82.146A	S82.236B
S72.445C	S73.005A	S82.013C	S82.102A	S82.146B	S82.236C
S72.446A	S73.006A	S82.014A	S82.102B	S82.146C	S82.241A
S72.446B	S73.011A	S82.014B	S82.102C	S82.151A	S82.241B
S72.446C	S73.012A	S82.014C	S82.109A	S82.151B	S82.241C
S72.451A	S73.013A	S82.015A	S82.109B	S82.151C	S82.242A
S72.451B	S73.014A	S82.015B	S82.109C	S82.152A	S82.242B
S72.451C	S73.015A	S82.015C	S82.111A	S82.152B	S82.242C
S72.452A	S73.016A	S82.016A	S82.111B	S82.152C	S82.243A
S72.452B	S73.021A	S82.016B	S82.111C	S82.153A	S82.243B
S72.452C	S73.022A	S82.016C	S82.112A	S82.153B	S82.243C
S72.453A	S73.023A	S82.021A	S82.112B	S82.153C	S82.244A
S72.453B	S73.024A	S82.021B	S82.112C	S82.154A	S82.244B
S72.453C	S73.025A	S82.021C	S82.113A	S82.154B	S82.244C
S72.454A	S73.026A	S82.022A	S82.113B	S82.154C	S82.245A
S72.454B	S73.031A	S82.022B	S82.113C	S82.155A	S82.245B
S72.454C	S73.032A	S82.022C	S82.114A	S82.155B	S82.245C
S72.455A	S73.033A	S82.023A	S82.114B	S82.155C	S82.246A
S72.455B	S73.034A	S82.023B	S82.114C	S82.156A	S82.246B
S72.455C	S73.035A	S82.023C	S82.115A	S82.156B	S82.246C
S72.456A	S73.036A	S82.024A	S82.115B	S82.156C	S82.251A
S72.456B	S73.041A	S82.024B	S82.115C	S82.161A	S82.251B
S72.456C	S73.042A	S82.024C	S82.116A	S82.162A	S82.251C
S72.461A	S73.043A	S82.025A	S82.116B	S82.169A	S82.252A
S72.461B	S73.044A	S82.025B	S82.116C	S82.191A	S82.252B
S72.461C	S73.045A	S82.025C	S82.121A	S82.191B	S82.252C
S72.462A	S73.046A	S82.026A	S82.121B	S82.191C	S82.253A
S72.462B	S77.00XA	S82.026B	S82.121C	S82.192A	S82.253B
S72.462C	S77.01XA	S82.026C	S82.122A	S82.192B	S82.253C
S72.463A	S77.02XA	S82.031A	S82.122B	S82.192C	S82.254A
S72.463B	S77.10XA	S82.031B	S82.122C	S82.199A	S82.254B
S72.463C	S77.11XA	S82.031C	S82.123A	S82.199B	S82.254C
S72.464A	S77.12XA	S82.032A	S82.123B	S82.199C	S82.255A
S72.464B	S79.001A	S82.032B	S82.123C	S82.201A	S82.255B
S72.464C	S79.002A	S82.032C	S82.124A	S82.201B	S82.255C
S72.465A	S79.009A	S82.033A	S82.124B	S82.201C	S82.256A
S72.465B	S79.011A	S82.033B	S82.124C	S82.202A	S82.256B
S72.465C	S79.012A	S82.033C	S82.125A	S82.202B	S82.256C
S72.466A	S79.019A	S82.034A	S82.125B	S82.202C	S82.261A
S72.466B	S79.091A	S82.034B	S82.125C	S82.209A	S82.261B
S72.466C	S79.092A	S82.034C	S82.126A	S82.209B	S82.261C
S72.471A	S79.099A	S82.035A	S82.126B	S82.209C	S82.262A
S72.472A	S79.101A	S82.035B	S82.126C	S82.221A	S82.262B
S72.479A	S79.102A	S82.035C	S82.131A	S82.221B	S82.262C
S72.491A	S79.109A	S82.036A	S82.131B	S82.221C	S82.263A
S72.491B	S79.111A	S82.036B	S82.131C	S82.222A	S82.263B
S72.491C	S79.112A	S82.036C	S82.132A	S82.222B	S82.263C
S72.492A	S79.119A	S82.041A	S82.132B	S82.222C	S82.264A
S72.492B	S79.121A	S82.041B	S82.132C	S82.223A	S82.264B
S72.492C	S79.122A	S82.041C	S82.133A	S82.223B	S82.264C
S72.499A	S79.129A	S82.042A	S82.133B	S82.223C	S82.265A
S72.499B	S79.131A	S82.042B	S82.133C	S82.224A	S82.265B
S72.499C	S79.132A	S82.042C	S82.134A	S82.224B	S82.265C
	S79.139A	S82.043A	S82.134B	S82.224C	S82.266A
	S79.141A	S82.043B	S82.134C	S82.225A	S82.266B

HAC 05: Falls and Trauma (continued)	S82.454C	S82.856C	S92.041B	S92.242B	T21.34XA
S82.266C	S82.455B	S82.861B	S92.042B	S92.243B	T21.35XA
S82.291A	S82.455C	S82.861C	S92.043B	S92.244B	T21.36XA
S82.291B	S82.456B	S82.862B	S92.044B	S92.245B	T21.37XA
S82.291C	S82.456C	S82.862C	S92.045B	S92.246B	T21.39XA
S82.292A	S82.461B	S82.863B	S92.046B	S92.251B	T21.70XA
S82.292B	S82.461C	S82.863C	S92.051B	S92.252B	T21.71XA
S82.292C	S82.462B	S82.864B	S92.052B	S92.253B	T21.72XA
S82.299A	S82.462C	S82.864C	S92.053B	S92.254B	T21.73XA
S82.299B	S82.463B	S82.865B	S92.054B	S92.255B	T21.74XA
S82.299C	S82.463C	S82.865C	S92.055B	S92.256B	T21.75XA
S82.301B	S82.464B	S82.866B	S92.056B	S92.301B	T21.76XA
S82.301C	S82.464C	S82.866C	S92.061B	S92.302B	T21.77XA
S82.302B	S82.465B	S82.871B	S92.062B	S92.309B	T21.79XA
S82.302C	S82.465C	S82.871C	S92.063B	S92.311B	T22.30XA
S82.309B	S82.466B	S82.872B	S92.064B	S92.312B	T22.311A
S82.309C	S82.466C	S82.872C	S92.065B	S92.313B	T22.312A
S82.311A	S82.491B	S82.873B	S92.066B	S92.314B	T22.319A
S82.312A	S82.491C	S82.873C	S92.101B	S92.315B	T22.321A
S82.319A	S82.492B	S82.874B	S92.102B	S92.316B	T22.322A
S82.391B	S82.492C	S82.874C	S92.109B	S92.321B	T22.329A
S82.391C	S82.499B	S82.875B	S92.111B	S92.322B	T22.331A
S82.392B	S82.499C	S82.875C	S92.112B	S92.323B	T22.332A
S82.392C	S82.51XB	S82.876B	S92.113B	S92.324B	T22.339A
S82.399B	S82.51XC	S82.876C	S92.114B	S92.325B	T22.341A
S82.399C	S82.52XB	S82.891B	S92.115B	S92.326B	T22.342A
S82.401B	S82.52XC	S82.891C	S92.116B	S92.331B	T22.349A
S82.401C	S82.53XB	S82.892B	S92.121B	S92.332B	T22.351A
S82.402B	S82.53XC	S82.892C	S92.122B	S92.333B	T22.352A
S82.402C	S82.54XB	S82.899B	S92.123B	S92.334B	T22.359A
S82.409B	S82.54XC	S82.899C	S92.124B	S92.335B	T22.361A
S82.409C	S82.55XB	S82.90XB	S92.125B	S92.336B	T22.362A
S82.421B	S82.55XC	S82.90XC	S92.126B	S92.341B	T22.369A
S82.421C	S82.56XB	S82.91XB	S92.131B	S92.342B	T22.391A
S82.422B	S82.56XC	S82.91XC	S92.132B	S92.343B	T22.392A
S82.422C	S82.61XB	S82.92XB	S92.133B	S92.344B	T22.399A
S82.423B	S82.61XC	S82.92XC	S92.134B	S92.345B	T22.70XA
S82.423C	S82.62XB	S89.001A	S92.135B	S92.346B	T22.711A
S82.424B	S82.62XC	S89.002A	S92.136B	S92.351B	T22.712A
S82.424C	S82.63XB	S89.009A	S92.141B	S92.352B	T22.719A
S82.425B	S82.63XC	S89.011A	S92.142B	S92.353B	T22.721A
S82.425C	S82.64XB	S89.012A	S92.143B	S92.354B	T22.722A
S82.426B	S82.64XC	S89.019A	S92.144B	S92.355B	T22.729A
S82.426C	S82.65XB	S89.021A	S92.145B	S92.356B	T22.731A
S82.431B	S82.65XC	S89.022A	S92.146B	S92.811B	T22.732A
S82.431C	S82.66XB	S89.029A	S92.151B	S92.812B	T22.739A
S82.432B	S82.66XC	S89.031A	S92.152B	S92.819B	T22.741A
S82.432C	S82.831B	S89.032A	S92.153B	S92.901B	T22.742A
S82.433B	S82.831C	S89.039A	S92.154B	S92.902B	T22.749A
S82.433C	S82.832B	S89.041A	S92.155B	S92.909B	T22.751A
S82.434B	S82.832C	S89.042A	S92.156B	T20.30XA	T22.752A
S82.434C	S82.839B	S89.049A	S92.191B	T20.311A	T22.759A
S82.435B	S82.839C	S89.091A	S92.192B	T20.312A	T22.761A
S82.435C	S82.841B	S89.092A	S92.199B	T20.319A	T22.762A
S82.436B	S82.841C	S89.099A	S92.201B	T20.32XA	T22.769A
S82.436C	S82.842B	S92.001B	S92.202B	T20.33XA	T22.791A
S82.441B	S82.842C	S92.002B	S92.209B	T20.34XA	T22.792A
S82.441C	S82.843B	S92.009B	S92.211B	T20.35XA	T22.799A
S82.442B	S82.843C	S92.011B	S92.212B	T20.36XA	T23.301A
S82.442C	S82.844B	S92.012B	S92.213B	T20.37XA	T23.302A
S82.443B	S82.844C	S92.013B	S92.214B	T20.39XA	T23.309A
S82.443C	S82.845B	S92.014B	S92.215B	T20.70XA	T23.311A
S82.444B	S82.845C	S92.015B	S92.216B	T20.711A	T23.312A
S82.444C	S82.846B	S92.016B	S92.221B	T20.712A	T23.319A
S82.445B	S82.846C	S92.021B	S92.222B	T20.719A	T23.321A
S82.445C	S82.851B	S92.022B	S92.223B	T20.72XA	T23.322A
S82.446B	S82.851C	S92.023B	S92.224B	T20.73XA	T23.329A
S82.446C	S82.852B	S92.024B	S92.225B	T20.74XA	T23.331A
S82.451B	S82.852C	S92.025B	S92.226B	T20.75XA	T23.332A
S82.451C	S82.853B	S92.026B	S92.231B	T20.76XA	T23.339A
S82.452B	S82.853C	S92.031B	S92.232B	T20.77XA	T23.341A
S82.452C	S82.854B	S92.032B	S92.233B	T20.79XA	T23.342A
S82.453B	S82.854C	S92.033B	S92.234B	T21.30XA	T23.349A
S82.453C	S82.855B	S92.034B	S92.235B	T21.31XA	T23.351A
S82.454B	S82.855C	S92.035B	S92.236B	T21.32XA	T23.352A
	S82.856B	S92.036B	S92.241B	T21.33XA	T23.359A

HAC 05: Falls and Trauma (continued)

T23.361A	T24.729A	T31.44	T32.61	T33.821A	T71.141A
T23.362A	T24.731A	T31.50	T32.62	T33.822A	T71.143A
T23.369A	T24.732A	T31.51	T32.63	T33.829A	T71.144A
T23.371A	T24.739A	T31.52	T32.64	T33.831A	T71.151A
T23.372A	T24.791A	T31.53	T32.65	T33.832A	T71.152A
T23.379A	T24.792A	T31.54	T32.66	T33.839A	T71.153A
T23.391A	T24.799A	T31.55	T32.70	T33.90XA	T71.154A
T23.392A	T25.311A	T31.60	T32.71	T33.99XA	T71.161A
T23.399A	T25.312A	T31.61	T32.72	T34.011A	T71.162A
T23.701A	T25.319A	T31.62	T32.73	T34.012A	T71.163A
T23.702A	T25.321A	T31.63	T32.74	T34.019A	T71.164A
T23.709A	T25.322A	T31.64	T32.75	T34.02XA	T71.191A
T23.711A	T25.329A	T31.65	T32.76	T34.09XA	T71.192A
T23.712A	T25.331A	T31.66	T32.77	T34.1XXA	T71.193A
T23.719A	T25.332A	T31.70	T32.80	T34.2XXA	T71.194A
T23.721A	T25.339A	T31.71	T32.81	T34.3XXA	T71.20XA
T23.722A	T25.391A	T31.72	T32.82	T34.40XA	T71.21XA
T23.729A	T25.392A	T31.73	T32.83	T34.41XA	T71.29XA
T23.731A	T25.399A	T31.74	T32.84	T34.42XA	T71.9XXA
T23.732A	T25.711A	T31.75	T32.85	T34.511A	T75.1XXA
T23.739A	T25.712A	T31.76	T32.86	T34.512A	
T23.741A	T25.719A	T31.77	T32.87	T34.519A	**HAC 06: Catheter**
T23.742A	T25.721A	T31.80	T32.88	T34.521A	**Associated Urinary**
T23.749A	T25.722A	T31.81	T32.90	T34.522A	**Tract Infection (UTI)**
T23.751A	T25.729A	T31.82	T32.91	T34.529A	Secondary diagnosis
T23.752A	T25.731A	T31.83	T32.92	T34.531A	not POA:
T23.759A	T25.732A	T31.84	T32.93	T34.532A	T83.511A
T23.761A	T25.739A	T31.85	T32.94	T34.539A	T83.518A
T23.762A	T25.791A	T31.86	T32.95	T34.60XA	
T23.769A	T25.792A	T31.87	T32.96	T34.61XA	**With or Without**
T23.771A	T25.799A	T31.88	T32.97	T34.62XA	Secondary diagnosis
T23.772A	T26.20XA	T31.90	T32.98	T34.70XA	(also not POA) of:
T23.779A	T26.21XA	T31.91	T32.99	T34.71XA	B37.41
T23.791A	T26.22XA	T31.92	T33.011A	T34.72XA	B37.49
T23.792A	T26.70XA	T31.93	T33.012A	T34.811A	N10
T23.799A	T26.71XA	T31.94	T33.019A	T34.812A	N11.9
T24.301A	T26.72XA	T31.95	T33.02XA	T34.819A	N12
T24.302A	T27.0XXA	T31.96	T33.09XA	T34.821A	N13.6
T24.309A	T27.1XXA	T31.97	T33.1XXA	T34.822A	N15.1
T24.311A	T27.2XXA	T31.98	T33.2XXA	T34.829A	N28.84
T24.312A	T27.3XXA	T31.99	T33.3XXA	T34.831A	N28.85
T24.319A	T27.4XXA	T32.10	T33.40XA	T34.832A	N28.86
T24.321A	T27.5XXA	T32.11	T33.41XA	T34.839A	N30.00
T24.322A	T27.6XXA	T32.20	T33.42XA	T34.90XA	N30.01
T24.329A	T27.7XXA	T32.21	T33.511A	T34.99XA	N34.0
T24.331A	T28.1XXA	T32.22	T33.512A	T67.0XXA	N39.0
T24.332A	T28.2XXA	T32.30	T33.519A	T69.021A	
T24.339A	T28.6XXA	T32.31	T33.521A	T69.022A	**HAC 07: Vascular**
T24.391A	T28.7XXA	T32.32	T33.522A	T69.029A	**Catheter Associated**
T24.392A	T31.10	T32.33	T33.529A	T70.3XXA	**Infection**
T24.399A	T31.11	T32.40	T33.531A	T71.111A	Secondary diagnosis
T24.701A	T31.20	T32.41	T33.532A	T71.112A	not POA:
T24.702A	T31.21	T32.42	T33.539A	T71.113A	T80.211A
T24.709A	T31.22	T32.43	T33.60XA	T71.114A	T80.212A
T24.711A	T31.30	T32.44	T33.61XA	T71.121A	T80.218A
T24.712A	T31.31	T32.50	T33.62XA	T71.122A	T80.219A
T24.719A	T31.32	T32.51	T33.70XA	T71.123A	
T24.721A	T31.33	T32.52	T33.71XA	T71.124A	
T24.722A	T31.40	T32.53	T33.72XA	T71.131A	
	T31.41	T32.54	T33.811A	T71.132A	
	T31.42	T32.55	T33.812A	T71.133A	
	T31.43	T32.60	T33.819A	T71.134A	

HAC 08: Surgical Site Infection of Mediastinitis Following Coronary Bypass Graft (CABG) Procedures

Secondary diagnosis not POA:
- J98.51
- J98.59

AND

Any of the following procedures:

0210083 Bypass Coronary Artery, One Artery from Coronary Artery with Zooplastic Tissue, Open Approach

0210088 Bypass Coronary Artery, One Artery from Right Internal Mammary with Zooplastic Tissue, Open Approach

0210089 Bypass Coronary Artery, One Artery from Left Internal Mammary with Zooplastic Tissue, Open Approach

021008C Bypass Coronary Artery, One Artery from Thoracic Artery with Zooplastic Tissue, Open Approach

021008F Bypass Coronary Artery, One Artery from Abdominal Artery with Zooplastic Tissue, Open Approach

021008W Bypass Coronary Artery, One Artery from Aorta with Zooplastic Tissue, Open Approach

0210093 Bypass Coronary Artery, One Artery from Coronary Artery with Autologous Venous Tissue, Open Approach

0210098 Bypass Coronary Artery, One Artery from Right Internal Mammary with Autologous Venous Tissue, Open Approach

0210099 Bypass Coronary Artery, One Artery from Left Internal Mammary with Autologous Venous Tissue, Open Approach

021009C Bypass Coronary Artery, One Artery from Thoracic Artery with Autologous Venous Tissue, Open Approach

021009F Bypass Coronary Artery, One Artery from Abdominal Artery with Autologous Venous Tissue, Open Approach

021009W Bypass Coronary Artery, One Artery from Aorta with Autologous Venous Tissue, Open Approach

02100A3 Bypass Coronary Artery, One Artery from Coronary Artery with Autologous Arterial Tissue, Open Approach

02100A8 Bypass Coronary Artery, One Artery from Right Internal Mammary with Autologous Arterial Tissue, Open Approach

02100A9 Bypass Coronary Artery, One Artery from Left Internal Mammary with Autologous Arterial Tissue, Open Approach

02100AC Bypass Coronary Artery, One Artery from Thoracic Artery with Autologous Arterial Tissue, Open Approach

02100AF Bypass Coronary Artery, One Artery from Abdominal Artery with Autologous Arterial Tissue, Open Approach

02100AW Bypass Coronary Artery, One Artery from Aorta with Autologous Arterial Tissue, Open Approach

02100J3 Bypass Coronary Artery, One Artery from Coronary Artery with Synthetic Substitute, Open Approach

02100J8 Bypass Coronary Artery, One Artery from Right Internal Mammary with Synthetic Substitute, Open Approach

02100J9 Bypass Coronary Artery, One Artery from Left Internal Mammary with Synthetic Substitute, Open Approach

02100JC Bypass Coronary Artery, One Artery from Thoracic Artery with Synthetic Substitute, Open Approach

02100JF Bypass Coronary Artery, One Artery from Abdominal Artery with Synthetic Substitute, Open Approach

02100JW Bypass Coronary Artery, One Artery from Aorta with Synthetic Substitute, Open Approach

02100K3 Bypass Coronary Artery, One Artery from Coronary Artery with Nonautologous Tissue Substitute, Open Approach

02100K8 Bypass Coronary Artery, One Artery from Right Internal Mammary with Nonautologous Tissue Substitute, Open Approach

02100K9 Bypass Coronary Artery, One Artery from Left Internal Mammary with Nonautologous Tissue Substitute, Open Approach

02100KC Bypass Coronary Artery, One Artery from Thoracic Artery with Nonautologous Tissue Substitute, Open Approach

02100KF Bypass Coronary Artery, One Artery from Abdominal Artery with Nonautologous Tissue Substitute, Open Approach

02100KW Bypass Coronary Artery, One Artery from Aorta with Nonautologous Tissue Substitute, Open Approach

02100Z3 Bypass Coronary Artery, One Artery from Coronary Artery, Open Approach

02100Z8 Bypass Coronary Artery, One Artery from Right Internal Mammary, Open Approach

02100Z9 Bypass Coronary Artery, One Artery from Left Internal Mammary, Open Approach

02100ZC Bypass Coronary Artery, One Artery from Thoracic Artery, Open Approach

02100ZF Bypass Coronary Artery, One Artery from Abdominal Artery, Open Approach

0210483 Bypass Coronary Artery, One Artery from Coronary Artery with Zooplastic Tissue, Percutaneous Endoscopic Approach

0210488 Bypass Coronary Artery, One Artery from Right Internal Mammary with Zooplastic Tissue, Percutaneous Endoscopic Approach

0210489 Bypass Coronary Artery, One Artery from Left Internal Mammary with Zooplastic Tissue, Percutaneous Endoscopic Approach

021048C Bypass Coronary Artery, One Artery from Thoracic Artery with Zooplastic Tissue, Percutaneous Endoscopic Approach

021048F Bypass Coronary Artery, One Artery from Abdominal Artery with Zooplastic Tissue, Percutaneous Endoscopic Approach

021048W Bypass Coronary Artery, One Artery from Aorta with Zooplastic Tissue, Percutaneous Endoscopic Approach

0210493 Bypass Coronary Artery, One Artery from Coronary Artery with Autologous Venous Tissue, Percutaneous Endoscopic Approach

0210498 Bypass Coronary Artery, One Artery from Right Internal Mammary with Autologous Venous Tissue, Percutaneous Endoscopic Approach

0210499 Bypass Coronary Artery, One Artery from Left Internal Mammary with Autologous Venous Tissue, Percutaneous Endoscopic Approach

021049C Bypass Coronary Artery, One Artery from Thoracic Artery with Autologous Venous Tissue, Percutaneous Endoscopic Approach

021049F Bypass Coronary Artery, One Artery from Abdominal Artery with Autologous Venous Tissue, Percutaneous Endoscopic Approach

021049W Bypass Coronary Artery, One Artery from Aorta with Autologous Venous Tissue, Percutaneous Endoscopic Approach

02104A3 Bypass Coronary Artery, One Artery from Coronary Artery with Autologous Arterial Tissue, Percutaneous Endoscopic Approach

02104A8 Bypass Coronary Artery, One Artery from Right Internal Mammary with Autologous Arterial Tissue, Percutaneous Endoscopic Approach

02104A9 Bypass Coronary Artery, One Artery from Left Internal Mammary with Autologous Arterial Tissue, Percutaneous Endoscopic Approach

02104AC Bypass Coronary Artery, One Artery from Thoracic Artery with Autologous Arterial Tissue, Percutaneous Endoscopic Approach

02104AF Bypass Coronary Artery, One Artery from Abdominal Artery with Autologous Arterial Tissue, Percutaneous Endoscopic Approach

02104AW Bypass Coronary Artery, One Artery from Aorta with Autologous Arterial Tissue, Percutaneous Endoscopic Approach

02104J3 Bypass Coronary Artery, One Artery from Coronary Artery with Synthetic Substitute, Percutaneous Endoscopic Approach

02104J8 Bypass Coronary Artery, One Artery from Right Internal Mammary with Synthetic Substitute, Percutaneous Endoscopic Approach

02104J9 Bypass Coronary Artery, One Artery from Left Internal Mammary with Synthetic Substitute, Percutaneous Endoscopic Approach

02104JC Bypass Coronary Artery, One Artery from Thoracic Artery with Synthetic Substitute, Percutaneous Endoscopic Approach

02104JF Bypass Coronary Artery, One Artery from Abdominal Artery with Synthetic Substitute, Percutaneous Endoscopic Approach

02104JW Bypass Coronary Artery, One Artery from Aorta with Synthetic Substitute, Percutaneous Endoscopic Approach

02104K3 Bypass Coronary Artery, One Artery from Coronary Artery with Nonautologous Tissue Substitute, Percutaneous Endoscopic Approach

02104K8 Bypass Coronary Artery, One Artery from Right Internal Mammary with Nonautologous Tissue Substitute, Percutaneous Endoscopic Approach

02104K9 Bypass Coronary Artery, One Artery from Left Internal Mammary with Nonautologous Tissue Substitute, Percutaneous Endoscopic Approach

02104KC Bypass Coronary Artery, One Artery from Thoracic Artery with Nonautologous Tissue Substitute, Percutaneous Endoscopic Approach

HAC 08: Surgical Artery Infection of Mediastinitis Following Coronary Bypass Graft (CABG) Procedures (continued)

02104KF Bypass Coronary Artery, One Artery from Abdominal Artery with Nonautologous Tissue Substitute, Percutaneous Endoscopic Approach

02104KW Bypass Coronary Artery, One Artery from Aorta with Nonautologous Tissue Substitute, Percutaneous Endoscopic Approach

02104Z3 Bypass Coronary Artery, One Artery from Coronary Artery, Percutaneous Endoscopic Approach

02104Z8 Bypass Coronary Artery, One Artery from Right Internal Mammary, Percutaneous Endoscopic Approach

02104Z9 Bypass Coronary Artery, One Artery from Left Internal Mammary, Percutaneous Endoscopic Approach

02104ZC Bypass Coronary Artery, One Artery from Thoracic Artery, Percutaneous Endoscopic Approach

02104ZF Bypass Coronary Artery, One Artery from Abdominal Artery, Percutaneous Endoscopic Approach

0211083 Bypass Coronary Artery, Two Arteries from Coronary Artery with Zooplastic Tissue, Open Approach

0211088 Bypass Coronary Artery, Two Arteries from Right Internal Mammary with Zooplastic Tissue, Open Approach

0211089 Bypass Coronary Artery, Two Arteries from Left Internal Mammary with Zooplastic Tissue, Open Approach

021108C Bypass Coronary Artery, Two Arteries from Thoracic Artery with Zooplastic Tissue, Open Approach

021108F Bypass Coronary Artery, Two Arteries from Abdominal Artery with Zooplastic Tissue, Open Approach

021108W Bypass Coronary Artery, Two Arteries from Aorta with Zooplastic Tissue, Open Approach

0211093 Bypass Coronary Artery, Two Arteries from Coronary Artery with Autologous Venous Tissue, Open Approach

0211098 Bypass Coronary Artery, Two Arteries from Right Internal Mammary with Autologous Venous Tissue, Open Approach

0211099 Bypass Coronary Artery, Two Arteries from Left Internal Mammary with Autologous Venous Tissue, Open Approach

021109C Bypass Coronary Artery, Two Arteries from Thoracic Artery with Autologous Venous Tissue, Open Approach

021109F Bypass Coronary Artery, Two Arteries from Abdominal Artery with Autologous Venous Tissue, Open Approach

021109W Bypass Coronary Artery, Two Arteries from Aorta with Autologous Venous Tissue, Open Approach

02110A3 Bypass Coronary Artery, Two Arteries from Coronary Artery with Autologous Arterial Tissue, Open Approach

02110A8 Bypass Coronary Artery, Two Arteries from Right Internal Mammary with Autologous Arterial Tissue, Open Approach

02110A9 Bypass Coronary Artery, Two Arteries from Left Internal Mammary with Autologous Arterial Tissue, Open Approach

02110AC Bypass Coronary Artery, Two Arteries from Thoracic Artery with Autologous Arterial Tissue, Open Approach

02110AF Bypass Coronary Artery, Two Arteries from Abdominal Artery with Autologous Arterial Tissue, Open Approach

02110AW Bypass Coronary Artery, Two Arteries from Aorta with Autologous Arterial Tissue, Open Approach

02110J3 Bypass Coronary Artery, Two Arteries from Coronary Artery with Synthetic Substitute, Open Approach

02110J8 Bypass Coronary Artery, Two Arteries from Right Internal Mammary with Synthetic Substitute, Open Approach

02110J9 Bypass Coronary Artery, Two Arteries from Left Internal Mammary with Synthetic Substitute, Open Approach

02110JC Bypass Coronary Artery, Two Arteries from Thoracic Artery with Synthetic Substitute, Open Approach

02110JF Bypass Coronary Artery, Two Arteries from Abdominal Artery with Synthetic Substitute, Open Approach

02110JW Bypass Coronary Artery, Two Arteries from Aorta with Synthetic Substitute, Open Approach

02110K3 Bypass Coronary Artery, Two Arteries from Coronary Artery with Nonautologous Tissue Substitute, Open Approach

02110K8 Bypass Coronary Artery, Two Arteries from Right Internal Mammary with Nonautologous Tissue Substitute, Open Approach

02110K9 Bypass Coronary Artery, Two Arteries from Left Internal Mammary with Nonautologous Tissue Substitute, Open Approach

02110KC Bypass Coronary Artery, Two Arteries from Thoracic Artery with Nonautologous Tissue Substitute, Open Approach

02110KF Bypass Coronary Artery, Two Arteries from Abdominal Artery with Nonautologous Tissue Substitute, Open Approach

02110KW Bypass Coronary Artery, Two Arteries from Aorta with Nonautologous Tissue Substitute, Open Approach

02110Z3 Bypass Coronary Artery, Two Arteries from Coronary Artery, Open Approach

02110Z8 Bypass Coronary Artery, Two Arteries from Right Internal Mammary, Open Approach

02110Z9 Bypass Coronary Artery, Two Arteries from Left Internal Mammary, Open Approach

02110ZC Bypass Coronary Artery, Two Arteries from Thoracic Artery, Open Approach

02110ZF Bypass Coronary Artery, Two Arteries from Abdominal Artery, Open Approach

0211483 Bypass Coronary Artery, Two Arteries from Coronary Artery with Zooplastic Tissue, Percutaneous Endoscopic Approach

0211488 Bypass Coronary Artery, Two Arteries from Right Internal Mammary with Zooplastic Tissue, Percutaneous Endoscopic Approach

0211489 Bypass Coronary Artery, Two Arteries from Left Internal Mammary with Zooplastic Tissue, Percutaneous Endoscopic Approach

021148C Bypass Coronary Artery, Two Arteries from Thoracic Artery with Zooplastic Tissue, Percutaneous Endoscopic Approach

021148F Bypass Coronary Artery, Two Arteries from Abdominal Artery with Zooplastic Tissue, Percutaneous Endoscopic Approach

021148W Bypass Coronary Artery, Two Arteries from Aorta with Zooplastic Tissue, Percutaneous Endoscopic Approach

0211493 Bypass Coronary Artery, Two Arteries from Coronary Artery with Autologous Venous Tissue, Percutaneous Endoscopic Approach

0211498 Bypass Coronary Artery, Two Arteries from Right Internal Mammary with Autologous Venous Tissue, Percutaneous Endoscopic Approach

0211499 Bypass Coronary Artery, Two Arteries from Left Internal Mammary with Autologous Venous Tissue, Percutaneous Endoscopic Approach

021149C Bypass Coronary Artery, Two Arteries from Thoracic Artery with Autologous Venous Tissue, Percutaneous Endoscopic Approach

021149F Bypass Coronary Artery, Two Arteries from Abdominal Artery with Autologous Venous Tissue, Percutaneous Endoscopic Approach

021149W Bypass Coronary Artery, Two Arteries from Aorta with Autologous Venous Tissue, Percutaneous Endoscopic Approach

02114A3 Bypass Coronary Artery, Two Arteries from Coronary Artery with Autologous Arterial Tissue, Percutaneous Endoscopic Approach

02114A8 Bypass Coronary Artery, Two Arteries from Right Internal Mammary with Autologous Arterial Tissue, Percutaneous Endoscopic Approach

02114A9 Bypass Coronary Artery, Two Arteries from Left Internal Mammary with Autologous Arterial Tissue, Percutaneous Endoscopic Approach

02114AC Bypass Coronary Artery, Two Arteries from Thoracic Artery with Autologous Arterial Tissue, Percutaneous Endoscopic Approach

02114AF Bypass Coronary Artery, Two Arteries from Abdominal Artery with Autologous Arterial Tissue, Percutaneous Endoscopic Approach

02114AW Bypass Coronary Artery, Two Arteries from Aorta with Autologous Arterial Tissue, Percutaneous Endoscopic Approach

02114J3 Bypass Coronary Artery, Two Arteries from Coronary Artery with Synthetic Substitute, Percutaneous Endoscopic Approach

02114J8 Bypass Coronary Artery, Two Arteries from Right Internal Mammary with Synthetic Substitute, Percutaneous Endoscopic Approach

02114J9 Bypass Coronary Artery, Two Arteries from Left Internal Mammary with Synthetic Substitute, Percutaneous Endoscopic Approach

02114JC Bypass Coronary Artery, Two Arteries from Thoracic Artery with Synthetic Substitute, Percutaneous Endoscopic Approach

HAC 08: Surgical Site Infection of Mediastinitis Following Coronary Bypass Graft (CABG) Procedures (continued)

02114JF   Bypass Coronary Artery, Two Arteries from Abdominal Artery with Synthetic Substitute, Percutaneous Endoscopic Approach

02114JW   Bypass Coronary Artery, Two Arteries from Aorta with Synthetic Substitute, Percutaneous Endoscopic Approach

02114K3   Bypass Coronary Artery, Two Arteries from Coronary Artery with Nonautologous Tissue Substitute, Percutaneous Endoscopic Approach

02114K8   Bypass Coronary Artery, Two Arteries from Right Internal Mammary with Nonautologous Tissue Substitute, Percutaneous Endoscopic Approach

02114K9   Bypass Coronary Artery, Two Arteries from Left Internal Mammary with Nonautologous Tissue Substitute, Percutaneous Endoscopic Approach

02114KC   Bypass Coronary Artery, Two Arteries from Thoracic Artery with Nonautologous Tissue Substitute, Percutaneous Endoscopic Approach

02114KF   Bypass Coronary Artery, Two Arteries from Abdominal Artery with Nonautologous Tissue Substitute, Percutaneous Endoscopic Approach

02114KW   Bypass Coronary Artery, Two Arteries from Aorta with Nonautologous Tissue Substitute, Percutaneous Endoscopic Approach

02114Z3   Bypass Coronary Artery, Two Arteries from Coronary Artery, Percutaneous Endoscopic Approach

02114Z8   Bypass Coronary Artery, Two Arteries from Right Internal Mammary, Percutaneous Endoscopic Approach

02114Z9   Bypass Coronary Artery, Two Arteries from Left Internal Mammary, Percutaneous Endoscopic Approach

02114ZC   Bypass Coronary Artery, Two Arteries from Thoracic Artery, Percutaneous Endoscopic Approach

02114ZF   Bypass Coronary Artery, Two Arteries from Abdominal Artery, Percutaneous Endoscopic Approach

0212083   Bypass Coronary Artery, Three Arteries from Coronary Artery with Zooplastic Tissue, Open Approach

0212088   Bypass Coronary Artery, Three Arteries from Right Internal Mammary with Zooplastic Tissue, Open Approach

0212089   Bypass Coronary Artery, Three Arteries from Left Internal Mammary with Zooplastic Tissue, Open Approach

021208C   Bypass Coronary Artery, Three Arteries from Thoracic Artery with Zooplastic Tissue, Open Approach

021208F   Bypass Coronary Artery, Three Arteries from Abdominal Artery with Zooplastic Tissue, Open Approach

021208W   Bypass Coronary Artery, Three Arteries from Aorta with Zooplastic Tissue, Open Approach

0212093   Bypass Coronary Artery, Three Arteries from Coronary Artery with Autologous Venous Tissue, Open Approach

0212098   Bypass Coronary Artery, Three Arteries from Right Internal Mammary with Autologous Venous Tissue, Open Approach

0212099   Bypass Coronary Artery, Three Arteries from Left Internal Mammary with Autologous Venous Tissue, Open Approach

021209C   Bypass Coronary Artery, Three Arteries from Thoracic Artery with Autologous Venous Tissue, Open Approach

021209F   Bypass Coronary Artery, Three Arteries from Abdominal Artery with Autologous Venous Tissue, Open Approach

021209W   Bypass Coronary Artery, Three Arteries from Aorta with Autologous Venous Tissue, Open Approach

02120A3   Bypass Coronary Artery, Three Arteries from Coronary Artery with Autologous Arterial Tissue, Open Approach

02120A8   Bypass Coronary Artery, Three Arteries from Right Internal Mammary with Autologous Arterial Tissue, Open Approach

02120A9   Bypass Coronary Artery, Three Arteries from Left Internal Mammary with Autologous Arterial Tissue, Open Approach

02120AC   Bypass Coronary Artery, Three Arteries from Thoracic Artery with Autologous Arterial Tissue, Open Approach

02120AF   Bypass Coronary Artery, Three Arteries from Abdominal Artery with Autologous Arterial Tissue, Open Approach

02120AW   Bypass Coronary Artery, Three Arteries from Aorta with Autologous Arterial Tissue, Open Approach

02120J3   Bypass Coronary Artery, Three Arteries from Coronary Artery with Synthetic Substitute, Open Approach

02120J8   Bypass Coronary Artery, Three Arteries from Right Internal Mammary with Synthetic Substitute, Open Approach

02120J9   Bypass Coronary Artery, Three Arteries from Left Internal Mammary with Synthetic Substitute, Open Approach

02120JC   Bypass Coronary Artery, Three Arteries from Thoracic Artery with Synthetic Substitute, Open Approach

02120JF   Bypass Coronary Artery, Three Arteries from Abdominal Artery with Synthetic Substitute, Open Approach

02120JW   Bypass Coronary Artery, Three Arteries from Aorta with Synthetic Substitute, Open Approach

02120K3   Bypass Coronary Artery, Three Arteries from Coronary Artery with Nonautologous Tissue Substitute, Open Approach

02120K8   Bypass Coronary Artery, Three Arteries from Right Internal Mammary with Nonautologous Tissue Substitute, Open Approach

02120K9   Bypass Coronary Artery, Three Arteries from Left Internal Mammary with Nonautologous Tissue Substitute, Open Approach

02120KC   Bypass Coronary Artery, Three Arteries from Thoracic Artery with Nonautologous Tissue Substitute, Open Approach

02120KF   Bypass Coronary Artery, Three Arteries from Abdominal Artery with Nonautologous Tissue Substitute, Open Approach

02120KW   Bypass Coronary Artery, Three Arteries from Aorta with Nonautologous Tissue Substitute, Open Approach

02120Z3   Bypass Coronary Artery, Three Arteries from Coronary Artery, Open Approach

02120Z8   Bypass Coronary Artery, Three Arteries from Right Internal Mammary, Open Approach

02120Z9   Bypass Coronary Artery, Three Arteries from Left Internal Mammary, Open Approach

02120ZC   Bypass Coronary Artery, Three Arteries from Thoracic Artery, Open Approach

02120ZF   Bypass Coronary Artery, Three Arteries from Abdominal Artery, Open Approach

0212483   Bypass Coronary Artery, Three Arteries from Coronary Artery with Zooplastic Tissue, Percutaneous Endoscopic Approach

0212488   Bypass Coronary Artery, Three Arteries from Right Internal Mammary with Zooplastic Tissue, Percutaneous Endoscopic Approach

0212489   Bypass Coronary Artery, Three Arteries from Left Internal Mammary with Zooplastic Tissue, Percutaneous Endoscopic Approach

021248C   Bypass Coronary Artery, Three Arteries from Thoracic Artery with Zooplastic Tissue, Percutaneous Endoscopic Approach

021248F   Bypass Coronary Artery, Three Arteries from Abdominal Artery with Zooplastic Tissue, Percutaneous Endoscopic Approach

021248W   Bypass Coronary Artery, Three Arteries from Aorta with Zooplastic Tissue, Percutaneous Endoscopic Approach

0212493   Bypass Coronary Artery, Three Arteries from Coronary Artery with Autologous Venous Tissue, Percutaneous Endoscopic Approach

0212498   Bypass Coronary Artery, Three Arteries from Right Internal Mammary with Autologous Venous Tissue, Percutaneous Endoscopic Approach

0212499   Bypass Coronary Artery, Three Arteries from Left Internal Mammary with Autologous Venous Tissue, Percutaneous Endoscopic Approach

021249C   Bypass Coronary Artery, Three Arteries from Thoracic Artery with Autologous Venous Tissue, Percutaneous Endoscopic Approach

021249F   Bypass Coronary Artery, Three Arteries from Abdominal Artery with Autologous Venous Tissue, Percutaneous Endoscopic Approach

021249W   Bypass Coronary Artery, Three Arteries from Aorta with Autologous Venous Tissue, Percutaneous Endoscopic Approach

02124A3   Bypass Coronary Artery, Three Arteries from Coronary Artery with Autologous Arterial Tissue, Percutaneous Endoscopic Approach

02124A8   Bypass Coronary Artery, Three Arteries from Right Internal Mammary with Autologous Arterial Tissue, Percutaneous Endoscopic Approach

02124A9   Bypass Coronary Artery, Three Arteries from Left Internal Mammary with Autologous Arterial Tissue, Percutaneous Endoscopic Approach

02124AC   Bypass Coronary Artery, Three Arteries from Thoracic Artery with Autologous Arterial Tissue, Percutaneous Endoscopic Approach

HAC 08: Surgical Site Infection of Mediastinitis Following Coronary Bypass Graft (CABG) Procedures (continued)

02124AF   Bypass Coronary Artery, Three Arteries from Abdominal Artery with Autologous Arterial Tissue, Percutaneous Endoscopic Approach

02124AW   Bypass Coronary Artery, Three Arteries from Aorta with Autologous Arterial Tissue, Percutaneous Endoscopic Approach

02124J3   Bypass Coronary Artery, Three Arteries from Coronary Artery with Synthetic Substitute, Percutaneous Endoscopic Approach

02124J8   Bypass Coronary Artery, Three Arteries from Right Internal Mammary with Synthetic Substitute, Percutaneous Endoscopic Approach

02124J9   Bypass Coronary Artery, Three Arteries from Left Internal Mammary with Synthetic Substitute, Percutaneous Endoscopic Approach

02124JC   Bypass Coronary Artery, Three Arteries from Thoracic Artery with Synthetic Substitute, Percutaneous Endoscopic Approach

02124JF   Bypass Coronary Artery, Three Arteries from Abdominal Artery with Synthetic Substitute, Percutaneous Endoscopic Approach

02124JW   Bypass Coronary Artery, Three Arteries from Aorta with Synthetic Substitute, Percutaneous Endoscopic Approach

02124K3   Bypass Coronary Artery, Three Arteries from Coronary Artery with Nonautologous Tissue Substitute, Percutaneous Endoscopic Approach

02124K8   Bypass Coronary Artery, Three Arteries from Right Internal Mammary with Nonautologous Tissue Substitute, Percutaneous Endoscopic Approach

02124K9   Bypass Coronary Artery, Three Arteries from Left Internal Mammary with Nonautologous Tissue Substitute, Percutaneous Endoscopic Approach

02124KC   Bypass Coronary Artery, Three Arteries from Thoracic Artery with Nonautologous Tissue Substitute, Percutaneous Endoscopic Approach

02124KF   Bypass Coronary Artery, Three Arteries from Abdominal Artery with Nonautologous Tissue Substitute, Percutaneous Endoscopic Approach

02124KW   Bypass Coronary Artery, Three Arteries from Aorta with Nonautologous Tissue Substitute, Percutaneous Endoscopic Approach

02124Z3   Bypass Coronary Artery, Three Arteries from Coronary Artery, Percutaneous Endoscopic Approach

02124Z8   Bypass Coronary Artery, Three Arteries from Right Internal Mammary, Percutaneous Endoscopic Approach

02124Z9   Bypass Coronary Artery, Three Arteries from Left Internal Mammary, Percutaneous Endoscopic Approach

02124ZC   Bypass Coronary Artery, Three Arteries from Thoracic Artery, Percutaneous Endoscopic Approach

02124ZF   Bypass Coronary Artery, Three Arteries from Abdominal Artery, Percutaneous Endoscopic Approach

0213083   Bypass Coronary Artery, Four or More Arteries from Coronary Artery with Zooplastic Tissue, Open Approach

0213088   Bypass Coronary Artery, Four or More Arteries from Right Internal Mammary with Zooplastic Tissue, Open Approach

0213089   Bypass Coronary Artery, Four or More Arteries from Left Internal Mammary with Zooplastic Tissue, Open Approach

021308C   Bypass Coronary Artery, Four or More Arteries from Thoracic Artery with Zooplastic Tissue, Open Approach

021308F   Bypass Coronary Artery, Four or More Arteries from Abdominal Artery with Zooplastic Tissue, Open Approach

021308W   Bypass Coronary Artery, Four or More Arteries from Aorta with Zooplastic Tissue, Open Approach

0213093   Bypass Coronary Artery, Four or More Arteries from Coronary Artery with Autologous Venous Tissue, Open Approach

0213098   Bypass Coronary Artery, Four or More Arteries from Right Internal Mammary with Autologous Venous Tissue, Open Approach

0213099   Bypass Coronary Artery, Four or More Arteries from Left Internal Mammary with Autologous Venous Tissue, Open Approach

021309C   Bypass Coronary Artery, Four or More Arteries from Thoracic Artery with Autologous Venous Tissue, Open Approach

021309F   Bypass Coronary Artery, Four or More Arteries from Abdominal Artery with Autologous Venous Tissue, Open Approach

021309W   Bypass Coronary Artery, Four or More Arteries from Aorta with Autologous Venous Tissue, Open Approach

02130A3   Bypass Coronary Artery, Four or More Arteries from Coronary Artery with Autologous Arterial Tissue, Open Approach

02130A8   Bypass Coronary Artery, Four or More Arteries from Right Internal Mammary with Autologous Arterial Tissue, Open Approach

02130A9   Bypass Coronary Artery, Four or More Arteries from Left Internal Mammary with Autologous Arterial Tissue, Open Approach

02130AC   Bypass Coronary Artery, Four or More Arteries from Thoracic Artery with Autologous Arterial Tissue, Open Approach

02130AF   Bypass Coronary Artery, Four or More Arteries from Abdominal Artery with Autologous Arterial Tissue, Open Approach

02130AW   Bypass Coronary Artery, Four or More Arteries from Aorta with Autologous Arterial Tissue, Open Approach

02130J3   Bypass Coronary Artery, Four or More Arteries from Coronary Artery with Synthetic Substitute, Open Approach

02130J8   Bypass Coronary Artery, Four or More Arteries from Right Internal Mammary with Synthetic Substitute, Open Approach

02130J9   Bypass Coronary Artery, Four or More Arteries from Left Internal Mammary with Synthetic Substitute, Open Approach

02130JC   Bypass Coronary Artery, Four or More Arteries from Thoracic Artery with Synthetic Substitute, Open Approach

02130JF   Bypass Coronary Artery, Four or More Arteries from Abdominal Artery with Synthetic Substitute, Open Approach

02130JW   Bypass Coronary Artery, Four or More Arteries from Aorta with Synthetic Substitute, Open Approach

02130K3   Bypass Coronary Artery, Four or More Arteries from Coronary Artery with Nonautologous Tissue Substitute, Open Approach

02130K8   Bypass Coronary Artery, Four or More Arteries from Right Internal Mammary with Nonautologous Tissue Substitute, Open Approach

02130K9   Bypass Coronary Artery, Four or More Arteries from Left Internal Mammary with Nonautologous Tissue Substitute, Open Approach

02130KC   Bypass Coronary Artery, Four or More Arteries from Thoracic Artery with Nonautologous Tissue Substitute, Open Approach

02130KF   Bypass Coronary Artery, Four or More Arteries from Abdominal Artery with Nonautologous Tissue Substitute, Open Approach

02130KW   Bypass Coronary Artery, Four or More Arteries from Aorta with Nonautologous Tissue Substitute, Open Approach

02130Z3   Bypass Coronary Artery, Four or More Arteries from Coronary Artery, Open Approach

02130Z8   Bypass Coronary Artery, Four or More Arteries from Right Internal Mammary, Open Approach

02130Z9   Bypass Coronary Artery, Four or More Arteries from Left Internal Mammary, Open Approach

02130ZC   Bypass Coronary Artery, Four or More Arteries from Thoracic Artery, Open Approach

02130ZF   Bypass Coronary Artery, Four or More Arteries from Abdominal Artery, Open Approach

0213483   Bypass Coronary Artery, Four or More Arteries from Coronary Artery with Zooplastic Tissue, Percutaneous Endoscopic Approach

0213488   Bypass Coronary Artery, Four or More Arteries from Right Internal Mammary with Zooplastic Tissue, Percutaneous Endoscopic Approach

0213489   Bypass Coronary Artery, Four or More Arteries from Left Internal Mammary with Zooplastic Tissue, Percutaneous Endoscopic Approach

021348C   Bypass Coronary Artery, Four or More Arteries from Thoracic Artery with Zooplastic Tissue, Percutaneous Endoscopic Approach

021348F   Bypass Coronary Artery, Four or More Arteries from Abdominal Artery with Zooplastic Tissue, Percutaneous Endoscopic Approach

021348W   Bypass Coronary Artery, Four or More Arteries from Aorta with Zooplastic Tissue, Percutaneous Endoscopic Approach

0213493   Bypass Coronary Artery, Four or More Arteries from Coronary Artery with Autologous Venous Tissue, Percutaneous Endoscopic Approach

0213498   Bypass Coronary Artery, Four or More Arteries from Right Internal Mammary with Autologous Venous Tissue, Percutaneous Endoscopic Approach

HAC 08: Surgical Site Infection of Mediastinitis Following Coronary Bypass Graft (CABG) Procedures (continued)

0213499	Bypass Coronary Artery, Four or More Arteries from Left Internal Mammary with Autologous Venous Tissue, Percutaneous Endoscopic Approach
021349C	Bypass Coronary Artery, Four or More Arteries from Thoracic Artery with Autologous Venous Tissue, Percutaneous Endoscopic Approach
021349F	Bypass Coronary Artery, Four or More Arteries from Abdominal Artery with Autologous Venous Tissue, Percutaneous Endoscopic Approach
021349W	Bypass Coronary Artery, Four or More Arteries from Aorta with Autologous Venous Tissue, Percutaneous Endoscopic Approach
02134A3	Bypass Coronary Artery, Four or More Arteries from Coronary Artery with Autologous Arterial Tissue, Percutaneous Endoscopic Approach
02134A8	Bypass Coronary Artery, Four or More Arteries from Right Internal Mammary with Autologous Arterial Tissue, Percutaneous Endoscopic Approach
02134A9	Bypass Coronary Artery, Four or More Arteries from Left Internal Mammary with Autologous Arterial Tissue, Percutaneous Endoscopic Approach
02134AC	Bypass Coronary Artery, Four or More Arteries from Thoracic Artery with Autologous Arterial Tissue, Percutaneous Endoscopic Approach
02134AF	Bypass Coronary Artery, Four or More Arteries from Abdominal Artery with Autologous Arterial Tissue, Percutaneous Endoscopic Approach
02134AW	Bypass Coronary Artery, Four or More Arteries from Aorta with Autologous Arterial Tissue, Percutaneous Endoscopic Approach
02134J3	Bypass Coronary Artery, Four or More Arteries from Coronary Artery with Synthetic Substitute, Percutaneous Endoscopic Approach
02134J8	Bypass Coronary Artery, Four or More Arteries from Right Internal Mammary with Synthetic Substitute, Percutaneous Endoscopic Approach
02134J9	Bypass Coronary Artery, Four or More Arteries from Left Internal Mammary with Synthetic Substitute, Percutaneous Endoscopic Approach
02134JC	Bypass Coronary Artery, Four or More Arteries from Thoracic Artery with Synthetic Substitute, Percutaneous Endoscopic Approach
02134JF	Bypass Coronary Artery, Four or More Arteries from Abdominal Artery with Synthetic Substitute, Percutaneous Endoscopic Approach
02134JW	Bypass Coronary Artery, Four or More Arteries from Aorta with Synthetic Substitute, Percutaneous Endoscopic Approach
02134K3	Bypass Coronary Artery, Four or More Arteries from Coronary Artery with Nonautologous Tissue Substitute, Percutaneous Endoscopic Approach
02134K8	Bypass Coronary Artery, Four or More Arteries from Right Internal Mammary with Nonautologous Tissue Substitute, Percutaneous Endoscopic Approach
02134K9	Bypass Coronary Artery, Four or More Arteries from Left Internal Mammary with Nonautologous Tissue Substitute, Percutaneous Endoscopic Approach
02134KC	Bypass Coronary Artery, Four or More Arteries from Thoracic Artery with Nonautologous Tissue Substitute, Percutaneous Endoscopic Approach
02134KF	Bypass Coronary Artery, Four or More Arteries from Abdominal Artery with Nonautologous Tissue Substitute, Percutaneous Endoscopic Approach
02134KW	Bypass Coronary Artery, Four or More Arteries from Aorta with Nonautologous Tissue Substitute, Percutaneous Endoscopic Approach
0213Z3	Bypass Coronary Artery, Four or More Arteries from Coronary Artery, Percutaneous Endoscopic Approach
0213Z8	Bypass Coronary Artery, Four or More Arteries from Right Internal Mammary, Percutaneous Endoscopic Approach
0213Z9	Bypass Coronary Artery, Four or More Arteries from Left Internal Mammary, Percutaneous Endoscopic Approach
0213ZC	Bypass Coronary Artery, Four or More Arteries from Thoracic Artery, Percutaneous Endoscopic Approach
0213ZF	Bypass Coronary Artery, Four or More Arteries from Abdominal Artery, Percutaneous Endoscopic Approach

HAC 09: Manifestations of Poor Glycemic Control

Secondary diagnosis not POA:

E08.00
E08.01
E08.10
E09.00
E09.01
E09.10
E10.10
E11.00
E11.01
E13.00
E13.01
E13.10
E15

HAC 10: Deep Vein Thrombosis (DVT) or Pulmonary Embolism (PE) with Total Knee or Hip Replacement

Secondary diagnosis not POA:

I26.02
I26.09
I26.92
I26.99
I82.401
I82.402
I82.403
I82.409
I82.411
I82.412
I82.413
I82.419
I82.421
I82.422
I82.423
I82.429
I82.431
I82.432
I82.433
I82.439
I82.441
I82.442
I82.443
I82.449
I82.491

I82.492
I82.493
I82.499
I82.4Y1
I82.4Y2
I82.4Y3
I82.4Y9
I82.4Z1
I82.4Z2
I82.4Z3
I82.4Z9

AND

Any of the following procedures:

0SR9019	Replacement of Right Hip Joint with Metal Synthetic Substitute, Cemented, Open Approach
0SR901A	Replacement of Right Hip Joint with Metal Synthetic Substitute, Uncemented, Open Approach
0SR901Z	Replacement of Right Hip Joint with Metal Synthetic Substitute, Open Approach
0SR9029	Replacement of Right Hip Joint with Metal on Polyethylene Synthetic Substitute, Cemented, Open Approach
0SR902A	Replacement of Right Hip Joint with Metal on Polyethylene Synthetic Substitute, Uncemented, Open Approach
0SR902Z	Replacement of Right Hip Joint with Metal on Polyethylene Synthetic Substitute, Open Approach
0SR9039	Replacement of Right Hip Joint with Ceramic Synthetic Substitute, Cemented, Open Approach
0SR903A	Replacement of Right Hip Joint with Ceramic Synthetic Substitute, Uncemented, Open Approach
0SR903Z	Replacement of Right Hip Joint with Ceramic Synthetic Substitute, Open Approach
0SR9049	Replacement of Right Hip Joint with Ceramic on Polyethylene Synthetic Substitute, Cemented, Open Approach
0SR904A	Replacement of Right Hip Joint with Ceramic on Polyethylene Synthetic Substitute, Uncemented, Open Approach
0SR904Z	Replacement of Right Hip Joint with Ceramic on Polyethylene Synthetic Substitute, Open Approach
0SR9069	Replacement of Right Hip Joint with Oxidized Zirconium on Polyethylene Synthetic Substitute, Cemented, Open Approach
0SR906A	Replacement of Right Hip Joint with Oxidized Zirconium on Polyethylene Synthetic Substitute, Uncemented, Open Approach
0SR906Z	Replacement of Right Hip Joint with Oxidized Zirconium on Polyethylene Synthetic Substitute, Open Approach
0SR907Z	Replacement of Right Hip Joint with Autologous Tissue Substitute, Open Approach
0SR90J9	Replacement of Right Hip Joint with Synthetic Substitute, Cemented, Open Approach
0SR90JA	Replacement of Right Hip Joint with Synthetic Substitute, Uncemented, Open Approach
0SR90JZ	Replacement of Right Hip Joint with Synthetic Substitute, Open Approach

HAC 10: Deep Vein Thrombosis (DVT) or Pulmonary Embolism (PE) with Total Knee or Hip Replacement (continued)

0SR90KZ Replacement of Right Hip Joint with Nonautologous Tissue Substitute, Open Approach

0SRA009 Replacement of Right Hip Joint, Acetabular Surface with Polyethylene Synthetic Substitute, Cemented, Open Approach

0SRA00A Replacement of Right Hip Joint, Acetabular Surface with Polyethylene Synthetic Substitute, Uncemented, Open Approach

0SRA00Z Replacement of Right Hip Joint, Acetabular Surface with Polyethylene Synthetic Substitute, Open Approach

0SRA019 Replacement of Right Hip Joint, Acetabular Surface with Metal Synthetic Substitute, Cemented, Open Approach

0SRA01A Replacement of Right Hip Joint, Acetabular Surface with Metal Synthetic Substitute, Uncemented, Open Approach

0SRA01Z Replacement of Right Hip Joint, Acetabular Surface with Metal Synthetic Substitute, Open Approach

0SRA039 Replacement of Right Hip Joint, Acetabular Surface with Ceramic Synthetic Substitute, Cemented, Open Approach

0SRA03A Replacement of Right Hip Joint, Acetabular Surface with Ceramic Synthetic Substitute, Uncemented, Open Approach

0SRA03Z Replacement of Right Hip Joint, Acetabular Surface with Ceramic Synthetic Substitute, Open Approach

0SRA07Z Replacement of Right Hip Joint, Acetabular Surface with Autologous Tissue Substitute, Open Approach

0SRA0J9 Replacement of Right Hip Joint, Acetabular Surface with Synthetic Substitute, Cemented, Open Approach

0SRA0JA Replacement of Right Hip Joint, Acetabular Surface with Synthetic Substitute, Uncemented, Open Approach

0SRA0JZ Replacement of Right Hip Joint, Acetabular Surface with Synthetic Substitute, Open Approach

0SRA0KZ Replacement of Right Hip Joint, Acetabular Surface with Nonautologous Tissue Substitute, Open Approach

0SRB019 Replacement of Left Hip Joint with Metal Synthetic Substitute, Cemented, Open Approach

0SRB01A Replacement of Left Hip Joint with Metal Synthetic Substitute, Uncemented, Open Approach

0SRB01Z Replacement of Left Hip Joint with Metal Synthetic Substitute, Open Approach

0SRB029 Replacement of Left Hip Joint with Metal on Polyethylene Synthetic Substitute, Cemented, Open Approach

0SRB02A Replacement of Left Hip Joint with Metal on Polyethylene Synthetic Substitute, Uncemented, Open Approach

0SRB02Z Replacement of Left Hip Joint with Metal on Polyethylene Synthetic Substitute, Open Approach

0SRB039 Replacement of Left Hip Joint with Ceramic Synthetic Substitute, Cemented, Open Approach

0SRB03A Replacement of Left Hip Joint with Ceramic Synthetic Substitute, Uncemented, Open Approach

0SRB03Z Replacement of Left Hip Joint with Ceramic Synthetic Substitute, Open Approach

0SRB049 Replacement of Left Hip Joint with Ceramic on Polyethylene Synthetic Substitute, Cemented, Open Approach

0SRB04A Replacement of Left Hip Joint with Ceramic on Polyethylene Synthetic Substitute, Uncemented, Open Approach

0SRB04Z Replacement of Left Hip Joint with Ceramic on Polyethylene Synthetic Substitute, Open Approach

0SRB069 Replacement of Left Hip Joint with Oxidized Zirconium on Polyethylene Synthetic Substitute, Cemented, Open Approach

0SRB06A Replacement of Left Hip Joint with Oxidized Zirconium on Polyethylene Synthetic Substitute, Uncemented, Open Approach

0SRB06Z Replacement of Left Hip Joint with Oxidized Zirconium on Polyethylene Synthetic Substitute, Open Approach

0SRB07Z Replacement of Left Hip Joint with Autologous Tissue Substitute, Open Approach

0SRB0J9 Replacement of Left Hip Joint with Synthetic Substitute, Cemented, Open Approach

0SRB0JA Replacement of Left Hip Joint with Synthetic Substitute, Uncemented, Open Approach

0SRB0JZ Replacement of Left Hip Joint with Synthetic Substitute, Open Approach

0SRB0KZ Replacement of Left Hip Joint with Nonautologous Tissue Substitute, Open Approach

0SRC069 Replacement of Right Knee Joint with Oxidized Zirconium on Polyethylene Synthetic Substitute, Cemented, Open Approach

0SRC06A Replacement of Right Knee Joint with Oxidized Zirconium on Polyethylene Synthetic Substitute, Uncemented, Open Approach

0SRC06Z Replacement of Right Knee Joint with Oxidized Zirconium on Polyethylene Synthetic Substitute, Open Approach

0SRC07Z Replacement of Right Knee Joint with Autologous Tissue Substitute, Open Approach

0SRC0J9 Replacement of Right Knee Joint with Synthetic Substitute, Cemented, Open Approach

0SRC0JA Replacement of Right Knee Joint with Synthetic Substitute, Uncemented, Open Approach

0SRC0JZ Replacement of Right Knee Joint with Synthetic Substitute, Open Approach

0SRC0KZ Replacement of Right Knee Joint with Nonautologous Tissue Substitute, Open Approach

0SRD069 Replacement of Left Knee Joint with Oxidized Zirconium on Polyethylene Synthetic Substitute, Cemented, Open Approach

0SRD06A Replacement of Left Knee Joint with Oxidized Zirconium on Polyethylene Synthetic Substitute, Uncemented, Open Approach

0SRD06Z Replacement of Left Knee Joint with Oxidized Zirconium on Polyethylene Synthetic Substitute, Open Approach

0SRD07Z Replacement of Left Knee Joint with Autologous Tissue Substitute, Open Approach

0SRD0J9 Replacement of Left Knee Joint with Synthetic Substitute, Cemented, Open Approach

0SRD0JA Replacement of Left Knee Joint with Synthetic Substitute, Uncemented, Open Approach

0SRD0JZ Replacement of Left Knee Joint with Synthetic Substitute, Open Approach

0SRD0KZ Replacement of Left Knee Joint with Nonautologous Tissue Substitute, Open Approach

0SRE009 Replacement of Left Hip Joint, Acetabular Surface with Polyethylene Synthetic Substitute, Cemented, Open Approach

0SRE00A Replacement of Left Hip Joint, Acetabular Surface with Polyethylene Synthetic Substitute, Uncemented, Open Approach

0SRE00Z Replacement of Left Hip Joint, Acetabular Surface with Polyethylene Synthetic Substitute, Open Approach

0SRE019 Replacement of Left Hip Joint, Acetabular Surface with Metal Synthetic Substitute, Cemented, Open Approach

0SRE01A Replacement of Left Hip Joint, Acetabular Surface with Metal Synthetic Substitute, Uncemented, Open Approach

0SRE01Z Replacement of Left Hip Joint, Acetabular Surface with Metal Synthetic Substitute, Open Approach

0SRE039 Replacement of Left Hip Joint, Acetabular Surface with Ceramic Synthetic Substitute, Cemented, Open Approach

0SRE03A Replacement of Left Hip Joint, Acetabular Surface with Ceramic Synthetic Substitute, Uncemented, Open Approach

0SRE03Z Replacement of Left Hip Joint, Acetabular Surface with Ceramic Synthetic Substitute, Open Approach

0SRE07Z Replacement of Left Hip Joint, Acetabular Surface with Autologous Tissue Substitute, Open Approach

0SRE0J9 Replacement of Left Hip Joint, Acetabular Surface with Synthetic Substitute, Cemented, Open Approach

0SRE0JA Replacement of Left Hip Joint, Acetabular Surface with Synthetic Substitute, Uncemented, Open Approach

0SRE0JZ Replacement of Left Hip Joint, Acetabular Surface with Synthetic Substitute, Open Approach

0SRE0KZ Replacement of Left Hip Joint, Acetabular Surface with Nonautologous Tissue Substitute, Open Approach

0SRR019 Replacement of Right Hip Joint, Femoral Surface with Metal Synthetic Substitute, Cemented, Open Approach

0SRR01A Replacement of Right Hip Joint, Femoral Surface with Metal Synthetic Substitute, Uncemented, Open Approach

0SRR01Z Replacement of Right Hip Joint, Femoral Surface with Metal Synthetic Substitute, Open Approach

HAC 10: Deep Vein Thrombosis (DVT) or Pulmonary Embolism (PE) with Total Knee or Hip Replacement (continued)

ØSRRØ39	Replacement of Right Hip Joint, Femoral Surface with Ceramic Synthetic Substitute, Cemented, Open Approach
ØSRRØ3A	Replacement of Right Hip Joint, Femoral Surface with Ceramic Synthetic Substitute, Uncemented, Open Approach
ØSRRØ3Z	Replacement of Right Hip Joint, Femoral Surface with Ceramic Synthetic Substitute, Open Approach
ØSRRØ7Z	Replacement of Right Hip Joint, Femoral Surface with Autologous Tissue Substitute, Open Approach
ØSRRØJ9	Replacement of Right Hip Joint, Femoral Surface with Synthetic Substitute, Cemented, Open Approach
ØSRRØJA	Replacement of Right Hip Joint, Femoral Surface with Synthetic Substitute, Uncemented, Open Approach
ØSRRØJZ	Replacement of Right Hip Joint, Femoral Surface with Synthetic Substitute, Open Approach
ØSRRØKZ	Replacement of Right Hip Joint, Femoral Surface with Nonautologous Tissue Substitute, Open Approach
ØSRSØ19	Replacement of Left Hip Joint, Femoral Surface with Metal Synthetic Substitute, Cemented, Open Approach
ØSRSØ1A	Replacement of Left Hip Joint, Femoral Surface with Metal Synthetic Substitute, Uncemented, Open Approach
ØSRSØ1Z	Replacement of Left Hip Joint, Femoral Surface with Metal Synthetic Substitute, Open Approach
ØSRSØ39	Replacement of Left Hip Joint, Femoral Surface with Ceramic Synthetic Substitute, Cemented, Open Approach
ØSRSØ3A	Replacement of Left Hip Joint, Femoral Surface with Ceramic Synthetic Substitute, Uncemented, Open Approach
ØSRSØ3Z	Replacement of Left Hip Joint, Femoral Surface with Ceramic Synthetic Substitute, Open Approach
ØSRSØ7Z	Replacement of Left Hip Joint, Femoral Surface with Autologous Tissue Substitute, Open Approach
ØSRSØJ9	Replacement of Left Hip Joint, Femoral Surface with Synthetic Substitute, Cemented, Open Approach
ØSRSØJA	Replacement of Left Hip Joint, Femoral Surface with Synthetic Substitute, Uncemented, Open Approach
ØSRSØJZ	Replacement of Left Hip Joint, Femoral Surface with Synthetic Substitute, Open Approach
ØSRSØKZ	Replacement of Left Hip Joint, Femoral Surface with Nonautologous Tissue Substitute, Open Approach
ØSRTØ7Z	Replacement of Right Knee Joint, Femoral Surface with Autologous Tissue Substitute, Open Approach
ØSRTØJ9	Replacement of Right Knee Joint, Femoral Surface with Synthetic Substitute, Cemented, Open Approach
ØSRTØJA	Replacement of Right Knee Joint, Femoral Surface with Synthetic Substitute, Uncemented, Open Approach
ØSRTØJZ	Replacement of Right Knee Joint, Femoral Surface with Synthetic Substitute, Open Approach
ØSRTØKZ	Replacement of Right Knee Joint, Femoral Surface with Nonautologous Tissue Substitute, Open Approach
ØSRUØ7Z	Replacement of Left Knee Joint, Femoral Surface with Autologous Tissue Substitute, Open Approach
ØSRUØJ9	Replacement of Left Knee Joint, Femoral Surface with Synthetic Substitute, Cemented, Open Approach
ØSRUØJA	Replacement of Left Knee Joint, Femoral Surface with Synthetic Substitute, Uncemented, Open Approach
ØSRUØJZ	Replacement of Left Knee Joint, Femoral Surface with Synthetic Substitute, Open Approach
ØSRUØKZ	Replacement of Left Knee Joint, Femoral Surface with Nonautologous Tissue Substitute, Open Approach
ØSRVØ7Z	Replacement of Right Knee Joint, Tibial Surface with Autologous Tissue Substitute, Open Approach
ØSRVØJ9	Replacement of Right Knee Joint, Tibial Surface with Synthetic Substitute, Cemented, Open Approach
ØSRVØJA	Replacement of Right Knee Joint, Tibial Surface with Synthetic Substitute, Uncemented, Open Approach
ØSRVØJZ	Replacement of Right Knee Joint, Tibial Surface with Synthetic Substitute, Open Approach
ØSRVØKZ	Replacement of Right Knee Joint, Tibial Surface with Nonautologous Tissue Substitute, Open Approach
ØSRWØ7Z	Replacement of Left Knee Joint, Tibial Surface with Autologous Tissue Substitute, Open Approach
ØSRWØJ9	Replacement of Left Knee Joint, Tibial Surface with Synthetic Substitute, Cemented, Open Approach
ØSRWØJA	Replacement of Left Knee Joint, Tibial Surface with Synthetic Substitute, Uncemented, Open Approach
ØSRWØJZ	Replacement of Left Knee Joint, Tibial Surface with Synthetic Substitute, Open Approach
ØSRWØKZ	Replacement of Left Knee Joint, Tibial Surface with Nonautologous Tissue Substitute, Open Approach
ØSU9ØBZ	Supplement Right Hip Joint with Resurfacing Device, Open Approach
ØSUAØBZ	Supplement Right Hip Joint, Acetabular Surface with Resurfacing Device, Open Approach
ØSUBØBZ	Supplement Left Hip Joint with Resurfacing Device, Open Approach
ØSUEØBZ	Supplement Left Hip Joint, Acetabular Surface with Resurfacing Device, Open Approach
ØSURØBZ	Supplement Right Hip Joint, Femoral Surface with Resurfacing Device, Open Approach
ØSUSØBZ	Supplement Left Hip Joint, Femoral Surface with Resurfacing Device, Open Approach

HAC 11: Surgical Site Infection Following Bariatric Surgery

Principal diagnosis of:
 E66.Ø1

AND

Secondary diagnosis not POA:
 K68.11
 K95.Ø1
 K95.81
 T81.4XXA

AND

Any of the following procedures:

ØD16Ø79	Bypass Stomach to Duodenum with Autologous Tissue Substitute, Open Approach
ØD16Ø7A	Bypass Stomach to Jejunum with Autologous Tissue Substitute, Open Approach
ØD16Ø7B	Bypass Stomach to Ileum with Autologous Tissue Substitute, Open Approach
ØD16Ø7L	Bypass Stomach to Transverse Colon with Autologous Tissue Substitute, Open Approach
ØD16ØJ9	Bypass Stomach to Duodenum with Synthetic Substitute, Open Approach
ØD16ØJA	Bypass Stomach to Jejunum with Synthetic Substitute, Open Approach
ØD16ØJB	Bypass Stomach to Ileum with Synthetic Substitute, Open Approach
ØD16ØJL	Bypass Stomach to Transverse Colon with Synthetic Substitute, Open Approach
ØD16ØK9	Bypass Stomach to Duodenum with Nonautologous Tissue Substitute, Open Approach
ØD16ØKA	Bypass Stomach to Jejunum with Nonautologous Tissue Substitute, Open Approach
ØD16ØKB	Bypass Stomach to Ileum with Nonautologous Tissue Substitute, Open Approach
ØD16ØKL	Bypass Stomach to Transverse Colon with Nonautologous Tissue Substitute, Open Approach
ØD16ØZ9	Bypass Stomach to Duodenum, Open Approach
ØD16ØZA	Bypass Stomach to Jejunum, Open Approach
ØD16ØZB	Bypass Stomach to Ileum, Open Approach
ØD16ØZL	Bypass Stomach to Transverse Colon, Open Approach
ØD16479	Bypass Stomach to Duodenum with Autologous Tissue Substitute, Percutaneous Endoscopic Approach
ØD1647A	Bypass Stomach to Jejunum with Autologous Tissue Substitute, Percutaneous Endoscopic Approach
ØD1647B	Bypass Stomach to Ileum with Autologous Tissue Substitute, Percutaneous Endoscopic Approach
ØD1647L	Bypass Stomach to Transverse Colon with Autologous Tissue Substitute, Percutaneous Endoscopic Approach
ØD164J9	Bypass Stomach to Duodenum with Synthetic Substitute, Percutaneous Endoscopic Approach
ØD164JA	Bypass Stomach to Jejunum with Synthetic Substitute, Percutaneous Endoscopic Approach
ØD164JB	Bypass Stomach to Ileum with Synthetic Substitute, Percutaneous Endoscopic Approach
ØD164JL	Bypass Stomach to Transverse Colon with Synthetic Substitute, Percutaneous Endoscopic Approach
ØD164K9	Bypass Stomach to Duodenum with Nonautologous Tissue Substitute, Percutaneous Endoscopic Approach
ØD164KA	Bypass Stomach to Jejunum with Nonautologous Tissue Substitute, Percutaneous Endoscopic Approach
ØD164KB	Bypass Stomach to Ileum with Nonautologous Tissue Substitute, Percutaneous Endoscopic Approach

HAC 11: Surgical Site Infection Following Bariatric Surgery (continued)

0D164KL	Bypass Stomach to Transverse Colon with Nonautologous Tissue Substitute, Percutaneous Endoscopic Approach
0D164Z9	Bypass Stomach to Duodenum, Percutaneous Endoscopic Approach
0D164ZA	Bypass Stomach to Jejunum, Percutaneous Endoscopic Approach
0D164ZB	Bypass Stomach to Ileum, Percutaneous Endoscopic Approach
0D164ZL	Bypass Stomach to Transverse Colon, Percutaneous Endoscopic Approach
0D16879	Bypass Stomach to Duodenum with Autologous Tissue Substitute, Via Natural or Artificial Opening Endoscopic
0D1687A	Bypass Stomach to Jejunum with Autologous Tissue Substitute, Via Natural or Artificial Opening Endoscopic
0D1687B	Bypass Stomach to Ileum with Autologous Tissue Substitute, Via Natural or Artificial Opening Endoscopic
0D1687L	Bypass Stomach to Transverse Colon with Autologous Tissue Substitute, Via Natural or Artificial Opening Endoscopic
0D168J9	Bypass Stomach to Duodenum with Synthetic Substitute, Via Natural or Artificial Opening Endoscopic
0D168JA	Bypass Stomach to Jejunum with Synthetic Substitute, Via Natural or Artificial Opening Endoscopic
0D168JB	Bypass Stomach to Ileum with Synthetic Substitute, Via Natural or Artificial Opening Endoscopic
0D168JL	Bypass Stomach to Transverse Colon with Synthetic Substitute, Via Natural or Artificial Opening Endoscopic
0D168K9	Bypass Stomach to Duodenum with Nonautologous Tissue Substitute, Via Natural or Artificial Opening Endoscopic
0D168KA	Bypass Stomach to Jejunum with Nonautologous Tissue Substitute, Via Natural or Artificial Opening Endoscopic
0D168KB	Bypass Stomach to Ileum with Nonautologous Tissue Substitute, Via Natural or Artificial Opening Endoscopic
0D168KL	Bypass Stomach to Transverse Colon with Nonautologous Tissue Substitute, Via Natural or Artificial Opening Endoscopic
0D168Z9	Bypass Stomach to Duodenum, Via Natural or Artificial Opening Endoscopic
0D168ZA	Bypass Stomach to Jejunum, Via Natural or Artificial Opening Endoscopic
0D168ZB	Bypass Stomach to Ileum, Via Natural or Artificial Opening Endoscopic
0D168ZL	Bypass Stomach to Transverse Colon, Via Natural or Artificial Opening Endoscopic
0DV64CZ	Restriction of Stomach with Extraluminal Device, Percutaneous Endoscopic Approach

HAC 12: Surgical Site Infection Following Certain Orthopedic Procedures of the Spine, Shoulder, and Elbow

Secondary diagnosis not POA:

K68.11
T81.4XXA
T84.60XA
T84.610A
T84.611A
T84.612A
T84.613A
T84.614A
T84.615A
T84.619A

T84.63XA
T84.69XA
T84.7XXA

AND

Any of the following procedures:

0RG0070	Fusion of Occipital-cervical Joint with Autologous Tissue Substitute, Anterior Approach, Anterior Column, Open Approach
0RG0071	Fusion of Occipital-cervical Joint with Autologous Tissue Substitute, Posterior Approach, Posterior Column, Open Approach
0RG007J	Fusion of Occipital-cervical Joint with Autologous Tissue Substitute, Posterior Approach, Anterior Column, Open Approach
0RG00A0	Fusion of Occipital-cervical Joint with Interbody Fusion Device, Anterior Approach, Anterior Column, Open Approach
0RG00AJ	Fusion of Occipital-cervical Joint with Interbody Fusion Device, Posterior Approach, Anterior Column, Open Approach
0RG00J0	Fusion of Occipital-cervical Joint with Synthetic Substitute, Anterior Approach, Anterior Column, Open Approach
0RG00J1	Fusion of Occipital-cervical Joint with Synthetic Substitute, Posterior Approach, Posterior Column, Open Approach
0RG00JJ	Fusion of Occipital-cervical Joint with Synthetic Substitute, Posterior Approach, Anterior Column, Open Approach
0RG00K0	Fusion of Occipital-cervical Joint with Nonautologous Tissue Substitute, Anterior Approach, Anterior Column, Open Approach
0RG00K1	Fusion of Occipital-cervical Joint with Nonautologous Tissue Substitute, Posterior Approach, Posterior Column, Open Approach
0RG00KJ	Fusion of Occipital-cervical Joint with Nonautologous Tissue Substitute, Posterior Approach, Anterior Column, Open Approach
0RG0370	Fusion of Occipital-cervical Joint with Autologous Tissue Substitute, Anterior Approach, Anterior Column, Percutaneous Approach
0RG0371	Fusion of Occipital-cervical Joint with Autologous Tissue Substitute, Posterior Approach, Posterior Column, Percutaneous Approach
0RG037J	Fusion of Occipital-cervical Joint with Autologous Tissue Substitute, Posterior Approach, Anterior Column, Percutaneous Approach
0RG03A0	Fusion of Occipital-cervical Joint with Interbody Fusion Device, Anterior Approach, Anterior Column, Percutaneous Approach
0RG03AJ	Fusion of Occipital-cervical Joint with Interbody Fusion Device, Posterior Approach, Anterior Column, Percutaneous Approach
0RG03J0	Fusion of Occipital-cervical Joint with Synthetic Substitute, Anterior Approach, Anterior Column, Percutaneous Approach

0RG03J1	Fusion of Occipital-cervical Joint with Synthetic Substitute, Posterior Approach, Posterior Column, Percutaneous Approach
0RG03JJ	Fusion of Occipital-cervical Joint with Synthetic Substitute, Posterior Approach, Anterior Column, Percutaneous Approach
0RG03K0	Fusion of Occipital-cervical Joint with Nonautologous Tissue Substitute, Anterior Approach, Anterior Column, Percutaneous Approach
0RG03K1	Fusion of Occipital-cervical Joint with Nonautologous Tissue Substitute, Posterior Approach, Posterior Column, Percutaneous Approach
0RG03KJ	Fusion of Occipital-cervical Joint with Nonautologous Tissue Substitute, Posterior Approach, Anterior Column, Percutaneous Approach
0RG0470	Fusion of Occipital-cervical Joint with Autologous Tissue Substitute, Anterior Approach, Anterior Column, Percutaneous Endoscopic Approach
0RG0471	Fusion of Occipital-cervical Joint with Autologous Tissue Substitute, Posterior Approach, Posterior Column, Percutaneous Endoscopic Approach
0RG047J	Fusion of Occipital-cervical Joint with Autologous Tissue Substitute, Posterior Approach, Anterior Column, Percutaneous Endoscopic Approach
0RG04A0	Fusion of Occipital-cervical Joint with Interbody Fusion Device, Anterior Approach, Anterior Column, Percutaneous Endoscopic Approach
0RG04AJ	Fusion of Occipital-cervical Joint with Interbody Fusion Device, Posterior Approach, Anterior Column, Percutaneous Endoscopic Approach
0RG04J0	Fusion of Occipital-cervical Joint with Synthetic Substitute, Anterior Approach, Anterior Column, Percutaneous Endoscopic Approach
0RG04J1	Fusion of Occipital-cervical Joint with Synthetic Substitute, Posterior Approach, Posterior Column, Percutaneous Endoscopic Approach
0RG04JJ	Fusion of Occipital-cervical Joint with Synthetic Substitute, Posterior Approach, Anterior Column, Percutaneous Endoscopic Approach
0RG04K0	Fusion of Occipital-cervical Joint with Nonautologous Tissue Substitute, Anterior Approach, Anterior Column, Percutaneous Endoscopic Approach
0RG04K1	Fusion of Occipital-cervical Joint with Nonautologous Tissue Substitute, Posterior Approach, Posterior Column, Percutaneous Endoscopic Approach
0RG04KJ	Fusion of Occipital-cervical Joint with Nonautologous Tissue Substitute, Posterior Approach, Anterior Column, Percutaneous Endoscopic Approach
0RG1070	Fusion of Cervical Vertebral Joint with Autologous Tissue Substitute, Anterior Approach, Anterior Column, Open Approach
0RG1071	Fusion of Cervical Vertebral Joint with Autologous Tissue Substitute, Posterior Approach, Posterior Column, Open Approach
0RG107J	Fusion of Cervical Vertebral Joint with Autologous Tissue Substitute, Posterior Approach, Anterior Column, Open Approach

HAC 12: Surgical Site Infection Following Certain Orthopedic Procedures of the Spine, Shoulder, and Elbow (continued)

ØRG10AØ Fusion of Cervical Vertebral Joint with Interbody Fusion Device, Anterior Approach, Anterior Column, Open Approach

ØRG10AJ Fusion of Cervical Vertebral Joint with Interbody Fusion Device, Posterior Approach, Anterior Column, Open Approach

ØRG10JØ Fusion of Cervical Vertebral Joint with Synthetic Substitute, Anterior Approach, Anterior Column, Open Approach

ØRG10J1 Fusion of Cervical Vertebral Joint with Synthetic Substitute, Posterior Approach, Posterior Column, Open Approach

ØRG10JJ Fusion of Cervical Vertebral Joint with Synthetic Substitute, Posterior Approach, Anterior Column, Open Approach

ØRG10KØ Fusion of Cervical Vertebral Joint with Nonautologous Tissue Substitute, Anterior Approach, Anterior Column, Open Approach

ØRG10K1 Fusion of Cervical Vertebral Joint with Nonautologous Tissue Substitute, Posterior Approach, Posterior Column, Open Approach

ØRG10KJ Fusion of Cervical Vertebral Joint with Nonautologous Tissue Substitute, Posterior Approach, Anterior Column, Open Approach

ØRG13770 Fusion of Cervical Vertebral Joint with Autologous Tissue Substitute, Anterior Approach, Anterior Column, Percutaneous Approach

ØRG1371 Fusion of Cervical Vertebral Joint with Autologous Tissue Substitute, Posterior Approach, Posterior Column, Percutaneous Approach

ØRG137J Fusion of Cervical Vertebral Joint with Autologous Tissue Substitute, Posterior Approach, Anterior Column, Percutaneous Approach

ØRG13AØ Fusion of Cervical Vertebral Joint with Interbody Fusion Device, Anterior Approach, Anterior Column, Percutaneous Approach

ØRG13AJ Fusion of Cervical Vertebral Joint with Interbody Fusion Device, Posterior Approach, Anterior Column, Percutaneous Approach

ØRG13JØ Fusion of Cervical Vertebral Joint with Synthetic Substitute, Anterior Approach, Anterior Column, Percutaneous Approach

ØRG13J1 Fusion of Cervical Vertebral Joint with Synthetic Substitute, Posterior Approach, Posterior Column, Percutaneous Approach

ØRG13JJ Fusion of Cervical Vertebral Joint with Synthetic Substitute, Posterior Approach, Anterior Column, Percutaneous Approach

ØRG13KØ Fusion of Cervical Vertebral Joint with Nonautologous Tissue Substitute, Anterior Approach, Anterior Column, Percutaneous Approach

ØRG13K1 Fusion of Cervical Vertebral Joint with Nonautologous Tissue Substitute, Posterior Approach, Posterior Column, Percutaneous Approach

ØRG13KJ Fusion of Cervical Vertebral Joint with Nonautologous Tissue Substitute, Posterior Approach, Anterior Column, Percutaneous Approach

ØRG1470 Fusion of Cervical Vertebral Joint with Autologous Tissue Substitute, Anterior Approach, Anterior Column, Percutaneous Endoscopic Approach

ØRG1471 Fusion of Cervical Vertebral Joint with Autologous Tissue Substitute, Posterior Approach, Posterior Column, Percutaneous Endoscopic Approach

ØRG147J Fusion of Cervical Vertebral Joint with Autologous Tissue Substitute, Posterior Approach, Anterior Column, Percutaneous Endoscopic Approach

ØRG14AØ Fusion of Cervical Vertebral Joint with Interbody Fusion Device, Anterior Approach, Anterior Column, Percutaneous Endoscopic Approach

ØRG14AJ Fusion of Cervical Vertebral Joint with Interbody Fusion Device, Posterior Approach, Anterior Column, Percutaneous Endoscopic Approach

ØRG14JØ Fusion of Cervical Vertebral Joint with Synthetic Substitute, Anterior Approach, Anterior Column, Percutaneous Endoscopic Approach

ØRG14J1 Fusion of Cervical Vertebral Joint with Synthetic Substitute, Posterior Approach, Posterior Column, Percutaneous Endoscopic Approach

ØRG14JJ Fusion of Cervical Vertebral Joint with Synthetic Substitute, Posterior Approach, Anterior Column, Percutaneous Endoscopic Approach

ØRG14KØ Fusion of Cervical Vertebral Joint with Nonautologous Tissue Substitute, Anterior Approach, Anterior Column, Percutaneous Endoscopic Approach

ØRG14K1 Fusion of Cervical Vertebral Joint with Nonautologous Tissue Substitute, Posterior Approach, Posterior Column, Percutaneous Endoscopic Approach

ØRG14KJ Fusion of Cervical Vertebral Joint with Nonautologous Tissue Substitute, Posterior Approach, Anterior Column, Percutaneous Endoscopic Approach

ØRG2070 Fusion of 2 or more Cervical Vertebral Joints with Autologous Tissue Substitute, Anterior Approach, Anterior Column, Open Approach

ØRG2071 Fusion of 2 or more Cervical Vertebral Joints with Autologous Tissue Substitute, Posterior Approach, Posterior Column, Open Approach

ØRG207J Fusion of 2 or more Cervical Vertebral Joints with Autologous Tissue Substitute, Posterior Approach, Anterior Column, Open Approach

ØRG20AØ Fusion of 2 or more Cervical Vertebral Joints with Interbody Fusion Device, Anterior Approach, Anterior Column, Open Approach

ØRG20AJ Fusion of 2 or more Cervical Vertebral Joints with Interbody Fusion Device, Posterior Approach, Anterior Column, Open Approach

ØRG20JØ Fusion of 2 or more Cervical Vertebral Joints with Synthetic Substitute, Anterior Approach, Anterior Column, Open Approach

ØRG20J1 Fusion of 2 or more Cervical Vertebral Joints with Synthetic Substitute, Posterior Approach, Posterior Column, Open Approach

ØRG20JJ Fusion of 2 or more Cervical Vertebral Joints with Synthetic Substitute, Posterior Approach, Anterior Column, Open Approach

ØRG20KØ Fusion of 2 or more Cervical Vertebral Joints with Nonautologous Tissue Substitute, Anterior Approach, Anterior Column, Open Approach

ØRG20K1 Fusion of 2 or more Cervical Vertebral Joints with Nonautologous Tissue Substitute, Posterior Approach, Posterior Column, Open Approach

ØRG20KJ Fusion of 2 or more Cervical Vertebral Joints with Nonautologous Tissue Substitute, Posterior Approach, Anterior Column, Open Approach

ØRG2370 Fusion of 2 or more Cervical Vertebral Joints with Autologous Tissue Substitute, Anterior Approach, Anterior Column, Percutaneous Approach

ØRG2371 Fusion of 2 or more Cervical Vertebral Joints with Autologous Tissue Substitute, Posterior Approach, Posterior Column, Percutaneous Approach

ØRG237J Fusion of 2 or more Cervical Vertebral Joints with Autologous Tissue Substitute, Posterior Approach, Anterior Column, Percutaneous Approach

ØRG23AØ Fusion of 2 or more Cervical Vertebral Joints with Interbody Fusion Device, Anterior Approach, Anterior Column, Percutaneous Approach

ØRG23AJ Fusion of 2 or more Cervical Vertebral Joints with Interbody Fusion Device, Posterior Approach, Anterior Column, Percutaneous Approach

ØRG23JØ Fusion of 2 or more Cervical Vertebral Joints with Synthetic Substitute, Anterior Approach, Anterior Column, Percutaneous Approach

ØRG23J1 Fusion of 2 or more Cervical Vertebral Joints with Synthetic Substitute, Posterior Approach, Posterior Column, Percutaneous Approach

ØRG23JJ Fusion of 2 or more Cervical Vertebral Joints with Synthetic Substitute, Posterior Approach, Anterior Column, Percutaneous Approach

ØRG23KØ Fusion of 2 or more Cervical Vertebral Joints with Nonautologous Tissue Substitute, Anterior Approach, Anterior Column, Percutaneous Approach

ØRG23K1 Fusion of 2 or more Cervical Vertebral Joints with Nonautologous Tissue Substitute, Posterior Approach, Posterior Column, Percutaneous Approach

ØRG23KJ Fusion of 2 or more Cervical Vertebral Joints with Nonautologous Tissue Substitute, Posterior Approach, Anterior Column, Percutaneous Approach

ØRG2470 Fusion of 2 or more Cervical Vertebral Joints with Autologous Tissue Substitute, Anterior Approach, Anterior Column, Percutaneous Endoscopic Approach

ØRG2471 Fusion of 2 or more Cervical Vertebral Joints with Autologous Tissue Substitute, Posterior Approach, Posterior Column, Percutaneous Endoscopic Approach

HAC 12: Surgical Site Infection Following Certain Orthopedic Procedures of the Spine, Shoulder, and Elbow (continued)

ØRG247J Fusion of 2 or more Cervical Vertebral Joints with Autologous Tissue Substitute, Posterior Approach, Anterior Column, Percutaneous Endoscopic Approach

ØRG24AØ Fusion of 2 or more Cervical Vertebral Joints with Interbody Fusion Device, Anterior Approach, Anterior Column, Percutaneous Endoscopic Approach

ØRG24AJ Fusion of 2 or more Cervical Vertebral Joints with Interbody Fusion Device, Posterior Approach, Anterior Column, Percutaneous Endoscopic Approach

ØRG24JØ Fusion of 2 or more Cervical Vertebral Joints with Synthetic Substitute, Anterior Approach, Anterior Column, Percutaneous Endoscopic Approach

ØRG24J1 Fusion of 2 or more Cervical Vertebral Joints with Synthetic Substitute, Posterior Approach, Posterior Column, Percutaneous Endoscopic Approach

ØRG24JJ Fusion of 2 or more Cervical Vertebral Joints with Synthetic Substitute, Posterior Approach, Anterior Column, Percutaneous Endoscopic Approach

ØRG24KØ Fusion of 2 or more Cervical Vertebral Joints with Nonautologous Tissue Substitute, Anterior Approach, Anterior Column, Percutaneous Endoscopic Approach

ØRG24K1 Fusion of 2 or more Cervical Vertebral Joints with Nonautologous Tissue Substitute, Posterior Approach, Posterior Column, Percutaneous Endoscopic Approach

ØRG24KJ Fusion of 2 or more Cervical Vertebral Joints with Nonautologous Tissue Substitute, Posterior Approach, Anterior Column, Percutaneous Endoscopic Approach

ØRG40070 Fusion of Cervicothoracic Vertebral Joint with Autologous Tissue Substitute, Anterior Approach, Anterior Column, Open Approach

ØRG40071 Fusion of Cervicothoracic Vertebral Joint with Autologous Tissue Substitute, Posterior Approach, Posterior Column, Open Approach

ØRG4007J Fusion of Cervicothoracic Vertebral Joint with Autologous Tissue Substitute, Posterior Approach, Anterior Column, Open Approach

ØRG400AØ Fusion of Cervicothoracic Vertebral Joint with Interbody Fusion Device, Anterior Approach, Anterior Column, Open Approach

ØRG400AJ Fusion of Cervicothoracic Vertebral Joint with Interbody Fusion Device, Posterior Approach, Anterior Column, Open Approach

ØRG400JØ Fusion of Cervicothoracic Vertebral Joint with Synthetic Substitute, Anterior Approach, Anterior Column, Open Approach

ØRG400J1 Fusion of Cervicothoracic Vertebral Joint with Synthetic Substitute, Posterior Approach, Posterior Column, Open Approach

ØRG400JJ Fusion of Cervicothoracic Vertebral Joint with Synthetic Substitute, Posterior Approach, Anterior Column, Open Approach

ØRG40KØ Fusion of Cervicothoracic Vertebral Joint with Nonautologous Tissue Substitute, Anterior Approach, Anterior Column, Open Approach

ØRG40K1 Fusion of Cervicothoracic Vertebral Joint with Nonautologous Tissue Substitute, Posterior Approach, Posterior Column, Open Approach

ØRG40KJ Fusion of Cervicothoracic Vertebral Joint with Nonautologous Tissue Substitute, Posterior Approach, Anterior Column, Open Approach

ØRG4370 Fusion of Cervicothoracic Vertebral Joint with Autologous Tissue Substitute, Anterior Approach, Anterior Column, Percutaneous Approach

ØRG4371 Fusion of Cervicothoracic Vertebral Joint with Autologous Tissue Substitute, Posterior Approach, Posterior Column, Percutaneous Approach

ØRG437J Fusion of Cervicothoracic Vertebral Joint with Autologous Tissue Substitute, Posterior Approach, Anterior Column, Percutaneous Approach

ØRG43AØ Fusion of Cervicothoracic Vertebral Joint with Interbody Fusion Device, Anterior Approach, Anterior Column, Percutaneous Approach

ØRG43AJ Fusion of Cervicothoracic Vertebral Joint with Interbody Fusion Device, Posterior Approach, Anterior Column, Percutaneous Approach

ØRG43JØ Fusion of Cervicothoracic Vertebral Joint with Synthetic Substitute, Anterior Approach, Anterior Column, Percutaneous Approach

ØRG43J1 Fusion of Cervicothoracic Vertebral Joint with Synthetic Substitute, Posterior Approach, Posterior Column, Percutaneous Approach

ØRG43JJ Fusion of Cervicothoracic Vertebral Joint with Synthetic Substitute, Posterior Approach, Anterior Column, Percutaneous Approach

ØRG43KØ Fusion of Cervicothoracic Vertebral Joint with Nonautologous Tissue Substitute, Anterior Approach, Anterior Column, Percutaneous Approach

ØRG43K1 Fusion of Cervicothoracic Vertebral Joint with Nonautologous Tissue Substitute, Posterior Approach, Posterior Column, Percutaneous Approach

ØRG43KJ Fusion of Cervicothoracic Vertebral Joint with Nonautologous Tissue Substitute, Posterior Approach, Anterior Column, Percutaneous Approach

ØRG4470 Fusion of Cervicothoracic Vertebral Joint with Autologous Tissue Substitute, Anterior Approach, Anterior Column, Percutaneous Endoscopic Approach

ØRG4471 Fusion of Cervicothoracic Vertebral Joint with Autologous Tissue Substitute, Posterior Approach, Posterior Column, Percutaneous Endoscopic Approach

ØRG447J Fusion of Cervicothoracic Vertebral Joint with Autologous Tissue Substitute, Posterior Approach, Anterior Column, Percutaneous Endoscopic Approach

ØRG44AØ Fusion of Cervicothoracic Vertebral Joint with Interbody Fusion Device, Anterior Approach, Anterior Column, Percutaneous Endoscopic Approach

ØRG44AJ Fusion of Cervicothoracic Vertebral Joint with Interbody Fusion Device, Posterior Approach, Anterior Column, Percutaneous Endoscopic Approach

ØRG44JØ Fusion of Cervicothoracic Vertebral Joint with Synthetic Substitute, Anterior Approach, Anterior Column, Percutaneous Endoscopic Approach

ØRG44J1 Fusion of Cervicothoracic Vertebral Joint with Synthetic Substitute, Posterior Approach, Posterior Column, Percutaneous Endoscopic Approach

ØRG44JJ Fusion of Cervicothoracic Vertebral Joint with Synthetic Substitute, Posterior Approach, Anterior Column, Percutaneous Endoscopic Approach

ØRG44KØ Fusion of Cervicothoracic Vertebral Joint with Nonautologous Tissue Substitute, Anterior Approach, Anterior Column, Percutaneous Endoscopic Approach

ØRG44K1 Fusion of Cervicothoracic Vertebral Joint with Nonautologous Tissue Substitute, Posterior Approach, Posterior Column, Percutaneous Endoscopic Approach

ØRG44KJ Fusion of Cervicothoracic Vertebral Joint with Nonautologous Tissue Substitute, Posterior Approach, Anterior Column, Percutaneous Endoscopic Approach

ØRG6070 Fusion of Thoracic Vertebral Joint with Autologous Tissue Substitute, Anterior Approach, Anterior Column, Open Approach

ØRG6071 Fusion of Thoracic Vertebral Joint with Autologous Tissue Substitute, Posterior Approach, Posterior Column, Open Approach

ØRG607J Fusion of Thoracic Vertebral Joint with Autologous Tissue Substitute, Posterior Approach, Anterior Column, Open Approach

ØRG60AØ Fusion of Thoracic Vertebral Joint with Interbody Fusion Device, Anterior Approach, Anterior Column, Open Approach

ØRG60AJ Fusion of Thoracic Vertebral Joint with Interbody Fusion Device, Posterior Approach, Anterior Column, Open Approach

ØRG60JØ Fusion of Thoracic Vertebral Joint with Synthetic Substitute, Anterior Approach, Anterior Column, Open Approach

ØRG60J1 Fusion of Thoracic Vertebral Joint with Synthetic Substitute, Posterior Approach, Posterior Column, Open Approach

ØRG60JJ Fusion of Thoracic Vertebral Joint with Synthetic Substitute, Posterior Approach, Anterior Column, Open Approach

ØRG60KØ Fusion of Thoracic Vertebral Joint with Nonautologous Tissue Substitute, Anterior Approach, Anterior Column, Open Approach

ØRG60K1 Fusion of Thoracic Vertebral Joint with Nonautologous Tissue Substitute, Posterior Approach, Posterior Column, Open Approach

ØRG60KJ Fusion of Thoracic Vertebral Joint with Nonautologous Tissue Substitute, Posterior Approach, Anterior Column, Open Approach

ØRG6370 Fusion of Thoracic Vertebral Joint with Autologous Tissue Substitute, Anterior Approach, Anterior Column, Percutaneous Approach

ØRG6371 Fusion of Thoracic Vertebral Joint with Autologous Tissue Substitute, Posterior Approach, Posterior Column, Percutaneous Approach

HAC 12: Surgical Site Infection Following Certain Orthopedic Procedures of the Spine, Shoulder, and Elbow (continued)

ØRG637J Fusion of Thoracic Vertebral Joint with Autologous Tissue Substitute, Posterior Approach, Anterior Column, Percutaneous Approach

ØRG63AØ Fusion of Thoracic Vertebral Joint with Interbody Fusion Device, Anterior Approach, Anterior Column, Percutaneous Approach

ØRG63AJ Fusion of Thoracic Vertebral Joint with Interbody Fusion Device, Posterior Approach, Anterior Column, Percutaneous Approach

ØRG63JØ Fusion of Thoracic Vertebral Joint with Synthetic Substitute, Anterior Approach, Anterior Column, Percutaneous Approach

ØRG63J1 Fusion of Thoracic Vertebral Joint with Synthetic Substitute, Posterior Approach, Posterior Column, Percutaneous Approach

ØRG63JJ Fusion of Thoracic Vertebral Joint with Synthetic Substitute, Posterior Approach, Anterior Column, Percutaneous Approach

ØRG63KØ Fusion of Thoracic Vertebral Joint with Nonautologous Tissue Substitute, Anterior Approach, Anterior Column, Percutaneous Approach

ØRG63K1 Fusion of Thoracic Vertebral Joint with Nonautologous Tissue Substitute, Posterior Approach, Posterior Column, Percutaneous Approach

ØRG63KJ Fusion of Thoracic Vertebral Joint with Nonautologous Tissue Substitute, Posterior Approach, Anterior Column, Percutaneous Approach

ØRG647Ø Fusion of Thoracic Vertebral Joint with Autologous Tissue Substitute, Anterior Approach, Anterior Column, Percutaneous Endoscopic Approach

ØRG6471 Fusion of Thoracic Vertebral Joint with Autologous Tissue Substitute, Posterior Approach, Posterior Column, Percutaneous Endoscopic Approach

ØRG647J Fusion of Thoracic Vertebral Joint with Autologous Tissue Substitute, Posterior Approach, Anterior Column, Percutaneous Endoscopic Approach

ØRG64AØ Fusion of Thoracic Vertebral Joint with Interbody Fusion Device, Anterior Approach, Anterior Column, Percutaneous Endoscopic Approach

ØRG64AJ Fusion of Thoracic Vertebral Joint with Interbody Fusion Device, Posterior Approach, Anterior Column, Percutaneous Endoscopic Approach

ØRG64JØ Fusion of Thoracic Vertebral Joint with Synthetic Substitute, Anterior Approach, Anterior Column, Percutaneous Endoscopic Approach

ØRG64J1 Fusion of Thoracic Vertebral Joint with Synthetic Substitute, Posterior Approach, Posterior Column, Percutaneous Endoscopic Approach

ØRG64JJ Fusion of Thoracic Vertebral Joint with Synthetic Substitute, Posterior Approach, Anterior Column, Percutaneous Endoscopic Approach

ØRG64KØ Fusion of Thoracic Vertebral Joint with Nonautologous Tissue Substitute, Anterior Approach, Anterior Column, Percutaneous Endoscopic Approach

ØRG64K1 Fusion of Thoracic Vertebral Joint with Nonautologous Tissue Substitute, Posterior Approach, Posterior Column, Percutaneous Endoscopic Approach

ØRG64KJ Fusion of Thoracic Vertebral Joint with Nonautologous Tissue Substitute, Posterior Approach, Anterior Column, Percutaneous Endoscopic Approach

ØRG7070 Fusion of 2 to 7 Thoracic Vertebral Joints with Autologous Tissue Substitute, Anterior Approach, Anterior Column, Open Approach

ØRG7071 Fusion of 2 to 7 Thoracic Vertebral Joints with Autologous Tissue Substitute, Posterior Approach, Posterior Column, Open Approach

ØRG707J Fusion of 2 to 7 Thoracic Vertebral Joints with Autologous Tissue Substitute, Posterior Approach, Anterior Column, Open Approach

ØRG70AØ Fusion of 2 to 7 Thoracic Vertebral Joints with Interbody Fusion Device, Anterior Approach, Anterior Column, Open Approach

ØRG70AJ Fusion of 2 to 7 Thoracic Vertebral Joints with Interbody Fusion Device, Posterior Approach, Anterior Column, Open Approach

ØRG70JØ Fusion of 2 to 7 Thoracic Vertebral Joints with Synthetic Substitute, Anterior Approach, Anterior Column, Open Approach

ØRG70J1 Fusion of 2 to 7 Thoracic Vertebral Joints with Synthetic Substitute, Posterior Approach, Posterior Column, Open Approach

ØRG70JJ Fusion of 2 to 7 Thoracic Vertebral Joints with Synthetic Substitute, Posterior Approach, Anterior Column, Open Approach

ØRG70KØ Fusion of 2 to 7 Thoracic Vertebral Joints with Nonautologous Tissue Substitute, Anterior Approach, Anterior Column, Open Approach

ØRG70K1 Fusion of 2 to 7 Thoracic Vertebral Joints with Nonautologous Tissue Substitute, Posterior Approach, Posterior Column, Open Approach

ØRG70KJ Fusion of 2 to 7 Thoracic Vertebral Joints with Nonautologous Tissue Substitute, Posterior Approach, Anterior Column, Open Approach

ØRG7370 Fusion of 2 to 7 Thoracic Vertebral Joints with Autologous Tissue Substitute, Anterior Approach, Anterior Column, Percutaneous Approach

ØRG7371 Fusion of 2 to 7 Thoracic Vertebral Joints with Autologous Tissue Substitute, Posterior Approach, Posterior Column, Percutaneous Approach

ØRG737J Fusion of 2 to 7 Thoracic Vertebral Joints with Autologous Tissue Substitute, Posterior Approach, Anterior Column, Percutaneous Approach

ØRG73AØ Fusion of 2 to 7 Thoracic Vertebral Joints with Interbody Fusion Device, Anterior Approach, Anterior Column, Percutaneous Approach

ØRG73AJ Fusion of 2 to 7 Thoracic Vertebral Joints with Interbody Fusion Device, Posterior Approach, Anterior Column, Percutaneous Approach

ØRG73JØ Fusion of 2 to 7 Thoracic Vertebral Joints with Synthetic Substitute, Anterior Approach, Anterior Column, Percutaneous Approach

ØRG73J1 Fusion of 2 to 7 Thoracic Vertebral Joints with Synthetic Substitute, Posterior Approach, Posterior Column, Percutaneous Approach

ØRG73JJ Fusion of 2 to 7 Thoracic Vertebral Joints with Synthetic Substitute, Posterior Approach, Anterior Column, Percutaneous Approach

ØRG73KØ Fusion of 2 to 7 Thoracic Vertebral Joints with Nonautologous Tissue Substitute, Anterior Approach, Anterior Column, Percutaneous Approach

ØRG73K1 Fusion of 2 to 7 Thoracic Vertebral Joints with Nonautologous Tissue Substitute, Posterior Approach, Posterior Column, Percutaneous Approach

ØRG73KJ Fusion of 2 to 7 Thoracic Vertebral Joints with Nonautologous Tissue Substitute, Posterior Approach, Anterior Column, Percutaneous Approach

ØRG7470 Fusion of 2 to 7 Thoracic Vertebral Joints with Autologous Tissue Substitute, Anterior Approach, Anterior Column, Percutaneous Endoscopic Approach

ØRG7471 Fusion of 2 to 7 Thoracic Vertebral Joints with Autologous Tissue Substitute, Posterior Approach, Posterior Column, Percutaneous Endoscopic Approach

ØRG747J Fusion of 2 to 7 Thoracic Vertebral Joints with Autologous Tissue Substitute, Posterior Approach, Anterior Column, Percutaneous Endoscopic Approach

ØRG74AØ Fusion of 2 to 7 Thoracic Vertebral Joints with Interbody Fusion Device, Anterior Approach, Anterior Column, Percutaneous Endoscopic Approach

ØRG74AJ Fusion of 2 to 7 Thoracic Vertebral Joints with Interbody Fusion Device, Posterior Approach, Anterior Column, Percutaneous Endoscopic Approach

ØRG74JØ Fusion of 2 to 7 Thoracic Vertebral Joints with Synthetic Substitute, Anterior Approach, Anterior Column, Percutaneous Endoscopic Approach

ØRG74J1 Fusion of 2 to 7 Thoracic Vertebral Joints with Synthetic Substitute, Posterior Approach, Posterior Column, Percutaneous Endoscopic Approach

ØRG74JJ Fusion of 2 to 7 Thoracic Vertebral Joints with Synthetic Substitute, Posterior Approach, Anterior Column, Percutaneous Endoscopic Approach

ØRG74KØ Fusion of 2 to 7 Thoracic Vertebral Joints with Nonautologous Tissue Substitute, Anterior Approach, Anterior Column, Percutaneous Endoscopic Approach

ØRG74K1 Fusion of 2 to 7 Thoracic Vertebral Joints with Nonautologous Tissue Substitute, Posterior Approach, Posterior Column, Percutaneous Endoscopic Approach

ØRG74KJ Fusion of 2 to 7 Thoracic Vertebral Joints with Nonautologous Tissue Substitute, Posterior Approach, Anterior Column, Percutaneous Endoscopic Approach

ØRG8070 Fusion of 8 or More Thoracic Vertebral Joints with Autologous Tissue Substitute, Anterior Approach, Anterior Column, Open Approach

ØRG8071 Fusion of 8 or More Thoracic Vertebral Joints with Autologous Tissue Substitute, Posterior Approach, Posterior Column, Open Approach

ØRG807J Fusion of 8 or More Thoracic Vertebral Joints with Autologous Tissue Substitute, Posterior Approach, Anterior Column, Open Approach

HAC 12: Surgical Site Infection Following Certain Orthopedic Procedures of the Spine, Shoulder, and Elbow (continued)

ØRG8ØAØ   Fusion of 8 or More Thoracic Vertebral Joints with Interbody Fusion Device, Anterior Approach, Anterior Column, Open Approach

ØRG8ØAJ   Fusion of 8 or More Thoracic Vertebral Joints with Interbody Fusion Device, Posterior Approach, Anterior Column, Open Approach

ØRG8ØJØ   Fusion of 8 or More Thoracic Vertebral Joints with Synthetic Substitute, Anterior Approach, Anterior Column, Open Approach

ØRG8ØJ1   Fusion of 8 or More Thoracic Vertebral Joints with Synthetic Substitute, Posterior Approach, Posterior Column, Open Approach

ØRG8ØJJ   Fusion of 8 or More Thoracic Vertebral Joints with Synthetic Substitute, Posterior Approach, Anterior Column, Open Approach

ØRG8ØKØ   Fusion of 8 or More Thoracic Vertebral Joints with Nonautologous Tissue Substitute, Anterior Approach, Anterior Column, Open Approach

ØRG8ØK1   Fusion of 8 or More Thoracic Vertebral Joints with Nonautologous Tissue Substitute, Posterior Approach, Posterior Column, Open Approach

ØRG8ØKJ   Fusion of 8 or More Thoracic Vertebral Joints with Nonautologous Tissue Substitute, Posterior Approach, Anterior Column, Open Approach

ØRG837Ø   Fusion of 8 or More Thoracic Vertebral Joints with Autologous Tissue Substitute, Anterior Approach, Anterior Column, Percutaneous Approach

ØRG8371   Fusion of 8 or More Thoracic Vertebral Joints with Autologous Tissue Substitute, Posterior Approach, Posterior Column, Percutaneous Approach

ØRG837J   Fusion of 8 or More Thoracic Vertebral Joints with Autologous Tissue Substitute, Posterior Approach, Anterior Column, Percutaneous Approach

ØRG83AØ   Fusion of 8 or More Thoracic Vertebral Joints with Interbody Fusion Device, Anterior Approach, Anterior Column, Percutaneous Approach

ØRG83AJ   Fusion of 8 or More Thoracic Vertebral Joints with Interbody Fusion Device, Posterior Approach, Anterior Column, Percutaneous Approach

ØRG83JØ   Fusion of 8 or More Thoracic Vertebral Joints with Synthetic Substitute, Anterior Approach, Anterior Column, Percutaneous Approach

ØRG83J1   Fusion of 8 or More Thoracic Vertebral Joints with Synthetic Substitute, Posterior Approach, Posterior Column, Percutaneous Approach

ØRG83JJ   Fusion of 8 or More Thoracic Vertebral Joints with Synthetic Substitute, Posterior Approach, Anterior Column, Percutaneous Approach

ØRG83KØ   Fusion of 8 or More Thoracic Vertebral Joints with Nonautologous Tissue Substitute, Anterior Approach, Anterior Column, Percutaneous Approach

ØRG83K1   Fusion of 8 or More Thoracic Vertebral Joints with Nonautologous Tissue Substitute, Posterior Approach, Posterior Column, Percutaneous Approach

ØRG83KJ   Fusion of 8 or More Thoracic Vertebral Joints with Nonautologous Tissue Substitute, Posterior Approach, Anterior Column, Percutaneous Approach

ØRG847Ø   Fusion of 8 or More Thoracic Vertebral Joints with Autologous Tissue Substitute, Anterior Approach, Anterior Column, Percutaneous Endoscopic Approach

ØRG8471   Fusion of 8 or More Thoracic Vertebral Joints with Autologous Tissue Substitute, Posterior Approach, Posterior Column, Percutaneous Endoscopic Approach

ØRG847J   Fusion of 8 or More Thoracic Vertebral Joints with Autologous Tissue Substitute, Posterior Approach, Anterior Column, Percutaneous Endoscopic Approach

ØRG84AØ   Fusion of 8 or More Thoracic Vertebral Joints with Interbody Fusion Device, Anterior Approach, Anterior Column, Percutaneous Endoscopic Approach

ØRG84AJ   Fusion of 8 or More Thoracic Vertebral Joints with Interbody Fusion Device, Posterior Approach, Anterior Column, Percutaneous Endoscopic Approach

ØRG84JØ   Fusion of 8 or More Thoracic Vertebral Joints with Synthetic Substitute, Anterior Approach, Anterior Column, Percutaneous Endoscopic Approach

ØRG84J1   Fusion of 8 or More Thoracic Vertebral Joints with Synthetic Substitute, Posterior Approach, Posterior Column, Percutaneous Endoscopic Approach

ØRG84JJ   Fusion of 8 or More Thoracic Vertebral Joints with Synthetic Substitute, Posterior Approach, Anterior Column, Percutaneous Endoscopic Approach

ØRG84KØ   Fusion of 8 or More Thoracic Vertebral Joints with Nonautologous Tissue Substitute, Anterior Approach, Anterior Column, Percutaneous Endoscopic Approach

ØRG84K1   Fusion of 8 or More Thoracic Vertebral Joints with Nonautologous Tissue Substitute, Posterior Approach, Posterior Column, Percutaneous Endoscopic Approach

ØRG84KJ   Fusion of 8 or More Thoracic Vertebral Joints with Nonautologous Tissue Substitute, Posterior Approach, Anterior Column, Percutaneous Endoscopic Approach

ØRGAØ7Ø   Fusion of Thoracolumbar Vertebral Joint with Autologous Tissue Substitute, Anterior Approach, Anterior Column, Open Approach

ØRGAØ71   Fusion of Thoracolumbar Vertebral Joint with Autologous Tissue Substitute, Posterior Approach, Posterior Column, Open Approach

ØRGAØ7J   Fusion of Thoracolumbar Vertebral Joint with Autologous Tissue Substitute, Posterior Approach, Anterior Column, Open Approach

ØRGAØAØ   Fusion of Thoracolumbar Vertebral Joint with Interbody Fusion Device, Anterior Approach, Anterior Column, Open Approach

ØRGAØAJ   Fusion of Thoracolumbar Vertebral Joint with Interbody Fusion Device, Posterior Approach, Anterior Column, Open Approach

ØRGAØJØ   Fusion of Thoracolumbar Vertebral Joint with Synthetic Substitute, Anterior Approach, Anterior Column, Open Approach

ØRGAØJ1   Fusion of Thoracolumbar Vertebral Joint with Synthetic Substitute, Posterior Approach, Posterior Column, Open Approach

ØRGAØJJ   Fusion of Thoracolumbar Vertebral Joint with Synthetic Substitute, Posterior Approach, Anterior Column, Open Approach

ØRGAØKØ   Fusion of Thoracolumbar Vertebral Joint with Nonautologous Tissue Substitute, Anterior Approach, Anterior Column, Open Approach

ØRGAØK1   Fusion of Thoracolumbar Vertebral Joint with Nonautologous Tissue Substitute, Posterior Approach, Posterior Column, Open Approach

ØRGAØKJ   Fusion of Thoracolumbar Vertebral Joint with Nonautologous Tissue Substitute, Posterior Approach, Anterior Column, Open Approach

ØRGA37Ø   Fusion of Thoracolumbar Vertebral Joint with Autologous Tissue Substitute, Anterior Approach, Anterior Column, Percutaneous Approach

ØRGA371   Fusion of Thoracolumbar Vertebral Joint with Autologous Tissue Substitute, Posterior Approach, Posterior Column, Percutaneous Approach

ØRGA37J   Fusion of Thoracolumbar Vertebral Joint with Autologous Tissue Substitute, Posterior Approach, Anterior Column, Percutaneous Approach

ØRGA3AØ   Fusion of Thoracolumbar Vertebral Joint with Interbody Fusion Device, Anterior Approach, Anterior Column, Percutaneous Approach

ØRGA3AJ   Fusion of Thoracolumbar Vertebral Joint with Interbody Fusion Device, Posterior Approach, Anterior Column, Percutaneous Approach

ØRGA3JØ   Fusion of Thoracolumbar Vertebral Joint with Synthetic Substitute, Anterior Approach, Anterior Column, Percutaneous Approach

ØRGA3J1   Fusion of Thoracolumbar Vertebral Joint with Synthetic Substitute, Posterior Approach, Posterior Column, Percutaneous Approach

ØRGA3JJ   Fusion of Thoracolumbar Vertebral Joint with Synthetic Substitute, Posterior Approach, Anterior Column, Percutaneous Approach

ØRGA3KØ   Fusion of Thoracolumbar Vertebral Joint with Nonautologous Tissue Substitute, Anterior Approach, Anterior Column, Percutaneous Approach

ØRGA3K1   Fusion of Thoracolumbar Vertebral Joint with Nonautologous Tissue Substitute, Posterior Approach, Posterior Column, Percutaneous Approach

ØRGA3KJ   Fusion of Thoracolumbar Vertebral Joint with Nonautologous Tissue Substitute, Posterior Approach, Anterior Column, Percutaneous Approach

ØRGA47Ø   Fusion of Thoracolumbar Vertebral Joint with Autologous Tissue Substitute, Anterior Approach, Anterior Column, Percutaneous Endoscopic Approach

HAC 12: Surgical Site Infection Following Certain Orthopedic Procedures of the Spine, Shoulder, and Elbow (continued)

ØRGA471 Fusion of Thoracolumbar Vertebral Joint with Autologous Tissue Substitute, Posterior Approach, Posterior Column, Percutaneous Endoscopic Approach

ØRGA47J Fusion of Thoracolumbar Vertebral Joint with Autologous Tissue Substitute, Posterior Approach, Anterior Column, Percutaneous Endoscopic Approach

ØRGA4AØ Fusion of Thoracolumbar Vertebral Joint with Interbody Fusion Device, Anterior Approach, Anterior Column, Percutaneous Endoscopic Approach

ØRGA4AJ Fusion of Thoracolumbar Vertebral Joint with Interbody Fusion Device, Posterior Approach, Anterior Column, Percutaneous Endoscopic Approach

ØRGA4JØ Fusion of Thoracolumbar Vertebral Joint with Synthetic Substitute, Anterior Approach, Anterior Column, Percutaneous Endoscopic Approach

ØRGA4J1 Fusion of Thoracolumbar Vertebral Joint with Synthetic Substitute, Posterior Approach, Posterior Column, Percutaneous Endoscopic Approach

ØRGA4JJ Fusion of Thoracolumbar Vertebral Joint with Synthetic Substitute, Posterior Approach, Anterior Column, Percutaneous Endoscopic Approach

ØRGA4KØ Fusion of Thoracolumbar Vertebral Joint with Nonautologous Tissue Substitute, Anterior Approach, Anterior Column, Percutaneous Endoscopic Approach

ØRGA4K1 Fusion of Thoracolumbar Vertebral Joint with Nonautologous Tissue Substitute, Posterior Approach, Posterior Column, Percutaneous Endoscopic Approach

ØRGA4KJ Fusion of Thoracolumbar Vertebral Joint with Nonautologous Tissue Substitute, Posterior Approach, Anterior Column, Percutaneous Endoscopic Approach

ØRGEØ4Z Fusion of Right Sternoclavicular Joint with Internal Fixation Device, Open Approach

ØRGEØ7Z Fusion of Right Sternoclavicular Joint with Autologous Tissue Substitute, Open Approach

ØRGEØJZ Fusion of Right Sternoclavicular Joint with Synthetic Substitute, Open Approach

ØRGEØKZ Fusion of Right Sternoclavicular Joint with Nonautologous Tissue Substitute, Open Approach

ØRGE34Z Fusion of Right Sternoclavicular Joint with Internal Fixation Device, Percutaneous Approach

ØRGE37Z Fusion of Right Sternoclavicular Joint with Autologous Tissue Substitute, Percutaneous Approach

ØRGE3JZ Fusion of Right Sternoclavicular Joint with Synthetic Substitute, Percutaneous Approach

ØRGE3KZ Fusion of Right Sternoclavicular Joint with Nonautologous Tissue Substitute, Percutaneous Approach

ØRGE44Z Fusion of Right Sternoclavicular Joint with Internal Fixation Device, Percutaneous Endoscopic Approach

ØRGE47Z Fusion of Right Sternoclavicular Joint with Autologous Tissue Substitute, Percutaneous Endoscopic Approach

ØRGE4JZ Fusion of Right Sternoclavicular Joint with Synthetic Substitute, Percutaneous Endoscopic Approach

ØRGE4KZ Fusion of Right Sternoclavicular Joint with Nonautologous Tissue Substitute, Percutaneous Endoscopic Approach

ØRGFØ4Z Fusion of Left Sternoclavicular Joint with Internal Fixation Device, Open Approach

ØRGFØ7Z Fusion of Left Sternoclavicular Joint with Autologous Tissue Substitute, Open Approach

ØRGFØJZ Fusion of Left Sternoclavicular Joint with Synthetic Substitute, Open Approach

ØRGFØKZ Fusion of Left Sternoclavicular Joint with Nonautologous Tissue Substitute, Open Approach

ØRGF34Z Fusion of Left Sternoclavicular Joint with Internal Fixation Device, Percutaneous Approach

ØRGF37Z Fusion of Left Sternoclavicular Joint with Autologous Tissue Substitute, Percutaneous Approach

ØRGF3JZ Fusion of Left Sternoclavicular Joint with Synthetic Substitute, Percutaneous Approach

ØRGF3KZ Fusion of Left Sternoclavicular Joint with Nonautologous Tissue Substitute, Percutaneous Approach

ØRGF44Z Fusion of Left Sternoclavicular Joint with Internal Fixation Device, Percutaneous Endoscopic Approach

ØRGF47Z Fusion of Left Sternoclavicular Joint with Autologous Tissue Substitute, Percutaneous Endoscopic Approach

ØRGF4JZ Fusion of Left Sternoclavicular Joint with Synthetic Substitute, Percutaneous Endoscopic Approach

ØRGF4KZ Fusion of Left Sternoclavicular Joint with Nonautologous Tissue Substitute, Percutaneous Endoscopic Approach

ØRGGØ4Z Fusion of Right Acromioclavicular Joint with Internal Fixation Device, Open Approach

ØRGGØ7Z Fusion of Right Acromioclavicular Joint with Autologous Tissue Substitute, Open Approach

ØRGGØJZ Fusion of Right Acromioclavicular Joint with Synthetic Substitute, Open Approach

ØRGGØKZ Fusion of Right Acromioclavicular Joint with Nonautologous Tissue Substitute, Open Approach

ØRGG34Z Fusion of Right Acromioclavicular Joint with Internal Fixation Device, Percutaneous Approach

ØRGG37Z Fusion of Right Acromioclavicular Joint with Autologous Tissue Substitute, Percutaneous Approach

ØRGG3JZ Fusion of Right Acromioclavicular Joint with Synthetic Substitute, Percutaneous Approach

ØRGG3KZ Fusion of Right Acromioclavicular Joint with Nonautologous Tissue Substitute, Percutaneous Approach

ØRGG44Z Fusion of Right Acromioclavicular Joint with Internal Fixation Device, Percutaneous Endoscopic Approach

ØRGG47Z Fusion of Right Acromioclavicular Joint with Autologous Tissue Substitute, Percutaneous Endoscopic Approach

ØRGG4JZ Fusion of Right Acromioclavicular Joint with Synthetic Substitute, Percutaneous Endoscopic Approach

ØRGG4KZ Fusion of Right Acromioclavicular Joint with Nonautologous Tissue Substitute, Percutaneous Endoscopic Approach

ØRGHØ4Z Fusion of Left Acromioclavicular Joint with Internal Fixation Device, Open Approach

ØRGHØ7Z Fusion of Left Acromioclavicular Joint with Autologous Tissue Substitute, Open Approach

ØRGHØJZ Fusion of Left Acromioclavicular Joint with Synthetic Substitute, Open Approach

ØRGHØKZ Fusion of Left Acromioclavicular Joint with Nonautologous Tissue Substitute, Open Approach

ØRGH34Z Fusion of Left Acromioclavicular Joint with Internal Fixation Device, Percutaneous Approach

ØRGH37Z Fusion of Left Acromioclavicular Joint with Autologous Tissue Substitute, Percutaneous Approach

ØRGH3JZ Fusion of Left Acromioclavicular Joint with Synthetic Substitute, Percutaneous Approach

ØRGH3KZ Fusion of Left Acromioclavicular Joint with Nonautologous Tissue Substitute, Percutaneous Approach

ØRGH44Z Fusion of Left Acromioclavicular Joint with Internal Fixation Device, Percutaneous Endoscopic Approach

ØRGH47Z Fusion of Left Acromioclavicular Joint with Autologous Tissue Substitute, Percutaneous Endoscopic Approach

ØRGH4JZ Fusion of Left Acromioclavicular Joint with Synthetic Substitute, Percutaneous Endoscopic Approach

ØRGH4KZ Fusion of Left Acromioclavicular Joint with Nonautologous Tissue Substitute, Percutaneous Endoscopic Approach

ØRGJØ4Z Fusion of Right Shoulder Joint with Internal Fixation Device, Open Approach

ØRGJØ7Z Fusion of Right Shoulder Joint with Autologous Tissue Substitute, Open Approach

ØRGJØJZ Fusion of Right Shoulder Joint with Synthetic Substitute, Open Approach

ØRGJØKZ Fusion of Right Shoulder Joint with Nonautologous Tissue Substitute, Open Approach

ØRGJ34Z Fusion of Right Shoulder Joint with Internal Fixation Device, Percutaneous Approach

ØRGJ37Z Fusion of Right Shoulder Joint with Autologous Tissue Substitute, Percutaneous Approach

ØRGJ3JZ Fusion of Right Shoulder Joint with Synthetic Substitute, Percutaneous Approach

ØRGJ3KZ Fusion of Right Shoulder Joint with Nonautologous Tissue Substitute, Percutaneous Approach

ØRGJ44Z Fusion of Right Shoulder Joint with Internal Fixation Device, Percutaneous Endoscopic Approach

ØRGJ47Z Fusion of Right Shoulder Joint with Autologous Tissue Substitute, Percutaneous Endoscopic Approach

ØRGJ4JZ Fusion of Right Shoulder Joint with Synthetic Substitute, Percutaneous Endoscopic Approach

ØRGJ4KZ Fusion of Right Shoulder Joint with Nonautologous Tissue Substitute, Percutaneous Endoscopic Approach

ØRGKØ4Z Fusion of Left Shoulder Joint with Internal Fixation Device, Open Approach

ØRGKØ7Z Fusion of Left Shoulder Joint with Autologous Tissue Substitute, Open Approach

ØRGKØJZ Fusion of Left Shoulder Joint with Synthetic Substitute, Open Approach

HAC 12: Surgical Site Infection Following Certain Orthopedic Procedures of the Spine, Shoulder, and Elbow (continued)

ØRGKØKZ Fusion of Left Shoulder Joint with Nonautologous Tissue Substitute, Open Approach

ØRGK34Z Fusion of Left Shoulder Joint with Internal Fixation Device, Percutaneous Approach

ØRGK37Z Fusion of Left Shoulder Joint with Autologous Tissue Substitute, Percutaneous Approach

ØRGK3JZ Fusion of Left Shoulder Joint with Synthetic Substitute, Percutaneous Approach

ØRGK3KZ Fusion of Left Shoulder Joint with Nonautologous Tissue Substitute, Percutaneous Approach

ØRGK44Z Fusion of Left Shoulder Joint with Internal Fixation Device, Percutaneous Endoscopic Approach

ØRGK47Z Fusion of Left Shoulder Joint with Autologous Tissue Substitute, Percutaneous Endoscopic Approach

ØRGK4JZ Fusion of Left Shoulder Joint with Synthetic Substitute, Percutaneous Endoscopic Approach

ØRGK4KZ Fusion of Left Shoulder Joint with Nonautologous Tissue Substitute, Percutaneous Endoscopic Approach

ØRGLØ4Z Fusion of Right Elbow Joint with Internal Fixation Device, Open Approach

ØRGLØ5Z Fusion of Right Elbow Joint with External Fixation Device, Open Approach

ØRGLØ7Z Fusion of Right Elbow Joint with Autologous Tissue Substitute, Open Approach

ØRGLØJZ Fusion of Right Elbow Joint with Synthetic Substitute, Open Approach

ØRGLØKZ Fusion of Right Elbow Joint with Nonautologous Tissue Substitute, Open Approach

ØRGL34Z Fusion of Right Elbow Joint with Internal Fixation Device, Percutaneous Approach

ØRGL35Z Fusion of Right Elbow Joint with External Fixation Device, Percutaneous Approach

ØRGL37Z Fusion of Right Elbow Joint with Autologous Tissue Substitute, Percutaneous Approach

ØRGL3JZ Fusion of Right Elbow Joint with Synthetic Substitute, Percutaneous Approach

ØRGL3KZ Fusion of Right Elbow Joint with Nonautologous Tissue Substitute, Percutaneous Approach

ØRGL44Z Fusion of Right Elbow Joint with Internal Fixation Device, Percutaneous Endoscopic Approach

ØRGL45Z Fusion of Right Elbow Joint with External Fixation Device, Percutaneous Endoscopic Approach

ØRGL47Z Fusion of Right Elbow Joint with Autologous Tissue Substitute, Percutaneous Endoscopic Approach

ØRGL4JZ Fusion of Right Elbow Joint with Synthetic Substitute, Percutaneous Endoscopic Approach

ØRGL4KZ Fusion of Right Elbow Joint with Nonautologous Tissue Substitute, Percutaneous Endoscopic Approach

ØRGMØ4Z Fusion of Left Elbow Joint with Internal Fixation Device, Open Approach

ØRGMØ5Z Fusion of Left Elbow Joint with External Fixation Device, Open Approach

ØRGMØ7Z Fusion of Left Elbow Joint with Autologous Tissue Substitute, Open Approach

ØRGMØJZ Fusion of Left Elbow Joint with Synthetic Substitute, Open Approach

ØRGMØKZ Fusion of Left Elbow Joint with Nonautologous Tissue Substitute, Open Approach

ØRGM34Z Fusion of Left Elbow Joint with Internal Fixation Device, Percutaneous Approach

ØRGM35Z Fusion of Left Elbow Joint with External Fixation Device, Percutaneous Approach

ØRGM37Z Fusion of Left Elbow Joint with Autologous Tissue Substitute, Percutaneous Approach

ØRGM3JZ Fusion of Left Elbow Joint with Synthetic Substitute, Percutaneous Approach

ØRGM3KZ Fusion of Left Elbow Joint with Nonautologous Tissue Substitute, Percutaneous Approach

ØRGM44Z Fusion of Left Elbow Joint with Internal Fixation Device, Percutaneous Endoscopic Approach

ØRGM45Z Fusion of Left Elbow Joint with External Fixation Device, Percutaneous Endoscopic Approach

ØRGM47Z Fusion of Left Elbow Joint with Autologous Tissue Substitute, Percutaneous Endoscopic Approach

ØRGM4JZ Fusion of Left Elbow Joint with Synthetic Substitute, Percutaneous Endoscopic Approach

ØRGM4KZ Fusion of Left Elbow Joint with Nonautologous Tissue Substitute, Percutaneous Endoscopic Approach

ØRQEØZZ Repair Right Sternoclavicular Joint, Open Approach

ØRQE3ZZ Repair Right Sternoclavicular Joint, Percutaneous Approach

ØRQE4ZZ Repair Right Sternoclavicular Joint, Percutaneous Endoscopic Approach

ØRQEXZZ Repair Right Sternoclavicular Joint, External Approach

ØRQFØZZ Repair Left Sternoclavicular Joint, Open Approach

ØRQF3ZZ Repair Left Sternoclavicular Joint, Percutaneous Approach

ØRQF4ZZ Repair Left Sternoclavicular Joint, Percutaneous Endoscopic Approach

ØRQFXZZ Repair Left Sternoclavicular Joint, External Approach

ØRQGØZZ Repair Right Acromioclavicular Joint, Open Approach

ØRQG3ZZ Repair Right Acromioclavicular Joint, Percutaneous Approach

ØRQG4ZZ Repair Right Acromioclavicular Joint, Percutaneous Endoscopic Approach

ØRQGXZZ Repair Right Acromioclavicular Joint, External Approach

ØRQHØZZ Repair Left Acromioclavicular Joint, Open Approach

ØRQH3ZZ Repair Left Acromioclavicular Joint, Percutaneous Approach

ØRQH4ZZ Repair Left Acromioclavicular Joint, Percutaneous Endoscopic Approach

ØRQHXZZ Repair Left Acromioclavicular Joint, External Approach

ØRQJØZZ Repair Right Shoulder Joint, Open Approach

ØRQJ3ZZ Repair Right Shoulder Joint, Percutaneous Approach

ØRQJ4ZZ Repair Right Shoulder Joint, Percutaneous Endoscopic Approach

ØRQJXZZ Repair Right Shoulder Joint, External Approach

ØRQKØZZ Repair Left Shoulder Joint, Open Approach

ØRQK3ZZ Repair Left Shoulder Joint, Percutaneous Approach

ØRQK4ZZ Repair Left Shoulder Joint, Percutaneous Endoscopic Approach

ØRQKXZZ Repair Left Shoulder Joint, External Approach

ØRQLØZZ Repair Right Elbow Joint, Open Approach

ØRQL3ZZ Repair Right Elbow Joint, Percutaneous Approach

ØRQL4ZZ Repair Right Elbow Joint, Percutaneous Endoscopic Approach

ØRQLXZZ Repair Right Elbow Joint, External Approach

ØRQMØZZ Repair Left Elbow Joint, Open Approach

ØRQM3ZZ Repair Left Elbow Joint, Percutaneous Approach

ØRQM4ZZ Repair Left Elbow Joint, Percutaneous Endoscopic Approach

ØRQMXZZ Repair Left Elbow Joint, External Approach

ØRUEØ7Z Supplement Right Sternoclavicular Joint with Autologous Tissue Substitute, Open Approach

ØRUEØJZ Supplement Right Sternoclavicular Joint with Synthetic Substitute, Open Approach

ØRUEØKZ Supplement Right Sternoclavicular Joint with Nonautologous Tissue Substitute, Open Approach

ØRUE37Z Supplement Right Sternoclavicular Joint with Autologous Tissue Substitute, Percutaneous Approach

ØRUE3JZ Supplement Right Sternoclavicular Joint with Synthetic Substitute, Percutaneous Approach

ØRUE3KZ Supplement Right Sternoclavicular Joint with Nonautologous Tissue Substitute, Percutaneous Approach

ØRUE47Z Supplement Right Sternoclavicular Joint with Autologous Tissue Substitute, Percutaneous Endoscopic Approach

ØRUE4JZ Supplement Right Sternoclavicular Joint with Synthetic Substitute, Percutaneous Endoscopic Approach

ØRUE4KZ Supplement Right Sternoclavicular Joint with Nonautologous Tissue Substitute, Percutaneous Endoscopic Approach

ØRUFØ7Z Supplement Left Sternoclavicular Joint with Autologous Tissue Substitute, Open Approach

ØRUFØJZ Supplement Left Sternoclavicular Joint with Synthetic Substitute, Open Approach

ØRUFØKZ Supplement Left Sternoclavicular Joint with Nonautologous Tissue Substitute, Open Approach

ØRUF37Z Supplement Left Sternoclavicular Joint with Autologous Tissue Substitute, Percutaneous Approach

ØRUF3JZ Supplement Left Sternoclavicular Joint with Synthetic Substitute, Percutaneous Approach

ØRUF3KZ Supplement Left Sternoclavicular Joint with Nonautologous Tissue Substitute, Percutaneous Approach

ØRUF47Z Supplement Left Sternoclavicular Joint with Autologous Tissue Substitute, Percutaneous Endoscopic Approach

ØRUF4JZ Supplement Left Sternoclavicular Joint with Synthetic Substitute, Percutaneous Endoscopic Approach

HAC 12: Surgical Site Infection Following Certain Orthopedic Procedures of the Spine, Shoulder, and Elbow (continued)

ØRUF4KZ Supplement Left Sternoclavicular Joint with Nonautologous Tissue Substitute, Percutaneous Endoscopic Approach

ØRUG07Z Supplement Right Acromioclavicular Joint with Autologous Tissue Substitute, Open Approach

ØRUG0JZ Supplement Right Acromioclavicular Joint with Synthetic Substitute, Open Approach

ØRUG0KZ Supplement Right Acromioclavicular Joint with Nonautologous Tissue Substitute, Open Approach

ØRUG37Z Supplement Right Acromioclavicular Joint with Autologous Tissue Substitute, Percutaneous Approach

ØRUG3JZ Supplement Right Acromioclavicular Joint with Synthetic Substitute, Percutaneous Approach

ØRUG3KZ Supplement Right Acromioclavicular Joint with Nonautologous Tissue Substitute, Percutaneous Approach

ØRUG47Z Supplement Right Acromioclavicular Joint with Autologous Tissue Substitute, Percutaneous Endoscopic Approach

ØRUG4JZ Supplement Right Acromioclavicular Joint with Synthetic Substitute, Percutaneous Endoscopic Approach

ØRUG4KZ Supplement Right Acromioclavicular Joint with Nonautologous Tissue Substitute, Percutaneous Endoscopic Approach

ØRUH07Z Supplement Left Acromioclavicular Joint with Autologous Tissue Substitute, Open Approach

ØRUH0JZ Supplement Left Acromioclavicular Joint with Synthetic Substitute, Open Approach

ØRUH0KZ Supplement Left Acromioclavicular Joint with Nonautologous Tissue Substitute, Open Approach

ØRUH37Z Supplement Left Acromioclavicular Joint with Autologous Tissue Substitute, Percutaneous Approach

ØRUH3JZ Supplement Left Acromioclavicular Joint with Synthetic Substitute, Percutaneous Approach

ØRUH3KZ Supplement Left Acromioclavicular Joint with Nonautologous Tissue Substitute, Percutaneous Approach

ØRUH47Z Supplement Left Acromioclavicular Joint with Autologous Tissue Substitute, Percutaneous Endoscopic Approach

ØRUH4JZ Supplement Left Acromioclavicular Joint with Synthetic Substitute, Percutaneous Endoscopic Approach

ØRUH4KZ Supplement Left Acromioclavicular Joint with Nonautologous Tissue Substitute, Percutaneous Endoscopic Approach

ØRUJ07Z Supplement Right Shoulder Joint with Autologous Tissue Substitute, Open Approach

ØRUJ0JZ Supplement Right Shoulder Joint with Synthetic Substitute, Open Approach

ØRUJ0KZ Supplement Right Shoulder Joint with Nonautologous Tissue Substitute, Open Approach

ØRUJ37Z Supplement Right Shoulder Joint with Autologous Tissue Substitute, Percutaneous Approach

ØRUJ3JZ Supplement Right Shoulder Joint with Synthetic Substitute, Percutaneous Approach

ØRUJ3KZ Supplement Right Shoulder Joint with Nonautologous Tissue Substitute, Percutaneous Approach

ØRUJ47Z Supplement Right Shoulder Joint with Autologous Tissue Substitute, Percutaneous Endoscopic Approach

ØRUJ4JZ Supplement Right Shoulder Joint with Synthetic Substitute, Percutaneous Endoscopic Approach

ØRUJ4KZ Supplement Right Shoulder Joint with Nonautologous Tissue Substitute, Percutaneous Endoscopic Approach

ØRUK07Z Supplement Left Shoulder Joint with Autologous Tissue Substitute, Open Approach

ØRUK0JZ Supplement Left Shoulder Joint with Synthetic Substitute, Open Approach

ØRUK0KZ Supplement Left Shoulder Joint with Nonautologous Tissue Substitute, Open Approach

ØRUK37Z Supplement Left Shoulder Joint with Autologous Tissue Substitute, Percutaneous Approach

ØRUK3JZ Supplement Left Shoulder Joint with Synthetic Substitute, Percutaneous Approach

ØRUK3KZ Supplement Left Shoulder Joint with Nonautologous Tissue Substitute, Percutaneous Approach

ØRUK47Z Supplement Left Shoulder Joint with Autologous Tissue Substitute, Percutaneous Endoscopic Approach

ØRUK4JZ Supplement Left Shoulder Joint with Synthetic Substitute, Percutaneous Endoscopic Approach

ØRUK4KZ Supplement Left Shoulder Joint with Nonautologous Tissue Substitute, Percutaneous Endoscopic Approach

ØRUL07Z Supplement Right Elbow Joint with Autologous Tissue Substitute, Open Approach

ØRUL0JZ Supplement Right Elbow Joint with Synthetic Substitute, Open Approach

ØRUL0KZ Supplement Right Elbow Joint with Nonautologous Tissue Substitute, Open Approach

ØRUL37Z Supplement Right Elbow Joint with Autologous Tissue Substitute, Percutaneous Approach

ØRUL3JZ Supplement Right Elbow Joint with Synthetic Substitute, Percutaneous Approach

ØRUL3KZ Supplement Right Elbow Joint with Nonautologous Tissue Substitute, Percutaneous Approach

ØRUL47Z Supplement Right Elbow Joint with Autologous Tissue Substitute, Percutaneous Endoscopic Approach

ØRUL4JZ Supplement Right Elbow Joint with Synthetic Substitute, Percutaneous Endoscopic Approach

ØRUL4KZ Supplement Right Elbow Joint with Nonautologous Tissue Substitute, Percutaneous Endoscopic Approach

ØRUM07Z Supplement Left Elbow Joint with Autologous Tissue Substitute, Open Approach

ØRUM0JZ Supplement Left Elbow Joint with Synthetic Substitute, Open Approach

ØRUM0KZ Supplement Left Elbow Joint with Nonautologous Tissue Substitute, Open Approach

ØRUM37Z Supplement Left Elbow Joint with Autologous Tissue Substitute, Percutaneous Approach

ØRUM3JZ Supplement Left Elbow Joint with Synthetic Substitute, Percutaneous Approach

ØRUM3KZ Supplement Left Elbow Joint with Nonautologous Tissue Substitute, Percutaneous Approach

ØRUM47Z Supplement Left Elbow Joint with Autologous Tissue Substitute, Percutaneous Endoscopic Approach

ØRUM4JZ Supplement Left Elbow Joint with Synthetic Substitute, Percutaneous Endoscopic Approach

ØRUM4KZ Supplement Left Elbow Joint with Nonautologous Tissue Substitute, Percutaneous Endoscopic Approach

ØSG0070 Fusion of Lumbar Vertebral Joint with Autologous Tissue Substitute, Anterior Approach, Anterior Column, Open Approach

ØSG0071 Fusion of Lumbar Vertebral Joint with Autologous Tissue Substitute, Posterior Approach, Posterior Column, Open Approach

ØSG007J Fusion of Lumbar Vertebral Joint with Autologous Tissue Substitute, Posterior Approach, Anterior Column, Open Approach

ØSG00A0 Fusion of Lumbar Vertebral Joint with Interbody Fusion Device, Anterior Approach, Anterior Column, Open Approach

ØSG00AJ Fusion of Lumbar Vertebral Joint with Interbody Fusion Device, Posterior Approach, Anterior Column, Open Approach

ØSG00J0 Fusion of Lumbar Vertebral Joint with Synthetic Substitute, Anterior Approach, Anterior Column, Open Approach

ØSG00J1 Fusion of Lumbar Vertebral Joint with Synthetic Substitute, Posterior Approach, Posterior Column, Open Approach

ØSG00JJ Fusion of Lumbar Vertebral Joint with Synthetic Substitute, Posterior Approach, Anterior Column, Open Approach

ØSG00K0 Fusion of Lumbar Vertebral Joint with Nonautologous Tissue Substitute, Anterior Approach, Anterior Column, Open Approach

ØSG00K1 Fusion of Lumbar Vertebral Joint with Nonautologous Tissue Substitute, Posterior Approach, Posterior Column, Open Approach

ØSG00KJ Fusion of Lumbar Vertebral Joint with Nonautologous Tissue Substitute, Posterior Approach, Anterior Column, Open Approach

ØSG0370 Fusion of Lumbar Vertebral Joint with Autologous Tissue Substitute, Anterior Approach, Anterior Column, Percutaneous Approach

ØSG0371 Fusion of Lumbar Vertebral Joint with Autologous Tissue Substitute, Posterior Approach, Posterior Column, Percutaneous Approach

ØSG037J Fusion of Lumbar Vertebral Joint with Autologous Tissue Substitute, Posterior Approach, Anterior Column, Percutaneous Approach

ØSG03A0 Fusion of Lumbar Vertebral Joint with Interbody Fusion Device, Anterior Approach, Anterior Column, Percutaneous Approach

HAC 12: Surgical Site Infection Following Certain Orthopedic Procedures of the Spine, Shoulder, and Elbow (continued)

ØSG03AJ   Fusion of Lumbar Vertebral Joint with Interbody Fusion Device, Posterior Approach, Anterior Column, Percutaneous Approach

ØSG03J0   Fusion of Lumbar Vertebral Joint with Synthetic Substitute, Anterior Approach, Anterior Column, Percutaneous Approach

ØSG03J1   Fusion of Lumbar Vertebral Joint with Synthetic Substitute, Posterior Approach, Posterior Column, Percutaneous Approach

ØSG03JJ   Fusion of Lumbar Vertebral Joint with Synthetic Substitute, Posterior Approach, Anterior Column, Percutaneous Approach

ØSG03K0   Fusion of Lumbar Vertebral Joint with Nonautologous Tissue Substitute, Anterior Approach, Anterior Column, Percutaneous Approach

ØSG03K1   Fusion of Lumbar Vertebral Joint with Nonautologous Tissue Substitute, Posterior Approach, Posterior Column, Percutaneous Approach

ØSG03KJ   Fusion of Lumbar Vertebral Joint with Nonautologous Tissue Substitute, Posterior Approach, Anterior Column, Percutaneous Approach

ØSG0470   Fusion of Lumbar Vertebral Joint with Autologous Tissue Substitute, Anterior Approach, Anterior Column, Percutaneous Endoscopic Approach

ØSG0471   Fusion of Lumbar Vertebral Joint with Autologous Tissue Substitute, Posterior Approach, Posterior Column, Percutaneous Endoscopic Approach

ØSG047J   Fusion of Lumbar Vertebral Joint with Autologous Tissue Substitute, Posterior Approach, Anterior Column, Percutaneous Endoscopic Approach

ØSG04A0   Fusion of Lumbar Vertebral Joint with Interbody Fusion Device, Anterior Approach, Anterior Column, Percutaneous Endoscopic Approach

ØSG04AJ   Fusion of Lumbar Vertebral Joint with Interbody Fusion Device, Posterior Approach, Anterior Column, Percutaneous Endoscopic Approach

ØSG04J0   Fusion of Lumbar Vertebral Joint with Synthetic Substitute, Anterior Approach, Anterior Column, Percutaneous Endoscopic Approach

ØSG04J1   Fusion of Lumbar Vertebral Joint with Synthetic Substitute, Posterior Approach, Posterior Column, Percutaneous Endoscopic Approach

ØSG04JJ   Fusion of Lumbar Vertebral Joint with Synthetic Substitute, Posterior Approach, Anterior Column, Percutaneous Endoscopic Approach

ØSG04K0   Fusion of Lumbar Vertebral Joint with Nonautologous Tissue Substitute, Anterior Approach, Anterior Column, Percutaneous Endoscopic Approach

ØSG04K1   Fusion of Lumbar Vertebral Joint with Nonautologous Tissue Substitute, Posterior Approach, Posterior Column, Percutaneous Endoscopic Approach

ØSG04KJ   Fusion of Lumbar Vertebral Joint with Nonautologous Tissue Substitute, Posterior Approach, Anterior Column, Percutaneous Endoscopic Approach

ØSG1070   Fusion of 2 or More Lumbar Vertebral Joints with Autologous Tissue Substitute, Anterior Approach, Anterior Column, Open Approach

ØSG1071   Fusion of 2 or More Lumbar Vertebral Joints with Autologous Tissue Substitute, Posterior Approach, Posterior Column, Open Approach

ØSG107J   Fusion of 2 or More Lumbar Vertebral Joints with Autologous Tissue Substitute, Posterior Approach, Anterior Column, Open Approach

ØSG10A0   Fusion of 2 or More Lumbar Vertebral Joints with Interbody Fusion Device, Anterior Approach, Anterior Column, Open Approach

ØSG10AJ   Fusion of 2 or More Lumbar Vertebral Joints with Interbody Fusion Device, Posterior Approach, Anterior Column, Open Approach

ØSG10J0   Fusion of 2 or More Lumbar Vertebral Joints with Synthetic Substitute, Anterior Approach, Anterior Column, Open Approach

ØSG10J1   Fusion of 2 or More Lumbar Vertebral Joints with Synthetic Substitute, Posterior Approach, Posterior Column, Open Approach

ØSG10JJ   Fusion of 2 or More Lumbar Vertebral Joints with Synthetic Substitute, Posterior Approach, Anterior Column, Open Approach

ØSG10K0   Fusion of 2 or More Lumbar Vertebral Joints with Nonautologous Tissue Substitute, Anterior Approach, Anterior Column, Open Approach

ØSG10K1   Fusion of 2 or More Lumbar Vertebral Joints with Nonautologous Tissue Substitute, Posterior Approach, Posterior Column, Open Approach

ØSG10KJ   Fusion of 2 or More Lumbar Vertebral Joints with Nonautologous Tissue Substitute, Posterior Approach, Anterior Column, Open Approach

ØSG1370   Fusion of 2 or More Lumbar Vertebral Joints with Autologous Tissue Substitute, Anterior Approach, Anterior Column, Percutaneous Approach

ØSG1371   Fusion of 2 or More Lumbar Vertebral Joints with Autologous Tissue Substitute, Posterior Approach, Posterior Column, Percutaneous Approach

ØSG137J   Fusion of 2 or More Lumbar Vertebral Joints with Autologous Tissue Substitute, Posterior Approach, Anterior Column, Percutaneous Approach

ØSG13A0   Fusion of 2 or More Lumbar Vertebral Joints with Interbody Fusion Device, Anterior Approach, Anterior Column, Percutaneous Approach

ØSG13AJ   Fusion of 2 or More Lumbar Vertebral Joints with Interbody Fusion Device, Posterior Approach, Anterior Column, Percutaneous Approach

ØSG13J0   Fusion of 2 or More Lumbar Vertebral Joints with Synthetic Substitute, Anterior Approach, Anterior Column, Percutaneous Approach

ØSG13J1   Fusion of 2 or More Lumbar Vertebral Joints with Synthetic Substitute, Posterior Approach, Posterior Column, Percutaneous Approach

ØSG13JJ   Fusion of 2 or More Lumbar Vertebral Joints with Synthetic Substitute, Posterior Approach, Anterior Column, Percutaneous Approach

ØSG13K0   Fusion of 2 or More Lumbar Vertebral Joints with Nonautologous Tissue Substitute, Anterior Approach, Anterior Column, Percutaneous Approach

ØSG13K1   Fusion of 2 or More Lumbar Vertebral Joints with Nonautologous Tissue Substitute, Posterior Approach, Posterior Column, Percutaneous Approach

ØSG13KJ   Fusion of 2 or More Lumbar Vertebral Joints with Nonautologous Tissue Substitute, Posterior Approach, Anterior Column, Percutaneous Approach

ØSG1470   Fusion of 2 or More Lumbar Vertebral Joints with Autologous Tissue Substitute, Anterior Approach, Anterior Column, Percutaneous Endoscopic Approach

ØSG1471   Fusion of 2 or More Lumbar Vertebral Joints with Autologous Tissue Substitute, Posterior Approach, Posterior Column, Percutaneous Endoscopic Approach

ØSG147J   Fusion of 2 or More Lumbar Vertebral Joints with Autologous Tissue Substitute, Posterior Approach, Anterior Column, Percutaneous Endoscopic Approach

ØSG14A0   Fusion of 2 or More Lumbar Vertebral Joints with Interbody Fusion Device, Anterior Approach, Anterior Column, Percutaneous Endoscopic Approach

ØSG14AJ   Fusion of 2 or More Lumbar Vertebral Joints with Interbody Fusion Device, Posterior Approach, Anterior Column, Percutaneous Endoscopic Approach

ØSG14J0   Fusion of 2 or More Lumbar Vertebral Joints with Synthetic Substitute, Anterior Approach, Anterior Column, Percutaneous Endoscopic Approach

ØSG14J1   Fusion of 2 or More Lumbar Vertebral Joints with Synthetic Substitute, Posterior Approach, Posterior Column, Percutaneous Endoscopic Approach

ØSG14JJ   Fusion of 2 or More Lumbar Vertebral Joints with Synthetic Substitute, Posterior Approach, Anterior Column, Percutaneous Endoscopic Approach

ØSG14K0   Fusion of 2 or More Lumbar Vertebral Joints with Nonautologous Tissue Substitute, Anterior Approach, Anterior Column, Percutaneous Endoscopic Approach

ØSG14K1   Fusion of 2 or More Lumbar Vertebral Joints with Nonautologous Tissue Substitute, Posterior Approach, Posterior Column, Percutaneous Endoscopic Approach

ØSG14KJ   Fusion of 2 or More Lumbar Vertebral Joints with Nonautologous Tissue Substitute, Posterior Approach, Anterior Column, Percutaneous Endoscopic Approach

ØSG3070   Fusion of Lumbosacral Joint with Autologous Tissue Substitute, Anterior Approach, Anterior Column, Open Approach

ØSG3071   Fusion of Lumbosacral Joint with Autologous Tissue Substitute, Posterior Approach, Posterior Column, Open Approach

Appendix J: Hospital Acquired Conditions

HAC 12: Surgical Site Infection Following Certain Orthopedic Procedures of the Spine, Shoulder, and Elbow (continued)

ØSG307J Fusion of Lumbosacral Joint with Autologous Tissue Substitute, Posterior Approach, Anterior Column, Open Approach

ØSG30A0 Fusion of Lumbosacral Joint with Interbody Fusion Device, Anterior Approach, Anterior Column, Open Approach

ØSG30AJ Fusion of Lumbosacral Joint with Interbody Fusion Device, Posterior Approach, Anterior Column, Open Approach

ØSG30J0 Fusion of Lumbosacral Joint with Synthetic Substitute, Anterior Approach, Anterior Column, Open Approach

ØSG30J1 Fusion of Lumbosacral Joint with Synthetic Substitute, Posterior Approach, Posterior Column, Open Approach

ØSG30JJ Fusion of Lumbosacral Joint with Synthetic Substitute, Posterior Approach, Anterior Column, Open Approach

ØSG30K0 Fusion of Lumbosacral Joint with Nonautologous Tissue Substitute, Anterior Approach, Anterior Column, Open Approach

ØSG30K1 Fusion of Lumbosacral Joint with Nonautologous Tissue Substitute, Posterior Approach, Posterior Column, Open Approach

ØSG30KJ Fusion of Lumbosacral Joint with Nonautologous Tissue Substitute, Posterior Approach, Anterior Column, Open Approach

ØSG3370 Fusion of Lumbosacral Joint with Autologous Tissue Substitute, Anterior Approach, Anterior Column, Percutaneous Approach

ØSG3371 Fusion of Lumbosacral Joint with Autologous Tissue Substitute, Posterior Approach, Posterior Column, Percutaneous Approach

ØSG337J Fusion of Lumbosacral Joint with Autologous Tissue Substitute, Posterior Approach, Anterior Column, Percutaneous Approach

ØSG33A0 Fusion of Lumbosacral Joint with Interbody Fusion Device, Anterior Approach, Anterior Column, Percutaneous Approach

ØSG33AJ Fusion of Lumbosacral Joint with Interbody Fusion Device, Posterior Approach, Anterior Column, Percutaneous Approach

ØSG33J0 Fusion of Lumbosacral Joint with Synthetic Substitute, Anterior Approach, Anterior Column, Percutaneous Approach

ØSG33J1 Fusion of Lumbosacral Joint with Synthetic Substitute, Posterior Approach, Posterior Column, Percutaneous Approach

ØSG33JJ Fusion of Lumbosacral Joint with Synthetic Substitute, Posterior Approach, Anterior Column, Percutaneous Approach

ØSG33K0 Fusion of Lumbosacral Joint with Nonautologous Tissue Substitute, Anterior Approach, Anterior Column, Percutaneous Approach

ØSG33K1 Fusion of Lumbosacral Joint with Nonautologous Tissue Substitute, Posterior Approach, Posterior Column, Percutaneous Approach

ØSG33KJ Fusion of Lumbosacral Joint with Nonautologous Tissue Substitute, Posterior Approach, Anterior Column, Percutaneous Approach

ØSG3470 Fusion of Lumbosacral Joint with Autologous Tissue Substitute, Anterior Approach, Anterior Column, Percutaneous Endoscopic Approach

ØSG3471 Fusion of Lumbosacral Joint with Autologous Tissue Substitute, Posterior Approach, Posterior Column, Percutaneous Endoscopic Approach

ØSG347J Fusion of Lumbosacral Joint with Autologous Tissue Substitute, Posterior Approach, Anterior Column, Percutaneous Endoscopic Approach

ØSG34A0 Fusion of Lumbosacral Joint with Interbody Fusion Device, Anterior Approach, Anterior Column, Percutaneous Endoscopic Approach

ØSG34AJ Fusion of Lumbosacral Joint with Interbody Fusion Device, Posterior Approach, Anterior Column, Percutaneous Endoscopic Approach

ØSG34J0 Fusion of Lumbosacral Joint with Synthetic Substitute, Anterior Approach, Anterior Column, Percutaneous Endoscopic Approach

ØSG34J1 Fusion of Lumbosacral Joint with Synthetic Substitute, Posterior Approach, Posterior Column, Percutaneous Endoscopic Approach

ØSG34JJ Fusion of Lumbosacral Joint with Synthetic Substitute, Posterior Approach, Anterior Column, Percutaneous Endoscopic Approach

ØSG34K0 Fusion of Lumbosacral Joint with Nonautologous Tissue Substitute, Anterior Approach, Anterior Column, Percutaneous Endoscopic Approach

ØSG34K1 Fusion of Lumbosacral Joint with Nonautologous Tissue Substitute, Posterior Approach, Posterior Column, Percutaneous Endoscopic Approach

ØSG34KJ Fusion of Lumbosacral Joint with Nonautologous Tissue Substitute, Posterior Approach, Anterior Column, Percutaneous Endoscopic Approach

ØSG704Z Fusion of Right Sacroiliac Joint with Internal Fixation Device, Open Approach

ØSG707Z Fusion of Right Sacroiliac Joint with Autologous Tissue Substitute, Open Approach

ØSG70JZ Fusion of Right Sacroiliac Joint with Synthetic Substitute, Open Approach

ØSG70KZ Fusion of Right Sacroiliac Joint with Nonautologous Tissue Substitute, Open Approach

ØSG734Z Fusion of Right Sacroiliac Joint with Internal Fixation Device, Percutaneous Approach

ØSG737Z Fusion of Right Sacroiliac Joint with Autologous Tissue Substitute, Percutaneous Approach

ØSG73JZ Fusion of Right Sacroiliac Joint with Synthetic Substitute, Percutaneous Approach

ØSG73KZ Fusion of Right Sacroiliac Joint with Nonautologous Tissue Substitute, Percutaneous Approach

ØSG744Z Fusion of Right Sacroiliac Joint with Internal Fixation Device, Percutaneous Endoscopic Approach

ØSG747Z Fusion of Right Sacroiliac Joint with Autologous Tissue Substitute, Percutaneous Endoscopic Approach

ØSG74JZ Fusion of Right Sacroiliac Joint with Synthetic Substitute, Percutaneous Endoscopic Approach

ØSG74KZ Fusion of Right Sacroiliac Joint with Nonautologous Tissue Substitute, Percutaneous Endoscopic Approach

ØSG804Z Fusion of Left Sacroiliac Joint with Internal Fixation Device, Open Approach

ØSG807Z Fusion of Left Sacroiliac Joint with Autologous Tissue Substitute, Open Approach

ØSG80JZ Fusion of Left Sacroiliac Joint with Synthetic Substitute, Open Approach

ØSG80KZ Fusion of Left Sacroiliac Joint with Nonautologous Tissue Substitute, Open Approach

ØSG834Z Fusion of Left Sacroiliac Joint with Internal Fixation Device, Percutaneous Approach

ØSG837Z Fusion of Left Sacroiliac Joint with Autologous Tissue Substitute, Percutaneous Approach

ØSG83JZ Fusion of Left Sacroiliac Joint with Synthetic Substitute, Percutaneous Approach

ØSG83KZ Fusion of Left Sacroiliac Joint with Nonautologous Tissue Substitute, Percutaneous Approach

ØSG844Z Fusion of Left Sacroiliac Joint with Internal Fixation Device, Percutaneous Endoscopic Approach

ØSG847Z Fusion of Left Sacroiliac Joint with Autologous Tissue Substitute, Percutaneous Endoscopic Approach

ØSG84JZ Fusion of Left Sacroiliac Joint with Synthetic Substitute, Percutaneous Endoscopic Approach

ØSG84KZ Fusion of Left Sacroiliac Joint with Nonautologous Tissue Substitute, Percutaneous Endoscopic Approach

XRG00F3 Fusion of Occipital-cervical Joint using Radiolucent Porous Interbody Fusion Device, Open Approach, New Technology Group 3

XRG1092 Fusion of Cervical Vertebral Joint using Nanotextured Surface Interbody Fusion Device, Open Approach, New Technology Group 2

XRG10F3 Fusion of Cervical Vertebral Joint using Radiolucent Porous Interbody Fusion Device, Open Approach, New Technology Group 3

XRG2092 Fusion of 2 or more Cervical Vertebral Joints using Nanotextured Surface Interbody Fusion Device, Open Approach, New Technology Group 2

XRG20F3 Fusion of 2 or more Cervical Vertebral Joints using Radiolucent Porous Interbody Fusion Device, Open Approach, New Technology Group 3

XRG4092 Fusion of Cervicothoracic Vertebral Joint using Nanotextured Surface Interbody Fusion Device, Open Approach, New Technology Group 2

XRG40F3 Fusion of Cervicothoracic Vertebral Joint using Radiolucent Porous Interbody Fusion Device, Open Approach, New Technology Group 3

HAC 12: Surgical Site Infection Following Certain Orthopedic Procedures of the Spine, Shoulder, and Elbow (continued)

XRG6092 Fusion of Thoracic Vertebral Joint using Nanotextured Surface Interbody Fusion Device, Open Approach, New Technology Group 2

XRG60F3 Fusion of Thoracic Vertebral Joint using Radiolucent Porous Interbody Fusion Device, Open Approach, New Technology Group 3

XRG7092 Fusion of 2 to 7 Thoracic Vertebral Joints using Nanotextured Surface Interbody Fusion Device, Open Approach, New Technology Group 2

XRG70F3 Fusion of 2 to 7 Thoracic Vertebral Joints using Radiolucent Porous Interbody Fusion Device, Open Approach, New Technology Group 3

XRG8092 Fusion of 8 or more Thoracic Vertebral Joints using Nanotextured Surface Interbody Fusion Device, Open Approach, New Technology Group 2

XRG80F3 Fusion of 8 or more Thoracic Vertebral Joints using Radiolucent Porous Interbody Fusion Device, Open Approach, New Technology Group 3

XRGA092 Fusion of Thoracolumbar Vertebral Joint using Nanotextured Surface Interbody Fusion Device, Open Approach, New Technology Group 2

XRGA0F3 Fusion of Thoracolumbar Vertebral Joint using Radiolucent Porous Interbody Fusion Device, Open Approach, New Technology Group 3

XRGB092 Fusion of Lumbar Vertebral Joint using Nanotextured Surface Interbody Fusion Device, Open Approach, New Technology Group 2

XRGB0F3 Fusion of Lumbar Vertebral Joint using Radiolucent Porous Interbody Fusion Device, Open Approach, New Technology Group 3

XRGC092 Fusion of 2 or more Lumbar Vertebral Joints using Nanotextured Surface Interbody Fusion Device, Open Approach, New Technology Group 2

XRGC0F3 Fusion of 2 or more Lumbar Vertebral Joints using Radiolucent Porous Interbody Fusion Device, Open Approach, New Technology Group 3

XRGD092 Fusion of Lumbosacral Joint using Nanotextured Surface Interbody Fusion Device, Open Approach, New Technology Group 2

XRGD0F3 Fusion of Lumbosacral Joint using Radiolucent Porous Interbody Fusion Device, Open Approach, New Technology Group 3

HAC 13: Surgical Site Infection (SSI) Following Cardiac Implantable Electronic Device (CIED) Procedures

Secondary diagnosis not POA:

K68.11
T81.4XXA
T82.6XXA
T82.7XXA

AND

Any of the following procedures:

02H43JZ Insertion of Pacemaker Lead into Coronary Vein, Percutaneous Approach

02H43KZ Insertion of Defibrillator Lead into Coronary Vein, Percutaneous Approach

02H43MZ Insertion of Cardiac Lead into Coronary Vein, Percutaneous Approach

02H63JZ Insertion of Pacemaker Lead into Right Atrium, Percutaneous Approach

02H63MZ Insertion of Cardiac Lead into Right Atrium, Percutaneous Approach

02H73JZ Insertion of Pacemaker Lead into Left Atrium, Percutaneous Approach

02H73MZ Insertion of Cardiac Lead into Left Atrium, Percutaneous Approach

02HK3JZ Insertion of Pacemaker Lead into Right Ventricle, Percutaneous Approach

02HL3JZ Insertion of Pacemaker Lead into Left Ventricle, Percutaneous Approach

02HN0JZ Insertion of Pacemaker Lead into Pericardium, Open Approach

02HN0MZ Insertion of Cardiac Lead into Pericardium, Open Approach

02HN3JZ Insertion of Pacemaker Lead into Pericardium, Percutaneous Approach

02HN3MZ Insertion of Cardiac Lead into Pericardium, Percutaneous Approach

02HN4JZ Insertion of Pacemaker Lead into Pericardium, Percutaneous Endoscopic Approach

02HN4MZ Insertion of Cardiac Lead into Pericardium, Percutaneous Endoscopic Approach

02PA0MZ Removal of Cardiac Lead from Heart, Open Approach

02PA3MZ Removal of Cardiac Lead from Heart, Percutaneous Approach

02PA4MZ Removal of Cardiac Lead from Heart, Percutaneous Endoscopic Approach

02PAXMZ Removal of Cardiac Lead from Heart, External Approach

02WA0MZ Revision of Cardiac Lead in Heart, Open Approach

02WA3MZ Revision of Cardiac Lead in Heart, Percutaneous Approach

02WA4MZ Revision of Cardiac Lead in Heart, Percutaneous Endoscopic Approach

0JH604Z Insertion of Pacemaker, Single Chamber into Chest Subcutaneous Tissue and Fascia, Open Approach

0JH605Z Insertion of Pacemaker, Single Chamber Rate Responsive into Chest Subcutaneous Tissue and Fascia, Open Approach

0JH606Z Insertion of Pacemaker, Dual Chamber into Chest Subcutaneous Tissue and Fascia, Open Approach

0JH607Z Insertion of Cardiac Resynchronization Pacemaker Pulse Generator into Chest Subcutaneous Tissue and Fascia, Open Approach

0JH608Z Insertion of Defibrillator Generator into Chest Subcutaneous Tissue and Fascia, Open Approach

0JH609Z Insertion of Cardiac Resynchronization Defibrillator Pulse Generator into Chest Subcutaneous Tissue and Fascia, Open Approach

0JH60PZ Insertion of Cardiac Rhythm Related Device into Chest Subcutaneous Tissue and Fascia, Open Approach

0JH634Z Insertion of Pacemaker, Single Chamber into Chest Subcutaneous Tissue and Fascia, Percutaneous Approach

0JH635Z Insertion of Pacemaker, Single Chamber Rate Responsive into Chest Subcutaneous Tissue and Fascia, Percutaneous Approach

0JH636Z Insertion of Pacemaker, Dual Chamber into Chest Subcutaneous Tissue and Fascia, Percutaneous Approach

0JH637Z Insertion of Cardiac Resynchronization Pacemaker Pulse Generator into Chest Subcutaneous Tissue and Fascia, Percutaneous Approach

0JH638Z Insertion of Defibrillator Generator into Chest Subcutaneous Tissue and Fascia, Percutaneous Approach

0JH639Z Insertion of Cardiac Resynchronization Defibrillator Pulse Generator into Chest Subcutaneous Tissue and Fascia, Percutaneous Approach

0JH63PZ Insertion of Cardiac Rhythm Related Device into Chest Subcutaneous Tissue and Fascia, Percutaneous Approach

0JH804Z Insertion of Pacemaker, Single Chamber into Abdomen Subcutaneous Tissue and Fascia, Open Approach

0JH805Z Insertion of Pacemaker, Single Chamber Rate Responsive into Abdomen Subcutaneous Tissue and Fascia, Open Approach

0JH806Z Insertion of Pacemaker, Dual Chamber into Abdomen Subcutaneous Tissue and Fascia, Open Approach

0JH807Z Insertion of Cardiac Resynchronization Pacemaker Pulse Generator into Abdomen Subcutaneous Tissue and Fascia, Open Approach

0JH808Z Insertion of Defibrillator Generator into Abdomen Subcutaneous Tissue and Fascia, Open Approach

0JH809Z Insertion of Cardiac Resynchronization Defibrillator Pulse Generator into Abdomen Subcutaneous Tissue and Fascia, Open Approach

0JH80PZ Insertion of Cardiac Rhythm Related Device into Abdomen Subcutaneous Tissue and Fascia, Open Approach

0JH834Z Insertion of Pacemaker, Single Chamber into Abdomen Subcutaneous Tissue and Fascia, Percutaneous Approach

0JH835Z Insertion of Pacemaker, Single Chamber Rate Responsive into Abdomen Subcutaneous Tissue and Fascia, Percutaneous Approach

0JH836Z Insertion of Pacemaker, Dual Chamber into Abdomen Subcutaneous Tissue and Fascia, Percutaneous Approach

0JH837Z Insertion of Cardiac Resynchronization Pacemaker Pulse Generator into Abdomen Subcutaneous Tissue and Fascia, Percutaneous Approach

0JH838Z Insertion of Defibrillator Generator into Abdomen Subcutaneous Tissue and Fascia, Percutaneous Approach

0JH839Z Insertion of Cardiac Resynchronization Defibrillator Pulse Generator into Abdomen Subcutaneous Tissue and Fascia, Percutaneous Approach

0JH83PZ Insertion of Cardiac Rhythm Related Device into Abdomen Subcutaneous Tissue and Fascia, Percutaneous Approach

0JPT0PZ Removal of Cardiac Rhythm Related Device from Trunk Subcutaneous Tissue and Fascia, Open Approach

0JPT3PZ Removal of Cardiac Rhythm Related Device from Trunk Subcutaneous Tissue and Fascia, Percutaneous Approach

0JWT0PZ Revision of Cardiac Rhythm Related Device in Trunk Subcutaneous Tissue and Fascia, Open Approach

0JWT3PZ Revision of Cardiac Rhythm Related Device in Trunk Subcutaneous Tissue and Fascia, Percutaneous Approach

HAC 14: Iatrogenic Pneumothorax with Venous Catheterization

Secondary diagnosis not POA:

J95.811

AND

Any of the following procedures:

02H633Z Insertion of Infusion Device into Right Atrium, Percutaneous Approach

02HK33Z Insertion of Infusion Device into Right Ventricle, Percutaneous Approach

02HS33Z Insertion of Infusion Device into Right Pulmonary Vein, Percutaneous Approach

02HS43Z Insertion of Infusion Device into Right Pulmonary Vein, Percutaneous Endoscopic Approach

02HT33Z Insertion of Infusion Device into Left Pulmonary Vein, Percutaneous Approach

02HT43Z Insertion of Infusion Device into Left Pulmonary Vein, Percutaneous Endoscopic Approach

02HV33Z Insertion of Infusion Device into Superior Vena Cava, Percutaneous Approach

02HV43Z Insertion of Infusion Device into Superior Vena Cava, Percutaneous Endoscopic Approach

05H033Z Insertion of Infusion Device into Azygos Vein, Percutaneous Approach

05H043Z Insertion of Infusion Device into Azygos Vein, Percutaneous Endoscopic Approach

05H133Z Insertion of Infusion Device into Hemiazygos Vein, Percutaneous Approach

05H143Z Insertion of Infusion Device into Hemiazygos Vein, Percutaneous Endoscopic Approach

05H333Z Insertion of Infusion Device into Right Innominate Vein, Percutaneous Approach

05H343Z Insertion of Infusion Device into Right Innominate Vein, Percutaneous Endoscopic Approach

05H433Z Insertion of Infusion Device into Left Innominate Vein, Percutaneous Approach

05H443Z Insertion of Infusion Device into Left Innominate Vein, Percutaneous Endoscopic Approach

05H533Z Insertion of Infusion Device into Right Subclavian Vein, Percutaneous Approach

05H543Z Insertion of Infusion Device into Right Subclavian Vein, Percutaneous Endoscopic Approach

05H633Z Insertion of Infusion Device into Left Subclavian Vein, Percutaneous Approach

05H643Z Insertion of Infusion Device into Left Subclavian Vein, Percutaneous Endoscopic Approach

05HM33Z Insertion of Infusion Device into Right Internal Jugular Vein, Percutaneous Approach

05HN33Z Insertion of Infusion Device into Left Internal Jugular Vein, Percutaneous Approach

05HP33Z Insertion of Infusion Device into Right External Jugular Vein, Percutaneous Approach

05HQ33Z Insertion of Infusion Device into Left External Jugular Vein, Percutaneous Approach

0JH63XZ Insertion of Vascular Access Device into Chest Subcutaneous Tissue and Fascia, Percutaneous Approach

Using the ICD-10-PCS tables construct the code that accurately represents the procedure performed.

Medical Surgical Section

	Procedure	Code
1.	Excision of malignant melanoma from skin of right ear	
2.	Laparoscopy with excision of endometrial implant from left ovary	
3.	Percutaneous needle core biopsy of right kidney	
4.	EGD with gastric biopsy	
5.	Open endarterectomy of left common carotid artery	
6.	Excision of basal cell carcinoma of lower lip	
7.	Open excision of tail of pancreas	
8.	Percutaneous biopsy of right gastrocnemius muscle	
9.	Sigmoidoscopy with sigmoid polypectomy	
10.	Open excision of lesion from right Achilles tendon	
11.	Open resection of cecum	
12.	Total excision of pituitary gland, open	
13.	Explantation of left failed kidney, open	
14.	Open left axillary total lymphadenectomy	
15.	Laparoscopic-assisted vaginal hysterectomy	
16.	Right total mastectomy, open	
17.	Open resection of papillary muscle	
18.	Total retropubic prostatectomy, open	
19.	Laparoscopic cholecystectomy	
20.	Endoscopic bilateral total maxillary sinusectomy	
21.	Amputation at right elbow level	
22.	Right below-knee amputation, proximal tibia/fibula	
23.	Fifth ray carpometacarpal joint amputation, left hand	
24.	Right leg and hip amputation through ischium	
25.	DIP joint amputation of right thumb	
26.	Right wrist joint amputation	
27.	Trans-metatarsal amputation of foot at left big toe	
28.	Mid-shaft amputation, right humerus	
29.	Left fourth toe amputation, mid-proximal phalanx	
30.	Right above-knee amputation, distal femur	
31.	Cryotherapy of wart on left hand	
32.	Percutaneous radiofrequency ablation of right vocal cord lesion	
33.	Left heart catheterization with laser destruction of arrhythmogenic focus, A-V node	
34.	Cautery of nosebleed	
35.	Transurethral endoscopic laser ablation of prostate	
36.	Percutaneous cautery of oozing varicose vein, left calf	

	Procedure	Code
37.	Laparoscopy with destruction of endometriosis, bilateral ovaries	
38.	Laser coagulation of right retinal vessel hemorrhage, percutaneous	
39.	Thoracoscopic pleurodesis, left side	
40.	Percutaneous insertion of Greenfield IVC filter	
41.	Forceps total mouth extraction, upper and lower teeth	
42.	Removal of left thumbnail	
43.	Extraction of right intraocular lens without replacement, percutaneous	
44.	Laparoscopy with needle aspiration of ova for in vitro fertilization	
45.	Nonexcisional debridement of skin ulcer, right foot	
46.	Open stripping of abdominal fascia, right side	
47.	Hysteroscopy with D&C, diagnostic	
48.	Liposuction for medical purposes, left upper arm	
49.	Removal of tattered right ear drum fragments with tweezers	
50.	Microincisional phlebectomy of spider veins, right lower leg	
51.	Routine Foley catheter placement	
52.	Incision and drainage of external anal abscess	
53.	Percutaneous drainage of ascites	
54.	Laparoscopy with left ovarian cystotomy and drainage	
55.	Laparotomy and drain placement for liver abscess, right lobe	
56.	Right knee arthrotomy with drain placement	
57.	Thoracentesis of left pleural effusion	
58.	Phlebotomy of left median cubital vein for polycythemia vera	
59.	Percutaneous chest tube placement for right pneumothorax	
60.	Endoscopic drainage of left ethmoid sinus	
61.	External ventricular CSF drainage catheter placement via burr hole	
62.	Removal of foreign body, right cornea	
63.	Percutaneous mechanical thrombectomy, left brachial artery	
64.	Esophagogastroscopy with removal of bezoar from stomach	
65.	Foreign body removal, skin of left thumb	
66.	Transurethral cystoscopy with removal of bladder stone	
67.	Forceps removal of foreign body in right nostril	
68.	Laparoscopy with excision of old suture from mesentery	
69.	Incision and removal of right lacrimal duct stone	
70.	Nonincisional removal of intraluminal foreign body from vagina	
71.	Right common carotid endarterectomy, open	
72.	Open excision of retained sliver, subcutaneous tissue of left foot	
73.	Extracorporeal shockwave lithotripsy (ESWL), bilateral ureters	

Procedure	Code
74. Endoscopic retrograde cholangiopancreatography (ERCP) with lithotripsy of common bile duct stone	
75. Thoracotomy with crushing of pericardial calcifications	
76. Transurethral cystoscopy with fragmentation of bladder calculus	
77. Hysteroscopy with intraluminal lithotripsy of left fallopian tube calcification	
78. Division of right foot tendon, percutaneous	
79. Left heart catheterization with division of bundle of HIS	
80. Open osteotomy of capitate, left hand	
81. EGD with esophagotomy of esophagogastric junction	
82. Sacral rhizotomy for pain control, percutaneous	
83. Laparotomy with exploration and adhesiolysis of right ureter	
84. Incision of scar contracture, right elbow	
85. Frenulotomy for treatment of tongue-tie syndrome	
86. Right shoulder arthroscopy with coracoacromial ligament release	
87. Mitral valvulotomy for release of fused leaflets, open approach	
88. Percutaneous left Achilles tendon release	
89. Laparoscopy with lysis of peritoneal adhesions	
90. Manual rupture of right shoulder joint adhesions under general anesthesia	
91. Open posterior tarsal tunnel release	
92. Laparoscopy with freeing of left ovary and fallopian tube	
93. Liver transplant with donor matched liver	
94. Orthotopic heart transplant using porcine heart	
95. Right lung transplant, open, using organ donor match	
96. Transplant of large intestine, organ donor match	
97. Left kidney/pancreas organ bank transplant	
98. Replantation of avulsed scalp	
99. Reattachment of severed right ear	
100. Reattachment of traumatic left gastrocnemius avulsion, open	
101. Closed replantation of three avulsed teeth, lower jaw	
102. Reattachment of severed left hand	
103. Right open palmaris longus tendon transfer	
104. Endoscopic radial to median nerve transfer	
105. Fasciocutaneous flap closure of left thigh, open	
106. Transfer left index finger to left thumb position, open	
107. Percutaneous fascia transfer to fill defect, right neck	
108. Trigeminal to facial nerve transfer, percutaneous endoscopic	
109. Endoscopic left leg flexor hallucis longus tendon transfer	
110. Right scalp advancement flap to right temple	

Procedure	Code
111. Bilateral TRAM pedicle flap reconstruction status post mastectomy, muscle only, open	
112. Skin transfer flap closure of complex open wound, left lower back	
113. Open fracture reduction, right tibia	
114. Laparoscopy with gastropexy for malrotation	
115. Left knee arthroscopy with reposition of anterior cruciate ligament	
116. Open transposition of ulnar nerve	
117. Closed reduction with percutaneous internal fixation of right femoral neck fracture	
118. Trans-vaginal intraluminal cervical cerclage	
119. Cervical cerclage using Shirodkar technique	
120. Thoracotomy with banding of left pulmonary artery using extraluminal device	
121. Restriction of thoracic duct with intraluminal stent, percutaneous	
122. Craniotomy with clipping of cerebral aneurysm	
123. Nonincisional, transnasal placement of restrictive stent in right lacrimal duct	
124. Catheter-based temporary restriction of blood flow in abdominal aorta for treatment of cerebral ischemia	
125. Percutaneous ligation of esophageal vein	
126. Percutaneous embolization of left internal carotid-cavernous fistula	
127. Laparoscopy with bilateral occlusion of fallopian tubes using Hulka extraluminal clips	
128. Open suture ligation of failed AV graft, left brachial artery	
129. Percutaneous embolization of vascular supply, intracranial meningioma	
130. Percutaneous embolization of right uterine artery, using coils	
131. Open occlusion of left atrial appendage, using extraluminal pressure clips	
132. Percutaneous suture exclusion of left atrial appendage, via femoral artery access	
133. ERCP with balloon dilation of common bile duct	
134. PTCA of two coronary arteries, LAD with stent placement, RCA with no stent	
135. Cystoscopy with intraluminal dilation of bladder neck stricture	
136. Open dilation of old anastomosis, left femoral artery	
137. Dilation of upper esophageal stricture, direct visualization, with Bougie sound	
138. PTA of right brachial artery stenosis	
139. Transnasal dilation and stent placement in right lacrimal duct	
140. Hysteroscopy with balloon dilation of bilateral fallopian tubes	
141. Tracheoscopy with intraluminal dilation of tracheal stenosis	
142. Cystoscopy with dilation of left ureteral stricture, with stent placement	
143. Open gastric bypass with Roux-en-Y limb to jejunum	
144. Right temporal artery to intracranial artery bypass using Gore-Tex graft, open	

Procedure	Code
145. Tracheostomy formation with tracheostomy tube placement, percutaneous	
146. PICVA (percutaneous in situ coronary venous arterialization) of single coronary artery	
147. Open left femoral-popliteal artery bypass using cadaver vein graft	
148. Shunting of intrathecal cerebrospinal fluid to peritoneal cavity using synthetic shunt	
149. Colostomy formation, open, transverse colon to abdominal wall	
150. Open urinary diversion, left ureter, using ileal conduit to skin	
151. CABG of LAD using left internal mammary artery, open off-bypass	
152. Open pleuroperitoneal shunt, right pleural cavity, using synthetic device	
153. Percutaneous placement of ventriculoperitoneal shunt for treatment of hydrocephalus	
154. End-of-life replacement of spinal neurostimulator generator, multiple array, in lower abdomen	
155. Percutaneous insertion of spinal neurostimulator lead, lumbar spinal cord	
156. Percutaneous replacement of broken pacemaker lead in left atrium	
157. Open placement of dual chamber pacemaker generator in chest wall	
158. Percutaneous placement of venous central line in right internal jugular, with tip in superior vena cava	
159. Open insertion of multiple channel cochlear implant, left ear	
160. Percutaneous placement of Swan-Ganz catheter in pulmonary trunk	
161. Bronchoscopy with insertion of Low Dose, Pd-103 brachytherapy seeds, right main bronchus	
162. Open insertion of interspinous process device into lumbar vertebral joint	
163. Open placement of bone growth stimulator, left femoral shaft	
164. Cystoscopy with placement of brachytherapy seeds in prostate gland	
165. Percutaneous insertion of Greenfield IVC filter	
166. Full-thickness skin graft to right lower arm, autograft (do not code graft harvest for this exercise)	
167. Excision of necrosed left femoral head with bone bank bone graft to fill the defect, open	
168. Penetrating keratoplasty of right cornea with donor matched cornea, percutaneous approach	
169. Bilateral mastectomy with concomitant saline breast implants, open	
170. Excision of abdominal aorta with Gore-Tex graft replacement, open	
171. Total right knee arthroplasty with insertion of total knee prosthesis	
172. Bilateral mastectomy with free TRAM flap reconstruction	
173. Tenonectomy with graft to right ankle using cadaver graft, open	

Procedure	Code
174. Mitral valve replacement using porcine valve, open	
175. Percutaneous phacoemulsification of right eye cataract with prosthetic lens insertion	
176. Transcatheter replacement of pulmonary valve using of bovine jugular vein valve	
177. Total left hip replacement using ceramic on ceramic prosthesis, without bone cement	
178. Aortic valve annuloplasty using ring, open	
179. Laparoscopic repair of left inguinal hernia with marlex plug	
180. Autograft nerve graft to right median nerve, percutaneous endoscopic (do not code graft harvest for this exercise)	
181. Exchange of liner in femoral component of previous left hip replacement, open approach	
182. Anterior colporrhaphy with polypropylene mesh reinforcement, open approach	
183. Implantation of CorCap cardiac support device, open approach	
184. Abdominal wall herniorrhaphy, open, using synthetic mesh	
185. Tendon graft to strengthen injured left shoulder using autograft, open (do not code graft harvest for this exercise)	
186. Onlay lamellar keratoplasty of left cornea using autograft, external approach	
187. Resurfacing procedure on right femoral head, open approach	
188. Exchange of drainage tube from right hip joint	
189. Tracheostomy tube exchange	
190. Change chest tube for left pneumothorax	
191. Exchange of cerebral ventriculostomy drainage tube	
192. Foley urinary catheter exchange	
193. Open removal of lumbar sympathetic neurostimulator lead	
194. Nonincisional removal of Swan-Ganz catheter from right pulmonary artery	
195. Laparotomy with removal of pancreatic drain	
196. Extubation, endotracheal tube	
197. Nonincisional PEG tube removal	
198. Transvaginal removal of brachytherapy seeds	
199. Transvaginal removal of extraluminal cervical cerclage	
200. Incision with removal of K-wire fixation, right first metatarsal	
201. Cystoscopy with retrieval of left ureteral stent	
202. Removal of nasogastric drainage tube for decompression	
203. Removal of external fixator, left radial fracture	
204. Trimming and reanastomosis of stenosed femorofemoral synthetic bypass graft, open	
205. Open revision of right hip replacement, with readjustment of prosthesis	
206. Adjustment of position, pacemaker lead in left ventricle, percutaneous	
207. External repositioning of Foley catheter to bladder	
208. Taking out loose screw and putting larger screw in fracture repair plate, left tibia	

Procedure	Code
209. Revision of totally implantable VAD port placement in chest wall, causing patient discomfort, open	
210. Thoracotomy with exploration of right pleural cavity	
211. Diagnostic laryngoscopy	
212. Exploratory arthrotomy of left knee	
213. Colposcopy with diagnostic hysteroscopy	
214. Digital rectal exam	
215. Diagnostic arthroscopy of right shoulder	
216. Endoscopy of maxillary sinus	
217. Laparotomy with palpation of liver	
218. Transurethral diagnostic cystoscopy	
219. Colonoscopy, discontinued at sigmoid colon	
220. Percutaneous mapping of basal ganglia	
221. Heart catheterization with cardiac mapping	
222. Intraoperative whole brain mapping via craniotomy	
223. Mapping of left cerebral hemisphere, percutaneous endoscopic	
224. Intraoperative cardiac mapping during open heart surgery	
225. Hysteroscopy with cautery of post-hysterectomy oozing and evacuation of clot	
226. Open exploration and ligation of post-op arterial bleeder, left forearm	
227. Control of post-operative retroperitoneal bleeding via laparotomy	
228. Reopening of thoracotomy site with drainage and control of post-op hemopericardium	
229. Arthroscopy with drainage of hemarthrosis at previous operative site, right knee	
230. Radiocarpal fusion of left hand with internal fixation, open	
231. Posterior spinal fusion at L1-L3 level with BAK cage interbody fusion device, open	
232. Intercarpal fusion of right hand with bone bank bone graft, open	
233. Sacrococcygeal fusion with bone graft from same operative site, open	
234. Interphalangeal fusion of left great toe, percutaneous pin fixation	
235. Suture repair of left radial nerve laceration	
236. Laparotomy with suture repair of blunt force duodenal laceration	
237. Perineoplasty with repair of old obstetric laceration, open	
238. Suture repair of right biceps tendon (upper arm) laceration, open	
239. Closure of abdominal wall stab wound	
240. Cosmetic face lift, open, no other information available	
241. Bilateral breast augmentation with silicone implants, open	
242. Cosmetic rhinoplasty with septal reduction and tip elevation using local tissue graft, open	
243. Abdominoplasty (tummy tuck), open	
244. Liposuction of bilateral thighs	
245. Creation of penis in female patient using tissue bank donor graft	

Procedure	Code
246. Creation of vagina in male patient using synthetic material	
247. Laparoscopic vertical (sleeve) gastrectomy	
248. Left uterine artery embolization with intraluminal biosphere injection	

Obstetrics

Procedure	Code
1. Abortion by dilation and evacuation following laminaria insertion	
2. Manually assisted spontaneous abortion	
3. Abortion by abortifacient insertion	
4. Bimanual pregnancy examination	
5. Extraperitoneal C-section, low transverse incision	
6. Fetal spinal tap, percutaneous	
7. Fetal kidney transplant, laparoscopic	
8. Open in utero repair of congenital diaphragmatic hernia	
9. Laparoscopy with total excision of tubal pregnancy	
10. Transvaginal removal of fetal monitoring electrode	

Placement

Procedure	Code
1. Placement of packing material, right ear	
2. Mechanical traction of entire left leg	
3. Removal of splint, right shoulder	
4. Placement of neck brace	
5. Change of vaginal packing	
6. Packing of wound, chest wall	
7. Sterile dressing placement to left groin region	
8. Removal of packing material from pharynx	
9. Placement of intermittent pneumatic compression device, covering entire right arm	
10. Exchange of pressure dressing to left thigh	

Administration

Procedure	Code
1. Peritoneal dialysis via indwelling catheter	
2. Transvaginal artificial insemination	
3. Infusion of total parenteral nutrition via central venous catheter	
4. Esophagogastroscopy with Botox injection into esophageal sphincter	
5. Percutaneous irrigation of knee joint	
6. Systemic infusion of recombinant tissue plasminogen activator (r-tPA) via peripheral venous catheter	
7. Transfusion of antihemophilic factor, (nonautologous) via arterial central line	
8. Transabdominal in vitro fertilization, implantation of donor ovum	
9. Autologous bone marrow transplant via central venous line	
10. Implantation of anti-microbial envelope with cardiac defibrillator placement, open	

Procedure	Code
11. Sclerotherapy of brachial plexus lesion, alcohol injection	
12. Percutaneous peripheral vein injection, glucarpidase	
13. Introduction of anti-infective envelope into subcutaneous tissue, open	

Measurement and Monitoring

Procedure	Code
1. Cardiac stress test, single measurement	
2. EGD with biliary flow measurement	
3. Right and left heart cardiac catheterization with bilateral sampling and pressure measurements	
4. Temperature monitoring, rectal	
5. Peripheral venous pulse, external, single measurement	
6. Holter monitoring	
7. Respiratory rate, external, single measurement	
8. Fetal heart rate monitoring, transvaginal	
9. Visual mobility test, single measurement	
10. Left ventricular cardiac output monitoring from pulmonary artery wedge (Swan-Ganz) catheter	
11. Olfactory acuity test, single measurement	

Extracorporeal or Systemic Assistance and Performance

Procedure	Code
1. Intermittent mechanical ventilation, 16 hours	
2. Liver dialysis, single encounter	
3. Cardiac countershock with successful conversion to sinus rhythm	
4. IPPB (intermittent positive pressure breathing) for mobilization of secretions, 22 hours	
5. Renal dialysis, 12 hours	
6. IABP (intra-aortic balloon pump) continuous	
7. Intra-operative cardiac pacing, continuous	
8. ECMO (extracorporeal membrane oxygenation), central	
9. Controlled mechanical ventilation (CMV), 45 hours	
10. Pulsatile compression boot with intermittent inflation	

Extracorporeal or Systemic Therapies

Procedure	Code
1. Donor thrombocytapheresis, single encounter	
2. Bili-lite phototherapy, series treatment	
3. Whole body hypothermia, single treatment	
4. Circulatory phototherapy, single encounter	
5. Shock wave therapy of plantar fascia, single treatment	
6. Antigen-free air conditioning, series treatment	
7. TMS (transcranial magnetic stimulation), series treatment	
8. Therapeutic ultrasound of peripheral vessels, single treatment	
9. Plasmapheresis, series treatment	
10. Extracorporeal electromagnetic stimulation (EMS) for urinary incontinence, single treatment	

Osteopathic

Procedure	Code
1. Isotonic muscle energy treatment of right leg	
2. Low velocity-high amplitude osteopathic treatment of head	
3. Lymphatic pump osteopathic treatment of left axilla	
4. Indirect osteopathic treatment of sacrum	
5. Articulatory osteopathic treatment of cervical region	

Other Procedures

Procedure	Code
1. Near infrared spectroscopy of leg vessels	
2. CT computer assisted sinus surgery	
3. Suture removal, abdominal wall	
4. Isolation after infectious disease exposure	
5. Robotic assisted open prostatectomy	
6. In vitro fertilization	

Chiropractic

Procedure	Code
1. Chiropractic treatment of lumbar region using long lever specific contact	
2. Chiropractic manipulation of abdominal region, indirect visceral	
3. Chiropractic extra-articular treatment of hip region	
4. Chiropractic treatment of sacrum using long and short lever specific contact	
5. Mechanically-assisted chiropractic manipulation of head	

Imaging

Procedure	Code
1. Noncontrast CT of abdomen and pelvis	
2. Intravascular ultrasound, left subclavian artery	
3. Fluoroscopic guidance for insertion of central venous catheter in SVC, low osmolar contrast	
4. Chest x-ray, AP/PA and lateral views	

Procedure	Code
5. Endoluminal ultrasound of gallbladder and bile ducts	
6. MRI of thyroid gland, contrast unspecified	
7. Esophageal videofluoroscopy study with oral barium contrast	
8. Portable x-ray study of right radius/ulna shaft, standard series	
9. Routine fetal ultrasound, second trimester twin gestation	
10. CT scan of bilateral lungs, high osmolar contrast with densitometry	
11. Fluoroscopic guidance for percutaneous transluminal angioplasty (PTA) of left common femoral artery, low osmolar contrast	

Nuclear Medicine

Procedure	Code
1. Tomo scan of right and left heart, unspecified radiopharmaceutical, qualitative gated rest	
2. Technetium pentetate assay of kidneys, ureters, and bladder	
3. Uniplanar scan of spine using technetium oxidronate, with first-pass study	
4. Thallous chloride tomographic scan of bilateral breasts	
5. PET scan of myocardium using rubidium	
6. Gallium citrate scan of head and neck, single plane imaging	
7. Xenon gas nonimaging probe of brain	
8. Upper GI scan, radiopharmaceutical unspecified, for gastric emptying	
9. Carbon 11 PET scan of brain with quantification	
10. Iodinated albumin nuclear medicine assay, blood plasma volume study	

Radiation Therapy

Procedure	Code
1. Plaque radiation of left eye, single port	
2. 8 MeV photon beam radiation to brain	
3. IORT of colon, 3 ports	
4. HDR brachytherapy of prostate using palladium-103	
5. Electron radiation treatment of right breast, with custom device	
6. Hyperthermia oncology treatment of pelvic region	
7. Contact radiation of tongue	
8. Heavy particle radiation treatment of pancreas, four risk sites	
9. LDR brachytherapy to spinal cord using iodine	
10. Whole body Phosphorus 32 administration with risk to hematopoetic system	

Physical Rehabilitation and Diagnostic Audiology

Procedure	Code
1. Bekesy assessment using audiometer	
2. Individual fitting of left eye prosthesis	

Procedure	Code
3. Physical therapy for range of motion and mobility, patient right hip, no special equipment	
4. Bedside swallow assessment using assessment kit	
5. Caregiver training in airway clearance techniques	
6. Application of short arm cast in rehabilitation setting	
7. Verbal assessment of patient's pain level	
8. Caregiver training in communication skills using manual communication board	
9. Group musculoskeletal balance training exercises, whole body, no special equipment	
10. Individual therapy for auditory processing using tape recorder	

Mental Health

Procedure	Code
1. Cognitive-behavioral psychotherapy, individual	
2. Narcosynthesis	
3. Light therapy	
4. ECT (electroconvulsive therapy), unilateral, multiple seizure	
5. Crisis intervention	
6. Neuropsychological testing	
7. Hypnosis	
8. Developmental testing	
9. Vocational counseling	
10. Family psychotherapy	

Substance Abuse Treatment

Procedure	Code
1. Naltrexone treatment for drug dependency	
2. Substance abuse treatment family counseling	
3. Medication monitoring of patient on methadone maintenance	
4. Individual interpersonal psychotherapy for drug abuse	
5. Patient in for alcohol detoxification treatment	
6. Group motivational counseling	
7. Individual 12-step psychotherapy for substance abuse	
8. Post-test infectious disease counseling for IV drug abuser	
9. Psychodynamic psychotherapy for drug dependent patient	
10. Group cognitive-behavioral counseling for substance abuse	

New Technology

Procedure	Code
1. Infusion of ceftazidime via peripheral venous catheter	

Answers to Coding Exercises

Medical Surgical Section

Procedure	Code
1. Excision of malignant melanoma from skin of right ear	ØHB2XZZ
2. Laparoscopy with excision of endometrial implant from left ovary	ØUB14ZZ
3. Percutaneous needle core biopsy of right kidney	ØTB03ZX
4. EGD with gastric biopsy	ØDB68ZX
5. Open endarterectomy of left common carotid artery	Ø3CJØZZ
6. Excision of basal cell carcinoma of lower lip	ØCB1XZZ
7. Open excision of tail of pancreas	ØFBGØZZ
8. Percutaneous biopsy of right gastrocnemius muscle	ØKBS3ZX
9. Sigmoidoscopy with sigmoid polypectomy	ØDBN8ZZ
10. Open excision of lesion from right Achilles tendon	ØLBNØZZ
11. Open resection of cecum	ØDTHØZZ
12. Total excision of pituitary gland, open	ØGTØØZZ
13. Explantation of left failed kidney, open	ØTT1ØZZ
14. Open left axillary total lymphadenectomy	Ø7T6ØZZ (RESECTION is coded for cutting out a chain of lymph nodes.)
15. Laparoscopic-assisted vaginal hysterectomy	ØUT9FZZ
16. Right total mastectomy, open	ØHTTØZZ
17. Open resection of papillary muscle	Ø2TDØZZ (The papillary muscle refers to the heart and is found in the *Heart and Great Vessels* body system.)
18. Total retropubic prostatectomy, open	ØVTØØZZ
19. Laparoscopic cholecystectomy	ØFT44ZZ
20. Endoscopic bilateral total maxillary sinusectomy	Ø9TQ8ZZ, Ø9TR8ZZ
21. Amputation at right elbow level	ØX6BØZZ
22. Right below-knee amputation, proximal tibia/fibula	ØY6HØZ1 (The qualifier *High* here means the portion of the tib/fib closest to the knee.)
23. Fifth ray carpometacarpal joint amputation, left hand	ØX6KØZ8 (A *complete* ray amputation is through the carpometacarpal joint.)
24. Right leg and hip amputation through ischium	ØY62ØZZ (The *Hindquarter* body part includes amputation along any part of the hip bone.)
25. DIP joint amputation of right thumb	ØX6LØZ3 (The qualifier *low* here means through the distal interphalangeal joint.)
26. Right wrist joint amputation	ØX6JØZØ (Amputation at the wrist joint is actually complete amputation of the hand.)
27. Trans-metatarsal amputation of foot at left big toe	ØY6NØZ9 (A *partial* amputation is through the shaft of the metatarsal bone.)
28. Mid-shaft amputation, right humerus	ØX68ØZ2

Procedure	Code
29. Left fourth toe amputation, mid-proximal phalanx	ØY6WØZ1 (The qualifier *High* here means anywhere along the proximal phalanx.)
30. Right above-knee amputation, distal femur	ØY6CØZ3
31. Cryotherapy of wart on left hand	ØH5GXZZ
32. Percutaneous radiofrequency ablation of right vocal cord lesion	ØC5T3ZZ
33. Left heart catheterization with laser destruction of arrhythmogenic focus, A-V node	Ø2583ZZ
34. Cautery of nosebleed	Ø95KXZZ
35. Transurethral endoscopic laser ablation of prostate	ØV5Ø8ZZ
36. Percutaneous cautery of oozing varicose vein, left calf	Ø65Y3ZZ
37. Laparoscopy with destruction of endometriosis, bilateral ovaries	ØU524ZZ
38. Laser coagulation of right retinal vessel hemorrhage, percutaneous	Ø85G3ZZ (The *Retinal Vessel* body-part values are in the *Eye* body system.)
39. Thoracoscopic pleurodesis, left side	ØB5P4ZZ
40. Percutaneous insertion of Greenfield IVC filter	Ø6HØ3DZ
41. Forceps total mouth extraction, upper and lower teeth	ØCDWXZ2, ØCDXXZ2
42. Removal of left thumbnail	ØHDQXZZ (No separate body-part value is given for thumbnail, so this is coded to *Fingernail*.)
43. Extraction of right intraocular lens without replacement, percutaneous	Ø8DJ3ZZ
44. Laparoscopy with needle aspiration of ova for in vitro fertilization	ØUDN4ZZ
45. Nonexcisional debridement of skin ulcer, right foot	ØHDMXZZ
46. Open stripping of abdominal fascia, right side	ØJD8ØZZ
47. Hysteroscopy with D&C, diagnostic	ØUDB8ZX
48. Liposuction for medical purposes, left upper arm	ØJDF3ZZ (The *Percutaneous* approach is inherent in the liposuction technique.)
49. Removal of tattered right ear drum fragments with tweezers	Ø9D77ZZ
50. Microincisional phlebectomy of spider veins, right lower leg	Ø6DY3ZZ
51. Routine Foley catheter placement	ØT9B7ØZ
52. Incision and drainage of external anal abscess	ØD9QXZZ
53. Percutaneous drainage of ascites	ØW9G3ZZ (This is drainage of the cavity and not the peritoneal membrane itself.)
54. Laparoscopy with left ovarian cystotomy and drainage	ØU914ZZ
55. Laparotomy and drain placement for liver abscess, right lobe	ØF91ØØZ
56. Right knee arthrotomy with drain placement	ØS9CØØZ
57. Thoracentesis of left pleural effusion	ØW9B3ZZ (This is drainage of the pleural cavity)
58. Phlebotomy of left median cubital vein for polycythemia vera	Ø59C3ZZ (The median cubital vein is a branch of the basilic vein)

Procedure	Code
59. Percutaneous chest tube placement for right pneumothorax	0W9930Z
60. Endoscopic drainage of left ethmoid sinus	099V4ZZ
61. External ventricular CSF drainage catheter placement via burr hole	009630Z
62. Removal of foreign body, right cornea	08C8XZZ
63. Percutaneous mechanical thrombectomy, left brachial artery	03C83ZZ
64. Esophagogastroscopy with removal of bezoar from stomach	0DC68ZZ
65. Foreign body removal, skin of left thumb	0HCGXZZ (There is no specific value for thumb skin, so the procedure is coded to *Hand*.)
66. Transurethral cystoscopy with removal of bladder stone	0TCB8ZZ
67. Forceps removal of foreign body in right nostril	09CKXZZ (Nostril is coded to the *Nasal mucosa and soft tissue* body-part value.)
68. Laparoscopy with excision of old suture from mesentery	0DCV4ZZ
69. Incision and removal of right lacrimal duct stone	08CX0ZZ
70. Nonincisional removal of intraluminal foreign body from vagina	0UCG7ZZ (The approach *External* is also a possibility. It is assumed here that since the patient went to the doctor to have the object removed, that it was not in the vaginal orifice.)
71. Right common carotid endarterectomy, open	03CH0ZZ
72. Open excision of retained sliver, subcutaneous tissue of left foot	0JCR0ZZ
73. Extracorporeal shockwave lithotripsy (ESWL), bilateral ureters	0TF6XZZ, 0TF7XZZ (The *Bilateral Ureter* body-part value is not available for the root operation FRAGMENTATION, so the procedures are coded separately.)
74. Endoscopic retrograde cholangiopancreatography (ERCP) with lithotripsy of common bile duct stone	0FF98ZZ (ERCP is performed through the mouth to the biliary system via the duodenum, so the approach value is *Via Natural or Artificial Opening Endoscopic*.)
75. Thoracotomy with crushing of pericardial calcifications	02FN0ZZ
76. Transurethral cystoscopy with fragmentation of bladder calculus	0TFB8ZZ
77. Hysteroscopy with intraluminal lithotripsy of left fallopian tube calcification	0UF68ZZ
78. Division of right foot tendon, percutaneous	0L8V3ZZ
79. Left heart catheterization with division of bundle of HIS	02883ZZ
80. Open osteotomy of capitate, left hand	0P8N0ZZ (The capitate is one of the carpal bones of the hand.)
81. EGD with esophagotomy of esophagogastric junction	0D948ZZ
82. Sacral rhizotomy for pain control, percutaneous	018R3ZZ
83. Laparotomy with exploration and adhesiolysis of right ureter	0TN60ZZ

Procedure	Code
84. Incision of scar contracture, right elbow	0HNDXZZ (The skin of the elbow region is coded to *Lower Arm*.)
85. Frenulotomy for treatment of tongue-tie syndrome	0CN7XZZ (The frenulum is coded to the body-part value *Tongue*.)
86. Right shoulder arthroscopy with coracoacromial ligament release	0MN14ZZ
87. Mitral valvulotomy for release of fused leaflets, open approach	02NG0ZZ
88. Percutaneous left Achilles tendon release	0LNP3ZZ
89. Laparoscopy with lysis of peritoneal adhesions	0DNW4ZZ
90. Manual rupture of right shoulder joint adhesions under general anesthesia	0RNJXZZ
91. Open posterior tarsal tunnel release	01NG0ZZ (The nerve released in the posterior tarsal tunnel is the tibial nerve.)
92. Laparoscopy with freeing of left ovary and fallopian tube	0UN14ZZ, 0UN64ZZ
93. Liver transplant with donor matched liver	0FY00Z0
94. Orthotopic heart transplant using porcine heart	02YA0Z2 (The donor heart comes from an animal [pig], so the qualifier value is *Zooplastic.*)
95. Right lung transplant, open, using organ donor match	0BYK0Z0
96. Transplant of large intestine, organ donor match	0DYE0Z0
97. Left kidney/pancreas organ bank transplant	0FYG0Z0, 0TY10Z0
98. Replantation of avulsed scalp	0HM0XZZ
99. Reattachment of severed right ear	09M0XZZ
100. Reattachment of traumatic left gastrocnemius avulsion, open	0KMT0ZZ
101. Closed replantation of three avulsed teeth, lower jaw	0CMXXZ1
102. Reattachment of severed left hand	0XMK0ZZ
103. Right open palmaris longus tendon transfer	0LX50ZZ
104. Endoscopic radial to median nerve transfer	01X64Z5
105. Fasciocutaneous flap closure of left thigh, open	0JXM0ZC (The qualifier identifies the body layers in addition to fascia included in the procedure.)
106. Transfer left index finger to left thumb position, open	0XXP0ZM
107. Percutaneous fascia transfer to fill defect, right neck	0JX43ZZ
108. Trigeminal to facial nerve transfer, percutaneous endoscopic	00XK4ZM
109. Endoscopic left leg flexor hallucis longus tendon transfer	0LXP4ZZ
110. Right scalp advancement flap to right temple	0HX0XZZ
111. Bilateral TRAM pedicle flap reconstruction status post mastectomy, muscle only, open	0KXK0Z6, 0KXL0Z6 (The transverse rectus abdominus muscle (TRAM) flap is coded for each flap developed.)
112. Skin transfer flap closure of complex open wound, left lower back	0HX6XZZ
113. Open fracture reduction, right tibia	0QSG0ZZ
114. Laparoscopy with gastropexy for malrotation	0DS64ZZ
115. Left knee arthroscopy with reposition of anterior cruciate ligament	0MSP4ZZ

Procedure	Code
116. Open transposition of ulnar nerve	01S40ZZ
117. Closed reduction with percutaneous internal fixation of right femoral neck fracture	0QS634Z
118. Trans-vaginal intraluminal cervical cerclage	0UVC7DZ
119. Cervical cerclage using Shirodkar technique	0UVC7ZZ
120. Thoracotomy with banding of left pulmonary artery using extraluminal device	02VR0CZ
121. Restriction of thoracic duct with intraluminal stent, percutaneous	07VK3DZ
122. Craniotomy with clipping of cerebral aneurysm	03VG0CZ (The clip is placed lengthwise on the outside wall of the widened portion of the vessel.)
123. Nonincisional, transnasal placement of restrictive stent in right lacrimal duct	08VX7DZ
124. Catheter-based temporary restriction of blood flow in abdominal aorta for treatment of cerebral ischemia	04V03DJ
125. Percutaneous ligation of esophageal vein	06L33ZZ
126. Percutaneous embolization of left internal carotid-cavernous fistula	03LL3DZ
127. Laparoscopy with bilateral occlusion of fallopian tubes using Hulka extraluminal clips	0UL74CZ
128. Open suture ligation of failed AV graft, left brachial artery	03L80ZZ
129. Percutaneous embolization of vascular supply, intracranial meningioma	03LG3DZ
130. Percutaneous embolization of right uterine artery, using coils	04LE3DT
131. Open occlusion of left atrial appendage, using extraluminal pressure clips	02L70CK
132. Percutaneous suture exclusion of left atrial appendage, via femoral artery access	02L73ZK
133. ERCP with balloon dilation of common bile duct	0F798ZZ
134. PTCA of two coronary arteries, LAD with stent placement, RCA with no stent	02703DZ, 02703ZZ (A separate procedure is coded for each artery dilated, since the device value differs for each artery.)
135. Cystoscopy with intraluminal dilation of bladder neck stricture	0T7C8ZZ
136. Open dilation of old anastomosis, left femoral artery	047L0ZZ
137. Dilation of upper esophageal stricture, direct visualization, with Bougie sound	0D717ZZ
138. PTA of right brachial artery stenosis	03773ZZ
139. Transnasal dilation and stent placement in right lacrimal duct	087X7DZ
140. Hysteroscopy with balloon dilation of bilateral fallopian tubes	0U778ZZ
141. Tracheoscopy with intraluminal dilation of tracheal stenosis	0B718ZZ
142. Cystoscopy with dilation of left ureteral stricture, with stent placement	0T778DZ
143. Open gastric bypass with Roux-en-Y limb to jejunum	0D160ZA
144. Right temporal artery to intracranial artery bypass using Gore-Tex graft, open	031S0JG
145. Tracheostomy formation with tracheostomy tube placement, percutaneous	0B113F4
146. PICVA (percutaneous in situ coronary venous arterialization) of single coronary artery	02103D4

Procedure	Code
147. Open left femoral-popliteal artery bypass using cadaver vein graft	041L0KL
148. Shunting of intrathecal cerebrospinal fluid to peritoneal cavity using synthetic shunt	00160J6
149. Colostomy formation, open, transverse colon to abdominal wall	0D1L0Z4
150. Open urinary diversion, left ureter, using ileal conduit to skin	0T170ZC
151. CABG of LAD using left internal mammary artery, open off-bypass	02100Z9
152. Open pleuroperitoneal shunt, right pleural cavity, using synthetic device	0W190JG
153. Percutaneous placement of ventriculoperitoneal shunt for treatment of hydrocephalus	00163J6
154. End-of-life replacement of spinal neurostimulator generator, multiple array, in lower abdomen	0JH80DZ (Taking out of the old generator is coded separately to the root operation *Removal*)
155. Percutaneous insertion of spinal neurostimulator lead, lumbar spinal cord	00HV3MZ
156. Percutaneous replacement of broken pacemaker lead in left atrium	02H73JZ (Taking out the broken pacemaker lead is coded separately to the root operation *Removal*.)
157. Open placement of dual chamber pacemaker generator in chest wall	0JH606Z
158. Percutaneous placement of venous central line in right internal jugular, with tip in superior vena cava	02HV33Z
159. Open insertion of multiple channel cochlear implant, left ear	09HE06Z
160. Percutaneous placement of Swan-Ganz catheter in pulmonary trunk	02HP32Z (The Swan-Ganz catheter is coded to the device value *Monitoring Device* because it monitors pulmonary artery output.)
161. Bronchoscopy with insertion of Low Dose Pd-103 brachytherapy seeds, right main bronchus	0BH081Z, DB11BB2
162. Open insertion of interspinous process device into lumbar vertebral joint	0SH00BZ
163. Open placement of bone growth stimulator, left femoral shaft	0QHY0MZ
164. Cystoscopy with placement of brachytherapy seeds in prostate gland	0VH081Z
165. Percutaneous insertion of Greenfield IVC filter	06H03DZ
166. Full-thickness skin graft to right lower arm, autograft (do not code graft harvest for this exercise)	0HRDX73
167. Excision of necrosed left femoral head with bone bank bone graft to fill the defect, open	0QR70KZ
168. Penetrating keratoplasty of right cornea with donor matched cornea, percutaneous approach	08R83KZ
169. Bilateral mastectomy with concomitant saline breast implants, open	0HRV0JZ
170. Excision of abdominal aorta with Gore-Tex graft replacement, open	04R00JZ
171. Total right knee arthroplasty with insertion of total knee prosthesis	0SRC0JZ
172. Bilateral mastectomy with free TRAM flap reconstruction	0HRV076
173. Tenonectomy with graft to right ankle using cadaver graft, open	0LRS0KZ

Appendix K: Coding Exercises and Answers

Procedure	Code
174. Mitral valve replacement using porcine valve, open	02RG08Z
175. Percutaneous phacoemulsification of right eye cataract with prosthetic lens insertion	08RJ3JZ
176. Transcatheter replacement of pulmonary valve using of bovine jugular vein valve	02RH38Z
177. Total left hip replacement using ceramic on ceramic prosthesis, without bone cement	0SRB03A
178. Aortic valve annuloplasty using ring, open	02UF0JZ
179. Laparoscopic repair of left inguinal hernia with marlex plug	0YU64JZ
180. Autograft nerve graft to right median nerve, percutaneous endoscopic (do not code graft harvest for this exercise)	01U547Z
181. Exchange of liner in femoral component of previous left hip replacement, open approach	0SUS09Z (Taking out of the old liner is coded separately to the root operation *Removal*)
182. Anterior colporrhaphy with polypropylene mesh reinforcement, open approach	0JUC0JZ
183. Implantation of CorCap cardiac support device, open approach	02UA0JZ
184. Abdominal wall herniorrhaphy, open, using synthetic mesh	0WUF0JZ
185. Tendon graft to strengthen injured left shoulder using autograft, open (do not code graft harvest for this exercise)	0LU207Z
186. Onlay lamellar keratoplasty of left cornea using autograft, external approach	08U9X7Z
187. Resurfacing procedure on right femoral head, open approach	0SUR0BZ
188. Exchange of drainage tube from right hip joint	0S2YX0Z
189. Tracheostomy tube exchange	0B21XFZ
190. Change chest tube for left pneumothorax	0W2BX0Z
191. Exchange of cerebral ventriculostomy drainage tube	0020X0Z
192. Foley urinary catheter exchange	0T2BX0Z (This is coded to *Drainage Device* because urine is being drained.)
193. Open removal of lumbar sympathetic neurostimulator lead	01PY0MZ
194. Nonincisional removal of Swan-Ganz catheter from right pulmonary artery	02PYX2Z
195. Laparotomy with removal of pancreatic drain	0FPG00Z
196. Extubation, endotracheal tube	0BP1XDZ
197. Nonincisional PEG tube removal	0DP6XUZ
198. Transvaginal removal of brachytherapy seeds	0UPH71Z
199. Transvaginal removal of extraluminal cervical cerclage	0UPD7CZ
200. Incision with removal of K-wire fixation, right first metatarsal	0QPN04Z
201. Cystoscopy with retrieval of left ureteral stent	0TP98DZ
202. Removal of nasogastric drainage tube for decompression	0DP6X0Z
203. Removal of external fixator, left radial fracture	0PPJX5Z
204. Trimming and reanastomosis of stenosed femorofemoral synthetic bypass graft, open	04WY0JZ
205. Open revision of right hip replacement, with readjustment of prosthesis	0SW90JZ
206. Adjustment of position, pacemaker lead in left ventricle, percutaneous	02WA3MZ
207. External repositioning of Foley catheter to bladder	0TWBX0Z

Procedure	Code
208. Taking out loose screw and putting larger screw in fracture repair plate, left tibia	0QWH04Z
209. Revision of totally implantable VAD port placement in chest wall, causing patient discomfort, open	0JWT0WZ
210. Thoracotomy with exploration of right pleural cavity	0WJ90ZZ
211. Diagnostic laryngoscopy	0CJS8ZZ
212. Exploratory arthrotomy of left knee	0SJD0ZZ
213. Colposcopy with diagnostic hysteroscopy	0UJD8ZZ
214. Digital rectal exam	0DJD7ZZ
215. Diagnostic arthroscopy of right shoulder	0RJJ4ZZ
216. Endoscopy of maxillary sinus	09JY4ZZ
217. Laparotomy with palpation of liver	0FJ00ZZ
218. Transurethral diagnostic cystoscopy	0TJB8ZZ
219. Colonoscopy, discontinued at sigmoid colon	0DJD8ZZ
220. Percutaneous mapping of basal ganglia	00K83ZZ
221. Heart catheterization with cardiac mapping	02K83ZZ
222. Intraoperative whole brain mapping via craniotomy	00K00ZZ
223. Mapping of left cerebral hemisphere, percutaneous endoscopic	00K74ZZ
224. Intraoperative cardiac mapping during open heart surgery	02K80ZZ
225. Hysteroscopy with cautery of post-hysterectomy oozing and evacuation of clot	0W3R8ZZ
226. Open exploration and ligation of post-op arterial bleeder, left forearm	0X3F0ZZ
227. Control of post-operative retroperitoneal bleeding via laparotomy	0W3H0ZZ
228. Reopening of thoracotomy site with drainage and control of post-op hemopericardium	0W3D0ZZ
229. Arthroscopy with drainage of hemarthrosis at previous operative site, right knee	0Y3F4ZZ
230. Radiocarpal fusion of left hand with internal fixation, open	0RGP04Z
231. Posterior spinal fusion at L1-L3 level with BAK cage interbody fusion device, open	0SG10AJ
232. Intercarpal fusion of right hand with bone bank bone graft, open	0RGQ0KZ
233. Sacrococcygeal fusion with bone graft from same operative site, open	0SG507Z
234. Interphalangeal fusion of left great toe, percutaneous pin fixation	0SGQ34Z
235. Suture repair of left radial nerve laceration	01Q60ZZ (The approach value is *Open*, though the surgical exposure may have been created by the wound itself.)
236. Laparotomy with suture repair of blunt force duodenal laceration	0DQ90ZZ
237. Perineoplasty with repair of old obstetric laceration, open	0WQN0ZZ
238. Suture repair of right biceps tendon (upper arm) laceration, open	0LQ30ZZ
239. Closure of abdominal wall stab wound	0WQF0ZZ
240. Cosmetic face lift, open, no other information available	0W020ZZ
241. Bilateral breast augmentation with silicone implants, open	0HV0JZ
242. Cosmetic rhinoplasty with septal reduction and tip elevation using local tissue graft, open	090K07Z
243. Abdominoplasty (tummy tuck), open	0W0F0ZZ

Procedure	Code
244. Liposuction of bilateral thighs	ØJØL3ZZ, ØJØM3ZZ
245. Creation of penis in female patient using tissue bank donor graft	ØW4NØK1
246. Creation of vagina in male patient using synthetic material	ØW4MØJØ
247. Laparoscopic vertical (sleeve) gastrectomy	ØDB64Z3
248. Left uterine artery embolization with intraluminal biosphere injection	04LF3DU

Obstetrics

Procedure	Code
1. Abortion by dilation and evacuation following laminaria insertion	10A07ZW
2. Manually assisted spontaneous abortion	10E0XZZ (Since the pregnancy was not artificially terminated, this is coded to *Delivery* because it captures the procedure objective. The fact that it was an abortion will be identified in the diagnosis code.)
3. Abortion by abortifacient insertion	10A07ZX
4. Bimanual pregnancy examination	10J07ZZ
5. Extraperitoneal C-section, low transverse incision	10D00Z2
6. Fetal spinal tap, percutaneous	10903ZA
7. Fetal kidney transplant, laparoscopic	10Y04ZS
8. Open in utero repair of congenital diaphragmatic hernia	10Q00ZK (Diaphragm is classified to the *Respiratory* body system in the *Medical and Surgical* section.)
9. Laparoscopy with total excision of tubal pregnancy	10T24ZZ
10. Transvaginal removal of fetal monitoring electrode	10P073Z

Placement

Procedure	Code
1. Placement of packing material, right ear	2Y42X5Z
2. Mechanical traction of entire left leg	2W6MXØZ
3. Removal of splint, right shoulder	2W5AX1Z
4. Placement of neck brace	2W32X3Z
5. Change of vaginal packing	2YØ4X5Z
6. Packing of wound, chest wall	2W44X5Z
7. Sterile dressing placement to left groin region	2W27X4Z
8. Removal of packing material from pharynx	2Y5ØX5Z
9. Placement of intermittent pneumatic compression device, covering entire right arm	2W18X7Z
10. Exchange of pressure dressing to left thigh	2WØPX6Z

Administration

Procedure	Code
1. Peritoneal dialysis via indwelling catheter	3E1M39Z
2. Transvaginal artificial insemination	3EØP7LZ
3. Infusion of total parenteral nutrition via central venous catheter	3EØ436Z
4. Esophagogastroscopy with Botox injection into esophageal sphincter	3EØG8GC (Botulinum toxin is a paralyzing agent with temporary effects; it does not sclerose or destroy the nerve.)
5. Percutaneous irrigation of knee joint	3E1U38Z
6. Systemic infusion of recombinant tissue plasminogen activator (r-tPA) via peripheral venous catheter	3EØ3317
7. Transfusion of antihemophilic factor, (nonautologous) via arterial central line	30263V1
8. Transabdominal in vitro fertilization, implantation of donor ovum	3EØP3Q1
9. Autologous bone marrow transplant via central venous line	30243GØ
10. Implantation of anti-microbial envelope with cardiac defibrillator placement, open	3EØ102A
11. Sclerotherapy of brachial plexus lesion, alcohol injection	3EØT3TZ
12. Percutaneous peripheral vein injection, glucarpidase	3EØ33GQ
13. Introduction of anti-infective envelope into subcutaneous tissue, open	3EØ102A

Measurement and Monitoring

Procedure	Code
1. Cardiac stress test, single measurement	4AØ2XM4
2. EGD with biliary flow measurement	4AØC85Z
3. Right and left heart cardiac catheterization with bilateral sampling and pressure measurements	4AØ23N8
4. Temperature monitoring, rectal	4A1Z7KZ
5. Peripheral venous pulse, external, single measurement	4AØ4XJ1
6. Holter monitoring	4A12X45
7. Respiratory rate, external, single measurement	4AØ9XCZ
8. Fetal heart rate monitoring, transvaginal	4A1H7CZ
9. Visual mobility test, single measurement	4AØ7X7Z
10. Left ventricular cardiac output monitoring from pulmonary artery wedge (Swan-Ganz) catheter	4A1239Z
11. Olfactory acuity test, single measurement	4AØ8XØZ

Extracorporeal or Systemic Assistance and Performance

	Procedure	Code
1.	Intermittent mechanical ventilation, 16 hours	5A1935Z
2.	Liver dialysis, single encounter	5A1C00Z
3.	Cardiac countershock with successful conversion to sinus rhythm	5A2204Z
4.	IPPB (intermittent positive pressure breathing) for mobilization of secretions, 22 hours	5A09358
5.	Renal dialysis, 12 hours	5A1D80Z
6.	IABP (intra-aortic balloon pump) continuous	5A02210
7.	Intra-operative cardiac pacing, continuous	5A1223Z
8.	ECMO (extracorporeal membrane oxygenation), central	5A1522F
9.	Controlled mechanical ventilation (CMV), 45 hours	5A1945Z
10.	Pulsatile compression boot with intermittent inflation	5A02115 (This is coded to the function value *Cardiac Output*, because the purpose of such compression devices is to return blood to the heart faster.)

Extracorporeal or Systemic Therapies

	Procedure	Code
1.	Donor thrombocytapheresis, single encounter	6A550Z2
2.	Bili-lite phototherapy, series treatment	6A601ZZ
3.	Whole body hypothermia, single treatment	6A4Z0ZZ
4.	Circulatory phototherapy, single encounter	6A650ZZ
5.	Shock wave therapy of plantar fascia, single treatment	6A930ZZ
6.	Antigen-free air conditioning, series treatment	6A0Z1ZZ
7.	TMS (transcranial magnetic stimulation), series treatment	6A221ZZ
8.	Therapeutic ultrasound of peripheral vessels, single treatment	6A750Z6
9.	Plasmapheresis, series treatment	6A551Z3
10.	Extracorporeal electromagnetic stimulation (EMS) for urinary incontinence, single treatment	6A210ZZ

Osteopathic

	Procedure	Code
1.	Isotonic muscle energy treatment of right leg	7W06X8Z
2.	Low velocity-high amplitude osteopathic treatment of head	7W00X5Z
3.	Lymphatic pump osteopathic treatment of left axilla	7W07X6Z
4.	Indirect osteopathic treatment of sacrum	7W04X4Z
5.	Articulatory osteopathic treatment of cervical region	7W01X0Z

Other Procedures

	Procedure	Code
1.	Near infrared spectroscopy of leg vessels	8E023DZ
2.	CT computer assisted sinus surgery	8E09XBG (The primary procedure is coded separately.)
3.	Suture removal, abdominal wall	8E0WXY8
4.	Isolation after infectious disease exposure	8E0ZXY6
5.	Robotic assisted open prostatectomy	8E0W0CZ (The primary procedure is coded separately.)
6.	In vitro fertilization	8E0ZXY1

Chiropractic

	Procedure	Code
1.	Chiropractic treatment of lumbar region using long lever specific contact	9WB3XGZ
2.	Chiropractic manipulation of abdominal region, indirect visceral	9WB9XCZ
3.	Chiropractic extra-articular treatment of hip region	9WB6XDZ
4.	Chiropractic treatment of sacrum using long and short lever specific contact	9WB4XJZ
5.	Mechanically-assisted chiropractic manipulation of head	9WB0XKZ

Imaging

	Procedure	Code
1.	Noncontrast CT of abdomen and pelvis	BW21ZZZ
2.	Intravascular ultrasound, left subclavian artery	B342ZZ3
3.	Fluoroscopic guidance for insertion of central venous catheter in SVC, low osmolar contrast	B5181ZA
4.	Chest x-ray, AP/PA and lateral views	BW03ZZZ
5.	Endoluminal ultrasound of gallbladder and bile ducts	BF43ZZZ
6.	MRI of thyroid gland, contrast unspecified	BG34YZZ
7.	Esophageal videofluoroscopy study with oral barium contrast	BD11YZZ
8.	Portable x-ray study of right radius/ulna shaft, standard series	BP0JZZZ
9.	Routine fetal ultrasound, second trimester twin gestation	BY4DZZZ
10.	CT scan of bilateral lungs, high osmolar contrast with densitometry	BB240ZZ
11.	Fluoroscopic guidance for percutaneous transluminal angioplasty (PTA) of left common femoral artery, low osmolar contrast	B41G1ZZ

Nuclear Medicine

Procedure	Code
1. Tomo scan of right and left heart, unspecified radiopharmaceutical, qualitative gated rest	C226YZZ
2. Technetium pentetate assay of kidneys, ureters, and bladder	CT631ZZ
3. Uniplanar scan of spine using technetium oxidronate, with first-pass study	CP151ZZ
4. Thallous chloride tomographic scan of bilateral breasts	CH22SZZ
5. PET scan of myocardium using rubidium	C23GQZZ
6. Gallium citrate scan of head and neck, single plane imaging	CW1BLZZ
7. Xenon gas nonimaging probe of brain	C050VZZ
8. Upper GI scan, radiopharmaceutical unspecified, for gastric emptying	CD15YZZ
9. Carbon 11 PET scan of brain with quantification	C030BZZ
10. Iodinated albumin nuclear medicine assay, blood plasma volume study	C763HZZ

Radiation Therapy

Procedure	Code
1. Plaque radiation of left eye, single port	D8Y0FZZ
2. 8 MeV photon beam radiation to brain	D0011ZZ
3. IORT of colon, 3 ports	DDY5CZZ
4. HDR brachytherapy of prostate using palladium-103	DV109BZ
5. Electron radiation treatment of right breast, with custom device	DM013ZZ
6. Hyperthermia oncology treatment of pelvic region	DWY68ZZ
7. Contact radiation of tongue	D9Y57ZZ
8. Heavy particle radiation treatment of pancreas, four risk sites	DF034ZZ
9. LDR brachytherapy to spinal cord using iodine	D016B9Z
10. Whole body Phosphorus 32 administration with risk to hematopoetic system	DWY5GFZ

Physical Rehabilitation and Diagnostic Audiology

Procedure	Code
1. Bekesy assessment using audiometer	F13Z31Z
2. Individual fitting of left eye prosthesis	F0DZ8UZ
3. Physical therapy for range of motion and mobility, patient right hip, no special equipment	F07L0ZZ
4. Bedside swallow assessment using assessment kit	F00ZHYZ
5. Caregiver training in airway clearance techniques	F0FZ8ZZ
6. Application of short arm cast in rehabilitation setting	F0DZ7EZ (Inhibitory cast is listed in the equipment reference table under E, *Orthosis*.)
7. Verbal assessment of patient's pain level	F02ZFZZ

Procedure	Code
8. Caregiver training in communication skills using manual communication board	F0FZJMZ (Manual communication board is listed in the equipment reference table under M, *Augmentative/ Alternative Communication*.)
9. Group musculoskeletal balance training exercises, whole body, no special equipment	F07M6ZZ (Balance training is included in the motor treatment reference table under *Therapeutic Exercise*.)
10. Individual therapy for auditory processing using tape recorder	F09Z2KZ (Tape recorder is listed in the equipment reference table under *Audiovisual Equipment*.)

Mental Health

Procedure	Code
1. Cognitive-behavioral psychotherapy, individual	GZ58ZZZ
2. Narcosynthesis	GZGZZZZ
3. Light therapy	GZJZZZZ
4. ECT (electroconvulsive therapy), unilateral, multiple seizure	GZB1ZZZ
5. Crisis intervention	GZ2ZZZZ
6. Neuropsychological testing	GZ13ZZZ
7. Hypnosis	GZFZZZZ
8. Developmental testing	GZ10ZZZ
9. Vocational counseling	GZ61ZZZ
10. Family psychotherapy	GZ72ZZZ

Substance Abuse Treatment

Procedure	Code
1. Naltrexone treatment for drug dependency	HZ94ZZZ
2. Substance abuse treatment family counseling	HZ63ZZZ
3. Medication monitoring of patient on methadone maintenance	HZ81ZZZ
4. Individual interpersonal psychotherapy for drug abuse	HZ54ZZZ
5. Patient in for alcohol detoxification treatment	HZ2ZZZZ
6. Group motivational counseling	HZ47ZZZ
7. Individual 12-step psychotherapy for substance abuse	HZ53ZZZ
8. Post-test infectious disease counseling for IV drug abuser	HZ3CZZZ
9. Psychodynamic psychotherapy for drug dependent patient	HZ5CZZZ
10. Group cognitive-behavioral counseling for substance abuse	HZ42ZZZ

New Technology

Procedure	Code
1. Infusion of ceftazidime via peripheral venous catheter	XW03321

Appendix L: Procedure Combination Tables

The tables below were developed to help simplify the relationship between ICD-10-PCS coding and MS-DRG assignment. The Centers for Medicare & Medicaid Services (CMS) has identified in the MS-DRG v35 Definitions Manual certain procedure combinations that must occur in order to assign a specific MS-DRG. There are many factors influencing MS-DRG assignment, including principal and secondary diagnoses, MCC or CC use, sex of the patient, and discharge status. These tables should be used only as a guide.

DRG 001-002 Heart Transplant or Implant of Heart Assist System

Heart Transplant
Replacement of Right and Left Ventricle   Ø2RKØJZ and Ø2RLØJZ

Insertion With Removal of Heart Assist System

Type of Heart Assist System	Code as appropriate Insertion by approach	Code also as appropriate Removal of Heart Assist System by approach
Biventricular External	Ø2HA[Ø,3,4]RS	Ø2PA[Ø,3,4]RZ
External	Ø2HA[Ø,4]RZ	Ø2PA[Ø,3,4]RZ

Revision With Removal of Heart Assist System

Type of Heart Assist System	Code as appropriate Revision by approach	Code also as appropriate Removal of Heart Assist System by approach
Implantable	Ø2WA[Ø,3,4]QZ	Ø2PA[Ø,3,4]RZ
External	Ø2WA[Ø,3,4]RZ	Ø2PA[Ø,3,4]RZ

DRG 008 Simultaneous Pancreas/Kidney Transplant

Transplanted Body Part Laterality	Code Transplant as appropriate by tissue type			Code also Pancreas Transplant as appropriate by tissue type		
	Allogeneic	Syngeneic	Zooplastic	Allogeneic	Syngeneic	Zooplastic
Kidney, Right	ØTYØØZØ	ØTYØØZ1	ØTYØØZ2	ØFYGØZØ	ØFYGØZ1	ØFYGØZ2
Kidney, Left	ØTY1ØZØ	ØTY1ØZ1	ØTY1ØZ2	ØFYGØZØ	ØFYGØZ1	ØFYGØZ2

DRG 023-027 Craniotomy

Site of Neurostimulator Lead	Code as appropriate Insertion of Lead by approach	Code also as appropriate Insertion of Device by type and subcutaneous site						
		Neuro-stimulator Generator	Stimulator Multiple Array Code as appropriate by approach			Stimulator Multiple Array, Rechargeable Code as appropriate by approach		
		Skull	Chest	Back	Abdomen	Chest	Back	Abdomen
Brain	ØØHØ[Ø,3,4]MZ	ØNHØØNZ	ØJH6[Ø,3]DZ	ØJH7[Ø,3]DZ	ØJH8[Ø,3]DZ	ØJH6[Ø,3]EZ	ØJH7[Ø,3]EZ	ØJH8[Ø,3]EZ
Cerebral Ventricle	ØØH6[Ø,3,4]MZ	ØNHØØNZ	ØJH6[Ø,3]DZ	ØJH7[Ø,3]DZ	ØJH8[Ø,3]DZ	ØJH6[Ø,3]EZ	ØJH7[Ø,3]EZ	ØJH8[Ø,3]EZ

DRG 028-030 Spinal Procedures

Generator Type	Insertion of Generator by Site			Code also as appropriate Insertion of Neurostimulator Lead by approach	
	Chest	Abdomen	Back	Spinal Canal	Spinal Cord
Single Array	ØJH6[Ø,3]BZ	ØJH8[Ø,3]BZ	ØJH7[Ø,3]BZ	ØØHU[Ø,3,4]MZ	ØØHV[Ø,3,4]MZ
Single Array, Rechargeable	ØJH6[Ø,3]CZ	ØJH8[Ø,3]CZ	ØJH7[Ø,3]CZ	ØØHU[Ø,3,4]MZ	ØØHV[Ø,3,4]MZ
Multiple Array	ØJH6[Ø,3]DZ	ØJH8[Ø,3]DZ	ØJH7[Ø,3]DZ	ØØHU[Ø,3,4]MZ	ØØHV[Ø,3,4]MZ
Multiple Array, Rechargable	ØJH6[Ø,3]EZ	—	ØJH7[Ø,3]EZ	ØØHU[Ø,3,4]MZ	ØØHV[Ø,3,4]MZ
Multiple Array, Rechargable	—	ØJH8[Ø,3]EZ	—	ØØHU[Ø,3,4]MZ	ØØHVØMZ
Multiple Array, Rechargable	—	ØJH8ØEZ	—	—	ØØHV[3,4]MZ

DRG 040-042 Peripheral and Cranial Nerve and Other Nervous System Procedures

Insertion of Neurostimulator Lead With Device

Site of Neurostimulator Lead	Code as appropriate Insertion by approach	Code also as appropriate Insertion of Device by type and subcutaneous site					
		Stimulator Single Array Code as appropriate by approach			Stimulator Single Array, Rechargeable Code as appropriate by approach		
		Chest	Back	Abdomen	Chest	Back	Abdomen
Cranial Nerve	00HE[0,3,4]MZ	0JH6[0,3]BZ	0JH7[0,3]BZ	0JH8[0,3]BZ	0JH6[0,3]CZ	0JH7[0,3]CZ	0JH8[0,3]CZ
Peripheral Nerve	01HY[0,3,4]MZ	0JH6[0,3]BZ	0JH7[0,3]BZ	0JH8[0,3]BZ	0JH6[0,3]CZ	0JH7[0,3]CZ	0JH8[0,3]CZ
Stomach	0DH6[0,3,4]MZ	0JH6[0,3]BZ	0JH7[0,3]BZ	0JH8[0,3]BZ	0JH6[0,3]CZ	0JH7[0,3]CZ	0JH8[0,3]CZ
Azygos vein	05H0[0,3,4]MZ	0JH6[0,3]BZ	0JH7[0,S]BZ	0JH8[0,3]BZ	0JH6[0,3]CZ	0JH7[0,S]CZ	0JH8[0,3]CZ
Innominate Vein, Right	05H3[0,3,4]MZ	0JH6[0,3]BZ	0JH7[0,S]BZ	0JH8[0,3]BZ	0JH6[0,3]CZ	0JH7[0,S]CZ	0JH8[0,3]CZ
Innominate Vein, Left	05H4[0,3,4]MZ	0JH6[0,3]BZ	0JH7[0,S]BZ	0JH8[0,3]BZ	0JH6[0,3]CZ	0JH7[0,S]CZ	0JH8[0,3]CZ
		Stimulator Multiple Array Code as appropriate by approach			Stimulator Multiple Array, Rechargeable Code as appropriate by approach		
		Chest	Back	Abdomen	Chest	Back	Abdomen
Cranial Nerve	00HE[0,3,4]MZ	0JH6[0,3]DZ	0JH7[0,3]DZ	0JH8[0,3]DZ	0JH6[0,3]EZ	0JH7[0,3]EZ	0JH8[0,3]EZ
Peripheral Nerve	01HY[0,3,4]MZ	0JH6[0,3]DZ	0JH7[0,3]DZ	0JH8[0,3]DZ	0JH6[0,3]EZ	0JH7[0,3]EZ	0JH8[0,3]EZ
Stomach	0DH6[0,3,4]MZ	0JH6[0,3]DZ	0JH7[0,3]DZ	0JH8[0,3]DZ	0JH6[0,3]EZ	0JH7[0,3]EZ	0JH8[0,3]EZ
Azygos vein	05H0[0,3,4]MZ	0JH6[0,3]DZ	0JH7[0,S]DZ	0JH8[0,3]DZ	0JH6[0,3]EZ	0JH7[0,S]EZ	0JH8[0,3]EZ
Innominate Vein, Right	05H3[0,3,4]MZ	0JH6[0,3]DZ	0JH7[0,S]DZ	0JH8[0,3]DZ	0JH6[0,3]EZ	0JH7[0,S]EZ	0JH8[0,3]EZ
Innominate Vein, Left	05H4[0,3,4]MZ	0JH6[0,3]DZ	0JH7[0,S]DZ	0JH8[0,3]DZ	0JH6[0,3]EZ	0JH7[0,S]EZ	0JH8[0,3]EZ

DRG 222-227 Cardiac Defibrillator Implant

Insertion of Generator With Insertion of Lead(s) into Coronary Vein, Atrium or Ventricle

Generator Type	Insertion of Generator by Site		Code also as appropriate Insertion of Leads by site				
	Chest	Abdomen	Coronary Vein	Atrium		Ventricle	
				Right	Left	Right	Left
Defibrillator	0JH6[0,3]8Z	0JH8[0,3]8Z	02H4[0,4]KZ	02H6[0,3,4]KZ	02H7[0,3,4]KZ	02HK[0,3,4]KZ	02HL[0,3,4]KZ
Cardiac Resynch Defibrillator Pulse Generator	0JH6[0,3]9Z	0JH8[0,3]9Z	02H4[0,3,4]KZ or 02H43[J,M]Z	02H6[0,3,4]KZ	02H7[0,3,4]KZ	02HK[0,3,4]KZ	02HL[0,3,4]KZ
Contractility Modulation Device	0JH6[0,3]AZ	0JH8[0,3]AZ	—	—	—	—	02HL[0,3,4]MZ

Insertion of Generator with Insertion of Lead(s) into Pericardium

Generator Type	Insertion of Generator by Site		Code also as appropriate Insertion of Leads by Type		
	Chest	Abdomen	Pericardium		
			Pacemaker	Defibrillator	Cardiac
Defibrillator	0JH6[0,3]8Z	0JH8[0,3]8Z	02HN[0,3,4]JZ	02HN[0,3,4]KZ	02HN[0,3,4]MZ
Cardiac Resynch Defibrillator Pulse Generator	0JH6[0,3]9Z	0JH8[0,3]9Z	02HN[0,3,4]JZ	02HN[0,3,4]KZ	02HN[0,3,4]MZ

DRG 326-328 Stomach, Esophageal and Duodenal Procedures

Site	Resection by Open Approach	Code also as appropriate Resection of Pancreas by Open Approach
Duodenum	0DT90ZZ	0FTG0ZZ

DRG 344-346 Minor Small and Large Bowel Procedures

Site	Repair by Open Approach	Code also as appropriate Repair by external approach of Abdominal Wall Stoma
Small Intestine	ØDQ8ØZZ	ØWQFXZ2
Duodenum	ØDQ9ØZZ	ØWQFXZ2
Jejunum	ØDQAØZZ	ØWQFXZ2
Ileum	ØDQBØZZ	ØWQFXZ2
Large Intestine	ØDQEØZZ	ØWQFXZ2
Large Intestine, Right	ØDQFØZZ	ØWQFXZ2
Large Intestine, Left	ØDQGØZZ	ØWQFXZ2
Cecum	ØDQHØZZ	ØWQFXZ2
Ascending Colon	ØDQKØZZ	ØWQFXZ2
Transverse Colon	ØDQLØZZ	ØWQFXZ2
Descending Colon	ØDQMØZZ	ØWQFXZ2
Sigmoid Colon	ØDQNØZZ	ØWQFXZ2

DRG 456-458 Spinal Fusion Except Cervical with Spinal Curvature/Malignancy/Infection or Extensive Fusions

Fusion of Thoracic and Lumbar Vertebra, Anterior Column

2 to 7 Thoracic Vertebra		Code also 2 or more Lumbar Vertebra	
ØRG[Ø,3,4][7,A,J,K,Z]Ø	XRG7ØF3	ØSG1[Ø,3,4][7,A,J,K,Z]Ø	XRGCØF3

Fusion of Thoracic and Lumbar Vertebra, Posterior Column

2 to 7 Thoracic Vertebra			Code also 2 or more Lumbar Vertebra		
Posterior Approach	Anterior Approach	New Technology	Posterior Approach	Anterior Approach	New Technology
ØRG7[Ø,3,4][7,J,K,Z]1	ØRG7[Ø,3,4][7,A,J,K,Z]J	XRG7Ø92 XRG7ØF3	ØSG1[Ø,3,4][7,J,K,Z]1	ØSG1[Ø,3,4][7,A,J,K,Z]J	XRGCØ92 XRGCØF3

DRG 466-468 Revision of Hip or Knee Replacement

Open Removal of Hip Joint Spacer, Liner, or Resurfacing Device With Supplement of Liner

Body Part	Removal Spacer/Liner/Resurfacing Device	Code also as appropriate Supplement of Body Part by Site		
		Joint	Acetabular Surface	Femoral Surface
Hip, RT	ØSP9Ø[8,9,B]Z	ØSU9Ø9Z	ØSUAØ9Z	ØSURØ9Z
Hip, LT	ØSPBØ[8,9,B]Z	ØSUBØ9Z	ØSUEØ9Z	ØSUSØ9Z

Open Removal of Hip Joint Spacer, Liner, Resurfacing Device, or Synthetic Substitute With Replacement

Body Part	Removal Spacer/Liner/Resurfacing Device/Synthetic Substitute	Code also as appropriate Replacement of Body Part by Device Type						
		Polyethylene	Metal	Metal on Poly	Ceramic	Ceramic on Poly	Oxidized Zirc on Poly	Synth Subst
Hip, RT	ØSP9Ø[8,9,B,J]Z	—	ØSR9Ø1[9,A,Z]	ØSR9Ø2[9,A,Z]	ØSR9Ø3[9,A,Z]	ØSR9Ø4[9,A,Z]	ØSR9Ø6[9,A,Z]	ØSR9ØJ[9,A,Z]
Hip, LT	ØSPBØ[8,9,B,J]Z	—	ØSRBØ1[9,A,Z]	ØSRBØ2[9,A,Z]	ØSRBØ3[9,A,Z]	ØSRBØ4[9,A,Z]	ØSRBØ6[9,A,Z]	ØSRBØJ[9,A,Z]
Acetabular Surface, RT	ØSP9Ø[8,9,B,J]Z	ØSRAØØ[9,A,Z]	ØSRAØ1[9,A,Z]	—	ØSRAØ3[9,A,Z]	—	—	ØSRAØJ[9,A,Z]
Acetabular Surface, LT	ØSPBØ[8,9,B,J]Z	ØSREØØ[9,A,Z]	ØSREØ1[9,A,Z]	—	ØSREØ3[9,A,Z]	—	—	ØSREØJ[9,A,Z]
Femoral Surface, RT	ØSP9Ø[8,9,B,J]Z	—	ØSRRØ1[9,A,Z]	—	ØSRRØ3[9,A,Z]	—	—	ØSRRØJ[9,A,Z]
Femoral Surface, LT	ØSPBØ[8,9,B,J]Z	—	ØSRSØ1[9,A,Z]	—	ØSRSØ3[9,A,Z]	—	—	ØSRSØJ[9,A,Z]

DRG 466-468 Revision of Hip or Knee Replacement   *(Continued)*

Percutaneous Endoscopic Removal of Hip Joint Spacer or Synthetic Substitute With Supplement of Liner

Body Part	Removal Spacer/Synthetic Substitute	Code also as appropriate Supplement of Body Part by Site		
		Joint	Acetabular Surface	Femoral Surface
Hip, RT	ØSP94[8,J]Z	ØSU909Z	ØSUA09Z	ØSUR09Z
Hip, LT	ØSPB4[8,J]Z	ØSUB09Z	ØSUE09Z	ØSUS09Z

Percutaneous Endoscopic Removal of Hip Joint Spacer or Synthetic Substitute With Replacement

Body Part	Removal Spacer/Synthetic Substitute	Code also as appropriate Replacement of Body Part by Device Type					
		Polyethylene	Metal	Metal on Poly	Ceramic	Ceramic on Poly	Synth Subst
Hip, RT	ØSP94[8,J]Z	—	ØSR901[9,A,Z]	ØSR902[9,A,Z]	ØSR903[9,A,Z]	ØSR904[9,A,Z]	ØSR90J[9,A,Z]
Hip, LT	ØSPB4[8,J]Z	—	ØSRB01[9,A,Z]	ØSRB02[9,A,Z]	ØSRB03[9,A,Z]	ØSRB04[9,A,Z]	ØSRB0J[9,A,Z]
Acetabular Surface, RT	ØSP94[8,J]Z	ØSRA00[9,A,Z]	ØSRA01[9,A,Z]	—	ØSRA03[9,A,Z]	—	ØSRA0J[9,A,Z]
Acetabular Surface, LT	ØSPB4[8,J]Z	ØSRE00[9,A,Z]	ØSRE01[9,A,Z]	—	ØSRE03[9,A,Z]	—	ØSRE0J[9,A,Z]
Femoral Surface, RT	ØSP94[8,J]Z	—	ØSRR01[9,A,Z]	—	ØSRR03[9,A,Z]	—	ØSRR0J[9,A,Z]
Femoral Surface, LT	ØSPB4[8,J]Z	—	ØSRS01[9,A,Z]	—	ØSRS03[9,A,Z]	—	ØSRS0J[9,A,Z]

Removal of Hip Joint Surface With Hip Joint Replacement

Body Part	Removal of Spacer/Liner/Resurfacing Device/Synthetic Substitute	Code also as appropriate Replacement of Hip Joint				
		Metal	Metal on Poly	Ceramic	Ceramic on Poly	Synth Subst
Acetabular Surface, RT	ØSPA[0,4]JZ	ØSR901[9,A,Z]	ØSR902[9,A,Z]	ØSR903[9,A,Z]	ØSR904[9,A,Z]	ØSR90J[9,A,Z]
Acetabular Surface, LT	ØSPE[0,4]JZ	ØSRB01[9,A,Z]	ØSRB02[9,A,Z]	ØSRB03[9,A,Z]	ØSRB04[9,A,Z]	ØSRB0J[9,A,Z]
Femoral Surface, RT	ØSPR[0,4]JZ	ØSR901[9,A,Z]	ØSR902[9,A,Z]	ØSR903[9,A,Z]	ØSR904[9,A,Z]	ØSR90J[9,A,Z]
Femoral Surface, LT	ØSPS[0,4]JZ	ØSRB01[9,A,Z]	ØSRB02[9,A,Z]	ØSRB03[9,A,Z]	ØSRB04[9,A,Z]	ØSRB0J[9,A,Z]

Removal of Hip Joint Surface with Replacement with New Joint Acetabular Surface

Body Part	Removal of Spacer/Liner/Resurfacing Device/Synthetic Substitute	Code also as appropriate Replacement of Acetabular Surface			
		Polyethylene	Metal	Ceramic	Synth Subst
Acetabular Surface, RT	ØSPA[0,4]JZ	ØSRA00[9,A,Z]	ØSRA01[9,A,Z]	ØSRA03[9,A,Z]	ØSRA0J[9,A,Z]
Acetabular Surface, LT	ØSPE[0,4]JZ	ØSRE00[9,A,Z]	ØSRE01[9,A,Z]	ØSRE03[9,A,Z]	ØSRE0J[9,A,Z]
Femoral Surface, RT	ØSPR[0,4]JZ	ØSRA00[9,A,Z]	ØSRA01[9,A,Z]	ØSRA03[9,A,Z]	ØSRA0J[9,A,Z]
Femoral Surface, LT	ØSPS[0,4]JZ	ØSRE00[9,A,Z]	ØSRE01[9,A,Z]	ØSRE03[9,A,Z]	ØSRE0J[9,A,Z]

Removal of Hip Joint Surface With Replacement with New Joint Femoral Surface

Body Part	Removal of Spacer/Liner/Resurfacing Device/Synthetic Substitute	Code also as appropriate Replacement of Femoral Surface		
		Metal	Ceramic	Synth Subst
Acetabular Surface, RT	ØSPA[0,4]JZ	ØSRR01[9,A,Z]	ØSRR03[9,A,Z]	ØSRR0J[9,A,Z]
Acetabular Surface, LT	ØSPE[0,4]JZ	ØSRS01[9,A,Z]	ØSRS03[9,A,Z]	ØSRS0J[9,A,Z]
Femoral Surface, RT	ØSPR[0,4]JZ	ØSRR01[9,A,Z]	ØSRR03[9,A,Z]	ØSRR0J[9,A,Z]
Femoral Surface, LT	ØSPS[0,4]JZ	ØSRS01[9,A,Z]	ØSRS03[9,A,Z]	ØSRS0J[9,A,Z]

Percutaneous Endoscopic Removal of Hip Joint Surface With Supplement of Liner

Body Part	Removal of Spacer/Liner/Resurfacing Device/Synthetic Substitute	Code also as appropriate Body Part by Site		
		Joint	Acetabular Surface	Femoral Surface
Acetabular Surface, RT	ØSPA4JZ	ØSU909Z	ØSUA09Z	ØSUR09Z
Acetabular Surface, LT	ØSPE4JZ	ØSUB09Z	ØSUE09Z	ØSUS09Z
Femoral Surface, RT	ØSPR4JZ	ØSU909Z	ØSUA09Z	ØSUR09Z
Femoral Surface, LT	ØSPS4JZ	ØSUB09Z	ØSUE09Z	ØSUS09Z

DRG 466-468 Revision of Hip or Knee Replacement

(Continued)

Removal of Knee Joint, Liner, With Replacement

Body Part	Removal of Liner	Code also as appropriate Replacement of Body Part				
		Joint	Oxidized Zirc on Poly	Unicondylar	Femoral Surface	Tibial Surface
Knee, RT	ØSPCØ9Z	ØSRCØJ[9,A,Z]	ØSRCØ6[9,A,Z]	ØSRCØL[9,A,Z]	ØSRTØJ[9,A,Z]	ØSRVØJ[9,A,Z]
Knee, LT	ØSPDØ9Z	ØSRDØJ[9,A,Z]	ØSRDØ6[9,A,Z]	ØSRDØL[9,A,Z]	ØSRUØJ[9,A,Z]	ØSRWØJ[9,A,Z]

Removal of Knee Joint, Spacer, With Replacement

Body Part	Removal of Spacer	Code also as appropriate Replacement of Body Part			
		Joint	Oxidized Zirc on Poly	Femoral Surface	Tibial Surface
Knee, RT	ØSPC[Ø,3,4]8Z	ØSRCØJ[9,A,Z]	ØSRCØ6[9,A,Z]	ØSRTØJ[9,A,Z]	ØSRVØJ[9,A,Z]
Knee, LT	ØSPD[Ø,3,4]8Z	ØSRDØJ[9,A,Z]	ØSRDØ6[9,A,Z]	ØSRUØJ[9,A,Z]	ØSRWØJ[9,A,Z]

Removal of Knee Joint, Synthetic Substitute, With Replacement

Body Part	Removal of Synthetic Substitute	Code also as appropriate Replacement of Body Part				
		Joint	Oxidized Zirc on Poly	Unicondylar	Femoral Surface	Tibial Surface
Knee, RT	ØSPC[Ø,4]JZ	ØSRCØJ[9,A,Z]	ØSRCØ6[9,A,Z]	ØSRCØL[9,A,Z]	ØSRTØJ[9,A,Z]	ØSRVØJ[9,A,Z]
Knee, LT	ØSPD[Ø,4]JZ	ØSRDØJ[9,A,Z]	ØSRDØ6[9,A,Z]	ØSRDØL[9,A,Z]	ØSRUØJ[9,A,Z]	ØSRWØJ[9,A,Z]

Open Removal of Knee Joint, Patellar Surface, With Replacement

Body Part	Removal of Patellar Surface	Code also as appropriate Replacement of Body Part			
		Joint	Oxidized Zirc on Poly	Femoral Surface	Tibial Surface
Knee, RT	ØSPCØJC	ØSRCØJ[9,A,Z]	ØSRCØ6[9,A,Z]	ØSRTØJ[9,A,Z]	ØSRVØJ[9,A,Z]
Knee, LT	ØSPDØJC	ØSRDØJ[9,A,Z]	ØSRDØ6[9,A,Z]	ØSRUØJ[9,A,Z]	ØSRWØJ[9,A,Z]

Percutaneous Endoscopic Removal of Knee Joint, Patellar Surface, With Replacement

Body Part	Removal of Patellar Surface	Code also as appropriate Replacement of Body Part	
		Joint	Oxidized Zirc on Poly
Knee, RT	ØSPC4JC	ØSRCØJ[9,A,Z]	ØSRCØ6[9,A,Z]
Knee, LT	ØSPD4JC	ØSRDØJ[9,A,Z]	ØSRDØ6[9,A,Z]

Removal of Knee Joint, Synthetic Substitute, With Replacement

Body Part	Removal of Synthetic Sustitute	Code also as appropriate Replacement of Body Part			
		Joint	Oxidized Zirc on Poly	Femoral Surface	Tibial Surface
Femoral Surface, RT	ØSPT[Ø,4]JZ	ØSRCØJ[9,A,Z]	ØSRCØ6[9,A,Z]	ØSRTØJ[9,A,Z]	ØSRVØJ[9,A,Z]
Femoral Surface, LT	ØSPU[Ø,4]JZ	ØSRDØJ[9,A,Z]	ØSRDØ6[9,A,Z]	ØSRUØJ[9,A,Z]	ØSRWØJ[9,A,Z]
Tibial Surface, RT	ØSPV[Ø,4]JZ	ØSRCØJ[9,A,Z]	ØSRCØ6[9,A,Z]	ØSRTØJ[9,A,Z]	ØSRVØJ[9,A,Z]
Tibial Surface, LT	ØSPW[Ø,4]JZ	ØSRDØJ[9,A,Z]	ØSRDØ6[9,A,Z]	ØSRUØJ[9,A,Z]	ØSRWØJ[9,A,Z]

DRG 485-489 Knee Procedures

Joint	Removal of Liner by open approach	Code also as appropriate Supplement of Tibial Surface by Site
Knee, RT	ØSPCØ9Z	ØSUVØ9Z
Knee, LT	ØSPDØ9Z	ØSUWØ9Z

DRG 515-517 Other Musculoskeletal System and Connective Tissue Procedures

Site	Reposition of Vertebra by percutaneous approach	Code also as appropriate Supplement With Synthetic Substitute by Percutaneous Approach at site of Repositioned Vertebra
Cervical	ØPS33ZZ	ØPU33JZ
Coccyx	ØQSS3ZZ	ØQUS3JZ
Lumbar	ØQSØ3ZZ	ØQUØ3JZ
Sacrum	ØQS13ZZ	ØQU13JZ
Thoracic	ØPS43ZZ	ØPU43JZ

DRG 518-52Ø Back and Neck Procedures, Except Spinal Fusion, or Disc Devices/Neurostimulators

Generator Type	Insertion of Generator by Site			Code also as appropriate Insertion Neurostimulator Lead by approach and Site	
	Chest	Abdomen	Back	Spinal Canal	Spinal Cord
Single Array	ØJH6[Ø,3]BZ	ØJH8[Ø,3]BZ	ØJH7[Ø,3]BZ	ØØHU[Ø,3,4]MZ	ØØHV[Ø,3,4]MZ
Single Array, Rechargeable	ØJH6[Ø,3]CZ	ØJH8[Ø,3]CZ	ØJH7[Ø,3]CZ	ØØHU[Ø,3,4]MZ	ØØHV[Ø,3,4]MZ
Multiple Array	ØJH6[Ø,3]DZ	ØJH8[Ø,3]DZ	ØJH7[Ø,3]DZ	ØØHU[Ø,3,4]MZ	ØØHV[Ø,3,4]MZ
Multiple Array, Rechargable	ØJH6[Ø,3]EZ	—	ØJH7[Ø,3]EZ	ØØHU[Ø,3,4]MZ	ØØHV[Ø,3,4]MZ
Multiple Array, Rechargable	—	ØJH8[Ø,3]EZ	—	ØØHU[Ø,3,4]MZ	ØØHVØMZ
Multiple Array, Rechargable	—	ØJH8ØEZ	—		ØØHV[3,4]MZ

DRG 582-583 Mastectomy for Malignancy

Site	Resection by Open approach	Code also as appropriate Resection of Lymph Nodes by Open approach by site			Code also as appropriate Resection of Thorax Muscle by Open approach	
		Axillary	Internal Mammary	Thorax	Right	Left
Breast, Right	ØHTTØZZ	Ø7T5ØZZ	Ø7T8ØZZ	Ø7T7ØZZ	ØKTHØZZ	—
Breast, Left	ØHTUØZZ	Ø7T6ØZZ	Ø7T9ØZZ	Ø7T7ØZZ	—	ØKTJØZZ
Breast, Bilateral	ØHTVØZZ	Ø7T5ØZZ and Ø7T6ØZZ	Ø7T8ØZZ and Ø7T9ØZZ	Ø7T7ØZZ	ØKTHØZZ	ØKTJØZZ

DRG 584-585 Breast Biopsy, Local Excision and Other Breast procedures

Resection of Breast With Resection of Lymph Nodes and Thorax Muscle

Site	Resection by Open approach	Code also as appropriate Resection of Lymph Nodes by Open approach by site			Code also as appropriate Resection of Thorax Muscle by Open approach	
		Axillary	Internal Mammary	Thorax	Right	Left
Breast, Right	ØHTTØZZ	Ø7T5ØZZ	Ø7T8ØZZ	Ø7T7ØZZ	ØKTHØZZ	—
Breast, Left	ØHTUØZZ	Ø7T6ØZZ	Ø7T9ØZZ	Ø7T7ØZZ	—	ØKTJØZZ
Breast, Bilateral	ØHTVØZZ	Ø7T5ØZZ and Ø7T6ØZZ	Ø7T8ØZZ and Ø7T9ØZZ	Ø7T7ØZZ	ØKTHØZZ	ØKTJØZZ

Replacement of Breast Tissue

Site	Replacement by Percutaneous approach with Autologous Tissue	Code also as appropriate Extraction of Subcutaneous Tissue by Percutaneous approach					
		Abdomen	Back	Buttock	Chest	Leg, Upper, Right	Leg, Upper, Left
Breast, Right	ØHRT37Z	ØJD83ZZ	ØJD73ZZ	ØJD93ZZ	ØJD63ZZ	ØJDL3ZZ	ØJDM3ZZ
Breast, Left	ØHRU37Z	ØJD83ZZ	ØJD73ZZ	ØJD93ZZ	ØJD63ZZ	ØJDL3ZZ	ØJDM3ZZ
Breast, Bilateral	ØHRV37Z	ØJD83ZZ	ØJD73ZZ	ØJD93ZZ	ØJD63ZZ	ØJDL3ZZ	ØJDM3ZZ

DRG 628-630 Other Endocrine, Nutritional and Metabolic Procedures

Open Removal of Hip Joint Spacer, Liner, Resurfacing Device, or Synthetic Substitute With Replacement

Body Part	Removal Spacer/Liner/Resurfacing Device/Synthetic Substitute	Code also as appropriate Replacement of Body Part by Device Type					
		Polyethylene	Metal	Metal on Poly	Ceramic	Ceramic on Poly	Synth Subst
Hip, RT	ØSP9Ø[8,9,B,J]Z	—	ØSR9Ø1[9,A,Z]	ØSR9Ø2[9,A,Z]	ØSR9Ø3[9,A,Z]	ØSR9Ø4[9,A,Z]	ØSR9ØJ[9,A,Z]
Hip, LT	ØSPBØ[8,9,B,J]Z	—	ØSRBØ1[9,A,Z]	ØSRBØ2[9,A,Z]	ØSRBØ3[9,A,Z]	ØSRBØ4[9,A,Z]	ØSRBØJ[9,A,Z]
Acetabular Surface, RT	ØSP9Ø[8,9,B,J]Z	ØSRAØØ[9,A,Z]	ØSRAØ1[9,A,Z]	—	ØSRAØ3[9,A,Z]	—	ØSRAØJ[9,A,Z]
Acetabular Surface, LT	ØSPBØ[8,9,B,J]Z	ØSREØØ[9,A,Z]	ØSREØ1[9,A,Z]	—	ØSREØ3[9,A,Z]	—	ØSREØJ[9,A,Z]
Femoral Surface, RT	ØSP9Ø[8,9,B,J]Z	—	ØSRRØ1[9,A,Z]	—	ØSRRØ3[9,A,Z]	—	ØSRRØJ[9,A,Z]
Femoral Surface, LT	ØSPBØ[8,9,B,J]Z	—	ØSRSØ1[9,A,Z]	—	ØSRSØ3[9,A,Z]	—	ØSRSØJ[9,A,Z]

Open Removal of Hip Joint Spacer, Liner, or Resurfacing Device With Supplement of Liner

Body Part	Removal Spacer/Liner/Resurfacing Device	Code also as appropriate Supplement of Body Part		
		Joint	Acetabular Surface	Femoral Surface
Hip, RT	ØSP9Ø[8,9,B]Z	ØSU9Ø9Z	ØSUAØ9Z	ØSURØ9Z
Hip, LT	ØSPBØ[8,9,B]Z	ØSUBØ9Z	ØSUEØ9Z	ØSUSØ9Z

Percutaneous Endoscopic Removal of Hip Joint Spacer or Synthetic Substitute With Replacement

Body Part	Removal Spacer/Synthetic Substitute	Code also as appropriate Replacement of Body Part by Device Type					
		Polyethylene	Metal	Metal on Poly	Ceramic	Ceramic on Poly	Synth Subst
Hip, RT	ØSP94[8,J]Z	—	ØSR9Ø1[9,A,Z]	ØSR9Ø2[9,A,Z]	ØSR9Ø3[9,A,Z]	ØSR9Ø4[9,A,Z]	ØSR9ØJ[9,A,Z]
Hip, LT	ØSPB4[8,J]Z	—	ØSRBØ1[9,A,Z]	ØSRBØ2[9,A,Z]	ØSRBØ3[9,A,Z]	ØSRBØ4[9,A,Z]	ØSRBØJ[9,A,Z]
Acetabular Surface, RT	ØSP94[8,J]Z	ØSRAØØ[9,A,Z]	ØSRAØ1[9,A,Z]	—	ØSRAØ3[9,A,Z]	—	ØSRAØJ[9,A,Z]
Acetabular Surface, LT	ØSPB4[8,J]Z	ØSREØØ[9,A,Z]	ØSREØ1[9,A,Z]	—	ØSREØ3[9,A,Z]	—	ØSREØJ[9,A,Z]
Femoral Surface, RT	ØSP94[8,J]Z	—	ØSRRØ1[9,A,Z]	—	ØSRRØ3[9,A,Z]	—	ØSRRØJ[9,A,Z]
Femoral Surface, LT	ØSPB4[8,J]Z	—	ØSRSØ1[9,A,Z]	—	ØSRSØ3[9,A,Z]	—	ØSRSØJ[9,A,Z]

Percutaneous Endoscopic Removal of Hip Joint Spacer or Synthetic Substitute With Supplement of Liner

Body Part	Removal Spacer/Synthetic Substitute	Code also as appropriate Supplement of Body Part by Site		
		Joint	Acetabular Surface	Femoral Surface
Hip, RT	ØSP94[8,J]Z	ØSU9Ø9Z	ØSUAØ9Z	ØSURØ9Z
Hip, LT	ØSPB4[8,J]Z	ØSUBØ9Z	ØSUEØ9Z	ØSUSØ9Z

Removal of Hip Joint Surface with Replacement with New Joint Acetabular Surface

Body Part	Removal of Spacer/Liner/Resurfacing Device/Synthetic Substitute	Code also as appropriate Replacement of Acetabular Surface			
		Polyethylene	Metal	Ceramic	Synth Subst
Acetabular Surface, RT	ØSPA[Ø,4]JZ	ØSRAØØ[9,A,Z]	ØSRAØ1[9,A,Z]	ØSRAØ3[9,A,Z]	ØSRAØJ[9,A,Z]
Acetabular Surface, LT	ØSPE[Ø,4]JZ	ØSREØØ[9,A,Z]	ØSREØ1[9,A,Z]	ØSREØ3[9,A,Z]	ØSREØJ[9,A,Z]
Femoral Surface, RT	ØSPR[Ø,4]JZ	ØSRAØØ[9,A,Z]	ØSRAØ1[9,A,Z]	ØSRAØ3[9,A,Z]	ØSRAØJ[9,A,Z]
Femoral Surface, LT	ØSPS[Ø,4]JZ	ØSREØØ[9,A,Z]	ØSREØ1[9,A,Z]	ØSREØ3[9,A,Z]	ØSREØJ[9,A,Z]

DRG 628-63Ø Other Endocrine, Nutritional and Metabolic Procedures *(Continued)*

Removal of Hip Joint Surface With Replacement with New Joint Femoral Surface

Body Part	Removal of Spacer/Liner/Resurfacing Device/Synthetic Substitute	Code also as appropriate Replacement of Femoral Surface		
		Metal	Ceramic	Synth Subst
Acetabular Surface, RT	ØSPA[Ø,4]JZ	ØSRRØ1[9,A,Z]	ØSRRØ3[9,A,Z]	ØSRRØJ[9,A,Z]
Acetabular Surface, LT	ØSPE[Ø,4]JZ	ØSRSØ1[9,A,Z]	ØSRSØ3[9,A,Z]	ØSRSØJ[9,A,Z]
Femoral Surface, RT	ØSPR[Ø,4]JZ	ØSRRØ1[9,A,Z]	ØSRRØ3[9,A,Z]	ØSRRØJ[9,A,Z]
Femoral Surface, LT	ØSPS[Ø,4]JZ	ØSRSØ1[9,A,Z]	ØSRSØ3[9,A,Z]	ØSRSØJ[9,A,Z]

Percutaneous Endoscopic Removal of Hip Joint Surface With Supplement of Liner

Body Part	Removal of Spacer/Liner/Resurfacing Device/Synthetic Substitute	Code also as appropriate Body Part by Site		
		Joint	Acetabular Surface	Femoral Surface
Acetabular Surface, RT	ØSPA4JZ	ØSU9Ø9Z	ØSUAØ9Z	ØSURØ9Z
Acetabular Surface, LT	ØSPE4JZ	ØSUBØ9Z	ØSUEØ9Z	ØSUSØ9Z
Femoral Surface, RT	ØSPR4JZ	ØSU9Ø9Z	ØSUAØ9Z	ØSURØ9Z
Femoral Surface, LT	ØSPS4JZ	ØSUBØ9Z	ØSUEØ9Z	ØSUSØ9Z

Removal of Knee Joint, Liner, With Replacement

Body Part	Removal of Liner	Code also as appropriate Replacement of Body Part			
		Joint	Unicondylar	Femoral Surface	Tibial Surface
Knee, RT	ØSPCØ9Z	ØSRCØJ[9,A,Z]	ØSRCØL[9,A,Z]	ØSRTØJ[9,A,Z]	ØSRVØJ[9,A,Z]
Knee, LT	ØSPDØ9Z	ØSRDØJ[9,A,Z]	ØSRDØL[9,A,Z]	ØSRUØJ[9,A,Z]	ØSRWØJ[9,A,Z]

Removal of Knee Joint, Patellar Surface, With Replacement

Body Part	Removal of Patellar Surface	Code also as appropriate Replacement of Body Part	
		Femoral Surface	Tibial Surface
Knee, RT	ØSPC[Ø,4]JC	ØSRTØJ[9,A]	ØSRVØJ[9,A]
Knee, LT	ØSPD[Ø,4]JC	ØSRUØJ[9,A]	ØSRWØJ[9,A,Z]

Removal of Knee Joint, Synthetic Substitute, With Replacement

Body Part	Removal of Synthetic Sustitute	Code also as appropriate Replacement of Body Part	
		Femoral Surface	Tibial Surface
Knee, RT	ØSPC[Ø,4]JZ	ØSRTØJ[9,A]	ØSRVØJ[9,A]
Knee, LT	ØSPD[Ø,4]JZ	ØSRUØJ[9,A]	ØSRWØJ[9,A,Z]
Femoral Surface, RT	ØSPT[Ø,4]JZ	ØSRTØJ[9,A]	ØSRVØJ[9,A]
Femoral Surface, LT	ØSPU[Ø,4]JZ	ØSRUØJ[9,A]	ØSRWØJ[9,A,Z]
Tibial Surface, RT	ØSPV[Ø,4]JZ	ØSRTØJ[9,A]	ØSRVØJ[9,A]
Tibial Surface, LT	ØSPW[Ø,4]JZ	ØSRUØJ[9,A]	ØSRWØJ[9,A,Z]

DRG 662-664 Minor Bladder Procedure

Repair of Bladder	Code also as appropriate Repair of Abdominal Wall	
	with Stoma	without Stoma
ØTQB[Ø,3,4]ZZ	ØWQFXZ2	ØWQFXZZ

DRG 665-667 Prostatectomy

Site	Resection by approach				Code also as appropriate Resection of Seminal Vesicles, Bilateral by approach	
	Open	Percutaneous Endoscopic	Via Natural or Artificial Opening	Via Natural or Artificial Opening Endoscopic	Open	Percutaneous Endoscopic
Prostate	ØVT00ZZ	ØVT04ZZ	ØVT07ZZ	ØVT08ZZ	ØVT30ZZ	ØVT34ZZ

DRG 707-708 Major Male Pelvic Procedures

Site	Resection by approach				Code also as appropriate Resection of Seminal Vesicles, Bilateral by approach	
	Open	Percutaneous Endoscopic	Via Natural or Artificial Opening	Via Natural or Artificial Opening Endoscopic	Open	Percutaneous Endoscopic
Prostate	ØVT00ZZ	ØVT04ZZ	ØVT07ZZ	ØVT08ZZ	ØVT30ZZ	ØVT34ZZ

DRG 734-735 Pelvic Evisceration, Radical Hysterectomy and Radical Vulvectomy

Pelvic Evisceration

Resection by Site						
Bladder	Cervix	Fallopian Tubes, Bilateral	Ovaries, Bilateral	Urethra	Uterus	Vagina
ØTTB0ZZ	ØUTC0ZZ	ØUT70ZZ	ØUT20ZZ	ØTTD0ZZ	ØUT90ZZ	ØUTG0ZZ

Radical Hysterectomy

Approach	Resection by Site		
	Cervix	Uterus	Uterine Support Structure
Vaginal	ØUTC[7,8]ZZ	ØUT9[7,8]ZZ	ØUT4[7,8]ZZ
Abdominal, Endoscopic	ØUTC4ZZ	ØUT9[4,F]ZZ	ØUT44ZZ
Abdominal, Open	ØUTC0ZZ	ØUT90ZZ	ØUT40ZZ

Radical Vulvectomy

Resection by Site	Code also as appropriate Excision of Inguinal Lymph Nodes by Approach	
Vulva	Right	Left
ØUTM[0,X]ZZ	07BH[0,4]ZZ	07BJ[0,4]ZZ

Non-OR procedure combinations

Note: The following table identifies procedure combinations that are considered Non-OR even though one or more procedures of the combination are considered valid DRG OR procedures

Dilation With Removal of Intraluminal Device - Via Natural or Artificial Opening

Code as appropriate Dilation by Site					Code also as appropriate Removal of Intraluminal Device by Site	
Hepatic Duct, Right	Hepatic Duct, Left	Cystic Duct	Common Bile Duct	Pancreatic Duct	Hepatobiliary Duct	Pancreatic Duct
ØF75[7,8]DZ	ØF76[7,8]DZ	ØF78[7,8]DZ	ØF79[7,8]DZ	ØF7D[7,8]DZ	ØFPB[7,8]DZ	ØFPD[7,8]DZ

Insertion With Removal of Intraluminal Device

Code as appropriate Insertion of Intraluminal Device into Hepatobiliary Duct	Code also as appropriate Removal of Intraluminal Device by Approach and Site			
	Via Natural or Artificial Opening		External	
	Hepatobiliary Duct	Pancreatic Duct	Hepatobiliary Duct	Pancreatic Duct
ØFHB[7,8]DZ	ØFPB[7,8]DZ	ØFPD[7,8]DZ	—	—
ØFHB7DZ	—	—	ØFPBXDZ	ØFPDXDZ

Notes

Notes

Notes

Notes